MW00844590

Advance Praise for

Comprehensive Textbook of Geriatric Psychiatry
Third Edition

"This is an outstanding book. It will be of use to all geriatricians, gero-psychiatrists, and all those who work with older persons. It was a joy to read."
—John E. Morley, M.B., B.Ch., Director of the Division of Geriatric Medicine, Saint Louis University School of Medicine

"The Third Edition of the *Comprehensive Textbook of Geriatric Psychiatry* is an instant classic. It is a must buy for fellows in geriatric psychiatry and medicine. This third edition will also be an indispensable reference for any health care professional hoping to stay current with the mental health needs of senior patients. The reviews are up to date and the section on the history of geriatrics and geriatric psychiatry is indeed comprehensive. The editors have achieved a near perfect balance in covering biomedical and psychosocial research, clinical practice, and public policy. This is truly an encyclopedia of geriatric mental health care divided into sections on the aging process, psychiatric evaluation, mental disorders of late life, and treatment with the medical-legal, ethical and financial issues combined in the financial sector."
—Gary J. Kennedy, M.D., Professor of Psychiatry, Montefiore Medical Center

"This is a comprehensive and up to date review of geriatric psychiatry. It will be helpful for the busy clinician and for the student studying for specialty exams."
—Peter V. Rabins, M.D., M.P.H., Johns Hopkins Schools of Medicine and Public Health

Praise for the Previous Editions of
Comprehensive Textbook of Geriatric Psychiatry

Comprehensive Textbook
of Geriatric Psychiatry

Comprehensive Textbook of Geriatric Psychiatry

Third Edition

Edited by

Joel Sadavoy, MD, FRCP(C)
Lissy F. Jarvik, MD, PhD
George T. Grossberg, MD
Barnett S. Meyers, MD

AAGP
American
Association
for Geriatric
Psychiatry

W. W. Norton and Company
New York London

Sponsored by the
American Association for
Geriatric Psychiatry

For information about permission to reproduce selections from this book, write to
Permissions, W. W. Norton & Company, Inc., 500 Fifth Avenue, New York, NY
10110

Production Manager: Jean Blackburn, Bytheway Publishing Services, Norwich, NY
Manufacturing by Quebecor Kingsport, Kingsport, TN

Library of Congress Cataloging-in-Publication Data

Comprehensive textbook of geriatric psychiatry. — 3rd ed. / edited by Joel
Sadavoy . . . [et al.].
   p. cm.
"A Norton professional book."
Rev. ed. of: Comprehensive review of geriatric psychiatry—II / edited by Joel Sadavoy
. . . [et al.]. 2nd ed. c1996.
Includes bibliographical references and index.
ISBN 0-393-70426-2
   1. Geriatric psychiatry. I. Sadavoy, Joel. II. Comprehensive review of
     geriatric psychiatry—II.
[DNLM: 1. Mental Disorders—Aged. WT 150 C7372 2004]
RC451.4.A5.C634 2004
618.97′689—dc22   2003064993

W. W. Norton & Company, Inc., 500 Fifth Avenue, New York, N.Y. 10110
www.wwnorton.com

W. W. Norton & Company Ltd., Castle House, 75/76 Wells St., London W1T 3QT

1 3 5 7 9 0 8 6 4 2

Contents

SECTION I: THE AGING PROCESS
Jeffrey Foster, MD, Section Editor

SECTION IV: TREATMENT
Ira Katz, MD, Section Editor

SECTION V: MEDICAL-LEGAL, ETHICAL, AND FINANCIAL ISSUES
Karen Blank, MD, Section Editor

Contributors

Robert C. Abrams, MD   Associate Professor of Clinical Psychiatry, Weill Medical College of Cornell University

Marc E. Agronin, MD   Director of Mental Health Services, Miami Jewish Home and Hospital for the Aged; Assistant Professor of Psychiatry, University of Miami School of Medicine

Cathy A. Alessi, MD   Associate Director of Clinical Programs, Geriatric Research, Education and Clinical Center–Sepulveda, VA Greater Los Angeles Healthcare System; Associate Professor, School of Medicine, Multicampus Program in Geriatric Medicine and Gerontology, University of California, Los Angeles

George S. Alexopoulos, MD   Professor of Psychiatry and Director, Weill–Cornell Institute of Geriatric Psychiatry, Weill Medical College of Cornell University

Roland M. Atkinson, MD   Professor of Psychiatry, Oregon Health and Science University–Portland

Stephen J. Bartels, MD, MS   Associate Professor of Psychiatry and Director of Aging Services Research, New Hampshire–Dartmouth Psychiatric Research Center, Department of Psychiatry, Dartmouth Medical School (Lebanon)

Ashok J. Bharucha, MD   Assistant Professor of Psychiatry, Western Psychiatric Institute and Clinic, University of Pittsburgh School of Medicine

Thomas D. Bird, MD   Professor of Neurology, Medical Genetics, and Psychiatry and Behavioral Sciences at the University of Washington; Staff physician, Geriatric Research Education and Clinical Center Veterans Administration, Puget Sound Health Care System, Seattle

Karen Blank, MD   Senior Research Psychiatrist, Braceland Center for Mental Health and Aging, Institute of Living; Associate Clinical Professor of Psychiatry, University of Connecticut School of Medicine, Hartford, Connecticut

Mihaela Boran, MD   State University of New York Downstate Medical Center, Brooklyn

Edith Ann Burns, MD   Associate Professor of Medicine, Section of Geriatrics, Department of Medicine Medical College of Wisconsin and Zablocki Veterans Administration Medical Center

Christine K. Cassel, MD, MACP   President and CEO, American Board of Internal Medicine

Harvey Max Chochinov, MD, PhD, FRCP (C)   Canada Research Chair in Palliative Care and Professor, Department of Psychiatry, Community Health Sciences, and Family Medicine, University of Manitoba and CancerCare Manitoba

C. Edward Coffey, MD   Chairman and Kathleen and Earl Ward Chair, Department of Psychiatry, Henry Ford Health System, Detroit, Michigan

Carl I. Cohen, MD   Professor of Psychiatry, State University of New York Downstate Medical Center, Brooklyn

Bertram J. Cohler, PhD   William Rainey Harper Professor, The College, the Committee on Human Development and the Departments of Psychology and Psychiatry, the University of Chicago

David K. Conn, MB, BCh, BAO, FRCP (C)   Psychiatrist-in-Chief, Baycrest Centre for Geriatric Care; Associate Professor of Psychiatry, University of Toronto; President, Canadian Academy of Geriatric Psychiatry

Aricca R. Dums, BA   Research Assistant, New Hampshire–Dartmouth Psychiatric Research Center and Department of Community and Family Medicine, Dartmouth Medical School (Lebanon)

Laura B. Dunn, MD   Assistant Professor of Psychiatry and Associate Director of Geriatric Psychiatry Fellowship, University of California, San Diego

Carl Eisdorfer, PhD, MD   Professor and Chairman of Psychiatry and Behavioral Sciences, University of Miami School of Medicine

Alastair J. Flint, MB, FRCP (C), FRANZCP   Professor of Psychiatry, University of Toronto and Head, Geriatric Psychiatry Program, University Health Network, Toronto

Linda Ganzini, MD, MPH   Professor of Psychiatry and Medicine, Oregon Health Sciences University; Director of Palliative Care Training Program, Veterans Affairs Medical Center, Portland, Oregon

Gary L. Gottlieb, MD, MBA   Professor of Psychiatry, Harvard Medical School; President, Brigham and Women's Hospital

Robert M. Greenberg, MD   Director of Geropsychiatry and ECT Services, Bon Secours Health System of New Jersey, Jersey City, New Jersey

George T. Grossberg, MD   Samuel W. Fordyce Professor and Director of Geriatric Psychiatry, St. Louis University School of Medicine

Barry J. Gurland, FRC Physicians (London), FRC Psychiatry   Sidney Katz Professor of Psychiatry and Director of Stroud Center for Study of Quality of Life, Columbia University

Nathan Herrmann, MD, FRCP (C)   Head of the Division of Geriatric Psychiatry and Associate Professor of Psychiatry, University of Toronto; Head of the Division of Geriatric Psychiatry, Sunnybrook and Women's Health Sciences Centre, Toronto

Daniel P. Holschneider, MD   Associate Professor, Departments of Psychiatry, Neurology, Cell and Neurobiology, University of Southern California, Los Angeles

Lissy F. Jarvik, MD, PhD   Professor Emerita of Psychiatry and Biobehavioral Sciences, University of California–Los Angeles School of Medicine; Distinguished Physician Emeritus, US Department of Veterans Affairs of the greater Los Angeles area

Dilip V. Jeste, MD   Professor of Psychiatry and Neuroscience, University of California, San Diego, and San Diego Veterans Affairs Medical Center

Ira R. Katz, MD, PhD   Professor of Psychiatry, University of Pennsylvania, Philadelphia VA Medical Center

Charles H. Kellner, MD   Professor and Chair, Department of Psychiatry, UMDNJ–New Jersey Medical School

Harold G. Koenig, MD   Associate Professor of Psychiatry and Medicine, Duke University Medical Center, Durham, North Carolina

Anand Kumar, MD   Professor of Psychiatry and Senior Research Scientist, Neuropsychiatric Institute, University of California, Los Angeles

Joseph Kwentus, MD   Professor of Psychiatry, University of Mississippi

Helen H. Kyomen, MD, MS   McLean Hospital, Division on Aging, Harvard Medical School

Lawrence W. Lazarus, MD, FAPA   Past President, AAGP; staff psychiatrist, Las Vegas Medical Center; visiting lecturer, Highlands University, Las Vegas, New Mexico

Barry Lebowitz, PhD   Chief, Adult and Geriatric Treatment and Preventive Interventions Research Branch, National Institute of Health

Molyn Leszcz, MD   Associate Professor of Psychiatry, University of Toronto; Head of Group Psychotherapy Program, Department of Psychiatry, University of Toronto

Andrew F. Leuchter, MD   Professor and Vice Chair of Psychiatry and Biobehavioral Sciences and Director of the Laboratory of Behavioral Pharmacology, UCLA Neuropsychiatric Institute

Elaine A. Leventhal, MD, PhD   Professor of Medicine Department of Medicine and Director of the Gerontological Institute, University of Medicine and Dentistry of New Jersey Robert Wood Johnson Medical School

Laurie A. Lindamer, PhD   Assistant Professor of Psychiatry, University of California, San Diego, and San Diego Veterans Affairs Medical Center

Benjamin Liptzin, MD   Chairman of Psychiatry, Baystate Health System, Springfield, Massachusetts; Professor and Deputy Chair of Psychiatry, Tufts University School of Medicine, Boston

David A. Loewenstein, PhD Professor of Psychiatry and Behavioral Sciences, University of Miami School of Medicine, and the Wien Center for Alzheimer's Disease and Memory Disorders, Mt. Sinai Medical Center, Miami Beach

Charles F. Longino, Jr, PhD Professor of Public Health Sciences, Wake Forest University School of Medicine, Winston-Salem, North Carolina

Francis J. McMahon, MD Chief of the Genetic Basis of Mood and Anxiety Disorders Program, National Institute of Mental Health, US Department of Health and Human Services; Associate Professor of Psychiatry, The Johns Hopkins University School of Medicine

Barnett S. Meyers, MD Professor of Psychiatry, Weill Medical College of Cornell University; Professor of Clinical Epidemiology, Graduate School of Health Sciences, Weill Medical College of Cornell University, New York Presbyterian Hospital–Westchester Division

Kristen Miller, MD Geriatric Fellow, Medical University of South Carolina

Jacobo Mintzer, MD Professor of Psychiatry, Neurology, Physiology and Neuroscience and Chief, Division of Geriatric Psychiatry, Medical University of South Carolina

Jeanne E. Nakamura, PhD Research Associate, The Claremont Graduate Center, Claremont, California

Jason T. Olin, PhD Associate Director, CNS and Clinical Development and Medical Affairs, Forest Research Institute, Jersey City, New Jersey

Thomas E. Oxman, MD Professor of Psychiatry and Community and Family Medicine, Director of Geriatric Psychiatry, Dartmouth Medical School, Lebanon, New Hampshire

Rona E. Pasternak, MD Associate Professor of Psychiatry and Human Behavior, Jefferson Medical College, Thomas Jefferson University, Philadelphia

Robert H. Payne, MD Family Psychiatry, Charleston Family Centre, Charleston, South Carolina

Sarah I. Pratt, PhD Research Associate, New Hampshire–Dartmouth Psychiatric Research Center and Department of Psychiatry, Dartmouth Medical School (Lebanon)

Sara A. Quandt, PhD   Professor, Section on Epidemiology, Department of Public Health Sciences, Wake Forest University School of Medicine

Stephen Read, MD   Associate Clinical Professor of Psychiatry and Biobehavioral Sciences, David Geffen School of Medicine at UCLA and the Greater Los Angeles Veterans Affairs Health Care System

Barry Reisberg, MD   Professor, Department of Psychiatry, New York University School of Medicine; Clinical Director, William and Sylvia Silberstein Aging and Dementia Research Center, New York University Medical Center

Stephanie S. Richards, MD   Assistant Professor of Psychiatry, Western Psychiatric Institute and Clinic, University of Pittsburgh School of Medicine

Jules Rosen, MD   Professor of Psychiatry, University of Pittsburgh School of Medicine, Chief of Longterm Care Services, Western Psychiatric Institute and Clinic, Pittsburgh, Pennsylvania

Barry W. Rovner, MD   Professor of Psychiatry and Human Behavior, Jefferson Medical College, The Farber Institute for Neurosciences, Thomas Jefferson University, Philadelphia

Mark P. Rubert, PhD   Research Assistant Professor of Psychiatry and Behavioral Sciences and the Center on Adult Development and Aging (D-101), University of Miami School of Medicine

Joel Sadavoy, MD, FRCP (C)   Professor and Pencer Chair in Applied General Psychiatry, University of Toronto; Psychiatrist-in-Chief, Mount Sinai Hospital

Muhammad Usman Saeed, MD   Clinical Research Fellow, William and Sylvia Silberstein Aging and Dementia Research Center, New York University Medical Center

Kenneth Sakauye, MD   Professor of Clinical Psychiatry and Director of Geriatric Psychiatry, Louisiana State University Health Science Center and Ochsner Foundation Hospital

Stephen R. Shuchter, MD   Professor of Clinical Psychiatry and Director, UCSD Outpatient Psychiatric Services, University of California, San Diego

Ivan L. Silver, MD, MEd, FRCP (C)   Professor of Psychiatry, Faculty of Medicine, University of Toronto, Sunnybrook and Women's College Health Sciences Centre

Clifford A. Smith, PhD   Assistant Professor of Psychology, Rush-Presbyterian-St. Luke's Medical Center, Chicago

Elliot Martin Stein, MD   Distinguished Fellow of the American Psychiatric Association; past President of the American Association for Geriatric Psychiatry

Joel E. Streim, MD   Associate Professor of Psychiatry, University of Pennsylvania, Philadelphia Veterans Administration Medical Center

Debby W. Tsuang, MD, MSc   Assistant Professor of Psychiatry and Behavioral Sciences and Adjunct Assistant Professor of Epidemiology, University of Washington; Staff physician, Mental Illness Research Education and Clinical Center, Veterans Administration, Puget Sound Health Care System, Seattle

Wilfred G. van Gorp, PhD, ABPP   Professor of Clinical Psychology, Department of Psychiatry, Columbia University College of Physicians and Surgeons

Jeff Victoroff, MD   Associate Professor of Clinical Neurology and Psychiatry, Keck School of Medicine, University of Southern California

Robert C. Young, MD   Professor of Psychiatry, Weill Medical College of Cornell University, New York Presbyterian Hospital–Westchester Division

Sidney Zisook, MD   Professor of Psychiatry and Director of Residency Training, University of California, San Diego

Preface

The third edition of this textbook has kept pace with the rapid advances in geriatric psychiatry. Many authors have returned with updated, revised chapters, and about half the book has been newly authored for this edition. Because of its comprehensive format and fully referenced material, the title of the book has been changed slightly to reflect its recognized status and purpose as a leading textbook in the field. We have endeavored to make this the best textbook of its kind, of use to students preparing for examinations and practitioners of all disciplines who treat psychiatric problems in the elderly. Every member of the multidisciplinary team that provides geriatric care, including psychiatrists, other physicians, psychogeriatricians, psychologists, nurses, social workers, occupational therapists, and other gerontologists, should find this textbook an in-depth reference resource. The self-assessment section is now in a separate companion volume meant to be used in conjunction with the textbook. Its format has been expanded to include annotations and referencing for each question to make it more useful for study purposes.

Producing a multiauthored book of this size and complexity is logistically challenging. The editors express their deep gratitude to Anne Marie Metelsky-Vico, Elvira Jimenez, Shushan Hovanesian, and Ruchi Kumar for their skill and dedication in keeping us organized and helping to ensure clear communication. We are grateful also to the section editors who so generously gave of their time and effort to bring this edition to fruition and to the reviewers whose expertise and hard work helped to enhance the quality of this volume. A substantial proportion of the chapters were reviewed by one or more independent outside reviewers. Their names are not listed because many of them requested anonymity. Finally, we express our sincere thanks to Deborah Malmud and Michael McGandy of our new publishers, W. W. Norton, for their support, understanding, and professionalism in producing this wonderful volume.

Introduction

The introduction for the third edition of this textbook builds on the introductions of previous editions. Gene Cohen and Sandy Finkel were the principle authors of the introductions for editions one and two, respectively, with contributions from Elliot Stein. Barnett Meyers is the principle author for the introduction to this third edition. The senior editors of this and previous editions, Joel Sadavoy, Lissy Jarvik, Lawrence Lazarus, and George Grossberg, have also contributed to all three versions.

Like the knowledge base of geriatric psychiatry itself, the introduction is a living document; each edition both synthesizes material from previous texts and summarizes more recent developments. Similarly, the next edition will build on this introduction to continue providing a historical perspective for our evolving knowledge base.

This introduction begins with a description of the underlying conceptual framework of the discipline of geriatric psychiatry, followed by a discussion of the academic underpinnings of the clinical discipline. The overview ends with the history of geriatric psychiatry from ancient times to the 21st century.

THE DISCIPLINE OF GERIATRIC PSYCHIATRY

Gerontology, geriatrics, and geriatric psychiatry have continued a rapid expansion that began in the second half of the 20th century. Changing demography and improvements in scientific methods have catalyzed this process. Whereas gerontology provides new information on normal and pathological aging generally, geriatrics focuses on clinical physical issues related to aging, and geriatric psychiatry concentrates on mental health and aging. Thus, geriatric psychiatry focuses on disorders (e.g., late-life affective disorders and Alzheimer's disease), interventions (e.g., psychotherapy and psychopharmacology), and service settings (e.g., geriatric assessment units and nursing homes) that are particularly relevant to later life. These areas of interest have developed into research-based specialized disciplines that are well integrated into academic medicine (Rowe et al., 1987).

Clinical geriatric psychiatry has five major conceptual themes: (1) the differentiation of changes of normal aging from symptoms of illness in later life; (2) the modifiability of illness in later life; (3) the modifiability of normal aging to improve functioning; (4) the capacity to change; and (5) distinguishing between changes in early-onset psychiatric disorders among individuals who have aged and those disorders that began de novo in later life, which provides the longitudinal perspective central to geriatric psychiatry.

Differentiation of Changes of Normal Aging
From Symptoms of Illness in Later Life

If one fails to distinguish illness from normal aging, then clinical symptoms are overlooked and dismissed as inevitable concomitants of the aging process; as a result, reversibility and treatment are not considered. As the sciences of gerontology and geriatrics developed in the mid-1970s, questions were raised about traditional views of normal aging as opposed to illness.

Alzheimer's disease is a prototype for this occurrence. The assumption that dementia is a natural consequence of growing old was captured by terms such as *senility* and *senile dementia*. However, two lines of evidence opened this assumption to question. First, accumulating longitudinal psychometric data began to document that many older persons maintained high levels of cognitive functioning. Normal aging was found to slow mental processes without resulting in qualitative decrements in cognitive functioning (Birren, 1964). When speed was not a factor, performance on some tests—especially when administered to healthy individuals—showed improvement during the responders' eighth decade. The second line of evidence came from discoveries made possible by improvements in neurochemistry and neuropathology. The demonstration that older persons who met premortem criteria for Alzheimer's-type dementia had histochemical and neuropathological deficiencies in the cholinergic system not present in age-matched controls was consistent with disease rather than normative aging as the cause of late-life cognitive deterioration (Cohen, 1989). Similarly, studies of late-life depression demonstrated that clinical depression is not a normal consequence of aging.

The Modifiability of Illness in Later Life

Recognition of the role of illness in the pathogenesis of some of the mental changes of later life led to a focus on modifiability and the treatment of underlying disorders. Growing clinical experience and new research methodologies showed that depression in elderly patients responded robustly to psychopharmacology and psychotherapy. Moreover, new views on treatment emerged for Alzheimer's disease with the demonstration that intervention could have an impact on the fundamental cognitive impairment and the excess disability resulting from comorbid conditions such as depression and delusions (Group for the Advancement of Psychiatry, Committee on Aging, 1988). The finding that cholinesterase inhibitors may improve the cognitive impairment of Alzheimer's disease and the development of criteria for diagnosing both psychosis (Jeste & Finkel, 2000) and depression associated with Alzheimer's disease (Olin et al., 2002) represent important advances toward finding effective treatments. In both cases, this psychopathology associated with Alzheimer's disease is considered reversible.

Modifiability of Normal Aging to Improve Functioning

The growth of understanding about how much functional decline in later life is attributable to disorders rather than to normal aging has made it easier to target specific treatments for specific illnesses. Nevertheless, evidence that even normal aging-related changes may be modified provides the opportunity to minimize decreases in functioning that may occur in the absence of disease. For example, even though reaction time is slowed with aging, the rate of reaction in later life can be improved with practice. Thus, elderly adults reported improvement in both the speed and the accuracy of responses to video game stimuli following a 7-week training program (Clark et al., 1987). Such research is relevant to the development of interventions that promote adaptation and improve the quality of later life.

The Capacity to Change and the Changing Attitudes Toward Later Life

Neither doubt about the value of time left nor skepticism about the capacity to change in later life has stood up to clinical experience. The significance of time and the capacity to change in old age were captured by Somerset Maugham (1938) in an observation on the behavior of the elder Cato approximately 20 centuries ago: "When I was young, I was amazed at Plutarch's statement that the elder Cato began, at the age of eighty to learn Greek. I am amazed no longer. Old age is ready to undertake tasks that youth shirked because they would take too long" (p. 297). With people older than 85 years representing the fastest-growing age group, most older adults do in fact have much time left for treatment and pleasure in their later years. This optimism is reflected in the potential for change that is evident in geriatric patients who undertake psychodynamically oriented psychotherapy late in life (Sadavoy & Leszcz, 1987).

Early-Onset Versus Late-Onset Disorders and the Longitudinal Perspective

The longitudinal perspective is central to geriatric psychiatry. The longitudinal approach enables geriatric psychiatry to contribute to the understanding of all age groups, including how aging affects basic psychological processes and how psychiatric disorders change across the life cycle. European psychiatrists utilized the longitudinal perspective to assess relationships between aging and the course and phenomenology of schizophrenia (Ciompi, 1972) and to distinguish late-life depression from neurological disorders that affect brain functioning (Roth, 1955). In the United States, comparisons of elderly patients with early-onset schizophrenia to those with onset in later life led to the delineation of a late-onset form of this disorder (Jeste et al., 1995; Pearlson et al., 1989).

These studies have provided information about the contributions of age of onset, aging, and chronicity to the phenomenology and treatment response of schizophrenia. For example, the demonstration that negative symptoms and affective blunting are less pronounced in late-onset than early-onset schizophrenia (Almeida et al., 1995; Jeste et al., 1995) may be explained by these phenomena occurring because of the chronicity of the disorder.

Another example comes from studies of geriatric depression. The hypothesis that depression results from central deficits of norepinephrine and serotonin in conjunction with evidence that activity of monoamine oxidase, an enzyme that metabolizes these neurotransmitters, increases with advancing years would suggest that the prevalence of major depression would increase during later life. However, epidemiological studies have demonstrated that this is not the case, and biological studies have not implicated neurotransmitter deficiencies in the pathogenesis of late-onset depression. Also, the intuitive notion that adverse life events related to aging explain the onset of geriatric depression is not always demonstrated, with many episodes appearing to develop "out of the blue" (Murphy, 1983). In contrast to the genetic predisposition seen in early-onset depression, chronic medical illness (Murphy, 1983) and disablement (Prince et al., 1998) appear to play causal roles for depression with onset in later life. Similarly, the suggestion that subclinical vascular disease contributes to the pathogenesis of late-onset depression (Alexopoulos et al., 1997; Krishnan et al., 1997) is based on studies using the longitudinal perspective of geriatric psychiatry.

Ideally, the longitudinal perspective requires following patients with diagnosable disorders for long periods of time. The study of geriatric patients offers a shortcut, albeit imperfect, to this process, providing a picture of the "whole person" in a biopsychosocial context (Jarvik, 1983). Also, longitudinal studies allow examination of factors that have an impact on mental health in later life. Utilizing this approach, Vaillant and Mukamal (2001) identified early life predictors of successful aging. Their longitudinal study of a cohort of male undergraduates demonstrated that factors present during young adulthood predicted mental health more than 60 years later. Depression was identified as the only factor, not under personal control, that predicted subjective and objective measures of successful aging; in contrast, uncontrollable factors such as childhood socioeconomic status and parental intimacy were not significant predictors.

GERIATRIC PSYCHIATRY AS AN ACADEMIC DISCIPLINE

The academic base of geriatric psychiatry has been essential to ensuring that clinical practice is based on empirical information and to providing the individual and institutional leadership required to carry out educational and research initiatives. The scientific underpinnings of modern geriatric psychiatry contributed to the development of the knowledge base required for recognition as a formally accredited discipline, the first new area of special competence in American psychiatry since the accreditation of child psychiatry some three decades earlier.

Several factors have contributed to this process. Dramatic growth in the number of people aged 65 years and older, who now comprise more than 12% of the population or more than 30 million people, provided a demographic imperative for this development. Increasing attention is given to the growing minority of older persons commonly referred to as the old-old. The number of people 85 years and older is expected to increase six- to sevenfold by the middle of the 21st century, at which time it will reach more than 15 million.

The American Board of Internal Medicine and the American Board of Family Practice recognized the impact of these demographic changes and the existence of sufficient empirically derived knowledge in geriatric medicine to justify recognition of geriatric medicine as meriting added qualifications in 1988. This led to the development of an examination to test competence for certification. A similar process occurred in psychiatry. By the late 1980s, the total number of American psychiatrists was approximately 35,000. Although relatively few psychiatrists had expressed interest in working with older adults a decade earlier, formal surveys taken during the 1980s found more than 5,000 psychiatrists providing active treatment to elderly persons, with the number of psychiatrists increasing steadily.

This interest in conjunction with an expanding empirically derived knowledge base led to rapid growth in the number of postresidency specialty training programs in geriatric psychiatry. The initial fellowship program established at Duke University in Durham, North Carolina, in 1965 remained the only one for more than a decade. But with the expansion of knowledge, especially since the 1980s, the number of postresidency programs in the United States has grown rapidly, with more than 60 postgraduate specialty residencies now approved by the American College of Graduate Medical Education. Similarly, every medical school in Canada provides 3 months of mandatory training in geriatric psychiatry to all psychiatric residents, with advanced training and fellowships available at several schools.

Accreditation has been a critical step to ensure the quality of the clinical and educational components of specialty training and the quality of clinicians who complete it. The American College of Graduate Medical Education, recognizing the need for formal training programs and for a method to document specialized knowledge, authorized certification of added qualifications in geriatric psychiatry during the late 1980s.

This step was strongly supported by the American Association of Geriatric Psychiatry (AAGP), which had grown rapidly during the 1980s. In anticipation of the examination, AAGP edited and published a syllabus of geriatric psychiatry (Lazarus, 1988) and the first edition of the *Comprehensive Review of Geriatric Psychiatry* (Sadavoy et al., 1991).

The American Board of Psychiatry and Neurology, which had the responsibility for developing an examination to assess this competency, administered the first added qualification examination in April 1991, which was 3 years after the first examination in geriatric medicine. Although initial examinees were eligible because of their clinical experience, eligibility now requires the completion of a year of postresidency training at an accredited program. In addition, a recertification examination has been developed for administration 10 years following initial certification.

DEVELOPMENT OF THE ACADEMIC DISCIPLINE:
THE ROLE OF FEDERAL SUPPORT

Although early geriatric psychiatrists were guided largely by clinical experience, the academic discipline has been built increasingly on a foundation of knowledge derived from systematic studies. In the United States, these studies and the development of investigators to conduct them resulted from major policy decisions made in Washington during the late 1970s to develop institutions that would jump-start the nascent discipline of geriatric psychiatry.

On a limited basis, the National Institute of Mental Health (NIMH) sponsored research between 1960 and the mid-1970s on the mental health of the aging (US Department of Health, Education, and Welfare, Public Health Service, 1977). In 1971, the second White House Conference on Aging took place and led to specific recommendations that catalyzed the formation of two institutions that would play critical roles in the development of academic geriatric psychiatry: the National Institute on Aging (NIA) of the National Institutes of Health and the Center for Studies on Aging within the NIMH.

The NIA, established in 1974, was assigned the responsibility for promoting, coordinating, and supporting psychological social and biological research about the normal aging process and diseases associated with aging. The Aging Branch of NIMH, established in 1975, became responsible for supporting research on the neurobiology, psychopathology, and treatment of late-life mental disorders.

Consistent with this dichotomization, support for studies of the pathophysiology, phenomenology, and treatment of Alzheimer's disease fell into the purview of NIA; studies of the psychiatric complications of this disorder are funded largely through NIMH. The appointment of Robert Butler, a geriatric psychiatrist with extensive clinical, research, and teaching experience, as the first NIA director acknowledged the importance of studies of mental health and aging. In its first decade, the NIA trained more than 100 new researchers (Butler, 1977). NIA research funds increased more than 10-fold after its establishment. NIA support focused on major studies of the pathophysiology, phenomenology, and treatment of Alzheimer's disease and of psychosocial and biological factors related to geriatric mental health.

Under the creative leadership of its first chief, Dr. Gene Cohen, the Aging Branch or NIMH Center for Studies of the Mental Health of the Aging grew rapidly as it carried out its mandate to support and coordinate research, clinical training projects, and research training. Research activities at NIA and NIMH were facilitated by additional government-sponsored reports in the late 1970s. In 1976, the Secretary of Health, Education, and Welfare appointed Eric Pfeiffer to establish an agenda on the needs of the mental health of older Americans. In 1977, President Carter established a task panel regarding mental health and mental illness in late life. Both reports were published in 1979 by the US Department of Health, Education, and Welfare, Federal Council on Aging.

Following Dr. Gene Cohen's appointment as deputy director of the NIA, Dr. Barry Lebowitz was appointed chief of the Aging Branch at NIMH. Earlier programs continued to flourish, and new ones were initiated as federal support for educational programs in mental health ended in the early 1980s, but funds for research increased. Programs designed initially to develop clinical educators were modified. The Academic Mental Health Award funding mechanism was used to train experienced geriatric clinician–educators in research methods and to train experienced general psychiatry investigators in clinical geriatric psychiatry. An emphasis was placed on recruiting and developing young investigators to pursue careers in academic geriatric psychiatry. The new cohort of clinical scholars and basic scientists assumed leadership roles in departments of psychiatry seeking to develop geriatric psychiatry training and research programs.

Support by NIMH is now limited to research, but includes grants for investigator development (K awards), investigator-initiated research projects (RO1s), and clinical research centers that focus on interventions. The fact that five major university-based geriatric psychiatry programs (Cornell University, Ithaca, NY; Duke University; University of Pennsylvania, Philadelphia; University of Pittsburgh; New York's University of Rochester; University of California at

In 1981, the Royal College of Physicians and Surgeons of Canada gave its first examination for certification in geriatric medicine; in 1983, the college mandated that all psychiatric training programs include psychogeriatric experience (Reichenfeld, 1987).

In 1988, the Royal College of Physicians in London, England, created its first examination for a diploma in geriatric medicine. The examination was not for geriatric specialists, but rather for physicians who were general practitioners and who wished to have special expertise in geriatric medicine. Consistent with these developments, an extensive psychogeriatric training program for medical students, physicians, nurses, and other health care professionals was established in Nottingham, United Kingdom, under the leadership of Tom Arie, a geriatric psychiatrist (Arie et al., 1985).

HISTORY OF GERIATRIC PSYCHIATRY

The Beginning

In the seventh century BC, the Maximes of PtahHaty (Loza & Milad, unpublished data, 1989) described cognitive impairment, perhaps associated with depression, that accompanied aging:

> Sovereign my master the old age is here, senility has descended in me, the weakness of my childhood is renewed, so I sleep all the time. The arms are weak, the legs have given up following the heart that has become tired. The mouth is mute, it can no longer speak, the eyes are weak, the ears are deaf, the nose is blocked, it can no longer breathe. The taste is completely gone. The spirit is forgetful. It can no longer remember yesterday. The bones ache in the old age, getting up and sitting down are both difficult. What was nice has become bad. What causes senility in men is bad in every way.

Examples of good mental health in the elders of ancient Egypt also exist (Loza & Milad, unpublished data, 1989). The statue of Nebenterou, son of the high priest of the 12th Dynasty (950–730 BC), bore the following engraving: "I have spent my life in happiness, without the worry of illness. . . . I have outlived my contemporaries. May this happen to you too." Evidence of attempts to treat dementia has been found in the Edwin Smith papyrus and the Magical Papyri.

The Bible offers a clinical description of an aging King David as suffering from a depression:

> Be gracious unto me, O Lord, for I am in distress;
> Mine eye wasted away with vexation, yea, my soul and my body.
> For my life is spent in sorrow, and my years is sighing;
> My strength faileth because of mine iniquity, and my bones are wasted away.

Because of all mine adversaries I am become a reproach, yea. . . .
I am forgotten as a dead man out of mind;
I am like useless vessel. (Psalms 31:9–12)

Both the absence of anxiety about dying and fears of disability and dementia were discussed by ancient philosophers. Plato observed that older people did not have increasing anxiety about death. He believed that reductions in the power of impulses led to the sense of tranquility and greater freedom to pursue philosophy and intellectual endeavors. In 44 BC, at the age of 62 years, Cicero wrote an essay on senescence (*De Senecute*) in which he described the problems and goals for older people. He acknowledged ageism in Roman society, but stressed the value of older people in administrative and intellectual pursuits. Cicero echoed Plato's ideas about diminishing sexual pleasure and greater acceptance of death in old age. He also described the severe regression that can occur with dementia, a condition he viewed with abhorrence.

During the Coptic era (Loza & Milad, unpublished data, 1989) (second to seventh centuries AD), Father Jean Cassien described a paranoid psychosis in a French monk in his book *Les Conferences des Peres du Desert*. In a delusional state, the monk ultimately killed himself.

Modern Geriatric Psychiatry to the Mid-20th Century

The ascension of rationalism and empiricism that occurred during the last three centuries was the foundation for advances in modern medicine. Esquirol, an 18th century descriptive psychiatrist recognized for his discussion of hallucinatory states, also differentiated dementia (loss of mental faculties) from amentia (mental retardation). He did not believe that dementia was an irreversible process, a view that was resurrected in that late 20th century. Berios differentiated depression and dementia in the 19th century based on his book, *Montpelier*.

In the United States, the first relevant treatise on geriatric psychiatry was written by Benjamin Rush in 1805: "An Account of the State of the Body and the Mind in Old Age; With Observation on Its Diseases and Remedies" (Butterfield, 1976). In the same year, Rush began an 8-year correspondence with his friend, the 70-year-old John Adams, that utilized their mutual reporting of dreams to help Adams cope with matters that "agitated" his state of mind (Schutz & Adair, 1966).

The late 19th and early 20th centuries were strongly influenced by the perspective brought by psychoanalysis. Based on his clinical experience with largely young adult patients, Freud was pessimistic about the application of psychoanalytic techniques to the treatment of "older people" (people older than 40 years). When Freud was 42 years old, he wrote "Sexuality in the Aetiology of the Neuroses," in which he stated: "With persons who are too far advanced in years, it [psychoanalytic method] fails because, owing to the accumulation of material, so much time would be required so that the end of the cure would be reached at a period of life in which much importance is no longer attached to nervous health" (1898/1953, p. 245). Subsequently, he recognized that his statements were based on his limited number of cases, predominantly of hysteria and obsessional neurosis; furthermore, this perspective is not consistent with the fundamental psychoanalytic precepts that basic psychodynamic conflicts develop during childhood, and that both these forces and the unconscious are timeless. This largely pessimistic "time running out" bias fails to recognize that the years an individual has remaining are the rest of that person's life.

Abraham (1927) described his more positive experience using psychoanalytic techniques in the treatment of older people: He said that it would seem incorrect today to deny the possibility of exercising a curative influence on the neurosis in the period of involution; rather, it is the task of psychoanalysis to inquire under which conditions the method of treatment can attain results in the later years.

Ferenczi (1955) described psychodynamic changes in later life, including decreased ability to sublimate, increased narcissism, and often a more negative and hostile approach to life. Ferenczi theorized that, in old age, there is a reversion to the discharge of pregenital impulses, including voyeurism, exhibitionism, and a tendency to masturbate, which he termed "underdistinguished" anal and urethral eroticism. Ferenczi did not address the contributions of diminished access to sexual partners and diminished potency in men to what he described as a regression to pregenital preoccupations in later life.

In addition to the blossoming of psychoanalysis, the 20th century brought an explosion of investigators taking the perspective of descriptive phenomenological psychiatry. In 1906, two revolutionary monographs were written. One was the classic description of dementia by Alzheimer (1987). The other was written by Gaupp (Barraclough, 1989), who differentiated dementias from nondementias (mainly depression). Although some nondementias ended in dementia, Gaupp observed that most did not. Gaupp's recognition that most psychiatric disorders in later life were not because of dementia and were not inherently progressive is a fundamental precept of modern geriatric psychiatry.

In 1922, G. Stanley Hall, who founded the first university psychology department in the United States at Johns Hopkins in Baltimore, Maryland, published *Senescence: The Last Half of Life*. Hall was one of the first scientists to use real data, responses to questionnaires, to support his observation that older people did not become more fearful of death, which supported Plato's observation made more than two millennia earlier. In 1914, Nascher published the textbook *Geriatrics: The Diseases of Old Age and Their Treatment*, thereby establishing a new name for the field. Nascher, who is considered the father of geriatrics in America, continued his interest in the field. His final article, "The Aging Mind," published in 1944, described the characteristics of chronic brain syndrome. Nascher posited that chronic brain syndrome had a genetic etiology.

Hitler's ascension to power in Germany prompted the relocation to the

United Kingdom of Felix Post and Sir Martin Roth, two of the fathers of modern geriatric psychiatry. These seminal contributors worked under Aubrey Lewis at the Maudsley Hospital. In 1946, Lewis decried the neglect of clinical geriatric psychiatry in view of the increasing number of older persons requiring psychiatry admissions (Lewis, 1946). Under the guidance and direction of Lewis, in 1947 Post assumed the first geriatric psychiatric position in England at the Bethlem Hospital. By 1950–1951, Post had developed an entire ward for people older than 60 years of age. Among his trainees were David Kay, who made major contributions to the understanding of the epidemiology and course of mental disorders in late life, and Raymond Levy and Tom Arie, who continued in Post's tradition.

Geriatric Psychiatry in the Second Half of the 20th Century

The end of World War II and the development of modern scientific methods facilitated a burgeoning in the number of investigators and the knowledge they generated. In the United States, a critical mass of investigators developed at Duke during the 1950s and 1960s under the leadership of Ewald Busse and launched the first academic program in geriatric psychiatry. These pioneers, including Carl Eisdorfer, Eric Pfeiffer, and Adrian Verwoerdt, went on to seed other programs and to train the next generation of investigators, which included Dan Blazer, Burton Reifler, and Murray Raskind. Results of the Duke longitudinal studies on aging began appearing in 1954. The Duke studies led to a series of books, many based on research findings from the longitudinal studies (Busse & Pfeiffer, 1969; Palmore, 1974, 1979).

Some 20 years later, Paul McHugh developed a group of investigators, including Marshall Folstein and Robert Robinson, at the Cornell Westchester Division. Their contributions included the Mini-Mental State Examination (Folstein et al., 1975), the concept of reversable dementia caused by depression, and seminal research on poststroke depression. The McHugh group moved on to Johns Hopkins before seeding other departments with geriatric psychiatry research expertise, leaving behind an infrastructure that would aid a new generation of investigators at Westchester.

In Great Britain, leadership was provided initially by psychiatrists at the Maudsley Hospital, but spread to Nottingham and other academic centers. The British longitudinal studies of elderly patients conducted by Post, Roth, Kay, and Hopkins and published in the 1950s and 1960s demonstrated empirically that the "organic psychoses" were distinguishable from functional psychiatric disorders that afflicted older persons, and that depressed patients without brain symptoms did not have an increased risk for developing them (Barraclough, 1989; Kay, 1962; Post, 1965; Roth, 1955). Roth's 1955 research led to the identification of a small proportion of hospitalized elders who had late-onset paranoid psychosis in an otherwise well-maintained personality. He described

this condition as late-life paraphrenia. Today, these individuals would be classified as suffering from either late-onset schizophrenia or delusional disorder,
depending on the presence of accompanying phenomena such as a disturbance
in thought processes or affect.

Kay's (1962) work demonstrated that patients with affective disorder were
more than twice as likely to die of cerebral vascular disease, a finding that has
been replicated by contemporary investigators. Also, the linking of cerebral
vascular disease to depression and of senile plaques to dementia (Blessed et al.,
1968; Roth, 1967) provided empirical evidence for the association between the
severity of Alzheimer's disease and the degree of abnormal neuropathology.
Diagnostic accuracy and determination of treatment response are inextricably
linked. The distinctions between organic and functional illnesses in later life
made through these longitudinal and neuropathological studies in the 1950s
and 1960s set the stage for the treatment studies and therapeutic optimism that
followed the introduction of effective pharmacological treatments (Kay, 1999).

T. K. Henderson of Edinburgh and Duncan McMillan of Nottingham
brought a mental health services perspective to working intensively with older
people with mental disorders. McMillan focused on the integration of services
with a strong social-psychiatric approach. He played a major role in the development of respite care to meet the need of families who had people with depression or dementia living with them. McMillan emphasized the importance
of ready access to an appropriate level and intensity of service based on the
patient's and family's needs. Nevertheless, recognition of the need for research
into the mental health services aspects of geriatric mental health care that
would complement improvements in the treatment of individual patients has
come late to geriatric psychiatry (Borson et al., 2001). Without improved continuity of care, elderly psychiatric patients suffering from chronic or highly recurrent psychiatric disorders will continue to run through the revolving door
of repeated hospital admissions because of the adverse effects of stigma and
physical disability on the delivery of effective postdischarge care.

The US–UK cross-national studies, initiated in the 1960s and led by John
Copeland in London and Barry Gurland in New York, were a major development in comparative epidemiology and led to the development of a standardized instrument, the Geriatric Mental State Schedule, for carrying out reliable
diagnostic assessments of geriatric patients. Development of the AGECAT by
Copeland et al. (1986) provided a computer-based method of diagnosis applicable for epidemiological and future cross-national studies.

The appointment of Raymond Levy as the first professor of the Department of Psychiatry of Old Age at Maudsley Hospital in 1984 and of Tom Arie
as chair of the Division of Health Care of the Aged at Nottingham formalized
British research structures devoted to the psychiatry of old age.

Similar developments occurred on the European continent and then spread
to Asia. In France, Jean-Marie Leger, professor and chair of the Department of
Psychiatry at the University of Limoges, started a psychogeriatric service in the

1970s. Soon, newly trained French psychiatrists developed satellites with similar services in other parts of France. In Switzerland, two psychogeriatric centers were established in French-speaking areas. After Junat established a substantial program in Geneva, Dr. Christian Mueller similarly established a service and academic component in Lausanne.

In the late 1960s, Kiloh emigrated from Newcastle in the United Kingdom to Sydney, Australia. Kiloh was a general psychiatrist with a special interest in electroencephalography. Dr. D. K. Henderson, a research psychiatrist, established a division of psychogeriatric research, and Edmund Chiu of Melbourne conducted research in dementias that are uncommonly seen.

Organized Geriatric Psychiatry:
The United States and Canada

The 1940s and 1950s saw rapid growth in institutions devoted to understanding mental health and aging. These organizations provided annual meetings at which investigators and clinicians could communicate about recent findings and led to the development of journals that disseminated knowledge. Such infrastructures were a step in developing a method for investigators to meet, discuss ideas and findings, and then generate the next series of studies. Institutions serving this function include sections devoted to geriatric mental health that were established within existing organizations and the development of new organizations formed specifically to address mental health in later life.

The American Geriatric Society, a multidisciplinary, clinically oriented organization founded in 1942, began to publish the *Journal of the American Geriatric Society* in 1953. The American Psychological Association developed a division devoted to the psychology of old age in 1946. The Gerontological Society of America was established in 1945 and included psychological sciences as one of its four principal sections. The Gerontological Society of America remains the major multidisciplinary organization in the United States devoted to the study of the various mental health aspects of aging, from the psychological and clinical to the sociological and economic. It began publishing the *Journal of Gerontology* in 1946.

The Group for the Advancement of Psychiatry (GAP) was founded in 1946 with the following goals: "to collect and appraise significant data in the field of psychiatry, mental health and human relations; to re-evaluate old concepts and to develop and test new ones; and to apply the knowledge thus obtained for the promotion of mental health in group human relations" (1950, p. 6). *The Problem of the Aged Patient in the Public Psychiatric Hospital* was GAP's first geropsychiatric monograph (1950). The GAP committee structure encourages specialized committees to develop and publish monographs related to their specific areas of expertise. The Committee on Aging, which was established in the early 1960s by Jack Weinberg, a future president of the American Psychiat-

San Diego) have competed successfully for NIMH support as clinical research centers during the last two decades testifies to the success of the discipline. By 1991, research in geriatric depression had produced a sufficient knowledge base to warrant an NIMH Consensus Conference on late-life depression. This was the first NIMH Consensus Conference to address a topic specific to geriatric psychiatry.

Between the 1960s and 1980s, the growth of academic geriatric psychiatry was marked by the publication of major texts on mental health and aging. Major textbooks appeared in the late 1980s and 1990s (Birren & Sloane, 1980; Busse & Blazer, 1980, 1996; Coffey & Cummings, 1994; Copeland et al., 1994; Sadavoy et al., 1991, 1996), and rapid growth in the knowledge base led to publication of an increasing number of specialty texts (Blazer, 1993; Cohen, 1988; Jenike, 1989; Sadavoy, 2004; Salzman, 1997; Salzman & Lebowitz, 1991; Szwabo & Grossberg, 1993). In addition, major peer-reviewed journals devoted primarily to geriatric psychiatry were created to publish the results of research findings, including the *International Journal of Geriatric Psychiatry*, the *Journal of Alzheimer's Disease and Related Disorders*, the *Journal of Psychiatry and Neurology*, *International Psychogeriatrics*, *American Journal of Geriatric Psychiatry*, and *Aging and Mental Health*. The growing number of high-quality scientific and clinical articles has led each of these journals to increase the number of issues published annually.

Despite the early success of investigators in geriatric mental health in competing for NIMH funding, developments have raised concerns about future research. Reorganization within NIMH has led to the end of a separate branch dedicated to aging research and of the Mental Disorders of Aging Review Committee. Thus, NIMH funding for geriatric research has leveled off despite the growing number of older persons and increasing knowledge about mental health problems related to aging and their responsiveness to treatment.

Geriatric psychiatry has advanced similarly in Canada and Great Britain. In these countries, recognition of geriatric medicine as a subspecialty also was followed by the development of academic training programs in geriatric psychiatry. The first North American professional association in geriatric psychiatry was founded in the Canadian province of Quebec in the 1940s. Early leaders and advocates for geriatric psychiatry in Canada included Drs. V. A. Kral, Martin Cole, and Hans Reichenfeld. The first Canadian division of geriatric psychiatry for the training of geriatric psychiatrists was established at the University of Toronto in 1978 under the leadership of Dr. Abraham Miller; subsequently, the program was led by Drs. Kenneth Shulman, Joel Sadavoy, and Nathan Herrmann. In 1991, the Canadian Academy of Geriatric Psychiatry, currently led by Dr. David Conn, was founded under the leadership of Dr. Joel Sadavoy (founding president), Dr. J. Kenneth LeClair, and Dr. Marie-France Tourigny-Rivard. The academy established a national fellowship program to develop leadership in geriatric psychiatry and set standards for resident and fellowship training that were adopted by medical schools throughout Canada.

ric Association (APA), has remained particularly active and is led currently by Kenneth Sakauye who succeeded Gene Cohen, the first editor of both *International Psychogeriatrics* and the *American Journal of Geriatric Psychiatry*. The GAP orientation has been toward sociological aspects of geriatric psychiatry, and this has led to publication of monographs and articles in peer-reviewed journals that address community mental health, the psychotherapy of Alzheimer's disease, and the homeless.

The Boston Society for Gerontologic Psychiatry (BSGP) was founded by a group of psychoanalytically oriented psychiatrists—Martin Berezin, Stanley Cath, David Blau, and Ralph Kahana, among others—with a special interest in developmental issues related to aging and the effects of aging on regulation of self-esteem. The BSGP's semiannual, half-day workshops became the primary source of intellectual stimulation for budding geriatric psychiatrists across the country. Articles from BSGP's symposia were published in three books in the 1960s (Berezin & Cath, 1965; Levin & Kahana, 1967; Zinberg & Kaufman, 1963). Subsequently, BSGP created the *Journal of Geriatric Psychiatry* in 1967 and stimulated the development of similar groups in Chicago, Houston, New York, and greater Washington, DC.

In the mid-1960s, the APA created a small component on aging, with particular interest in community geriatric psychiatry, under the leadership of Alexander Simon. It was not until 1979, however, that APA initiated the Council on Aging (COA), which was to develop position papers on aging and mental health for the parent organization and to serve a liaison function with non-APA organizations devoted to geriatric psychiatry. The COA developed and published numerous important articles on topics such as psychiatric services, reimbursement, Alzheimer's disease, the interface of medicine and psychiatry in geriatrics, models of care, postgraduate education, nursing homes, geriatric psychiatry in the public sector, minorities, forensic psychiatric issues, and psychotropic medication for older people (Baker et al., 1985; Finkel et al., 1981; Moak et al., 1989). Early COA leaders included many of the "founding fathers" of geriatric psychiatry, such as Ewald Busse, Jack Weinberg, George Pollock, Charles Gaitz, Charles Wells, Sanford Finkel, Charles Shamoian, Gene Cohen, Jerome Yesavage, and Burton Reifler.

By 1978, there was a clear need for an American organization with a specific focus on geriatric psychiatry. Although the field had been developing significantly since the late 1940s, the increasing number of older people, the concomitant number of older persons with psychiatric disorders (particularly depressions and dementias), and the larger base of knowledge mandated the establishment of a forum in which to exchange ideas (Finkel, 1979). To accomplish this end, Sanford Finkel assembled a group of 15 nationally recognized leaders in the field of geriatric psychiatry to discuss the establishment of a national organization, the AAGP. This organizational meeting occurred initially at the 1978 annual meeting of the APA, the theme of which was aging. The initial goals of AAGP were

- To provide a focus for dissemination of information to the psychiatrists who care for the elderly. (A primary mechanism would be the publication of a newsletter that would provide information regarding mental health issues and elderly people.)
- To increase the attention of APA on the field of aging, with particular reference to services, training, research, and policy development. (AAGP also wished to advocate the establishment of a significant component on aging in APA.)
- To encourage local societies concerned with mental health aspects of aging. The first AAGP newsletter included "The Rationale for the Creation of an American Psychiatric Association Council on Aging" (Finkel, 1978).

In its first year, discussions between AAGP and Alan Stone, president-elect of APA, led to the establishment, on February 23, 1979, of the COA, effective September 1979. Also, Congress held the first national legislative conference on the mental health of older Americans in 1979.

AAGP began publishing a newsletter six times per year and instituted educational and research symposia at its annual meetings in addition to supporting more limited regional programs. A liaison relationship with APA was established. AAGP presidents in the 1980s included Sanford Finkel, Eric Pfeiffer, Alvin Levenson, Lissy Jarvik, Elliott Stein, Charles Shamoian, Lawrence Lazarus, and George Grossberg.

AAGP continued its membership growth during the late 1980s and 1990s, with over 1,300 members by 1995 and over 1,500 in 2000. After a decade of debate about designing a role of nonpsychiatric mental health professions in AAGP, a trial program was initiated to accept a limited number of nonpsychiatrists as affiliate members. During the early 1990s, under the presidential leadership of Jonathan Lieff, Barnett Meyers, Alan Siegal, Gary Gottlieb, and Ira Katz, AAGP undertook reorganization to streamline operations and facilitate the develop of the administrative infrastructure needed to expand activities beyond delivering direct services to its members and providing support for the annual meeting. The first full-time executive director was recruited in 1994.

During the late 1980s and 1990s, collaboration between AAGP and both the COA and its parent organization, the APA, increased. In the early 1990s, a permanent rotating seat on the Council was created for this purpose for the AAGP immediate past president. Previously, Ken Sakauye and Jerome Yesavage had served this liaison function informally while serving as COA chairs and participating at AAGP board meetings. AAGP was also invited by APA to appoint a member to represent the organization in an ex officio capacity at the APA assembly meetings. APA and its COA have collaborated with AAGP on the development of positions on parity in reimbursement for mental disorders, the appropriate application of guidelines for use of pharmacotherapeutic medications in the nursing home, the impact of managed care on psychiatric services to older persons, and the debate concerning national health care reform.

AAGP has continued to promote research and the development of young investigators. Formation of the Research Committee in 1991, with Dilip Jeste as its first chair, was a critical step in this process. Presentation of the Member-in-Training, Junior Investigator, and Senior Investigator Awards, made through the Research Committee, became a mechanism for acknowledging the work of investigators at different levels and of recognizing the scientific foundation on which knowledge disseminated at the annual meeting rests. The Summer Research Institute in Geriatric Psychiatry, supported through NIMH funding, has provided a 1-week program of intensive mentoring and didactic teaching that develops the scientific skills of young investigators who are selected through a competitive process. The program has already borne fruit by generating clinical investigators who have competed successfully for NIMH career development (K) awards. In addition, an AAGP-supported 1-day premeeting workshop is held for current K awardees to facilitate the development of their research skills. Another premeeting workshop, Stepping Stones, was initiated to introduce psychiatric residents to geriatric psychiatry.

Developments in Canada have largely paralleled those in the United States. The Canadian Psychiatric Association developed a division on aging in the 1970s, and the Canadian Geriatric Association was developed during the same decade. These institutions have continued to be active. The Canadian Academy of Geriatric Psychiatry was founded to establish, promote, and develop excellence in geriatric psychiatry in Canada. In contrast to the AAGP, this subspecialty organization required formal training or attainment of specified criteria for practice in geriatric psychiatry as a condition for membership. The academy's newsletter, website, annual scientific meeting, and national fellowship programs have been used to continue the education of its membership. In 2002 the CAGP spearheaded the formation of a National Nursing Home Coalition of over 60 organizations to address standards of institutional care for elders.

Organized Geriatric Psychiatry: Beyond the United States and Canada

The International Association of Gerontology was organized in Liege, Belgium, in 1950 and has supported regularly scheduled and well-attended multidisciplinary conferences around the world. These conferences addressed multiple issues related to aging, including mental health and mental illness (Shock, 1988).

The World Health Organization (WHO) has had a longstanding interest in psychogeriatrics; it published an early monograph (1972a) that elaborated the extent of the potential problems of psychopathology in later life, organizational services, research, epidemiology, and training (Henderson & MacFadyen,

1985). WHO has made efforts to stimulate the production of self-help guides and has developed monographs on drugs and senile dementia as well as mental health care (WHO, 1972b, 1983, 1984, 1985). Other areas of exploration in psychogeriatrics include assessing mental health care needs in the community and attention to diagnostic classification. WHO has given increasing attention to the problems of dementia, depression, and disablement and has contributed to the development of instruments for cross-cultural assessment, including the WHO Disablement Assessment Scale (WHODAS) (Epping-Jordan & Usten, 2000), which is used to assess relationships between late-life mental disorders and disablement.

International geriatric psychiatry also grew rapidly through other organizations. The World Psychiatric Association section on geriatric psychiatry increased its visibility with meetings in Europe and North America during the 1970s and 1980s with representation by leading academic geriatric psychiatrists such as Carl Eisdorfer, who served as chair of the section, and Raymond Levy, who served as secretary.

A major thrust for international collaboration in psychogeriatrics came with the foundation of the International Psychogeriatric Association (IPA) in the early 1980s. The fledgling organization began as the Nottingham 1980 Club, which followed an annual psychogeriatric conference for psychiatrists, internists, and general practitioners who worked with older patients. The 2-week course was devised and supervised by Tom Arie. Shortly after the 1980 meeting, two Canadians, Imre Fejer and Hans Reichenfeld, sought to establish an international organization. Dr. Sanford Finkel, the first president of AAGP, applied his leadership experience to the IPA and served as its first president.

After collaboration with Dr. A. Ashour of Ains Shams Medical School in Egypt, Cairo became the site of the first meeting of the IPA, the International Conference for the Mental Health of the Elderly. As a result of the meeting, the Egyptian medical schools in Cairo incorporated geriatrics into their training, and the Egyptian Medical Association developed a special committee on geriatrics.

Under the strong leadership of presidents Sanford Finkel, Manfred Bergener, Gustav Bucht, and Kazuo Hasegawa and with publication of a newsletter and later the journal *International Psychogeriatrics*, IPA has grown rapidly and played an important role in founding national psychogeriatric societies in Japan, Italy, and Sweden. IPA continued the growth of its membership and the number of countries represented. *International Psychogeriatrics* has expanded to a quarterly publication cycle, with special supplements devoted to important cross-cultural topics such as delirium, dementia, and late-life suicide. IPA joined the World Psychiatric Association in 1992, although it maintains its separate structure and functions.

Asia and Latin America are in many ways the next frontiers for geriatric psychiatry, and strong leadership groups have emerged in Hong Kong, Japan, Korea, and Brazil. It is expected that the Pacific Rim College of Psychiatrists, an organization founded in the late 1970s and comprised primarily of academic psychiatrists based in Asian countries, will develop a subsection devoted to geriatric psychiatry. Formation of the International College of Geriatric Neuropsychopharmacology in 2000 as an offshoot of the American College of Neuropsychopharmacology, with Dilip Jeste as its first president, has provided a venue for integrating the findings of leading clinical investigators with those of basic science researchers across the world.

REIMBURSEMENT FOR PSYCHIATRIC SERVICES TO OLDER PERSONS

The 1960s marked the US inception of several Great Society programs, including Medicare and Medicaid, which allowed more older people to receive inpatient psychiatric services. Initially, outpatient services were severely limited by a $250 annual cap, which remained until 1988. The limited Medicare coverage of outpatient services for the 95% of older adults who live in the community discouraged elderly persons from using mental health services and practitioners from providing them. The low visibility of geriatric psychiatry and a tradition of stigmatization interfered with attempts to secure improved patient benefits, but they gradually improved. Psychologists became eligible for reimbursement under certain conditions. In addition, under the leadership of Margaret Heckler, Secretary of Health and Human Services, Alzheimer's disease centers in various sections of the country were created, and psychiatrists treating elderly patients with dementia were reimbursed without an annual maximum when providing medical therapy and medication.

The 1981 White House Conference on Aging made further recommendations to increase funding for research and treatment based on the multidisciplinary Mini-Conference on the Mental Health of Older Americans (White House Conference on Aging, 1981). The action group to implement the recommendations investigated community mental health centers and the general problems of underservice to older persons (Fleming et al., 1984). Improved mental health benefits were finally approved in 1988. Although there are no longer annual limits on reimbursement of outpatient mental health services through Medicare, the 50% copayment remains a particular problem for indigent older persons living on fixed incomes who do not have coinsurance. The improvements in Medicare coverage that have occurred were presumably because of changes in public and political opinion that resulted from increased public awareness of the knowledge and skills of practitioners of geriatric psychiatry and of the effectiveness of treatments for late-life mental disorders.

THE GROWTH OF CONSUMER ORANIZATIONS

The 1980s marked the substantial growth of lay organizations that serve as advocacy groups for elderly persons and the beginning of dialogues between these organizations and leadership of geriatric psychiatry. The growth of consumer advocacy groups and their gradual recognition that mental health problems are not stigmatizing have been a major factor in the growth of public awareness of and support for improved geriatric mental health services. Growth of the American Association for Retired Persons (AARP), the National Council on Aging, and the Alzheimer's Disease and Related Disorders Association (ADRDA) continued to meet the needs of an increasing number of older persons.

The ADRDA pursues the goals of better serving persons with Alzheimer's disease and other forms of dementia and of their families through supporting research to improve diagnosis and treatment. ADRDA goals include the development of local networks to provide information to caregivers, initiate family support groups, sponsor educational programs, and publish a newsletter to keep caregivers informed of research developments. Leading geriatric psychiatrists, including Peter Rabins, who wrote *The 36-Hour Day* with Nancy Mace (1981), and Lissy Jarvik, who wrote *Parent Care: A Common Sense Guide for Adult Children* with Gary Small (1988), have made major contributions to ADRDA. Nevertheless, the establishment of formal liaisons between ADRDA and organized geriatric psychiatry has been limited by concerns about possible stigmatization of Alzheimer's patients and the initial perception that geriatric psychiatry condones the use of psychiatric medications in long-term care for the purpose of chemical restraint.

Overcoming similar concerns about the potential for stigmatizing later life as a time of deteriorating mental health has also slowed the development of ongoing relationships between organized geriatric psychiatry and consumer groups such as AARP. Nevertheless, meetings held between AAGP leadership and AARP in the late 1980s and early 1990s set the stage for collaborative initiatives and mutual support. The delivery of the keynote address at the 1991 Orlando AAGP annual meeting by Horace Deets, executive director of AARP, was evidence of the shared concerns of these organizations. Gene Cohen has continued to provide consultation to AARP on mental health issues, and Nathan Billig has had a similar role with the National Council on Aging. The October 2001 Consensus Conference, Unmet Needs in Diagnosis and Treatment of Mood Disorders in Late Life, sponsored by the National Depressive and Manic-Depressive Association, further demonstrated recognition by a major advocacy group of advances in geriatric psychiatry and the work that remains to be done.

Although much has been accomplished, more must be achieved during the early 21st century for geriatric psychiatry to reach its next plateau. High-priority issues include:

- The institution of new initiatives for research on prevention, treatment, and mental health services related to late-life mental disorders
- The expansion of knowledge about the pathogenesis and prevention of Alzheimer's disease and other psychiatric disorders of later life

- The delineation of psychiatric complications of dementia as potential targets for treatment
- The achievement of greater visibility for geriatric psychiatry among the general public, policymakers, and advocacy groups that represent older persons
- The undertaking of initiatives involving collaboration between organized geriatric psychiatry and consumer advocacy groups to improve mental health in later life
- The achievement of parity, particularly under Medicare, to ensure that older persons receive the same benefits for the treatment of mental health problems that they receive for physical health conditions
- Provision of a balance between the shorter hospital stays required to control heath care spending and the development of the more integrated and comprehensive mental health care system required by frail older persons

The chapters that follow provide state-of-the-art knowledge in the growing field of psychogeriatrics as well as cutting-edge findings that can be expected to improve the clinical mental health care of older persons in the years ahead.

REFERENCES

Abraham K. The applicability of psychoanalytic treatment to patients at an advanced age. In: Abraham K, ed. *Selected Papers on Psychoanalysis*. London, England: Hogarth Press; 1927:312–331.

Alexopoulos GS, Meyers BS, Young RC, Kakuma T, Silbersweig D, Charlson M. Clinically defined vascular depression. *Am J Psychiatry*. 1997;154:562–565.

Almeida O, Howard R, Levy R, David AS. Psychotic states arising in late life (late paraphrenia): psychopathology and nosology. *Br J Psychiatry*. 1995;166:205–214.

Alzheimer A. A characteristic disease of the cerebral cortex. In: Bick K, Amaducci L, Pepeu G, eds. *The Early Story of Alzheimer's Disease*. New York, NY: Raven Press; 1987.

Arie T, Jones R, Smith C. The educational potential of old age psychiatric services. In: Arie T, ed. *Recent Advances in Psychogeriatrics*. Edinburgh, Scotland: Churchill Livingstone; 1985.

Baker FN, Pen IN, Yesavage JY. *An Overview of Legal Issues in Geriatric Psychiatry*. Washington, DC: American Psychiatric Press; 1985.

Barraclough B. Conversations with Felix Post: part II. *Psychiatr Bull*. 1989;13:114–119.

Berezin MA, Cath SH, eds. *Geriatric Psychiatry: Grief, Loss and Emotional Disorders in the Aging Process*. New York, NY: International University Press; 1965.

Birren JE. Neural basis of personal adjustment in aging. In: *Age With a Future*. Copenhagen, Denmark: Munkegaard; 1964.

Birren J, Sloane B. *Handbook of Mental Health and Aging*. Englewood Cliffs, NJ: Prentice-Hall; 1980.

Blazer DG. *Depression in Late Life*. St. Louis, MO: CV Mosby; 1993.

Blessed G, Tomlinson BE, Roth M. The association between quantitative measures of dementia and of senile change in the cerebral grey matter of elderly subjects. *Br J Psychiatry.* 1968;114:797–811.

Borson S, Bartels SJ, Colenda CC, Gottlieb GL, Meyers B. Geriatric mental health services research: strategic plan for an aging population: report of the Health Services Work Group of the American Association for Geriatric Psychiatry. *Am J Geriatr Psychiatry.* 2001;9(3):191–204.

Busse EW, Blazer DG, eds. *Handbook of Geriatric Psychiatry.* New York, NY: Van Nostrand Reinhold; 1980.

Busse EW, Blazer DG, eds. *Textbook of Geriatric Psychiatry.* Washington, DC: American Psychiatric Press; 1996.

Busse EW, Pfeiffer E, eds. *Behavior and Adaptation in Late Life.* Boston, MA: Little, Brown; 1969.

Butler RN. Mission of the National Institution on Aging. *J Am Geriatr Soc.* 1977;25: 97–103.

Butterfield LH. Benjamin Rush, the American Revolution and the American millennium. *Harvard Med Alumni Bull.* 1976;50:16–22.

Ciompi L. The outcome of late life psychiatric disorders. *J Geriatr Psychiatry.* 1972;39: 789–794.

Clark JE, Lanphear AK, Riddick CC. The effects of videogame playing on the response selection processing of elderly adults. *J Gerontol.* 1987;4:82–85.

Coffey CE, Cummings JL, eds. *Textbook of Geriatric Neuropsychiatry.* Washington, DC: American Psychiatric Press; 1994.

Cohen GD. *The Brain in Human Aging.* New York, NY: Springer; 1988.

Cohen GD. The movement toward subspecialty status for geriatric psychiatry in the United States. *Int Psychogeriatr.* 1989;1:201–205.

Copeland JRM, Abou-Saleh MT, Blazer DG, eds. *Principles and Practice of Geriatric Psychiatry.* London: Wiley; 1994.

Copeland JRM, Dewey ME, Griffiths-Jones. A computerized psychiatric diagnostic and case nomenclature for elderly subjects. *Psychol Med.* 1984;23:88–99.

Epping-Jordan JA, Ustun TB. The WHODAS-II: levelling the playing field for all disorders. *WHO Ment Health Bull.* 2000;6:5–6.

Ferenczi S. A contribution to the understanding of the psychoneuroses of the age of involution. In: Balint M, ed. *Selected Papers: Problems and Methods of Psychoanalysis, Vol. 3: Final Contributions to the Problems and Methods of Psychoanalysis.* New York, NY: Basic Books; 1955.

Finkel SI. The rationale for the creation of an American Psychiatric Council on Aging. *AAGP Newsletter.* 1978;1:5.

Finkel SI. Experience of a private practice psychiatrist working with the elderly in the community. *Int J Ment Health.* 1979;8:147–172.

Finkel SI, Borson S, Shamoian C, et al. *The American Psychiatric Association Task Force Report on the 1981 White House Conference on Aging.* Washington, DC: American Psychiatric Association; 1981.

Fleming AS, Buchanan JG, Santos JF. *Report on the Survey of Community Health Centers by the Action Committee to Implement the Mental Health Recommendations of the 1981 White House Conference on Aging.* Chicago, IL: The Retirement Research Foundation; 1984.

Folstein M, Folstein S, McHugh PR. Mini-Mental State: a practical method of grading the cognitive state of patients for the clinician. *J Psychiatr Res.* 1975;12:189–198.

Freud S. My view on the past plagued by sexuality in the aetiology of the neuroses. In: Jones E, ed. *The Complete Psychological Works of Sigmund Freud*. Vol. 6. London: Hogarth Press; 1953. (Original work published 1898)

Group for the Advancement of Psychiatry. *The Problem of the Aged Patient in the Public Psychiatric Hospital*. New York, NY: Group for Advancement of Psychiatry; 1950. GAP Report 14.

Group for the Advancement of Psychiatry, Committee on Aging. *The Psychiatric Treatment of Alzheimer's Disease*. New York, NY: Brunner/Mazel; 1988.

Hall GS. *Senescence: The Last Half of Life*. New York, NY: Appleton; 1922.

Henderson JH, MacFadyen DM. Psychogeriatrics and the programmes of the World Health Organization. In: Arie T, ed. *Recent Advances in Psychogeriatrics*. Edinburgh, Scotland: Churchill Livingstone; 1985.

Jarvik L. The impact of immediate life situations on depression, illness, and loss. In: Bresla D, Haig MR, eds. *Depression and Aging*. New York, NY: Springer; 1983: 114–120.

Jarvik LF, Small GW. *Parent Care: A Common Sense Guide for Adult Children*. New York, NY: Crown Publishers; 1988.

Jenike MA. *Geriatric Psychiatry and Psychopharmacology*. St. Louis, MO: Mosby–Year Book, 1989.

Jeste DV, Finkel SI. Psychosis of Alzheimer disease and related dementias. Diagnostic criteria for a distinct syndrome. *Am J Geriatr Psychiatry*. 2000;8:29–34.

Jeste DV, Harris MJ, Krull A, Kuck J, McAdams LA, Heaton R. Clinical and neuropsychological characteristics of patients with late-onset schizophrenia. *Am J Psychiatry*. 1995;152:722–730.

Kay DW. Geriatric psychiatry in the 1950s and 1960s: recollections. *Int Psychogeriatr*. 1999;11:363–365.

Kay DWK. Outcome and causes of death in mental disorders of old age: a long-term follow-up of functional and organic psychosis. *Acta Psychiatr Scand*. 1962;38:249–276.

Krishnan KRR, Hays JC, Blazer DG. MRI-defined vascular depression. *Am J Psychiatry*. 1997;154:497–501.

Lazarus LW, ed. *Essentials of Geriatric Psychiatry*. New York, NY: Springer; 1988.

Levin S, Kahana RJ. *Psychodynamic Studies on Aging, Creativity, Reminiscing, and Dying*. New York, NY: International Universities Press; 1967.

Lewis A. Aging and senility: a major problem of psychiatry. *J Ment Sci*. 1946;92:150–170.

Mace NL, Rabins PV. *The 36-Hour Day*. Baltimore, MD: Johns Hopkins University Press; 1981.

Maugham S. *The Summing Up*. London, England: William Heinemann; 1938.

Moak GS, Stein EM, Rubin JEV. *The Over-50 Guide to Psychiatric Medications*. Washington, DC: American Psychiatric Press; 1989.

Murphy E. The prognosis of depression in old age. *Br J Psychiatry*. 1983;142:111–119.

Nascher IL. *Geriatrics: The Diseases of Old Age and Their Treatment*. Philadelphia, PA: P. Blokiston's Son; 1914.

Nascher IL. The aging mind. *Med Record*. 1944;157–669.

Olin JT, Schneider LS, Katz IR, et al. National Institute of Mental Health—provisional diagnostic criteria for depression of Alzheimer's disease. *Am J Geriatr Psychiatry*. 2002;10:125–128.

Palmore E, ed. *Normal Aging II.* Durham, NC: Duke University Press; 1974.

Palmore E. Predictors of successful aging. *Gerontologist.* 1979;19:427–431.

Pearlson GD, Kreger L, Rabins PV, et al. A chart review study of late-onset and early onset schizophrenia. *Am J Psychiatry.* 1989;146:1568–1574.

Post F. *The Clinical Psychiatry of Late Life.* Oxford, UK: Pergamon; 1965.

Prince MJ, Harwood RH, Mann TA. A prospective population-based cohort study of the effects of disablement and social milieu on the onset and maintenance of late-life depression. The Gospel Oak Project VII. *Psychol Med.* 1998;28:337–350.

Reichenfeld HF. Geriatric psychiatry north of the border. *AAGP Newsletter.* 1987;9: 11–12.

Roth M. The natural history of mental disorders in old age. *J Ment Sci.* 1955;101: 281–301.

Roth M. The relationship between quantitative measures of dementia and degenerative changes in the cerebral grey matter of elderly subjects. *Proc R Soc Med.* 1967;60: 254.

Rowe JW, Grossman E, Bond E. The Institute of Medicine Committee on Leadership for Academic Geriatric Medicine: academic geriatrics for the year 2000. *N Engl J Med.* 1987;316:1425–1428.

Sadavoy J, *Psychotropic Drugs and the Elderly: Fast Facts.* New York:

Sadavoy J, Lazarus LW, Jarvik L, eds. *Comprehensive Review of Geriatric Psychiatry.* Washington, DC: American Psychiatric Press; 1991.

Sadavoy J, Lazarus L, Jarvik L, Grossberg G, eds. *Comprehensive Review of Geriatric Psychiatry.* 2nd ed. Washington, DC: American Psychiatric Press; 1996.

Sadavoy J, Leszcz M. *Treating the Elderly With Psychotherapy: The Scope for Change in Later Life.* New York, NY: International Universities Press; 1987.

Salzman C. *Clinical Geriatric Psychopharmacology.* Philadelphia, PA: Lippincott, Williams & Wilkins; 1997.

Salzman C, Lebowitz BD, eds. *Anxiety in the Elderly.* New York, NY: Springer; 1991.

Schutz JA, Adair D, eds. *The Spur of Fame: Dialogues of John Adams and Benjamin Rush, 1805–1813.* San Marino: Liberty Fund; 1966.

Shock NW. *The International Association of Gerontology: A Chronicle—1950 to 1986.* New York, NY: Springer; 1988.

Szwabo PA, Grossberg GT, eds. *Problem Behaviors in Long-Term Care.* New York, NY: Springer; 1993.

US Department of Health, Education, and Welfare, Federal Council on Aging. *Mental Health and the Elderly—Recommendations for Action. The Reports of the President's Commission on Mental Health: Task Panel on the Elderly and the Secretary's Committee on Mental Health and Illness of the Elderly.* Washington, DC: US Government Printing Office; 1979. DHEW Publication 80–20960.

US Department of Health, Education, and Welfare, Public Health Service. *National Institute of Mental Health Research on the Mental Health of Aging—1960–1976.* Rockville, MD: 1977.

Vaillant GE, Mukamal K. Successful aging. *Am J Psychiatry.* 2001;158:839–847.

White House Conference on Aging. *Report of the Mini-Conference on the Mental Health of Older Americans (Mer-16).* Washington, DC: US Government Printing Office; 1981.

World Health Organization. *Drugs and the Elderly.* Copenhagen, Denmark: World Health Organization; 1985.

World Health Organization. *Mental Health Care of the Elderly: Report on a Working Group.* Copenhagen, Denmark: World Health Organization Regional Office for Europe; 1983.

World Health Organization. *Psychogeriatrics. Report of a World Health Organization Scientific Group.* Geneva, Switzerland: World Health Organization; 1972a. Technical Report Series 507.

World Health Organization. *Self Health Care and Older People: A Manual for Public Policy and Programme Development.* Copenhagen, Denmark: World Health Organization; 1984.

World Health Organization. *Senile Dementia: Report of a Scientific Group.* Geneva, Switzerland: World Health Organization; 1972b.

Zinberg NE, Kaufman I. *Normal Psychology of the Aging Process.* New York, NY: International Universities Press; 1963.

Comprehensive Textbook
of Geriatric Psychiatry

SECTION I

The Aging Process

1

Epidemiology of Psychiatric Disorders

Barry J. Gurland, FRC Physicians (London), FRC Psychiatry

E pidemiology can contribute to learning about psychiatric problems in aging by the study of the variation in the frequency and course of psychiatric problems across subgroups of aging persons. Frequency may be expressed as *prevalence*, usually the number of cases found in a defined population during a specific period of time such as a day (point prevalence) or a longer period of a month or a year (period prevalence), or *incidence* (usually new cases emerging during a period of time, typically a year). Variation in frequency can be linked to group characteristics such as age, gender, education, ethnicity, other demographic classes, or other accompaniments or precedents of interest (e.g., life events, social supports, medical illness, or genetic inheritance). Such relationships can indicate who is vulnerable to developing a disorder and what are the potential causes of the disorder. Longitudinal studies can determine the duration of a disorder and range of outcomes that occur in general or in special circumstances (e.g., location in a community or in an institution or types and use of available health services). Psychiatric problems in epidemiological reports are often taken to mean diagnostic groups, usually restricted to those meeting criteria in a nomenclature, such as the *Diagnostic and Statistical Manual of*

Owing to the large number of citations, references prior to 1990 are cited in the chapter on epidemiology in the first and second editions of this book.

Mental Disorders, Fourth Edition (*DSM-IV*; American Psychiatric Association [APA], 1994), but may also refer to symptom syndromes that are of clinical interest or are linked to serious consequences.

EPIDEMIOLOGICAL STRATEGIES

Epidemiological studies can produce descriptive accounts of the frequency and distribution of psychiatric disorders. For example, it may be found in the older population that there are more women than men with depression, and that the proportion of women with depression is greater than the corresponding proportion of men. However, epidemiology makes little sense if it is restricted to mustering subgroups and counting problems; it is the analysis of the circumstances surrounding variation that carries etiologic, clinical, and service implications. To investigate what makes women appear more susceptible to (i.e., at greater risk for) depression, then analytic epidemiology must be used (Hendrie, 1997). This will involve, in this instance, measuring and evaluating the relative importance of the many candidate influences on rates of depression that might occur more often in women because of their distinctive gender-related biological characteristics or because of their unique social and psychological experiences and situations. Longitudinal studies generally yield more informative data for analytic approaches than do cross-sectional studies.

Interpreting Epidemiological Findings

Given the inevitable inexactitudes of survey procedures (e.g., measurement error, missing data because of nonresponders, limitations in generalizing), it is desirable to compare several related studies and exercise good judgment in reaching inferences from survey findings. It is also important to interpret epidemiological evidence on the course and outcome of a disorder in the light of information on the proportion of cases in contact with health care resources, receiving appropriate treatment, and with access to informal sources of care. It is also necessary to take into consideration the extent to which course and outcomes are determined by overlap between psychiatric disorder and comorbidity with other psychiatric, medical, and social problems.

Epidemiological comparisons across different studies may be confounded by diversity in methods of information collection and case ascertainment (i.e., differences in the wording of questionnaires, training of interviewers, use of informants, diagnostic nosologies, period of ascertainment) (Lepine & Bouchez, 1998). Various standard techniques, such as computerized diagnoses (e.g., AGECAT; Copeland et al., 1990) can be set to obtain consistent designation of psychiatric disorders. Nevertheless, the information obtained from a given questionnaire (e.g., on cognition) may be influenced not only by the nature of a psychiatric disorder, but also by variations in the gender, education, and social class composition of the comparison groups (Burvill, 1990).

Milder or earlier cases are probably less reliably diagnosed than well-established cases. A comparison of five operational methods for diagnosis of mild dementia among elderly patients showed a considerable influence of "non-dementia" factors. In a follow-up study of community residents with minimal dementia, only 6 of 29 survivors after 1 year showed progressive intellectual deterioration, and 13 were reclassified as normal (O'Connor & Roth, 1990). In a representative sample of elderly people aged 70 years and older residing in a community, prevalence rates for mild dementia varied widely according to the criteria used.

Epidemiological data may be derived from subjective and objective measures in field interviews, expert evaluation, or laboratory investigations. Subjective or self-report information may introduce uncertainty about the degree to which positive responses are determined by the tendency of the subject to report the condition. Expert evaluation is open to the emphases of a particular professional training background. Laboratory tests may have a high rate of nonresponders. The greater the variety of sources and types of information converging on a given condition and its associations, the greater the confidence that can be placed in the findings. Epidemiological findings carry relevant messages for clinical practice, public health responses, and research directions, for example, estimating the extent and location of the need for preventive and active treatment to reduce risks of onset, persistence, or relapse of psychiatric disorders; identifying likely causes; and gauging the effects of age on the frequency and course of psychiatric disorders.

Estimating the Extent and Location of the Need for Treatment of Psychiatric Disorders

The distribution of psychiatric disorders among elders may vary considerably with the care setting, region, and time period (Sandberg et al., 1998). Orienting distributions to care settings is helpful for health policy formation, planning of clinical services, and setting clinical practice standards, but results from any particular setting must be cautiously interpreted in the light of possible regional and period variation.

SPECIFIC DISORDERS

Depression

RATES Reported rates of depression will vary depending on the level of severity of depression that is designated as fulfilling the criteria for diagnosis, so rates may vary widely across sites of study (Ayuso-Mateos et al., 2001). In samples representative of all noninstitutionalized persons aged 65 years or older in a defined geographic area, depressions conforming to *DSM-III* or *DSM-IV* (APA,

1980, 1994) criteria (mainly major depression and dysthymia) have been reported to be present in 2% and 4% (McConnell et al., 2002; Weissman et al., 1991) of the population, with major depression accounting for less than 1%. Subsyndromal (or subthreshold) depressions, which do not meet criteria for *DSM* diagnoses because the symptoms are fewer or shorter in duration (Mulsant & Ganguli, 1999; Papassotiropoulos & Heun, 1999; Schotte & Cooper, 1999) are more common than major depressions and dysthymias and account for substantial psychosocial impairment and risk of developing major depression and of suicide (Sadek & Bona, 2000). Persons aged 65 years and older comprise 6.3% of all individuals with major depression and dysthymia and 12.9% of those with subclinical depression (Johnson et al., 1992).

Some community studies have found considerably higher rates of depression among elders (e.g., a prevalence rate of 9% for major depression in cognitively intact elderly community subjects). Moreover, if persons with all depressive symptomatology of clinical interest are included, the reported rates rise to 10%, 15%, or even higher (Kennedy et al., 1990; Livingston et al., 1990), and incidence rates have been reported as high as 11.2% over 2 years. Clinical significance (i.e., warranting psychiatric attention) may include major depression, dysthymia, atypical depressions, and subthreshold affective disorders.

Among short-stay psychiatric inpatients, depressions that meet *DSM-III* or *DSM-IV* (APA, 1980, 1994) criteria are common. In many such settings, one half of all admissions may conform to the criteria for major depression. An admixture of anxiety symptoms with varying degrees of prominence is common. Residents in nursing homes and congregate apartment residences have been found to have a 15.7% prevalence of major depression and a 16.5% prevalence for minor depressive symptoms; with an incidence of major depression at the end of 1 year of 6.6% and even higher in persons with preexisting minor depression (Parmelee et al., 1992).

In ambulatory medical settings, anxiety and depressive disorders are common, especially atypical, rather than major, depressions, largely because depression is increased in both acute and chronic medical disorders. Depression as a nosological entity and as a symptom syndrome that does not meet diagnostic criteria is the most frequently encountered psychiatric condition in primary medical care (Blacker & Clare, 1988; Katon & Sullivan, 1990), with major depression in about 5% to 10% of primary care patients (Katon & Schulberg, 1992). Dysthymias in elders are mostly found in primary care settings (Kirby, Bruce et al., 1999). Among patients admitted to an acute geriatric care unit, 10% had a depressive illness, and a further 30% had some milder, but clinically significant, symptoms (Finch et al., 1992).

COURSE   Clinically significant depression in elders tends to be chronic (especially in women), with half the cases remaining depressed for lengthy periods of time (Livingston et al., 1997) and perhaps only 20% remaining depression free over a few years (Sharma et al., 1998). Few of these elderly receive adequate treatment, although treated cases remit sooner than do earlier onset cases (Reynolds et al., 1998). Among the reported consequences of depression are social withdrawal and desolation, excess service use, and suicide (Palsson & Skoog, 1997). Moreover, depression has been reported to increase mortality rates (Sharma et al., 1998), although some studies suggest that this relationship disappears once the associated disability is taken into account. There is a corresponding controversy as to whether depression causes acceleration of life-shortening conditions, such as cognitive and physical deterioration, the converse, or both (reciprocal effects) (Parmelee et al., 1998).

The outcome of depression appears to be altered by the size, functioning, and perceived helpfulness and warmth of the patient's social network; the quality of social exchanges is more salient than the mere quantity of social interactions. Adequacy of emotional support is most protective, but also relevant are tangible support (help with tasks), confidants, and visits from children. Infrequency and other deficits in the extent and closeness of the person's social contacts, the expectation of help from that network, and the paucity of club or religious membership correlate with a higher risk of depression (Norris & Murrell, 1990; Russell & Cutrona, 1991; Stallones et al., 1990). It may be that stress precipitates relapse of depression in the presence of weak social supports. The risk of relapse and recurrence of treated major depression in elders may be determined also by impairment of executive function (initiation and perseveration) (Alexopoulos et al., 2000).

INFLUENCES   Risk of depression is increased by female gender, prior history of depression, bereavement, living alone, weak social supports, caregiver burden, nursing home admission, cognitive decline, anxiety, alcohol abuse, medications, medical conditions, physical function deficits, and limitation of activities (Jorm, 1995; Lepine & Bouchez, 1998; Mulsant & Ganguli, 1999; Schoevers et al., 2000). In a study drawn from general practitioner lists, the incidence of depression (depressive psychosis and neurosis together; more or less equivalent to *DSM-III* [APA, 1980] major depression and dysthymia) was predicted most powerfully by lack of satisfaction with life, loneliness, smoking, female gender, and recent bereavement (Green et al., 1992). Higher rates of depression in older women than older men have been widely reported (Palinkas et al., 1990), with as much as a two-fold gender difference (Burt & Stien, 2002; Dewey et al., 1993). The excess rates in women are a consistent finding (Ustun, 2000) and may have emerged in those born after World War II (Murphy et al., 2000). Depression in women may be related to transitions in reproductive and hormonal events.

Depression is associated with the accumulation of life events and constant strain and is moderated by higher levels of mastery and social support. Life events, including loss of a spouse and change in functional ability, have been observed to influence the outcome of depression in elderly patients (Oxman et al., 1992). Cumulative life events and chronic strain have independent effects on depression, although older subjects may have a more constricted set of sa-lient life events than younger persons. Negative life events, particularly be-reavement, often precipitate episodes of depression in the form of a disorder or clinically severe dysphoria (Livingston et al., 1990).

Higher rates of depression have been noted in certain socioeconomically disadvantaged older groups (George et al., 1991). The effect of social patterns on depression may work through the sense of control persons have over their lives, on the perception of receiving support, and the nature of problem-solving communication at times of crisis or through preventive actions. Conversely, in-effective help from others and failures in giving encouragement and assistance where and when needed may expose the older person not only to the more immediate effects of stress, but also to the depressing influence of sustained daily hassles over a long period of time (Russell & Cutrona, 1991). Social relationships can induce both health-promoting and health-damaging effects, possibly through the medium of hormonal, cardiovascular, and immune path-ways (Seeman, 2000). Social supports in the period preceding aging can have a powerful influence on the onset and persistence of psychiatric problems, such as depression, during the period of transition into the older age brackets (Vail-lant et al., 1998).

For older persons, death of a spouse is often more depressing than death of a parent or child (Norris & Murrell, 1990). Elevated levels of depression have been found in widows preceding, and for up to 2 years following, be-reavement; a majority of widows had high scores on depression rating scales soon after bereavement, but most of the high scorers returned to prebereave-ment levels at 12 months (Harlow et al., 1991). Symptoms of self-limiting grief are hard to distinguish from diagnostic criteria for depressive disorder in the first 3 months after a loss (Zisook & Schuchter, 1991), although feelings of guilt and worthlessness are much less prominent than in nonbereaved persons with depression. Small social networks (e.g., fewer children in contact, living alone, and lack of active membership in clubs or religious circles) and small size of the friendship network increase vulnerability to depression during be-reavement. Friends have a longer term influence on adjustment to single living, whereas families seemed to be a bigger help soon after bereavement. Depres-sion several months before bereavement can predict postbereavement depres-sion and identify caregivers who might benefit from early intervention (Harlow et al., 1991).

AGE Depression rates do not appear to rise with age (Christensen et al., 1999; Dewey et al., 1993), although there is lack of agreement on this. A peak in depression rates has been noted in women before 60 years of age, with a secondary peak after age 65, although no such pattern was seen in men (Wu & Anthony, 2000). Depression in older age groups has possibly been undercounted in surveys. There may be a low degree of agreement between survey methods of diagnosis and clinical evaluation of major depression, with the survey missing cases for which subjects, especially older subjects, under-reported symptoms attributed to life crises and medical conditions (Eaton et al., 2000). Depression screening scales may be rendered less efficient by the overlap between depressive and physical impairment symptoms (Vahle et al., 2000) because of the confounds of physical comorbidity and age-specific pre-sentation of symptoms (Gottfries, 1998; Snowdon, 1990). Some reports suggest that depression may be expressed not as sadness, but as unexplained somatic symptoms, slowed movement, lack of interest in personal care, sleep distur-bance, or limitations of activities (Gallo & Rabins, 1999). Also, studies so far include relatively small numbers of subjects who are very old.

If risk factors are controlled, rates of depression (and anxiety) may even tend to decrease with age beyond that which can be explained by attrition because of institutional admission and mortality (Jorm, 2000). Perhaps older persons are able to cope well with physical illness and other age-related insults. Some studies have suggested that elderly people are less prone to blame them-selves regarding their disability and more likely to receive calmly the reality or possibility of a life-threatening illness such as cancer. Older adults may be viewed as a band of survivors who have learned to cope with adverse circumstances. Moreover, events such as physical illness tend with aging to become more chronic than acute and perhaps are less stressful for that reason (Kennedy et al., 1990). Other explanations that have been offered include a selective vulner-ability to premature death or institutionalization in earlier onset depressions or the receipt of treatment that prevents new episodes from occurring in later life. Perhaps neurobiological changes with age make the older person less vulnera-ble to depression. Moreover, the incidence and prevalence of mania arguably decrease with age (McDonald, 2000).

RECOGNITION The opportunity to detect depression in medical settings is particu-larly important because of the associated suffering and the risk of suicide. Depression as a syndrome or diagnosable disorder in medical settings is often chronic, although potentially responsive to antidepressants (Katon et al., 1993). Patients in primary medical care, judged by research evaluation to be suitable for a trial of antidepressants, nonetheless often go untreated (Katon et al., 1992). Even major depression is underrecognized and undertreated, perhaps because physicians do not distinguish depressive from physical symptoms or because patients minimize their symptoms or attribute them to a physical cause (Pin-cus & Pettit, 2001). Information from screening instruments has been shown to increase recognition and treatment of depression by the primary care physician (Magruder-Habib et al., 1990), and efforts have been made to raise awareness of practitioners and patients about the opportunities to effectively treat depres-sive disorders.

COMORBIDITY OF PHYSICAL ILLNESS AND DEPRESSION Depression of all types, including clinically significant depression, is increased in the presence of a wide variety of functional impairments and physical illnesses (Wells et al., 1993). The risk for depression in the physically ill older patient is increased up to threefold. This association holds true not only for the symptoms and syndromes of depression, but also for depression diagnoses such as major depression. Increasing disability and deterioration in health are stronger predictors of depression than number of medical conditions, social support, and stress. Affective and anxiety disorders are associated with both acute and chronic illness and limitations of physical functioning.

The causal direction between physical illness and depression is uncertain and has been argued both ways (Wells et al., 1992). Depression may amplify (i.e., increase the severity, awareness, and reporting of) the symptoms of physical illness. With some exceptions, the links between physical illness and depression are general and multiple rather than specific. Reciprocal influences between depression and physical illness or dysfunction could also operate through the personal meanings of lost health and functioning, noncompliance with treatment, stress imposed by symptoms, suppression of immune processes, concurrent aging effects on physical illness and neurotransmitter levels controlling mood, consequences of constricted lives and erosion of independence, increased sensitivity in awareness of physical symptoms, and side effects of medications.

There are some especially depressogenic medical conditions, for example, stroke, particularly left hemisphere lesions; Parkinson's disease (Zesiewicz & Hauser, 2002) (for which the depression is related to severity of the condition) (Tom & Cummings, 1998); cancer (Chochinov, 2001); and endocrine disorders (Finch et al., 1992). Cushing's syndrome predisposes not only to major depression, but also to mania, anxiety disorders, and cognitive decline and may respond better to inhibitors of corticosteroid production than to specific treatments of the psychiatric symptoms (Sonino & Fava, 2001). Some studies reported that depression rates are increased in epilepsy, especially of the temporal lobe type and left sided (Harden, 2002). Gender differences have been reported in response to disability and physical illness, with depression tending to be a reaction to pain in women and to functional impairment in men. In African Americans, depression has been associated with cardiovascular disorders, a number of comorbid conditions, and a number of medications for chronic illness (Okwumabua et al., 1997).

The acuity or chronicity of the course of the physical condition also modifies its effect on depression. Depression occurring after stroke is associated with aggravation of functional and cognitive impairment and increased risk of death (Whyte & Mulsant, 2002). Depression tends to improve as physical status improves (von Korff et al., 1990). More than one third of major depressions found in one community study were associated with medication use, pointing to the need to avoid nonessential medications.

Somatic symptoms could potentially confound the diagnosis of major depression, especially if the primary care patient emphasizes the somatic rather than the mood symptoms of depression or complains principally about the symptoms of an accompanying physical illness. Multiplicity of pains raises the likelihood that a depressive disorder is present (Dworkin et al., 1990).

Complicating these relationships is the finding that hypochondriasis, a fearful preoccupation with disease and related physical sensations that has a prevalence in primary medical care of 0.8% to 4.5%, is associated with increased rates of depression or anxiety (Magarinos et al., 2002). Somatization disorder occurs in approximately 5% to 10% of primary care patients and is frequently accompanied by a depressive disorder. Among elders in a residential facility, chronic fatigue was almost universal, but the intensity varied with depression symptoms, pain, and numbers of medications (Liao & Ferrell, 2000). Chronic fatigue syndromes differ in construct from depression and anxiety (Hadzi-Pavlovic et al., 2000). However, the risk of a new onset of chronic fatigue is increased by an episode of depression; fatigue predicts a later depression syndrome (Addington et al., 2001).

SUICIDE Rates of completed suicide are particularly high in older groups (Pritchard, 1992), especially white males (Dennis & Lindesay, 1995), although suicidal ideation occurs more frequently in women than in men (Hintikka et al., 2001). Distinctions between predictors of suicide attempts and completions are not marked in elderly people. With advancing age, a higher proportion of suicide attempts succeed (Hawton & Fagg, 1990). Older adults attempting suicide are at high risk for a later completed suicide (Merrill & Owens, 1990). Suicidal ideation in a general population of elders has been reported at 5.4% for the wish to die and 1% for suicidal thoughts or actions (Barnow & Linden, 2000). Studies in both the United Kingdom and the United States have shown that adults aged 65 years or older constitute approximately 4% to 6% of people who have attempted suicide and have been referred for treatment.

The great majority of older people who have completed suicide had a preceding psychiatric condition, usually major depression with a late onset, often the first episode (Conwell et al., 1991; Draper, 1994). In addition to the effects of depressive disorders, risk of suicide attempts and completions is accentuated in older adults who are divorced, alcoholic (Draper, 1994), recently bereaved, have a sense of loneliness and isolation, or are seriously physically ill (Conwell et al., 1990; Nowers, 1993), particularly if the illness is painful (Lindesay, 1991b). Lifelong traits, such as incapacity for intimacy, feelings of helplessness, or intolerance for change may heighten vulnerability (Lindesay, 1991b). Risk of suicide peaks in women at about the time of menopause.

Public health measures to reduce access to means of suicide are important. Suicide from drug overdose remains high in the older age groups and highest in men older than 75 years (37.7 deaths per million), most often from paracetamol, benzodiazepines, antidepressants, and opiates (in descending order of frequency) (Shah et al., 2002). The individual who intends suicide is often physically ill and hence is in contact with a physician (Osuna et al., 1997), thus offering an opportunity for prevention. In addition, because over 80% of elders with suicidal ideation were diagnosed with a psychiatric disorder, this raises a caution in assessing the appropriateness of physician-assisted suicide.

Anxiety Disorders

Anxiety disorders usually take the form of generalized anxiety or phobias, especially agoraphobia without panic attacks (Flint, 1998, 1999). The spectrum of anxiety disorders also includes panic, obsessional, and somatization disorders. Generalized anxiety and social phobias are associated with a level of impairment comparable to, and independent of, major depression (Shah et al., 2002) and tend to be persistent if untreated (den Boer, 2000; Faravelli et al., 2000; Hidalgo et al., 2001; Wittchen & Fehm, 2001). Yet, persons with generalized anxiety tend not to seek professional treatment (Kessler et al., 2001), and social phobias are underrecognized and undertreated in primary care (Hidalgo et al., 2001).

Anxiety disorders in elders are reported to decrease with age (Forsell & Winblad, 1998; Regier et al., 1990), at least in the very old (Schaub & Linden, 2000), although this has been questioned (Fuentes & Cox, 1997; Palmer et al., 1997; Spinhoven et al., 1997; van Balkom et al., 2000). Anxiety disorders in elders usually began earlier in life and are precipitated by stressful events and chronic disease.

However, anxiety symptoms, such as those associated with depression and dementia, may remain at a level frequency until an advanced age. Agoraphobia in elderly people is commonly of late onset, often precipitated by comorbid physical illness or other traumatic incident (Lindesay, 1991a). Specific fears are more often of early onset and less disabling. Obsessive-compulsive disorder may increase in older women (Eaton et al., 1991). Posttraumatic stress syndrome is less frequent in older than younger populations (Creamer et al., 2001).

Rates of anxiety disorders range from upward of 4% of community-residing elders (Blazer et al., 1991; Karno & Golding, 1991; McConnell et al., 2002; Swartz et al., 1991). Anxiety symptoms have been reported in close to 40% of those treated in inpatient and outpatient geriatric services. Prevalence of phobic disorders in a community survey of urban elderly people in the United Kingdom was 10%. Those who were phobic in this community survey had multiple fears and an increased prevalence of other neurotic symptoms. Rates of social phobias are higher in women than in men (Hidalgo et al., 2001; Krasucki et al., 1999; Sinoff et al., 1999).

Relationships between phobic disorder and physical illness might arise from the anxiety occasioned by the stress of physical illness; by virtue of the depressive effects of physical illness; through specific pathways associated with, for example, cardiovascular disorder, respiratory illness, or inner ear dysfunction; and through common roots in social class deprivations.

The anxiety disorders are commonly secondary to, and frequent (about 1 in 4) concomitants of, depressive disorder in elders (Banazak, 1997; Lenze et al., 2000; Lepine, 2001). Many of the risk factors for anxiety are common to depression. However, twin studies showed that the environmental determinants and sociodemographic predictors of generalized anxiety and major depression are different (Kessler et al., 2001). Risks of anxiety disorder in first-degree relatives are increased four to six times for a proband's diagnosis of panic disorder, generalized anxiety disorder, phobias, and obsessive-compulsive disorder, but environmental influences are also significant (Hettema et al., 2001).

Dementias

RATES Determining the incidence and prevalence of dementia has been described as an inexact science (Kukull & Bowen, 2002). The criteria chosen for an epidemiological study may substantially determine the results. With that reserve stated, around 5% to 8% of all older adults have progressive dementias; about two thirds of these patients reside in the community (Hanninen et al., 2002; Livingston et al., 1990; Ravaglia et al., 2002). This latter proportion can drop to one half or less when the capacity of long-term care facilities is large. Rates are doubled if milder cases are included (Hendrie, 1998).

Complaints of memory problems are common in elderly people residing in a community, but most of those who complain have neither dementia nor depression. Nevertheless, a substantial proportion (around 20%) of persons with mild cognitive impairment (sometimes defined as more than 1.5 SD below mean cognitive scores or Clinical Dementia Rating (CDR) 0.5, but not meeting criteria for dementia) have an onset of diagnosable dementia within a few years, and most have associated depression or physical illness (Ritchie et al., 2000). Only 13% with recent observable change in cognitive functioning have a benign and transient syndrome. Cognitive impairment not diagnosable as dementia has a prevalence rate of 23.4% in African Americans 65 years and older (12.5% medically unexplained, 4.0% from medical illness, 3.6% from stroke, 1.5% from alcohol abuse). Among this group, 26% became demented within 18 months of diagnosis (Unverzagt et al., 2001).

The great majority of dementias are reported as caused by Alzheimer's disease (AD), Lewy body dementia, or frontotemporal dementia. A vascular origin caused by multiinfarcts or other cerebrovascular disorder is a somewhat less common cause (Aguero-Torres et al., 1999; Copeland et al., 1992; Jellinger, 1999; Launer & Hofman, 1992; Letenneur et al., 1993), although there are also studies that showed relatively high rates for vascular dementias (Ravaglia et al., 2002). Alzheimer's or related dementias and vascular subtypes may be present together, and it may be difficult to establish which predominates. Perhaps Alzheimer's or related dementias alone account for about 60% of cases of dementia, an additional 10% might be because of multiinfarct dementia, and another 15% might be caused by both. The residual group of about 15% includes dementias associated with well-recognized neurological diseases (e.g., Huntington's chorea or parkinsonism) and a variety of causes that may be treatable (e.g., increased intracranial pressure; systemic effects from metabolic, toxic, or anoxic conditions; altered mood). Of patients with a dementia syndrome in contact with medical providers, 18% have an incidence of a dementia syndrome that meets *DSM-IV* (APA, 1994) criteria for vascular dementia (Knopman et al., 2002).

AGE   Rates of dementia rise steeply with age, doubling every 5 years (McDowell, 2001). Close to roughly half of all elders 85 years and older may be affected (Forsell & Winblad, 1997; Gallo & Lebowitz, 1999). The prevalence of Alzheimer's disease and other dementias increases even through the most advanced ages (Fratiglioni et al., 1991). Incidence varies from less than 1% annually at age 70 years to about 4% annually at 85 years of age. Rates of vascular dementia follow the same steep age gradient (Leys et al., 1998). The moderate degree of cognitive impairment also increases with age: 27.6% for ages 75 to 84 years and 38.0% for ages 85 years and older (Unverzagt et al., 2001).

What has been called the "demographic clock" suggests that, as the aging population expands, cases of dementia will correspondingly increase and place unparalleled demands on health and personal care services (DeKosky, 2001). Lifetime risk is about one in three for men who survive to age 85 years and probably in the same range for women. Disability-adjusted life years for women with dementia have been reported in the range between 1,050 and 1,404 per 100,000 women (Essink-Bot et al., 2002).

CULTURE AND EDUCATION   Low education appears to be associated with a higher risk for developing dementia of the Alzheimer and vascular subtypes (Li et al., 1991) and for increased rates of alcoholic dementia. The educational relationship is not fully explained by occupation, life habits, hypertension, or cardiovascular disease (Ravaglia et al., 2002). A question about the interpretation of these results is raised by the possible effect of education on tests of cognitive status (Murden et al., 1991). Education-specific norms for cut scores have been proposed for middle school, high school, and college graduates (Uhlmann et al., 1991). Educational achievement probably has a widespread nonspecific effect on the mental health of elders (Kubzansky et al., 1998), as well as a specific effect on predisposition to dementia.

Rates of dementia in Nigeria have been reported to be low relative to those in Western countries. A comparison of Nigerian elders in Ibadan and African Americans in Indianapolis, Indiana, showed rates for dementia and Alzheimer's disease as 2.29% and 1.41% respectively in Ibadan versus 8.24% and 6.24% in Indianapolis (Ogunniyi et al., 2000). Apolipoprotein E (APOE) ε4 was associated with dementia only in Indianapolis, and vascular risk factors were lower in Nigeria, suggesting that environmental factors may be at work. An alternative set of explanations invokes differential survival rates, hiding of cases by relatives, perception of the illness as normal aging, reluctance to seek medical treatment, or defective case-finding techniques (Ineichen, 2000).

Among community residents aged 65 years and older, the prevalence of dementia, the proportion of vascular dementias, and a history of heart attacks, high blood pressure, diabetes, and stroke have been found to be higher in blacks than in whites (Heyman et al., 1991). The cumulative risk of dementia by age 85 years in first-degree biological relatives of African Americans has been reported as 43.7%, and for whites, the risk was 26.9% (Green et al., 2002); there was no ethnic difference in relation to APOE (APOE ε4 allele) genotype. Especially high rates of dementia of the Alzheimer type have also been found in Latino groups (Gurland et al., 1999).

The proportions of subtypes of dementia may vary depending on the ethnic, racial, and cultural characteristics of the population. Rates of dementia, particularly of the Alzheimer's disease type, are reported as relatively low in certain Asian groups (Chiu et al., 1998; Fukunishi et al., 1991; Silverman et al., 1992). The prevalence and incidence of multiinfarct dementia was higher than primary degenerative dementia in elderly Beijing residents (Li et al., 1991). These rates are low, and the subtype ratio is reversed compared with British and American studies. However, the comparative results are not uniformly confirmed. Alzheimer's disease was less common than vascular dementia before 1990, but has since become almost twice as common in Korea, Japan, and China, possibly as a result of a shifting interaction of changing mortality and incidence rates (Suh & Shah, 2001).

In these cross-cultural studies, there may be confounds arising from the alteration by low education, illiteracy, and other group characteristics of the sensitivity and specificity of screening and diagnostic procedures (Chandra et al., 1998). Modern psychometric theory (e.g., item response theory) examines differential item functioning to detect items biased by education and other demographic factors to improve culture fairness of screening and neuropsychological tests (Teresi et al., 2000).

INFLUENCES   Often reported risk factors for Alzheimer's disease and related dementias include age, APOE ε4 allele presence, family history, and Down syndrome; inconsistently reported are female gender, low education, depression (probably prodromal), head injury, aluminum in water, hypertension, older fathers, and coal-mining fathers (Whalley, 2001). Risks might be lowered by nonsteroidal antiinflammatory agents, estrogen in the postmenopausal period, physical activity, B_6, B_{12}, folate, and red wine in modest quantities, although data for each of these are best viewed as tentative and often conflicting. Gene-environmental interactions appear to be important.

Age-sex incidence rates of AD and other dementias were comparable between the genders in most US studies, but several European and Asian populations showed an excess in women (Edland et al., 2002). Female gender has been associated with a higher prevalence of dementias even after educational controls and across cultural groups (Giampaoli, 2000; Li et al., 1989). Women are purportedly more prone not only to develop dementia, but also to survive more often to extreme old age, for which the risk of developing dementia is highest. Men may have higher rates of multiinfarct dementia.

Since the advent of antiretroviral therapy, a longer life expectancy for persons infected with human immunodeficiency virus (HIV) and changing mores are leading to a rising prevalence among the elderly population of this group and their accompanying cognitive deficits, from mild complaints to frank dementia (Hinkin et al., 2001). An encephalopathy or dementia is associated with raised serum aluminum levels during the course of renal dialysis (Rob et al., 2001).

Chronic use of benzodiazepines has been observed to increase the risk of cognitive decline (Paterniti et al., 2002). The use of benzodiazepines is probably a marker of unspecified psychiatric disorders or symptoms in elders and is a known hazard for falls and accidents (Kirby, Denihan et al., 1999). Neuroleptics are displacing benzodiazepines, with much of the neuroleptics given to persons 65 years or older (Linden & Thiels, 2001).

The broader concept of vascular cognitive impairment has replaced multiinfarct dementia (Haring, 2002). Rates of vascular dementias are increased by stroke, hypertension, heart disease, alcoholism, inactivity, excess fat intake, nicotine, and elevated blood glucose and triglycerides (Leys et al., 1998; Rob et al., 2001). About a quarter of patients who have had a stroke are demented (Van Kooten & Koudstaal, 1998). Untreated hypertension is a particular risk for vascular dementia (Tzourio et al., 1999); conversely, rates of vascular dementia are declining, probably because of preventive treatment of hypertension (Dartigues, 1999). In this respect, cognitive decline was greater in elders using calcium channel blockers than in those using other antihypertensives (Maxwell et al., 1999).

COURSE   Characteristic consequences of dementia include premature death, disability, dependence, intellectual and physical deterioration, institutional admission, and fractures and falls (Rose & Maffulli, 1999). Depressive symptoms in dementia are common, with subsyndromal depression the most common type (Thorpe & Groulx, 2001), especially among those with the multiinfarct and Parkinson's disease subtypes of dementia. Except for extreme apathy, symptoms of depression in dementia in community-dwelling elders are similar to those of cognitively intact elderly patients with major depression.

COMORBIDITY OF DEMENTIA AND DEPRESSION   Major depression is found in cases of Alzheimer's disease and related dementias at high rates, up to 30% in some series. Subsyndromal depression is particularly common in dementia and is very distressing in patients with these mixed conditions. The cognitive impairment component usually follows a progressively deteriorating course despite improvement in depression in response to treatment.

Pioneering studies found no increased risk of dementia in patients with late-onset depression; however, in about 10% of major depressions, a syndrome resembling dementia was noted to arise and be resolved when the depression remitted. This syndrome was earlier known as depressive pseudodementia and later as reversible dementia or depressive dementia, but could justly be viewed as depression in probable dementia. Only about 5% of cases referred for investigation of dementia improve cognitively, at least temporarily, with antidepressive treatment. Of these, from 20% to 50% or more (depending on the length of follow-up) relapse into cognitive deterioration. A conservative position is that the prognosis of depression is guarded if cognitive impairment is concurrent.

Confusional States

A confusional state or delirium is usually caused by factors surrounding medical illness and dementia and is therefore common in acute medical settings and nursing homes. Delirium (confusional state) is found in at least 10% to 15% of patients in acute medical and surgical settings and postoperatively (Bucht et al., 1999) and has been noted in as many as 25% of general medical inpatients and rehabilitation inpatients. It may occur even more commonly in neurology service populations. Although almost half of elderly medical or surgical inpatients have some form of psychiatric morbidity, hospital stay has been lengthened primarily by cognitive impairment (Fulop et al., 1998). Symptoms of delirium may be mistaken for dementia, but are distinguishable, and the underlying condition is usually treatable.

Schizophrenia

RATES Schizophrenia and conditions related to schizophrenia, such as paranoid disorder or paraphrenia, may occur for the first time in late adulthood (45–64 years of age) or old age (Jeste, 1993). Early studies reported that a small minority of patients who were first admitted to inpatient units after the age of 60 years had late-onset symptoms closely related to schizophrenia. It later was recognized that a substantial minority of patients with schizophrenia have an onset after 40 years of age (late-onset schizophrenia) or after 60 years of age (very late onset schizophrenialike psychosis) (Howard et al., 2000).

The prevalence of schizophrenia is about 1.4 to 4.6 per 1,000 in the general population (Jablensky, 2000). Active symptoms among individuals with schizophrenia who have grown old, together with late-onset persistent paranoid states, are noted in less than 0.5% of the community population (Keith et al., 1991), although obtrusive behaviors may leave the impression of a more frequent presence. It has been claimed that, with highly sensitive measures, paranoid features can be found in as many as 11% of elderly patients.

AGE-RELATED SYNDROMES Early- and late-onset types of schizophrenia overlap in clinical presentation and outcome. Late-onset schizophrenia, generally regarded as schizophrenia altered by age (Roth & Kay, 1998), is characterized by relatively good premorbid functioning and milder negative or thought disorder symptoms (Wynn Owen & Castle, 1999). A paranoid picture may predominate. The term *paranoia* has historically referred to well-organized delusional states with an onset late in life and without evident hallucinations or deterioration of thought processes, affect, or personality; *late paraphrenia* refers to a similar syndrome, but with hallucinations (Grief & Eastwood, 1993). It has been suggested that elderly patients with paranoia have strikingly more neurological disorders and are less responsive to treatment than paraphrenics (Flint et al., 1991). Late-onset types have been reported to have a higher frequency of distinctive brain abnormalities and neuropsychological deficits and a higher female-to-male ratio than in younger groups (Almeida et al., 1992).

The majority of individuals with schizophrenia will achieve old age even though they have a higher death rate than the general population. Most will be left with impaired functioning, including up to two thirds of cases who become chronic (an der Heiden & Hafner, 2000). However, about one third of the survivors to old age will have recovered virtually completely. The functional and social outcomes of schizophrenia in elders are worse if the symptoms are of the negative type or if cognitive impairment exists (McGurk et al., 2000). There is no increased risk for Alzheimer's disease, either clinically or at autopsy (Jellinger & Gabriel, 1999; Lindenmayer et al., 1997; Murphy et al., 1998), but the coexistence of cognitive impairment increases the chances of institutional admission (Evans et al., 1999).

The symptoms of early-onset schizophrenia tend to become less vivid and disturbing to the patient and others as age advances (e.g., fewer positive symptoms). Schizophrenia follows a course of progressive amelioration over time, resulting in increasing intervals before rehospitalization (Eaton et al., 1992). Older schizophrenic subjects tend to have insight into their difficulty in taking initiatives, giving emotional support, and dealing with conflict (Semple et al., 1999).

Possible explanations (Soni & Mallik, 1993) for the more favorable course of the late-onset types of schizophrenia range from changes in administrative practice to improved patient compliance with medications, early recognition of impending relapse, better family relationships, biological changes with age (Sandyk & Awerbuch, 1993), improved adaptation and coping, and diminished metabolic degradation of psychotropic medications.

LONG-TERM CARE SETTINGS In three developed countries, cohorts first discharged from psychiatric hospitals in the late 1960s to early 1970s had a prevalence of the onset of schizophrenia after age 40 years of around 25% to 44% and after 60 years of age of around 6% to 12%. Between 1970 and 1986, the proportion of patients with schizophrenia who were elderly admitted to state hospitals did not change substantially (Thompson et al., 1993). At the beginning of the decade starting in 1980, long-stay psychiatric centers contained a disproportionate number of elderly patients, as many as half the resident population, and a substantial proportion (35%–60%) of these elderly patients were first admitted during early adulthood with a diagnosis of schizophrenia.

Since that time, there have been large changes in the location of patients owing to policies of reducing the inpatient population. Patients with schizophrenia aged 65 years or older who have aged in long-stay public hospitals are characterized by deficit states with negative symptoms and thought disorder. These features are in large part determined by selective retention, although poor self-care and decreased social interaction might be aggravated by a long-term institutional effect. Downsizing of public psychiatric hospitals has left some inpatients who are not able to survive in the community with the generally inadequate available level of support. These patients typically have hard-to-manage behavioral problems: hostility, impulsiveness, agitation, suspiciousness, and psychotic symptoms (White et al., 1997).

INFLUENCES Lifelong isolation is characteristic of patients with late-onset schizophrenia; the sufferers are often unmarried or have few children, although they usually manage an independent existence fairly well. An abnormal personality (cold and querulous) and an unfavorable social milieu are often a long prelude to the emergence of frank paranoid symptoms in old age. Hearing impairment that affects receptive communication in social situations and beginning many years before the onset of paranoid symptoms is more frequent, about threefold, in older persons with a late-onset paranoid disorder than in age-matched controls or patients with affective disorder.

Schizophrenia is genetically complex, and the predictive value of individual genes is low (Hallmayer, 2000). Nonspecific background factors catalyze the actions of genetically mediated pathways (Jablensky, 2000). Certain psychopathological syndromes and personality traits form a spectrum of genetically related disorders (Lichtermann et al., 2000). The complexities of genetics of risk in schizophrenia remain to be unraveled (Hyman, 2000).

Alcoholism

RATES Alcohol abuse and dependence are detected by community surveys in about 1% to 2% of elderly people; the rate is higher than this in men and lower in women (Liberto et al., 1992). The prevalence and incidence of alcohol abuse decrease with age (Atkinson, 1994). However, new cases do continue to occur; one third to one half of elderly patients with problem drinking have an onset in middle or late life (Atkinson, 1994; Lakhani, 1997; Liberto et al., 1992; Rigler, 2000; Teesson et al., 2000). Alcohol abuse may increase again in very old men (Eaton et al., 1991).

Rates of excess alcohol consumption and associated problems for samples of patients aged 60 years and older can be as high as 44% in admissions to psychiatrically oriented units and around 5% in a primary medical care setting

(Liberto et al., 1992). In as many as one third of elderly patients ill enough to be admitted to an acute psychiatric ward, alcohol abuse was previously unde-tected by medical staff (Mears & Spice, 1993). Nevertheless, there are method-ological problems that tend to lead to an underestimation of alcohol use (and illicit drug consumption) in surveys of older adults (Mishara & McKim, 1993).

INFLUENCES Late-onset alcoholism probably does not stem from an underlying associated psychiatric disorder any more often than is the case for early-onset alcoholism (Atkinson et al., 1990; Schonfeld & Dupree, 1991). There is no personality profile of vulnerability specific to alcoholism as opposed to other psychiatric conditions (Mulder, 2002). However, bereavement may tend to precede hospital admission for elderly patients with problem drinking, and trauma and psychiatric symptoms increase the burden of alcoholism (Parry et al., 2002). Sons of alcoholics are at greater risk (Mulder, 2002). Gene-environ-ment interactions are implicated (Moran, 1999).

Alcohol and substance abuse are frequent in posttraumatic stress disorder, which is usually primary, but withdrawal symptoms may exacerbate the stress and provoke a vicious cycle (Parry et al., 2002). Very low rates found in some surveys may be caused by the poor economic status of the particular elderly population under study and the limit that restricted income imposes on the ability to obtain quantities of alcohol (Livingston & King, 1993). Higher eco-nomic status increases the likelihood of a late onset of alcoholism.

Rates are increased by availability and social customs (Hishinuma et al., 2000). Alcoholism may become more common in the geriatric range as cohorts with at-risk patterns of drinking get older (Reid & Anderson, 1997). Among community-residing persons aged 45 years and older, 15% were found to be severe drinkers (Nakamura et al., 1990). The majority of admissions to detoxi-fication centers used to be older white males, but these centers now have in-creased admissions of women, African Americans, and Hispanics; there has been a shift from alcoholism to cocaine and heroin use (McCarty et al., 2000). It is predicted that there will be an increased presence of comorbid alcoholism among elders in health services (Johnson, 2000).

COURSE Excess alcohol consumption remains a problem in the older age group, especially among single or divorced men (Lakhani, 1997; Teesson et al., 2000), many of whom do not recognize the adverse effects of heavy drinking (Ruchlin, 1997). Alcoholism increases inappropriate health care use, including excessive emergency room visits (Holroyd et al., 1997). As many as 24% of emergency clinic admissions in an urban center were alcoholic; those admitted tended to be unemployed, male, homeless, and abusers of other drugs (Whiteman et al., 2000). Elders with an early onset of alcoholism have the additional problems associated with long-term toxicity (Rigler, 2000).

Alcoholic problems may be responsible in elderly persons for falls, amne-sia, incontinence, injuries from accidents in the home, and behavioral problems

(Weyerer et al., 1999). Cognitive deterioration may occur, but mainly when a genetic predisposition, such as APOE genotype, also exists (Dufouil et al., 2000). Well-publicized reports of a protective action against coronary artery disease by light or moderate drinking might encourage more older adults to begin drinking (Shaper, 1990). Length of the alcoholic history is directly related to the effects on general health (Graham & Schmidt, 1998). In Veterans Affairs nursing homes, almost a third of the residents may have a history of alcohol abuse sometime in their lives, and many of these individuals show improved functioning during their hospital stay, especially if the abuse was of recent onset (Oslin et al., 1997).

AGE   The course and outcome of alcoholism are somewhat better for late-onset than for early-onset alcoholism, with milder symptoms and more frequent spontaneous recovery (Moos et al., 1991). Patients with late onset of alcoholism, matched for age with patients with early onset cases, are less frequently intoxicated, less likely to have delirium tremens, and more often compliant with treatment (Schonfeld & Dupree, 1991). Similarly, among drivers arrested for drinking, elders are more likely to complete treatment successfully (Fitzgerald & Mulford, 1992). Older compared with younger American Indians have a higher rate of abstinence from alcohol (May & Gossage, 2001).

NURSING HOMES

The great majority of nursing home residents have psychiatric problems, mainly depression or dementia or a behavioral disturbance. The need for suitably trained staff in these locations is pressing. It has been calculated by extrapolation from a national survey that only 33% of residents had no mental disorder (Eichmann et al., 1992). Half or more of the long-stay residents in nursing homes have Alzheimer's disease or related dementia; this rate is higher in urban than rural settings (Magaziner et al., 2000). Delirium is a common complication (Bucht et al., 1999). Individuals with schizophrenia may be placed in nursing homes, especially if chronic medical problems have supervened. A diagnosis of schizophrenia, based on information obtained from staff and records, has been reported in about 6% of nursing home residents (average age 79 years). Compared with their community-residing counterparts, residents with a psychiatric disorder in nursing homes tend to be more aggressive, isolated, and cognitively and functionally impaired (Bartels et al., 1997).

The US Omnibus Budget Reconciliation Act of 1987 (OBRA 87) attempted sweeping changes in admission and retention criteria for residents in Medicare- or Medicaid-certified nursing homes (Smith & Jensen, 1990) seeking to divert patients with mental illness to other sites with better access to appropriate treatment. Only a very small proportion of elderly people in nursing homes and with a mental disorder were actually receiving mental health treatment at the time of the 1985 National Nursing Home Survey (Burns et al.,

1993). Nevertheless, it was noted that, given the high rates of depression and anxiety among those eligible for residency by virtue of dependencies (three or more impairments in activities of daily living [ADLs]) and the frequency of behaviors such as aggression and screaming, those who would remain in nursing homes after OBRA 87 might still include about one third whose diagnosis mandated them to receive mental health care. OBRA 87 was implemented in 1990 and led to several changes in the profile of residents and in responsive initiatives. There has been a reduction in resident elders with schizophrenia (who usually are physically independent) (Sherrell et al., 1998); cases of depression and dementia, which are associated with physical functional deficits, have increased (Mechanic & McAlpine, 2000).

OBRA 87 also required the reduction of unnecessary use of antipsychotic drugs, previously reported to be administered to about one fifth of nursing home residents, mostly for control of the disturbing behaviors of dementia. Through education of staff in the use of behavioral techniques, the number of days on which antipsychotic medications were given to the residents was greatly reduced, whereas days of application of physical restraints were also decreased; behavioral problems did not increase in frequency as antipsychotic medication was withdrawn (Ray et al., 1993).

CAREGIVERS

Caregivers of persons with dementia, especially those who seek help, are prone to develop clinically diagnosable depression in many cultures (Mintzer & Macera, 1992). The stress on an older person caring for a dependent spouse may double the risk of suffering a depressive disorder (Denihan et al., 1998). Depression may not be relieved for many months after a spouse is placed in an institution, even though social activities are resumed by the caregiver (Matsuda et al., 1997). Both younger and older persons alike may become depressed in facing the duties of caregiving (Kubota et al., 2000).

EFFECTS OF AGING ON PSYCHIATRIC DISORDERS

The context in which people live changes over time, and its influence on psychiatric disorders in aging changes accordingly. Each new generation or cohort may arrive at old age with a distinctive profile of age-related predispositions and resistances to psychiatric disorder, and aging itself may acquire new stressors and supports. Thus, the psychiatric epidemiology of older persons may be a moving picture produced variously by aging and cohort effects.

Cohort Effects

There is some evidence that rates of depression have been increasing among older persons (Bland, 1997), and that there will be an increase in suicide of older persons in the next few decades (Bharucha & Satlin, 1997). Cohort effects are probably the main determinants of age variation in alcohol consumption and associated problems; rates of alcohol abuse are also likely to increase as the baby boomers age (Reid & Anderson, 1997; Stoltenberg et al., 1999). Smoking is currently associated with functional psychiatric disorders in younger, but not older, age groups, possibly because of changing norms and motivations in choosing to smoke; as the younger cohort ages, they may carry that risk into older age (Jorm, 1999).

Context of Aging

Psychiatric problems in elderly patients occur in the context of physical, mental, and social aging. The effect of age itself must be separated from that of accompanying difficulties, such as changes in health and social supports. Aging adds distinctive characteristics not only to the nature, presentation, and treatment of psychiatric problems, but also to the social milieu, a vital aspect of treatment. One third of older adults live alone, but most have someone, usually a daughter or daughter-in-law, who assists in the support and management of treatment (Albert & Cattell, 1994).

Among the population aged 65 years and older, a majority have at least one chronic physical disorder, and a minority are impaired in mobility or capacity to carry out the daily tasks of independent living (e.g., self-care and household chores) (Verbrugge, 1990). Only about 5% of all older adults need to live in highly sheltered residences such as nursing homes, although this percentage increases sharply in those older than 80 years. There are changes in the speed and style of intellectual activities and slowing of the rate of new learning, but the great majority of older adults remain mentally active and competent. Those are the normal standards against which the causes, presentation, and consequences of psychiatric disorders at older ages are evaluated.

It is evident from the prevalence data that psychiatric problems are frequent during the period conventionally designated as containing the older age groups (starting at age 65 years). Repeated complaints of mental distress among adults are associated with disability payments, lost productivity, excess use of social services, and premature death (Centers for Disease Control and Prevention, 1998). Psychoses in elders have a tendency to increase in frequency with age-related conditions such as physical illness, cognitive decline, social isolation, polypharmacy, and sensory deficits (Targum & Abbott, 1999). Visual hallucinations arising for the first time in elders are most likely because of organic disorders, although they can occur in schizophrenia or severe depression (Paulson, 1997). Somatization is probably not a result of aging, but of underlying depression or physical illness (Sheehan & Banerjee, 1999). Memory complaints, of course, may be caused by an established dementia, but also occur as a symptom of depression (Derouesne et al., 1999). Remission of episodes of psychiatric disorder vary with aging, increasing (improving) for antisocial disorders, decreasing (worsening) for panic and obsessive compulsive disorders, and remaining unaffected for major depression and phobias (Bland et al., 1997).

For certain psychiatric disorders, the increased contribution of biological deficits arising from wear and tear may reduce the determining effects of genetic predisposition (Henderson & Kay, 1997) or may interact with these determining effects. Gene-environmental interactions are becoming clearer in major psychiatric disorders, but a more general genetic susceptibility to stress may be at play in common psychiatric syndromes (Cooper, 2001).

CONCLUSION: SERVICE ACTIONS SUGGESTED BY EPIDEMIOLOGY

Epidemiological perspectives highlight the need for specially skilled professionals to care for elderly patients with psychiatric problems. Age-relevant epidemiology adds understanding of diagnosis, evaluation of causes, administration of treatment, and longer term management. The epidemiological perspective can guide the acts of scouting for opportunities to reduce the risk of onset, persistence, and relapse of psychiatric problems. The discovery of precursors of a condition can suggest opportunities for preventive interventions. Treatable problems are frequently encountered in the older population in the community and in the spectrum of clinical and residential settings. Life-threatening behavioral emergencies in elders include confusion, suicide risks, homicide risk, aggression, and abuse (Tueth & Zuberi, 1999).

The complex set of relations connecting depression and physical illness opens up several evident opportunities for intervention in gaining compliance, minimizing medication effects, enhancing motivation, strengthening physiological and physical functioning, and improving quality of life. Epidemiological data show that depression impedes recovery of function in medical conditions such as ischemic heart disease, stroke, and disability from a variety of causes. Treating the depression may be a means of secondarily preventing the prolongation of the physical illness just as treating the physical illness may relieve a depression.

Older persons with psychiatric problems do seek help, although not necessarily appropriately or from psychiatrists. Psychotropic medications are actively dispensed to the older patient by primary care physicians, who are often the sole providers of professional care for patients with mental health problems. Depression is among the most frequent diagnoses among older patients referred to a psychiatrist. However, elderly patients are less likely than younger patients to be evaluated and treated by a mental health specialist, even if specialist referrals are available.

Depressive syndromes account for a greater proportion of service use than do the diagnostic categories. Major depression and dysthymia and subclinical depressive syndromes are associated with increased use of psychoactive medications and treatment for emotional problems in medical and emergency department settings.

Lifetime prevalence of any mental disorder has been reported by consistent diagnostic measures in seven countries (Canada, United States, Brazil, Mexico, Germany, the Netherlands, and Turkey) as varying from over 40% to as low as 12%, with chronicity common ("Cross-National Comparisons," 2000). Depending on the type of service, the likelihood of contact may be higher or lower for individuals with depressive symptoms than for those with diagnosable depression, but the size of the former group overshadows that of the latter and accounts for the disproportion in aggregate use of services.

If personal characteristics are prodromal signs of an eventual psychotic disorder, they may offer a means of intervention for high-risk groups. For example, long-range possibilities for prevention of some late-onset paranoid states are raised by epidemiological findings, and the prediction of postbereavement status by depression several months prior to bereavement could be applied to selecting vulnerable caregivers for early intervention.

Although the dementias are, for the most part, not yet markedly amenable to preventive strategies, consideration of the relative rates of the dementia subtypes and of conditions that can mimic dementia keep the issue of prevention open. In the near future, new treatments may make early detection of dementia a therapeutic necessity.

The compelling importance of the field of geriatric psychiatry stems not only from the growing number and proportion of elderly patients, especially the very old, but also equally from gains in longevity and active life expectancy. This change in the life span means that old age occupies a larger proportion of the average life. Consequently, the quality of life in old age and the influence of psychiatric problems on that quality are growing in relevance to a person's entire life. Prevention and treatment of psychiatric disorders can help older adults fully enjoy their added years.

REFERENCES

Addington AM, Gallo JJ, Ford DE, Eaton WW. Epidemiology of unexplained fatigue and major depression in the community: the Baltimore ECA follow-up, 1981–1994. *Psychol Med.* 2001;31:1037–1044.

Aguero-Torres H, Winblad B, Fratiglioni L. Epidemiology of vascular dementia: some results despite research limitations. *Alzheimer Dis Assoc Dis.* 1999;13(Suppl 3): S15–S20.

Albert SM, Cattell MG. *Old Age in Global Perspective.* New York, NY: G. K. Hall; 1994:87.

Alexopoulos GS, Meyers BS, Young RC, et al. Executive dysfunction and long-term outcomes of geriatric depression. *Arch Gen Psychiatry.* 2000;57:285–290.

Almeida OP, Howard R, Forstl H, et al. Late paraphrenia: a review. *Int J Geriatr Psychiatry.* 1992;7:543–548.

American Psychiatric Association. *Diagnostic and Statistical Manual of Mental Disorders*. 3rd ed. Washington, DC: American Psychiatric Association; 1980.

American Psychiatric Association. *Diagnostic and Statistical Manual of Mental Disorders*. 4rth ed. Washington, DC: American Psychiatric Association; 1994.

an der Heiden W, Hafner H. The epidemiology of onset and course of schizophrenia. *Eur Arch Psychiatry Clin Neurosci*. 2000;250(6):292–303.

Atkinson RM. Late onset problem drinking in older adults. *Int J Geriatr Psychiatry*. 1994;9:321–326.

Atkinson RM, Tolson RL, Turner JA. Late versus early onset problem drinking in older men. *Alcohol Clin Exp Res*. 1990;14:574–579.

Ayuso-Mateos JL, Vazquez-Barquero JL, Dowrick C, et al. ODIN Group Depressive Disorders Europe: prevalence figures from the ODIN study. *Br J Psychiatry*. 2001; 179:308–316.

Banazak DA. Anxiety disorders in elderly patients. *J Am Board Fam Pract*. 1997;10: 280–289.

Barnow S, Linden M. Epidemiology and psychiatric morbidity of suicidal ideation among the elderly. *Crisis J Crisis Interv Suicide*. 200;21(4):171–180.

Bartels SJ, Mueser KT, Miles KM. A comparative study of elderly patients with schizophrenia and bipolar disorder in nursing homes and the community. *Schizophr Res*. 1997;27:181–190.

Bharucha AJ, Satlin A. Late-life suicide: a review. *Harv Rev Psychiatry*. 1997;5(2): 55–65.

Blacker CV, Clare AW. The prevalence and treatment of depression in general practice. *Psychopharmacology*. 1988;95:S14–S17.

Bland RC. Epidemiology of affective disorders: a review. *Can J Psychiatry*. 1997;42: 367–377.

Bland RC, Newman SC, Orn H. Age and remission of psychiatric disorders. *Can J Psychiatry*. 1997;42:722–729.

Blazer DG, Hughes D, George LK. Generalized anxiety disorder. In: Robins LN, Regier DA, eds. *Psychiatric Disorders in America: The Epidemiologic Catchment Area Study*. New York, NY: Free Press; 1991:180–203.

Bucht G, Gustafson Y, Sandberg O. Epidemiology of delirium. *Dement Geriatr Cogn Disord*. 1999;10:315–318.

Burns BJ, Wagner HR, Taube JE, et al. Mental health service use by the elderly in nursing homes. *Am J Public Health*. 1993;83:331–337.

Burt VK, Stien K. Epidemiology of depression throughout the female life cycle. *J Clin Psychiatry*. 2002;63(Suppl 7):9–15.

Burvill PW. The impact of criteria selection on prevalence rates. Fifth Congress of the International Federation of Psychiatric Epidemiology (1990, Montreal, Canada). *Psychiat J Univ Ottowa*. 1990;15:194–199.

Centers for Disease Control and Prevention. Self reported frequent mental distress among adults—United States, 1993–1996. *MMWR Morb Mortal Wkly Rep*. 1998; 47:326–331.

Chandra V, Ganguili M, Ratcliff G, et al. Practical issues in cognitive screening of elderly illiterate populations in developing countries. The Indo-US Cross-National Dementia Epidemiology Study. *Aging (Milano)*. 1998;10:349–357.

Chiu HF, Lam LC, Chi I, et al. Prevalence of dementia in Chinese elderly in Hong Kong. *Neurology*. 1998;50:1002–1009.

Chochinov HM. Depression in cancer patients. *Lancet Oncol.* 2001;2:499–505.

Christensen H, Jorm AF, Mackinnon AJ, et al. Age differences in depression and anxiety symptoms: a structural equation modeling analysis of data from a general population sample. *Psychol Med.* 1999;29:325–339.

Conwell Y, Olsen K, Caine ED, et al. Suicide in later life: psychological autopsy findings. *Int Psychogeriatr.* 1991;3:59–66.

Conwell Y, Rotenberg M, Caine ED. Completed suicide at age 50 and over. *J Am Geriatr Soc.* 1990;38:640–644.

Cooper B. Nature, nurture and mental disorder: old concepts in the new millennium. *Br J Psychiatry Suppl.* 2001;40:s91–s101.

Copeland JR, Dewey ME, Griffiths-Jones HM. Dementia and depression in elderly persons: AGECAT compared with *DSM-III* and pervasive illness. *Int J Geriatr Psychiatry.* 1990;5:47–51.

Copeland JRM, Dewey ME, Davidson IA, et al. Geriatric Mental State AGECAT: prevalence, incidence and long-term outcome of dementia and organic disorders in the Liverpool Study of Continuing Health in the Community. *Neuroepidemiology.* 1992;11:84–87.

Creamer M, Burgess P, McFarlane AC. Post-traumatic stress disorder: findings from the Australian National Survey of Mental Health and Well-being. *Psychol Med.* 2001; 31:1237–1247.

Cross-national comparisons of the prevalences and correlates of mental disorders. WHO International Consortium in Psychiatric Epidemiology. *Bull World Health Organ.* 2000;78:413–426.

Dartigues JF. Dementia: epidemiology, intervention and concept of care. *Z Gerontol Geriatr.* 1999;32:407–411.

DeKosky ST. Epidemiology and pathophysiology of Alzheimer's disease. *Clin Cornerstone.* 2001;3(4):15–26.

den Boer JA. Social anxiety disorder/social phobia: epidemiology, diagnosis, neurobiology, and treatment. *Compr Psychiatry.* 2000;41:405–415.

Denihan A, Bruce I, Coakley D, Lawlor BA. Psychiatric morbidity in cohabitants of community-dwelling elderly depressives. *Int J Geriatr Psychiatry.* 1998;13:691–694.

Dennis MS, Lindesay J. Suicide in the elderly: the United Kingdom perspective. *Int Psychogeriatr.* 1995;7:263–274.

Derouesne C, Lacomblez L, Thibault S, LePoncin M. Memory complaints in young and elderly subjects. *Int J Geriatr Psychiatry.* 1999;14:291–301.

Dewey ME, de la Camara C, Copeland JRM, et al. Cross-cultural comparison of depression and depressive symptoms in older people. *Acta Psychiatr Scand.* 1993;87:369–373.

Draper BM. The elderly admitted to a general hospital psychiatry ward. *Aust N Z J Psychiatry.* 1994;28:288–297.

Dufouil C, Tzourio C, Brayne C, Berr C, Amouyel P, Alperovitch A. Influence of apolipoprotein E genotype on the risk of cognitive deterioration in moderate drinkers and smokers. *Epidemiology.* 2000;11:280–284.

Dworkin SF, von Korff M, LeResche L. Multiple pains and psychiatric disturbance: an epidemiologic investigation. *Arch Gen Psychiatry.* 1990;7:239–244.

Eaton WW, Bilker W, Haro JM, et al. Long-term course of hospitalization for schizophrenia. II. Change with passage of time. *Schizophr Bull.* 1992;18:229–241.

Eaton WW, Dryman A, Weissman MM. Panic and phobia. In: Robins LN, Regier DA, eds. *Psychiatric Disorders in America: The Epidemiologic Catchment Area Study.* New York, NY: Free Press; 1991:155–179.

Eaton WW, Neufeld K, Chen LS, Cia G. A comparison of self-report and clinical diagnostic interview for depression: diagnostic interview schedule and schedules for clinical assessment in neuropsychiatry in the Baltimore Epidemiology Catchment Area follow-up. *Arch Gen Psychiatry.* 2000;57:217–222.

Edland SD, Rocca WA, Peterson RC, Cha RH, Kokmen E. Dementia and Alzheimer disease incidence rates do not vary by sex in Rochester, Minn. *Arch Neurol.* 2002; 59:1589–1593.

Eichmann MA, Griffin BP, Lyons JS, et al. An estimation of the impact of OBRA-87 on nursing home care in the United States. *Hosp Community Psychiatry.* 1992;43: 781–789.

Essink-Bot ML, Pereira J, Packer C, Schwarzinger M, Burstrom K. Cross-national comparability of burden of disease estimates: the European Disability Weights Project. *Bull World Health Organ.* 2002;80:644–652.

Evans JD, Negron AE, Palmer BW, Paulsen JS, Heaton RK, Jeste DV. Cognitive deficits and psychopathology in institutionalized versus community-dwelling elderly schizophrenia. *J Geriatr Psychiatry Neurol.* 1999;12:11–15.

Faravelli C, Zucchi T, Viviani B, et al. Epidemiology of social phobia: a clinical approach. *Eur Psychiatry.* 2000;15:17–24.

Finch EJL, Ramsay R, Katona CLE. Depression and physical illness in the elderly. *Clin Geriatr Med.* 1992;8:275–287.

Fitzgerald JL, Mulford HA. Elderly vs. younger problem drinker "treatment" and recovery experiences. *Br J Addict.* 1992;87:1281–1291.

Flint AJ. Management of anxiety in late life. *J Geriatr Psychiatry Neurol.* 1998;11:194–200.

Flint AJ. Anxiety disorders in late life. *Can Fam Physician.* 1999;45:2672–2679.

Flint AJ, Rifat SL, Eastwood MR. Latent onset paranoia: distinct from paraphrenia? *Int J Geriatr Psychiatry.* 1991;6:103–109.

Forsell Y, Winblad B. Feelings of anxiety and associated variables in a very elderly population. *Int J Geriatr Psychiatry.* 1998;13:454–458.

Forsell Y, Winblad B. Psychiatric disturbances and the use of psychotropic drugs in a population of nonagenarians. *Int J Geriatr Psychiatry.* 1997;12:533–536.

Fratiglioni L, Grut M, Forsell Y, et al. Prevalence of Alzheimer's disease and other dementias in an elderly urban population: relationship with age, sex, and education. *Neurology.* 1991;41:1886–1892.

Fuentes K, Cox BJ. Prevalence of anxiety disorders in elderly adults: a critical analysis. *J Behav Ther Exp Psychiatry.* 1997;28:269–279.

Fukunishi I, Hayabara T, Hosokawa K. Epidemiological surveys of senile dementia in Japan. *Int J Soc Psychiatry.* 1991;37:51–56.

Fulop G, Strain JJ, Fahs MC, Schmeidler J, Snyder S. A prospective study of the impact of psychiatric comorbidity on length of hospital stays of elderly medical-surgical inpatients. *Psychomatics.* 1998;39:273–280.

Gallo JJ, Lebowitz BD. The epidemiology of common late-life mental disorders in the community: themes for the new century. *Psychiatr Serv.* 1999;50:1158–1166.

Gallo JJ, Rabins PV. Depression without sadness: alternative presentations of depression in late life. *Am Fam Physician.* 1999;60:820–826.

George LK, Linderman R, Blazer DG, et al. Cognitive impairment. In: Robins LN, Regier DA, eds. *Psychiatric Disorders in America: The Epidemiologic Catchment Area Study.* New York, NY: Free Press; 1991:291–327.

Giampaoli S. Epidemiology of major age-related disease in women compared to men. *Aging (Milano).* 2000;12:93–105.

Gottfries CG. Is there a difference between elderly and younger patients with regard to the symptomatology and aetiology of depression? *Int Clin Psychopharmacol.* 1998; 13(Suppl 5):S13–S18.

Graham K, Schmidt G. The effects of drinking on health of older adults. *Am J Drug Alcohol Abuse.* 1998;24:465–481.

Green BH, Copeland JRM, Dewey ME, et al. Risk factors for depression in elderly people: a prospective study. *Acta Psychiatr Scand.* 1992;86:213–217.

Green RC, Cupples LA, Go R, et al. MIRAGE Study Group. Risk of dementia among white and African American relatives of patients with Alzheimer disease. *JAMA.* 20020;287:329–336.

Grief C, Eastwood RM. Paranoid disorders in the elderly. *Int J Geriatr Psychiatry.* 1993; 8:681–684.

Gurland BJ, Wilder DE, Lantigua R, et al. Rates of dementia in three ethnoracial groups. *Int J Geriatr Psychiatry.* 1999;14:481–493.

Hadzi-Pavlovic D, Hickie IB, Wilson AJ, Davenport TA, Lloyd AR, Wakefield D. Screening for prolonged fatigue syndromes: validation of the SOFA scale. *Soc Psychiatry Psychiatr Epidemiol.* 2000;35:471–479.

Hallmayer J. The epidemiology of the genetic liability for schizophrenia. *Aust N Z J Psychiatry.* 2000;34(Suppl):S47–S55, discussion S56–S57.

Hanninen T, Hallikainen M, Tuomainen S, Vanhanen M, Soininen H. Prevalence of mild cognitive impairment: a population-based study in elderly subjects. *Acta Neurol Scand.* 2002;106:148–154.

Harden CL. The co-morbidity of depression and epilepsy: epidemiology, etiology, and treatment. *Neurology.* 2002;59(6, Suppl 4):S48–S55.

Haring HP. Cognitive impairment after stroke. *Curr Opin Neurol.* 2002;15:79–84.

Harlow SD, Goldberg EL, Comstock GW. A longitudinal study of risk factors for depressive symptomatology in elderly widowed and married women. *Am J Epidemiol.* 1991;134:526–538.

Hawton K, Fagg J. Deliberate self-poisoning and self-injury in older people. *Int J Geriatr Psychiatry.* 1990;5:367–373.

Henderson AS, Kay DW. The epidemiology of functional psychoses of late onset. *Eur Arch Psychiatry Clin Neurosci.* 1997;247:176–189.

Hendrie HC. Epidemiology of Alzheimer's disease. *Geriatrics.* 1997;52(Suppl 2):S4–S8.

Hendrie HC. Epidemiology of dementia and Alzheimer's disease. *Am J Geriatr Psychiatry.* 1998;6(2, Suppl 1):S3–S18.

Hettema JM, Neale MC, Kendler KS. A review and meta-analysis of the genetic epidemiology of anxiety disorders. *Am J Psychiatry.* 2001;158:1568–1578.

Heyman A, Fillenbaum G, Prosnitz B, Raiford K, Burchett B, Clark C. Estimated prevalence of dementia among elderly black and white community residents. *Arch Neurol.* 1991;48:594–598.

Hidalgo RB, Barnett SD, Davidson JR. Social anxiety disorder in review: two decades of progress. *Int J Neuropsychopharmacol.* 2001;4:279–289.

Hinkin CH, Castellon SA, Atkinson JH, Goodkin K. Neuropsychiatric aspects of HIV infection among older adults. *J Clin Epidemiol.* 2001;54(Suppl 1):S44–S52.

Hintikka J, Pesonen T, Saarinen P, Tanskanen A, Lehtonen J, Viinamaki H. Suicidal ideation in the Finnish general population. A 12 month follow-up study. *Soc Psychiatry Psychiatr Epidemiol.* 2001;36:590–594.

Hishinuma ES, Nishimura ST, Miyamoto RH, Johnson RC. Alcohol use in Hawaii. *Hawaii Med J.* 2000;59:329–335.

Holroyd S, Currie L, Thompson-Heisterman A, Abraham I. A descriptive study of elderly community-dwelling alcoholic patients in the rural south. *Am J Geriatr Psychiatry.* 1997;5:221–228.

Howard R, Rabins PV, Seeman MV, Jeste DV. Late-onset schizophrenia and very-late-onset schizophrenia-like psychosis: an international consensus. The International Late-Onset Schizophrenia Group. *Am J Psychiatry.* 2000;157:172–178.

Hyman SE. The genetics of mental illness: implications for practice. *Bull World Health Organ.* 2000;78:455–463.

Ineichen B. The epidemiology of dementia in Africa: a review. *Soc Sci Med.* 2000;50: 1673–1677.

Jablensky A. Epidemiology of schizophrenia: the global burden of disease and disability. *Eur Arch Psychiatry Clin Neurosci.* 2000;250:274–285.

Jellinger KA. What is new in degenerative dementia disorders? *Wien Klin Wochenschr.* 1999;111:682–704.

Jellinger KA, Gabriel E. No increased incidence of Alzheimer's disease in elderly schizophrenics. *Acta Neuropathol.* 1999;97:165–169.

Jeste DV. Late-onset schizophrenia. *Int J Geriatr Psychiatry.* 1993;8:283–285.

Johnson I. Alcohol problems in old age: a review of recent epidemiological research. *Int J Geriatr Psychiatry.* 2000;15:575–581.

Johnson J, Weissman MM, Klerman GL. Service utilization and social morbidity associated with depressive symptoms in the community. *JAMA.* 1992;267:1478–1483.

Jorm AF. The epidemiology of depressive states in the elderly: implications for recognition, intervention and prevention. *Soc Psychiatry Psychiatr Epidemiol.* 1995;30(2): 53–59.

Jorm AF. Association between smoking and mental disorders: results from an Australian National Prevalence Survey. *Aust N Z J Public Health.* 1999;23:245–248.

Jorm AF. Does old age reduce the risk of anxiety and depression? A review of epidemiological studies across the adult life span. *Psychol Med.* 2000;30:11–22.

Karno M, Golding JM. Obsessive compulsive disorder. In: Robins LN, Regier DA, eds. *Psychiatric Disorders in America: The Epidemiologic Catchment Area Study.* New York, NY: Free Press; 1991:204–219.

Katon VAT, von Korff M, Lin F, et al. Adequacy and duration of antidepressant treatment in primary care. *Med Care.* 1992;30:67–76.

Katon W, Schulberg HC. Epidemiology of depression in primary care. Special section: developing guidelines for treating depressive disorders in the primary care setting. *Gen Hosp Psychiatry.* 1992;14:237–247.

Katon W, Sullivan M. Depression and chronic medical illness. *J Clin Psychiatry.* 1990; 51:3–11.

Katon W, Sullivan M, Russo J, et al. Depressive symptoms and measures of disability: a prospective study. *J Affect Disord.* 1993;27:245–254.

Keith SJ, Regier DA, Rae DS. Schizophrenic disorders. In: Robins LN, Regier DA, eds. *Psychiatric Disorders in America: The Epidemiologic Catchment Area Study.* New York, NY: Free Press; 1991:33–52.

Kennedy GJ, Kelman HR, Thomas C. The emergence of depressive symptoms in late life: the importance of declining health and increasing disability. *J Community Health.* 1990;15:93–104.

Kessler RC, Keller MB, Wittchen HU. The epidemiology of generalized anxiety disorder. *Psychiatr Clin North Am.* 2001;24:19–39.

Kirby M, Bruce I, Coakley D, Lawlor BA. Dysthymia among the community-dwelling elderly. *Int J Geriatr Psychiatry.* 1999;14:440–445.

Kirby M, Denihan A, Bruce I, Radic A, Coakley D, Lawlor BA. Benzodiazepine use among the elderly in the community. *Int J Geriatr Psychiatry.* 1999;14:280–284.

Knopman DS, Rocca WA, Cha RH, Edland SD, Kokmen E. Incidence of vascular dementia in Rochester, Minn, 1985–1989. *Arch Neurol.* 2002;59:1605–1610.

Krasucki C, Ryan P, Ertan T, Howard R, Lindesay J, Mann A. The FEAR: a rapid screening instrument for generalized anxiety in elderly primary care attenders. *Int J Geriatr Psychiatry.* 1999;14:60–68.

Kubota M, Babazono A, Aoyama H. Women's anxiety in old age and long-term care provision for the elderly. *Acta Med Okayama.* 2000;54:75–83.

Kubzansky LD, Berkman LF, Glass TA, Seeman TE. Is educational attainment associated with shared determinants of health in the elderly? Findings from the MacArthur Studies of Successful Aging. *Psychosom Med.* 1998;60:578–585.

Kukull WA, Bowen JD. Dementia epidemiology. *Med Clin North Am.* 2002;86:573–590.

Lakhani N. Alcohol use amongst community-dwelling elderly people: a review of the literature. *J Adv Nurs.* 1997;25:1227–1232.

Launer LJ, Hofman A. Studies on the incidence of dementia: the European perspective. *Neuroepidemiology.* 1992;11:127–134.

Lenze EJ, Mulsant BH, Shear MK, et al. Comorbid anxiety disorders in depressed elderly patients. *Am J Psychiatry.* 2000;157:722–728.

Lepine JP. Epidemiology, burden, and disability in depression and anxiety. *J Clin Psychiatry.* 2001;62(Suppl 13):4–10, discussion 11–12.

Lepine JP, Bouchez S. Epidemiology of depression in the elderly. *Int Clin Psychopharmacol.* 1998;13(Suppl 5):S7–S12.

Lester D. Attempts to explain changing elderly suicide rate: a comment on Pritchard [letter to the editor]. *Int J Geriatr Psychiatry.* 1993;8:435.

Letenneur L, Fabrigoule D, Dartigues JF. Incidence and premonitory symptoms of dementia. *Ann Med Psychol.* 1993;151:670–672.

Leys D, Pasquier F, Parnetti L. Epidemiology of vascular dementia. *Haemostasis.* 1998;28:134–150.

Li G, Shen YC, Chen CH, et al. A three-year follow-up study of age-related dementia in an urban area of Beijing. *Acta Psychiatr Scand.* 1991;83:99–104.

Li G, Shen YC, Chen CH, et al. An epidemiological survey of age-related dementia in an urban area of Beijing. *Acta Psychiatr Scand.* 1989;79:557–563.

Liao S, Ferrell BA. Fatigue in an older population. *J Am Geriatr Soc.* 2000;48:426–430.

Liberto JG, Oslin DW, Ruskin PE. Alcoholism in older persons: a review of the literature. *Hosp Community Psychiatry.* 1992;43:975–984.

Lichtermann D, Karbe E, Maier W. The genetic epidemiology of schizophrenia and of schizophrenia spectrum disorders. *Eur Arch Psychiatry Clin Neurosci.* 2000;250:304–310.

Linden M, Thiels C. Epidemiology of prescriptions for neuroleptic drugs: tranquilizers rather than antipsychotics. *Pharmacopsychiatry.* 2001;34:150–564.

Lindenmayer JP, Negron AE, Shah S, et al. Cognitive deficits and psychopathology in elderly schizophrenic patients. *Am J Geriatr Psychiatry.* 1997;5:31–42.

Lindesay J. Phobic disorders in the elderly. *Br J Psychiatry.* 1991a;159:531–541.

Lindesay J. Suicide in the elderly. *Int J Geriatr Psychiatry.* 1991b;6:355–361.

Livingston BM, Kim K, Leaf PJ, et al. Depressive disorders and dysphoria resulting from conjugal bereavement in a prospective community sample. *Am J Psychiatry.* 1990; 147:608–611.

Livingston G, Hawkins A, Graham N, et al. The Gospel Oak Study: prevalence rates of dementia, depression and activity limitation among elderly residents in inner London. *Psychol Med.* 1990;20:137–146.

Livingston G, King M. Alcohol abuse in an inner city elderly population: the Gospel Oak Survey. *Int J Geriatr Psychiatry.* 1993;8:511–514.

Livingston G, Watkin V, Milne B, Manela MV, Katona C. The natural history of depression and the anxiety disorders in older people: the Islington community study. *J Affect Disord.* 1997;46:255–262.

Magarinos M, Zafar U, Nissenson K, Blanco C. Epidemiology and treatment of hypochondriasis. *CNS Drugs.* 2002;16:9–22.

Magaziner J, German P, Zimmerman SI, et al. The prevalence of dementia in a statewide sample of new nursing home admissions aged 65 and older: diagnosis by expert panel. Epidemiology of Dementia in Nursing Homes Research Group. *Gerontologist.* 2000;40:663–672.

Magruder-Habib K, Zung WWK, Feussner JR. Improving physicians' recognition and treatment of depression in general medical care. *Med Care.* 1990;28:239–250.

Matsuda O, Hasebe N, Ikehara K, Futatsuya M, Akahane N. Longitudinal study of the mental health of caregivers caring for elderly patients with dementia: effect of institutional placement on mental health. *Psychiatry Clin Neurosci.* 1997;51:289–293.

Maxwell CJ, Hogan DB, Ebly EM. Calcium-channel blockers and cognitive function in elderly people: results from the Canadian Study of Health and Aging. *CMAJ.* 1999; 161:501–506.

May PA, Gossage P. New data on the epidemiology of adult drinking and substance use among American Indians of the northern states: male and female data on prevalence, patterns, and consequences. *Am Indian Alsk Native Ment Health Res.* 2001; 10(2):1–26.

McCarty D, Caspi Y, Panas L, Krakow M, Mulligan DH. Detoxification center: who's in the revolving door? *J Behav Health Serv Res.* 2000;27:245–256.

McConnell P, Bebbington P, McClelland R, Gillespie K, Houghton S. Prevalence of psychiatric disorder and the need for psychiatric care in Northern Ireland. Population study in the District of Derry. *Br J Psychiatry.* 2002;181:214–219.

McDonald WM. Epidemiology, etiology, and treatment of geriatric mania. *J Clin Psychiatry.* 2000;61(Suppl 13):3–11.

McDowell I. Alzheimer's disease: insight from epidemiology. *Aging (Milano).* 2001; 13(3):143–162.

McGurk SR, Moriarty PJ, Harvey PD, Parrella M, White L, Davis KL. The longitudinal relationship of clinical symptoms, cognitive functioning, and adaptive life in geriatric schizophrenia. *Schizophr Res.* 2000;42:47–55.

Mears HJ, Spice C. Screening for problem drinking in the elderly: a study in the elderly mentally ill. *Int J Geriatr Psychiatry.* 1993;8:319–326.

Mechanic D, McAlpine DD. Use of nursing homes in the care of persons with severe mental illness: 1985 to 1995. *Psychiatr Serv.* 2000;51:354–358.

Merrill J, Owens J. Age and attempted suicide. *Acta Psychiatr Scand.* 1990;82:385–388.

Mintzer JE, Macera CA. Prevalence of depressive symptoms among white and African-American caregivers of demented patients. *Am J Psychiatry.* 1992;149:575–576.

Mishara BL, McKim W. Methodological issues in surveying older persons concerning drug use. *Int J Addict.* 1993;28:305–326.

Moos RH, Brennan PL, Moos JS. Short-term processes of remission and non remission among late-life problem drinkers. *Alcohol Clin Exp Res.* 1991;15:948–955.

Moran P. The epidemiology of antisocial personality disorder. *Soc Psychiatry Psychiatr Epidemiol.* 1999;34:231–242.

Mulder RT. Alcoholism and personality. *Aust N Z J Psychiatry.* 2002;36:44–52.

Mulsant BH, Ganguli M. Epidemiology and diagnosis of depression in late life. *J Clin Psychiatry.* 1999;60(Suppl 20):9–15.

Murden RA, McRae TD, Kaner S, et al. Mini-Mental State Exam scores vary with education in blacks and whites. *J Am Geriatr Soc.* 1991;39:149–155.

Murphy GM Jr, Lim KO, Wieneke M, et al. No neuropathologic evidence for an increased frequency of Alzheimer's disease. *Biol Psychiatry.* 1998;43:205–209.

Murphy JM, Laird NM, Monson RR, Sobol AM, Leighton AH. Incidence of depression in the Stirling County Study: historical and comparative perspective. *Psychol Med.* 2000;30:505–514.

Nakamura CM, Molgaard CA, Stanford EP, et al. A discriminant analysis of severe alcohol consumption among older persons. *Alcohol Alcohol.* 1990;25:75–80.

Norris FH, Murrell SA. Social support, life events, and stress as modifiers of adjustment to bereavement by older adults. *Psychol Aging.* 1990;5:429–436.

Nowers M. Deliberate self-harm in the elderly: a survey of one London borough. *Int J Geriatr Psychiatry.* 1993;8:609–614.

O'Connor DW, Roth M. Coexisting depression and dementia in a community survey of the elderly. *Int Psychogeriatr.* 1990;2:45–53.

Ogunniyi A, Baiyewu O, Gurege O, et al. Epidemiology of dementia in Nigeria: results from the Indianapolis-Ibadan study. *Eur J Neurol.* 2000;7:485–490.

Okwumabua JO, Baker FM, Wong SP, Pilgram BO. Characteristics of depressive symptoms in elderly urban and rural African Americans. *J Gerontol A Biol Sci Med Sci.* 1997;52:M241–M246.

Oslin DW, Streim JE, Parmelee P, Boyce AA, Katz IR. Alcohol abuse: a source of reversible functional disability among residents of a VA nursing home. *Int J Geriatr Psychiatry.* 1997;12:825–832.

Osuna E, Perez-Carceles MD, Conejero J, Abenza JM, Luna A. Epidemiology of suicide in elderly people in Madrid, Spain (1990–1994). *Forens Sci Int.* 1997;87:73–80.

Oxman TE, Berkman LF, Kasl S, et al. Social support and depressive symptoms in the elderly. *Am J Epidemiol.* 1992;135:356–368.

Palinkas LA, Wingard DL, Barrett-Connor E. Chronic illness and depressive symptoms in the elderly: a population-based study. *J Clin Epidemiol.* 1990;43:1131–1141.

Palmer BW, Jeste DV, Sheikh JI. Anxiety disorders in the elderly: *DSM-IV* and other barriers to diagnosis and treatment. *J Affect Disord.* 1997;46:183–190.

Palsson S, Skoog I. The epidemiology of affective disorders in the elderly: a review. *Int Clin Psychopharmacol.* 1997;12(Suppl 7):S3–S13.

Papassotiropoulos A, Heun R. Detection of subthreshold depression and subthreshold anxiety in the elderly. *Int J Geriatr Psychiatry.* 1999;14:643–650.

Parmelee PA, Katz IR, Lawton MP. Incidence of depression in long-term care settings. *J Gerontol Med Sci.* 1992;47:M189–M196.

Parmelee PA, Lawton, MP, Katz IR. The structure of depression among elderly institution residents: affective and somatic correlates of physical frailty. *J Gerontol A Biol Sci Med Sci.* 1998;53:M155–M162.

Parry CD, Bhana A, Pluddemann A, et al. The South African Community Epidemiology Network on Drug Use (SACENDU): description, findings (1997–99) and policy implications. *Addiction.* 2002;97:969–976.

Paterniti S, Dufouil C, Alperovitch A. Long-term benzodiazepine use and cognitive decline in the elderly: the Epidemiology of Vascular Aging Study. *J Clin Psychopharmacol.* 2002;22:285–293.

Paulson GW. Visual hallucinations in the elderly. *Gerontology.* 1997;43:255–260.

Pincus HA, Pettit AR. The societal costs of chronic major depression. *J Clin Psychiatry.* 2001;62(Suppl 6):5–9.

Pritchard C. Changes in elderly suicides in the USA and the developed world 1974–87: comparison with current homicide. *Int J Geriatr Psychiatry.* 1992;7:125–134.

Ravaglia G, Forti P, Maioli F, et al. Education, occupation, and prevalence of dementia: findings from the Conselice study. *Dement Geriatr Cogn Disord.* 2002;14(2):90–100.

Ray WA, Taylor JA, Meador KG, et al. Reducing antipsychotic drug use in nursing homes: a controlled trial of provider education. *Arch Intern Med.* 1993;153:713–721.

Regier DA, Narrow WE, Rae DS. The epidemiology of anxiety disorders: the Epidemiologic Catchment Area (ECA) experience. *J Psychiatr Res.* 1990;24:314.

Reid MC, Anderson PA. Geriatric substance use disorder. *Med Clin North Am.* 1997; 81:999–1016.

Reynolds CF 3rd, Dew MA, Frank E, et al. Effects of age at onset of first lifetime episode of recurrent major depression on treatment response and illness course in elderly patients. *Am J Psychiatry.* 1998;155:795–799.

Rigler SK. Alcoholism in the elderly. *Am Fam Physician.* 2000;61:1710–1716, 1883–1884, 1887–1888, passim.

Ritchie K, Ledesert B, Touchon J. Subclinical cognitive impairment: epidemiology and clinical characteristics. *Comp Psychiatry.* 2000;41(2, Suppl 1):61–65.

Rob PM, Neiderstatd C, Reusche E. Dementia in patients undergoing long-term dialysis: aetiology, differential diagnoses, epidemiology and management. *CNS Drugs.* 2001;15:691–699.

Rose S, Maffulli N. Hip fractures. An epidemiological review. *Bull Hosp Joint Dis.* 1999;58:197–201.

Roth M, Kay DW. Late paraphrenia: a variant of schizophrenia manifest in late life or an organic clinical syndrome: a review of recent evidence. *Int J Geriatr Psychiatry.* 1998;13:775–784.

Ruchlin HS. Prevalence and correlates of alcohol use among older adults. *Prev Med.* 1997;26(Pt 1):651–657.

Russell DW, Cutrona CE. Social support, stress, and depressive symptoms among the elderly: test of a process model. *Psychol Aging.* 1991;6:190–201.

Sadek N, Bona J. Subsyndromal symptomatic depression: a new concept. *Depression Anxiety.* 2000;12:30–39.

Sandberg O, Gustafson Y, Brannstrom B, Bucht G. Prevalence of dementia, delirium and psychiatric symptoms in various care settings for the elderly. *Scand J Soc Med.* 1998;26:56–62.

Sandyk R, Awerbuch GI. Late-onset schizophrenia: relationship to awareness of abnormal involuntary movements and tobacco addiction. *Int J Neurosci.* 1993;71:9–19.

Schaub RT, Linden M. Anxiety and anxiety disorders in the old and very old—results from the Berlin Aging Study (BASE). *Compr Psychiatry* 2000;41(2, Suppl 1):48–54.

Schoevers RA, Beekman AT, Deeg DJ, Geerlings MI, Jonker C, Van Tilburg W. Risk factors for depression in later life; results of a prospective community based study (AMSTEL). *J Affect Disord.* 2000;59:127–137.

Schonfeld L, Dupree LW. Antecedents of drinking for early- and late-onset elderly alcohol abusers. *J Stud Alcohol.* 1991;52:587–592.

Schotte K, Cooper B. Subthreshold affective disorders: a useful concept in psychiatric epidemiology? *Epidemiol Psichiatr Soc.* 1999;8:255–261.

Seeman TE. Health promoting effects of friends and family on health outcomes in older adults. *Am J Health Promot.* 2000;14:362–370.

Semple SJ, Patterson TL, Shaw WS, Grant I, Moscona S, Jeste DV. Self perceived interpersonal competence in older schizophrenia patients: the role of patient characteristics and psychosocial factors. *Acta Psychiatr Scand.* 1999;100(2):126–135.

Shah R, Uren Z, Baker A, Majeed A. Trends in suicide from drug overdose in the elderly in England and Wales, 1993–1999. *Int J Geriatr Psychiatry.* 2002;17:416–421.

Shaper AG. Alcohol and mortality: a review of prospective studies. *Br J Addict.* 1990; 85:837–847.

Sharma VK, Copeland JR, Dewey ME, Lowe D, Davidson I. Outcome of the depressed elderly living in the community in Liverpool: a 5 year follow up. *Psychol Med.* 1998;28:1329–1337.

Sheehan B, Banerjee S. Review: somatization in the elderly. *Int J Geriatr Psychiatry.* 1999;14:1044–1049.

Sherrell K, Anderson R, Buckwalter K. Invisible residents: the chronically mentally ill elderly in nursing homes. *Arch Psychiatr Nurs.* 1998;12:131–139.

Silverman JM, Li G, Schear S, et al. A cross-cultural family history study of primary progressive dementia in relatives of non demented elderly Chinese, Italians, Jews and Puerto Ricans. *Acta Psychiatr Scand.* 1992;85:211–217.

Sinoff G, Ore L, Zlotorgorsky D, Tamir A. Short Anxiety Screening Test—a brief instrument for detecting anxiety in the elderly. *Int J Geriatr Psychiatry.* 1999;14:1062–1071.

Smith DA, Jensen S. OBRA—its effect on the mentally ill in South Dakota nursing homes. *S D J Med.* 1990;43:13–14.

Snowdon J. The prevalence of depression in old age. *Int J Geriatr Psychiatry.* 1990;5: 141–144.

Soni SD, Mallik A. The elderly chronic schizophrenic inpatient: a study of psychiatric morbidity in "elderly graduates." *Int J Geriatr Psychiatry.* 1993;8:665–673.

Sonino N, Fava GA. Psychiatry disorders associated with Cushing's syndrome: epidemiology, pathophysiology and treatment. *CNS Drugs.* 2001;15:361–373.

Spinhoven P, Ormeel J, Sloekers PP, Kempen GI, Speckens AE, Van Hemert AM. A validation study of the Hospital Anxiety and Depression Scale (HADS) in different groups of Dutch subjects. *Psychol Med.* 1997;27:363–370.

Stallones L, Marx MB, Garrity TF. Prevalence and correlates of depressive symptoms among older US adults. *Am J Prev Med.* 1990;6:295–303.

Stoltenberg SF, Hill EM, Mudd SA, Blow FC, Zucker RA. Birth cohort difference in features of antisocial alcoholism among men and women. *Alcohol Clin Exp Res.* 1999;23:1884–1891.

Suh GH, Shah A. A review of the epidemiological transition in dementia—cross-national comparisons of the indices related to Alzheimer's disease and vascular dementia. *Acta Psychiatr Scand.* 2001;104:4–11.

Swartz M, Landerman R, George LK, et al. Somatization disorder. In: Robins LN, Regier DA, eds. *Psychiatric Disorders in America: The Epidemiologic Catchment Area Study.* New York, NY: Free Press; 1991:220–257.

Targum SD, Abbott JL. Psychoses in the elderly: a spectrum of disorders [review]. *J Clin Psychiatry.* 1999;60(Suppl 8):4–10.

Teesson M, Hall W, Lynskey M, Degenhardt L. Alcohol- and drug-use disorders in Australia: implications of the National Survey of Mental Health and Well Being. *AustN Z J Psychiatry.* 2000;34:206–213.

Teresi JA, Kleinman M, Ocepek-Welikson K. Modern psychometric method for detection of differential item functioning: application to cognitive assessment measures. *Stat Med.* 2000;19:1651–1683.

Thompson JW, Belcher JR, DeForge BR, et al. Changing characteristics of schizophrenic patients admitted to state hospitals. *Hosp Community Psychiatry.* 1993;44:231–235.

Thorpe L, Groulx B. Canadian Centres for Clinical Cognitive Research. Depressive syndromes in dementia. *Can J Neurol Sci.* 2001;28(Suppl 1):S83–S95.

Tom T, Cummings JL. Depression in Parkinson's disease: pharmacological characteristics and treatment. *Drugs Aging.* 1998;12:55–74.

Tueth MJ, Zuberi P. Life-threatening psychiatric emergencies in the elderly: overview. *J Geriatr Psychiatry Neurol.* 1999;12:60–66.

Tzourio C, Dufouil C, Ducimetiere P, Alperovitch A. Cognitive decline in individuals with high blood pressure: a longitudinal study in the elderly. EVA Study Group. Epidemiology of Vascular Aging. *Neurology.* 1999;53:1948–1952.

Uhlmann RF, Larson EB. Effect of education on the Mini-Mental State Examination as a screening test for dementia. *J Am Geriatr Soc.* 1991;39:876–880.

Unverzagt FW, Gao S, Baiyewu O, et al. Prevalence of cognitive impairment: data from the Indianapolis Study of Health and Aging. *Neurology.* 2001;57:1655–1662.

Ustun TB. Cross-national epidemiology of depression and gender. *J Gender-Specific Med.* 2000;3(2):54–58.

Vahle VJ, Anderson EM, Hagglund KJ. Depression measures in outcomes research. *Arch Phys Med Rehab.* 2000;81(12 Suppl 2):S53–S62.

Vaillant GE, Meyer SE, Mukamal K, Soldz S. Are social supports in late midlife a cause or a result of successful physical ageing? *Psychol Med.* 1998;28:1159–1168.

van Balkom AJ, Beekman AT, de Beurs E, Deeg DJ, van Dyck R, van Tilburg W. Comorbidity of the anxiety disorders in a community-based older population in the Netherlands. *Acta Psychiatr Scand.* 2000;101:37–45.

Van Kooten F, Koudstaal PJ. Epidemiology of post stroke dementia. *Haemostasis.* 1998;28(3–4):124–133.

Verbrugge LM. Longer life but worsening health? In: Lee PR, Estes CL, eds. *The Nation's Health.* 3rd ed. Boston, MA: Jones and Bartlett; 1990:14–34.

von Korff M, Dworkin S, Le Resche L. Graded chronic pain status: an epidemiological evaluation. *Pain.* 1990;40:279–291.

Weissman MM, Bruse ML, Leaf PJ, et al. Affective disorders. In: Robins LN, Regier DA, eds. *Psychiatric Disorders in America: The Epidemiologic Catchment Area Study.* New York, NY: Free Press; 1991:53–80.

Wells KS, Burnam MA, Rogers W, et al. The course of depression in adult outpatients: results from the Medical Outcomes Study. *Arch Gen Psychiatry.* 1992;49:788–794.

Wells KS, Rogers W, Burnam MA, et al. Course of depression in patients with hypertension, myocardial infarction, or insulin-dependent diabetes. *Am J Psychiatry.* 1993; 150:632–638.

Weyerer S, Schaufele M, Zimber A. Alcohol problems among residents in old age homes in the city of Manheim, Germany. *Aust N Z J Psychiatry.* 1999;33:825–830.

Whalley LJ. Early-onset Alzheimer's disease in Scotland: environmental and familial factors. *Br J Psychiatry Suppl.* 2001;40:s53–s59.

White L, Parrella M, McCrystal-Simon J, Harvey PD, Masiar SJ, Davidson M. Characteristics of elderly psychiatric patients retained in a state hospital during downsizing: a prospective study with replication. *Int J Geriatr Psychiatry.* 1997;12:474–480.

Whiteman PJ, Hoffman RS, Goldfrank LR. Alcoholism in the emergency department: an epidemiologic study. *Acad Emerg Med.* 2000;7:14–20.

Whyte EM, Mulsant BH. Post stroke depression: epidemiology, pathophysiology, and biological treatment. *Biol Psychiatry.* 2002;52:253–264.

Wittchen HU, Fehm L. Epidemiology, pattern of comorbidity, and associated disabilities of social phobia. *Psychiatr Clin North Am.* 2001;24:617–641.

Wu LT, Anthony JC. The estimated rate of depression mood in US adults: recent evidence for a peak in later life. *J Affect Disord.* 2000;60:159–171.

Wynn Owen PA, Castle DJ. Late onset schizophrenia: epidemiology, diagnosis, management and outcomes. *Drugs Aging.* 1999;15(2):81–89.

Zesiewicz TA, Hauser RA. Depression in Parkinson's disease. *Curr Psychiatry Rep.* 2002;4:69–73.

Zisook S, Schuchter SR. Depression through the first year after the death of a spouse. *Am J Psychiatry.* 1991;148:1346–1352.

2

Genetics of Dementia

Debby W. Tsuang, MD, MSc
Thomas D. Bird, MD

The past decade has seen a tremendous explosion of new information on the genetics of a variety of dementing disorders. It is critical that geriatric psychiatrists keep updated on these findings so they can properly diagnose and manage patients. We briefly review fundamental concepts in human genetics by describing the most common modes of inheritance and the fundamental tools of molecular genetics.

We selected seven of the most prominent examples of dementing disorders for which genes have been identified, and we summarize the clinical, genetic, epidemiological, and molecular genetic findings on these disorders. Our goal is to provide a succinct description of the latest genetic findings on these important disorders so geriatric psychiatrists can more effectively diagnose and manage these conditions in their patients.

MODES OF INHERITANCE

Inheritance patterns for various genetic disorders are summarized in Table 2-1. Excellent references include *Principles of Medical Genetics* (Gelehrter & Collins, 1990) and *Thompson and Thompson Genetics in Medicine* (Thompson et al., 1991).

Autosomal dominant inheritance occurs in multiple generations, affecting both males and females (see Figure 2-1). Each offspring of affected individuals

TABLE 2-1. Inheritance patterns

	Risk to offspring	Father-to-son transmission	Father-to-daughter transmission	Affected generations
Autosomal dominant	50%, regardless of sex	Yes	Yes	Multiple
Autosomal recessive	25%, regardless of sex	Yes	Yes	One (unless inbreeding involved)
X-linked recessive	50% of sons of carrier female are affected 50% of daughters of carrier female are carriers 100% of daughters of carrier male are carriers	No	100% of daughters of carrier male are carriers	Multiple
Multifactoral	Based on empiric risk	Yes	Yes	Multiple; risks vary depending on degree of relatedness to affected proband

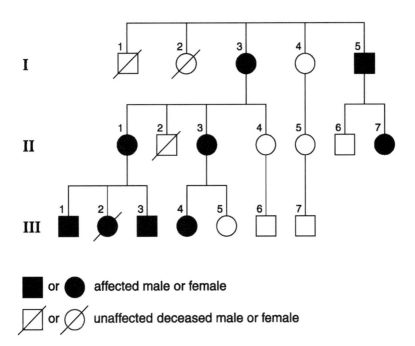

■ or ● affected male or female

▱ or ⊘ unaffected deceased male or female

FIGURE 2-1. Autosomal dominant inheritance in multiple generations.

has a 50% risk of inheriting the disease gene. Huntington's disease (HD) and familial Alzheimer's disease (FAD) are examples of autosomal dominant inheritance. However, autosomal dominant inheritance may also be associated with variable expressivity and reduced penetrance. *Variable expressivity* refers to variability of the phenotype, that is, the extent to which the genetic mutation is expressed. For example, in neurofibromatosis type 1 (NF1), the clinical features may be as mild as cafe-au-lait skin spots or as severe as mental retardation and brain tumors. The gene is the same in all affected individuals (the *NF1* gene on chromosome 17), but at least 40 known mutations are associated with NF. Related symptoms may vary substantially, and some of this variability may be associated with the specific mutation in the *NF1* gene. However, there is no clear phenotype-genotype correlation. *Penetrance*, on the other hand, is an all-or-nothing phenomenon that refers to whether a genotype is expressed. Penetrance usually refers to dominant traits in heterozygotes. If a condition is expressed in less than 100% of gene carriers, it is said to have reduced penetrance. Some individuals may carry the mutated gene, but remain asymptomatic throughout their lives. These individuals can still pass the mutated gene to their offspring.

Autosomal recessive inheritance usually occurs in a single sibship in only one generation (see Figure 2-2). Sibship consists of all brothers and sisters in one generation. Parents who are carriers of one copy of the disease gene are

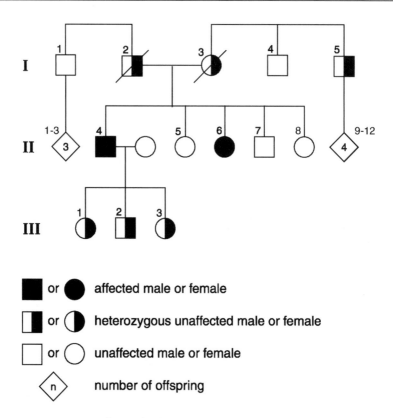

FIGURE 2-2. Autosomal recessive inheritance.

called *heterozygotes*. Two carrier parents have a 25% chance of having a child who is a *homozygote*. A homozygote has two copies of the disease gene and will thus manifest the disease. Carriers are relatively infrequent in the general population, so autosomal recessive conditions are rare and are more likely to occur in inbred populations. Disorders consistent with recessive inheritance include cystic fibrosis and phenylketonuria. Carriers of autosomal recessive genes are not usually clinically recognizable, but estimates of carrier frequency for a recessive condition are important for purposes of genetic counseling. Because an autosomal recessive condition has to be inherited through both parents, the risk that any carrier will have an affected child depends on the carrier frequency in the general population or in the specific ethnic group of the parents. Although recessive models are often used in molecular linkage studies of psychiatric disorders, no particular psychiatric disorders are known to strictly follow this mode of inheritance.

X-linked recessive inheritance refers to a pattern of transmission involving genes on the X chromosome (see Figure 2-3). The X and Y chromosomes, which are responsible for sex determination, are usually distributed so that males in-

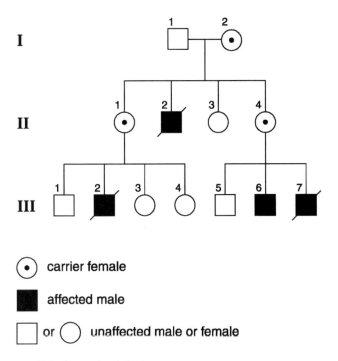

FIGURE 2-3. X-linked recessive inheritance.

herit one X and one Y chromosome; females inherit two X chromosomes. Pheno-types determined by genes on the X chromosome have a characteristic sex distribution and pattern of inheritance. As an example, consider the case of an X-linked recessive disease. In this case, only males develop the disorder because they have only one X chromosome. Females are typically unaffected because they have a normal gene on their other X chromosome; however, they may carry the mutated gene and can pass it on to their sons and daughters. For X-linked recessive diseases, sons of an affected male do not inherit the gene be-cause they inherit the Y (not X) chromosome from their father. However, the daughters of affected males have a 100% chance of inheriting the X disease gene from their father. Hemophilia A is an example of an X-linked recessive disorder.

Mitochondrial inheritance is an example of nonclassical single-gene inheri-tance. The peculiarity of mitochondrial gene inheritance is that the patients are always related through the maternal line, and no affected male transmits the disease (see Figure 2-4). Mitochondria can be found only in the cytoplasm of the egg. Both sons and daughters of affected mothers are at risk for inheritance of abnormal mitochondria. There is significant variable expressivity in mito-chondrial diseases. There have been reports of families with bipolar disorder that show excessive maternal transmission; however, no specific mitochondrial

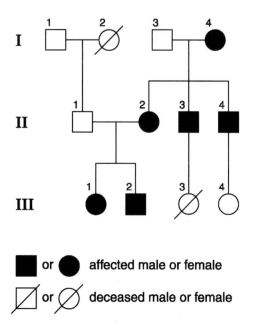

FIGURE 2-4. Mitochondrial inheritance.

mutation has yet been identified for these families. Well-established associations between mitochondrial DNA and disease include such rare neurological diseases as Leber's optic atrophy.

Multifactorial inheritance refers to disorders that result from a combination of environmental and genetic factors, each making a relatively small contribution to the development of the disease. Both polygenic and oligogenic inheritance fall under the larger umbrella of multifactorial inheritance. The term *polygenic inheritance* has a more limited definition, suggesting inheritance of a large number of genes with small and additive effects. This mode of inheritance accounts for inherited normal traits such as height and intelligence. *Oligogenic inheritance* refers to the interactions of a small number of major genes (e.g., epistatic interaction), that result in a disorder. These genes may have varying effects on the susceptibility to disease expression. This type of model allows for *epistasis*, which is the interaction of numerous genes with one another. Multifactorial inheritance may recur in a population, but this pattern may not be readily apparent in individual families.

Because the concordance rates for most psychiatric disorders are considerably less than 100% among monozygotic twins (Tsuang et al., 1995), it has been suggested that environmental factors contribute to the development of such disorders. One model to account for this observation proposes a genetic liability with a genetic liability threshold. Genetically liable individuals, if exposed to the necessary environmental factors, will develop the disease.

Recurrence risks in multifactorial disorders are estimates averaged from a collection of families (Faraone et al., 1999). Risks to first-degree relatives of affected persons are more for single-gene autosomal dominant or recessive disorders than for multifactorial disorders. The multifactorial genetic risk to first-degree relatives is usually on the magnitude of 1- to 10-fold higher than the incidence found in the general population, but this risk decreases rapidly in second-degree relatives. The recurrence risk is higher when more than one family member is affected. Multiple cases in some families suggest that the degree of liability can be variable among different families. The actual risk for an individual family may be higher or lower than the average.

The threshold model assumes that affected individuals fall to the extreme right of the continuum. Therefore, first-degree relatives, who share one half of their genes with the affected individual, will have a distribution of genetic liability shifted to the right of that of the general population (see Figure 2-5). Second-degree relatives, who share one fourth of their genes with the affected individuals, will have a distribution that is closer to the mean of the general population. Third-degree relatives, who share only one eighth of their genes, will have a liability much closer to that of the general population and will therefore have only a slightly increased risk of developing the disorder compared to the general population. Examples of multifactorial inheritance include some forms of late-onset Alzheimer's disease (AD), diabetes mellitus, hypertension, schizophrenia, and affective disorder. However, until specific causative genes are identified, it remains impossible to identify other genetic and environmental risk factors that contribute to these disorders.

GENETIC TESTING

DNA testing is the newest technique to test for the presence or absence of hereditary disorders. This technique involves direct examination of the DNA molecule itself, typically obtained from blood. This may involve sequencing of the disease gene, such as determination of the number of CAG repeats in the 5′ region of the Huntington's disease gene. Other tests detect metabolic by-products (e.g., techniques to detect phenylalanine in patients with phenylketonuria) and chromosomal microdeletions through microscopic examination of fluorescent chromosomes (e.g., fluorescent in situ hybridization techniques to detect the deletion in patients with velocardiofacial syndrome). Genetic tests are used in many ways, including

- Presymptomatic testing for prediction of adult-onset disorders
- Diagnostic testing for symptomatic individuals
- Prenatal diagnostic testing
- Newborn screening
- Carrier screening
- Forensic testing

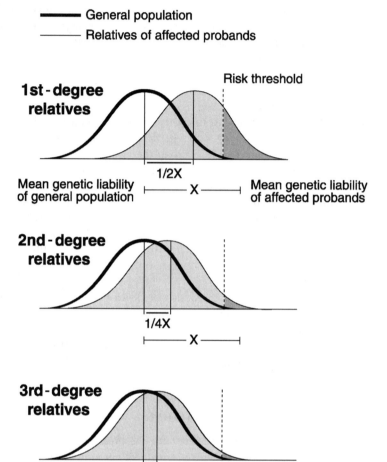

FIGURE 2-5.   Shift of genetic liability distribution according to the threshold model.

Among these types, geriatric psychiatrists are most likely to encounter pre-symptomatic testing and diagnostic testing.

For many at-risk individuals, the availability of direct, DNA-based genetic tests gives them the opportunity to clarify any uncertainty about their risks and to plan better. For a small subset of individuals with early-onset Alzheimer's disease, genetic testing is available (McConnell et al., 1999). At present, three genes have been identified in rare autosomal dominant, early-onset AD families; these genes are on chromosomes 1, 14, and 21 (Levy-Lahad et al., 1998; St. George-Hyslop, 2000). These three genes account for less than 5% of all cases of AD. Genetic testing for the *presenilin 1 (PS1)* gene is available on a commercial basis; *presenilin 2 (PS2)* gene and amyloid precursor protein (APP) mutation screening are only available on a research basis. Individuals who test positive may benefit from closer surveillance. The benefits of presymptomatic treatment with cholinesterase inhibitors remain unclear at this time.

For individuals from the small number of high-risk early-onset AD families, DNA tests are highly accurate. However, for most individuals, only age-adjusted risk estimates can be provided.

For the general population, the cumulative risk of AD is approximately 2% to 5% at age 70 years. This risk increases approximately 0.5% to 1% per year after 70 years of age. For individuals with a first-degree relative with AD, the same 2% to 5% risk is observed earlier in life (at approximately 60 to 65 years old) (Heston, 1992). Risk to family members is higher if multiple family members are affected. Like most other psychiatric disorders, multiple genes and environmental factors are presumed to be involved. Therefore, testing for susceptibility genes is likely to be much more difficult to interpret and may actually lead to more uncertainty (Welch & Burke, 1998). Although the apolipoprotein E *(APOE)* ε4 allele is strongly associated with late-onset AD (Corder et al., 1993; Saunders et al., 1993), presymptomatic testing for AD using *APOE* genotyping is not recommended because of its limited sensitivity and specificity (American College, 1995; Knopman et al., 2001).

Diagnostic genetic testing in symptomatic individuals also presents some challenges. *APOE* ε4 homozygotes constitute 2% to 3% of the general population and 15% to 20% of patients with AD. However, approximately 35% to 50% of AD patients do not carry an ε4 allele. Therefore, other etiological factors exist. Genetic counseling (described below) is a time-consuming process, but pre- and posttest counseling are critical to ensure the best outcome.

More information about currently available DNA diagnostic tests can be obtained from GeneTests (www.genetests.org). Information on genetic counseling in a variety of dementing disorders (e.g., Alzheimer's disease, Huntington's disease) can be obtained from GeneClinics (www.geneclinics.org).

The discovery of new disease genes occurs weekly. However, tests for these disease genes are not always readily available because it often takes months or years to confirm initial research findings, to determine the frequency of these mutations in clinical samples, and to determine the penetrance (the probability of developing the disease given the presence of a mutation) of these genes. This delay in test availability can be very frustrating for at-risk individuals and their families.

In addition, different mutations (in the same or a different gene) can result in the same disease. Conversely, the same mutation may manifest itself differently in some families. Many genes have many different causative mutations, all of which can result in disease. Commercially available genetic tests for some disorders may not screen for all known mutations, just the most common ones. In most cases, negative results are informative. However, in cases of rare mutations, negative results may be misleading. Clinicians need to understand the limitations of specific laboratory tests to avoid false reassurance.

GENETIC COUNSELING

Genetic counseling is a well-established medical subspecialty that helps to communicate genetic risks to patients and their family members. We provide here the general principles of genetic counseling. We then discuss the potential adverse consequences and the ethical implications raised by the availability of genetic testing. We discuss guidelines that may be applicable to neuropsychiatric disorders (Bird & Bennett, 1995; Huggins et al., 1990; Quaid, 1992).

Once the correct diagnosis has been made, genetic counseling involves educating the patient's family about the clinical and genetic aspects of the disease. Much of the counseling may involve recurrence risk estimates. The recurrence risks for the various modes of inheritance are presented in Table 2-1. Autosomal dominant inheritance is fairly straightforward, but the other modes of inheritance can be confusing.

The counseling process can be improved using diagrams and drawings. In addition, the concept of probabilities can be demonstrated by flipping a coin 10 times. This will help illustrate that each conception (or coin toss) and the associated risk are independent of previous conceptions and their associated risks (Faraone et al., 1999).

Genetic counseling educates those seeking counseling (the *consultands*) and provides them with relevant information concerning the disorder of interest. Multiple visits may be necessary. Genetic counseling must be tailored to the specific disease and to the needs of the individual and his or her family.

Following the initial evaluation of the consultand, further evaluation of family members may be indicated. Detailed assessments may be necessary to confirm the diagnosis of the affected individual. Genetic testing may be available to determine if a presymptomatic person (presymptomatic testing) or if a symptomatic person (diagnostic testing) carries the mutation. Genetic testing may also be available for the disease of interest.

It is often critical to provide follow-up counseling for additional questions, as well as for reassessment of the psychological state of the consultands. In addition, it is important to provide families with names and addresses of local and national support groups. Finally, because the diagnosis of an individual has implications for his or her family members, providers must be ready to deal with the repercussions of the new knowledge for various relatives. Other references provide details regarding genetic counseling in psychiatric disorders (Harper, 1998; Hodgkinson et al., 2001; Tsuang et al., 2001).

ETHICAL ISSUES IN GENETIC TESTING

The guiding principle in the ethics of clinical practice and genetics research (see also Chapter 38) is obtaining informed consent. Consultands choosing genetic testing for clinical reasons should be thoroughly informed of the risks and benefits of the procedure and should always have the option to terminate at any time. Part of the consent process should describe the confidentiality of the data; however, the genetic counselor should inform the consultands that the genetic information will be part of their medical record (Billings et al., 1992).

To compute the costs of health and life insurance, actuaries take into account many factors known to predict disease and death. Few people argue with the fact that smokers pay higher health insurance premiums than nonsmokers. However, is the use of genetic information by insurance companies justified? Theoretically, insurance companies could have access to the genetic profiles of individuals who apply for insurance. Should those who are at risk for an untreatable or chronically debilitating disorder pay higher insurance premiums? Should the insurance company have the right to deny coverage? The answers to these questions are unclear.

Like insurance companies, employers may want to know their employees' risk for genetic disorders. Because potential employees may eventually be less productive and may increase health care costs, some employers might discriminate based on genetic testing results. Although this may be unjustifiable to some, others may argue that, in occupations that involve the safety of the general public (e.g., commercial airline pilots, physicians, police), genetic tests for disorders that may impair judgment and job performance indeed should be used by the employer.

The implications of the Human Genome Project have not escaped the attention of legislators. In the United States, several states have already enacted genetic privacy laws (Herstek, 1999; Rothstein, 1998). In general, these laws limit the use of genetic data by insurance companies. However, the idea that genetic data should be treated differently from other clinical data has been hotly debated. We can anticipate the ethical and legal debates over genetic testing will continue. Indeed, they are likely to intensify if and when the capability to predict some types of behavioral and personality traits becomes possible. For additional information, refer to the Ethical, Legal, and Social Implications (ELSI) Research Program Web site (http://www.nhgri.nih.gov/ELSI/).

The Human Genome Project will undoubtedly provide an abundance of data that researchers may use to help identify genes that contribute to human behavioral disorders. With the "working draft" of the human genome in hand, identification of genes associated with behavior continues. The implications of the use of genetic data for diagnosis and treatment of psychiatric disorders remain unclear. As psychiatric genetics enters the gene identification era, the clinical applications of genetic testing will increase (Rutter & Plomin, 1997). This will raise many questions about the legal, ethical, and social implications of genetic tests.

PRIMER IN MOLECULAR GENETICS

The human genome includes 3 billion nucleotides and approximately 30,000 genes. It is currently not feasible to examine these genes one at a time, even if the search could be limited to just the genes expressed in the human brain. Thus, finding a causative gene for a particular disease is like finding a needle in a haystack. Currently, approximately 9,000 genetic diseases have been described, and genes for over 800 genetic disorders have been identified. Diagnostic tests are available for many of these disorders. The chain of research in molecular genetic studies is as follows: (1) Where are the disease genes located? (2) Which genes cause which diseases? (3) How does the disruption of a gene lead to the development of certain diseases?

DNA is composed of nucleotide bases, deoxyribose, and phosphate groups. There are two types of nucleotide bases: the purines, adenine (A) and guanine (G); and the pyrimidines, thymine (T) and cytosine (C). The intertwining of two strands of DNA ensures base pairing of the strands. This pairing provides a means for accurate replication because one strand serves as the template for the creation of a new strand. In addition, the system contains several means for error correction. The complementary structure of DNA has important implications for molecular research. For example, to identify a DNA fragment with a particular sequence of DNA, its complementary sequence can be used to find the molecule of interest (see Figure 2-6).

Genes encode information for the production of functional proteins. Genomic DNA undergoes transcription, yielding *messenger RNA* (mRNA). Small parts of the genome (3%) form mRNA transcripts, which in turn form sequences called *exons*.

Interspersed noncoding DNA sequences are called *introns*. Introns are spliced out when the mature mRNA is formed. However, introns are necessary for the regulation of mRNA formation and for maintaining the structure of the chromosome. After modification, mRNA is transported out of the nucleus into the cytoplasm. The information is then translated into amino acid sequences and synthesized into a protein.

In addition to the DNA in the nucleus, mitochondria in the cytoplasm also contain their own DNA (mtDNA). This is a closed, circular DNA molecule that replicates separately from the rest of the genome. Heritable errors leading to mitochondrial dysfunction can arise from mutations in mitochondrial DNA. The discovery of mitochondrial mutations has led to a better understanding of mitochondrial molecular biology.

The human genome is extremely large, but highly repetitive. For detailed analyses, the DNA has to be cleaved into pieces of a particular size in a sequence-specific fashion. Then individual DNA fragments are isolated, produced in large quantities, and further analyzed. This is possible through the techniques of recombinant technology using cloning vectors and poly merase chain reactions. Detailed molecular biology techniques are beyond the scope of this book; for detailed descriptions and protocols, refer to molecular biology textbooks such as *Human Molecular Genetics* (Strachan & Reed, 1999) and *Molecular Biology of the Cell* (Alberts et al., 2002).

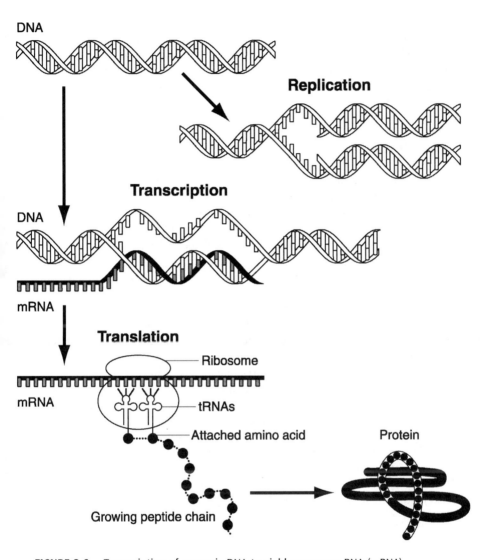

FIGURE 2-6. Transcription of genomic DNA to yield messenger RNA (mRNA).

GENETICS OF DEMENTIA

In the following sections, we discuss seven of the most prominent examples of dementing disorders for which genes have been identified. These disorders comprise the most common causes of dementia in the elderly. Identification of rare mutations in several genes has resulted in the discovery of novel proteins associated with each disorder. Interestingly, all of these mutant proteins result in abnormal aggregation and deposit that are pathological hallmarks of each condition (e.g., α-synuclein in Lewy bodies [LBs] of Parkinson's disease [PD] and peptide αβ in the neuritic plaques of Alzheimer's disease) (Taylor et al., 2002). The list of conditions discussed in this chapter is not exhaustive. *Neurogenetics* (Pulst, 2000) and *Alzheimer's Disease* (Terry et al., 1999) provide detailed descriptions regarding specific disorders.

Alzheimer's Disease

CLINICAL FEATURES   Alzheimer's disease is the most common cause of dementia (Adams & Victor, 2001). It is a slowly progressive disease that initially presents with short-term memory loss and other cognitive changes (e.g., difficulties in calculation, getting lost). Additional symptoms include executive dysfunction, confusion, aphasia, gait, and behavioral disturbances. Typically, the age of onset is older than 65 years. The duration of illness may range from 4 to 20 years. More women than men are affected, even after adjustment for the greater longevity of females.

PATHOLOGICAL FEATURES   Pathologically, there is diffuse cerebral atrophy with β-amyloid (Aβ) senile neuritic plaques, neurofibrillary tangles (NFTs), and amyloid angiopathy as first described by Alois Alzheimer in 1907 (Alzheimer, 1907). Neuritic plaques are complex structures that consist primarily of a core of abnormal aggregates of a small protein molecule known as Aβ. Neurofibrillary tangles are dense bundles of helically wound abnormal fibers composed of a modified form of a normally occurring neuronal protein, the microtubule-associated protein tau. The presence of either senile plaques or neurofibrillary tangles is not pathognomic of AD (Adams & Duchen, 1992). They are known to occur in other neurodegenerative disorders and in normal aging. The clinical history of progressive memory loss and other cognitive deficits (McKhann et al., 1984) and a high density of these lesions in specific brain regions are currently considered to confirm the diagnosis of AD (National Institute on Aging, 1997).

EPIDEMIOLOGY   The risk for AD increases with advancing age. Approximately 10% of the Caucasian population older than 70 years have dementia, and over half of them have AD (Seshadri et al., 1997). After age 85, approximately 20% to 40% of the general population have clinically significant dementia.

The next most important risk factor for AD is family history. Epidemiological studies show that individuals who have an affected first-degree relative with AD have an approximately fourfold increased risk of developing AD and a total lifetime risk of 38% (Lautenschlager et al., 1996; Rocca et al., 1986), although more recent European studies do not report such high estimates (Launer et al., 1999). To date, reports on monozygotic (MZ) and dizygotic (DZ) twin pairs have suggested higher concordance rates in MZ than in DZ twins (Bergem et al., 1997). Although the numbers of twins studied were small, these studies suggest that genetic components play an important role in the development of AD. However, the lack of complete concordance in MZ twins suggests that environmental components are also important in the etiology of AD (Figure 2-7).

The risk for AD is even higher if there are individuals in more than one generation with the disease, especially when the disease is early onset (younger than age 65). Early evidence of a genetic basis for AD was the observation that all persons with trisomy 21 (Down syndrome) who survive beyond age 40 invariably demonstrate the neuropathological features of AD (Mann, 1993). These observations led to the discovery of mutations in the amyloid precursor protein (*APP*) gene on chromosome 21, the first documented genetic cause of AD (Goate et al., 1991). Although there are fewer than 20 families worldwide with APP mutations, the discovery of these mutations confirmed that genetic factors are important in AD.

FAMILIAL ALZHEIMER'S DISEASE   Although there is no universally accepted definition of FAD, our working definition is the presence of three or more affected first-degree relatives (with at least one individual's diagnosis confirmed by autopsy). The clinical features of FAD are typically indistinguishable from nonfamilial

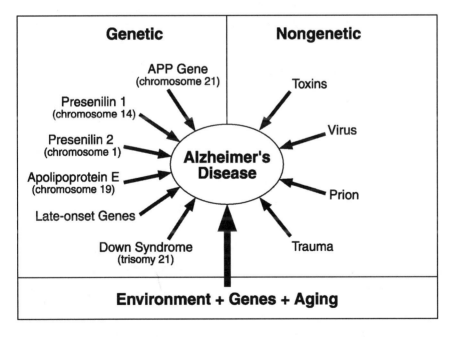

FIGURE 2-7. Complexity of neurodegenerative diseases (APP, amyloid precursor protein).

(or sporadic) AD (Bird et al., 1989). Disease duration is usually 6 to 10 years (but can range from 2 to longer than 20 years). Familial AD is typically divided into early onset (younger than 65 years) and late onset (older than 65 years). In some of these rare families, AD occurs as a single-gene autosomal dominant trait. Thus far, three causative genes have been found in early-onset families (Levy-Lahad and Bird, 2000). Although they account for less than 2% of all individuals with AD, the discovery of these gene mutations has been critical in designing studies to investigate the underlying pathophysiology in AD. A fourth gene, the *APOE ε4* is a major risk factor for both early- and late-onset AD. Other important genetic and environmental risk factors remain to be discovered.

AMYLOID PRECURSOR PROTEIN   The *APP* gene maps to the long arm of chromosome 21. It encodes for a precursor protein that is proteolytically cleaved to form β-amyloid protein (Aβ). Aβ is a peptide with 39–43 amino acids that is the major component of the neuritic plaque, one of the neuropathological hallmarks of AD. Two proteolytic pathways for APP processing have been shown to occur normally (see Figure 2-8). The first is cleavage within the Aβ sequence by a protease referred to as α-secretase (Sisodia et al., 1990). Aβ is destroyed by this cleavage; thus, this process does not contribute to Aβ formation.

The second cleavage is on either side of the Aβ sequence. Enzymes called β- and γ-secretase cleave APP to form the N (amino) and C (carboxy) termini of Aβ-peptide, respectively. β-Secretase cleaves APP first, followed by γ-secretase cleavage, which can result in Aβ peptides of different lengths (Selkoe, 1998). Two β-secretases have been identified, BACE (B-site APP-cleaving enzyme) 1 and 2 (Nunan & Small, 2000).

γ-Secretase cleavages occur within the predicted transmembrane domain of APP, resulting in the Aβ40 and Aβ42 species. The predominant species, Aβ40,

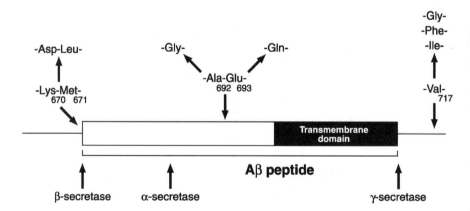

FIGURE 2-8. Normally occurring proteolytic pathways for amyloid precursor protein.

is formed by cleavage after the 40th amino acid of Aβ. Aβ42 only accounts for 10% of the totally secreted Aβ. It is hypothesized that Aβ42 is the pathogenic species in FAD because the proportion of Aβ42 is increased in FAD, and it is the major constituent of the amyloid plaques (Selkoe, 1998). These two (β- and γ-secretases) enzymes are potential therapeutic targets because inhibition of their activity would decrease Aβ production.

In 1990, a mutation in the *APP* gene was first discovered to be associated with a rare condition, cerebral hemorrhagic amyloidosis of the Dutch type (Van Broeckhoven et al., 1990). Because cerebral amyloidosis is also a hallmark of AD, this led to the search for *APP* mutations in FAD. In 1991, it was discovered that a valine-to-isoleucine substitution existed at codon 717 (Val717Ile) in two families (Goate et al., 1991). Subsequently, more than 20 different families have been identified with disease-causing *APP* mutations.

APP mutations are a very rare cause of early-onset FAD (which is itself uncommon). They most likely account for less than 10% of early-onset FAD. Clinically, *APP* mutations result in autosomal dominant early-onset AD that is typically fully penetrant by the early 60s. In the Val717Ile mutation, age of onset ranges from 41 to 64 years (mean 50 years). There is no evidence that APP mutations are responsible for late-onset FAD.

PRESENILIN 1/CHROMOSOME 14 GENE   In 1992, genetic linkage of FAD to a chromosome 14 locus was established and confirmed (Schellenberg et al., 1992). The gene *PS1* was subsequently discovered in 1995 (Sherrington et al., 1995). This gene is predicted to encode a protein with 467 amino acids and with 7 to 10 hydrophobic transmembrane domains (see Figure 2-9). More than 70 different

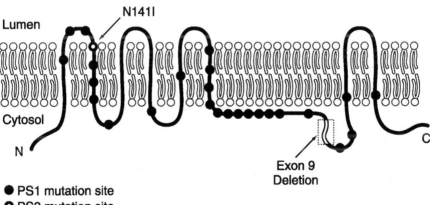

FIGURE 2-9. Gene mutation sites.

mutations in the *PS1* gene have been identified worldwide (Cruts & Van Broeckhoven, 1998). The majority of these mutations are missense mutations (i.e., one base pair change that results in a single amino acid substitution). However, most of the mutations do not result in a truncated normal protein, suggesting that the mutations likely cause a gain in protein function rather than a loss of function. The function of *PS1* remains unknown, but it may have γ-secretase-like activity (Selkoe, 2001; Selkoe & Wolfe, 2000).

Of the three genes known to cause FAD, *PS1* mutations are associated with the earliest age of onset and cause the most rapidly progressing course of disease. Disease onset ranges from 35 to 55 years of age. Penetrance is nearly complete by age 65 years. Disease duration is usually short, ranging from 5.8 to 6.8 years.

The clinical picture is typically characterized by severe dementia associated with language disturbances and myoclonus, which appear relatively early in the disease course (Haltia et al., 1994; Lampe et al., 1994). One mutation (an exon 9 deletion) is often associated with early spasticity (see arrow in Figure 2-9).

PS1 mutations are more common than *APP* mutations and are responsible for about 30% to 60% of early-onset FAD and less than 5% of all AD (Levy-Lahad et al., 1998). A commercial test is available for *PS1* mutations. However, it is critical that genetic counseling take place prior to genetic testing in asymptomatic individuals.

PRESENILIN 2/CHROMOSOME 1 GENE   The third AD gene was discovered shortly after the discovery of the *PS1* gene. It was found in FAD kindreds with Volga German (VG) ancestry (Levy-Lahad, Wasco et al., 1995). These families are ethnic Germans who migrated to Russia but remained separated from the native Russian population. Many of these families subsequently immigrated to the United States, and eight of these families were found to have FAD, presumably based on a genetic founder effect (i.e., a single common affected ancestor). The *PS2* gene was cloned because of its genetic similarity (homology) with the *PS1* gene (Levy-Lahad, Wasco et al., 1995; Levy-Lahad, Wijsman et al., 1995; Levy-Lahad et al., 1996). It was also referred to as STM-2 (seven-transmembrane domains); however, the exact number of transmembrane domains remains unknown.

PS2 is predicted to encode a protein with 448 amino acids that is 67% identical to *PS1* (see Figure 2-9). The highest degree of conservation is within the hydrophobic/transmembrane domains, suggesting that these regions are important in the normal functioning of the protein. Furthermore, the genomic similarity between *PS1* and *PS2* suggests that they arose by duplication. To date, only four or five mutations in *PS2* have been discovered (Cruts & Van Broeckhoven, 1998). A single mutation (N141I) occurs in all VG pedigrees, consistent with the founder effect hypothesis. Like most *PS1* mutations, all *PS2* mutations are also missense mutations.

Clinical features associated with *PS2* mutations have been reported primarily in the Volga Germans. Mean age of onset in these families is 54.9 ± 8.5 years, and mean disease duration is 7.6 ± 3.2 years. However, within the VG families, there is high variability in age of onset, ranging from 40 to 75 years (Bird et al., 1996). The *PS2* mutation is highly penetrant (>95%). The dementia in *PS2* AD is clinically and neuropathologically indistinguishable from sporadic AD.

ROLE OF PRESENILIN 1 AND PRESENILIN 2 IN THE PATHOGENESIS OF ALZHEIMER'S DISEASE   Both the *PS1* and the *PS2* genes are normally expressed ubiquitously within the brain, although the expression is entirely neuronal (Kovacs et al., 1996; McMillan et al., 1996). The presenilins may be involved in intracellular trafficking of APP. Neuronal cultures derived from *PS1* knockout mice embryos show lack of cleavage of APP by γ-secretase and a decrease in Aβ production. This suggests that *PS1* normally functions to promote the cleavage and subsequent clearance of Aβ amyloid (Selkoe, 1998). There is evidence to suggest that *PS1* may be the γ-secretase (Selkoe, 2001; Selkoe & Wolfe, 2000) and that *PS1* mutations specifically affect γ-secretase, resulting in globally increased Aβ42 production (Vassar & Citron, 2000). Patients with *PS1* and *PS2* mutations have elevated Aβ, and their skin fibroblasts produce increased amounts of Aβ. Interested readers should refer to other references for more details (St. George-Hyslop, 2000).

APOLIPOPROTEIN E   The *APOE* gene was initially identified as a genetic risk factor for AD by genetic linkage analysis of late-onset FAD pedigrees on 19q13.2 (Pericak-Vance et al., 1991). Because *APOE* was known to be present in amyloid plaques and neurofibrillary tangles, these observations made *APOE* a plausible candidate gene. A strong allelic association between *APOE* ε4 and AD was established in 1993 (Saunders et al., 1993) and was rapidly confirmed in autopsy-proven sporadic and familial late-onset AD cases.

AD risk associated with *APOE* is dose dependent (Corder et al., 1993; Tsai et al., 1994). Compared to the most common *APOE* genotype (ε3/ε3), odds ratios range from 2.8 to 4.4 for AD subjects with one ε4 allele; the odds ratio increases from 7.0 to 19.3 for subjects with two ε4 alleles (Kukull et al., 1996; Mayeux et al., 1993). These risk estimates are not as strongly observed in African Americans or Hispanics (Farrer et al., 1997), although Hispanics with one or two ε4 alleles and African Americans who are ε4 homozygotes remain at increased risk for developing AD (Tang et al., 1996).

Studies suggest a different ε4 allele effect in males compared to females. In males, only ε4/ε4 homozygotes have a younger age at onset; in females, one ε4 allele is sufficient to reduce the age of onset (Payami et al., 1994). The *APOE* ε4 risk seems to be more pronounced in females than males (Breitner et al., 1999; Farrer et al., 1997) (see Figure 2-10). The Breitner study reported that women with the ε4/ε4 genotype (approximately 1% of the general population) have a 40% risk of developing AD by the age of 73 years. However, not all

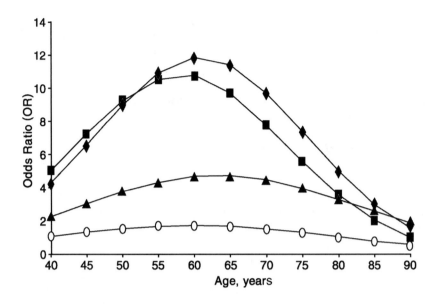

O Men ε3/ε4
▲ Women ε3/ε4
■ Men ε4/ε4
♦ Women ε4/ε4

FIGURE 2-10.   Apolipoprotein E ε4 risk.

studies support these findings. In addition, a few studies suggest a reduced frequency of the *APOE* ε2 allele in AD patients (Corder et al., 1994; Panza et al., 2000).

GENETIC TESTING It has been stated that genetic testing is not appropriate for routine use in the evaluation of most patients with dementia (Knopman et al., 2001). PS1, PS2, and APP mutations are rarely present, even in families with early-onset FAD (Cruts & Van Broeckhoven, 1998). Therefore, genetic testing for these mutations should not be routinely ordered (Steinbart et al., 2001). Furthermore, *APOE* genotyping is not recommended for the diagnosis of AD because the presence of the ε4 allele is not highly predictive of the presence of neuropathological AD. Some have advocated *APOE* testing as an adjunct in the diagnostic evaluation of demented persons (Roses & Saunders, 1997), but a community-based study suggested that it only adds a small amount of certainty to diagnostic accuracy (Tsuang et al., 1999).

LATE-ONSET ALZHEIMER'S DISEASE Over 50 genes have been tested as candidate genes in the search for late-onset FAD genes. It has been reported that several of these genes are linked to late-onset FAD. Linkage studies suggest that chromosome 12 contains candidate genes such as α-2 macroglobulin (A2M) (Blacker et al., 1998) and low-density lipoprotein receptor-related proteins (LRPs) (Lendon et al., 1997). However, neither has been clearly established as an AD gene (Blennow et al., 2000; Rudrasingham et al., 1999). Other studies have suggested the involvement of genes on chromosome 10 in late-onset AD (Bertram et al., 2000; Ertekin-Taner et al., 2000), but this will require further evaluation. Numerous association studies have implicated other potential genetic factors in AD, but most have not been confirmed or replicated. These include interleukin-6, HLA (human leukocyte antigen), α-1-antichymotrypsin, and angiotensin-converting enzyme (Bertram & Tanzi, 2001; Myers & Goate, 2001; Schellenberg et al., 2000). Further studies are ongoing.

Frontotemporal Dementia

CLINICAL FEATURES Initially, Pick described a clinical syndrome with dementia, progressive aphasia, and frontal cortical atrophy (Adams & Victor, 2001). Later, neuronal cytoplasmic inclusions (Pick bodies) were observed on neuropathological study of some cases. However, because most patients with dementia and prominent frontal lobe dysfunction do not have Pick bodies, confusion has reigned in the nosology of frontotemporal dementia (FTD). Terminology has included Pick's disease, Pick complex, non-AD dementia, disinhibition-dementia-parkinsonism-amyotrophy complex (DDPAC), and frontal-lobe degeneration with spinal motor degeneration (FLDMD). In the 1980s, clinical and pathological studies helped solidify consensus diagnostic criteria for FTD (Brun, 1987; Neary et al., 1988, 1993).

The typical clinical presentation is a personality or behavioral change (often disinhibition) with relatively intact memory. Later, there may be marked confusion, mutism, or parkinsonian features. There are at least three subtypes of FTD, including progressive aphasia, semantic dementia, and frontal lobe degeneration (Snowden et al., 1996). Patients with progressive aphasia have progressively nonfluent speech with agraphia, alexia, and acalculia, yet word meaning is preserved. Patients with semantic dementia have predominantly temporal lobe abnormalities with progressive loss of word meaning, but have a preserved ability to read and write regular words. Patients with frontal lobe degeneration have a marked loss of personal and social awareness with hyperorality, distractibility, and task impersistence. In general, patients with inferior frontal lobe degeneration tend to be more disinhibited; patients with lesions in the dorsolateral-frontal lobes tend to be abulic.

PATHOLOGICAL FEATURES Pathologically, there is lobar frontal or temporal atrophy. Many individuals have only gliosis and neuronal loss without distinctive features. Other individuals have cytoplasmic inclusions that may be typical Pick bodies or another variety of τ-positive material, sometimes resembling neuro-fibrillary tangles. Classic Pick's disease with Pick bodies is considered a subtype of FTD. Some individuals also have anterior horn cell loss in the spinal cord.

EPIDEMIOLOGY   Incidence and prevalence studies in FTD are not well established, partly because of its clinical heterogeneity. The only available sample estimating the incidence was based on clinician referrals. In one study (Stevens et al., 1998), the prevalence rose from 1.2 to 28 per 1 million from the third to the sixth decade. This is probably an underestimate. Among all patients with dementia, FTD is thought to comprise approximately 10% of cases and probably even a larger percentage in younger age groups.

FTD is the most common syndrome with prominent frontal lobe degeneration. It is commonly misdiagnosed as Alzheimer's disease, dementia with Lewy bodies, or AD with vascular disease. In the Consortium to Establish a Registry for Alzheimer's Disease (CERAD) neuropathological studies, FTD-like pathology was observed in 3% to 9% of patients with a clinical diagnosis of AD (Gearing et al., 1995). The frequency of FTD in autopsy series of dementia varies from 0% to 15% (Kosunen et al., 1996).

GENETICS   Familial aggregation was the first feature of FTD which suggested that there may be underlying genetic etiology. Several groups reported a positive family history in FTD patients in 10% to 60% of cases (Gustafson, 1987; Stevens et al., 1998). Segregation analyses suggested that first-degree relatives of FTD patients are 3.5 times more likely to develop dementia compared to first-degree relatives of normal controls. It was also suggested that age of onset in relatives of FTD patients was on the average 11 years younger than in other dementia patients (Stevens et al., 1998). There are a few large families with multiple affected individuals in which FTD appears to segregate in a highly penetrant, autosomal dominant fashion. The success in gene identification (see next section) in families with atypical dementia not only confirmed the genetic basis of FTD, but also established it as a distinct clinical and pathological entity.

FRONTOTEMPORAL DEMENTIA AND PARKINSONISM LINKED TO CHROMOSOME 17   The first systematic linkage study of FTD families mapped the gene to chromosome 17 (Wilhelmsen et al., 1994). Subsequently, many other families with FTD-like features also showed linkage to the same region. Interestingly, several other clinically distinct syndromes also mapped to 17q21–22, including patients with parkinsonism (Wszolek et al., 1992) and schizophreniform features (Sumi et al., 1992).

At the consensus meeting on chromosome 17–linked dementia in 1996, these syndromes were classified as frontotemporal dementia and parkinsonism linked to chromosome 17 (FTDP-17) (Foster et al., 1997). Even though many clinical differences existed, pathological similarities between the various syndromes included tau protein aggregates in the absence of amyloid plaques. Some of these aggregates had morphology similar to the NFTs seen in AD.

Because tau is a major component of NFTs and the *TAU* gene was in the critical region, it was considered an important candidate gene for FTDP-17. After some failed attempts to identify mutations in this gene, the first tau mutation was identified in a family with familial presenile dementia with psychosis (Poorkaj et al., 1998). Currently, over 20 tau mutations have been identified in FTDP-17 families (Wilhelmsen, 1998). However, other families with problems not linked to chromosome 17 (and without *TAU* mutations) have been identified, and linkage to chromosome 3 has been reported in one such family (Brown et al., 1995). The causative gene in this disease is yet to be identified.

TAU GENE The modified product of the *TAU* gene is a major component of NFTs seen in AD. The *TAU* gene is large, with 100,000 base pairs of DNA and 15 exons (see Figure 2-11, top). During transcription, it undergoes complex splicing (see Figure 2-11, middle). There are commonly six alternatively spliced isoforms of the *TAU* gene involving exons 2, 3, and 10 (shaded regions). The large bold arrow in Figure 2-11 points to the first *TAU* mutation (V337M) discovered to be associated with FTD (Poorkaj et al., 1998).

All but one of the currently identified mutations affect microtubule binding domains. Most of these mutations are missense, appearing both in the coding regions and in the noncoding regions (introns). Some mutations are believed to cause disease by producing functional changes that interfere with the normal binding of microtubules; other mutations change the ratio of tau isoforms in the brain (3 and 4 repeat tau).

The discovery of *TAU* mutations in families with FTDP-17 has confirmed the fact that genetics play a role in a subgroup of FTD cases. More work needs to be done to determine the range of *TAU* mutations in FTD and related disorders. In other conditions with tau aggregate pathology, such as Guamanian ALS (amyotrophic lateral sclerosis), Parkinson's dementia complex, and progressive supranuclear palsy, there is genetic association data to suggest that *TAU* plays a role in this disease (Baker et al., 1999; Higgins et al., 1998; Poorkaj, Tsuang, et al., 2001b). Most cases of FTD are sporadic and are not associated with *TAU* mutations (Houlden et al., 1999; Poorkaj, Grossman, et al., 2001a). If FTD is clearly familial and the affected individuals have tau-related neuropathology, then the frequency of *TAU* mutations increases to as high as 30% to 40%.

Explanations for the various clinical, pathological, and molecular findings will be necessary to understand better the role of tau and the frontal lobes in behavior and cognition. Understanding the in vivo processing of the tau gene will be important in the eventual development of therapeutic treatments.

Parkinson's Disease

CLINICAL FEATURES Parkinson's disease is a common neurodegenerative disorder in the aging population. The clinical symptoms of PD include resting tremor, rigidity, bradykinesia, and postural instability. The typical age of onset is in

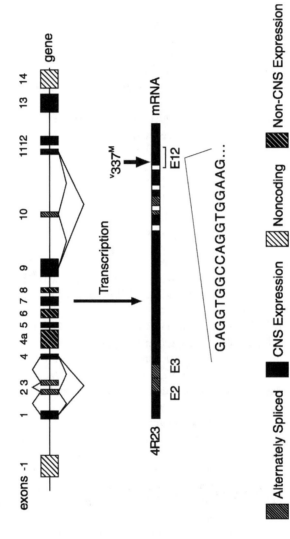

FIGURE 2-11. The *TAU* gene is large, with 100,000 base pairs of DNA and 15 exons; during transcription, it undergoes complex splicing. (*Note:* Intron distances are not to scale; CNS, central nervous system.)

the 60s. About 20% to 30% of PD patients develop dementia in the course of illness (Arsland & Larsen, 1998). The neuropathological features of PD include the presence of Lewy bodies (LBs; see Figure 2-12), intracytoplasmic neuronal inclusions, and neuronal loss in the substantia nigra.

EPIDEMIOLOGY The major risk factors identified to date for PD include positive family history, age, and rural living. Nearly one third of all instances of PD are familial, a small subset of which follow autosomal dominant inheritance. However, the majority of cases appear to be "sporadic." In addition, the incidence of PD increases with age.

The genetics of the common form of PD appear complex, potentially involving multiple susceptibility genes in the development of PD (Payami & Zareparsi, 1998). The contribution of environmental factors also may be substantial. The observation that numerous young patients who used street drugs contaminated with 1-methyl-4-phenyl-1,2,5,6-tetrahydropyridine (MPTP) and subsequently developed classical PD led to the development of an animal model for PD. Toxicology is now an active area of research investigating additional risk factors and mechanisms by which toxic agents cause PD.

The first descriptions of familial PD date to the 19th century, when Gowers (1888) first reported that up to 15% of PD patients may have a positive family history of PD. However, subsequent studies, including twin studies, in which concordance rates did not differ between monozygotic and dizygotic twins (Marsden, 1987) failed to demonstrate strong evidence for the genetic basis of PD.

The role of genetic factors in the etiology of PD has gained renewed atten-

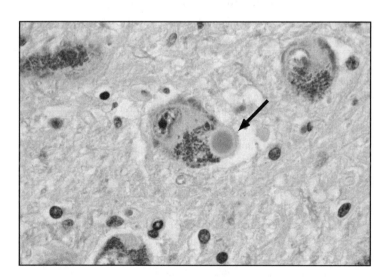

FIGURE 2-12. Lewy body.

tion. Several epidemiological surveys show an increased risk for PD in relatives of affected individuals, with first-degree relatives having a risk two to three times higher of developing PD than relatives of normal controls (Marder et al., 1996; Payami et al., 1994; Vieregge & Heberlein, 1995). In addition, twin studies that utilized positron emission tomography to identify presymptomatic individuals reported a higher concordance rate (up to 45%) in monozygotic twins (Piccini et al., 1997).

FAMILIAL PARKINSON'S DISEASE   Families in which PD is clearly inherited have been reported (Golbe et al., 1996). The mapping of the α-synuclein gene in one of these families (Polymeropoulos et al., 1996) was an important step in identifying the genetic contribution to familial PD. The discovery of a second disease-causing gene, *parkin* (Matsumine et al., 1997), confirmed the role of genetic factors in PD. There is genetic heterogeneity in PD; these two genes have been identified and a third has been mapped to chromosome 2 (Gasser et al., 1998).

α-SYNUCLEIN MUTATIONS   α-Synuclein was the first causative gene identified in familial PD. The initial family identified with autosomal dominant PD included affected individuals with typical idiopathic PD (in both clinical and neuropathological features). However, the age of onset was relatively early (46 ± 13 years). In this family and in three Greek families with familial PD, a mutation in the α-synuclein gene on chromosome 4 was shown to cosegregate with the disease (Polymeropoulos et al., 1997). A single base-pair change results in the substitution of alanine by threonine at position 53 (A53T). The pathogenic effect of this mutation remains unclear. Another α-synuclein mutation (A30P) has been reported (Kruger et al., 1998), but there is no evidence of α-synuclein mutations in many other multigenerational families with PD (Polymeropoulos, 2000). As such, α-synuclein mutations are a very rare cause of familial PD.

α-Synuclein protein is found in presynaptic nerve terminals and is a component of the neuritic amyloid plaque in AD. Antibodies for α-synuclein strongly stain Lewy bodies (Spillantini et al., 1997), which are pathological hallmarks of PD. α-Synuclein protein is widely expressed in the brain. It has been hypothesized that the aggregation of α-synuclein is critical to the pathogenesis of PD. This hypothesis is supported by the observation that α-synuclein aggregates in vitro, and that introduction of pathogenic mutations in recombinantly expressed proteins prompts aggregation. This remains an active area of investigation.

α-Synuclein transgenic mice carrying the A53T missense mutation have neuronal features strikingly similar to those in human brains with Lewy body pathology, neuronal degeneration, and motor defects (van der Putten et al., 2000). This and other data suggest that mutant α-synuclein interferes with synaptic maintenance (Duda et al., 2000). Further development of these mouse models will provide a means to assess the pathophysiology underlying PD as well as to test potential therapeutic strategies.

PARKIN MUTATIONS   Early-onset PD has been defined as Parkinson's disease with an age of onset younger than 40 years. In a few early-onset cases, the same Lewy bodies typically observed in idiopathic and familial PD have been described. Other families with a recessive form of parkinsonism do not have Lewy bodies. This last group was initially described in Japanese families and is called *autosomal recessive juvenile parkinsonism*. Onset is usually in the teens or twenties. Patients are responsive to levodopa (L-dopa), but show severe levodopa-induced dyskinesias and other motor complications. However, the entire spectrum of this disease remains to be defined. The genetic locus for autosomal recessive juvenile parkinsonism has been mapped to chromosome 6, with mutations in a large gene called *parkin* (Abbas et al., 1999; Kitada et al., 1998). This is a novel gene with unknown function; however, it appears to code an ubiquitin protein ligase.

OTHER PARKINSON'S DISEASE LOCI   Another genetic locus in familial parkinsonism has been identified by linkage analysis on chromosome 2 (Gasser et al., 1998). Individuals affected in these families have clinical features most closely resembling sporadic PD, including age of onset (mean 59 years). Based on the observation of a common haplotype in two of the linked families, a founder effect appears likely. Analysis of unaffected family members suggests that there is reduced penetrance (40%) of the disease allele.

GENETIC FACTORS IN SPORADIC PARKINSON'S DISEASE   For most PD, there is no clear family history of parkinsonism. It is generally assumed that genetic susceptibility combined with environmental factors cause PD. A possible clue to the interaction of genetic and environmental factors is the discovery of polymorphisms in the *CYP2D6* gene, which codes for debrisoquine 4-hydroxylase and is associated with a higher risk for developing PD. This gene encodes an enzyme involved in the detoxification of a number of endogenous and exogenous compounds. The B allele of this gene is associated with decreased metabolism of the enzyme and is hypothesized to play a role in PD. Although confirmed in several independent studies, this association is not conclusive. Several multicenter studies are under way using affected sib pairs to confirm these findings and to identify additional PD susceptibility loci. In summary, the common forms of PD appear to be multifactorial (i.e., the result of a complex interplay between genetic and environmental factors).

FAMILIAL PARKINSONISM PLUS SYNDROMES   Some PD families exhibit additional neurological features, such as pyramidal tract dysfunction, dementia, or amyotrophy (Wszolek et al., 1993). Therefore, these families are classified as familial parkinsonism plus syndromes. The relationship between these familial cases and sporadic idiopathic PD remains unclear. In some of these families, dementia is predominant, and neuropathology is consistent with diffuse Lewy body disease (Wakabayashi et al., 1998; Waters & Miller, 1994). However, genetic linkage studies in these families have been inconclusive.

DEMENTIA WITH LEWY BODIES   The dementia with LB (DLB) diagnostic entity (Mc-Keith et al., 1996) encompasses any individual who exhibits clinical dementia and has Lewy bodies on autopsy, thereby including diffuse Lewy body disease (DLBD) and the Lewy body variant of AD. As anticipated, there is substantial clinical overlap of DLB with AD and PD. Clinically, DLB is characterized by progressive and fluctuating cognitive impairment, parkinsonism (either de novo or neuroleptic induced), and psychosis with prominent visual hallucinations. Over half of the individuals with autopsy-proven DLB had hallucinations or systematized delusions during the course of illness (Ballard et al., 1999). Behavioral disturbances (e.g., systematized delusions or hallucinations) require neuroleptic treatment, which worsens parkinsonian signs and symptoms. These cases present therapeutic challenges for geriatric psychiatrists.

Neuropathologically, DLB is characterized by the presence of LBs, which are also the hallmark of PD. However, the distribution of LBs differs between DLB and idiopathic PD. In DLB, LBs are widely distributed throughout the paralimbic and neocortical regions of the brain. In PD, they occur predominantly in the substantia nigra. In addition, 50% to 70% of individuals with neocortical LBs also have substantial AD pathology, namely, Aβ deposition (Ballard et al., 1999). The boundaries of DLB are still far from a clear definition because of its shared clinical and neuropathological features with both PD and AD.

Although the majority of individuals with DLB are considered sporadic cases, there are several reports in which it appears to be familial (Denson et al., 1997; Ohara et al., 1999). No genes have been identified that cause DLB. Additional genetic and neuropathological studies are necessary to investigate further the role of genetic factors in DLB.

Vascular Dementia

CLINICAL FEATURES   Binswanger (1894) and Alzheimer (1911) described behavioral disorders related to arteriosclerosis. Initially, these conditions were categorized as subcortical arteritis and later as Binswanger's disease. With newer neuroimaging techniques, small-vessel ischemic disease is now commonly observed in geriatric patients. The contribution of small-vessel atherosclerotic disease to clinical dementia remains controversial. Vascular dementia typically does not have a distinct genetic risk factor, although multiple cerebrovascular risk factors are heritable (such as hyperlipidemia and hypertension). The genetics of vascular dementia are likely multifactorial. As a result, assessing the genetic contributions of each of the risk factors is extremely complicated. We focus on a rare cerebrovascular disease associated with dementia for which a gene has been discovered.

An autosomal dominant syndrome of hereditary multiinfarct dementia has been described with subsequent gene identification (Salloway & Hong, 1998). This disorder is named cerebral autosomal dominant arteriopathy with subcortical infarcts and leukoencephalopathy (CADASIL). Although this is a rare form of vascular dementia, it is the first genetic form of geriatric dementia with depression to be identified. Therefore, this disorder should be considered in the differential diagnosis of geriatric patients presenting with these symptoms.

Clinically, patients with CADASIL can have dementia (80%), depression (30%–50%), and migraine with an aura (30%) during their course of illness. The typical age of onset is in the 50s or 60s, and typical age at death is 64.5 years. Cognitive impairment in CADASIL is best characterized as frontal lobe disturbance with inattention, perseveration, apathy, and pseudobulbar affect.

On T-2 weighted magnetic resonance imaging (MRI), patients with CADASIL have areas of high signal in the periventricular and deep white matter and the basal ganglia. These abnormalities may be observed when patients are in their 20s and are asymptomatic. These individuals present similarly to patients with multiple sclerosis. Hyperintensities increase over the next two decades of life until confluent areas of high signal appear in the subcortical white matter. Transient ischemic attacks begin to occur in the late 40s and 50s, sometimes with extensive lacunar infarcts. The patients often are not hypertensive. Pathologically, there is a narrowing of small arteries throughout the brain because of smooth muscle layer hypertrophy, with electron microscopy showing osmophilic densities in the arteriolar media. The diagnosis can sometimes be confirmed by skin biopsies that show the arteriolar pathology.

NOTCH3   Linkage analysis mapped the CADASIL gene to the short arm of chromosome 19p13.22 (Tournier-Lasserve et al., 1993). Mutations in the NOTCH3 gene were first reported in 1996. According to subsequent studies, these mutations may be present in individuals without a positive family history (Joutel et al., 2000). The frequency of NOTCH3 mutations in sporadic and familial cases with vascular dementia remains unclear, but appears to be rare. Mutations in the APP and cystatin-β genes are also very rare causes of cerebral amyloid angiopathy and hemorrhagic strokes. Regardless of their prevalence, the discovery of these mutations provides an opportunity to explore the genetics of cerebrovascular disease.

The interaction of the multiple risk factors related to stroke is extremely complex. Additional knowledge regarding the genetic and environmental risk factors related to conditions such as atherosclerosis, diabetes mellitus, and hypertension may result in future prevention of and intervention in dementia associated with cerebrovascular disease.

Huntington's Disease

CLINICAL FEATURES First described in 1872 (Huntington, 1872), clear familial aggregation was noted in Huntington's disease (HD). The clinical triad in HD includes chorea, dementia, and behavioral disturbances. Chorea is the main motor sign in HD. These involuntary movements are present during waking hours, typically cannot be voluntarily suppressed, and actually increase with stress. Some patients may develop bradykinesia, rigidity, or dystonia. Aspiration secondary to dysphagia is the most common cause of mortality and morbidity. The typical pattern of cognitive decline includes slowness of thought, impaired ability to integrate new knowledge (particularly new motor skills), and lack of awareness of one's own disability. Visuospatial memory is particularly affected, while verbal memory remains preserved until late in the course of the illness. Changes in mood and personality are common, ranging from irritability and depression to psychosis (Folstein, 1997). Suicide is more common in HD than in the general population. Psychiatric symptoms may precede the first motor signs and symptoms by many years and do not necessarily relate to the severity of chorea or dementia. Other symptoms commonly observed include apathy, aggressive behavior, sexual disinhibition, and alcohol abuse.

The diagnosis of HD is indicated by the presence of a positive family history of an autosomal dominant neurodegenerative disorder consistent with HD, presence of progressive motor disability (including both voluntary and involuntary movements), cognitive decline, and behavioral disturbances. Caudate atrophy on computed tomography (CT) or MRI provides additional support for the diagnosis. Finally, DNA analysis confirms the diagnosis. The mean age of onset in HD is about 40 years (Harper, 1991), although the age of onset ranges from 2 to 80 years. The duration of HD is typically 15 years, with mean age of death from 51 to 63 years.

PATHOLOGICAL FEATURES The primary pathology of HD is in the corpus striatum, where neuronal loss occurs first in the caudate and later in the globus pallidus. Caudate atrophy is evident on MRI, with characteristic concavity of the ventrolateral aspect of the lateral ventricles. A neuropathological grading system rates the macroscopic and microscopic appearance of the striatum (Vonsattel et al., 1985). The neuronal loss appears to be selective, with the medium spiny neurons preferentially lost. Neurons containing GABA (γ-aminobutyric acid) and enkephalin are most severely affected, and the most consistent neurochemical findings are low levels of these two neurotransmitters. The discovery of intranuclear inclusions that contain the protein encoded by the HD gene (called *huntingtin*) (Davies et al., 1997) in the brains of those with HD has resulted in new avenues of animal research. Whether these inclusions interfere with nuclear function or are markers for neurodegeneration remains unknown.

EPIDEMIOLOGY Many epidemiological studies have been performed worldwide. There is general agreement that the prevalence of HD in western European countries is between 3 and 10 per 100,000 persons; in the United States, the prevalence ranges from 4 to 5 per 100,000 persons. The prevalence of HD is the highest in those aged 40 to 59 (approximately 12.5 per 100,000). The rates are lower in Japan, China, and Finland and in African blacks.

GENETICS HD is inherited as an autosomal dominant trait. In 1983, HD became the first genetic disorder to be linked by restriction fragment length polymorphism (RFLP) markers to a locus on chromosome 4 (Gusella et al., 1993). Ten years later, an international research consortium reported the successful cloning and sequencing of the HD gene (Huntington's Disease Collaborative Research Group, 1993), a novel gene containing a trinucleotide repeat. The trinucleotide repeat includes three nucleotides cytosine-adenine-guanine (CAG) that is repeated beyond the normal range is associated with HD. This highly polymorphic CAG repeat is located on the 5' region of the HD gene (see Figure 2-13). Genetic markers are indicated on the top of Figure 2-13. D4S10 was the initial marker linked to HD. The bold lines in Figure 2-13 indicate the HD gene, named Interesting Transcript 15 (IT15).

Individuals who have more than 36 CAG repeats in the HD gene may develop symptomatic HD. The majority of individuals with adult-onset HD have 38 to 45 CAG repeats. Individuals with more repeats (>60) are more likely to have juvenile-onset illness. A significant correlation between the number of CAG repeats and age of onset in HD has been demonstrated (Andrew et al., 1993; Duyao et al., 1993; Norremolle et al., 1993; Snell et al., 1993). The association was the highest in individuals with large numbers of CAG repeats (>60) who tended to have a younger age of onset. However, the number of CAG repeats is not useful for predicting the age of onset or type of symptoms at presentation in individual patients.

HD is the first of numerous neurodegenerative disorders associated with a trinucleotide repeat expansion. Several other neuropsychiatric disorders (e.g., fragile X mental retardation and hereditary ataxias) that exhibit anticipation (described in the next paragraph) are also trinucleotide repeat disorders (Margolis et al., 1999).

Interestingly, the discovery of dynamic repeat mutations helps account for the long-observed clinical phenomenon of *anticipation*, which is the observation that a disease becomes more severe and appears earlier with each successive generation. Similar to the other trinucleotide repeat disorders, this is because of the unstable expansion of the CAG repeats when they are passed from parent to offspring. In addition, paternal HD alleles are more likely to undergo significant expansion than maternal alleles, resulting in the observation that those with larger repeat sizes are more likely to have affected fathers.

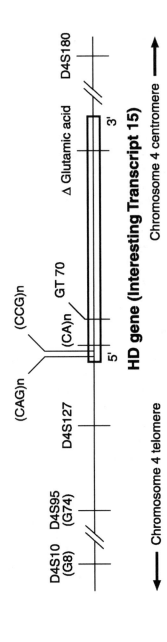

HD gene (Interesting Transcript 15)

Normal gene: 10 - 27 CAG repeats
Affected gene: > 36 CAG repeats

FIGURE 2-13. Genetic markers of Huntington's disease.

Prion Disease

Although prion diseases are relatively uncommon, they exemplify transmissible and heritable forms of dementia. What we now know as prion diseases were first described in the 1800s with reports of scrapie in sheep. Scrapie was shown to be experimentally transmissible in 1936 (Cuille & Chelle, 1936). Human prion diseases were recognized in the 1920s by Creutzfeldt and Jakob and were referred to as spongiform encephalopathies (Creutzfeldt, 1920; Jakob, 1921). In the 1960s, kuru (a deadly neurodegenerative disorder transmitted through ritualistic cannibalism) was recognized as similarly transmissible (Gajdusek et al., 1966). In the 1990s, the occurrence of bovine spongiform encephalopathy (BSE, mad cow disease) further increased the recognition of these disorders. The prevalence of Creutzfeldt-Jakob disease (CJD) is approximately 1 case per 1 million persons.

Prions are small proteinaceous particles that resist inactivation by the conventional method of proteinases (Diener et al., 1982). The normal cellular prion protein PrP^c is a membrane protein primarily expressed in astrocytes (Kretzschmar et al., 1986; Manson et al., 1992; Moser et al., 1995). The mechanisms by which PrP^c coverts to the scrapie isoform of the prion protein PrP^{Sc} remain unclear, but the protein structure does undergo a three-dimensional configuration change.

Six human diseases associated with prions have been described, including kuru, CJD, Gerstmann-Sträussler-Scheinker (GSS) syndrome, fatal familial insomnia (FFI), atypical prion disease, and new variant CJD (nvCJD; see Figure 2-14).

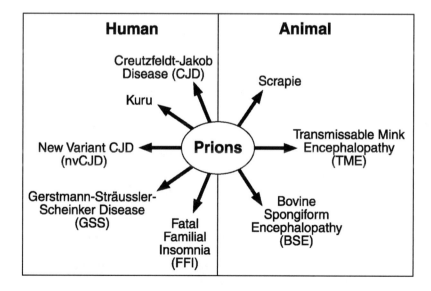

FIGURE 2-14. Human diseases associated with prions.

The identification of the prion protein (*PRNP*) gene on chromosome 20 that encodes PrP has rapidly transformed neurobiological and genetic research in this area (Prusiner, 1996) and resulted in Stanley Prusiner winning the Nobel prize. Although some families have mutations in the *PRNP* gene that are transmitted in an autosomal dominant fashion and other cases are caused by known exposure to contaminated tissue, most sporadic cases have no known cause. Interestingly, some prion diseases (such as CJD and nvCJD) can be both vertically (heritable) and horizontally (infectious) transmitted. In this section, we review the genetics of CJD, GSS, and FFI. Current nosology may in the future be replaced by specific DNA mutations, such as "familial prion disease with a P102L mutation and predominant ataxia."

CREUTZFELDT-JAKOB DISEASE   Sporadic CJD most often affects patients in their 50s and 60s. The typical clinical presentation includes rapid progressive cognitive decline (less than 2 years to death) accompanied by a variety of neurological signs (most commonly rigidity, ataxia, and myoclonus) and characteristic synchronous spikes on electroencephalogram (EEG) in an afebrile individual. However, these classical symptoms occur in less than 60% of cases. Other clinical features may include psychotic symptoms resembling schizophrenia, as well as extrapyramidal and cerebellar dysfunction or akinetic mutism.

The diagnosis of CJD should be entertained in individuals with rapidly progressive neuropsychiatric disorders. Clinical diagnostic criteria were established by a large CJD surveillance group in Europe (Concerted Action of the EU, 1993–1994); however, a definitive diagnosis can only be made on neuropathological or biochemical examination of the brain. A cerebrospinal fluid test for the 14-3-3 protein has been diagnostically useful. However, false positives as well as false negatives have been reported (Burkhard et al., 2001).

The neuropathological hallmarks of CJD include spongiform degeneration, neuronal loss, and astrocytic gliosis. The scrapie isoform of the prion-positive kuru plaques and other PrP-containing amyloid plaques are pathognomic of prion disease. However, they are found almost exclusively in familial CJD cases with *PRNP* mutations and only in a small minority of sporadic cases. Several different types of mutations that cause familial CJD are known.

PrP MUTATIONS   The human *PRNP* gene is located on the short arm of chromosome 20. This gene is highly conserved throughout many species, suggesting that its function is critical. However, the cellular function of the PrP^{Sc} remains unknown. In families with inherited prion diseases, more than 15 types of mutations have been described (Mastrianni, 1998). There are no systematic studies that provide frequency estimates of known mutations in different patient samples.

The most common PrP mutation associated with familial prion disease is the E200K mutation (glutamic acid to lysine). This mutation has been found in more than 50 families worldwide. Up to 50% of those with familial cases have this mutation. The largest known cluster is among Libyan Jews living in Israel, who have an incidence of CJD 100-fold greater than the population worldwide (Gabizon et al., 1993).

Another missense mutation (D178N) in the *PRNP* gene has been reported in a number of different families. Surprisingly, the phenotype depends heavily on the genotype present at an entirely different codon (codon position 129). In families with the D178N mutation and valine at position 129, the presentation is fairly typical CJD, with memory loss, ataxia, and myoclonus. The age of onset is in the 50s and 60s, with the disease duration ranging from 9 months to 4 years. The EEG shows generalized slowing rather than periodic triphasic waves. Brain pathology shows diffuse spongiform degeneration in the cerebral cortex and the basal ganglia with relative sparing of the thalamus.

Alternately, in families with the same D178N mutation but with methionine at position 129, the phenotype is FFI. These patients often present with insomnia and dysautonomia. They may later show signs of ataxia, dysarthria, myoclonus, and pyramidal tract dysfunction. In later stages, patients exhibit complete insomnia, dementia, rigidity, dystonia, and mutism. The duration of illness is very short (an average of 13 months).

Neuropathologically, FFI is characterized by neuronal loss and astrocytic gliosis that preferentially affects the thalamus. At least 21 families with FFI-D178N mutations have been reported (Gambetti & Lugaresi, 1998). It is unclear why the codon 129 genotype dramatically influences the phenotype associated with the D178N mutation, but presumably it affects the prion protein three-dimensional structure.

Another phenotype, GSS syndrome, is caused by several different mutations in the *PRNP* gene (Windl & Kretzschmar, 2000). Clinical symptoms include early ataxia, dementia, dysphagia, dysarthria, and hyporeflexia. Patients with GSS are more likely to exhibit ataxia than patients with CJD. On the other hand, patients with CJD are more likely to have dementia and myoclonus. However, clinical symptoms often overlap and do not always "breed true" within families. Family members with the same *PRNP* mutation may have either phenotype. GSS is always considered genetic and often has a longer disease duration than CJD. Neuropathologically, GSS is distinct from CJD in that GSS is characterized by the presence of large multicentric PrP-containing amyloid plaques with variable spongiform changes.

The most common mutation associated with GSS is the P102L mutation. More than 30 affected families with this mutation in the Northern hemisphere have been described (Young et al., 1995). This was the first mutation formally linked to a human prion disease and is also the causative mutation originally described by Gerstmann, Sträussler, and Scheinker (Hsiao et al., 1989).

The clinical and neuropathological characteristics in these families are indistinguishable from those in sporadic CJD. Interestingly, when infected brain tissue from CJD-E200K patients was injected into primates, the disease was transmitted in most trials, but transmission has not been demonstrated in other families with different mutations (Chapman et al., 1992). This finding is similar to results observed in experiments using brains of those with sporadic CJD.

PSYCHIATRIC DISORDERS AND *PRNP* MUTATIONS   In several families, nvCJD cases presented with psychiatric symptoms (Samaia et al., 1997; Will et al., 1996). In a Brazilian family (Samaia et al., 1997), there were six individuals with schizophrenia or schizoaffective disorder and three individuals with possible psychiatric symptoms. In one of the affected individuals, a missense mutation in the *PRNP* gene was isolated. This patient exhibited persecutory delusions, auditory hallucinations, and severe depression, with suicide attempts, over a 10-year period. Neurological symptoms such as ataxia, dementia, or EEG findings were absent. Lifelong severe psychiatric disorders with prominent psychotic symptoms, depressive features, and dementia were present in four of five mutation carriers. However, the frequency of *PRNP* mutations in patients with familial psychiatric disorders remains unknown.

Mitochondrial Disorders

Mitochondrial disorders are clinically diverse and are defined by structural or functional abnormalities in the mitochondria or the mitochondrial DNA. Because mtDNA has a poorly developed repair system, mutations are most often not repaired. Although rare, an increasing number of mtDNA mutations have been described in several neurological disorders. The characteristics of inherited mitochondrial disorders include maternal inheritance, heteroplasmy, mitotic segregation, and the threshold effect. Because mtDNA is almost exclusively maternally inherited, all mtDNA mutations are passed on by mothers. Because of the clinical heterogeneity associated with mitochondrial disorders, analysis of large families is often necessary to establish the pattern of maternal inheritance.

Heteroplasmy refers to the mixture of both mutant and wild-type molecules within mitochondria. In normal cells, all mtDNA molecules are identical. As heteroplasmic cells undergo cell division, the proportions of mutant and normal mtDNA allocated to daughter cells shift. Therefore, some clinical symptoms may improve as a child ages. *Mitotic segregation* also explains the markedly different levels of mutant mtDNA in members of the same family, as well as among different tissues within an individual. *Threshold effect* is the observation that a certain level of mutant mtDNA must be surpassed before a cell expresses a defect. The variability in onset and severity of clinical manifestations depend on a balance between the energy supply and oxidative demands of different organ systems.

Mitochondrial disorders have been implicated in prevalent neurodegenerative disorders (such as AD), as well as in normal aging itself, but the evidence is controversial. Aging is associated with an increase in mtDNA mutations.

These are not specifically germline mutations, but rather accumulating mutations that may occur over time in any organ, including the brain. The precise effects of these mutations are not known. These mutations are not genetically transmitted to the next generation, but may cause abnormal functioning of the organs in which they occur. It has been hypothesized that several different mutations may ultimately contribute to functional impairment.

There is evidence that mtDNA mutations may be involved in neurodegenerative conditions such as AD. It is postulated that mtDNA mutations in AD may lower the oxidative efficiency of critical neuronal populations early in life (Bonilla et al., 1999). An increase in oxidative damage to mtDNA in the brains of those with AD has been reported. In addition, younger (<75 years) patients with AD are more likely to have an increased level of a common mtDNA deletion and mutation than age-matched controls.

However, the data need to be confirmed. It remains unclear if these observations are the consequences of the disease or if they contribute to the pathophysiology. Screening for mtDNA mutations is not recommended for these common neurodegenerative disorders until the frequency of the mutations has been established (Chinnery et al., 2001).

Molecular genetic tests are available for the best-understood inherited mitochondrial disorders. However, absence of these mutations does not preclude mtDNA defects. Chapter 15 in Pulst's *Neurogenetics* (2000) provides additional details.

SUMMARY

Many neurodegenerative diseases are complex disorders. Our understanding of the genetic basis of these disorders (such as Alzheimer's disease) has made tremendous advances in the past decade. One common characteristic of these disorders is the existence of rare families in which the disease is inherited as a Mendelian trait. Identification of rare mutations in these families has led to the discovery of novel proteins associated with each disorder. In this chapter, we reviewed the genetics of several common neurodegenerative disorders associated with cognitive or behavioral disturbances and for which causative genes have been identified.

Further genetic analysis will clarify the roles of the known genes in the pathogenesis of common sporadic forms of disease. Investigation of the normal and aberrant functions of these genes will provide insights into the underlying mechanisms of these disorders. Ongoing molecular genetic and molecular biologic research will lead to new strategies for therapeutic interventions.

Although molecular genetics has helped clarify the etiology of these disorders, clinicians have played a critical role in careful identification and classification of many families who were involved in the eventual mapping and cloning of causative mutations. The role of the clinician should not be underestimated.

Future clinical and molecular genetics findings hold many clinical implications for geriatric psychiatry. It is likely that new diagnostic, therapeutic, and preventive strategies for dementing disorders are on the horizon.

ACKNOWLEDGMENTS

We want to thank Lillian DiGiacomo for editorial assistance and Molly Wamble for technical assistance.

REFERENCES

Abbas N, Lucking CB, Ricard S, et al. A wide variety of mutations in the parkin gene are responsible for autosomal recessive parkinsonism in Europe. French Parkinson's Disease Genetics Study Group and the European Consortium on Genetic Susceptibility in Parkinson's Disease. *Hum Mol Genet.* 1999;8:567–574.

Adams JH, Duchen LW, eds. *Greenfield's Neuropathology.* New York, NY: Oxford University Press; 1992.

Adams R, Victor M. *Principles of Neurology.* New York, NY: McGraw-Hill; 2001.

Alberts B, Bray D, Lewis J, et al. *Molecular Biology of the Cell.* New York, NY: Garland; 1994.

Alberts B, Johnson A, Lewis L, et al. *Molecular Biology of the Cell.* New York, NY: Garland Science; 2002.

Alzheimer A. Uber eine eigenartige Erkankung der Hirnrinde. *Allg Z Psychiatr.* 1907; 64:146.

Alzheimer A. Uber eigenartigen Krankheitsfalle des spateren Alters. *Zentralblatt Gesamte Neurologie Psychiatrie.* 1911;4:356–358.

American College of Medical Genetics/American Society of Human Genetics Working Group on ApoE and Alzheimer disease. Statement on use of apolipoprotein E testing for Alzheimer disease. American College of Medical Genetics/American Society of Human Genetics Working Group on ApoE and Alzheimer disease. *JAMA.* 1995; 274:1627–1629.

Andrew S, Goldberg Y, Kremer B, et al. The relationship between trinucleotide (CAG) repeat length and clinical features of Huntington's disease. *Nat Genet.* 1993;4:398–403.

Arsland D, Larsen JP. Emotional and cognitive disorders in Parkinson disease. *Tidsskr Nor Laegeforen.* 1998;118:3959–3963.

Baker M, Litvan I, Houlden H, et al. Association of an extended haplotype in the tau gene with progressive supranuclear palsy. *Hum Mol Genet.* 1999;8:711–715.

Ballard C, Holmes C, McKeith I, et al. Psychiatric morbidity in dementia with Lewy bodies: a prospective clinical and neuropathological comparative study with Alzheimer's disease. *Am J Psychiatry.* 1999;156:1039–1045.

Bergem AL, Engedal K, Kringlen E. The role of heredity in late-onset Alzheimer disease and vascular dementia. A twin study. *Arch Gen Psychiatry.* 1997;54:264–270.

Bertram L, Blacker D, Mullin K, et al. Evidence for genetic linkage of Alzheimer's disease to chromosome 10q. *Science.* 2000;290:2302–2303.

Bertram L, Tanzi RE. Dancing in the dark? The status of late-onset Alzheimer's disease genetics. *J Mol Neurosci.* 2001;17:127–136.

Billings PR, Kohn MA, de Cuevas M, et al. Discrimination as a consequence of genetic testing. *Am J Hum Genet.* 1992;50:476–482.

Binswanger O. Die Abgrenzung des allgemeinen progressiven Paralysie. *Berl Klin Wochenschr.* 1894;31:1103–1105, 1137–1139, 1180–1186.

Bird T, Sumi S, Nemens E. Phenotypic heterogeneity of familial Alzheimer's disease: a study of 24 kindreds. *Ann Neurol.* 1989;24:12–25.

Bird TD, Bennett RL. Why do DNA testing? Practical and ethical implications of new neurogenetic tests. *Ann Neurol.* 1995;38:141–146.

Bird TD, Levy-Lahad E, Poorkaj P, et al. Wide range in age of onset for chromosome 1-related familial Alzheimer's disease. *Ann Neurol.* 1996;40:932–936.

Blacker D, Wilcox MA, Laird N, et al. Alpha-2 macroglobulin is genetically associated with Alzheimer disease. *Nat Genet.* 1998;1998:357–360.

Blennow K, Ricksten A, Prince JA, et al. No association between the alpha-2 macroglobulin (A2M) deletion and Alzheimer's disease, and no change in A2M mRNA, protein, or protein expression. *J Neural Transm.* 2000;107:1065–1079.

Bonilla E, Tanji K, Hirano M, et al. Mitochondrial involvement in Alzheimer's disease. *Biochim Biophys Acta.* 1999;1410:171–182.

Breitner JC, Wyse BW, Anthony JC, et al. APOE-epsilon4 count predicts age when prevalence of AD increases, then declines: the Cache County Study. *Neurology.* 1999; 53:321–331.

Brown J, Ashworth A, Gydesen S, et al. Familial non-specific dementia maps to chromosome 3. *Hum Mol Genet.* 1995;4:1625–1628.

Brun A. Frontal lobe degeneration of non-Alzheimer type. I. Neuropathology. *Arch Gerontol Geriatr.* 1987;6:193–208.

Burkhard PR, Sanchez JC, Landis T, et al. CSF detection of the 14-3-3 protein in unselected patients with dementia. *Neurology.* 2001;56:1528–1533.

Chapman J, Brown P, Rabey J, et al. Transmission of spongiform encephalopathy from a familial Creutzfeldt-Jakob disease patient of Jewish Libyan origin carrying the PRNP codon 200 mutation. *Neurology.* 1992;42:1249–1250.

Chinnery PF, Taylor GA, Howell N, et al. Point mutations of the mtDNA control region in normal and neurodegenerative human brains. *Am J Hum Genet.* 2001;68:529–532.

Concerted Action of the EU. *Surveillance of Creutzfeldt-Jakob Disease in the European Community.* Rome, Italy: Concerted Action of the EU; 1993–1994.

Corder E, Saunders A, Strittmatter W, et al. Gene dose of apolipoprotein E type 4 allele and the risk of Alzheimer's disease in late onset families. *Science.* 1993;261:921–923.

Corder EH, Saunders AM, Risch NJ, et al. Protective effect of apolipoprotein E type 2 allele for late onset Alzheimer disease. *Nat Genet.* 1994;7:180–184.

Creutzfeldt HG. Uber eine eigenartige herdformige Erkrankung des Zentralnervensystems. *Z Ges Neurol Psychiatrie.* 1920;57:1–18.

Cruts M, Van Broeckhoven C. Presenilin mutations in Alzheimer's disease. *Hum Mutat.* 1998;11:183–190.

Cuille J, Chelle P-L. La maladie dite tremblante du mouton est-elle inoculable? *C R Acad Sci III.* 1936;203:1552–1554.

Davies SW, Turmaine M, Cozens BA, et al. Formation of neuronal intranuclear inclusions underlies the neurological dysfunction in mice transgenic for the HD mutation. *Cell.* 1997;90:537–548.

Denson MA, Wszolek ZK, Pfeiffer RF, et al. Familial parkinsonism, dementia, and Lewy body disease: study of family G. *Ann Neurol.* 1997;42:638–643.

Diener TO, McKinley MP, Prusiner SB. Viroids and prions. *Proc Natl Acad Sci USA.* 1982;79:5220–5224.

Duda JE, Lee VE, Trojanowski JQ. Neuropathology of synuclein aggregates. *J Neurosci Res.* 2000;61:121–127.

Duyao M, Ambrose C, Myers R, et al. Trinucleotide repeat length instability and age of onset in Huntington's disease. *Nat Genet.* 1993;4:387–392.

Ertekin-Taner N, Graff-Radford N, Younkin LH, et al. Linkage of plasma Abeta42 to a quantitative locus on chromosome 10 in late-onset Alzheimer's disease pedigrees. *Science.* 2000;290:2303–2304.

Faraone S, Tsuang M, Tsuang D. *Genetics of Mental Disorders: A Guide for Students, Clinicians, and Researchers.* New York, NY: Guilford Press; 1999.

Farrer LA, Cupples LA, Haines JL, et al. Effects of age, sex, and ethnicity on the association between apolipoprotein E genotype and Alzheimer disease: a meta-analysis. APOE and Alzheimer Disease Meta Analysis Consortium. *JAMA.* 1997;278:1349–1356.

Folstein MF. Differential diagnosis of dementia: the clinical process. *Psychiatr Clin North Am.* 1997;20:45–57.

Foster NL, Wilhelmsen K, Sima AA, et al. Frontotemporal dementia and parkinsonism linked to chromosome 17: a consensus conference. Conference Participants. *Ann Neurol.* 1997;41:706–715.

Gabizon R, Rosenmann H, Meiner Z, et al. Mutation and polymorphism of the prion protein gene in Libyan Jews with Creutzfeldt-Jakob disease (CJD). *Am J Hum Genet.* 1993;53:828–835.

Gajdusek DC, Gibbs CJ, Alpers M. Experimental transmission of a Kuru-like syndrome to chimpanzees. *Nature.* 1966;209:794–796.

Gambetti P, Lugaresi E. Conclusions of the symposium. *Brain Pathol.* 1998;8:571–575.

Gasser T, Muller-Myhsok B, Wszolek ZK, et al. A susceptibility locus for Parkinson's disease maps to chromosome 2p13. *Nat Genet.* 1998;18:262–265.

Gearing M, Mirra SS, Hedreen JC, et al. The Consortium to Establish a Registry for Alzheimer's Disease (CERAD). Part X. Neuropathology confirmation of the clinical diagnosis of Alzheimer's disease. *Neurology.* 1995;45:461–466.

Gelehrter TD, Collins FS. *Principles of Medical Genetics.* Baltimore, MD: Williams and Wilkins; 1990.

Goate A, Chartier-Harlin MC, Mullan M, et al. Segregation of a missense mutation in the amyloid precursor protein gene with familial Alzheimer's disease. *Nature.* 1991; 349:704–706.

Golbe LI, Di Iorio G, Sanges G, et al. Clinical genetic analysis of Parkinson's disease in the Contursi kindred. *Ann Neurol.* 1996;40:767–775.

Gowers WR. *A Manual of Diseases of the Nervous System.* Philadelphia, PA: Blakiston's; 1888.

Gusella JF, MacDonald ME, Ambrose CM, et al. Molecular genetics of Huntington's disease. *Arch Neurol.* 1993;50:1157–1163.

Gustafson L. Frontal lobe degeneration of non-Alzheimer type. II. Clinical picture and differential diagnosis. *Arch Gerontol Geriatr.* 1987;6:209–223.

Haltia M, Viitanen M, Sulkava R, et al. Chromosome 14-encoded Alzheimer's disease: genetic and clinicopathological description. *Ann Neurol.* 1994;36:362–367.

Harper P. *Practical Genetic Counseling*. London, England: Reed Educational and Professional Publishing; 1998.

Harper PS. *Huntington's Disease*. London, England: Saunders; 1991.

Herstek J. Finance issue brief: genetic testing. *Issue Brief Health Policy Track Serv.* 1999; Jun 25:1–10.

Heston L. Alzheimer's disease. In: King R, Rotter J, Motulsky A, eds. *Genetics of Common Diseases*. New York, NY: Oxford University Press; 1992:792–800.

Higgins I, Litvan I, Pho L, et al. Progressive supranuclear gaze palsy in linkage disequilibrium with tau and not the α-synuclein gene. *Neurology*. 1998;50:270–273.

Hodgkinson KA, Murphy J, O'Neill S, et al. Genetic counselling for schizophrenia in the era of molecular genetics. *Can J Psychiatry*. 2001;46:123–130.

Houlden H, Baker M, Adamson J, et al. Frequency of tau mutations in three series of non-Alzheimer's degenerative dementia. *Ann Neurol*. 1999;46:243–248.

Hsiao K, Baker HF, Crow TJ, et al. Linkage of a prion protein missense variant to Gerstmann-Straussler syndrome. *Nature*. 1989;338:342–345.

Huggins M, Bloch M, Kanani S, et al. Ethical and legal dilemmas arising during predictive testing for adult-onset disease: the experience of Huntington disease. *Am J Hum Genet*. 1990;47:4–12.

Huntington G. On chorea. *Med Surg Rep*. 1872;26:320–321.

Huntington's Disease Collaborative Research Group. A novel gene containing a trinucleotide repeat that is expanded and unstable on Huntington's disease chromosomes. The Huntington's Disease Collaborative Research Group. *Cell*. 1993;72: 971–983.

Jakob A. Uber eigenartige Erkrankungen des Zentralnervensystems mit bemerkenswertem anatomischem Befunde (spastische Pseudosklerose-Encephalomyelopathie mit disseminierten Degenerationsherden). *Dtsch Z Nervenheilkd*. 1921;70:132–146.

Joutel A, Dodick DD, Parisi JE, et al. De novo mutation in the Notch3 gene causing CADASIL. *Ann Neurol*. 2000;47:388–391.

Kitada T, Asakawa S, Hattori N, et al. Mutations in the parkin gene cause autosomal recessive juvenile parkinsonism. *Nature*. 1998;392:605–608.

Knopman D, DeKosky S, Cummings J, et al. Practice parameter: diagnosis of dementia (an evidence-based review). Report of the Quality Standards Subcommittee of the American Academy of Neurology. *Neurology*. 2001;56:1143–1153.

Kosunen O, Soininen H, Paljarvi L, et al. Diagnostic accuracy of Alzheimer's disease: a neuropathological study. *Acta Neuropathol*. 1996;91:185–193.

Kovacs DM, Fausett HJ, Page KJ, et al. Alzheimer-associated presenilins 1 and 2: neuronal expression in brain and localization to intracellular membranes in mammalian cells. *Nat Med*. 1996;2:224–229.

Kretzschmar HA, Prusiner SB, Stowring LE, et al. Scrapie prion proteins are synthesized in neurons. *Am J Pathol*. 1986;122:1–5.

Kruger R, Kuhn W, Muller T, et al. Ala30Pro mutation in the gene encoding α-synuclein in Parkinson's disease. *Nat Genet*. 1998;18:106–108.

Kukull WA, Schellenberg GD, Bowen JD, et al. Apolipoprotein E in Alzheimer's disease risk and case detection: a case-control study. *J Clin Epidemiol*. 1996;49:1143–1148.

Lampe TH, Bird TD, Nochlin D, et al. Phenotype of chromosome 14-linked familial Alzheimer's disease in a large kindred. *Ann Neurol*. 1994;36:368–378.

Launer LJ, Andersen K, Dewey ME, et al. Rates and risk factors for dementia and Alzheimer's disease: results from EURODEM pooled analyses. EURODEM Incidence

Research Group and Work Groups. European Studies of Dementia. *Neurology.* 1999;52:78–84.

Lautenschlager NT, Cupples LA, Rao VS, et al. Risk of dementia among relatives of Alzheimer's disease patients in the MIRAGE study: what is in store for the oldest old? *Neurology.* 1996;46:641–650.

Lendon C, Talbot C, Craddock N, et al. Genetic association studies between dementia of the Alzheimer's type and three receptors of apolipoprotein E in a Caucasian population. *Neurosci Lett.* 1997;222:187–190.

Levy-Lahad E, Bird T. Alzheimer's disease: genetic factors. In: Pulst S, ed. *Neurogenetics.* Oxford, UK: Oxford University Press; 2000:317–333.

Levy-Lahad E, Poorkaj P, Wang K, et al. Genomic structure and expression of STM2, the chromosome 1 familial Alzheimer disease gene. *Genomics.* 1996;34:198–204.

Levy-Lahad E, Tsuang D, Bird TD. Recent advances in the genetics of Alzheimer's disease. *J Geriatr Psychiatry Neurol.* 1998;11:42–54.

Levy-Lahad E, Wasco W, Poorkaj P, et al. Candidate gene for the chromosome 1 familial Alzheimer's disease locus. *Science.* 1995;269:973–977.

Levy-Lahad E, Wijsman EM, Nemens E, et al. A familial Alzheimer's disease locus on chromosome 1. *Science.* 1995;269:970–973.

Mann DMA. Association between Alzheimer's disease and Down syndrome: neuropathological observations. In: Berg JM, Karlinksy J, Holland AJ, eds. *Alzheimer Disease, Down Syndrome, and Their Relationship.* Oxford, UK: Oxford University Press; 1993:71–92.

Manson J, West JD, Thomson V, et al. The prion protein gene: a role in mouse embryogenesis? *Development.* 1992;115:117–122.

Marder K, Tang MX, Mejia H, et al. Risk of Parkinson's disease among first-degree relatives: a community-based study. *Neurology.* 1996;47:155–160.

Margolis RL, McInnis MG, Rosenblatt A, et al. Trinucleotide repeat expansion and neuropsychiatric disease. *Arch Gen Psychiatry.* 1999;56:1019–1031.

Marsden CD. Parkinson's disease in twins. *J Neurol Neurosurg Psychiatry.* 1987;50:105–106.

Mastrianni JA. The prion diseases: Creutzfeldt-Jakob, Gerstmann-Straussler-Scheinker, and related disorders. *J Geriatr Psychiatry Neurol.* 1998;11:78–97.

Matsumine H, Saito M, Shimoda-Matsubayashi S, et al. Localization of a gene for an autosomal recessive form of juvenile Parkinsonism to chromosome 6q25.2-27. *Am J Hum Genet.* 1997;60:588–596.

Mayeux R, Stern Y, Ottman R, et al. The apolipoprotein epsilon 4 allele in patients with Alzheimer's disease. *Ann Neurol.* 1993;34:752–754.

McConnell L, Koenig B, Greely H, et al. Genetic testing and Alzheimer disease: recommendations of the Stanford Program in Genomics, Ethics, and Society. *Genet Test.* 1999;3:3–12.

McConnkey EH. *Human Genetics: The Molecular Revolution.* Sudbury, UK: Jones and Bartlett; 1993.

McKeith IG, Galasko D, Kosaka K, et al. Consensus guidelines for the clinical and pathologic diagnosis of dementia with Lewy bodies (DLB): report of the consortium on DLB international workshop. *Neurology.* 1996;47:1113–1124.

McKhann G, Drachman D, Folstein M, et al. Clinical diagnosis of Alzheimer's disease: report of the NINCDS-ADRDA Work Group under the auspices of Department of

Health and Human Services Task Force on Alzheimer's Disease. *Neurology.* 1984; 34:939–944.

McMillan PJ, Leverenz JB, Poorkaj P, et al. Neuronal expression of STM2 mRNA in human brain is reduced in Alzheimer's disease. *J Histochem Cytochem.* 1996;44: 1215–1222.

Moser M, Colello RJ, Pott U, et al. Developmental expression of the prion protein gene in glial cells. *Neuron.* 1995;14:509–517.

Myers AJ, Goate AM. The genetics of late-onset Alzheimer's disease. *Curr Opin Neurol.* 2001;14:433–440.

National Institute on Aging. Consensus recommendations for the postmortem diagnosis of Alzheimer's disease. The National Institute on Aging, and Reagan Institute Working Group on Diagnostic Criteria for the Neuropathological Assessment of Alzheimer's Disease. *Neurobiol Aging.* 1997;18:S1–S2.

Neary D, Snowden JS, Mann DM. Familial progressive aphasia: its relationship to other forms of lobar atrophy. *J Neurol Neurosurg Psychiatry.* 1993;56:1122–1125.

Neary D, Snowden JS, Northen B, et al. Dementia of frontal lobe type. *J Neurol Neurosurg Psychiatry.* 1988;51:353–361.

Norremolle A, Riess O, Epplen J, et al. Trinucleotide repeat elongation in the Huntingtin gene in Huntington Disease patients from 71 Danish families. *Hum Mol Genet.* 1993;2:1475–1476.

Nunan J, Small DH. Regulation of APP cleavage by alpha-, beta- and gamma-secretases. *FEBS Lett.* 2000;483:6–10.

Ohara K, Takauchi S, Kokai M, et al. Familial dementia with Lewy bodies (DLB). *Clin Neuropathol.* 1999;18:232–239.

Panza F, Solfrizzi V, Torres F, et al. Apolipoprotein E in Southern Italy: protective effect of epsilon 2 allele in early- and late-onset sporadic Alzheimer's disease. *Neurosci Lett.* 2000;292:79–82.

Payami H, Larsen K, Bernard S, et al. Increased risk of Parkinson's disease in parents and siblings of patients. *Ann Neurol.* 1994;34:659–661.

Payami H, Montee KR, Kaye JA, et al. Alzheimer's disease, apolipoprotein E4, and gender. *JAMA.* 1994;271:1316–1317.

Payami H, Zareparsi S. Genetic epidemiology of Parkinson's disease. *J Geriatr Psychiatry Neurol.* 1998;11:1–9.

Pericak-Vance MA, Bebout JL, Gaskell PC Jr, et al. Linkage studies in familial Alzheimer disease: evidence for chromosome 19 linkage. *Am J Hum Genet.* 1991;48:1034–1050.

Piccini P, Morrish P, Turjanski N, et al. Dopaminergic function in familial Parkinson's disease: a clinical and 18F-dopa positron emission tomography study. *Ann Neurol.* 1997;41:222–229.

Polymeropoulos MH. Genetics of Parkinson's disease. *Ann N Y Acad Sci.* 2000;920: 28–32.

Polymeropoulos MH, Higgins JJ, Golbe LI, et al. Mapping of a gene for Parkinson's disease to chromosome 4q21-q23. *Science.* 1996;274:1197–1199.

Polymeropoulos MH, Lavedan C, Leroy E, et al. Mutation in the alpha-synuclein gene identified in families with Parkinson's disease. *Science.* 1997;276:2045–2047.

Poorkaj P, Bird TD, Wijsman E, et al. Tau is a candidate gene for chromosome 17 frontotemporal dementia. *Ann Neurol.* 1998;43:815–825.

Poorkaj P, Grossman M, Steinbart E, et al. Frequency of tau gene mutations in familial and sporadic cases of non-Alzheimer dementia. *Arch Neurol.* 2001;58:383–387.

Poorkaj P, Tsuang D, Wijsman E, et al. TAU as a susceptibility gene for amyotropic lateral sclerosis-parkinsonism dementia complex of Guam. *Arch Neurol.* 2001;58: 1871–1878.

Prusiner S. Molecular biology and genetics of prion diseases. *Cold Spring Harb Symp Quant Biol.* 1996;61:473–493.

Pulst SM. *Neurogenetics.* Oxford, UK: Oxford University Press; 2000.

Quaid K. Presymptomatic testing for HD: recommendations for counseling. *J Genet Couns.* 1992;1:277–302.

Rocca WA, Amaducci LA, Schoenberg BS. Epidemiology of clinically diagnosed Alzheimer's disease. *Ann Neurol.* 1986;19:415–424.

Roses AD, Saunders AM. Apolipoprotein E genotyping as a diagnostic adjunct for Alzheimer's disease. *Int Psychogeriatr.* 1997;9:277–88, discussion 317–321.

Rothstein MA. Genetic privacy and confidentiality: why they are so hard to protect. *J Law Med Ethics.* 1998;26:178, 198–204.

Rudrasingham V, Wavrant-De Vrieze F, Lambert JC, et al. Alpha-2 macroglobulin gene and Alzheimer disease. *Nat Genet.* 1999;22:17–91, discussion 21–22.

Rutter M, Plomin R. Opportunities for psychiatry from genetic findings. *Br J Psychiatry.* 1997;171:209–219.

Salloway S, Hong J. CADASIL syndrome: a genetic form of vascular dementia. *J Geriatr Psychiatry Neurol.* 1998;11:71–77.

Samaia HB, Mari JJ, Vallada HP, et al. A prion-linked psychiatric disorder. *Nature.* 1997;390:241.

Saunders A, Strittmatter W, Schmechel D, et al. Association of apolipoprotein E allele epsilon 4 with late-onset familial and sporadic Alzheimer's disease. *Neurology.* 1993;43:1467–1472.

Schellenberg GD, Bird TD, Wijsman EM, et al. Genetic linkage evidence for a familial Alzheimer's disease locus on chromosome 14. *Science.* 1992;258:668–671.

Schellenberg GD, D'Souza I, Poorkaj P. The genetics of Alzheimer's disease. *Curr Psychiatry Rep.* 2000;2:158–164.

Selkoe D, Wolfe M. In search of gamma-secretase: presenilin at the cutting edge. *Proc Natl Acad Sci U S A.* 2000:5690–5692.

Selkoe DJ. The cell biology of beta-amyloid precursor protein and presenilin in Alzheimer's disease. *Trends Cell Biol.* 1998;8:447–453.

Selkoe DJ. Alzheimer's disease: genes, proteins, and therapy. *Physiol Rev.* 2001;81:741–766.

Seshadri S, Wolf PA, Beiser A, et al. Lifetime risk of dementia and Alzheimer's disease: the impact of mortality on risk estimates in the Framingham Study. *Neurology.* 1997;49:1498–1504.

Sherrington R, Rogaev E, Liang Y, et al. Cloning of a gene bearing missense mutations in early-onset familial Alzheimer's disease. *Nature.* 1995;375:754–760.

Sisodia SS, Koo EH, Beyreuther K, et al. Evidence that beta-amyloid protein in Alzheimer's disease is not derived by normal processing. *Science.* 1990;248:492–495.

Snell R, MacMillan J, Cheadle J, et al. Relationship between trinucleotide repeat expansion and phenotypic variation in Huntington's disease. *Nat Genet.* 1993;4:393–397.

Snowden JS, Neary D, Mann DMA. *Fronto-Temporal Lobar Degeneration: Fronto-*

Temporal Dementia, Progressive Aphasia Semantic Dementia. New York, NY: Churchill Livingstone; 1996.

Spillantini MG, Schmidt ML, Lee VM, et al. Alpha-synuclein in Lewy bodies. *Nature.* 1997;388:839–840.

Steinbart EJ, Smith CO, Poorkaj P, et al. Impact of DNA testing for early-onset familial Alzheimer disease and frontotemporal dementia. *Arch Neurol.* 2001;58:1828–1831.

Stevens M, van Duijn CM, Kamphorst W, et al. Familial aggregation in frontotemporal dementia. *Neurology.* 1998;50:1541–1545.

St. George-Hyslop PH. Molecular genetics of Alzheimer's disease. *Biol Psychiatry.* 2000; 47:183–199.

Strachan T, Read A. *Human Molecular Genetics 2.* New York, NY: Wiley-Liss; 1999.

Sumi SM, Bird TD, Nochlin D, et al. Familial presenile dementia with psychosis associated with cortical neurofibrillary tangles and degeneration of the amygdala. *Neurology.* 1992;42:120–127.

Tang MX, Maestre G, Tsai WY, et al. Relative risk of Alzheimer disease and age-at-onset distributions, based on APOE genotypes among elderly African Americans, Caucasians, and Hispanics in New York City. *Am J Hum Genet.* 1996;58:574–584.

Taylor JP, Hardy J, Fischbeck KH. Toxic proteins in neurodegenerative disease. *Science.* 2002;296:1991–1995.

Terry RD, Katzman R, Bick KL, et al., eds. *Alzheimer Disease.* Philadelphia, PA: Lippincott, Williams, and Wilkins; 1999.

Thompson MW, McInnes RR, Willard HF. *Thompson and Thompson Genetics in Medicine.* Philadelphia, PA: Saunders; 1991.

Tournier-Lasserve E, Joutel A, Melki J, et al. Cerebral autosomal dominant arteriopathy with subcortical infarcts and leukoencephalopathy maps to chromosome 19q12. *Nat Genet.* 1993;3:256–259.

Tsai MS, Tangalos EG, Petersen RC, et al. Apolipoprotein E: risk factor for Alzheimer disease. *Am J Hum Genet.* 1994;54:643–649.

Tsuang D, Larson EB, Bowen J, et al. The utility of apolipoprotein E genotyping in the diagnosis of Alzheimer disease in a community-based case series. *Arch Neurol.* 1999;56:1489–1495.

Tsuang DW, Faraone SV, Tsuang MT. Genetic counseling for psychiatric disorders. *Curr Psychiatry Rep.* 2001;3:138–143.

Tsuang MT, Tohen M, Zahner GEP, eds. *Textbook in Psychiatric Epidemiology.* New York, NY: Wiley; 1995.

Van Broeckhoven C, Haan J, Bakker E, et al. Amyloid β protein precursor gene and hereditary cerebral hemorrhage with amyloidosis (Dutch). *Science.* 1990;248: 1120–1122.

van der Putten H, Wiederhold KH, Probst A, et al. Neuropathology in mice expressing human alpha-synuclein. *J Neurosci.* 2000;20:6021–6029.

Vassar R, Citron M. Abeta-generating enzymes: recent advances in beta- and gamma-secretase research. *Neuron.* 2000;27:419–422.

Vieregge P, Heberlein I. Increased risk of Parkinson's disease in relatives of patients. *Ann Neurol.* 1995;37:685.

Vonsattel J-P, Myers R, Stevens T, et al. Neuropathological classification of Huntington's disease. *J Neuropathol Exp Neurol.* 1985;44:559–577.

Wakabayashi K, Hayashi S, Ishikawa A, et al. Autosomal dominant diffuse Lewy body disease. *Acta Neuropathol (Berl)*. 1998;96:207–210.

Waters C, Miller C. Autosomal dominant Lewy body parkinsonism in a four-generation family. *Ann Neurol*. 1994;35:59–64.

Welch H, Burke W. Uncertainties in genetic testing for chronic disease. *JAMA*. 1998; 280:1525–1527.

Wilhelmsen K, Lynch T, Pavlou E, et al. Localization of disinhibition-dementia-parkinsonism-amyotrophy complex to 17q21-22. *Am J Hum Genet*. 1994;55:1159–1165.

Wilhelmsen KC. Frontotemporal dementia genetics. *J Geriatr Psychiatry Neurol*. 1998; 11:55–60.

Will RG, Ironside JW, Zeidler M, et al. A new variant of Creutzfeldt-Jakob disease in the UK. *Lancet*. 1996;347:921–925.

Windl O, Kretzschmar HA. Prion diseases. In: Pulst SM, ed. *Neurogenetics*. Oxford, UK: Oxford University Press; 2000:191\n218.

Wszolek ZK, Cordes M, Calne DB, et al. Hereditary Parkinson disease: report of 3 families with dominant autosomal inheritance. *Nervenarzt*. 1993;64:331–335.

Wszolek ZK, Pfeiffer RF, Bhatt MH, et al. Rapidly progressive autosomal dominant parkinsonism and dementia with pallido-ponto-nigral degeneration. *Ann Neurol*. 1992;32:312–320.

Young K, Jones CK, Piccardo P, et al. Gerstmann-Straussler-Scheinker disease with mutation at codon 102 and methionine at codon 129 of PRNP in previously unreported patients. *Neurology*. 1995;45:1127–1134.

3

Genetics of Mood Disorders and Associated Psychopathology

Francis J. McMahon, MD

INTRODUCTION

Primary affective disorders, which are largely genetic in origin, were traditionally felt to occur mainly in young people, while secondary or symptomatic affective disorders predominated in the elderly. This view fits with the general idea that genetic contributions to disease tend to diminish with age (Childs & Scriver, 1986). In practice, however, affective disorders in the elderly are a mixture of persistent, early-onset diseases and incident, late-onset diseases, which creates a complex mix of primary and secondary cases.

Most episodes of affective disorder in the elderly represent the persistence or episodic recurrence of primary mood disorders that began much earlier in life. A genetic contribution to these early-onset disorders is clear, although environmental factors also play a role. On the other hand, a greater proportion of affective disorders in the elderly, compared to younger patient groups, occurs in the context of preexisting or concomitant vascular, neurological, or other disease. Genetic forms of such diseases are being recognized with increasing frequency. In this sense, so-called secondary affective disorders in the elderly may often have a genetic basis, albeit one that leads to a broader clinical picture, or phenotype, than the so-called primary affective disorders are generally felt to encompass.

In this chapter, the genetics of affective disorders in the elderly are reviewed. This review encompasses the genetics of primary or idiopathic affective disorders that typically begin early in life, but still account for a large proportion of affective disorders in the aging population. The main findings of the major twin, family, adoption, and linkage studies are summarized, and their methods are reviewed. The genetics of the so-called secondary or symptomatic affective disorders that form an important part of the clinical picture of genetic disorders that occur later in life are also reviewed. Finally, the genetics of substance abuse, anxiety disorders, and other conditions that have often been associated with mood disorders are reviewed.

TERMS AND METHODS

Because the science of genetics still remains somewhat specialized, a brief review of terms and methods is in order. Human genetics, to paraphrase McKusick (1993), is the science of human variation in the broadest sense. Thus, the methods of human genetics range from those of epidemiology and population genetics on the macroscopic scale to those of single-nucleotide variation on the microscopic scale. From the standpoint of genetic methodology, there is no fundamental difference between diseases, such as mood disorders, and other traits, such as height and eye color. Generally, the word *disease* is used here, but from the standpoint of the methods, it should be understood that *trait* could easily be used instead.

Genetic epidemiology forms the foundation for genetic investigation because it establishes the importance of genetics in the etiology of a disease. Genetic epidemiological investigation takes the form of family, twin, and adoption studies. As with all epidemiological investigation, the methods of ascertainment (i.e., the ways in which subjects are identified and enrolled in the study) are crucial. Diagnostic methods and criteria are also important, as are the statistical methods employed. The power of genetic epidemiology lies in the ability to parse genetic and nongenetic factors, but it is important to remember that genetic epidemiology is an observational rather than experimental science. This limits the kinds of conclusions that can be drawn from genetic epidemiological data.

In twin studies, the relative genetic contribution to a trait or illness, its heritability, is estimated by comparing identical (monozygotic) twins with fraternal (dizygotic) twins. Because monozygotic twins share all genes while dizygotic twins share on average only 50% of genes, monozygotic twins are expected to be more alike, or concordant, for a trait with a significant genetic basis. Because they directly control for the degree of genetic similarity among subjects, twin studies can also shed light on nongenetic contributions to traits or disease. Indeed, given a sufficient sample size, twin methods provide quantitative estimates of the degree to which genes and environment contribute to a trait or disease and can even parse the environmental contribution into components that are shared by twins and those that are not.

Despite their unique strengths, twin studies cannot definitively establish a genetic etiology for a disease. There are two main reasons for this. Monozygotic twins usually share the placenta, look very much alike, and are similar for many traits. Thus, they may experience a more similar environment than dizygotic twins, confounding the influence of genes and environment in human study designs. Some studies suggest that this is not a major problem in practice (Kendler et al., 1993b), but even subtle violations of the "equal environment assumption" could have a significant impact in behavioral studies. The other problem with twin studies is that heritability, because it is not a direct measure of genetic effects, varies across populations and time, further diminishing the ability to establish genetic etiology by twin studies alone.

Family studies reveal aspects of the familial nature of disease: its mode of inheritance, the range of clinical or phenotypic expression within the family, and the intergenerational differences that result from dynamic genes and environments. The classical family study design calls for the collection of a large sample of unrelated cases, or probands, followed by the systematic evaluation of relatives. Depending on the study design, the kinds of relatives included can vary from first-degree relatives only (as in sibling-pair designs) all the way to distant cousins (as in extended kinship designs). It is important to ascertain relatives systematically, without regard to their expected phenotype, and to evaluate relatives through direct examination because reports from relatives often greatly underestimate the presence of psychiatric phenotypes (Mendlewicz et al., 1975; Orvaschel et al., 1982).

A properly collected family sample is valuable for many kinds of studies. In segregation analysis, the pattern of illness transmission through the family is studied in an attempt to model the mode of inheritance. For example, autosomal dominant diseases tend to appear in all generations of a family, among the offspring of both affected mothers and fathers, while X-linked recessive diseases appear only in males who are related to other affected males through the maternal lineage. Studies of the rates of illness among relatives are another valuable use of family data. When certain traits are observed more often than expected among the relatives of an affected proband, this suggests that the traits belong to the range of clinical expression for the disease, often referred to as the phenotypic spectrum. For such studies, a sample of unaffected probands and their relatives, collected and evaluated in the same way as the affected probands and their relatives, forms an important control group.

Family data are also useful for studying differences in affected phenotypes between generations. For example, most diseases caused by expansion of triplet repeat DNA sequences, such as Huntington's disease, show decreased age at onset and a more severe phenotype in successive generations of a family, a phenomenon known as anticipation. Cohort effects are another phenomenon that can contribute to differences in phenotypes between generations in a population, although these differences are attributable to environmental factors common to a particular range of birth years rather than to any genetic changes.

Because many familial traits, such as food preferences, are not genetic, the genetic basis of a familial trait is best demonstrated by other kinds of studies. Adoption studies offer the best opportunity in human genetics to unravel the relative contributions of genes and environment to disease. In the simplest adoption study, the rates of a disease are compared in the biological and adoptive parents of adoptees affected by that disease. Diseases that depend more on genetic influences will tend to occur more in biological parents of the adoptees, while those more dependent on environmental influences will not. Adoption study designs are the best way to control for environmental influences, but are not immune to them. Adoptees may be placed out of the birth parents' home at differing ages, and even those adopted at birth are exposed to the intrauterine environment of the biological mother. For this reason, people born of surrogate mothers, who carry a donated ovum to term then give the baby to adoptive parents, may form a valuable population for adoption studies in the future.

Epidemiological studies can help determine the importance of genetics in disease, but they cannot shed much light on the specific genes involved. At this point, molecular genetic studies come into play. These studies encompass much of the field of human genetics, but can be conveniently grouped into studies of linkage, association, and gene expression. In linkage studies, the transmission of a disease within a family is compared to the transmission of easily measurable genetic markers with locations on each chromosome that are known with some precision. Because parental chromosomes can recombine, exchanging genetic material with each other during transmission from parents to offspring, diseases that are consistently transmitted together with a particular chromosomal segment are likely to be caused by a gene residing in that same chromosomal segment. Classical genetic markers were themselves clinical traits, such as color blindness, but linkage studies are now performed using thousands of densely spaced molecular markers that are scored using essentially automated methods, allowing virtually any chromosomal segment to be tracked precisely from generation to generation in a family. The final localization of the sought-for gene then depends on a potentially laborious process of elimination, studying each gene in the linked segment for evidence of changes associated with disease.

It is at the stage of pinpointing a particular disease gene that association studies come into play. Unlike linkage studies, which determine the cotransmission of marker and disease in families, association studies look for the co-occurrence of marker and disease in populations. Association studies can be used to evaluate the potential role of a particular known gene in a disease, as in candidate gene studies. Association studies are also useful for the fine mapping of disease genes. This is because association signals, unlike linkage signals, which are demarcated only by the few recombination events that occur in the families studied, extend just a short distance across a chromosome in most populations. Most modern association studies use single-nucleotide polymorphisms (SNPs), an abundant form of genetic variation that encompasses both nonfunctional marker SNPs and functional SNPs that can play a direct role in determining disease susceptibility (Figure 3-1).

Association studies are often performed in a sample of cases and controls. Such a design can be powerful (Teng & Risch, 1999), but is subject to spurious findings due to genetic differences between cases and controls unrelated to the disease of interest, a phenomenon known as population stratification (for review, see Greenberg et al., 1998). For this reason, family-based designs that determine the proportion of marker alleles transmitted by heterozygous parents to affected offspring are often preferred (Cervino & Hill, 2000; Spielman et al., 1993). Unless association testing leads to an obvious genetic lesion (such as a stop codon or massively expanded triplet repeat), association analysis usually cannot alone demonstrate definitively which gene (or genes) in an associated region truly determines disease susceptibility. For this, direct studies of gene expression and function are usually necessary.

Gene expression studies have benefited enormously from the introduction of microarray technology. Using this technology, a complete set of expressed genes (cDNAs) from a organism are spotted onto a solid surface, such as a

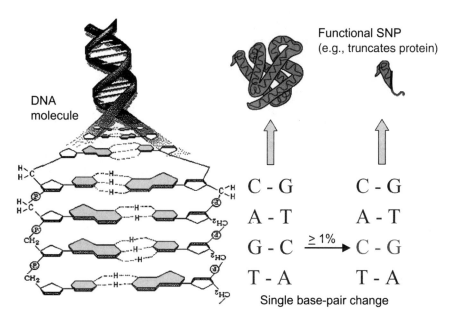

FIGURE 3-1. Single-nucleotide polymorphism (SNP) can play a direct role in determination of disease susceptibility. (Modified from http://www.nhgri.nih.gov/DIR/VIP/Learning_Tools/genetic_illustrations.html.)

glass chip, 1 gene per spot, then exposed to mRNA from the tissue of interest (Figure 3-2). Highly sensitive tags allow precise determination of the relative degree of hybridization between the test mRNA molecules and each cDNA molecule. In this way, the full range of genes represented on the chip can be tested for increased or decreased expression in the tissue of interest. Gene expression arrays have already expanded our understanding of gene function in cancer because cancerous tissue is readily available and can be easily compared to the noncancerous tissue from the same person. The lack of a similarly accessible source of tissue limits the use of gene expression arrays in psychiatry using current technology, but studies of tissue not from the central nervous system and of postmortem brain tissue may ultimately prove valuable.

THE GENETICS OF EARLY-ONSET AFFECTIVE DISORDER

Twin Studies

As discussed above, twin studies are a valuable method for estimating the heritability of a disease. There are several well-known twin studies of affective disorders. Those based on the Danish Twin Register (Kyvik et al., 1996) and those based on the Virginia Twin Registry (Kendler et al., 1992) have contributed much of what we now understand about the heritability of bipolar and unipolar affective disorder. These registries are large, systematic samples of twins that have been assessed longitudinally using standardized diagnostic methods blind to the diagnosis of the co-twin. Thus, they overcome many of the methodological shortcomings of other samples.

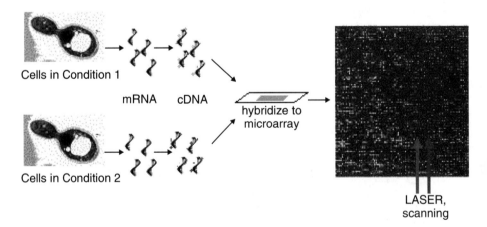

FIGURE 3-2. Use of microarray technology for gene expression studies. (From Brazma A, Parkinson J, Schlitt T, Shojatalab M. A quick introduction to elements of biology—cells, molecules, genes, functional genomes, microarrays. European Bioinformatics Institute. Available at http://www.ebi.ac.uk/microarray/biology_intro.html.)

The Danish Twin Register is a complete listing of all same-sex twins born in Denmark between the years 1870 and 1920. By cross-referencing this listing with centralized medical records, official suicides, and persons who reported a psychiatric hospital admission, Bertelsen and colleagues (1977) identified 110 twin pairs in which at least 1 individual had been diagnosed with an affective disorder. These twins were directly examined by psychiatrists and assigned a diagnosis. Among monozygotic twins diagnosed with bipolar disorder, 67% of their co-twins were also diagnosed with bipolar or unipolar disorder, compared to 20% among dizygotic twin pairs. This demonstrates that bipolar disorder and unipolar disorder are genetically related, and that most of the liability to develop these illnesses is genetically determined. The main drawback of this study is that it only included twin pairs in which at least 1 twin had been treated for or had died of suicide. Because people who seek treatment for a psychiatric illness or die of suicide tend to be more ill than those with the same illness who do not, the Danish Twin Study is best for estimating the heritability of the more severe cases of major affective disorder, typical of what would be seen in the clinic. For heritability estimates more typical of what would be seen in the community, the Virginia Twin Registry is valuable.

The Virginia Twin Registry is a population-based listing of 1,721 female twins. Kendler and colleagues (1993a) sent questionnaires to all women on the registry and directly interviewed both members of 742 pairs, asking them about a variety of psychiatric symptoms. They found that a lifetime history of major depression had a heritability of 40% to 70%. Other major twin studies, which also included men in the sample, reached similar conclusions (Lyons et al., 1998; McGuffin et al., 1996).

Family Studies

The familial nature of affective disorders has been recognized since antiquity. Although family studies cannot in themselves establish genetic etiology, they provide a naturalistic glimpse of the range of psychopathology among relatives. Family studies of affective disorders were first undertaken in the late 19th century, at a time when epidemiological and diagnostic methods in psychiatry were relatively undeveloped. The family studies performed in the 1970s and 1980s form the basis of our modern understanding of affective disorders as familial illnesses.

The main finding from several decades of family studies is clear: affective disorder in a proband predicts elevated rates of specific illnesses in the relatives (for review, see McMahon & DePaulo, 1998). Relatives of probands with unipolar disorder have about a 2-fold greater risk for unipolar or bipolar disorder, but most studies detect no increased risk for schizophrenia. Relatives of probands with bipolar disorder have about a 4-fold greater risk of unipolar disorder and a 10-fold to 15-fold greater risk of bipolar disorder, but again no increased risk for schizophrenia. These findings are typically interpreted as indicating that affective disorders and schizophrenia do not share overlapping genetic determinants, but a significant increase of both bipolar and unipolar disorders among the relatives of probands with schizophrenia contributes to a lingering controversy over this issue (Henn et al., 1995).

Another consistent finding is that the gender of the affected proband does not significantly affect the rates of mood disorder among the proband's relatives. By contrast, some studies have shown that the risk or age at onset of mood disorder in the offspring depends on the gender of the parent who apparently transmits the illness (Grigoroiu-Serbanescu et al., 1998; McMahon et al., 1995).

Findings from family studies are the basis of the classical multiple threshold model of affective disorders (Falconer, 1965; Reich et al., 1972). Under this model, which was borrowed and adapted from the realm of quantitative genetics, individuals are thought to be distributed along a continuum of liability, determined by their genetic endowment. At various points along this continuum, thresholds are passed, and disease results. The form of the disease (unipolar, bipolar, schizoaffective) is determined by the degree of genetic loading and the consequent position of the individual along the liability continuum. The threshold model is still influential in psychiatric genetics, but awaits direct testing by the discovery of the genes involved and study of their patterns of transmission in families.

Segregation analyses, an attempt to determine which mode of inheritance is most consistent with the pattern of illness transmission in families, have not yielded definitive results. Most have been unable to distinguish between *multifactorial* models, under which genetic and nongenetic factors both play a significant role in causing illness, and Mendelian or major gene models with reduced or incomplete penetrance (i.e., in which many of those carrying the disease gene do not express it).

Segregation analysis as a method does not deal well with samples in which a variety of different modes of inheritance act in different families, a very likely reality with affective disorders. Nevertheless, segregation data reveal an important difference between Mendelian and other kinds of genetic effects, a difference that rests on the rate at which illness risk declines with each step of relatedness away from the proband (e.g., to parents and siblings, aunts, uncles, grandparents, etc.).

With Mendelian diseases, the rates of illness decline by a factor of 2 with each step of relatedness, while more rapid declines are typical of multigenic or multifactorial diseases (Risch, 1990). While few family studies have systematically evaluated second-degree and third-degree relatives, illness rates appear to decline rapidly among the relatives of probands with affective disorder, by a factor of 3 to 5 with each step of relatedness. This means that the parents, siblings, and offspring of someone with affective disorder are at a measurably increased risk of affective disorder themselves, while their cousins, nieces, and nephews are not. This suggests that more than 1 and perhaps several genes, acting together, determine the liability to bipolar disorder in a family.

Family data have also been useful for studying nontraditional forms of inheritance, such as anticipation and genomic imprinting. Anticipation is the term applied to a pattern of inheritance characterized by earlier onset or worsening of symptoms across successive generations within a family. The first modern demonstration of anticipation in bipolar disorder (McInnis et al., 1993) was followed by several studies with similar results (e.g., Engstrom et al., 1995; Ohara et al., 1998). Penrose (1948) pointed out the often-subtle biases that can lead to the false appearance of anticipation in families, but the consistent observation of anticipation in virtually all samples studied indicates that at least some anticipation characterizes the transmission of affective disorder (for review, see McInnis, 1996). In the case of Mendelian diseases, anticipation is regarded as the hallmark of a particular kind of mutation arising in repetitive DNA sequences, known as trinucleotide repeats, that actually expand (or occasionally contract) in repeat number when transmitted from generation to generation in a family. Whether anticipation in affective disorder indicates trinucleotide expansion is unknown, but several attempts to detect expanded trinucleotide repeats in patients with mood disorders have failed to identify pathogenic expansions (Goossens et al., 2001; Guy et al., 1997).

Adoption Studies

Adoption studies demonstrate that the familiality of affective disorders has a genetic basis. The best-known adoption studies of affective disorders have been based on the affected adoptee design. Scientists examined the biological and adoptive parents of adults who were adopted as infants and later developed an affective disorder. Most of these studies found that mood disorders are increased 3-fold to 5-fold among the biological, but not the adoptive, parents of adoptees with mood disorders (Mendlewicz & Rainer, 1977; Wender et al., 1986). In other words, the tendency to develop mood disorders travels with the adoptee to the adoptive environment and cannot be attributed to exposure to the biological parent's mood disorder.

The main criticism of the adoption studies of affective disorders is that the sample sizes were small. Indeed, the classic study of Mendlewicz and Rainer (1977) was based on only 29 adoptees with bipolar disorder, and the other adoption studies were not much larger. This reflects the difficulty in collecting large samples that depend on the "natural experiment" of adoption and the adult onset of affective disorder occurring in the same person. Still, the magnitude of the effects leaves little doubt as to the importance of genetic factors in determining the liability to major mood disorders.

Linkage Studies

Close to 100 genetic linkage studies of mood disorders have been published since the landmark Amish study in 1987 (Egeland et al., 1987). This study seemed to have uncovered strong evidence of linkage to chromosome 11p, but this finding was reversed after more data were gathered (Kelsoe et al., 1989). Although linkage methodology has become much more robust since 1987, the field has continued to be troubled by difficulties in consistently replicating linkage findings. Because linkage methods are efficient only when genes of major effect are present, it is perhaps not surprising that the several small-effect to moderate-effect genes that likely underlie mood disorders have been difficult to spot consistently with linkage methods.

Despite these difficulties, at least a few linkages have been detected in multiple studies. These include regions on chromosomes 4p, 8p, 12q, 13q, 18p and 18q, 21q, 22q, and Xq (Figure 3-3; for a review, see Prathikanti & McMahon, 2001). Chromosome 18 is notable because one region or another of this small chromosome has been linked to bipolar disorder by some 20 studies (reviewed in Van Broeckhoven & Verheyen, 1999). The regions linked to bipolar disorder are large and are not demonstrable in all samples studied, perhaps due to differences in the genes that play the most important etiological role in different

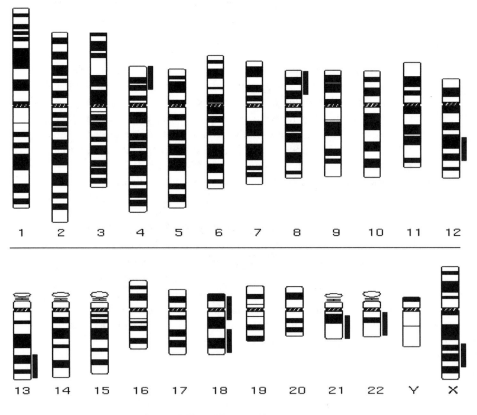

FIGURE 3-3. Linkages detected in multiple studies.

study samples (i.e., genetic heterogeneity). Because different susceptibility genes may occur more often in certain populations, even subtle differences in family ascertainment could have a large impact on which linkage signals can be detected in a given sample.

Efforts to identify the genes that reside within these linked regions have been dramatically accelerated by the mapping and sequencing efforts of the Human Genome Project. These resources, and the growing number of families volunteering for linkage studies, make it likely that one or more susceptibility genes will be identified in the linked regions in the near future.

Association Studies

Many association studies of candidate genes have been completed, but no particular association finding has been widely accepted by the field. The reasons for this are many. Genes have so far been chosen for study based on a plausible hypothesis connecting the known function of the gene to some currently accepted idea about the biology of mood disorders. It is possible that our current knowledge of the biology of mood disorders and of the underlying genes is still too sketchy to provide a reliable means for selecting candidate genes for study. It is also possible that methodological limitations, such as sample size, informativeness of the markers studied, or highly heterogeneous samples, have obscured true findings with false-positive and false-negative results. Linkage signals in specific regions of the genome may ultimately prove to be a more systematic way to select genes for study by association. Studies of genes known to play an important role in complex diseases, such as cardiovascular disease, suggest that extensive study of all genetic variation in and around the gene of interest in large samples is probably needed to evaluate fully any potential association between alleles of that gene and a common disease phenotype.

THE GENETICS OF LATE-ONSET AFFECTIVE DISORDER

Psychiatrists in the 19th century believed that there was an important difference between mood disorders beginning early in life and those first occurring late in life: the early-onset cases were attributed to heredity, while the late-onset cases were seen as the result of vascular disease. We now appreciate the importance of nonhereditary factors in early-onset mood disorders, particularly major depression. On the other hand, the growing recognition of a variety of hereditary diseases of late life that characteristically include mood disorders in the clinical picture suggests that the importance of hereditary factors in late-onset mood disorders may have been underestimated. Still, the broad strokes of the 19th century view find support in modern epidemiology.

Family studies usually show that the proportion of relatives affected with a mood disorder increases with decreasing age at onset in the proband (Loranger & Levine, 1995; Weissman & Wickramaratne, 2000). This has generally been interpreted as a sign of the greater burden of susceptibility genes in families with early-onset mood disorders. The view that late-onset cases have a predominantly vascular etiology finds support in neuroimaging studies. For example, several studies have reported increases in subcortical white matter hyperintensities detectable by magnetic resonance imaging in the brains of people with late-onset mood disorders (Dupont et al., 1990; Krishnan et al., 1997; Lenze et al., 1999). Thus, it does appear that, in general, early-onset and late-onset mood disorders may differ in their predominant etiology.

There is no universal agreement as to what age distinguishes early-onset from late-onset cases. Most studies simply divide the sample at some arbitrary age, usually between 35 and 45 years. Studies of age at onset generally do not support such an arbitrary cutoff, instead finding a relatively smooth distribution of ages at onset, peaking in the late teens and early 20s, but extending from late adolescence through life (McMahon et al., 1994; McMahon & DePaulo, 1996). Some studies do detect a second peak in the onset curve, typically around age 60–70 years, suggesting that something typically occurring in this age range can cause or at least trigger episodes of mood disorder in some people.

Neurological Disease

There is increasing recognition of the importance of mood disorders complicating, or resulting from, neurological disease (Lyketsos et al., 2002). Several inherited, adult-onset neurological diseases that can present as mood disorder are shown in Table 3-1. Mood disorders may precede other signs of these conditions by months or years, and many of these conditions are probably underdiagnosed.

Some 20% to 30% of patients with the degenerative neurological condition known as CADASIL (cerebral autosomal dominant arteriopathy with subcortical infarcts and leukoencephalopathy) have a mood disorder, including depressive, manic, and suicidal presentations (Chabriat et al., 1995; Dichgans et al., 1998; Harris & Filley, 2001). Patients with frontotemporal dementia (FTD) commonly develop depressive symptoms, and the hypersexuality and disinhibition seen with FTD can be mistaken for mania (Lynch et al., 1994). Alzheimer's disease is often complicated by major depression (Bozeat et al., 2000; Groves et al., 2000), sometimes significantly preceding cognitive impairment (Geerlings et al., 2000). Huntington's disease can present with manic or depressive symptoms (Cummings, 1995; Shiwach, 1994) and is strongly associated with suicide (Di Maio et al., 1993). More than one disease gene or allele underlie most of these disorders, but it is currently unknown whether mood disorder presentations are associated with particular disease alleles. More details on the molecular genetics of these conditions can be found in Chapter 2 of this volume.

TABLE 3-1. Adult-onset diseases that can present with mood disorder

Disease	OMIM number	Other names/ related conditions	Distinguishing features	Mode of inheritance	Genetic lesion
Hereditary multiinfarct dementia	125310	CADASIL	Multiple, deep white matter infarcts; migraine; TIAs	AD	*NOTCH3* mutations
Alzheimer's disease	104300		Prominent memory loss, other cognitive changes	complex, but rare AD forms exist	Several, associated with *APOE-4*
Frontotemporal dementia	600274/ 601630	Pick's disease; disinhibition-dementia-parkinsonism-amyotrophy complex	Impulsive behavior; muscle wasting and weakness	AD	Mutations in the gene encoding *tau* protein
Familial multiple sclerosis	126200		Focal central nervous system hyperintensities; elevated CSF myelin basic protein	Complex	Unknown; associated with *HLA-DR2*
Familial Parkinson's disease	168600		Tremor; rigidity; anosmia; early onset	Complex, but rare Mendelian forms may exist	Unclear; associated with genes encoding *parkin* and *α-synuclein*
Huntington's disease	143100	DRLPA	Choreiform movements; ataxia	AD	Trinucleotide expansion in gene encoding *huntingtin*
Parkinsonism with alveolar hypoventilation	16805	Perry's disease	Decreased CSF taurine; respiratory failure	AD	Unknown

AD, autosomal dominant; CADASIL, cerebral autosomal dominant arteriopathy with subcortical infarcts and leukoencephalopathy; CSF, cerebrospinal fluid; DRLPA, dentatorubral and pallidoluysian atrophy; OMIM, Online Mendelian Inheritance in Man; TIAs, transient ischemic attacks.

Cardiovascular Disease

There appears to be an important, two-way relationship between mood disorders and cardiovascular disease. Many studies suggest that major depression increases the risk of cardiovascular disease even after controlling for cardiac risk factors, such as smoking, that may be more prevalent in those suffering from a mood disorder (Anda et al., 1993). On the other hand, several studies have shown that about one fifth of patients develop major depression following a myocardial infarction (MI), and that these patients are several times more likely to die than those who do not develop major depression (for review, see Glassman & Shapiro, 1998). It is unknown whether this association is mediated by the physical or psychological sequelae of a myocardial infarction. Changes in the autonomic nervous system and platelets may play a major role. It is also possible that this association reflects unidentified susceptibility genes that both mood disorders and cardiovascular disease share.

Cancers

Recognition of the substantial contribution of genetics to cancer has led to groundbreaking discoveries such as *BRCA1*, a gene that dramatically increases the risk of breast cancer, and P53, a cell cycle regulator linked to a large variety of cancers. Cancer patients often suffer from demoralization and major depression, which should be treated aggressively. Despite this understandable association between life-threatening illness and depressive symptoms, however, there is little evidence that cancer (with the possible exception of pancreatic cancer) is a significant contributor to mood disorders in late life. The converse idea that mood disorders might somehow predispose to cancer has been dealt a blow by a large, population-based survey in Denmark that showed no increased incidence of breast cancer among some 67,000 women admitted to psychiatric units in Denmark for treatment of mood disorders (Hjerl et al., 1999).

GENETICS OF ASSOCIATED CONDITIONS

Substance Abuse

Substance abuse and dependence are difficult to study genetically because they are behaviors and are inherently dependent on exposure to the abused substance, a variable that is largely culturally determined. Substance abuse and dependence among the elderly in Western societies has been limited almost entirely to alcohol, nicotine, and prescription drugs (this will likely change as people born after World War II grow older). Of these, only alcohol has been studied extensively in the elderly.

Family and twin studies suggest that genes account for approximately 40%

to 60% of the risk for alcoholism, but multiple genes appear to be involved (for review, see Schuckit, 2000). Individual variation in alcohol-metabolizing enzymes, behavioral response to alcohol, and electrophysiological measures— all genetically influenced—together with comorbid conditions such as mood disorders may account for much of the individual variation in risk for alcoholism. Association studies have indicated that alleles of the alcohol-metabolizing enzymes alcohol dehydrogenase (ADH) and aldehyde dehydrogenase (ALDH) strongly reduce the risk of alcoholism in Asian populations. Other association and linkage studies are under way, but with no definitive results so far.

Alcoholism is frequently accompanied by other kinds of substance abuse and dependence. Family data indicate that alcohol, marijuana, and cocaine dependence and habitual smoking are all familial, but that some of the familial factors are specific to the type of substance abused (Bierut et al., 1998). This could reflect family-specific exposure to particular drugs in a shared familial environment (e.g., cocaine in US cities) or specific genetic factors.

Anxiety Disorders

The anxiety disorders encompass panic disorder with and without agoraphobia, obsessive-compulsive disorder, specific phobias, and generalized anxiety disorder. Of these, obsessive-compulsive disorder appears to be rare in the elderly, and the genetics of specific phobias and generalized anxiety have been little studied. In contrast, panic disorder is not rare in the elderly and has been the subject of several twin, family, and linkage studies.

Twin studies consistently have found a high heritability for panic disorder and for CO_2-induced panic attacks, thought to be a related phenotype. The largest such study was based on the Virginia Twin Registry, all females. The results best fit with a model in which genes jointly influence the risk of phobia, bulimia nervosa, and panic disorder and in which the expression of a particular disease in a particular person is largely determined by individual environmental factors (Kendler et al., 1995).

The pioneering family study of panic disorder (then known as neurocirculatory asthenia) found an increased rate of panic disorder and alcoholism in the relatives of affected probands and concluded that the apparent transmission pattern was most consistent with autosomal dominant inheritance (Cohen et al., 1951). While modern studies support the strong familiality of panic disorder, no consistent evidence for a particular mode of inheritance has emerged (Hopper et al., 1987; Pauls et al., 1980).

Linkage and association studies of panic disorder are still in the early phases. Several genetic linkage studies of panic disorder are under way, but the 3 published genomewide screens were all inconclusive (Crowe et al., 2001; Gelernter et al., 2001; Knowles et al., 1998). Association studies have focused on genes with a function that can be plausibly related to panic attacks. The serotonin transporter has been implicated by some association studies (Lesch et al., 1996) and may play a more general role in trait anxiety (Mazzanti et al., 1998).

Suicide

Suicide almost always occurs in the setting of mental illness, usually a major mood disorder, so the genetics of suicide coincide to a certain extent with the genetics of the major mood disorders. That mood disorder genetics provide an incomplete account of the genetics of suicide is revealed by two phenomena. First, an unacceptable 15% of all people with a major mood disorder may ultimately die of suicide (Wyatt & Henter, 1995). How do those who die of suicide differ from the 85% with major mood disorder who die of other causes? Do at least some of these differences have a genetic basis? Second, several studies suggest that suicide clusters in families, and that this is not merely the result of more severe major mood disorder in those families (Egeland & Sussex, 1985). Twin studies suggest that suicidal behavior is significantly heritable, even when mood disorder is taken into account (Statham et al., 1998), but the strong correlation between suicide and major mood disorders makes it difficult to untangle the genetic contribution to suicide independent of the genetic contribution to mood disorder (Roy et al., 1999). Finally, several studies have suggested that polymorphisms in the tryptophan hydroxylase (TPH) gene, which encodes the rate-limiting enzyme in the synthesis of serotonin, may be involved in suicidal behavior, particularly of an impulsive, violent nature (Nielsen et al., 1998). A definitive role for tryptophan hydroxylase in suicide has not been established.

CONCLUSION

When encountering an older patient with major depression or bipolar disorder, bear in mind that genetic etiology and influences are not confined to the young. Whether the patient is young or old, primary and secondary mood disorders and related conditions appear to be under substantial genetic influences throughout life. Ongoing identification of the specific genes involved will greatly enhance diagnosis and treatment.

REFERENCES

Anda RF, Williamson DF, Jones D, et al. Depressed affect, hopelessness, and the risk of ischemic heart disease in a cohort of US adults. *Epidemiology*. 1993;4:285–294.

Bertelsen A, Harvald B, Hauge M. A Danish twin study of manic depressive disorders. *Br J Psychiatry*. 1977;130:330–351.

Bierut LJ, Dinwiddie SH, Begleiter H, et al. Familial transmission of substance dependence: alcohol, marijuana, cocaine, and habitual smoking: a report from the Collaborative Study on the Genetics of Alcoholism. *Arch Gen Psychiatry.* 1998;55:982–988.

Bozeat S, Gregory CA, Ralph MA, et al. Which neuropsychiatric and behavioural features distinguish frontal and temporal variants of frontotemporal dementia from Alzheimer's disease? *J Neurol Neurosurg Psychiatry.* 2000;69:178–186.

Cervino AC, Hill AV. Comparison of tests for association and linkage in incomplete families. *Am J Hum Genet.* 2000;67:120–132.

Chabriat H, Vahedi K, Iba-Zizen MT, et al. Clinical spectrum of CADASIL: a study of 7 families. *Lancet.* 1995;346:934–939.

Childs B, Scriver C. Age at onset and causes of disease. *Perspect Biol Med.* 1986;29:437–460.

Cohen ME, Badal DW, Kilpatrick A, Reed EW, White PD. The high familial prevalence of neurocirculatory asthenia (anxiety neurosis, effort syndrome). *Am J Hum Genet.* 1951;3:126–158.

Crowe RR, Goedken R, Samuelson S, Wilson R, Nelson J, Noyes R Jr. Genomewide survey of panic disorder. *Am J Med Genet.* 2001;105:105–109.

Cummings JL. Behavioral and psychiatric symptoms associated with Huntington's disease. *Adv Neurol.* 1995;65:179–186.

Dichgans M, Mayer M, Uttner I, et al. The phenotypic spectrum of CADASIL: clinical findings in 102 cases. *Ann Neurol.* 1998;44:731–739.

Di Maio L, Squitieri F, Napolitano G, et al. Suicide risk in Huntington's disease. *J Med Genet.* 1993;30:293–295.

Dupont R, Jernigan T, Butters N, et al. Subcortical abnormalities detected in bipolar affective disorder using magnetic resonance imaging. Clinical and neuropsychological significance. *Arch Gen Psychiatry.* 1990;47:55–59.

Egeland J, Sussex JN. Suicide and family loading for affective disorders. *JAMA.* 1985;254:915–918.

Egeland JA, Gerhard DS, Pauls DL, et al. Bipolar affective disorders linked to DNA markers on chromosome 11. *Nature.* 1987;325:783–787.

Engstrom C, Thornlund AS, Johansson EL, et al. Anticipation in unipolar affective disorder. *J Affect Dis.* 1995;35:31–40.

Falconer D. The inheritance of liability to certain diseases, estimated from the incidence among relatives. *Ann Hum Genet.* 1965;29:51–76.

Geerlings MI, Schmand B, Braam AW, et al. Depressive symptoms and risk of Alzheimer's disease in more highly educated older people. *J Am Geriatr Soc.* 2000;48:1092–1097.

Gelernter J, Bonvicini K, Page G, Goodson S. Linkage genome scan for loci predisposing to panic disorder or agoraphobia. *Am J Med Genet.* 2001;105:548–557.

Glassman AH, Shapiro PA. Depression and the course of coronary artery disease. *Am J Psychiatry.* 1998;155:4–11.

Goossens D, Del-Favero J, Van Broeckhoven C. Trinucleotide repeat expansions: do they contribute to bipolar disorder? *Brain Res Bull.* 2001;56:243–257.

Greenberg B, McMahon F, Murphy D. Serotonin transporter candidate gene studies in affective disorders and personality: promises and potential pitfalls. *Mol Psychiatry.* 1998;3:186–189.

Grigoroiu-Serbanescu M, Martinez M, Nothen M, et al. Patterns of parental transmission and familial aggregation models in bipolar affective disorder. *Am J Med Genet (Neuropsychiatr Genet).* 1998;81:397–404.

Groves WC, Brandt J, Steinberg M, et al. Vascular dementia and Alzheimer's disease: is there a difference? A comparison of symptoms by disease duration. *J Neuropsychiatry Clin Neurosci.* 2000;12:305–315.

Guy C, Bowen T, Daniels JK, et al. Exclusion of expansion of 50 CAG/CTG trinucleotide repeats in bipolar disorder. *Am J Psychiatry.* 1997;154:1146–1147.

Harris JG, Filley CM. CADASIL: neuropsychological findings in three generations of an affected family. *J Int Neuropsychol Soc.* 2001;7:768–774.

Henn S, Bass N, Shields G, et al. Affective illness and schizophrenia in families with multiple schizophrenic members—independent illness or variant gene(s). *Eur Neuropsychopharmacol.* 1995;5:31–36.

Hjerl K, Andersen EW, Keiding N, et al. Breast cancer risk among women with psychiatric admission with affective or neurotic disorders: a nationwide cohort study in Denmark. *Br J Cancer.* 1999;81:907–911.

Hopper JL, Judd FK, Derrick PL, Burrows GD. A family study of panic disorder. *Genet Epidemiol.* 1987;4:33–41.

Kelsoe JR, Ginns EI, Egeland JA, et al. Re-evaluation of the linkage relationship between chromosome 11p loci and the gene for bipolar affective disorder in the Old Order Amish. *Nature.* 1989;342:238–243.

Kendler KS, Neale MC, Kessler RC, et al. The lifetime history of major depression in women. *Arch Gen Psychiatry.* 1993a;50:863–870.

Kendler KS, Neale MC, Kessler RC, Heath AC, Eaves LJ. A population-based twin study of major depression in women: the impact of varying definitions of illness. *Arch Gen Psychiatry.* 1992;49:257–266.

Kendler KS, Neale MC, Kessler RC, Heath AC, Eaves LJ. A test of the equal-environment assumption in twin studies of psychiatric illness. *Behav Genet.* 1993b;23: 21–27.

Kendler KS, Walters EE, Neale MC, Kessler RC, Heath AC, Eaves LJ. The structure of the genetic and environmental risk factors for six major psychiatric disorders in women. Phobia, generalized anxiety disorder, panic disorder, bulimia, major depression, and alcoholism. *Arch Gen Psychiatry.* 1995;52:374–383.

Knowles JA, Fyer AJ, Vieland VJ, et al. Results of a genome-wide genetic screen for panic disorder. *Am J Med Genet.* 1998;81:139–147.

Krishnan KR, Hays JC, Blazer DG. MRI-defined vascular depression. *Am J Psychiatry.* 1997;154:497–501.

Kyvik KO, Christensen K, Skytthe A, Harvald B, Holm NV. The Danish Twin Register. *Dan Med Bull.* 1996;43:467–470.

Lenze E, Cross D, McKeel D, et al. White matter hyperintensities and gray matter lesions in physically healthy depressed subjects. *Am J Psychiatry.* 1999;156:1602–1607.

Lesch K-P, Bengel D, Heils A, et al. Association of anxiety-related traits with a polymorphism in the serotonin transporter gene regulatory region. *Science.* 1996;274:1527–1530.

Loranger AW, Levine PM. Age at onset of bipolar affective illness. *Arch Gen Psychiatry.* 1978;35:1345–1348.

Lyketsos CG, Lopez O, Jones B, Fitzpatrick AL, Breitner J, DeKosky S. Prevalence of neuropsychiatric symptoms in dementia and mild cognitive impairment: results from the cardiovascular health study. *JAMA.* 2002;288:1475–1483.

Lynch T, Sano M, Marder KS, et al. Clinical characteristics of a family with chromosome 17-linked disinhibition-dementia-parkinsonism-amyotrophy complex. *Neurology*. 1994;44:1878–1884.

Lyons MJ, Eisen SA, Goldberg J, et al. A registry-based twin study of depression in men. *Arch Gen Psychiatry*. 1998;55:468–472.

Mazzanti CM, Lappalainen J, Long JC, et al. Role of the serotonin transporter promoter polymorphism in anxiety-related traits. *Arch Gen Psychiatry*. 1998;55:936–940.

McGuffin P, Katz R, Watkins S, Rutherford J. A hospital-based twin register of the heritability of *DSM-IV* unipolar depression. *Arch Gen Psychiatry*. 1996;53:129–136.

McInnis MG. Anticipation: an old idea in new genes. *Am J Hum Genet*. 1996;59:973–979.

McInnis MG, McMahon FJ, Chase G, et al. Anticipation in bipolar affective disorder. *Am J Hum Genet*. 1993;53:385–390.

McKusick VA. Medical genetics. A 40-year perspective on the evolution of a medical specialty from a basic science. *JAMA*. 1993;270:2351–2356.

McMahon FJ, Chase GA, Simpson SG, et al. Clinical subtype, sex, and lineality influence onset age of major affective disorder in a family sample. *Am J Psychiatry*. 1994;151:210–215.

McMahon FJ, DePaulo JR. *Affective disorders*. In: Jamison JL, ed. *Principles of Molecular Medicine*. Totowa, NJ: Humana; 1998.

McMahon FJ, DePaulo JR. Genetics and age at onset. In: Shulman KI, Tohen M, Kutcher S, eds. *Mood Disorders Throughout the Lifespan*. New York, NY: Wiley-Liss; 1996.

McMahon FJ, Stine OC, Meyers DA, et al. Patterns of maternal transmission in bipolar affective disorder. *Am J Hum Genet*. 1995;56:1277–1286.

Mendlewicz J, Fleiss JL, Cataldo M, et al. Accuracy of the family history method in affective illness. Comparison with direct interviews in family studies. *Arch Gen Psychiatry*. 1975;32:309–314.

Mendlewicz J, Rainer JD. Adoption study supporting genetic transmission in manic-depressive illness. *Nature*. 1977;268:327–329.

Nielsen DA, Virkkunen M, Lappalainen J, et al. A tryptophan hydroxylase gene marker for suicidality and alcoholism. *Arch Gen Psychiatry*. 1998;55:593–602.

Ohara K, Suzuki Y, Ushimi Y, et al. Anticipation and imprinting in Japanese familial mood disorders. *Psychiatry Res*. 1998;79:191–198.

Orvaschel H, Thompson WD, Belanger A, et al. Comparison of the family history method to direct interview. *J Affect Dis*. 1982;4:49–59.

Pauls DL, Bucher KD, Crowe RR, Noyes R Jr. A genetic study of panic disorder pedigrees. *Am J Hum Genet*. 1980;32:639–644.

Penrose LS. The problem of anticipation in pedigrees of dystrophia myotonica. *Ann Eugenics*. 1948;14:125–132.

Prathikanti S, McMahon FJ. Genome scans for susceptibility genes in bipolar affective disorder. *Ann Med*. 2001;33:257–262.

Reich T, James JW, Morris CA. The use of multiple thresholds in determining the mode of transmission of semi-continuous traits. *Ann Hum Genet*. 1972;36:163–184.

Risch N. Linkage strategies for genetically complex traits. *Am J Hum Genet*. 1990;46:229–241.

Roy A, Nielsen D, Rylander G, et al. Genetics of suicide in depression. *J Clin Psychiatry*. 1999;60(suppl 2):12–17.

Schuckit MA. Genetics of the risk for alcoholism. *Am J Addict.* 2000;9:103–112.

Shiwach R. Psychopathology in Huntington's disease patients. *Acta Psychiatr Scand.* 1994;90:241–246.

Spielman RS, McGinnis RE, Ewens WJ. Transmission test for linkage disequilibrium: the insulin gene region and insulin-dependent diabetes mellitus (IDDM). *Am J Hum Genet.* 1993;52:506–516.

Statham DJ, Heath AC, Madden PA, et al. Suicidal behaviour: an epidemiological and genetic study. *Psychol Med.* 1998;28:839–855.

Teng J, Risch N. The relative power of family-based and case-control designs for linkage disequilibrium studies of complex human diseases. II. Individual genotyping. *Genome Res.* 1999;9:234–241.

Van Broeckhoven C, Verheyen G. Report of the chromosome 18 workshop. *Am J Med Genet.* 1999;88:263–270.

Weissman MM, and Wickramaratne P. Age of onset and familial risk in major depression [letter; comment]. *Arch Gen Psychiatry.* 2000;57:513–514.

Wender PH, Kety SS, Rosenthal D, et al. Psychiatric disorders in the biological and adoptive families of adopted individuals with affective disorders. *Arch Gen Psychiatry.* 1986;43:923–929.

Wyatt RJ, Henter I. An economic evaluation of manic-depressive illness—1991. *Soc Psychiatry Psychiatr Epidemiol.* 1995;30:213–219.

4

The Biology of Aging

Elaine A. Leventhal, MD, PhD
Edith Ann Burns, MD

Development, maturation, and aging are observed in all living organisms. "Normal" aging or *senescence* is associated with declines in actual number of active metabolic cells and cellular functions over the life span. Many theories have been proposed to explain these continuously changing processes of the life cycle. Senescence has been hypothesized to result from the accumulation of cellular and nuclear mutations after exposure to free-oxygen radicals, lipoperoxidases, decreased protein turnover, and a loss of regenerative ability ("wear-and-tear" theories of aging) (Jazwinski, 1996; Kirkwood, 1996). Another attractive current theory assumes that progressive shortening of telomeres limits the cell's ability to perform mitosis, thus leading to programmed death or apoptosis, a process that allows cells to be replaced. If cells have undergone cellular and nuclear mutations and are unable to repair the DNA damage, they may become resistant to apoptotic signaling, accumulate damaged DNA, and thus have decreased responses to stress and an increased incidence of disease (Harman, 1991; Semsei, 2000; Warner et al., 1997).

Over time, variability in genetic predisposition to disease and unique history of environmental and behavioral insults in any given individual lead to the differences that produce the heterogeneity between individual elderly. Thus, significant biological and psychological changes occur at different rates within and between aging individuals. The ability to respond to stress becomes compromised, yet in the absence of significant chronic disease, functional independence can be maintained well into the ninth decade.

Many observable physical and psychological senescent changes are the result of illness that may or may not be alterable and not because of aging per se. Some changes occur gradually; others present acutely. When such conditions do occur, they can introduce unexpected and unwelcome changes in self-perceptions of health, functionality, and vulnerability. Illness, whether gradual or sudden, brings dysfunction, and efforts to overcome functional losses can lead to unexpected and sometimes undesirable treatments (e.g., prescribing of medications with high toxicity and potentially limited efficacy). Illness-induced functional decline can produce actual and perceived stigmatization and can lead to withdrawal from social roles and reductions in earning capacity. In addition, illness often requires participation in complex and unfamiliar institutional and social structures while dealing with personal physical dysfunction (Leventhal et al., 1999).

GENERAL BODY AGING

Some of the changes in body composition commonly seen with aging are decreases in stature, lean body mass, total body water (10%–15%), and bone mineral density. In general, there is a quantitative loss of cells and many of the enzymatic activities within cells. These "microscopic" changes result in macroscopic alterations in body composition, with up to an 80% decrease in overall muscle mass and average 35% increase in total body fat, with a central redistribution of adipose tissue. Fat deposition accumulates around and within the viscera, but there is a loss of fat subcutaneously. Thus, older people lose "insulation" and are more sensitive to extremes of ambient temperature than are younger people.

Circadian rhythm timing changes across the life span, affecting sleep patterns and the secretion of hormones, such as the gonadotropins, thyrotropin, and melatonin. The significance of these changes is not yet well understood. It is interesting to note that the MacArthur studies on successful aging have demonstrated that individuals with higher nocturnal secretion of cortisol and catecholamines experienced greater declines in cognitive and physical function during follow-up periods of 3 years (Rowe & Kahn, 1998).

Each organ system is reviewed in turn, concluding with a discussion of changes in sleep patterns with age. Changes in the major organ systems are reviewed.

SKIN

Aging of the skin is a reflection not only of physical changes, but also of environmental exposure (e.g., solar-induced photoaging). The skin as a whole atrophies, with loss of the subcutaneous cushion of fat. There may be fewer immunologically active Langerhans cells and shrinkage of dermal appendages, including sweat and sebaceous glands. With fewer sebaceous and eccrine glands, the skin becomes dry or xerotic. Cold temperatures and the low humidity of heated rooms exacerbate the condition, producing itching and occasional cracking. There are fewer blood vessels in the skin, and the rate of skin healing slows. Elastin, the structural element responsible for the "stretch" in tissues, fragments with age. Nails grow more slowly.

However, not all these normal age-related changes represent cell or tissue loss or deterioration. Collagen accumulates, as evidenced by increased interstitial matrix formation. Examples of the effects of such age-related changes in elastin and collagen can be seen in wrinkling (Kligman et al., 1985; Yaar, 1990).

Excessive tanning has significant effects on the skin, accelerating both normal senescent changes and also producing pathology because there is loss of skin melanocytes, leading to a decrease in pigmentation and increased vulnerability to sun damage. Sun exposure produces the senile changes that accelerate fragmentation of skin elastin and encourage increased collagen deposition. People with prolonged tanning exposure have more wrinkles at earlier ages as well as a greater incidence of malignant neoplasms such as the actinic keratoses, basal and squamous cell cancers, and malignant melanomas. Benign neoplasms are also common, although of still-unknown etiology. They include the waxy or rough-surfaced, pigmented seborrheic keratoses. In addition, as the skin thins and dermal appendages become atrophic, vascular structures are more easily visualized and spider veins can crop up. Senile purpuric lesions also become increasingly common as the thinning dermis cannot lend support to fragile blood vessels, which then become vulnerable to minimal trauma.

CARDIOVASCULAR SYSTEM

Feelings of being old are often associated with loss of energy and easy fatigability. There are many potential causes for these nonspecific symptoms, and they are frequently attributed to an aging cardiovascular system. Indeed, the cardiovascular system may be a major factor, if not the primary source, of decreased tolerance for exercise and loss of conditioning. Normal aging changes in the cardiovascular system are detailed in Table 4-1.

With time, the ventricular myocardium thickens, the ventricular cavities become smaller, and the amount of blood pumped per contraction decreases. Heart rate also slows with time as cells in the sinus node decline by up to 90%. The decrease in rate may also be related to "downregulation" or decreased responsiveness of adrenergic receptors on heart muscle even though synthesis and clearance of epinephrine does not change. As a result, the maximum heart rate in response to increased activity and stress diminishes. The anatomic changes in the vascular system affect function by causing declines in cardiac output and therefore a decrease in response to work demands (Arking, 1998; Folkow & Svanborg, 1993; Lakatta, 1987, 1985; Marin, 1995; Morley & Reese, 1989; Rodeheffer et al., 1984).

TABLE 4-1. Cardiovascular system changes with normal aging

Cellular and structural level	Function
Increased size of myocytes	Decreased protein synthesis
Decreased number of myocytes	Decreased adaptation
Increased degenerative products (lipid, collagen, lipofuscin, amyloid)	Increased rate of relaxation
	Increased duration of contraction
Elongation/tortuosity of aorta	Increased systolic blood pressure
Increased thickening	Decreased compliance of peripheral vessels
Increased fibrosis	
Increased left atrial dimension	Increased stroke volume
Increased left ventricular wall thickness	Decreased cardiac output with stress; no change in cardiac output at rest
Aortic sclerosis and mitral annular calcification	

Blood vessels narrow as endothelial linings thicken and smooth muscle mass declines. In the elderly, it becomes increasingly common for calcium to be deposited in vessel walls in the presence of medial necrosis. The blood vessels become more rigid, contributing to the slow elevation in blood pressure with aging in the absence of cardiovascular disease. These senescent vascular changes may never reach a pathological range, but it is rare for an individual to be very old without hypertensive disease. When coronary artery disease is present along with normal cardiac aging, function is further compromised.

Women appear to enjoy a slower rate of progression of atherosclerotic disease before the menopause. This advantage is reflected in the lower incidence of coronary artery disease in premenopausal women (Anderson et al., 1997). However, cardiovascular disease becomes the major killer in postmenopausal women, and it can present with atypical symptoms and be more lethal than in men. The musculoskeletal system and the lungs also play a major role in exercise tolerance, adding another dimension to the senescent changes in the heart chambers, blood vessels, and valves.

RESPIRATORY SYSTEM

The aging changes in the cardiovascular system are mirrored by an even more rapid rate of functional decline in the respiratory system. Based on observations in healthy older adults without chronic illness, all parts of the pulmonary system age. This includes changes in lung tissue as well as the muscles, ribs, and vertebrae of the thoracic cage. This is summarized in Table 4-2. Total lung capacity does not change over time, but residual volume increases because of greater closing volume. Ventilatory control becomes compromised as the responses to hypoxemia and hypercapnia decline. Smooth muscle in the bronchi, diaphragm, and chest wall becomes weakened because of excess deposition

TABLE 4-2.   Respiratory system changes in normal aging

Structural	Functional
Increased chest wall stiffness	Increased elastic work of breathing
Increased muscle atrophy	Decreased maximum ventilatory volume (MVV)
Decreased anterior-posterior diameter	Decreased lung surface area (P_aO_2)
Increased terminal alveoli	Decreased vital capacity (VC) flow rates
Decreased elasticity	(average decrease of 18% between 20 and 80 years of age)
Collagen rearrangement	Increased residual volume
Decreased ciliary function	Decreased cough effectiveness

of collagen and fragmentation of elastin fibers, resulting in diminished work capacity.

Although arterial blood gas measurements do not show changes in pH and PCO_2, the oxygen content and PO_2 decline. The decrease in arterial PO_2 is approximately 3 mm Hg per decade. The anatomic basis for the change is the enlargement of alveolar ducts with loss in elastic tissue, resulting in a decreased surface area for gas exchange. The alveolar septae are critical as the exchange sites for the gases oxygen and carbon dioxide. Old lungs have scattered areas of fibrosis or disruptions in the septae that interfere with gaseous exchange.

These manifestations of senile emphysema, although asymptomatic at rest, may limit the amount of exercise and energy that can be expended even more than functional changes in the cardiovascular system described above (Rossi et al., 1996; Tockman, 1994). They also limit ventilatory reserve and predispose to dyspnea when comorbid stressors are present, such as congestive heart failure, pleural effusions, interstitial processes, and the like. Airways in dependent portions of the lung stay closed at higher volumes, and more airways are closed during part or all of the respiratory cycle.

Even though the lower portions of the lung are better perfused regardless of age, the higher closing volume increases ventilation-perfusion mismatch and accounts for declining PO_2 seen with advancing age. The older person's PO_2 is lower in the supine than in the sitting position because of changes in thoracic mechanics. Dynamic pulmonary function peaks at 30 years of age, and this peak determines the likelihood of future compromise from such age-related changes as decreased peak expiratory flow (because of reduced muscle function), decreased forced expiratory volume in 1 second (FEV_1) (because of increased lung compliance), and decreased forced vital capacity (FVC). Cough becomes less vigorous, and mucociliary clearance is slowed so that the most distal portions of the lungs are less efficiently cleared.

These anatomic and functional age-related changes in the respiratory system lead to decreased maximum oxygen utilization. Additional changes in respiratory mechanics include reduced chest wall compliance because of calcification of costochondral cartilages, decreased compliance of lungs because of loss of elastic recoil, and increased dependence on abdominal breathing. The ability to fully expand the chest begins to diminish; by 40 years of age, full expansion does not occur in the supine position, and by 65 years of age, full expansion does not occur while sitting. In addition, disturbances in swallowing function with disorganized esophageal contractions can predispose the elderly person to aspiration and serious pulmonary complications. These are discussed in the section on the gastrointestinal tract.

There are clear gender differences in thoracic cage aging. This may result from a higher incidence of spinal osteoporosis and spontaneous compression fractures of the vertebral bodies and muscle mass loss, which compromise the size of the thoracic cage in females. Thus, women exhibit a diminished exercise capacity along with the vulnerability to fractures and a greater possibility for immobilization.

Moreover, it is difficult to determine how much of the respiratory functional decline observed is age-related senile emphysema and how much is environmentally induced because most individuals are exposed to some degree of air pollution. There are no studies on nonsmokers living in nonpolluted environments, but it must be expected that use of cigarettes or other inhaled substances exaggerates the aging changes just described. Smoking accelerates fibrotic and disruptive changes in the alveolar walls, leading to decreased diffusion capacity, increased secretions, and an increased rate of chronic infection. Coughing is less vigorous, and mucociliary clearance is slower. The pathological conditions of bronchitis and emphysema mimic and accelerate the changes seen with normal aging. Cigarette smoking also is toxic for osteoblasts and is a major determinant of secondary osteoporosis, especially in male smokers.

MUSCULOSKELETAL SYSTEM

Aging of the skeleton is probably responsible for generating the most common physical complaints of age and has the largest responsibility for limiting job-related and recreational activities and functions of daily living. The symptoms of stiffness and joint and muscle aches because of arthritis are frequently ascribed to "getting old." Although some skeletal and joint aging is unavoidable because of wear and tear, diseases, nutritional differences, and history of trauma contribute to the heterogeneity seen between individuals. Although it can be difficult to separate the effects of all these factors, some changes appear to occur generally with age, and there are distinct gender differences in aging involving the bones, muscles, ligaments, and tendons.

On average, men display greater musculoskeletal strength after pubescence, although they lose significant muscle mass with time, as do women. In both genders, the loss is neither linear nor uniform, but accelerates with increasing age. Type II muscle fibers show the greatest declines, in both number and size of the myofibrils, resulting in shrinking muscle bundles. There are fewer motor units, and innervation appears less stable. Contractions take a longer time to reach peak tension and have a slower relaxation phase. Strength also declines, although it is maintained relatively longer in the upper than in the lower extremities.

Cartilage-bound water content declines, as does proteoglycan monomer content, and there is increased linkage protein fragmentation. Keratin sulfate and hyaluronic acid levels increase; the amount of synovial fluid decreases. The changes in water content, combined with the biochemical changes described, correlate with a decrease in the tensile strength of articular cartilage.

Mineralization of the skeleton declines at a rate of about 0.8% to 1.0% per year between the ages of 30 and 90 years for both men and women. However, women become osteopenic at an accelerated rate (between 8% and 10% per year) around the menopause. This represents an approximate 10-year advantage for men. The gender-specific rate of demineralization is particularly complex, with the effects of circulating hormones varying by location. For example, the effect of estrogens and progesterone is most pronounced in the maintenance of vertebral trabecular bone. By contrast, calcium, vitamin D, and weight-bearing activities appear to be more critical for the remodeling of the cortical bones of the extremities. Thus, postmenopausal women are more vulnerable to fractures of the vertebral spine than men of the same age. Both men and women are at risk for fractures of the long bones, but women are fracture prone 10 years earlier than men of the same cohort (Kenny, 2000; Raiz, 1997). Comorbid diseases can accelerate and exaggerate bone loss and osteoporosis in both men and women.

GASTROINTESTINAL TRACT

Mouth and Upper Intestinal Tract

Aging changes are obvious in the mouth. With time, the teeth show reduced dentine production, shrinkage and fibrosis of root pulp, gingival retraction, and loss of bone density in the alveolar ridges, especially after tooth loss. The gums recede, and enamel and dentine wear down. There is an increase in caries, especially of the root, that appears to be correlated with changes in bacterial content of the mouth and increased colonization with gram-positive facultative cocci, which replace gram-negative anaerobic rods; the population of fusospirochetal organisms remains unchanged. There are modest age-related changes in the salivary glands, with a small decrease in the number of acinar cells and slight decreases in saliva production. These changes generally cause no more than minor symptoms. However, because of these changes, older adults are at higher risk of developing xerostomia, or dry mouth, which is caused by such conditions as nasal obstruction, diseases that lead to mouth breathing, drugs, or autoimmune diseases such as Sjogren's syndrome (Loesche et al., 1995).

Esophageal function is largely preserved. Primary aging changes are related to smooth muscle weakness and manifested by decreased amplitude of peristaltic movements as the number of cells in the myenteric ganglia declines (Sallout et al., 1999).

The stomach shows evidence of impaired secretory capacity, with maximal stimulated gastric acid production decreasing by 5 mEq per hour each decade. Serum gastrin levels increase, and intrinsic factor levels decrease. These changes can lead to vitamin B_{12} malabsorption. Atrophic gastritis is common, appearing in 28% to 96% of elderly. Gastric emptying appears to be impaired only slightly.

There is minimal change in the small intestine and only a marginal reduction in mesenteric and splanchnic blood flow in the absence of vascular disease. One age-related process that has been observed is a decrease in absorptive surface area with concomitant loss of microvilli of the brush border and associated enzymatic activities. The overall weight of the small intestine decreases with, as noted above, significant decreases in mucosal surface area, yet without overall decreases in level of function. Xylose, iron, and folate absorption have generally been considered to remain normal (although some reports indicate decline); lipid and calcium absorption declines and is probably related to decreases in vitamin D availability and activity. Some lipid-soluble compounds (e.g., vitamins A and K and cholesterol) are absorbed more rapidly. There is a reduction in the number of Peyer's patches and lymphoid follicles within the patches. Absorption is largely preserved, but some deficits do exist and, when combined with poor intake and disease, can lead to malnutrition (Blechman & Gelb, 1999; Nagar & Roberts, 1999).

Liver

The liver decreases in weight and size, from 4% to 2% of total body weight. Hepatic blood flow shows a 1.5% decrease per year, so that there will be a 50% reduction in flow over the life span. Hepatocyte numbers decline, but the individual hepatocytes become larger. The synthesis of clotting factors dependent on vitamin K is decreased. All ingested drugs and metabolites absorbed from the small intestine and stomach pass through the liver. Some are unchanged; others undergo metabolic detoxification by microsomal enzymes into water-soluble substances for renal excretion.

With decreases in liver mass, losses in cellular microsomal enzyme activity (primarily cytochrome P-450) are seen, and along with a decrease in blood flow, there is a decrease in the rate of biotransformation. Thus, oxidation or phase I of hepatic microsomal enzyme synthesis is the principal metabolic pathway that diminishes with age, particularly in men.

These functional changes result in prolongation in the half-life of many drugs and metabolites that are inactivated by the liver and thus increased bioavailability of those drugs that undergo extensive first-pass liver metabolism. Conjugation or phase II metabolism remains largely unchanged (i.e., glucuronidation is not altered) (Altman, 1990; Varanasi et al., 1999). There are changes in the biliary ducts; the proximal common duct dilates, and the preampullary common duct narrows. Gallbladder function is preserved, but changes in bile composition increase the risk of gallstone formation (Affronti, 1999).

Large Intestine

Although the large bowel experiences alterations in flora and transit time is generally unchanged in healthy elderly persons, colonic transit time has been implicated in the common problem of constipation in older people. Subtle anatomic changes include mucosal atrophy, glandular degeneration, hypertrophy of the muscularis mucosa, and atrophy of the muscularis externa.

ENDOCRINE SYSTEM

Thyroid

The normal thyroid secretes a relatively inactive molecule, thyroxine (T_4), which is converted peripherally to the active 3,5,3'-triiodothyronine (T_3). The secretory rate is under feedback control mediated by the secretion of thyroid-stimulating hormone (TSH) from the anterior pituitary. Thus, when insufficient T_4 is produced or there is inadequate conversion of T_4 to T_3 in peripheral tissues, the pituitary responds by putting out more TSH in an attempt to stimulate the thyroid to be more active.

There are age-related changes in circulating hormone levels, with a gradual decline seen in circulating T_3 concentrations, especially in late old age, even though T_4 does not appear to change across the life span. The inactive reverse T_3 may be elevated, but the physiological significance of the increase remains unknown. Elevated TSH secretion has been reported in persons older than 60 years of age (Mooradian & Wong, 1994; Sawin et al., 1979), but this finding is not consistent (see Chapter 11, this volume, for more discussion of thyroid disease).

Pancreas

The pancreas exhibits some moderate anatomic changes, with fat deposition and shrinkage of islet cells, but no reduction in amount or content of pancreatic fluid (Kreel & Sandin, 1973). These changes include ductal epithelial hyperplasia and intralobular fibrosis. There continues to be controversy about changes in pancreatic enzyme production, although most studies have shown no changes in the absence of disease (Martin & Ulrich, 1999).

Age-related impairment in glucose metabolism has been recognized for more than 60 years, but the mechanisms have just begun to be investigated. Most studies showed that healthy elderly respond to oral or intravenous glucose challenges with modest impairments in glucose and insulin clearance. Insulin levels are equivalent or slightly higher than those from younger challenged individuals, and peripheral insulin resistance is increasingly common because of free fatty acid deposition in muscles. These changes play a significant role in carbohydrate intolerance and the development of type 2 diabetes in aging. There is no evidence to support changes in basal hepatic glucose production or changes in insulin receptor numbers or affinity (see Table 4-3).

There continues to be controversy concerning the relative contributions of aging, obesity, genetic factors (family history of diabetes), physical exercise, diet, and diabetes-inducing drugs in senescent carbohydrate intolerance and emergence of latent diabetes. Thus, it is reasonable to assume that the observed clearance abnormalities and insulin resistance in older people may be related to many factors other than biological aging and may be influenced substantially by diet or exercise. There is also accumulating evidence that insulin resistance and abnormal triglyceride metabolism are genetically determined risk factors that, if diagnosed and treated before overt hyperglycemia is present (as early as childhood), could delay the appearance of this disease (Sinha et al., 2002).

THE NERVOUS SYSTEM

The aging nervous system is discussed in Chapter 5. Given the complexity of the nervous system, it is to be expected that there will be significant variability in the functional changes that mirror anatomic changes of aging. In general, these observations are based on cross-sectional studies and thus are open to criticism. It appears that the cognitive functions that change minimally from ages 25 to 75 years include vocabulary, information accrual, and comprehension and digit forward pass. There is a subtle change in hand two-point discrimination and minimal touch sensation loss in the fingers and toes. A greater than 20% decline is seen in "dexterity areas," including hand-foot tapping and tandem stepping. The ability to rise from a chair also decreases; however, these tasks reflect muscle as well as nervous system function and may be confounded by joint disease. Arthritic changes in the hands will produce difficulty in dexterous activities such as cutting with a knife, zipping, and buttoning. Thus, studies of function using activities of daily living (ADL) types of activities may significantly confound aging with the effects of chronic illness (Park et al., 2002).

Research has shown that there is much less neuronal loss than previous-

TABLE 4-3. Endocrine system changes in normal aging

Decreased	Increased
Insulin secretion	Insulin levels (or unchanged)
Insulin clearance	Adipose tissue with age and with obesity
Peripheral glucose utilization	Insulin resistance
No change in glucagon	

ly assumed, although brain weight declines significantly with age, and blood flow is decreased by about 20% in the absence of vascular disease. In addition, decrements are seen in cerebral autoregulation. Cells disappear randomly throughout the cortex, but in other brain areas, there is clustered loss (i.e., disproportionately greater loss of cells in the cerebellum, the locus ceruleus, and the substantia nigra). The hypothalamus, pons, and medulla have modest age-related losses (Anglade et al., 1997).

Myelin decreases primarily in the white matter of the cortex (Mielke et al., 1998; Saunders et al., 1999; Sjobeck et al., 1999). Evidence points to the role of apoptosis in brain neuron death (Sastry & Rao, 2000). Although there is cellular dropout, new synapses continue to form throughout the life span (Aamodt & Constantine-Paton, 1999). The number of spinal cord motor neurons remains essentially unchanged until about the sixth decade of life, after which losses occur in the anterior horn cells (Cruz-Sanchez et al., 1998). Vibratory and tactile thresholds decrease, and the thermal threshold in the fingers increases.

Changes in the ability to learn include decline in cognitive functions such as fluid or working memory, speed of processing, and the like; crystallized and experiential knowledge do not change. In fact, domain-specific knowledge among the intact elderly may exceed that for younger adults when different age cohorts are compared (Figure 4-1). This "wisdom" can translate into unique sources of health information and behaviors for themselves and others within their network of influence.

In the emotional domain, reductions in physical function and participation in daily activities caused by aging and disease are associated with increases in negative affect and declines in positive affect and also result in reduced assessments of health (Benyamini et al., 1999). In their meta-analysis, Benyamini and Idler (1999) showed that these reductions, in association with lowered expectations of functional ability and life expectancy, can affect the use of medical care.

IMMUNE SYSTEM

Many studies have explored the effect of aging on immune system function, often yielding conflicting results. There is general agreement that, with increasing age, there is a shift in cell populations such that the total number of immune cells does not change, but there are decreases in the number of uncommitted or "virgin" cells and increases in the number of memory cells. This occurs in most subsets of T cells (Table 4-4). Old T cells and B cells also have alterations in the density and expression of cell surface markers and immunoglobulin markers.

The functional changes in immunity with aging are much more impressive than the quantitative ones. The ability of all types of lymphocytes to grow and proliferate in response to most types of stimuli is lower in aged compared to

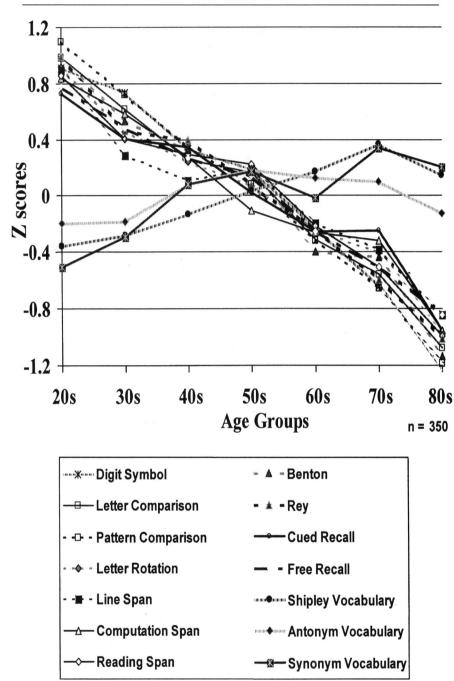

FIGURE 4-1. Processing and knowledge measures across the life span. (Adapted from Park et al., 2002.)

TABLE 4-4.   Changes in lymphocytes with age

Decreased	Increased
Number of virgin (reactive) T cells	Number of memory (inert) T cells
Number of mitogen-responsive cells	T-cell help for nonspecific antibody pro-
Stem cell generation of T cells	duction
Proliferative response	Antiidiotypic antibody production
Expression of early activation genes	Number of natural killer cells
Sensitivity to activating signals	
Cytotoxic cell target binding	
Suppressor cell function	
Help for generation of cytotoxic effector cells	
T-cell help for specific antibody production	
B-cell surface major histocompatibility complex class II molecular expression	
Number of B cells capable of clonal expansion	
Number of bone marrow B-cell precursors	
Specific antibody production	
B-cell potency	
B-cell antigen recognition	
Affinity of antibody for targets	

young individuals. One of the earliest steps in initiation of proliferation is the production of interleukin 2 (IL-2). There is impaired IL-2 production by T cells from aged individuals, reduced density of IL-2 receptors on cell surfaces, and reduced affinity of the receptors for IL-2 (Table 4-5). These declines are likely because of age-related defects in the function of various genes necessary for cell activation or signal transduction.

Changes in the production of many other interleukins have also been described in older adults, although it is unclear if these are dependent or independent of the changes in signal transduction. The result is less-than-optimal activation of the immune cascade, leading to impaired T cell helper and effector activity, fewer B cells recruited to produce antibody, and production of defective antibodies. All these changes result in reduced in vitro and in vivo antibody-dependent reactions and cell-mediated toxicity. Thus, aged individuals display less-vigorous reactions to delayed-sensitivity skin testing, decreased responses to protective immunizations, and increased susceptibility to viral and bacterial infections (Burns & Goodwin, 1997).

Theories about the causes of age-related changes in immunity have changed and developed over the years, but there still is no evidence for any one major underlying cause. Because of the marked changes in T cell function, early

TABLE 4-5.   Changes in interleukins with age

Decreased	Increased or unchanged
Expression of IL-2 mRNA	In vivo levels of IL-6
Proportion of cells expressing IL-2R	Nonspecific stimulation of T-cell IL-4 and
High-affinity binding sites for IL-2	IL-6
T cell production/secretion of IL-2	Nonspecific stimulation of T-cell IFN-γ
T cell proliferative response to IL-2	and IFN-γ mRNA
Memory T cell production of IL-4	Memory T cell production of IL-2
Sensitivity to IL-4	Lymphocyte production of IL-1 in MLC
B cell sensitivity to IL-4	Possibly lymphocyte production of IL-5
Nonspecific stimulation of lymphocyte-	Lymphocyte production of IL-10
produced IL-8	
Monocyte secretion of IL-1	
IL-2-stimulated NK cell production of IFN	
IF-12 production in tuberculosis-infected	
mouse lungs	

IFN, interferon; IL, interleukin; IL-2R, IL-2 receptor; MLC, mixed lymphocyte culture; mRNA, messenger RNA; NK, natural killer.

theories focused on the role of the thymus in maintaining immune function. The thymus gland begins to involute during adolescence, with a gradual decline in mass and thymic hormone production. By the age of 60 years, thymic hormones are undetectable in most adults. A number of studies have shown at least partial restoration of immune functions for a brief time by exposing lymphocytes from elderly adults to thymic hormones or giving elderly adults thymic hormone supplements.

Several other hormonal substances that decline with age have been studied because of their potential to reverse some of the immune declines described above. These include melatonin (Burns & Goodwin, 1997); growth hormone and its precursor, insulinlike growth factor 1 (Saito et al., 1996); and the adrenal hormone dehydroepiandrosterone (Araneo et al., 1995; Danenberg et al., 1995). However, the clinical use of these substances is controversial, and it is unlikely that thymic involution alone or changes in any one hormone are responsible for the immunological changes as there is great variability from person to person in all these parameters and in the age-related deterioration in immune function (Burns & Goodwin, 1997).

Other possible contributors to impaired immunity with aging include deficits in a variety of nutritional factors that are common in the aged. For example, the reversal of protein-calorie malnutrition and antioxidant vitamin deficiency can result in restoration of immune activity, improved vaccine response, and fewer days of illness (Chandra & Puri, 1985). However, their clinical use is still controversial. Enhanced immune responses and improved clinical outcomes have also been reported in healthy older adults given antioxidant vitamin supplements (Chandra, 1992). Aspirin and other nonsteroidal anti-inflammatory drugs have been shown to significantly improve specific immune responses because they inhibit immune-suppressing prostaglandins in adults over the age of 75 years (Meydani et al., 1994).

Investigators in the field of physiological psychology have described complex and direct links between the perceptual capabilities of the central nervous system (CNS) and the immune system. A series of elegant taste-aversion learning experiments in rats demonstrated that it is possible to elicit specific immune responses with sensory cues (Ader & Cohen, 1981). The neurohumorally mediated effects of stress on the immune system have also been well demonstrated in carefully controlled experiments with rodents and primates (Borysenko & Borysenko, 1982; Rosenberg et al., 1982). Studies in humans have demonstrated similar effects, although it is impossible to achieve the same degree of control as in the animal studies.

Health surveys have reported clusters of illness (from the common cold to cancer) occurring around the time of major life changes (Minter & Patterson-Kimball, 1978). Other studies have found strong correlations between loneliness and decreased proliferative responses of lymphocytes, decreased natural killer cell activity, and impaired DNA splicing and repair in lymphocytes (Glaser, Thorn, et al., 1985). The stress of final examinations has been correlated with rises in serum antibody titers against the herpes simplex type I virus and recurrence of cold sores (Glaser, Kiecolt-Glaser, et al., 1985) and decreased proliferation of memory T cells (Glaser et al., 1993).

Healthy adults over the age of 60 years with a strong social support system (e.g., a close confidant) have significantly greater total lymphocyte counts and stronger proliferation of lymphocytes than those without such a relationship (Thomas et al., 1989). Persons experiencing the stress of caregiving for a spouse with dementia have poorer antibody responses to influenza vaccination than matched control subjects, and their lymphocytes make less interleukin 1β and interleukin 2 when stimulated with virus in vitro (Kielcolt-Glaser et al., 1996). These caregivers also display delayed wound healing after punch biopsy of the skin compared to noncaregiving, age-matched controls (Kiecolt-Glaser et al., 1995).

Stress-induced suppression of immunity has been reversed with psychological interventions, such as writing about traumatic events and simple relaxation exercises, although the duration of the effect is unknown (Kiecolt-Glaser et al., 1985; Pennebaker et al., 1988). The mechanisms that underlie such associations, and the modulating effects of age, are not fully understood. It is also probable that nonimmune factors may affect intrinsic compartments of the immune system. For example, immunosuppression may result either from increased output of corticotropin or the gonadotropins, leading to the release of suppressive hormones such as cortisol. Lymphoid cells possess receptors for neuropeptides and other hormones, such as growth hormone, insulin, calcitonin, thyroxin, and steroids (e.g., cortisol) (Fabris, 1981). These findings suggest a number of pathways by which psychiatric illness could potentially influence immune function and so lead to clinical pathology and illness, providing a challenging area for further research.

KIDNEYS

The kidneys are one of the two major excretory systems and function via passive glomerular filtration, active tubular secretion, and reabsorption and passive tubular diffusion. Age-related changes are summarized in Table 4-6. Creatinine clearance and glomerular filtration rate decline by 40% to 50% across the lifetime. There is a modest reduction in the capacity to conserve sodium and increased osmoreceptor sensitivity, producing more vasopressin and water retention. Thus, the elderly are prone to develop the syndrome of inappropriate antidiuretic hormone (SIADH) secretion.

Normal creatinine levels in an elderly patient may be misleading because the decline of muscle mass with aging may lead to a decline in serum creatinine despite loss of kidney function (Table 4-7). Although blood urea nitrogen (BUN) and creatinine may be elevated very late in life because of age-related declines in renal function (Rowe et al., 1976; Wesson, 1969), when circulating levels of BUN and creatinine rise before the ninth decade, it can be assumed there is significant pathology along with age-related changes in kidney function. If BUN is elevated alone, this may represent prerenal failure indicative of other illness-related processes without renal dysfunction (Clark, 2000). The decline in renal function has serious implications for drug prescribing patterns in the elderly (Finch & Schneider, 1985; Kenney, 1989).

TABLE 4-6.   Renal system changes with aging

Normal aging	Disease related
Decreased creatinine clearance (7.5–10 mL/min/decade)	Decreased efficiency of drug clearance
Decreased renal blood flow	Prolonged drug half-life
Decreased maximum urine osmolality	Higher circulating drug levels
Decreased acidification and handling of acid load	
Decreased renin response to volume depletion or low sodium	
Decreased hydroxylation of vitamin D	
Decreased metabolism of parathyroid hormone, calcitonin, glucagon	

TABLE 4-7.   Normal aging and renal function

Age (years)	CrCl (mL/min/1.73 m^2)	Serum Cr (mg/100 mL)
25–34	140 ± 2.5	0.81 ± 0.01
35–44	133 ± 1.8	0.81 ± 0.01
45–54	127 ± 1.4	0.83 ± 0.01
55–64	120 ± 1.7	0.84 ± 0.01
65–74	110 ± 2.0	0.83 ± 0.01
75–84	97 ± 2.9	0.84 ± 0.02

Source: Modified from Rowe et al. (1976).
Cr, creatinine; CrCl, creatinine clearance.

THE REPRODUCTIVE SYSTEM

Changes in Women

Aging of the ovary begins in utero and continues throughout the life span. Potential germ cells reach maturation in the ovaries during gestation and undergo massive attrition prior to birth, declining from a population of 10×10^6 cells at the organogenesis of the ovary to 10^6 at parturition. This steady decline in functional cell number continues until pubescence, when there remains a population of about 10,000 cells available for impregnation. The attrition of these cells continues, but at a slower rate, throughout the female's reproductive period with its monthly cyclicity and interruptions for pregnancy (Nicosia, 1983).

The maturation of germ cells and the production of ovarian hormones are controlled by a positive-feedback loop between the brain and the gonads; hormones (luteinizing hormone [LH] and follicular-stimulating hormone [FSH]) secreted by the anterior pituitary regulate the follicular ripening of ova and the production of the ovarian hormones estrogen and progesterone. These hormones in turn exert negative feedback to the pituitary, controlling production of gonadotropins. Follicles containing the mature ovum and capable of synthesizing estrogen and progesterone continue to decrease in number, so that at the climacteric, there are too few remaining to produce adequate circulating hormones to stimulate not only the gonad-dependent end organs such as the breasts and genitalia (and trabecular bone of the vertebrae), but also to participate in the negative-feedback cycling with the pituitary. As estrogenic stimulation declines, females begin to experience the effects of hormonal deficiency, including atrophy of the breasts and genitalia and vasomotor instability.

The reduction in estrogen and progesterone results, finally, in the cessation of menstruation or the menopause and an uninhibited production of the pituitary gonadotropic hormones. All women show elevations in circulating pituitary gonadotropic hormones (LH and FSH) after they enter the perimenopausal period between the ages of 40 and 55, the physiological significance of which is not clear (Barbo, 1987; Mastroianni & Paulsen, 1986). After the menopause, with loss of the protective effects of estrogen and progesterone, there is greater vulnerability to stroke, coronary artery disease, and osteoporosis-associated diseases (Greendale & Judd, 1993).

Changes in Men

Men show significantly less attrition of testicular structures compared to the decline of the ovaries in females, and slower declines in hormonal synthesis and secretion. The potential sperm cells remain at a primitive level into adulthood, arrested at the spermatogonium stage within the testis. The process of maturation to mature sperm continues throughout the lifetime of most men, although sperm production decreases, and those found in older testes have a greater frequency of chromosomal abnormalities. Degeneration also occurs in the seminiferous tubules; there are fewer Leydig cells, and more aberrant nuclei are seen in Sertoli cells.

Total, free, and bioavailable testosterone levels decrease because sex-hormone-binding globulin increases with age, causing some degree of testicular failure. In many men, the negative-feedback loop between the testes and the anterior pituitary is unchanged until the eighth decade; elevated gonadotropic hormones are rarely seen before the age of 70 and, if elevated, LH may be less bioactive. Thus, in males, the pattern is somewhat analogous to the age-related changes in the thyroid described above. TSH and LH both increase without corresponding changes in T_4 and testosterone, respectively. FSH generally follows a pattern similar to that of LH. In the normal population, a few individuals in their late 40s and 50s have elevated levels of FSH, but the majority do not have increased levels until their 70s (Rowland et al., 1993; Stearns et al., 1974).

SEXUAL FUNCTION

The mature adult's need for intimacy, affection, and social interaction does not diminish with time, and interest in sexual activity remains a major component of the quality in life. Declines in sexual activity are related directly to physical and mental health status or availability of a partner.

Female Sexuality

The relationship of sexuality to the menopause is not clear. Estrogen deficiency does produce significant changes in the vaginal tissues, with increased fragility and decreased elasticity, lubrication, and vaginal blood flow. These changes can lead to dyspareunia and bleeding and thus decreased interest in intercourse. There is reduced vaginal vasocongestion and breast engorgement during excitation, fewer uterine contractions during orgasm, and more rapid return to the unaroused state. However, these changes are less marked in sexually active women. A study of midlife women demonstrated an increase in sexual behavior after menopause; this was associated with reduced fear of pregnancy and stable relationships (Gelfand, 2000; Kingsberg, 2000).

Male Sexuality

Sexual activity and enjoyment extend throughout the life span. In the original studies of sexual behavior by Masters and Johnson (1966), there was no upper age limit for sexual function, although many studies of aging men report a decline in frequency of intercourse, with satisfaction confounded by social, psychological, physiological, and cultural factors (Bortz et al., 1999). Age-related alterations in the sexual response cycle may include delayed erection during the excitement phase, reductions in scrotal tensing and vasocongestion, prolongation of the plateau phase, and reduced preejaculatory secretion. The orgasm tends to be shorter, contractions and ejaculatory force are reduced, and the resolution phase is more rapid. There may be increased cross linkages in the penile collagenous tissues, reducing the compliance of the corpus cavernosa and decreasing venous occlusion. Testosterone levels are important for libido and affect; thus, males with early hypogonadism report impotence, erectile dysfunction, fatigue, and irritability. Although most common after the age of 80 years, testosterone deficiency can be seen in younger males in the absence of chronic illness (Morley & Perry, 1999).

AGING CHANGES IN SLEEP PATTERNS

Sleep is defined by sleep structure (stages of sleep), sleep patterns (amount and timing of sleep), and subjective reports. There appear to be at least two rhythmic patterns that control sleep. One is represented by light-dependent, calendar-associated circadian rhythms that may be responsive to exogenous and endogenous melatonin; the second is represented by innate CNS-mediated sleep cycle changes. Aging changes occur in both of these. In normal aging, the stages of sleep change dramatically. Older adults take longer to fall asleep and awaken more frequently during sleep cycles; their overall time asleep is decreased, and their sleep efficiency and the depth of sleep are both reduced.

Comparisons of tracings of sleep electroencephalograms (EEGs) between different age cohorts showed that neonates sleep nearly all the time, they have few and short periods of rapid eye movement (REM), and they awaken or are aroused rarely, for short periods, primarily for feeding and when physically uncomfortable. Infants spend most of their time in stage IV or deep sleep. As an individual matures to young adulthood (adolescence through 30 or 40 years of age), a second sleep EEG pattern predominates. There is significantly less stage IV deep sleep, more REM, and mostly sleep at stage II, with few arousal periods (Dijk, 1999).

The pattern for a healthy, elderly individual is significantly different. Stage IV sleep is essentially absent, replaced by stage II. There is both a reduction in REM and a dramatic increase in arousal periods throughout the sleep cycle (Ficca, 1999). This may represent a functional change based on loss of cells in the locus ceruleus (Dement et al., 1985).

These alterations in sleep patterns are a source of much concern for up to 50% of persons 60 years and older, with 12% of an epidemiological sample of persons older than 65 years reporting significant and chronic insomnia. Aging individuals believe they do not sleep very well and insist they are up all night. Indeed, they are frequently aroused, but the total amount of sleep that occurs during the night is essentially unchanged. Up to half of community-dwelling elderly persons use either over-the-counter or prescription sleeping medications. Those that have been studied have been shown to have sleep aberrations on monitoring. On the other hand, older women appear to have better preservation of slow-wave sleep than older men (Fukuda, 1999).

Severe insomnia is associated with chronic illness: congestive heart failure, obstructive airway disease, prostate problems, systemic hypertension, diabetes, rheumatic diseases (Katz & McHorney, 1998). Insomnia is associated with an increased use of medical services (Benca & Quintas, 1997; Lavie, 1981). Compared to good sleepers, insomniacs visit their primary physicians and other health professionals significantly more often, use more treatments or medications (cardiovascular, CNS, gastrointestinal, and urogenital), and are hospitalized more than twice as often (Léger et al., 2002).

Clinicians are well aware of the strong association between depression and sleep problems (insomnia or hypersomnia). The presence of insomnia or hypersomnia is one of the diagnostic criteria of the *Diagnostic and Statistical Manual of Mental Disorders*, Fourth Edition (*DSM-IV*; American Psychiatric Association, 1994) for depressive episodes and major depression. But, in the United States, few primary care physicians inquire about their patients' sleep and, when presented with a problem of insomnia, most do not inquire about potential causes (Everit & Avorn, 1990; Simon et al., 1996). And, most health professionals (general practitioners, nurses, specialists) lack basic knowledge, training, and updates on sleep disorders (Kryger et al., 1999).

As a result, insomnia is often mistreated. Medical guidelines for the treatment of insomnia recommend prescribing benzodiazepines (BDZs) for about 4 weeks (Consensus Conference, 1984); however, most BDZ and other hypnotic use is chronic. In the United States, the chronic use of hypnotics was estimated to range from 10% to 30% (Gallup Organization, 1991). The likelihood of chronic use of BDZs was significantly higher in insomniacs than in other BDZ users (Simon et al., 1996).

Less than 4 weeks of treatment with hypnotics is recommended for acute transient insomnias. However, most patients with chronic insomnia assume that treatment is acceptable on a chronic basis, and transient and acute periods often go untreated. Excessive prescribing of hypnotic medications is common for older patients and can increase vulnerability to confusion and delirium as well as addiction. Thus, it may be inappropriate to prescribe hypnotics except in times of extreme stress or during hospitalization or sickness.

Other nonpharmacological interventions to facilitate good "sleep hygiene" need to be utilized to treat this maladaptive response to normal aging. For chronic primary insomnia, as well as for drug-dependency insomnia, behavioral-cognitive treatments (BCTs) address strategies to eliminate perpetuating factors (for example, dysfunctional sleep hygiene). In studies that have looked at pharmacological treatments in comparison to BCT, the clinical gains on BCT are greater for total sleep time; tolerance, rebound insomnia, and dependence are often reported, but have not been documented. Although the treatment is more time consuming and costly and gains are slower with BCTs, improvements last longer after the end of treatment, and there are no known side effects. Positive results of BCT in the elderly have been documented (e.g., Morin, 1993; Morin et al., 1994, 1999).

SUMMARY

Significant cell- and organ-specific biological changes occur at different rates within and between aging individuals; these changes lead to functional decline. The ability to respond to stress becomes compromised, yet in the absence of significant chronic disease, functional independence can be maintained well into the ninth decade. Understanding these aging patterns is particularly relevant for the psychiatrist, who must appreciate the limited reserve of the older patients, the fragility of the immune response, and the increased vulnerability to medications of all types and yet respect the remarkable resilience of the elderly "survivor."

REFERENCES

Aamodt SM, Constantine-Paton M. The role of neural activity in synaptic development and its implications for adult brain function. *Adv Neurol.* 1999;79:133–144.

Ader R, Cohen N. Conditioned immunopharmacologic responses. In: Ader R, ed. *Psychoneuroimmunology.* Orlando, FL: Academic Press; 1981:281–317.

Affronti J. Biliary disease in the elderly patient. *Clin Geriatr Med.* 1999;15:571–572.

Altman DF. Changes in gastrointestinal, pancreatic, biliary and hepatic function with aging. *Gastroenterol Clin North Am.* 1990;19:227–234.

American Psychiatric Association. *Diagnostic and Statistical Manual of Mental Disorders.* 4th ed. Washington, DC: American Psychiatric Association; 1994.

Anderson RN, Kochanek KD, Murphy SI. Report of final mortality statistics, 1995. *Monthly Vital Stat Rep.* 1997;45(11 supp 2).

Reference entries preceded by an asterisk are recommended reading.

Anglade P, Vyas S, Hirsch EC, Agid Y. Apoptosis in dopaminergic neurons of the human substantia nigra during normal aging. *Histol Histopathol.* 1997;12:603–610.

Araneo B, Dowell T, Woods ML, et al. DHEAS as an effective vaccine adjuvant in elderly humans. Proof-of-principle studies. *Ann N Y Acad Sci.* 1995;774:232–248.

Arking R. *Biology of Aging: Observations and Principles.* 2nd ed. Sunderland, MA: Sinauer Associates; 1998.

Barbo, DM. The physiology of the menopause in the postmenopausal woman. *Med Clin North Am,* 1987;71:11–22.

*Benca R, Quintas J. Sleep and host defenses: a review. *Sleep.* 1997;20:1027–1037.

Benyamini Y, Idler EL. Community studies reporting association between self-rated health and mortality: additional studies, 1995 to 1998. *Res Aging.* 1999;21:392–401.

Benyamini Y, Leventhal EA, Leventhal H. Self-assessments of health: what do people know that predicts their mortality? *Res Aging.* 1999;21:477–500.

Blechman MB, Gelb AM. Aging and gastrointestinal physiology. *Clin Geriatr Med.* 1999;15:429–438.

Bortz WM 2nd, Wallace DH, Wiley D. Sexual function in 1,202 aging males: differentiating aspects. *J Gerontol A Biol Sci Med Sci.* 1999;54:M237–M241.

Borysenko M, Borysenko J. Stress, behavior and immunity: animal models and mediating mechanisms. *Gen Hosp Psychiatry.* 1982;4:59–67.

*Burns EA, Goodwin JS. Immunodeficiency of aging. *Drugs Aging.* 1997;11:374–397.

Chandra RK. Effect of vitamin and trace-element supplementation on immune responses and infection in elderly subjects. *Lancet.* 1992;340:1124–1127.

Chandra RK, Puri S. Nutritional support improves antibody response to influenza vaccine in the elderly. *BMJ.* 1985;291:709.

*Clark B. Biology of renal aging in humans. *Adv Ren Replace Ther.* 2000;7:11–21.

Cruz-Sanchez FF, Moral A, Tolosa E, de Belleroche J, Rossi ML. Evaluation of neuronal loss, astrocytosis and abnormalities of cytoskeletal components of large motor neurons in the human anterior horn in aging. *J Neural Transm.* 1998;105:689–701.

Danenberg HD, Ben-Yehuda A, Zakay-Rones Z, et al. DHEA treatment reverses the impaired immune response of old mice to influenza vaccination and protects from influenza infection. *Vaccine.* 1995;13:1445–1448.

*Dement W, Richardson G, Prinz P, Carskadon M, Kripke D, Czeisler C. Changes of sleep and wakefulness with age. In: Finch C, Schneider EL, eds. *Handbook of the Biology of Aging.* 2nd ed. New York, NY: Van Nostrand Reinhold; 1985:692–720.

Diabetes Prevention Program Research Group (DPPRG). Reduction in the incidence of type 2 diabetes with lifestyle intervention or metformin. *N Engl J Med.* 2002;346:393–403.

Dijk DJ. Circadian regulation of human sleep and age-related changes in its timing consolidation and EEG characteristics. *Ann Med.* 1999;31:130–140.

*Consensus Conference. Drugs and insomnia: the use of medications to promote sleep. *JAMA.* 1984;251:2410–2414.

Everitt DE, Avorn J. Clinical decision-making in the evaluation and treatment of insomnia. *Am J Med.* 1990;89:357–362.

Fabris N. Body homeostatic mechanisms and aging of the immune system. In: Kay M, Makinodan T, eds. *CRC Handbook of Immunology in Aging.* Boca Raton, FL: CRC Press; 1981.

Ficca G. The organization of rapid eye movement activity during rapid eye movement sleep is impaired in the elderly. *Neurosci Lett.* 1999;275:219–221.

Finch CE, Schneider EL. *Handbook of Biology of Aging.* Vol. 2. 2nd ed. New York, NY: Van Nostrand Reinhold; 1985.

Folkow B, Svanborg A. Physiology of cardiovascular aging. *Physiol Rev.* 1993;73:725–764.

Fukuda N. Gender difference of slow wave sleep in middle aged and elderly subjects. *Psychiatry Clin Neurosci.* 1999;53:151–153.

Gallup Organization. *Sleep in America: 1991.* Princeton, NJ: Gallup Organization; 1991.

Gelfand MM. Sexuality among older women. *J Womens Health Gend Based Med.* 2000; 9(suppl 1):S15–S20.

Glaser R, Kiecolt-Glaser JK, Speicher CE, et al. The relationship of stress and loneliness and changes in herpes virus latency. *J Behav Med.* 1985;8:249–260.

Glaser R, Pearson GR, Bonneau RH, et al. Stress and the memory T cell response to the Epstein-Barr virus in healthy medical students. *Health Psychol.* 1993;12:435–442.

Glaser R, Thorn BE, Tarr KL, et al. Effects of stress on methyltransferase synthesis: an important DNA repair enzyme. *Health Psychol.* 1985;4:403–412.

Greendale GA, Judd HL. The menopause: health implications and clinical management. *J Am Geriatr Soc.* 1993;41:426–436.

*Harman D. The aging process: major risk factor for disease and death. *Proc Natl Acad Sci U S A.* 1991;88:5360–5363.

Jazwinski SM. Longevity, genes, and aging. *Science.* 1996;273:54–59.

Katz DA, McHorney C. Clinical correlates of insomnia in patients with chronic illnesses. *Arch Intern Med.* 1998;158:1099–1107.

*Kenney AR. *Physiology of Aging: A Synopsis.* 2nd ed. Chicago, IL: Year Book Medical Publishers; 1989.

Kenny AM. Osteoporosis. Pathogenesis. *Rheum Dis Clin North Am.* 2000;26;569–591.

Kielcolt-Glaser JK, Glaser R, Gravenstein S, Malarkey WB, Sheridan J. Chronic stress alters the immune response to influenza virus vaccine in older adults. *Proc Natl Acad Sci U S A.* 1996;93:3043–3047.

Kiecolt-Glaser JK, Glaser R, Williger D, et al. Psychosocial enhancement of immuno-competence in a geriatric population. *Health Psychol.* 1985;4:25–41.

Kiecolt-Glaser JK, Marucha PT, Malarkey WH, et al. Slowing of wound healing by psychological stress. *Lancet.* 1995;346:1194–1196.

Kingsberg SA. The psychological impact of aging on sexuality and relationships. *J Womens Health Gend Based Med.* 2000;9(suppl 1):S33–S38.

Kirkwood TBL. Human senescence. *Bioessays.* 1996;18:1009–1016.

Kligman AM, Grove GL, Balin AK. Aging of human skin. In Finch CE, Schneider EL, eds. *Handbook of Biology of Aging*, Vol. 2. 2nd ed. New York, NY: Van Nostrand Reinhold; 1985:820–841.

Kreel L, Sandin B. Changes in pancreatic morphology associated with aging. *Gut.* 1973; 14:962.

Kryger M, Lavie P, Rosen R. Recognition and diagnosis of insomnia. *Sleep.* 1999; 22(supp 3):S421–S426.

*Lakatta EG. Cardiovascular function and age. *Geriatrics.* 1987;42;84–94.

Lakatta EG. Heart and circulation. In: Finch CE, Schneider EL, eds. *Handbook of Biol-*

ogy of Aging. Vol. 2. 2nd ed. New York, NY: Van Nostrand Reinhold; 1985: 377–414.

Lavie P. Sleep habits and sleep disturbances in industrial workers in Israel: main findings and some characteristics of workers complaining of excessive daytime sleepiness. *Sleep.* 1981;4;147–158.

Léger D, Guilleminault C, Biol DS, Bader G, Levy E, Paiiard M. Medical and socio-professional impact of insomnia. *Sleep.* 2002;25:625–629.

*Leventhal EA, Burns EA. Immune dysfunction in the elderly and the occurrence of cancer: aging and the insults of a lifetime of living. In: Dammacco F, ed. *Tumor Immunology and Immunoregulation by Thymic Hormones.* Milan, Italy: Masson; 1987:41–56.

*Leventhal H, Idler EL, Leventhal EA. The impact of chronic illness on the self system. In: Contrada RJ, Ashmore RD, eds. *Self, Social Identity and Physical Health: Influences of Illness on Self and Identity.* Oxford, UK: Oxford University Press; 1999: 185–208.

Loesche WJ, Bromberg J, Terpenning MS, et al. Xerostomia, xerogenic medications and food avoidances in selected geriatric groups. *J Am Geriatr Soc.* 1995;43:401–407.

Marin J. Age-related changes in vascular responses: a review. *Mech Ageing Dev.* 1995; 79:71–114.

Martin SP, Ulrich CD. Pancreatic disease in the elderly. *Clin Geriatr Med.* 1999;15: 579–580.

Masters WH, Johnson VE. *Human Sexual Response.* Boston, MA: Little, Brown; 1966.

Mastrioanni L, Paulsen CA. *The Climacteric.* New York, NY: Plenum Press; 1986.

Meydani SN, Leka L, Loszewski R. Long-term vitamin E supplementation enhances immune response in healthy elderly. *FASEB J.* 1994;8:A274.

Mielke R, Kessler J, Szelies B, Herholz K, Wienhard K, Heiss WD. Normal and pathological aging—findings of positron-emission tomography. *J Neural Transm.* 1998; 105:821–837.

Minter RE, Patterson-Kimball C. Life events and illness onset: a review. *Psychosomatics.* 1978;19:334–339.

Mooradian AD, Wong NC. Age-related changes in thyroid hormone action. *Eur J Endocrinol.* 1994;131(15):451–461.

Morin C. *Insomnia: Psychological Assessment and Management.* New York, NY: Guilford Press; 1993.

Morin CM, Culbert JP, Schwartz SM. Nonpharmacological intervention for insomnia: a meta-analysis of treatment efficacy. *Am J Psychiatry.* 1994;151;1172–1180.

*Morin M, Colecchi C, Stone J, Sood R, Brimk D. Behavioral and pharmacological therapies for late-life insomnia: a randomized controlled trial. *JAMA.* 1999;281: 991–999.

Morley JE, Perry HM 3rd. Androgen deficiency in aging men. *Med Clin North Am.* 1999;83:vii, 1279–1289.

Morley JE, Reese SS. Clinical implications of the aging heart. *Am J Med.* 1989;86: 77–86.

Nagar A, Roberts IM. Small bowel diseases in the elderly. *Clin Geriatr Med.* 1999;15: 473–478.

Nicosia SV. Morphological changes in the human ovary throughout life. In: Serra GB, ed. *The Ovary.* New York, NY: Raven Press; 1983:57–81.

*Park DC, Lautenschlager G, Hedden T, Davidson NS, Smith AD, Smith PK. Models of visuospatial and verbal memory across the adult life span. *Psychol Aging.* 2002;17: 299–320.

Pennebaker JW, Kiecolt-Glaser JK, Glaser R. Disclosure of traumas and immune function: health implications for psychotherapy. *J Consult Clin Psychol.* 1988;56:239–245.

Raiz LG. The osteoporosis revolution. *Ann Intern Med.* 1997;126:458–462.

Rodeheffer RJ, Gerstenblith G, Becker LC, Fleg JL, Weisfeldt ML, Lakatta EG. Exercise cardiac output is maintained with advancing age in healthy human subjects: cardiac dilatation and increased stroke volume compensate for a diminished heart rate. *Circulation.* 1984;69:203–213.

Rosenberg LT, Coe CL, Levine S. Complement levels in the squirrel monkey. *Lab Anim Sci.* 1982;32:371–372.

Rossi A, Ganassini A, Tantucci C, et al. Aging and the respiratory system. *Aging (Milano).* 1996;8(3):143–161.

Rowe JW, Andres R, Tobin JD, Norris AH, Shock NW. The effect of age on creatinine clearance in man: a cross-sectional and longitudinal study. *J Gerontol.* 1976;31: 155–163.

Rowe JW, Kahn RL. *Successful Aging.* New York, NY: Pantheon Press; 1998.

Rowland DL, Greenleaf WJ, Dorfman LJ, et al. Aging and sexual function in men. *Arch Sex Behav.* 1993;22:545–557.

Saito H, Inoue T, Fukatsu K, et al. Growth hormone and the immune response to bacterial infection. *Hormone Res.* 1996;45:50–54.

Sallout H, Mayoral W, Benjamin SB. The aging esophagus. *Clin Geriatr Med.* 1999:15: 439–456.

Sastry PS, Rao KS. Apoptosis and the nervous system. *J Neurochem.* 2000;74:1–20.

Saunders DE, Howe FA, van den Boogaart A, Griffiths JR, Brown MM. Aging of the adult human brain: in vivo quantitation of metabolite content with proton magnetic resonance spectroscopy. *J Magn Reson Imaging.* 1999;9:711–716.

Sawin CT, Chopra D, Azizi F, Mannix JE, Bacharach P. The aging thyroid: increased prevalence of elevated serum thyrotropin levels in the elderly. *JAMA.* 1979;242: 247–250.

Semsei I. On the nature of aging. *Mech Ageing Dev.* 2000;117:93–108.

Simon G, Von Korff M, Barlow W, Pabiniak C, Wagner E. Predictors of chronic BDZ use in a health maintenance organization sample. *J Clin Epidemiol.* 1996;9:1067–1073.

Sinha R, Fisch G, Teague B, et al. Prevalence of impaired glucose tolerance among children and adolescents with marked obesity. *N Engl J Med.* 2002;346:802–810.

Sjobeck M, Dahlen S, Englund E. Neuronal loss in the brainstem and cerebellum—part of the normal aging process? A morphometric study of the vermis cerebelli and inferior olivary nucleus. *J Gerontol A Biol Sci Med Sci.* 1999;54:B363–B368.

Stearns EL, MacDonnell JA, Kaufman BJ, et al. Declining testicular function with age. *Am J Med.* 1974;57:761–766.

Thomas PD, Goodwin JM, Goodwin JS. Effect of social support on stress-related changes in cholesterol level, uric acid level and immune function in an elderly sample. *Am J Psychiatry.* 1985;142:735–737.

Tockman MS. Aging of the respiratory system. In: Hazzard WR, Andres R, Bierman EL, Blass JP. *Principles of Geriatric Medicine and Gerontology.* 3rd ed. New York, NY: McGraw-Hill; 1994:555–564.

Varanasi RV, Varanasi SG, Howell CD. Liver diseases. *Clin Geriatr Med.* 1999;15:559–561.

Warner HR, Hodes RJ, Pocinki K. What does cell death have to do with aging? *J Am Geriatr Soc.* 1997;45:1140–1146.

Wesson LG. *Physiology of the Human Kidney.* New York, NY: Grune and Stratton; 1969.

Yaar M. Cellular and molecular mechanisms of cutaneous aging. *J Dermatol Surg Oncol.* 1990;16:915–922.

5

Normal Aging: Changes in Cognitive Abilities

Mark P. Rubert, PhD
David A. Loewenstein, PhD
Carl Eisdorfer, PhD, MD

What is normal aging? The answer to this question has been changing as the average life span has continued to lengthen throughout the last century (National Center for Health Statistics, 1993). Now advertisements show active older adults enjoying their lives because they drink Sustacal, and older couples tell us how Viagra has improved their sex lives. It has been suggested that the aging of the baby boom generation is behind some of this shift in the societal view of aging, and that this trend will accelerate as the baby boomers attempt to stave off the physical and psychological changes associated with aging because the early boomers are growing close to 60 years old.

In part, the changes that occur with aging are the result of gradual decline in the function of various organ systems, with many organ systems losing function at the rate of about 1% per year after 30 years of age. However, the effects of aging are not solely the result of biological changes. Increasing age is also associated with changes in cognitive function as a result of reduction of the number of neurons within the brain, particularly in the hippocampus, frontal-striatal regions, and specific areas of the cerebral cortex. In addition, increased stress on organ systems vital to blood circulation may affect cognition and decrease sensory and perceptual abilities.

As a person grows older, all five senses decline in acuity (Carman, 1997; Zarit & Zarit, 1987). Vision and auditory loss are frequently the most problematic for older persons (Loewenstein & Eisdorfer, 1992; Orr, 1991). For example, a reduction in visual acuity can result in decreased independence by affecting the person's ability to drive an automobile and navigate familiar and unfamiliar locations. As vision worsens, the individual may lose the ability to read and to pursue hobbies such as needlepoint. In a similar manner, decreased hearing can pose substantial problems with regard to the individual's autonomy and can lead to increased isolation from others. Such changes lead to alterations in vision, taste, and cognitive capacity; these changes occur to a lesser extent than is commonly believed and may be at least somewhat mitigated by initial ability, practice, exercise, medication, or other lifestyle changes (Finch & Tanzi, 1997; La Rue, 1999; Loewenstein & Eisdorfer, 1992; Zarit & Zarit, 1987).

The psychological changes associated with aging are the product of alterations in anatomy and physiology as well as changes in social status (e.g., retirement) and interpersonal factors (e.g., loss of friends or widowhood). In addition, certain physiological insults or trauma show cumulative effects with age and may directly or indirectly affect performance (e.g., occupational noise exposure is associated with hearing loss). Certain environmental stressors, such as financial problems, crime, reduced standard of living, and other life stage problems (e.g., moving to a new living situation), are also more likely to occur as one grows older. Further, factors such as exercise, diet, health care utilization, and other socioeconomic and cultural differences between older and younger adults result in lifestyle differences and cohort effects that appear as age-related changes in late life. Generalizations about age-related changes can be made, but care must be taken as individual differences also increase with age (Eisdorfer & Mintzer, 1988).

COGNITIVE ABILITIES

The study of the intellectual changes resulting from normal psychological aging is challenging. For example, longitudinal studies with the elderly are difficult because the majority of the subjects in a study may have risk factors associated with cognitive decline, such as hypertension (Cullum et al., 2000). In addition, educational attainment (Ardilla et al., 2000), health and nutrition as an infant and child (Leon, 1998; Sorensenson, 1997), and even exposure to certain illnesses make it difficult to study individuals in different age and ethnocultural groups because cohort effects may confound or bias many of the dependent measures due to an enhanced probability of disease and an increased likelihood of attrition through illness or death (Loewenstein & Eisdorfer, 1992; Schaie, 1988).

These difficulties not withstanding, the results of research indicate that many of the intellectual declines associated with aging are a function of psychomotor slowing and declines in sensory-perceptual abilities. In addition, increased anxiety may cause poor performance in some older persons in formal testing situations (Wetherell et al., 2002).

Intellectual Functions

The extensive literature on changes in intellectual performance with aging indicates that abilities peak in the 30s, plateau through the 50s or early 60s, and then begin a slow, but increasingly rapid, decline in the late 70s (Botwinick, 1977; Cunningham, 1987; Schaie, 1980). However, changes in intelligence as a function of age may be confounded by cohort effects as many of these studies had cross-sectional designs (Loewenstein & Eisdorfer, 1992; Rabbitt, 1979). Studies that looked at change longitudinally showed marked individual variability and suggested that decline in functioning may be the result of factors such as depression and other physical maladies rather than the result of normal aging (Cullum et al., 2000; Hassing et al., 2002; Jarvik & Bank, 1983; Rabbit et al., 2002).

Despite the belief that older adults are unable to learn new information, or the "you can't teach an old dog new tricks" hypothesis, research has shown that older adults are able to learn and can benefit from the use of encoding strategies. They also can benefit from longer exposure to the to-be-remembered stimuli and may benefit from techniques designed to enhance their motivation. Spar and La Rue (2002) concluded that cognitive functions such as attention span; everyday communication skills; lexical, phonological, and syntactic knowledge; discourse comprehension; and simple visual perception remain preserved in older adults. On the other hand, selective attention, cognitive flexibility and the ability to shift cognitive sets, naming objects, verbal fluency, more complex visuoconstructive skills, and logical analysis may decrease with age.

Cross-sectional data on the intellectual functioning of 1,628 community-dwelling individuals, who were typically well educated, with good jobs, with middle incomes, and with ages that ranged from 29 to 88 years, were reported by Schaie and Willis (1993). Age-related performance declines began around age 50 years for inductive reasoning, spatial orientation, verbal memory, and perceptual speed. Differences in numeric and verbal abilities appeared in the later 60s, and performance on all tasks declined in the 80s, with the largest performance decline in the perceptual speed tasks and the least in the vocabulary tasks. Hultsch and colleagues (1992) found age-related declines in working memory, verbal fluency, and world knowledge, even when cohort effects were controlled statistically.

A two-factor model of intelligence has been used to account for the differential decline in intellectual skills by distinguishing between crystallized and fluid abilities (Horn & Cattell, 1967; Horn & Donaldson, 1976). Crystallized abilities are represented by knowledge acquired during the person's lifetime; as indicated above, several studies indicated that these abilities improve or remain consistent until late in life. In contrast, fluid abilities are represented by the ability to solve new tasks by the acquisition of new knowledge and new skills. Salthouse (1999) reported a significant decline in many fluid abilities between the ages of 25 and 75 years, but crystallized abilities remained stable or improved until well into the 80s.

Such differences in types of abilities can also help explain the lack of consistent findings on the relationship of age to work performance. Given the declines in inductive reasoning, spatial orientation, verbal memory, and perceptual speed, it could be expected that the work performance of the older person would decline. However, both a review of the literature (Rhodes, 1983) and a meta-analysis of 65 studies (McEvoy & Cascio, 1989) failed to find a clear relationship between age and work performance, although those studies generally did not discriminate between the nature of the job and the years of experience the individual had performing that job. Years of job experience lead to the crystallization of abilities such that they do not decline much with age and, in fact, may demonstrate improvement with age due to the years of practice.

Jobs that demand more fluid abilities should demonstrate more impairment in the performance of the older worker. One example of how this change in fluid ability may have an impact on an older person's life was seen when women from 25 to 70 years were asked to learn a computer-based task. Increased age was associated with longer response times and more errors, and the older women felt the task was more difficult and more tiring (Czaja & Sharit, 1993). Another study found that skilled older typists did not show age-related slowing in their motor performance, but that unskilled older typists (fluid ability) were slower than younger unskilled typists (Bosman, 1993).

The concept of brain reserve capacity that has been used to account for intraindividual differences in response to head injury and dementia may also be relevant to the study of normal aging. It has been noted by many researchers that there are large individual differences in response to aging, both in the biological and cognitive systems. The concepts of reserve capacity and threshold in dementia are taken from the Newcastle studies, which first raised the possibility of individual differences to account for differences between postmortem findings and other measures of dementia (Blessed et al., 1968; Roth et al., 1967). Satz (1993) reviewed the research in brain reserve capacity and found that bright, well-educated patients—factors that are presumably reflective of higher levels of reserve capacity—retained more of their abilities in the face of organic impairments relative to less-educated patients.

Salthouse and Ferrer-Caja (2003) suggested that age-related declines in processing speed, memory, and reasoning may reflect different underlying structural changes. This may help explain why interindividual variability in performance on intelligence and memory tasks increases with advancing age (Christensen et al., 1994) and why factors other than age have been found to account for much of the variance in test performance (Avolio & Waldman, 1994). Other studies of normal older adults found that chronological age is probably a variable that mediates the presentation of other disorders, such as dementia, and that it has minimal independent predictive power (Piquet et al., 2002). This suggests that the intellectual declines associated with aging may be the result of other influences (e.g., ethnoracial, social, and environmental variables) that disturb and disrupt an individual's cognitive/intellectual functioning in middle and old age.

Memory Functions

When older adults complain about their cognitive functions, they most often cite difficulties with memory (Guterman et al., 1993; Williams et al., 1983). While there are changes in memory associated with aging, the actual deterioration among healthy adults is not nearly as extensive as once thought (Zarit & Zarit, 1987), and it may be that the brain makes changes that can help compensate for declines in memory performance (Grady & Craik, 2000). The failure to appreciate that memory impairment was the result of neurodegenerative diseases or other medical or neuropsychiatric conditions (Cullum et al., 2000; Hassing et al., 2002) led to the erroneous belief in the past that significant memory problems were a normal result of aging. Therefore, it is quite important to avoid overinterpretation of small changes in memory (La Rue, 1999).

Those individuals who have subjective memory complaints but have no objective impairments in neuropsychological performance tend to demonstrate relatively stable performance in the next couple of years if they remain in good health (Youngjohn & Crook, 1993). Another group of older adults exhibit memory complaints, demonstrate memory performance that is 1 standard deviation or more below the performance of younger normal adults, and do not have any intellectual or other cognitive impairments. This may be referred to as age-associated memory impairment or age-related cognitive change; it was previously defined as benign senescent forgetfulness and is usually not associated with longitudinal decline (Hannien & Soininen, 1997). On the other hand, individuals with memory impairments of 1.5 standard deviations or more below expected levels relative to age and education-related peers, without general cognitive impairment, who participate in normal activities of daily living, and who are without dementia may have mild cognitive impairment that may represent an early sign of degenerative dementia such as Alzheimer's disease. When these subjects are followed longitudinally, they had a reported conversion rate of 10% to 15% per year to probable Alzheimer's disease (Peterson, 2000; Peterson et al., 1997). Outside the United States, similar types of criteria include age-associated cognitive decline (American Psychiatric Association [APA], 1994) or cognitive impairment with no dementia (Tuokko & Frerichs, 2000).

It should be noted, however, that these conversion rates may reflect sampling bias because most reports were based on studies of patients referred for clinical evaluation. In fact, the diagnosis of mild cognitive impairment based on cognitive testing in the general community is much less stable than in clinic-based samples, with many persons obtaining unimpaired scores on follow-up (Larrieu et al., 2002; Ritchie et al., 2001). For persons residing in the community, cognitive areas other than memory are likely to be affected because various medical conditions are more prevalent in the general population of older adults (e.g., diabetes, cerebrovascular disease, and other general medical conditions).

Memory is a very complex entity that is not yet fully understood. In general, distinctions are made between encoding, storage/consolidation, and retrieval. Provided that there are no primary hearing or visual deficits, the ability to encode sensory and auditory information as well as to briefly hold information in memory does not appear to decline as a function of age (see Sugar & McDowd, 1992). Further, remote memory for overlearned events in the distant past or procedural memory (overlearned procedural abilities with a motor component) does not appear to be particularly susceptible to the effects of normal aging and is often intact in the mild stages of neurodegenerative diseases such as Alzheimer's disease (Craik & Salthouse, 1992; La Rue, 1999; Loewenstein & Mogosky, 1999).

In contrast, most older adults experience a decline in secondary memory, particularly episodic memory for recent events. For example, older adults are usually more sensitive to distractors on divided attention tasks (Craik, 1977), quick pacing of material (Monge & Hultsch, 1971), and the amount of material presented to them at one time (Light et al., 1982). It has been hypothesized that this reduction in the ability to learn new material may in part be related to degeneration of the hippocampus, frontal lobe, and related executive systems and a decrease in the efficacy or abundance of neurotransmitters such as acetylcholine (de Leon et al., 1996; La Rue, 1992).

Although older persons generally evidence significant improvement in performance when provided with memory encoding strategies that appear to be typically employed by younger subjects, it appears that the initial benefits afforded by these strategies are not permanent because older adults tend to stop employing the techniques that they have learned (Anschutz et al., 1987; Scogin & Bienas, 1988). There is some evidence that training in cognitive skills and problem-solving strategies can be beneficial (Baltes et al., 1989). In any case, tools to enhance the efficacy of encoding may be beneficial in creating a greater sense of personal control, self-efficacy, and the reassurance that occasional memory lapses are normal (La Rue, 1992).

Boyarsky and Eisdorfer (1972) have shown that learning in older persons may be less efficient in that older subjects are more likely to learn peripheral and nonrelevant material, while younger subjects are more task oriented. It should be noted, however, that there is considerable variability among individuals according to the familiarity and salience of the material to be remembered, the educational attainment of the individual, the type of organizational strategy employed, and whether the material is to be recognized rather than recalled (Hultsch & Dixon, 1990).

It has also been proposed that a reduction in overall processing speed may result in some of the cognitive difficulties encountered in normal aging (Salthouse, 1985, 1999) or a decrease in the ability to inhibit irrelevant information (Hasher & Zacks, 1988). In fact, Loewenstein and coworkers (2003) demonstrated that the early manifestations of Alzheimer's disease may involve not only deficits in delayed recall and rate of forgetting, but also susceptibility to proactive (and sometimes retroactive) interference of semantically similar targets presented during learning trials. The effects of proactive and retroactive interference will require further research in both normal elderly populations and those with early neurodegenerative disease to understand these effects.

CULTURAL DIFFERENCES

The findings reported in the section on cognition are largely the result of research on populations without minority subjects. However, many investigators have shown that the results of intelligence tests are influenced by the cultural background of the individual being tested (Pick, 1980). Despite the importance of cultural variables, surprisingly few studies have addressed the patterns of cognitive decline among elders in various ethnic and cultural groups (Loewenstein et al., 1994; Loewenstein & Quiroga, 1998; Loewenstein & Rubert, 1992; Valle, 1989).

Furthermore, applying traditional normative data to these populations may be seriously misleading because measures of semantic memory and language may be biased against those individuals for whom English is a second language (Argüelles & Loewenstein, 1997; Loewenstein et al., 1994; Lopez & Taussig, 1991). For example, normal, healthy, Spanish-speaking elderly living in the community in the United States evidenced lower performance on certain tests of verbal fluency, such as the Controlled Word Association Test (Benton & Hamsher, 1977), even when the test was administered in the patient's native language (Loewenstein & Rubert, 1992; Taussig et al., 1992), perhaps because the relative frequency of a word beginning with a certain letter of the alphabet is not equivalent in English and Spanish or because Spanish speakers must also decide whether a phonologically correct word also begins with the correct letter. Even a test that involves only numbers (Digit Span) has been shown to be biased against Hispanic older adults (Argüelles et al., 2001; La Rue et al., 1999), but this bias can be greatly minimized by employing a paradigm by which digits are presented as groups rather than singly (Argüelles et al., 2001).

A major challenge facing researchers is the establishment of normative databases that take education, gender, age, sociological and cultural background, and the applicability of tests, testing situations, and test administrators into account (Loewenstein & Quiroga, 1998; Loewenstein & Rubert, 1992). However, even with normative data for a given measure that appears to be adequate, the measure may still not be valid. Different cultural and language groups may be unwilling to participate in normative studies; even when they do, it is often extremely difficult to account adequately for the impact of the immigration experience and sociopolitical influences such as discriminatory laws and practices.

Loewenstein and associates (Argüelles & Loewenstein, 1997; Loewenstein et al., 1993, 1994) contended that a measure may be culturally biased because (1) a measure developed for an English-speaking population may not be salient or meaningful to other populations and (2) the frequency of "correct" responses may vary based on the cultural background of the group studied. In addition, immigrant cultural groups may vary from similar groups in the native homeland, and Geisinger (1992) has recommended the inclusion of formal measures of acculturation when individuals from other cultures are assessed with psychological tests.

FUNCTIONAL CHANGES

Although the age-related changes in sensation and perception, intellectual abilities, and memory are significant in and of themselves, the ability to perform those functions necessary for personal care (activities of daily living, ADLs) and those functions necessary for maintaining an independent residence (instrumental activities of daily living, IADLs) are critical indicators of an individual's ability to live independently (Loewenstein & Mogosky, 1999; Loewenstein & Rubert, 1992).

Loewenstein and colleagues (1989) developed the Direct Assessment of Functional Status, a measure that directly assesses an older person's ability to perform several instrumental activities of daily living (e.g., telling time, orientation to date, using the telephone, preparing a letter for mailing, writing a check, making change, shopping for groceries) and activities of daily living (e.g., eating, dressing, and grooming). Older adults typically do not have any difficulties performing the IADLs and ADLs that they have successfully performed in the past unless they have significant cognitive deterioration caused by conditions such as Alzheimer's disease, significantly impaired physical or mental health, or significant perceptual impairments (Loewenstein et al., 1992). A number of informant and performance-based measures have also been developed for the functional assessment of older adult populations (see Loewenstein & Mogosky, 1999, for a review).

Crimmins and Saito (1993) examined the determinants of functional change over 2 years in 3,169 noninstitutionalized elderly who were 70 years of age or older. At the initial assessment, they found that less than 10% of their subjects reported difficulty in performing their IADLs (range 3.1%–9.3%), and with the exception of reporting difficulty walking, less than 8% reported difficulty in performing their ADLs (range 1.0%–7.6%). Two years later, the reported increase in difficulty performing IADLs ranged from 3.3% to 6.0%. For ADLs, the reported increase ranged from 2.1% to 6.9%, except for difficulty walking, which increased by 9.9%. Over a period of only 1 year, Myers and colleagues (1993) found increases in the time it took for a person to open bottles with safety tops (line up the arrows and push down/pull up before turning), remove a pill from a blister pack, boil water for soup, put away a bowl, and walk a distance of 12 feet.

Why are we concerned about these declines in functional performance? Studies have shown that declines in functional status are significantly associated with death and nursing home placement (Messinger-Rapport et al., 2003; Ribbon et al., 1992).

EXERCISE AND AGING

Mobility is also likely to decline as a person grows older, regardless of whether the person has a chronic disease (Visser et al., 2002). Physicians are now told to encourage their older patients to adopt a program of regular exercise (Hall, 1992) as several studies have documented that participation in a regular program of aerobic exercise can slow or reverse age-related declines in cardiovascular function and musculoskeletal fitness (Evans & Campbell, 1993; Warren et al., 1993). High levels of cardiovascular fitness may even protect cognitive functions (Barnes et al., 2003), and aerobic exercise is a good way to improve cardiorespiratory fitness, perhaps even if you are over 80 (Vaitkevicius et al., 2002). Aerobic exercise has also been associated with beneficial changes in performance on cognitive tasks, such as performance on simple and choice reaction time tasks (Bashore, 1989; Spirduso & Clifford, 1978). These benefits may not extend to memory processes (Blumenthal & Madden, 1988; Madden et al., 1989), but exercise can improve the memory of depressed older adults (Khatri et al., 2001).

One area of cognitive function for which age-related differences in performance have been found is attentional capacity. Attentional capacity is typically assessed by divided attention tasks; subjects are required to perform two tasks simultaneously. Hawkins and coworkers (1992) evaluated the effect of exercise on attentional processes. First, they compared the performances of young (20–35 years old) and older adults (65–74 years old) on a time-sharing task (subjects must switch attention between two sequential tasks). Young adults were more efficient on the time-shared task and able to switch their attention more rapidly compared to the older adults. Next, the same tasks were given to 37 older subjects, 18 of whom were assigned to a 10-week aerobic exercise program. The older exercisers performed significantly better on the time-sharing and attentional tasks compared to the control subjects. The authors suggested that these changes may be the result of enhanced cardiovascular sufficiency.

SUCCESSFUL AGING

Rowe and Kahn (1998) defined successful aging as the maintenance of three key personal characteristics: (1) low risk of disease and disability due to disease, (2) high mental and physical functioning, and (3) active engagement with

life. However, older adults with chronic health problems and functional limitations certainly can age successfully, and Rowe and Kahn presented such notable examples as Stephen Hawking, Franklin Roosevelt, and Mother Teresa.

Rowe and Kahn (1998) also addressed the outcomes of the MacArthur
study. Participants in the MacArthur study cohort ($N = 1,189$) were selected
to represent the top third of their age group (70–79 years) in terms of their
physical and cognitive functioning. This meant that they had no difficulties
performing their daily activities, little difficulty getting around physically, and
grossly intact memory and cognition. The participants completed a battery of
tests assessing their cognitive and physical abilities, and their physical health
and mental health status were also evaluated. Based on these evaluations, three
factors were found to promote productivity in old age: (1) health and overall
ability to function, (2) friendships and other social relationships, and (3) other
personal characteristics, such as being better educated and having a sense of
mastery (feeling able to cope with the challenges of life). As they noted, the
elements are obviously interrelated because staying in good health and maintaining physical and mental functioning makes it easier to remain socially active and engaged in life.

Another way to study successful aging is to evaluate the characteristics of
long-lived, community-dwelling individuals who are in relatively good health
and functioning. This is the approach used by the Georgia Centenarian Study
(Poon, Clayton et al., 1992; Poon, Martin et al., 1992). Three cohorts of 88
participants were recruited; the cohorts were 100 to 109 years old, 80 to 89
years old, and 60 to 65 years old. The participants' cognitive and physical
abilities, physical and mental health status, and personality and life satisfaction
were evaluated. It was found that cognitive resources were necessary for successful aging in that cognitive dysfunction meant that everyday functioning
could not be maintained. More important, they found that, despite a decline
in cognitive abilities, there was no age-related decline in the ability to solve
everyday problems; this ability is one that is, arguably, important for survival.
In terms of their personality characteristics, the centenarians were higher on
dominance, suspiciousness, and imagination. Martin et al. (1992) suggested
that these personality traits may be protective in later adulthood.

A final area that some would define as successful aging would be to become wiser with age. Some of the more significant studies on wisdom have
been performed by Baltes and colleagues (see Baltes, 1993, for a review of this
work). They postulated that wisdom is related to crystallized intelligence, and
that wisdom-related knowledge, especially expertise-related knowledge, is established and refined during the life span by the tasks of life management, life
planning, and life review. Smith and Baltes (1990) compared younger and older
adults on wisdom-related tasks and found no significant differences in their
performance. Similarly, Baltes (1993) studied older persons nominated for their
wisdom. No negative effects for age were found, but there was also little evidence of increased wisdom among those nominated for their wisdom compared
to the control subjects. However, age-related increases in wisdom were re-

ported in another study that defined wisdom in terms of the ability to solve problems faced in everyday life (Cornelius & Caspi, 1987), similar to the results of the Georgia Centenarian Study (Poon, Martin et al., 1992).

CONCLUSION

In this chapter, we examined a number of the normal psychological changes that appear associated with aging. Sensory-perceptual changes that result in diminished visual and auditory acuity are problematic for older adults. The ability to shift cognitive set rapidly, psychomotor speed, reaction time, verbal fluency, complex visuoconstructive skills, and logical analysis skills appear to decrease with age. While older adults may have more difficulty with novel tasks, especially tasks that require quick psychomotor responses, the notion that increasing age is associated with the loss of all intellectual and memory abilities is simply incorrect. Several longitudinal studies have shown that significant memory problems are a sign of neurodegenerative disease or other medical or neuropsychiatric conditions.

Much of the research has a cross-sectional design, and the longitudinal studies have to deal with the potential confound of cohort effects. Many of the measures are not adequately validated for older adults and suffer from cultural bias. This is particularly problematic given the rapid rate of growth of ethnoracial minority groups, particularly in the older adults, in the United States (US Bureau of the Census, 1995).

Poor physical health has a significant negative impact on cognitive functioning, but cardiovascular fitness and mood can be significantly improved in the older person by appropriate interventions, including programs of regular aerobic exercise. Improvement in cardiovascular function and mood may result in improvements in cognition.

Now, we have begun to strive for successful aging, rather than "usual aging." Rowe and Kahn (1998) defined successful aging as (1) low risk of disease and disability due to disease, (2) high mental and physical functioning, and (3) active engagement with life. The Georgia Centenarian Study concluded that the ability to solve everyday problems is an important indicator of successful aging; interestingly, this has been used as a definition for wisdom. The follow-up assessments of the MacArthur study cohort and similar studies of older adults will doubtless become a major factor in helping the baby boom generation avoid morbidity and delay mortality as they become older adults.

REFERENCES

American Psychiatric Association. *Diagnostic and Statistical Manual of Mental Disorders.* 4th ed. Washington, DC: American Psychiatric Association; 1994.

Anschutz L, Camp CJ, Markley RP, Kramer JJ. Remembering mnemonics: a three-year follow-up on the effects of mnemonics training in elderly adults. *Exp Aging Res.* 1987;13:141–143.

Ardilla A, Ostrosky-Solis F, Rosselli M, Gomez C. Age-related cognitive decline during normal aging: the complex effects of education. *Arch Clin Neuropsychol.* 2002;15: 495–513.

Argüelles T, Loewenstein DA. Research says "Sí" to the development of culturally appropriate cognitive assessment tools. *Generations.* 1997;21:30–31.

Argüelles T, Loewenstein DA, Argüelles S. The impact of the native language of Alzheimer's disease and normal elderly individuals on their ability to recall digits. *Aging Ment Health.* 2001;5:358–365.

Avolio BJ, Waldman DA. Variations in cognitive, perceptual, and psychomotor abilities across the working life span: examining the effects of race, sex, experience, education, and occupational type. *Psychol Aging.* 1994;9:430–442.

Baltes PB. The aging mind: potential and limits. *Gerontologist.* 1993;33:580–594.

Baltes PB, Sowarka D, Kliegl R. Cognitive training research on fluid intelligence in old age: what can older adults achieve by themselves? *Psychol Aging.* 1989;4:217–221.

Barnes DE, Yaffe K, Satariano WA, Tager IB. A longitudinal study of cardiorespiratory fitness and cognitive function in healthy older adults. *J Am Geriatr Soc.* 2003;51: 459–465.

Bashore T. Age, physical fitness and mental processing speed. In: Lawton MP, ed. *Annual Review of Gerontology and Geriatrics.* New York, NY: Springer; 1989:120–144.

Benton A, Hamsher K. *Multilingual Aphasia Examination.* Iowa City: University of Iowa; 1977.

Blessed G, Tomlinson BE, Roth M. Association between quantitative measures of dementing and senile change in the cerebral grey matter of elderly subjects. *Br J Psychiatry.* 1968;114:797–811.

Blumenthal JA, Madden DJ. Effects of aerobic exercise training, age, and physical fitness on memory search performance. *Psychol Aging.* 1988;3:280–285.

Bosman EA. Age-related differences in the motoric aspects of transcription typing skill. *Psychol Aging.* 1993;8:87–102.

Botwinick J. Intellectual abilities. In: Birren JE, Schaie KW, eds. *Handbook of the Psychology of Aging.* New York, NY: Van Nostrand Reinhold; 1977:580–605.

Boyarsky RE, Eisdorfer C. Forgetting in older persons. *J Gerontol.* 1972;27:254–258.

Carman MB. The psychology of normal aging. *Psychiatr Clin North Am.* 1997;20: 15–24.

Christensen H, Mackinnon A, Jorm AF, Henderson AS, Scott LR, Korten AE. Age differences and interindividual variation in cognition in community-dwelling elderly. *Psychol Aging.* 1994;9:381–390.

Cornelius SW, Caspi A. Everyday problem-solving in adulthood and old age. *Psychol Aging.* 1987;2:144–153.

Craik FIM. Age differences in human memory. In Birren JE, Schaie KW, eds. *Handbook of the Psychology of Aging.* New York, NY: Van Nostrand Reinhold; 1977:384–420.

Craik FIM, Salthouse TA, eds. *The Handbook of Aging and Cognition.* Hillsdale, NJ: Erlbaum; 1992.

Crimmins EM, Saito Y. Getting better and getting worse: transitions in functional status among older Americans. *J Aging Health.* 1993;5:3–36.

Cullum S, Huppert FA, McGee M, et al. Decline across different domains of cognitive function in normal aging: results of a longitudinal population-based study using CAMCOG. *Int J Geriatr Psychiatry.* 2000;15:853–862.

Cunningham WR. Intellectual abilities and age. In: Schaie KW, ed. *Annual Review of Gerontology and Geriatrics*. New York, NY: Springer; 1987:117–134.

Czaja SJ, Sharit J. Age differences in the performance of computer-based work. *Psychol Aging*. 1993;8:59–67.

de Leon MJ, Cnvit A, George AE, et al. In vitro studies of the hippocampus in normal aging and in incipient Alzheimer's disease. *Ann NY Acad Sci*. 1996;777:1–13.

Eisdorfer C, Mintzer J. Performance and aging: an intergrative biopsychosocial paradigm. In: Bergener M, Ermini M, Stahelin HB, eds. *Crossroads in Aging*. London, England: Academic Press; 1988:189–203.

Evans WJ, Campbell WW. Sarcopenia and age-related changes in body composition and functional capacity. *J Nutr*. 1993;123:465–468.

Finch CE, Tanzi RE. Genetics of aging. *Science*. 1997;278:407–411.

Geisinger KF. Fairness and selected psychometric issues in psychological testing of hispanics. In: Geisinger KF, ed. *Psychological Testing of Hispanics*. Washington, DC: American Psychological Association; 1992:17–42.

Grady CL, Craik FIM. Change in memory processing with age. *Curr Opin Neurobiol*. 2000;10:224–231.

Guterman A, Loewenstein D, Gamez E, Lermo M, Weinberg G, Kotler K. Stressful life experiences in the early detection of Alzheimer's disease: potential limitations associated with the estimation of illness duration. *Behav Health Aging*. 1993;3:43–49.

Hall NK. Health maintenance and promotion. In: Ham RJ, Sloane PD, eds. *Primary Care Geriatrics: A Case-Based Approach*. 2nd ed. St. Louis, MO: Mosby—Year Book; 1992:95–118.

Hannien T, Soininen H. Age-associated memory impairment: normal aging or warning of dementia? *Drugs Aging*. 1997;11:480–489.

Hasher L, Zacks RT. Working memory, comprehension and aging: a review and new view. In: Bower GH, ed. *The Psychology of Learning and Motivation*. Vol. 22. San Diego, CA: Academic Press; 1988:193–225.

Hassing LB, Johansson B, Berg S, et al. Terminal decline and markers of cerebro- and cardiovascular disease: findings from a longitudinal study of the oldest old. *J Gerontol B Psychol Sci Soc Sci*. 2002;57:P268–P276.

Hawkins HL, Kramer AF, Capaldi D. Aging, exercise, and attention. *Psychol Aging*. 1992;7:643–653.

Horn JL, Cattell RB. Age differences in fluid and crystallized intelligence. *Acta Psychol*. 1967;26:107–129.

Horn JL, Donaldson G. On the myth of intellectual decline in adulthood. *Am Psychol*. 1976;31:701–719.

Hultsch DF, Dixon RA. Learning and memory in aging. In: Birren JE, Shaie KW, eds. *Handbook of the Psychology of Aging*. 3rd ed. New York, NY: Academic Press; 1990:258–274.

Hultsch DF, Hertzog C, Small BJ, McDonald-Miszczak L, Dixon RA. Short-term longitudinal change in cognitive performance in later life. *Psychol Aging*. 1992;7:571–584.

Jarvik LF, Bank L. Aging twins: longitudinal psychometric data. In: Schaie KW, ed. *Longitudinal Studies of Adult Psychological Development*. New York, NY: Guilford Press; 1983:40–63.

Khatri P, Blumenthal JA, Babyak MA, et al. Effects of exercise training on cognitive functioning among depressed older men and women. *J Aging Phys Activ*. 2001;9:43–57.

Larrieu A, Letenneur L, Orgogozo J, et al. Incidence and outcome of mild cognitive impairment in a population-based prospective cohort. *Neurology.* 2002;59:1594–1599.

La Rue A. *Aging and Neuropsychological Assessment.* New York, NY: Plenum Press; 1992.

La Rue A. Geriatric neuropsychology: principles of assessment. In: Lichtenberg P, ed. *Handbook of Assessment in Clinical Gerontology.* New York, NY: Wiley; 1999:381–416.

La Rue A, Romero LJ, Ortiz IE, Liang HC, Lindeman RD. Neuropsychological performance of Hispanic and non-Hispanic older adults: an epidemiologic survey. *Clin Neuropsychol.* 1999;13d:474–486.

Leon DA. Reduced fetal growth rate and increased risk of death from ischemic heart disease: a cohort study of 15,000 Swedish men and women 1915 to 1929. *BMJ.* 1998;317:241–245.

Light LL, Zelinski EM, Moore M. Adult age differences in reasoning from new information. *J Exp Psychol Learn Mem Cogn.* 1982;8:435–447.

Loewenstein DA, Acevedo A, Schram L, et al. Semantic interference in mild Alzheimer's disease: preliminary findings. *Am J Geriatr Psychiatry.* 2003;11:252–255.

Loewenstein DA, Amigo E, Duara R, et al. A new scale for the assessment of functional status in Alzheimer's disease and related disorders. *J Gerontol.* 1989;44:114–121.

Loewenstein DA, Argüelles T, Argüelles S, Linn-Fuentes P. Potential cultural bias in the neuropsychological assessment of the older adult. *J Clin Exp Neuropsychol.* 1994; 16:623–629.

Loewenstein DA, Argüelles T, Barker WW, Duara R. A comparative analysis of neuropsychological test performance of Spanish-speaking and English-speaking patients with Alzheimer's disease. *J Gerontol.* 1993;48:P142–P149.

Loewenstein DA, Eisdorfer CE. Issues in geriatric research. In: George LK, Hsu G, Hersen M, eds. *Research in Psychiatry: Issues, Strategies and Methods.* New York, NY: Plenum Press; 1992:427–443.

Loewenstein DA, Mogosky B. The functional assessment of the older adult patient. In: Lichtenberg P, ed. *Handbook of Assessment in Clinical Gerontology.* New York, NY: Wiley; 1999:529–554.

Loewenstein D, Quiroga M. Neuropsychological assessment of Alzheimer's disease: an examination of the important issues underlying current practice. In: Kumar V, Eisdorfer C, eds. *Advances in the Diagnosis and Treatment of Alzheimer's Disease.* New York, NY: Springer, 1998:152–169.

Loewenstein DA, Rubert MP. The NINCDS-ADRDA neuropsychological criteria for the assessment of dementia: limitations of current diagnostic guidelines. *Behav Health Aging.* 1992;2:113–121.

Loewenstein DA, Rubert MP, Berkowitz-Zimmer N, Guterman A, Morgan R, Hayden S. Neuropsychological test performance and prediction of functional capacities in dementia. *Behav Health Aging.* 1992;2:149–158.

Lopez SR, Taussig FM. Cognitive-intellectual functioning of Spanish-speaking impaired and nonimpaired elderly: implications for culturally sensitive assessment. *Psychol Assess J Consul Clin Psychol.* 1991;3:448–454.

Madden DJ, Blumenthal JA, Allen PA, Emery CF. Improving aerobic capacity in healthy older adults does not necessarily lead to improved cognitive function. *Psychol Aging.* 1989;4:307–320.

Martin P, Poon LW, Clayton GM, Lee HS, Fulks JS. Personality, life events and coping in the oldest-old. *Int J Aging Hum Dev.* 1992;34:19–30.

McEvoy GM, Cascio WF. Cumulative evidence of the relationship between employee age and job performance. *J Appl Psychol.* 1989;74:11–17.

Messinger-Rapport B, Snader CEP, Blackstone EH, Yu D, Lauer MS. Value of exercise capacity and heart rate recovery in older people. *J Am Geriatr Soc.* 2003;51:63–68.

Monge R, Hultsch D. Paired associate learning as a function of adult age and the length of anticipation and inspection intervals. *J Gerontol.* 1971;26:157–162.

Myers AM, Holliday PJ, Harvey KA, Hutchinson KS. Functional performance measures: are they superior to self-assessments? *J Gerontol Med Sci.* 1993;48:M196–M206.

National Center for Health Statistics. *Advance Report of Final Mortality Statistics, 1990.* Hyattsville, MD: National Center for Health Statistics, 1993.

Orr AL. The psychosocial aspects of aging and vision loss. *J Gerontol Soc Work.* 1991; 17:1–14.

Peterson RC. Mild cognitive impairment: transition between aging and Alzheimer's disease. *Neurologia.* 2000;15:93–101.

Peterson RC, Smith GE, Waring SC, Ivnik RJ, Kokmen E, Tangelos EG. Aging, memory and cognitive impairment. *Int Psychogeriatr.* 1997;9:65–69.

Pick AD. Cognition: psychological perspectives. In: Trandis HC, Lonner W, eds. *Handbook of Cross-Cultural Psychology: Basic Processes.* Vol. 3. Boston, MA: Allyn and Bacon; 1980:117–153.

Piguet O, Grayson DA, Broe GA, et al. Normal aging and executive functions in "old-old" community dwellers: poor performance is not an inevitable outcome. *Int Psychogeriatr.* 2002;14:139–159.

Poon LW, Clayton GM, Martin P, et al. The Georgia Centenarian Study. *Int J Aging Hum Dev.* 1992;34:1–18.

Poon LW, Martin P, Clayton GM, Messner SA, Noble CA. The influence of cognitive resources on adaptation and old age. *Int J Aging Hum Dev.* 1992;34:31–46.

Rabbitt P, Watson P, Donlan C, et al. Effects of death within 11 years on cognitive performance in old age. *Psychol Aging.* 2002;17:468–481.

Rabbitt PMA. Some experiments and a model for changes in attentional selectivity with old age. In: Hoffmeister F, Muller C, eds. *Brain Function in Old Age.* Berlin, Germany: Springer-Verlag; 1979.

Rhodes SR. Age-related differences in work attitudes and behavior: a review and conceptual analysis. *Psychol. Bull.* 1983;93:328–367.

Ribbon DB, Si AL, Kimpau S. The predictive validity of self-report and performance-based measures of function and health. *J Gerontol Med Sci.* 1992;47:M106–M110.

Ritchie K, Artero S, Touchon J. Classification criteria for mild cognitive impairment: a population-based validation study. *Neurology.* 2001;56:37–42.

Roth M, Tomlinson BE, Blessed G. The relationship between quantitative measures of dementia and of degenerative changes in the cerebral grey matter of elderly subjects. *Proc R Soc Med.* 1967;60:254–260.

Rowe JW, Kahn RL. *Successful Aging.* New York, NY: Pantheon Books; 1998.

Salthouse TA. *Theory of Cognitive Aging.* New York, NY: Elsevier Science; 1985.

Salthouse TA. Theories on cognition. In: Bengston VL, Warner Schaie K, eds. *Handbook of Theories of Aging.* New York, NY: Springer; 1999.

Salthouse TA, Ferrer-Caja E. What needs to be explained to account for age-related effects on multiple cognitive variables? *Psychol Aging.* 2003;18:91–110.

Satz P. Brain reserve capacity on symptom onset after brain injury: a formulation and review of the evidence for threshold theory. *Neuropsychology.* 1993;7:273–295.

Schaie KW. Intelligence and problem solving. In: Birren JE, Schaie KW, eds. *Handbook of the Psychology of Aging.* New York, NY: Van Nostrand Reinhold; 1980:39–58.

Schaie KW. Internal validity threats in studies of adult cognitive development. In: Howe

ML, Brainerd CJ, eds. *Cognitive Development in Adulthood: Progress in Cognitive Development Research.* New York, NY: Springer-Verlag; 1988:241–272.

Schaie KW, Willis SL. Age difference patterns of psychometric intelligence in adulthood: generalizability within and across ability domains. *Psychol Aging.* 1993;8:44–55.

Scogin F, Bienas JL. A three-year follow-up of older adult participants in memory skills training program. *Psychol Aging.* 1988;3:334–337.

Smith J, Baltes PB. Wisdom-related knowledge: age/cohort differences in response to life-planning problems. *Dev Psychol.* 1990;26:494–505.

Sorensenson HT. Birth weight and cognition: a historical cohort study. *BMJ.* 1997;315: 401–403.

Spar JE, La Rue A. *Concise Guide to Geriatric Psychiatry.* 3rd ed. Washington, DC: American Psychiatric Publishing; 2002.

Spirduso WW, Clifford P. Replication of age and physical activity effects on reaction time and movement time. *J Gerontol.* 1978;43:23–30.

Sugar JA, McDowd JM. Memory, learning, and attention. In: Birren JE, Sloane RB, Cohen GD, eds. *Handbook of Mental Health and Aging.* 2nd ed. New York, NY: Academic Press; 1992:307–337.

Taussig IM, Henderson VW, Mack W. Spanish translation and validation of a neuropsychological battery: performance of Spanish- and English-speaking Alzheimer's disease patients and normal comparison subjects. In: Brink TL, ed. *Hispanic Aged Mental Health.* Binghamton, NY: Haworth Press; 1992:95–108.

Tuokko H, Frerichs R. Cognitive impairment with no dementia (CIND): longitudinal studies, findings, and the issues. *Clin Neuropsychol.* 2000;14:504–525.

US Bureau of the Census. *Current Population Reports, Series P23–189. Population Profile of the United States.* Washington, DC: US Government Printing Office; 1995.

Vaitkevicius PV, Ebersold C, Shah MS, et al. Effects of aerobic exercise training in community based subjects aged 80 and older: a pilot study. *J Am Geriatr Soc.* 2002; 50:2009–2013.

Valle R. Cultural and ethnic issues in Alzheimer's disease family research. In: Light E, Lebowitz BD, eds. *Alzheimer's Disease Treatment and Family Stress: Directions for Research.* Washington, DC: Dept. of Health and Human Services; 1989:122–154. DHHS Publication (ADM) 89-1569.

Visser M, Pluijm SMF, Stel VS, Bosscher RJ, Deeg DJH. Physical activity as a determinant of change in mobility performance: the longitudinal aging study Amsterdam. *J Am Geriatr Soc.* 2002;50:1774–1781.

Warren BJ, Nieman DC, Dotson RG, et al. Cardiorespiratory responses to exercise training in septuagenarian women. *Int J Sports Med.* 1993;14:60–65.

Wetherell JL, Reynolds CA, Gatz M, Pedersen NL. Anxiety, cognitive performance and cognitive decline in normal aging. *J Gerontol B Psychol Sci Soc Sci.* 2002;57:P246–P255.

Williams A, Denney NW, Schadler M. Elderly adults' perception of their own cognitive development during the adult years. *Int J Aging Hum Dev.* 1983;16:147–158.

Youngjohn JR, Crook TH III. Stability of everyday memory in age-associated memory impairment: a longitudinal study. *Neuropsychology.* 1993;7:406–416.

Zarit JM, Zarit SH. Molar aging: the physiology and psychology of normal aging. In: Carstensen LL, Edelstein BA, eds. *Handbook of Clinical Gerontology.* New York, NY: Pergamon Press; 1987:18–32.

6

Sociodemographic Aspects of Aging

Charles F. Longino, Jr, PhD
Sara A. Quandt, PhD

Sociodemographic aspects of mental health and mental illness are particularly important in geriatric psychiatry as a social context for individual cases. Concurrent with biologically based changes in health, old age brings many important socially induced changes that have the potential for producing negative or positive effects on both the physical and the mental well-being of older persons. These social changes include altered marriage and family patterns, living arrangements, work behaviors, economic status, and social support. Neither the psychiatric therapist nor the researcher can afford to ignore the sociodemographic aspects of old age when considering the older patient, client, or subject. To do so is to ignore the setting in which the condition is nurtured and the epidemiological connections to age, gender, race, ethnicity, work, economic status, and marital and residential relationships. These are the primary social factors that condition health and mental health. The physical and mental conditions that make illness more or less likely and that make coping more or less successful are rooted partly in sociodemographic factors.

INTERACTIONS OF THE SOCIOCULTURAL ENVIRONMENT AND HEALTH STATUS

A number of lines of inquiry point to the interaction of the sociocultural environment and health. The fact that married persons, particularly males, live longer and exhibit healthier lifestyles than nonmarried persons is interpreted

147

as evidence for the benefits of social interaction and social support. There is increasing recognition, however, that the mere presence of a social network does not always indicate a high level of support. Interactions with spouse, children, and neighbors can be negative, aversive, and even abusive. In addition, social contacts must be mobilized into emotional or instrumental assistance for them to be supportive. Rapp and coworkers (1998) argued that some older individuals are more resourceful than others in producing support from their social networks.

Some environments make social contact outside the household difficult. Rural elders, in the face of increasing disability, often face significant challenges in maintaining social interaction due to distances between residences and lack of transportation (Quandt & Arcury, 2001). Loss of kin and friends through death and the loss of proximity through geographic out-migration results in diminished social contacts for many rural elders. In the absence of other organizations, rural churches and senior centers are important institutions for maintaining social relations. Older adults also can be isolated in some urban neighborhoods due to fear of crime or disability. However, the number of services and associations available to urban and suburban elders is generally high.

Throughout this review, disparities in health by gender, ethnicity, and socioeconomic status recur, indicating the cumulative effects on health of lack of physical and social resources over the life course. Individuals in minority ethnic groups and with lower incomes and levels of educational attainment are less exposed to health education, are more exposed to environmental stressors, and are more constrained in their ability to access preventive and acute medical services. While average life expectancy for the population as a whole has increased dramatically and health care for older adults has become more available, ethnic minorities still have higher rates of disability and disease.

SOCIAL AND DEMOGRAPHIC CHARACTERISTICS

There are several sources of current statistics on the older population. Unless otherwise specified, however, this review and summary of social and demographic characteristics was drawn from a 1996 report jointly produced by the US Bureau of the Census and the National Institute on Aging, titled 65+ *in the United States*, and *Elderly Americans*, published by the Population Reference Bureau (Himes, 2001). The perspectives in this chapter, therefore, are focused on North America, especially the United States.

Age and Aging

At the beginning of the 20th century, fewer than 1 in 25 Americans were aged 65 years or older. By 2000, 1 in 8 were at least 65 years old. With each passing decade before 1990, there were over 20% more persons aged 65 years or older in the US population. In the 1990s and in the first decade of the 21st century, however, this growth slowed to about 12% because of the low fertility rate during the Great Depression in the 1930s. This older part of the population will more than double after 2010 because of the entrance of baby boomers (those born between 1946 and 1964). By 2030, there will be as many persons older than 65 years as younger than 18 years (about one fifth of the total population each), and the median age of all Americans is expected to be 43 years. The proportion of the US population older than 85 years will grow from 1% in 1990 to 5% in 2050. More people are surviving into their 10th and 11th decades as well.

The US Census Bureau estimates that there were about 50,000 persons aged 100 years or older in 1994, and their number will increase for half a century more. If current students of geriatric psychiatry have a 30-year career, the proportion and number of older persons in the US population will have doubled by the time they retire from practice. Even if the proportion of older persons seeking psychiatric services remains constant during this period, the number of patients or clients will more than double. The major surge, however, will not occur until after 2010.

Although the overall number of older adults in the United States is growing, not all sex, race, and ethnic categories are equally represented in the total population of older persons. Women continue to live longer than men, so the ratio of women to men varies dramatically with age. In 2000, there were 3 women for every 2 men 65 years or older, and the sex ratio favoring females is even more skewed in progressively older groups (Himes, 2001). In 2000, the population 65 years or older contained 84% whites, 8% African Americans, 4% persons from other races, and 5% Hispanics. However, when racial, nationality, and language categories are compared, it is important to remember that these categories have heterogeneous populations as well. Immigration is one of the forces increasing the ethnic heterogeneity in the American population.

The overall aging of the US population is, of course, related to increased life expectancy. A child born in 1900 had a life expectancy of 47 years; in 1960, this figure had grown to 69 years, and in 2000, it was 76.9 years (79.5 for women and 74.1 for men). The increases in life expectancy during the first five decades of the last century were due largely to the decreased infant mortality rate and reduced mortality from infectious diseases. By contrast, the increases in life expectancy since the 1960s are due largely to lower mortality rates among middle-aged and older individuals. Persons who were 65 years of age in 2000 could expect to live, on average, an additional 17.9 years. The gap in life expectancy for men and women, which grew in the 1970s and 1980s, appears to have stopped growing by the new century (Himes, 2001). White women outlive African American women by about 5 years; the difference is 7 years for men. These differences narrow, however, at advanced ages and fall to zero at 85 years and older (Himes, 2001).

As the baby boomers retire, the population older than 65 years will expand greatly, to 54 million in 2020. By 2060, the number is expected to approach 90 million (Himes, 2001). Older Americans are increasingly active, healthy, and able to take on new roles. Because of their numbers, however, there will also be an increase in those who will need assistance with housing, health care, and other services.

Work and Retirement

As people live longer, they spend more time in several of life's major phases, most notably education, work, and retirement. Before World War II, retirement was the domain of a privileged few, but it has now become an institutionalized expectation, and there appears to be increasing acceptance of it as a desired social status (Atchley, 1994).

On the whole, labor force and retirement patterns have been different for men and women. Since 1900, the average time spent by women in the labor force has increased from 6.3 to 29.4 years. Retirement is an issue for a growing number of women, and the proportion of women entering retirement will increase dramatically with the aging of the baby boom generation in this century.

Retirement is not a single concept. Age 65 has been considered the "normal retirement age" in the United States since the Social Security Act was passed in 1935. Perhaps it should be moved to 62, the year that Social Security is first available (on an actuarially reduced basis) because, since 1950, fewer than half (46%) of all men were still working at 64 years of age. By 2000, the proportion had fallen to 19% (Himes, 2001). In addition, most private pensions provide benefits for eligible employees before 65 years of age, a trend that accelerated in the 1960s and 1970s (US Department of Labor, Bureau of Labor Statistics, 1989). Normal age of retirement may increase in the future, however, as the age requirement for Social Security benefits slowly increases from 65 to 67 years. At the other extreme, many people continue to work full or part time after they begin receiving retired worker benefits. Are these individuals retired? The younger an individual is at retirement (except for those who retire because of a disability), the more likely it is that he or she will continue to work (Ullmann et al., 1991). In 1993, 54% of older workers were working part time, allowing them to have a flexible activity agenda in retirement.

Studies have indicated that people retire for a variety of reasons, although most workers retire when they feel they can afford to do so (Quinn & Burkhauser, 1990). Thus, persons without pensions, savings, or assets, including a home, are likely to remain in the labor force longer than persons who have such resources.

As a result of these factors, professionals and self-employed persons have greater variation in their age at retirement than workers employed by businesses and corporations. More individuals in the first two groups (especially self-employed persons) can more often afford early retirement. At the same time, among professionals, job satisfaction is often high, encouraging phased-in retirement or retirement at a later age. Physicians often do this by simply not accepting new patients. Corporation workers who seek earlier retirement are more frequently motivated by health problems. Understanding retirement requires understanding the links between persons and their jobs (Atchley, 1994; Ullmann et al., 1991).

Economic Resources, Income, and Expenditures

Older persons in America tend to have lower incomes than those younger than 65 years old because income drops in retirement, usually by at least one third. Moreover, the median income decreases with increasing age. Older Americans should not be characterized as affluent or poor. They are both. The income gains of the 1990s were not shared equally within subgroups of the elderly population, so it may be misleading only to talk about the total elderly population.

Surveys of income adequacy showed that high proportions of older persons feel that their income is adequate, even when objectively it is low (Streib, 1985). Liang and Fairchild (1979) found, in an analysis of six national samples of elderly people, that feelings of relative deprivation affected their financial satisfaction more than their actual income. The sense of income adequacy was strengthened when comparisons were made between themselves and others their age who had less adequate incomes.

Older adults are slightly less likely than younger adults to live in households in which the income is below the poverty level. To keep poverty rates in perspective, however, it should be remembered that the poverty rate in the households of elderly individuals declined from 28.5% in 1966, to 14.6% in 1974 and 11.4% in the 1980s, to 10.2% in 2000. The highest poverty rates are associated with minority women living alone. In 2000, of elderly black women living alone, 43% had incomes below the poverty level, reflecting the fact that more older women and persons of color live below the poverty level than men and white persons (Himes, 2001).

Elderly individuals generally consume fewer goods and services than non-elderly individuals, although they spend slightly higher proportions of their budgets on essentials. Persons aged 65 years and older spend more of their consumption dollars on housing, food, and medical care compared to the amount spent by younger persons on these items. Health care is the one service or commodity that elderly persons spend more on in actual dollars and as a percentage of total expenditures than the nonelderly. The major health expense for elderly households is health insurance, including Medicare. Even though they had lower incomes and fewer household members, elderly individuals spend more than twice as much as their younger counterparts on health insurance, prescription drugs, and medical supplies.

Education Level

At one time, older people were at a real educational disadvantage compared to the young. Today, however, recently retired Americans (65–74 years old) are the best-educated generation of seniors ever. Two thirds finished high school, contrasted with just over half of those aged 75 years and older. Future generations of older Americans will fare even better (Treas & Longino, 1997).

Rising educational attainment has been a very positive development because people with more education are at an advantage in many different ways (Treas, 1995). Even taking account of their higher incomes, people with more education have fewer disabilities, avoid the early onset of chronic disease, and enjoy lower death rates. It is likely that better educated seniors have greater access to information about how to promote health, how to recognize illness, and how to get treatment. Schooling also shapes lifestyle preferences. Every year, tens of thousands of well-educated seniors attend "emeriti college" courses across the United States and have made some college towns popular retirement communities.

Economic and educational resources strongly influence the quality of life of persons in their later years, as they do for all individuals. The combination of economic resources and living arrangement, however, determines adequate or inadequate support in later life.

Marital Status and Living Arrangements

Marital status, family patterns, and living arrangements vary greatly between men and women aged 65 years and older. In 2001, most older men (75%) live in family settings; the proportion for women living in such settings is much lower (44%). According to the March 2001 current population survey, nearly one half (45%) of all women 65 years and older were widows (Himes, 2001). The gender gap in life expectancy, however, has narrowed about a year in the past decade, probably due to falling heart disease rates among men. The number of divorced persons entering retirement will increase with the emergence of baby boomer retirement in the next decade (Himes, 2001). One implication of these trends is that older people who are socially isolated seek professional and institutional care earlier than those with stronger social support ties.

A trend away from intergenerational living arrangements has increased the proportion of individuals living alone even among the very old. The proportion of persons older than 85 years living with children declined in the 1980s to about 10% and has remained low. During that decade, the percentage in this advanced age category living alone rose from 29.7% to 36.8% (Longino, 1994). Because so many are widowed, more older women live alone than older men. The presence of "assisted living facilities" allows many of these persons in their eighth decade to live alone. This option, featuring one-room and two-room apartments, is not new, but its availability greatly expanded during the

1990s, offering dining room meals, reminders to take medications, and other services. Assisted living of this sort is a functional alternative to living with relatives when one can no longer live alone without some assistance. African Americans and Hispanics are much more likely to live in three-generation arrangements than are whites.

Housing

Most older people, about 80% in 2000 (Himes, 2001), own their own homes. Furthermore, about three quarters live in single-family homes. Home ownership is lowest among low-income groups, and low income is more pronounced in some racial and ethnic categories. Immigration obviously compounds this picture. The houses occupied by older persons, on average, are older than those occupied by persons in younger age categories; it would be surprising if it were otherwise. Although the housing of the elderly is older, it is basically sound. Over four fifths own their homes free and clear.

Geographic Mobility

Older individuals tend to remain where they have spent most of their adult lives. A few move after retirement. Of those who move, about half move short distances, within their counties. About 5% of all persons 60 years and older make long-distance interstate moves in any 5-year period.

Interstate migration is focused. Of the nearly 1.9 million Americans 60 years and older who moved out of state between 1985 and 1990, nearly half (49%) went to 1 of 7 states, in the following order: Florida, California, Arizona, Texas, North Carolina, Pennsylvania, and New Jersey. Florida is in a class by itself, receiving nearly one fourth of all interstate migrants 60 years and older. Florida's homestead tax exemption and lower rates of inheritance tax have been traditional draws, but the link to previous vacationing patterns is a more powerful motivator. Most long-distance moves soon after retirement are lifestyle motivated.

Much smaller migration streams in the reverse direction have been detected, with retirees returning from the Sunbelt to the major "sending" states. Migrants in these counterstreams tend to be, on average, a few years older, widowed, more often living dependently or in institutions after their arrival, and more often returning to their states of birth than migrants to the major destination states such as Florida.

Older people move for different reasons at different times. Early moves tend to be amenity seeking; later ones are more often health or social support related (Longino, 1995). Naturalized citizens can, and sometimes do, bring their parents to this country. However, there seems to be a selectivity process at work so that older people who make this strenuous change of cultural landscape tend to be healthier than people of the same age who do not move.

Political Participation

Voter turnout for presidential elections began to fall around the mid-1960s for the general population and reached its lowest level in 1988. That year, overall voter turnout in the US presidential election was 57%, compared with 69% in 1964. More than 3 in 5 registered voters over age 65 years have voted in presidential elections since 1964. Older people are more likely to vote than any younger age group. This gives older individuals, collectively, considerable political clout. Among persons of retirement age, those aged 65–74 years are the most likely to vote. Health issues limit many forms of social participation, including voting, and such limitations tend to increase with age.

During the late 1960s and early 1970s, many baby boomers were vocal and active politically, supporting numerous causes and movements. As a birth cohort, they also registered the greatest disillusionment due to the Watergate scandal. Political cynicism increased as participation plummeted among baby boomers. Their participation is expected to rise as they continue to age, but the size of that increase is not known at this time. As a consequence, there is likely to be a dip in the political participation of the elderly in the 2010s and 2020s.

HEALTH CHARACTERISTICS AND HEALTH BEHAVIORS

This section focuses on health in the older population. Its purpose is to give health professionals a perspective within which to understand individual patients. The information on mortality and morbidity, disability, and health risk behaviors was drawn, unless otherwise indicated, from national surveillance sources cited by the National Center for Health Statistics (1999) and Centers for Disease Control and Prevention (CDC; 1999). All data, unless otherwise indicated, refer to noninstitutionalized older adults.

Mortality and Morbidity

The five leading causes of death of persons 65 years of age and older are heart disease (33%), cancer (22%), stroke (8%), chronic obstructive pulmonary disease (6%), and pneumonia or influenza, which are tied with diabetes at 3% (Himes, 2001). Among both men and women aged 65–74 years, cancer is the leading cause of death. Alzheimer's disease (3%) follows diabetes as the seventh leading cause of death among persons of aged 65 years and older in the general population.

Chronic conditions are a substantial burden on the health of older adults, as well as on the economic status and quality of life of elders and their families. Those conditions common among the elderly include arthritis, hypertension, respiratory illnesses, heart disease, diabetes, stroke, and cancer. Among noninstitutionalized persons 70 years and older, 79% report one or more of these conditions. The majority of older adults have arthritis, with the level higher in women than men (63% vs. 50%). Hypertension affects 40% of women 70 years and older and 32% of men.

Ethnic disparities in diabetes morbidity mirror those of mortality. Hypertension is 1.5 times more frequently reported by African American older adults than by elders who are non-Hispanic whites. There is increasing recognition of the link between diabetes and cardiovascular disease, the large number of persons with undiagnosed diabetes, and the greater burden of diabetic complications (e.g., renal disease) among minority elders. Minority adults and those with lower education levels also are less likely to receive preventive care services (such as foot examinations, glucose self-monitoring, and glycosylated hemoglobin monitoring) that may help prevent diabetic complications (CDC, 2000). Having health insurance is associated with greater receipt of preventive services for diabetes, of course.

The self-report of health as excellent, very good, good, fair, or poor represents a cumulative measure of physical, mental, and social aspects of health. It is strongly predictive of mortality and of declines in physical functioning independent of medical conditions. The proportion of adults who consider themselves to be in fair or poor health increases with age for both men and women. At 85 years and older, over one third of adults rate their health as only fair or poor, while two thirds say that their health is good, very good, or excellent. More minority elders rate their health as fair or poor at every age than do whites, and self-rated health varies with income and educational attainment. These findings reflect disparities in objectively assessed health, as well as cultural differences in the interpretation of health status.

Disability

Disability is defined as limitation in the ability to care for oneself without assistance, particularly to perform basic (e.g., bathing, toileting, dressing, eating) and instrumental (e.g., shopping, cleaning, making meals, and bill paying) activities of daily living (ADLs; instrumental ADLs [IADLs]). Among persons 70 years and older, 20% had difficulty performing one or more ADL items, and 10% had difficulty with one or more IADL items. Disability is greater among women than men, and it increases with age. When physical functioning is assessed with specific tests, women also display greater disability. Women 70 years and older were more likely than men to be unable to climb a flight of stairs (11% vs. 6%) or walk a quarter mile unassisted (18% vs. 12%). Blacks report greater disability across all age groups than whites do. Regionally, older adults in the South report the greatest impairment to physical functioning.

Visual and hearing impairments are a significant source of disability in the older population, affecting a substantial proportion of older persons. Of community-dwelling adults 70 years and older, 18% report visual impairment (full or partial blindness or other trouble seeing), 33% hearing impairment, and 9% both. Older adults with sensory impairments are 2 to 3 times more likely to report difficulty walking, getting outside, and performing IADL items. They also report more falls and less participation in social activities.

The proportion of older adults reporting almost all forms of disability has decreased over the last decade, an indicator of more successful aging and perhaps a reflection of cohort effects of greater availability of medical and preventive care. Nevertheless, the absolute numbers of disabled older adults continue to increase due to rising life expectancy, and many of the disparities in disability by ethnicity, gender, and socioeconomic status continue.

Health Risk Behaviors

Health risk behaviors such as smoking and physical inactivity are leading contributors to disability, reduced quality of life, morbidity, and premature mortality in the United States. Nationwide, 13% of persons 65 to 74 years of age report smoking, compared to 7% among persons 75 years and older. The number of current smokers has remained stable over time, while the number of former smokers has tripled over the last three decades, reflective of improved rates of smoking cessation. Overall, smoking is more prevalent among men than women, among African Americans than whites or Hispanics, and among those with lower income and educational attainment. One would reasonably expect the incidence of smoking to decline further in the future as a result of cohort succession.

Leisure time physical inactivity increases with age. Approximately 35% of persons 65 to 74 years old report no strenuous physical activity; the rate rises to 46% among those 75 years and older. Women tend to report lower levels of physical activity than men. Blacks report less activity than whites. Regional differences are apparent for both blacks and whites. Rates of physical inactivity are highest in the South and lowest in the West. These gender, ethnic, and regional differences in physical inactivity are paralleled by rates of overweight and obesity. Again, there should be an increase in the value of exercise among those reaching early retirement age in the next two decades.

Religion

A growing number of studies have associated religiosity and religious practices with better mental and physical health in old age (Koenig, 1995). This association has been attributed to religion promoting healthier lifestyles, offering a sense of belonging and tangible support, and providing a framework within which to understand the meaning and purpose of one's life in times of crisis. National data show that the current cohort of older adults is more religious than younger people, with 76% rating religion as "very important" in their lives, compared with only 44% of those younger than 30 years. Also, 52%

attend religious services at least once per week, more than any other age group (Princeton Religious Research Center, 1994).

There is considerable variation in religious belief and practices. Even within single denominations (e.g., Lutheran, Presbyterian, Baptist), there are extremely conservative, as well as more liberal, subgroups. Studies of nonorganized religious activities (e.g., prayer, scripture reading) and religious belief (e.g., in miracles and healing) demonstrate the variation in its importance across ethnic and cultural groups (Levin et al., 1994), with greater importance attributed to religion and a more personal involvement in religion demonstrated by older African American than white adults (Gesler et al., 2000).

REFERENCES

Atchley RC. Social Forces and Aging, 7th ed. Belmont, CA: Wadsworth; 1994.

Centers for Disease Control and Prevention. CDC surveillance summaries, December 17, 1999. MMWR Morb Mortal Wkly Rep. 1999;48(SS-8):51–88.

Centers for Disease Control and Prevention. Levels of diabetes-related preventive-care practices—United States, 1997–1999. MMWR Morb Mortal Wkly Rep. 2000;49: 954–958.

Gesler W, Arcury TA, Koenig HG. An introduction to three studies of rural elderly people: effect of religion and culture on health. J Cross-Cultural Gerontol. 2000; 15:1–12.

Himes CL. Elderly Americans. Washington, DC: Population Reference Bureau; 2001.

Koenig HG. Religion and health in later life. In: Kimble MA, McFadden SH, Ellor JW, Seeber JJ, eds. Aging, Spirituality, and Religion: A Handbook. Minneapolis, MN: Fortress Press; 1995:9–29.

Levin JS, Taylor RJ, Chatters LM. Race and gender differences in religiosity among older adults: findings from four national surveys. J Gerontol. 1994;49:S137–S145.

Liang J, Fairchild TJ. Relative deprivation and perception of financial adequacy among the aged. J Gerontol. 1979;34:746–759.

Longino CF. Retirement Migration in America. Houston, TX: Vacation Publications; 1995.

Longino CF. State Profiles of the Oldest Americans in 1990: Decade Cohort Changes and the Disabled. Final Report Submitted to the American Association of Retired Persons Andrus Foundation. Winston-Salem, NC: Reynolds Gerontology Program, Wake Forest University; December 1994.

National Center for Health Statistics. Health, United States, 1999 with Health and Aging Chartbook. Hyattsville, MD: US Dept. of Health and Human Services; 1999.

Princeton Religious Research Center. Importance of religion climbing again. Emerg Trends. 1994;16:1–4.

Quandt SA, Arcury TA. The rural elderly. In: Lesnoff-Caravaglia G, ed. Aging and Public Health. Springfield, IL: Charles C Thomas; 2001:124–126.

Quinn JF, Burkhauser RV. Work and retirement. In: Binstock RH, George LK, eds. Handbook on Aging and the Social Sciences. Orlando, FL: Academic Press; 1990: 307–327.

Rapp SR, Shumaker S, Schmidt S, et al. Social resourcefulness: its relationship to social support and wellbeing among caregivers of dementia victims. *Aging Ment Health.* 1998;2:40–48.

Streib GF. Social stratification and aging. In: Binstock RH, Shanas E, eds. *Handbook of Aging and the Social Sciences.* 2nd ed. New York, NY: Van Nostrand Reinhold; 1985:339–368.

Treas, J. Older Americans in the 1990s and beyond. *Popul Bull.* 1995;50:1–45.

Treas J, Longino CF. Demography of aging in the United States. In: Ferraro K, ed. *Gerontology: Perspectives and Issues.* New York, NY: Springer; 1997:19–50.

Ullmann SG, Holtmann AG, Longino CF. *Early Retirement: A Descriptive and Analytical Study. Final Report Submitted to the American Association of Retired Persons Andrus Foundation.* Coral Gables, FL: Center on Adult Development, University of Miami; June 1991.

US Bureau of the Census. *65+ in the United States.* Washington, DC: US Government Printing Office; 1996. Current Population Reports: Special Studies, P23-190.

US Department of Labor, Bureau of Labor Statistics. *Labor Market Problems of Older Workers.* Washington, DC: US Dept of Labor; 1989.

7

Self, Morale, and the Social World of Older Adults

Jeanne E. Nakamura, PhD
Bertram J. Cohler, PhD

The study of personality across the second half of life has been marked by two concerns: the extent to which changes taking place in psychological functions across later life may lead to increased problems managing the tasks of everyday life and the extent to which the daily round continues to support the experience of morale and personal integrity or coherence. Missing in much of this discussion is a view of aging as a part of the expectable course of life. At least in part, emphasis on issues of "successful" aging reflects concern more generally in our culture with continued personal mobility and maintenance of interpersonal autonomy. Increasing need to depend on others to complete such activities of everyday living as grocery shopping is a major source of lowered morale in later life. Concern with successful aging may also be a consequence of the linear manner in which the course of life is understood.

This chapter considers aging in terms of the course of life as a whole, focusing on expectable changes in experience of self and others that serve as the background against which to understand both psychopathology and directed psychotherapeutic intervention. It is particularly important to view the second half of life in terms of expectable changes that occur both within lives over time and within the larger context of our culture. Our culture has portrayed the course of life as linear, with a beginning, middle, and end. Within this linear life story, later life is often assumed to be a time of decline, perhaps marked by struggle, accompanying the loss of such formerly sustaining activities as pursuit of a career. Just as in stories, in which the conclusion is expected to resolve the conflict posed within the plot, later life is assumed to resolve concerns enduring across a lifetime and to provide enhanced coherence or integrity, making possible a "good" death.

However, recent study has suggested that this portrait of age and decline does not well represent the lives of older adults in contemporary society. This chapter reviews evidence which suggests that later life is marked by its own achievements and problems, and that, at least until very late life, health and activity provide important sources of satisfaction and morale for many elders.

AGING, SOCIAL TIMING, AND THE COURSE OF LIFE

An alternative to the reductionist perspective of much of developmental psychology may be found in the emergence of a life-course perspective in the social sciences that recognizes that the meanings we make of experiences over a lifetime are interwoven with shared understandings and expectations. From this perspective, it is difficult to view the course of life apart from our shared understanding of expectable continuities and discontinuities from earliest childhood to oldest age. We share understandings within our culture regarding the significance of such role entrances and exits as assumption of the roles of parent and grandparent, retirement, and widowhood; these shared meanings are the foundation for experiences of particular persons as they encounter these transitions.

The term *aging* is often equated in our culture with a negative state of decline and senescence, implying loss, infirmity, and limitation. Viewing the second half of life from this perspective, some investigators have sought examples of older adults who are apparently more resilient even as confronted with the presumed negative impact of aging. Discussions of successful aging such as those of Rowe and Kahn (1987, 1998) or Baltes and Baltes (1990) focus on means used to resist presumed experience of decline and deficit. However, expectable changes that take place across the second half of life are not different in kind from those that take place at other points in the course of life. There is little discussion of "successful" adolescence, although it is often claimed that this period is accompanied by a particular sense of personal crisis (Erikson, 1950/1963; Freud, 1965). Study of the expectable course of adolescence (Csikszentmihalyi & Larson, 1984; Offer & Offer, 1975; Offer & Sabshin, 1984) shows that a crisis view of adolescence conflicts with the reality reported by adolescents. In a similar manner, a view of later life as a time of decline and infirmity conflicts with reports on the lives of older adults (Bengtson et al., 1985; Clausen, 1993; Schaie, 1981).

Viewed from a life-course perspective, aging refers to the socially constructed and psychologically experienced passage of time. Birren and Renner (1977) defined aging as "regular changes that occur in mature genetically representative organisms living under representative environmental conditions as they advance in chronological age" (p. 4).

The important aspect of this definition is that aging is a process that begins in early adulthood and continues across the course of life. As Birren and Renner (1977) noted, age may be understood in terms of (1) biological-functional changes in capacity relevant to the length of the life span; (2) psychological-functional age, or capacity to maintain continued adaptation to the environment; and (3) social age, or place in a shared definition of lives over time.

THE ORDER OF LIFE CHANGES

Since Durkheim's (1912/1963) discussion of the social origins of thought, it has been acknowledged that experiences of particular persons cannot be understood apart from the larger social order that structures and gives meaning to such experiences. It is precisely the social definition of the course of life that transforms the study of the life span or life cycle into the study of the life course. There is explicit recognition that changes with age are governed by shared definitions of expectable life events. Expected changes at particular ages are a function of the shared understandings of the length of lives and of the required progression or transitions through institutionally and informally defined social roles (Elder & Rockwell, 1979; Neugarten & Hagestad, 1976; Sorokin & Merton, 1937). Role transitions may be on time, too early, or too late in terms of the shared timetable.

Normative and eruptive changes or events both must be understood in a larger sociohistorical context (Hultsch & Plemons, 1979). To a great extent, particular adverse events that affect many people, such as the Great Depression (Elder, 1974, 1979; Elder & Rockwell, 1979), natural disasters, or social cataclysms such as wars or assassinations of national leaders, lead to feelings of shared participation in social experiences, which creates social bonds, distinguishing persons who have endured these events from those who have not. Further, these sociohistorical events color responses to subsequent events (Elder, 1974, 1979, 1996, 1997).

The sense of being "on time" or "off time" is always relative to that of other members of the same cohort, although there is a biological ceiling on the course of life engendered by the biosocial facts of the human life cycle. As both men and women come to marry later in adulthood, the sense of the expectable age at which one becomes a parent shifts. Retirement during a person's late 60s or early 70s may be viewed increasingly as appropriate, but retirement before a person's mid-60s (characteristic of Japanese society; Plath, 1980a, 1980b) would be considered off time across successive cohorts within US society.

As contrasted with on-time or expectable role transitions, off-time events may lead to decreased morale. In the case of some events, such as marriage, the event may happen late, while other events, such as widowhood, may happen early. In general, it is those events that take place unexpectedly early, such as adolescent pregnancy or widowhood in early-to-middle life, which are particularly likely to lower morale. By their very nature, these events occur suddenly and provide little opportunity for advance preparation. Discovery of a life-threatening illness in a spouse or offspring may provide some opportunity for preparing for loss and change. However, the absence of peers who are experiencing similar losses, at the same point in the life course, makes the anticipatory grief more difficult.

Even when understood as changes taking place across the second half of life, including the long period of life following retirement, there is little evidence that older adulthood is uniformly and inevitably characterized by experience of decline and decrement in personal and intellectual functioning (George, 1980; Perlmutter, 1983; Salthouse, 1989, 1990; Schaie, 1990, 1993, 1996). For example, cognitive changes with age show considerable individual differences; changes in functioning vary widely across cognitive abilities for any particular person; and in the absence of dementia, learning can continue into very old age (Baltes & Mayer, 1999; Schaie, 1994). Butler and Lewis (1977) documented the problems posed in understanding aging that stem from a view of the second half of life as a period of decline and infirmity. It is important to understand the second half of life in terms of the expectable course of life and to focus on factors that determine response to both expectable and eruptive life changes most characteristic of this particular point in the course of life.

Having attained a characteristic adult role portfolio (Hagestad, 1974), eruptive and normative events continue to interact with events resulting from the vicissitudes of adult roles, within particular cohorts, changing across the course of life. For example, with the advent of late life, the number of possible role transitions diminishes, leading to a reduction in the number of expectable normative transitions. Older persons are more at risk for some kinds of expectable losses, such as the death of longtime friends and relatives. Losses at older ages may be particularly poignant, remaining adverse life changes may be at least as painful as that adversity already experienced, and loss of morale may occur due to unexpected adverse events happening among friends and kindred. At the same time, there generally are fewer unexpected adverse life events to serve as sources of distress among older adults, with some adverse events having already occurred and others an expectable part of old age (Goldberg & Comstock, 1980; Lazarus & DeLongis, 1983; Lowenthal et al., 1975; Uhlenhuth et al., 1974). Findings regarding the age-related prevalence of stressful life events must be understood within particular sociohistorical circumstances and recognizing the changing significance of a past loss across the course of life.

CONTINUITY AND CHANGE WITHIN LIVES

Much of the study of personality and adult lives has been founded on a reading of Freud's epigenetic psychology, which presumes to show that experiences from earliest childhood are formative in later personality development and change. Freud was much influenced by 19th century science (Sulloway, 1979), primarily Darwin's report on evolution and Schliemann's reports on the excavation of ancient Troy. These reports emphasized the extent to which earlier structures continued to underlie later changes, influencing these later developments. This epigenetic approach, systematized in psychoanalysis by Abraham (1921/1953a, 1924/1953b) and Erikson (1950/1963), received apparent support from animal studies of "critical periods" or moving windows in development when the occurrence or absence of events (e.g., imprinting in ducks) permanently affects functions of the evolving organism (Lorenz, 1937/1957; Tinbergen, 1951). The concept was generalized to human development without empirical evidence. In the same manner, both social learning approaches and Piaget's genetic epistemology emphasize the developmental primacy of early over later experiences (Miller & Dollard, 1941; Murphy, 1947/1966).

The existence of a necessary, causal connection between earlier and later states has been called into question by both clinical and systematic empirical studies of lives over time. For example, imprinting plays a minimal role in human learning and development (Berenthal & Campos, 1987; Colombo, 1982; Emde, 1981; Kagan et al., 1978). Longitudinal studies of personality from childhood through middle and late life indicate that lives are less continuous and predictably ordered than is assumed in epigenetic models (Clarke & Clarke, 1981; Emde, 1981, 1985; Gergen, 1980, 1982; Kagan, 1980; Neugarten, 1969, 1979).

Much of the evidence supporting a view of lives as continuous and predictable over time has come from systematic trait studies founded on paper-and-pencil personality measures administered to different age groups (Leon et al., 1979; Stevens & Truss, 1985; Wiggins, 1997). Costa, McCrae, and colleagues (Costa et al., 1998; Costa & McCrae, 1980, 1985, 1989, 1994, 1997) provided findings based on a self-report instrument designed to measure five traits or factors claimed to remain stable across adulthood: neuroticism, extroversion, openness to experience, agreeableness, and conscientiousness (Wiggins, 1996; Wiggins & Trapnell, 1997).

Relying largely on cross-sectional study and test-retest correlations over a 10-year time span, Costa and McCrae claim that such study provides evidence that personality dispositions show little change over the course of adult lives (at least after 30 years of age). Costa and McCrae's claim has elicited some critical comments based on their research approach and additional critique based on the very question posed.

In the first place, paper-and-pencil measures of personality may tell us more about cultural conceptions of person than about the subjectivities of persons dealing with adult experiences (Shweder, 1975, 1977). From this perspective, findings of trait consistency would show little more than that adults agree on what constitute salient dispositions within our culture. Further, the psychologist Mischel (1968) contended that personality dispositions as studied by Costa, McCrae, and colleagues reflect primarily the present situation and response to it rather than some inherent "internal" psychological disposition. Moreover, Haan and coworkers (1986) noted that a test-retest approach to demonstration of personality stability over time presumes that persons of different ages agree on the meaning of a particular personality attribute. These authors report findings from a longitudinal study which suggest that some points in the course of life may show more change, while other points show relative stability. Overall, "childhood and adolescence were times of stability and systematic development in personality, whereas the adult years were times of greater experiential change . . . substantial changes still seem to be occurring up to late maturity, especially for the women" (p. 230).

Consistent with the report of Haan and colleagues (1986) and with others' critiques (e.g., Gergen, 1977; Harré, 1998; Mischel & Shoda, 1995; Ricoeur, 1992), Cervone and Shoda (1999) raised the fundamental question of the basis for assuming continuity in personality dispositions over a lifetime. Assessments of consistency and change within lives must be founded on study of the manner in which adults experience their lives and the meanings they make of lived experience. Reliance on trait constructs measured through paper-and-pencil inventories does not permit such understanding and focuses rather on statistical averages. Test-retest stability tells us little about the extent to which adults are able to maintain a coherent life story.

Cervone and Shoda (1999) suggested that Costa and McCrae's (1980, 1997) approach confuses description with explanation. Of even greater significance for study of consistency and change in adult lives, Cervone and Shoda maintained that focus on personality dispositions as a means for the study of adult lives has been superseded by a focus on the manner and extent to which adults are able to maintain a sense of self-coherence. Cervone and Shoda also observed that persons not only react in particular ways to particular environments, but are also proactive, working to create change, actively working to create coherence, and competently and effectively managing their lives. Studies of lives that use dispositional constructs are unable to capture this proactive aspect of development or self-efficacy (Bandura, 1982, 1997). Development across the course of life must be understood as a continuing effort at maintaining a coherent narrative or life story of a presently experienced past, lived present, and anticipated future that reflects a dialectic with both historical and social change (Riegel, 1979; Wertsch, 1998).

Systematic study of lives from childhood through middle and later life suggests that change rather than continuity may be the most interesting focus in understanding the course of lives over time. Further, developmental psychologists Kagan (1980, 1998) and Lewis (1997) and child psychiatrist Emde (1981, 1985) have reviewed findings from longitudinal and other research, including the Berkeley longitudinal studies and the work of psychiatrist and developmental psychopathologist Rutter. They view change and discontinuity as characterizing lives over time and found that much of what happens to us is a function of life experience after early childhood. There is little reason to presume that adverse experiences that take place earlier in life irrevocably determine the forward course of development or need necessarily influence the manner in which adults manage such expectable transitions as work to retirement or such unexpected adversity as early off-time death of a spouse. Writing about conditions that facilitate the capacity to overcome adversity, Lewis (1997) observed that "the search for precursors or causes of later behavior may be a noble but impossible task" (p. 97). Further, as Werner showed in a continuing study of a group of children followed from birth in Hawaii (Werner, 1985, 1990; Werner et al., 1971; Werner & Smith, 1977, 1982, 1992), factors leading to enhanced resilience at one point in the course of life may not be good predictors of resilience at another point in the course of life. As Lewis (1997) so sagely observed: "While the idea of the continuous course of development can be taken as a premise, it must, after fifty years of intensive study, remain just that, a world view . . . in its place we must find something else" (p. 97).

THE DILEMMA OF "SUCCESSFUL AGING" AND MAINTENANCE OF SENSE OF EFFECTANCE

Writing at a time when psychoanalytic psychology appeared to portray human behavior largely as reactive to intractable, destructive wishes, the psychologist White (1959) suggested that desire to attain competence or mastery in dealing with the environment, or "sense of effectance" must also be considered in the effort to understand motivation. White's call for study of competence or ego strengths was consistent with the psychoanalyst Hartmann's (1939/1959) view of psychological health in which wishes were not founded on biological desire (Rapaport & Gill, 1959). Bandura, a psychologist, echoed a similar theme in his social learning theory, a response to the reductionist, drive-centered learning theory of Hull (1943). Bandura (1982, 1989, 1997) termed his perspective *self-efficacy,* observing that beliefs regarding personal agency or capacity to effect change and control events are central in maintaining morale. Variation in sense of self-efficacy was presumed to have implications for both thought and action.

To the extent that persons believe they are able to control their environment, they are more likely to persevere when confronted with obstacles in their life and to realize enhanced personal resilience. As Lachman and coworkers (1994) noted, sense of personal control, that one can take charge of what happens in life in terms of both personal efficacy and control of the external environment, is associated with better health, enhanced socioeconomic success, and higher level of intellectual functioning into later life. Together with maintenance of social support, a continued sense of personal efficacy is among the most important factors contributing to longevity and well-being into later life (Rodin, 1986; Rowe & Kahn, 1987). However, correlations between subjective and objectively assessed sense of control are at best moderate. While Lachman and colleagues (1994) maintained that subjective elements of this belief are important, Baltes and Baltes (1990) primarily emphasized an objectively evaluated sense of control.

This concept of self-efficacy has been important in studies of adaptation to the challenges of later life. Following Rowe and Kahn's (1987) initial statement of so-called successful aging, psychologists Baltes and Baltes (1990) elaborated on the importance that self-efficacy, understood as a sense of personal control, holds for the study of successful aging. This concern with the dynamic of personal control followed from their research program, which viewed aging as further development rather than decline and emphasized the significance of adaptive mechanisms of selection, optimization, and compensation in fostering morale and continued sense of effectance through later life.

The concept of self-efficacy and the closely related dimension of sense of personal control have informed two of the most important studies of aging over the past two decades, that by the MacArthur Foundation Research Network on successful aging (Berkman et al., 1993) and the closely allied Berlin Aging Study, which focused on many of the themes elaborated in the Mac-Arthur Network research (Baltes et al., 1999; Baltes & Smith, 1997; Lindenberger et al., 1999). In a multisite study of community-living elders in their eighth decade of life who varied in physical and cognitive functioning, the Mac-Arthur Network group focused on strengths rather than problems associated with aging and reported important social status and personal control belief differences between high- and low-functioning groups of older adults. Those elders showing higher levels of physical and social functioning were likely to have been more economically successful in their lives, to have realized higher levels of educational attainment, and to have had better health habits and fewer symptoms of psychiatric distress. They reported greater sense of self-efficacy and were more likely than their low-functioning counterparts to be active in their community.

Particularly relevant for the present discussion of self-efficacy, two reports supported by the MacArthur Network study (Lang et al., 1997; Seeman et al., 1999) focused on this dimension of well-being. Lang and colleagues reported on findings from study of a group of elders living in a retirement community, who were aged 56 to 88 years and not a part of the core MacArthur Network study. Lang and coworkers focused on the reciprocal relationship between reported social ties and short-term fluctuation in self-efficacy beliefs concerning social relationships.

Those older adults who maintained a higher sense of self-efficacy also showed greater stability of this attribute over time, particularly when they felt affirmed and supported by others. Sense of control over the social environment is enhanced by being part of a social world; fluctuation over short periods is influenced by access to others. Consistent with Antonucci and Jackson's (1987) report on the importance of social ties for affirming sense of efficacy, continued threats to the social network may undermine middle-aged and older adults' belief in personal control in the domain of social ties. While enhanced belief in effectance in social relationships is sustaining over times when others are less likely to be available, aspects of the social surroundings are able to facilitate this sense of effectance within the social domain. There is also a reciprocal relationship between sense of self-efficacy and health (Lachman et al., 1994, pp. 224–225).

A second study, based on the core multisite MacArthur sample (Seeman et al., 1999), reported on the salience of strong sense of self-efficacy in maintaining morale even when experiencing physical disability. Measures of the perception of interpersonal and instrumental self-efficacy and evaluations of activities of daily living and performance of physical tasks over a period of more than 2 years were analyzed. Men and, to a somewhat lesser extent, women who expressed enhanced beliefs regarding self-efficacy within the instrumental domain, but not within the interpersonal domain, were better able to withstand any possible decrement in health and capacity for managing the daily round over the period of study. Self-efficacy beliefs predicted variations in functional disability independent of underlying physical capacities, suggesting that persons experiencing a weaker sense of effectance in mastering the tasks of everyday living lose morale and put forth less effort to overcome adversity. These adults may lose their sense of hope and determination, which in turn affects the impact of health setbacks on morale. This finding suggests that fostering enhanced self-effectance in the instrumental realm may lead to better physical function and health. The group of men and women selected for the core MacArthur study were by and large well functioning across the period of study. Following Bandura's (1989) observation, the salience of self-efficacy may become important only when there is significant challenge to functioning; the decrement reported for this group of elders may not have been sufficient to test the significance of self-efficacy beliefs as a protective measure when encountering adversity.

In the Berlin Aging Study, a probability sample of more than 500 older men and women living in then West Berlin completed a battery of measures in a cross-sectional study based on decade of life. Smith and Baltes (1999) reported little relationship between sense of control over one's life and sense of being controlled by others. Older adults within this group were more likely to maintain that others played an increasingly important role in their lives. This heightened sense of external control is of course realistic, recognizing that among the oldest old (over age 85 years), most adults have some significant health problems and necessarily become more dependent on others for assistance with the tasks of everyday living.

Consistent with findings reported by Lachman and Leff (1989), aging-related changes and decrements in health and physical mobility inevitably do influence the sense of personal control as shaped more by environment than by personal efforts. In sum, as in the MacArthur findings, experience plays an important role in the sense of effectance in later life. The loss through death or residential relocation of persons important in a person's social network and in providing personal resources is a real and definite challenge that may affect the sense of effectance within the interpersonal and instrumental domains alike. At the same time, findings from the (West) Berlin study showed that even elders were able to maintain a positive self-concept over time and maintained a sense of control over both their lives and the larger social world. Finally, it should be noted that adversity and obstacles encountered in later life may actually lead to increased determination to overcome this adversity, and that a sense of self-efficacy may not necessarily decline (Krause, 1999). Prior commitment to an important domain of life may lead to continued struggle and commitment rather than resignation if older adults are able to maintain positive morale and self-esteem.

To date, contributions from the study of self-efficacy in later life have underlined the importance of studying competence rather than decline and disability. While the concept of successful aging poses problems of value, presuming that a good old age is one merely continuous with earlier life, emphasizing continued high levels of intellectual activity and participation in a wide range of activities, it does serve as an important qualification to more traditional views of aging as necessarily a time of decline. According to Gergen and Gergen (1986), the traditional view

> holds the individual's deteriorating bodily system as central to understanding his or her conduct. This extended script invites the individual to speak critically about self, to make fewer claims to self-worth, to speak disparagingly about well-being . . . to seek dependency in relationships with others, to seek reliance on medical support systems, and so on. (p. 8)

At the same time, both the decline view and the concepts of successful aging and self-efficacy are very much culture bound to the bourgeois West. Kakar, a South Asian psychoanalyst (1978, 1979/1992), for example, noted that the expectable course in Hindu society of South Asia is for older adults to withdraw from the world and spend increased time in meditation and spiritual growth. As social psychologists Gergen and Gergen (1986) commented, self-efficacy is a particular way of talking about oneself and one's relation to the real world.

PERSONAL ADJUSTMENT AND LIFE CHANGES

Across the adult years, transition into and out of expectable adult roles appears to have less impact on morale than is commonly assumed. Neugarten and Datan (1974) and Datan and coworkers (1981) showed that expectable or on-time menopause among women has little impact on personal adjustment. Bengtson and Robertson (1985) showed that continuing intergenerational contact, even when in the context of caregiving, need not adversely impact morale. Numerous studies have shown that the transition from work to retirement does not necessarily adversely affect the morale or the physical health of most workers

(Kasl, 1984; Wan, 1984), even though some of those employed anticipate that they will worry more about their health after they retire (Ekerdt & Bosse, 1982).

Studies of widowhood yield a complex picture. Lieberman and Peskin (1992), Strobe and Strobe (1987), and Mendes de Leon and colleagues (1994) reported that on-time, expectable transition to widowhood has little long-term impact on the mental health of widows, while both women and, particularly, men widowed off time early reported prolonged struggles with an overwhelming sense of loss (Glick et al., 1974; Heyman & Gianturco, 1973; Lichtenstein et al., 1996; Wortman & Silver, 1987, 1990).

On the other hand, Wortman and Silver (1990) reported that, while there is some recovery of morale over the short term, recovery might extend over a decade or two following the death of the spouse. In a related study, Carr and coworkers (2000) reported that findings regarding adjustment following widowhood must be qualified in terms of marital adjustment and satisfaction. Enhanced dependence on a spouse, assumption of significant new responsibilities following the death of the spouse, and (contrary to common clinical wisdom) particular warmth and closeness to the spouse all predict elevated levels of distress.

While Carr and colleagues found few gender differences in personal distress accompanying widowhood, other research suggests that gender must be considered in understanding this life-course transition. Women widowed at an expectable age (mid-to-late 70s) seem to recover from the immediate loss within a period of about a year, whereas older men do not show a similar capacity to recover from grief. Further, Lichtenstein and colleagues (1996), taking advantage of a Swedish study of adult twins raised together and apart and followed over the adult years, reported that much of the depression observed to accompany widowhood may have been initiated well prior to the spouse's death in anticipation of this loss. Using the unique comparison of a still-married identical (monozygotic) twin, Lichtenstein and colleagues showed that there is some lasting impact of depression consequent to the advent of widowhood for women when considering baseline scores on depression prior to loss of the spouse.

The manner in which persons cope with these events often changes their personal significance (Fisseni, 1985; Maas, 1985). Much less is known about the factors that permit persons to remain resilient, even when confronted by adversity, than about those factors that may lead to distress and psychopathology (Cohler, 1987; Cohler et al., 1995; Vaillant, 1993). Whitbourne (1985) reviewed findings regarding the interplay of social timing and life changes; this study emphasized the multiple factors, from social circumstances and family values to the unique life history, that enter into both present understanding and response to adversity. Whitbourne's review stressed the significance of considering life changes across the course of life in terms of resources presently available for withstanding the impact of adverse life changes. This approach, closely identified with empirical studies by Lowenthal and coworkers (1975), Lazarus and Folkman (1984), and Vaillant (1993), focuses on the manner in which problems are approached and the extent to which persons are able to accurately evaluate and appropriately respond to challenges.

However, one possible problem with this approach, when understood from the perspective of the second half of life, is that it assumes an active, problem-centered mode of response that may be more appropriate to life changes taking place across middle age than to those associated with later life. While Folkman and Lazarus (1980), McCrae and Costa (1990), and Lazarus and DeLongis (1983) maintained that coping processes are stable across the adult years and not affected by age, both the mode of measurement and the restricted age range (only up to 65 years of age) qualify the assertion that age and coping approach are unrelated. Indeed, findings reported by Lieberman and Falk (1971), Cohler and Lieberman (1980), Hultsch and Plemons (1979), and Brim and Ryff (1980) suggested that older adults might respond to adversity in ways qualitatively different from those of younger adults.

Middle-aged adults tend to use reminiscence about the past in an effort to solve problems, while older adults use reminiscence to make peace with present reality and to cope with adversity using emotion-focused rather than problem-focused solutions (Lazarus & Folkman, 1984). Older adults tend somewhat more to look inward or to depend on a confidante rather than family members such as offspring in the effort to resolve problems in their present life. Indeed, even Lazarus and DeLongis (1983) recognized that there are changes with age in the experience of life changes; older adults may become less distressed than younger counterparts when confronting health crises due to the interplay of place in the course of life and a shifting perspective on the very concept of mortality. Older adults are apparently better able to confront these issues of mortality than their younger counterparts (Zweibel & Cassel, 1989; Zweibel & Lydens, 1990).

When there is little to be attained by active coping efforts, efforts to manage life circumstances may be less effective than renewed focus on the personal significance of this experience. Indeed, Kohut (1978) suggested that increased use of reminiscence and other modes of providing self-comfort and integrity might be the most effective response to surgery and other hospitalizations. Effectively using reminiscence and other so-called emotion-focused modes of coping with adversity and distress (Lazarus & Folkman, 1984) appears to be somewhat less difficult for older persons than for their younger counterparts. From the time of Butler's (1963) initial formulation, much of the literature has shown that the capacity to use reminiscence as a mode of comforting is particularly characteristic of later life (Haight, 1991).

Further, as Thomae (1990) observed, accepting the reality of present life circumstances does not necessarily imply passivity. Consistent with Janis's (1958) findings regarding denial and recovery from surgery, when confronted by a painful present reality that is beyond personal control, the best alternative may be to accept the present situation and to rely on memory of the past as consolation. Emphasis on active, problem-centered coping reflects life circumstances more relevant to the young-old than to the old-old. Reminiscence is particularly significant as a coping technique in later life because it provides a means of solace that fosters adjustment to a reality that is often physically and emotionally painful (Cohler & Galatzer-Levy, 1990; Elson, 1987; McMahon & Rhudick, 1964, 1967).

TIME, MEMORY, AND THE COURSE OF ADULT LIFE

Across the course of life, there are marked changes in the use of time and memory. For young children, the primary focus is the present, with a growing awareness of the past across the preschool years. The shift from early to middle childhood is marked by principal concern with the present, while that from childhood to adolescence is marked by changes in sense of time and organization of memory of the past (Cottle, 1977; Cottle & Klineberg, 1974; Greene, 1986, 1990) to include not only past and present, but also a connected future. Adolescent use of time shifts from a focus on the present, with an imagined future posed in terms of some idealized person or group, to more realistic appraisal of what may be attained over time. The adolescent and young adult looks forward, planning and anticipating, coping with uncertainty regarding next steps in terms of available opportunities; the middle-aged adult begins to turn to the past as a source of guidance during periods of personal distress (Lieberman & Falk, 1971). Indeed, across the course of the second half of life, the past may become mythologized, organized in a particular manner to provide meaning for particular present experiences and guidance in coping with problems. There may be a fourth transformation as well, associated with moving from middle to later life; this is sometimes known as the *crisis of survivorship*. Again, time and memory increasingly become reorganized as, with the death of spouse and friends, reminiscence replaces relationships as the source of present experience.

The Finitude of Life

One particularly significant feature of the second half of life concerns shared understandings of the very finitude of life (Munnichs, 1966) and of one's present position in terms of expectable longevity. Neugarten (1979) and Neugarten and Datan (1974) portrayed the experience, generally occurring during the fifth decade of life, of realizing that there is less time to be lived than has been lived already. This crisis of finitude is a consequence of the comparison of the trajectory of life with shared expectations concerning the duration of life. Awareness of finitude is heightened by increased acquaintance with mortality through experience of the deaths of parents and other family members and, increasingly, consociates (Plath, 1980a) or members of the same sociohistorical cohort (Jaques, 1965, 1980; Pollock, 1971, 1980, 1981).

This heightened awareness of mortality, portrayed by Munnichs (1966) as increased "awareness of the finitude of life" and elaborated by Marshall (1975, 1981, 1986), Jaques (1965, 1980), Neugarten (1979), and Sill (1980), results in a transformation in emphasis in temporal orientation from time already lived to that remaining to be lived and transformation in memory to increased preoccupation with the past and reminiscence. At first, this reminiscence is used actively in the service of coping with life changes associated with career and family (Lieberman & Falk, 1971; Lieberman & Tobin, 1983). At some point during the late 40s or early 50s, persons begin to look backward to the past for inspiration and meaning, rather than finding such meaning through anticipation of the future. For women and, especially, men, marked distress accompanied this transformation to midlife in a systematic study reported by Lieberman and Tobin (1983) and Cohler and Lieberman (1979). Men in their early 50s and women in their late 50s were particularly likely to express feelings of lowered morale, increased concerns about health, and increased feelings of anxiety and depression. This sense of disharmony and self-search has been reflected in the popular culture as the "midlife crisis." At least in part, these heightened concerns appear to account for a first hospitalization for psychiatric illness (Gutmann et al., 1982).

As a consequence of this increased personalization of death and awareness of finitude, persons begin to develop a more inward orientation, portrayed by Jung (1933) as introversion and by Neugarten (1973, 1979) as interiority. This midlife transformation is characterized by increasing preoccupation with the meaning of life, reviewing the past, and taking stock of personal accomplishments and disappointments (Butler, 1963; Kaminsky, 1984b; Moody, 1984); decreased interest in a wide variety of interdependent ties with kindred, particularly those that are obligatory rather than voluntary (Cohler, 1983; Cohler & Grunebaum, 1981; Pruchno et al., 1984; Rook, 1984); and decreased interest in taking on new challenges. It should be noted that this psychological transformation need not be reflected in the changing patterns of social ties suggested in discussions of disengagement (Cumming & Henry, 1961; Hochschild, 1975; Neugarten, 1973).

Findings reported by Back (1974), Gutmann (1975, 1977, 1987), and Sinnott (1982) also suggest that there may be gender-related differences across the years of middle and later life in the expression of interiority, the timing of the transformation to midlife, and the significance of this transformation for continued adjustment. Men at midlife become increasingly concerned with issues of personal comfort and with seeking succor from others, moving away from reliance on active mastery in solving problems at home and at work. Women may become somewhat more oriented toward active mastery and instrumental-executive activities, moving away from their earlier involvement in caring for others as wife, mother, and kin-keeper (Cohler & Grunebaum, 1981; Firth et al., 1970; Gilligan, 1982; Gutmann, 1987) and beginning to see themselves more in terms of present involvements beyond home and family (Back, 1974).

As a consequence of increased awareness of the finitude of life, both men and women appear to show increased concern with self and decreased patience for demands on time and energy that, increasingly, are in short supply (Back, 1974; Cohler & Grunebaum, 1981; Cohler & Lieberman, 1980; Erikson, 1980/ 1989; Erikson et al., 1986; Neugarten, 1979; Hazan, 1980; Lowenthal et al., 1975; Kernberg, 1980; Rook, 1984). Concern with realization of goals and with reworking the presently understood story of the course of life to maintain a sense of personal coherence become particularly salient in later middle age and require time and energy, which is then less available for other pursuits. The ability to mourn goals not attained and to accept the finitude of life without despair provides some evidence of the successful realization of this effort (Pollock, 1981).

The sense of a life foreshortened requires changes in the manner in which time is used in the ordering of this account. As a consequence, there may be a transformation in the experience of time and the use of memory (Cohler & Freeman, 1993; Lieberman & Falk, 1971; Lieberman & Tobin, 1983) that poses unique problems for the maintenance of a sense of personal integrity. At least some older adults deal with the increased sense of finitude of life by focusing on day-to-day issues rather than worrying about the future. In the words of one man in his 90s: "I take each day as it comes; who can predict the future" (Galatzer-Levy & Cohler, 1993, p. 321). While relying on the presently experienced past as a source of solace at times of distress and as guidance in resolving problems, the course of daily life is much more structured around the present than the future.

Reminiscence in Later Life

Erikson and colleagues (1986) described well the significance of reminiscence in later life as a source of the comfort and solace once available through relationships with others. Over time, with the death of friends and relatives (Kohut, 1974/1978, 1975, 1977, 1982; Horton, 1981; Horton et al., 1988), memory increasingly serves the functions previously realized through being with others. Reminiscence serves the dual function of comfort and storehouse of memories continually reordered over time to preserve sense of meaning and purpose even as confronted by adversity and social dislocation. Across the course of later life, reminiscence is increasingly used in the service of life review (Butler, 1963; Kaufman, 1986; Tobin, 1991), settling accounts with the entire prior course of life (Lieberman & Falk, 1971). Life review fosters the increased introspective activity occasioned by intensified awareness of finitude across later life, assisting in the process of maintaining sense of purpose into oldest age, as long as memory is accessible regarding the past (Benedek, 1959/1973).

Erikson's observation regarding the significance of reminiscence and personal review of the life story points out the importance of the remembered past for the maintenance of morale in later life (Myerhoff, 1978, 1992). Butler

(1963) noted the significance of the life review for the reintegration of the remembered past as a part of making sense of life as lived. As Myerhoff (1992) observed: "The integration with earlier states of being surely provides the sense of continuity and completeness that may be counted as an essential developmental task of old age. It may not yield wisdom . . . it does give what [Erikson] would consider ego integrity, the opposite of disintegration" (p. 239).

At the same time, memory itself may be painful, as among those older adults experiencing memory loss, such as patients in the early stage of Alzheimer's disease. Forgetting names, dates, and places is personally mortifying and deprives older adults of the very source of solace and comfort that is sustaining even as they are confronted by the reality of loss. It interferes with the ability to foster a sense of a continuing, coherent narrative of the course of life. The depressive affect often observed across the early-to-middle phase of Alzheimer's disease (Lazarus et al., 1987) may be a reflection of the loss of the narrative capacity, essential in preserving meaning and personal integration, that results from the impairment of memory.

SOCIAL TIES IN LATER LIFE

Recalling the past through recounting the presently experienced life story, as in the life of the aging Dr. Borg, the protagonist in Ingmar Bergman's 1957 film *Wild Strawberries*, contributes to personal well-being across the second half of life in ways that may be quite different from the use of the past either in early adulthood or middle-age (Lieberman & Falk, 1971; Lieberman & Tobin, 1983). Cohler and Galatzer-Levy (1990) have suggested that memories of the past may largely replace interpersonal contact as a source of solace during times of distress. The reality of the loss through death of spouse and close friends, problems in moving about, and limitations on personal energy all contribute to increased preference for memory of times spent with others rather than spending time with them in the present (although many older persons prefer to live by taking each day as it comes, solace is found in recollection and reminiscence of the past). Remembering and recounting the life story replaces contact with others as an essential or evoked other and are essential in maintaining a sense of personal integrity and morale.

Relations with Family and Friends

This perspective on the intrapsychic significance of social ties differs from perspectives that emphasize the significance of attaining interpersonal autonomy in realizing personal maturity. Those perspectives include the ethological-attachment group, portrayed by Bowlby (1982) and extended to the study of adult social relations by Antonucci (1990), Marris (1974/1986), and others, and the separation-individuation paradigm formulated by Mahler and coworkers (1975) and extended in consecutive panels to the study of middle childhood, adolescence and adulthood, and aging ("Experience of Separation-Individuation," 1973a, 1973b, 1973c). All tend to describe a level of ideal personal autonomy that is beyond that achieved by most adults.

In contrast, self-psychological perspectives emphasize the meaning of social ties over time, as revealed in the psychoanalytic interview (Kohut, 1971). Such experience-focused, phenomenological rather than behavioral perspectives regarding self emphasize the meaning that others hold for the individual rather than merely demonstrating that adults maintain important social ties and reporting on the aggregation of number and nature of ties with others. Much literature on the significance of social ties for adult adjustment has focused on the positive relationship between morale and size of self-reported social network (Adams, 1989; Antonucci, 1990). The social network or convoy of social support is believed to reduce the otherwise stressful effects of adverse life changes, buffering the individual from mental and physical ill health (Aneshensel & Stone, 1982; Antonucci, 1990; Caplan & Killilea, 1976; Dean & Lin, 1977; Eckenrode & Gore, 1981; Greenblatt et al., 1982; Kahn, 1979, 1994; Kahn & Antonucci, 1980; Killilea, 1982; Parkes and Weiss, 1983; Schultz & Rau, 1985; Turner, 1981; Weiss, 1982).

Very little study has focused on the manner in which social ties foster morale across the course of life or has explored the possibility that the very meaning of the experience of being with others changes across the life course. Pinquart and Sörenson (2000) reported on a meta-analysis of nearly 300 studies concerned with the association between aspects of social ties and self-reported well-being among older adults. Of particular relevance for the present discussion, these authors reported that, with advancing age, concern with the quality of social ties or "socioemotional selectivity" (Carstensen, 1991; Lansford et al., 1998) continues together with assurance of sufficient social ties that are qualitatively satisfying (Lang et al., 1998) in maintaining a sense of well-being. As older adults experience a thinning of their social network due to the death of friends, there appears to be increasing concern that there will be enough companions for socializing. Older adults prefer a smaller network of more intimate others than younger adults do, and they prefer friends and confidantes, rather than offspring, for social support (Fung et al., 1999; Lee, 1979; Martire et al., 1999). However, as Pinquart and Sörenson (2000) reported, relations with adult offspring do continue to be an important source of well-being as long as this contact does not impose undue strictures on time and personal resources of the older parent. This meta-analysis confirms Rosenmayr and Kockeis's (1963) finding that older adults prefer relations with offspring to reflect "intimacy at a distance."

Across the second half of life, brothers and sisters are likely to play a particularly important role in provision of support and assistance and in maintenance of morale for each other (Cicirelli, 1990, 1992). It has been difficult for those studying the family of the second half of life to shift from concern with relations of parents and children to a larger focus on brothers and sisters and other relatives as important for morale and adjustment (Cohler & Alter-gott, 1995).

Much research has focused on receipt of support or care not just outside the experience of receiving such care, but also outside the experiential world of those providing care. As a result of focusing on the recipient, studies tend to report on the benefits to young adults of receiving care, rather than the costs to their middle-aged parents of providing such care. Cohler (1983), Cohler and Lieberman (1980), Cohler and Grunebaum (1981), Pruchno and coworkers (1984), and Rook (1984) all emphasized the interdependent nature of care provided. When an individual experiences adversity, family members are expected to pro-vide assistance. The impact of adversity and its sequelae radiate outward from the immediate family to a large sphere of relatives. Family members are bound together by ties of "invisible loyalty" (Boszormenyi-Nagy & Spark, 1973) and do provide assistance for each other in times of distress. Further, as both the Harris and Associates (1975) survey on aging and the Berlin Aging Study (Wagner et al., 1999) showed, reciprocal exchange of resources continues into oldest age, including with own kindred.

Older family members have a larger number of younger relatives demand-ing care than elders who may be looked to for understanding and solace at time of need. They differentially become providers of care. While such care may have supportive and comforting implications for younger members of the family, it means an increased burden for older family members (Rosenmayr & Kockeis, 1963). For example, Robertson (1977), Szinovacz and colleagues (1999), Wood and Robertson (1978), Cohler and Grunebaum (1981), Cherlin and Furstenberg (1986), and Thomas (1990) all reported on grandparents who were resentful of the demands made on them for babysitting by their young adult offspring. At the same time, particularly among middle-aged grand-parents, their aging parents increasingly seek care and comfort rather than pro-viding it. Caring for dependent parents, while often a source of role strain, nevertheless may be somewhat less a source of distress for the generation in the middle than caring for young adults and their offspring. Those in middle and late life share a view of the life course that explicitly recognizes the finitude of life that is not shared by young adult offspring (Bromberg, 1983; Cohler et al., 1988).

The "generation in the middle" (Brody, 1966, 1970, 1981, 1985), particu-larly women in the family, are expected to provide care both upward and downward across the generations, often leading to feelings of dissatisfaction with social ties (Rook, 1984, 1989). Women have been socialized since early childhood into the roles of kin-keeping and child care (Chodorow, 1978; Firth et al., 1970). Women in the middle-aged generation are particularly likely to report feelings of being overburdened by demands of the social network or convoy and associated feelings of lowered morale. Further, having finished ac-tive parenting, middle-aged mothers may return to school or start working and feel their child's demands to be an intrusion on their own time and schedule.

Indeed, feelings of role strain and overload may be a greater problem than feelings of social isolation among late middle-aged women in our society (Dunkel-Schetter & Wortman, 1981).

The middle-aged person's response to the increased number of demands is also made difficult by the inward turn that occurs across the second half of life. Energy is deployed differently; persons experiencing the midlife transformation are likely to seek more time for self and to become increasingly preoccupied with their experience of aging. Indeed, there is an enhanced preference for solitude that is too often assumed to reflect social isolation in later life.

Loneliness and Being Alone

It is significant that studies of older persons found no greater report of feelings of loneliness than earlier in life (Fiske, 1980; Lowenthal, 1964; Lowenthal & Robinson, 1976; Mancini, 1979; Mancini et al., 1980; Townsend, 1957), although one study suggested decreased feelings of loneliness among still-married elderly couples (Wagner et al., 1999), and others reported increased loneliness among widowed men (Elwell & Maltbie-Crannell, 1981) or among women who had lived with a spouse for many years as contrasted with women living alone (Essex & Nam, 1987). Bankoff (1983) reported that increased distress is associated with the period immediately following widowhood. If widowhood happens approximately on time, much of this loneliness appears to diminish with time.

As Fiske (1980) and colleagues noted in their studies of middle and later life, there is a difference between being alone and being lonely. Successively across the second half of life, with the deaths of family members and friends, there is diminished access to familiar forms of social support. At the same time, as noted above, the use of reminiscence increases. Being alone both provides time for reminiscence and requires reminiscence as a means of ensuring meaning.

THE EXPERIENCE OF HEALTH IN LATER LIFE

Health in general is increasingly a concern across the second half of life. Middle age brings a greater sense of physical vulnerability, and "body monitoring" may intensify (Neugarten, 1968). Whitbourne (1987) discussed the intended and unintended consequences for health of the various strategies that individuals employ as they seek to maintain continuity of identity in the face of the mental and physical changes that accompany aging. For adults of all ages, the largest category of fears for the self concerns physical condition—health, appearance, weight. In later life, these fears appear to become more vivid and concrete (Cross & Markus, 1991). Of the "feared selves" that older adults report, those related to health tend to be dreaded most (Hooker, 1992).

In studies concerning the impact of health on morale, quality of life, and experience of self in later life, the focus has been on health status as subjectively perceived. Older adults' global evaluations of their health are associated with physician ratings and specific health indices (Fillenbaum, 1979; LaRue et al., 1979). The latter have been assumed to be more reliable measures, but there is some evidence that subjective health may be a more sensitive predictor of mortality (Hooker & Siegler, 1992; Idler & Kasl, 1991; Kaplan et al., 1988; Mossey & Shapiro, 1982). Continued physical mobility appears central to the older adult's subjective perception of health (Borawski et al., 1996; Shanas et al., 1968). Illness that does not affect the ability to remain active is less likely to lead to lowered morale or reduced social contact, and mobility may be even more important than income level in fostering sense of personal well-being (Kaufman, 1986; Larson, 1978; Zautra & Hempel, 1984).

Stolar and colleagues (1992) reported that health problems most clearly affecting morale may be those that cannot be integrated within a coherent life story (Antonovsky, 1987). Older adults' overall satisfaction with life was less affected by chronic illnesses such as arthritis and diabetes, which were experienced as understandable and manageable, than by health problems such as bladder trouble, vertigo, or difficulty walking, with causes and treatment that were experienced as less clear-cut. The last problems are likely to be unpredictably disruptive of everyday activities and social contacts.

In spite of health worries and ailments, older adults tend to describe their health as being very good. Indeed, among those over 65 years of age, there does not appear to be an increase with age in the proportion who regard their health as poor, even though the incidence of health problems does rise (Ferraro, 1980; Shanas et al., 1968). Cockerham and coworkers (1983) reported that older adults describe their general health in more positive terms than do younger adults. Older adults' tendency to report that they are in good health may reflect comparison of self-perceptions with that of age peers rather than present objective health status or comparison with health earlier in life. Further, as consociates begin to die, survival itself may be taken as an indication that one enjoys reasonably good health. Across very late life, the daily routine becomes less physically demanding, with increased enjoyment of solitude and reminiscence. Even diminished mobility may be adequate for sustaining morale (Cockerham et al., 1983; Cohler, 1993).

WISDOM AND CREATIVITY ACROSS
THE SECOND HALF OF LIFE

The search for a view of aging that challenges the notion of later life as a time of decline has encouraged attention to the expression of wisdom and creativity across the second half of life. In relation to wisdom, Gutmann (1987) noted the respect accorded to elders in traditional society; the longer life experience that accompanies the passage of years is presumed to lead to a perspective on self and others that is less self-interested and to an enlarged understanding of the nature of life.

It should be noted that study of wisdom has become caught up in larger contemporary social and political issues, such as those regarding the presence of gender and age bias across the course of life. Scholarly study has sometimes been designed in an effort to prove the worth of older adults in a society too often preoccupied with masculinity and youth (Kaminsky, 1993; Kastenbaum, 1993; McCullough, 1993; Moody, 1986, 1993; Orwoll & Achenbaum, 1993).

The Wise Elder as the Ideal Type

Erikson's (1950/1963, 1960, 1968) epigenetic model portrays wisdom as an attitude of detached concern optimally attained in later life. Faced with finitude, a fragmenting sense of despair—rooted in regrets about the life one has lived, frustration with limitations in the present, and fear and uncertainty about one's future—counters the development of a sense of wholeness, coherence, or integrity through coming to terms with one's life. In successful resolution of the issue of integrity, sense of despair is transformed with a sense of wholeness (Erikson, 1979) rather than denied through desperate optimism (Erikson et al., 1986), creation of a too-coherent life story (Manheimer, 1992), or some other form of what Erikson called pseudointegrity. Tobin (1991) suggested that, over time, Erikson increasingly focused discussions of integrity and wisdom on use of reminiscence, with a sense of wholeness attained through review of one's life. Processes that Erikson identifies with attainment of wisdom have been explored in the literature on reminiscence, life review, and life story. In a relevant empirical study, individuals nominated by others as wise appeared to show greater acceptance of the personal past (Orwoll & Perlmutter, 1990).

The growing attention to wisdom outside the tradition pioneered by Erikson (Sternberg, 1990a) can be traced to concern in our time with successful aging. Viewed from this perspective, wisdom seems an especially promising focus of attention, constituting a gain in functioning that is distinctively associated with later life. Heckhausen and colleagues (1989) found that, of 100 desirable psychological attributes, *wise* and *dignified* were the only ones expected to emerge in old age.

One focus of recent study has been to identify folk notions of wisdom by eliciting characteristics of the prototypical wise person (Chandler & Holliday, 1990; Clayton & Birren, 1980; Holliday & Chandler, 1986; Sternberg, 1990b). As Chandler and Holliday (1990) observed, the recurrence of essentially the same set of descriptors across studies suggests that a distinguishable folk concept of wisdom persists (Cole et al., 1993). The concept is multidimensional. The wise individual understands self and others; is perceptive, intuitive, empathic, knowledgeable, measured, and experienced; and recognizes essences, contexts, consequences, and multiple perspectives. This definition may be cul-

ture specific to at least some degree. Takahashi and Bordia (2000) elicited similarity judgments for a set of personality descriptors from college students in
different cultures; while Americans associated *wise* with *knowledgeable* and
experienced, their Indian and Japanese counterparts associated it with *discreet*.

In proposing definitions of wisdom, recent theorists have drawn on these
commonsense understandings, treatments of wisdom within philosophy, and contemporary conceptions of personality, development, and especially cognition
(Chandler & Holliday, 1990). A thread running through many of these discussions is the notion of recognition of and response to human limitation and
doubt about the truth of what one knows (Meacham, 1990; Taranto, 1989).
Baltes and colleagues, who viewed the wise person as possessing high levels of
knowledge about life, encompassed within this an awareness of life's uncertainties, social context, and relativity, as well as factual and procedural knowledge
about living (Baltes et al., 1990; Baltes & Smith, 1990; Baltes & Staudinger,
2000; Clayton, 1982). Invoking the distinction between fluid intelligence,
which may decline in late life, and crystallized intelligence, which does not,
they conceptualized wisdom as a form of expertise that makes possible good
judgment, sound advice, and special insight concerning "important but uncertain" life matters. In a series of studies, they presented a hypothetical person's
life dilemma, asked how the person might respond, and evaluated the degree
of knowledge about life—the wisdom—reflected in the proposed responses.

Although Erikson's identification of wisdom as the defining ego strength
of old age might imply that it is a normative developmental achievement, Erikson and coworkers (1986) acknowledged that many of the older adults they
interviewed had not achieved it. Consistent with this view, Baltes and colleagues reported that few adults of any age provided commentary reflective of
wisdom in response to hypothetical life problems (e.g., Smith & Baltes, 1990).
By this measure at least (Bandura, 1997, cautioned that wisdom is enacted and
modeled as well as dispensed, and that measures need to take this into account), wisdom appears to be rare. Clayton (1975) outlined contemporary cultural forces that may work against development or appreciation of wisdom
as defined by Erikson, including contemporary preoccupation with youth and
mundane, worldly activity.

From the perspective of successful aging, interest in wisdom rests on the
assumption that, however rarely attained, it is a late-life accomplishment. The
evidence is mixed. In terms of perception of self, older adults believe that their
adaptation to the successes and disappointments met in life and their acceptance of the personal past as "inevitable, appropriate, and meaningful" have
increased with age (Ryff & Heincke, 1983). Both young and middle-aged
adults projected they would experience a greater sense of integrity in late life
than they attributed to themselves in the present, suggesting that there is a
shared expectation that the sense of integrity increases across the life course
(Ryff & Heincke, 1983).

Further, adults of various ages tend to nominate older adults when asked to identify someone wise (Orwoll & Perlmutter, 1990). There is some evidence that women tend to identify kin, and that men call on experiences at work in nominating wise persons (Sowarka, 1989, cited in Sternberg, 1990a), although this may reflect cohort-specific gender differences in both meaning and participation within the world of work. In addition, a small sample of older adults outperformed young adults on a task requiring the ability to make attributions about inner states of self and others, potentially a component of wisdom (Happé et al., 1998). Older adults appeared to draw on social interaction more effectively than their younger counterparts when performing wisdom tasks (Baltes & Staudinger, 2000).

On the other hand, while young and middle-aged adults associate wisdom with old age (Clayton & Birren, 1980), older adults associate wisdom less closely with being old than do younger adults, and they view themselves as no wiser than younger adults see themselves (Clayton & Birren, 1980; Orwoll & Perlmutter, 1990). From some perspectives (e.g., Meacham, 1990), this might be viewed as itself evidence of wisdom, a knowledge that one does not know. Alternatively, perhaps wisdom is not a function of age.

Several studies conducted by Baltes and colleagues with adults aged 20 to 80 years showed no age differences favoring older adults (Staudinger, 1999). Even life review tasks, theoretically more familiar to older than to younger adults, have not shown consistent increases in performance with age, although older adults certainly were represented among those few whose responses were judged most indicative of wisdom (Baltes & Staudinger, 2000; Staudinger et al., 1992). Evaluation of responses to life-planning tasks led Baltes's group to propose that wisdom may not be global and cumulative. Instead, adults may possess most "expert knowledge" about life matters specific to their place in historical time and in the life course (Smith & Baltes, 1990).

For different reasons, Meacham (1990) also rejected a cumulative view of change in wisdom. Meacham argued provocatively that, because accumulation of knowledge and power tends to undermine an attitude of doubt concerning what one knows, the expectable course of wisdom is one of decline with age. The young can be wise: Meacham invoked Anne Frank as an example of youthful wisdom. Perhaps the image of the wise elder represents most of all a source of solace and hope for young and middle-aged adults (Galatzer-Levy & Cohler, 1993; Meacham, 1990).

The nature of experiences that might foster development of wisdom is not well understood. For many current theorists, and perhaps in folk conceptions as well, wisdom is associated with old age because it is seen as something gained through long experience. If wisdom connotes a sense of coherence, it again is normatively tied to the second half of life when "coherence work" (Moody, 1993) intensifies in response to awareness of finitude (Taranto, 1989). If wisdom is expertise about life's uncertainties (Baltes & Smith, 1990), its acquisition is favored by broad and extensive life experience and nurturance by experts. Work-related experience with life planning, life management, and life review is conducive to wisdom-related performance. From the perspective of knowledge acquisition, it is understandable that young adults today might be more expert than older adults in some areas, particularly problems related to the meaning of work, positive health habits, and quality of life, which are salient in early adulthood for present cohorts, but possibly less salient for older adults. In addition to creating areas of knowledge that are unfamiliar to older cohorts, rapid cultural change may render portions of their store of knowledge obsolete (Rowe & Kahn, 1998).

For the most part, recent research has not been concerned with the inner experience of the wise adult. One exception is Ardelt's (1997) analysis of Berkeley Guidance Study data, which led Ardelt to view wisdom as a personal resource contributing to morale in later life. Defining wisdom as the integration of cognitive, affective, and reflective qualities (cf. Clayton & Birren, 1980), encompassing depth of understanding, compassion, and the transcendence of one's subjectivity and projections, Ardelt found that, for both older women and older men, wisdom has a significant positive relationship to life satisfaction independent of objective conditions such as health and income. This is consistent with the view of wisdom as a source of comfort, understanding, and compassion (Erikson, 1979; Erikson et al., 1986). Orwoll and Achenbaum (1993) suggested that wisdom may be experienced differently by men and women, expressed principally in the interpersonal realm by women and manifested in communal concerns, and expressed in the intrapersonal realm by men and evident as agentic concerns (Gutmann, 1987).

Expression of Creativity Across Middle and Later Life

Because involvement in creative activity is perceived as one means of maintaining vitality into oldest age (e.g., Erikson et al., 1986), much of the recent interest in late-life creativity has been spurred by efforts to counteract the "aging-as-decline" perspective (Cole, 1992; Cole et al., 1993). However, psychometric research on creative potential and study of changes in creative productivity across the adult years—two established lines of research bearing on late-life creativity—in fact have been preoccupied with the narrow question of whether creativity decreases across the second half of life.

Older adults appear to perform less well than younger adults on paper-and-pencil measures of creative ability (Alpaugh & Birren, 1977; McCrae et al., 1987). It is not clear whether test performance in any way indexes real-life creativity or whether group differences of the magnitude found hold real-world significance (Romaniuk & Romaniuk, 1981; Schaie, 1984, 1990, 1996; Schaie et al., 1973; Simonton, 1990c). Use of this paradigm to study aging and creativity is problematic.

A separate research tradition ensures study of real-life creativity by adopting a historiometric approach. Change in creative productivity across the life course is measured by analyzing historical records of the career output of eminent artists, scientists, and scholars. With some qualifications (e.g., Dennis, 1956, 1966), the studies suggest that, on average, output (both of major and of minor works) rises at successive ages until it reaches a peak, with lower output thereafter (Lehman, 1953, 1956; Simonton, 1990a, 1990b, 1990c). As Kastenbaum (1992) points out, however, the meaning and causes of this pattern have yet to be understood. Waning capacities constitute only one possible explanation; social, cultural, and other nonendogenous factors may be important (Hendricks, 1999).

Although it might be inferred that creative achievement inevitably declines in late adulthood, Lehman and Simonton noted the many counterexamples of artists, scientists, and others whose major creative contributions occurred late in life (cf. Kastenbaum, 1991). In addition, age at peak output and steepness of decline both vary greatly by domain. One eminent translator of classical languages observed that it is impossible to attain a good working knowledge of Greek and do a decent job of translating classical Greek texts until the eighth or ninth decade of life. Simonton (1998) concluded that a major work can be produced at any point in a particular creator's career, and that "creativity of the highest caliber can continue until a person's final days" (pp. 14–15).

Whereas much research on creativity has focused on the late-career productivity of great artists and scientists, from the standpoint of the experience of self over the life course, it is the impact of creative activity on the person rather than on the culture that holds greatest interest. Creative pursuits may constitute a means of warding off boredom or responding to an experienced imperative to stay active (Lieberman & Lieberman, 1983). When the imperative to keep busy or get involved is counter to the person's preferences, creative arts—like other externally motivated activities—may be experienced largely as an unwelcome imposition (Pruyser, 1987) and can adversely affect morale. Indeed, busyness may interfere with other less visible forms of creative activity, such as life review (Butler, 1963; Kastenbaum, 1992; Tobin, 1991). When freely embraced, however, creative pursuits can contribute to a sense of efficacy, purpose, and continuing growth for older adults, fostering well-being by providing a means of connecting with others, forgetting aches and pains, and deriving satisfaction from involvement in an enjoyed activity (Fisher & Specht, 1999).

For lifelong artists and scientists, creative activity has become a core element of the self and key way of engaging the world and represents a continuing source of meaning and morale in late adulthood (Csikszentmihalyi, 1996). The inward turn in later adulthood, and the effort to integrate and make sense of experience, may also contribute to a distinctive old age style for at least some great artists, encompassing such qualities as introspection and a "cultivated passivity" (Cohen-Shalev, 1989, p. 33). Creative activities also may be newly and distinctively engaging in late life as older adults become increasingly concerned with their experiences and strive to construct accounts of their lives that preserve a sense of coherence (Cohler, 1993). Francis (1992) described a group of retirees whose art either represented scenes from their work life or incorporated skills and materials drawn from their work world. Through the visual arts, these older adults variously evoked, memorialized, reworked, sought to justify, or struggled to come to terms with and integrate the personal past. For other older adults, creative writing appears to provide the medium for life review (Kaminsky, 1984a).

Artistic activity is associated with health and well-being in later life, whether the activity is pursued throughout the adult years or is deferred during middle adulthood (Erikson et al., 1986; Lorenzen-Huber, 1991; Torrance, 1977). Vaillant (1993, 2001) reported that, in two major longitudinal studies, men and women who had been creative at midlife expressed higher morale and reported greater physical vigor in old age than their less-creative counterparts.

In part because of the perception that creative activity contributes to well-being in later life, there is strong interest in enabling participation in the arts by older adults (e.g., Hickson & Housley, 1997). From a life course perspective, it is important to realize that adults who reach later life during different historical periods will have had very different experiences regarding their artistic activity and will have encountered different cultural attitudes toward it. Krantz (1977) and Osherson (1980) studied career change in midlife; they described men who were seeking to leave organizational careers that had offered little opportunity or support for creativity and personal expression. The offspring of this generation grew up in the child- and then youth-centered expressive culture of the mid-20th century. Interviewing the offspring at early middle age, Leinberger and Tucker (1991) repeatedly heard declarations of frustrated desire for a career in the arts, a personal history likely to foster interest in artistic activity as this baby boom generation reaches later life.

CONCLUSION

Study of older adulthood within the context of the course of life as a whole marks an important departure for both psychiatry and the social sciences. With as much as one third of the life span to be lived after retirement in contemporary society, it is essential that earlier conceptions of the place of the second half of life within the course of life as a whole be reconsidered. It is largely as a consequence of shared understandings of the significance of particular chronological ages that particular ages are imbued with meanings. Understanding of health is also subjectively constructed; regardless of so-called objective indices of illness, as long as older adults are able to retain independent functioning and manage tasks of daily life, positive morale is maintained that mitigates against otherwise presumed interference by illness in well-being. At the present time, with those over 85 years old the most rapidly growing age group within the population, it is important to reconsider views of personal change and capacity for continued adaptation to social change across later life and to plan more effectively for the social and health needs of this group of older adults across the 21st century.

Reconsideration of previous findings has shown the limitations arising from the study of a particular generation or cohort of adults across the second half of life. Older adults, at least until about age 65 years, are as healthy as younger counterparts and show little of the personal rigidity and decrement in cognitive functioning earlier believed to characterize the later years. Improved health across the course of life and greater education and subsequent continued immersion in activities that foster cognitive competence through oldest age have contributed to a generation of particularly effective older adults. While areas of creative contribution may change over time, there is sustained capacity for creative activity across the years of middle and later life. Active and involved in both family and community, more than half of persons older than 85 years continue to live independently; indeed, continued autonomy and capacity for managing everyday life activities characterizes the largest number of older adults and is critically important for maintaining morale and adjustment. Consistent with this portrait of older adults as competent and contributing members of the community who are creative and involved in a complex network of relationships with both friends and family, present cohorts of older adults show little of the self-preoccupation earlier assumed to characterize personality in later life (Silverstone, 1996).

Implications of this new view of competence and health across the second half of life are important in considering issues of intervention, particularly with the aging of the baby boomers (Cornman & Kingson, 1996). While those individuals who require psychiatric intervention highlight problems confronted by older adults, to date there has been little of the consideration of primary prevention with older adults that has characterized study and intervention across the years of childhood and adolescence. Creative reconsideration is needed of issues such as housing that supports intergenerational living, including that among families of choice; home-based health care, which fosters positive morale by enabling continued independent living; and the significant role of both friends and siblings as sources of care and support. All of these are important in forestalling the cycle of personal disorganization that ultimately requires psychiatric intervention. Increased attention to issues of quality of life across the life course remains a concern of highest priority for psychiatry and the social sciences.

REFERENCES

Abraham K. Contribution to a discussion on tic. In: *Selected Papers on Psychoanalysis* (Bryan D, Strachey A, trans.). New York, NY: Basic Books; 1953a:323–325. (Original work published 1921.)

Abraham K. A short study on the development of the libido, viewed in the light of mental disorders. In: *Selected Papers on Psychoanalysis*. New York, NY: Basic Books; 1953b:418–501. (Original work published 1924.)

Adams R. Conceptual and methodological issues in studying friendships of older adults. In: Adams R, Blieszner R, eds. *Older Adult Friendship: Structure and Process*. Newbury Park, CA: Sage; 1989:17–41.

Alpaugh PK, Birren JE. Variables affecting creative contributions across the adult life span. *Hum Dev.* 1977;20:240–248.

Aneshensel C, Stone J. Stress and depression: a test of the buffering model of social support. *Arch Gen Psychiatry.* 1982;39:1392–1396.

Antonovsky A. *Unraveling the Mystery of Health: How People Manage Stress and Stay Well*. San Francisco, CA: Jossey-Bass; 1987.

Antonucci T. Social supports and social relationships. In: Binstock R, George LK, eds. *Handbook of Aging and the Social Sciences*. 3rd ed. New York, NY: Academic Press; 1990:205–227.

Antonucci TC, Jackson JS. Social support, interpersonal efficacy, and health. In: Carstensen L, Edelstein BA, eds. *Handbook of Clinical Gerontology*. New York, NY: Pergamon Press; 1987:291–311.

Ardelt M. Wisdom and life satisfaction in old age. *J Gerontol.* 1997;52B:P15–P27.

Back KW. Transition to aging and the self image. In: Palmore E, ed. *Normal Aging: II*. Durham, NC: Duke University Press; 1974:207–216.

Baltes P, Baltes M. Psychological perspectives on successful aging: the model of selective optimization with compensation. In: Baltes B, Baltes M, eds. *Successful Aging: Perspectives From the Behavioral Sciences*. Cambridge, UK: Cambridge University Press; 1990:1–34.

Baltes PB, Mayer KU, eds. *The Berlin Aging Study: Aging From 70 to 100*. New York, NY: Cambridge University Press; 1999.

Baltes PB, Mayer KU, Helmchen H, Steinhagen-Thiessen E. The Berlin Aging Study (BASE): sample, design and overview of measures. In: Baltes PB, Mayer KU, eds. *The Berlin Aging Study: Aging From 70 to 100*. New York, NY: Cambridge University Press; 1999:15–55.

Baltes PB, Smith J. Toward a psychology of wisdom and its ontogenesis. In: Sternberg R, ed. *Wisdom: Its Nature, Origins, and Development*. New York, NY: Cambridge University Press; 1990:87–120.

Baltes PB, Smith J. A systematic-holistic view of psychological functioning in very old age: introduction to a collection of articles from the Berlin Aging Study. *Psychol Aging.* 1997;12:395–409.

Baltes PB, Smith J, Staudinger UM, Sowarka D. Wisdom: one facet of successful aging? In: Perlmutter M, ed. *Late Life Potential*. Washington, DC: Gerontological Society of America; 1990:63–81.

Baltes PB, Staudinger UM. A metaheuristic (pragmatic) to orchestrate mind and virtue toward excellence. *Am Psychol.* 2000;55:122–136.

Bandura A. Self-efficacy mechanism in human agency. *Am Psychol.* 1982;37:122–147.

Bandura A. Human agency in social cognitive theory. *Am Psychol.* 1989;44:1175–1184.

Bandura A. *Self-efficacy: The Exercise of Control*. New York, NY: Freeman; 1997.

Bankoff E. Social support and adaptation to widowhood. *J Marriage Family.* 1983;45:827–839.

Benedek T. Parenthood as a developmental phase: a contribution to the theory of the libido (with discussion). In: *Psychoanalytic Investigations: Selected Papers by The-rese Benedek*. New York, NY: Quadrangle Books; 1973:377–407. (Original work published 1959.)

Bengtson V, Reedy M, Gordon C. Aging and self-conceptions: Personality processes and social contexts. In: Birren J, Schaie KW, eds. *Handbook of the Psychology of Aging*. New York, NY: Van Nostrand-Reinhold; 1985:544–593.

Bengtson V, Robertson J, eds. *Grandparenthood*. Newbury Park, CA: Sage; 1985.

Berenthal B, Campos J. New directions in the study of early experience. *Child Dev*. 1987;58:560–567.

Berkman LF, Seeman TE, Albert M, et al. High, usual, and impaired functioning in community-dwelling older men and women: findings from the MacArthur Foundation Research Network on successful aging. *J Clin Epidemiol*. 1993;10:1129–1140.

Birren J, Renner V. Research on the psychology of aging: principles and explanation. In: Birren J, Schaie KW, eds. *Handbook of the Psychology of Aging*. New York, NY: Van Nostrand-Reinhold; 1977:3–38.

Borawski EA, Kinney JM, Kahana E. The meaning of older adults' health appraisals: congruence with health status and determinant of mortality. *J Gerontol*. 1996;54B:S157–S170.

Boszormenyi-Nagy I, Spark C. *Invisible Loyalties: Reciprocity in Intergenerational Family Therapy*. New York, NY: Harper & Row; 1973.

Bowlby J. Attachment and loss: retrospect and prospect. *Am J Orthopsychiatry*. 1982;52:664–678.

Brim OG, Jr, Ryff C. On the properties of life events. In: Baltes P, Brim OG, Jr, eds. *Life-span Development and Behavior*. Vol. 3. New York, NY: Academic Press; 1980:368–388.

Brody E. The aging family. *Gerontologist*. 1966;6:201–206.

Brody E. The etiquette of filial behavior. *Int J Aging Hum Dev*. 1970;1:87–97.

Brody E. "Women in the middle" and family help to older people. *Gerontologist*. 1981;21:471–480.

Brody E. Parent care as a normative family stress. *Gerontologist*. 1985;25:19–29.

Bromberg E. Mother-daughter relationships in later life: the effect of quality of relationship upon mutual aid. *J Gerontol Soc Work*. 1983;6:75–79.

Butler R. The life review: an interpretation of reminiscence in the aged. *Psychiatry*. 1963;26:65–76.

Butler R, Lewis M. *Aging and Mental Health: Positive Psychosocial Approaches*. St. Louis, MO: Mosby; 1977.

Caplan G, Killilea M, eds. *Support Systems and Mutual Help: Multidisciplinary Explorations*. New York, NY: Grune & Stratton; 1976.

Carr D, House JS, Kessler RC, et al. Marital quality and psychological adjustment to widowhood among older adults: a longitudinal analysis. *J Gerontol Soc Sci*. 2000;55B:S197–S207.

Carstensen L. Selectivity theory: social activity in life-span context. *Annu Rev Gerontol Geriatr*. 1991;11:195–217.

Cervone D, Shoda Y. Beyond traits in the study of personality coherence. *Curr Direct Psychol Sci*. 1999;8:27–32.

Chandler M, Holliday S. Wisdom in a post apocalyptic age. In: Sternberg R, ed. *Wisdom: Its Nature, Origins, and Development*. New York, NY: Cambridge University Press; 1990:121–141.

Cherlin A, Furstenberg F, Jr. *The New American Grandparent: A Place in the Family, a Life Apart.* New York, NY: Basic Books; 1986.

Chodorow N. *The Reproduction of Mothering.* Berkeley: University of California Press; 1978.

Cicirelli V. Family support in relation to health problems of the elderly. In: Brubaker T, ed. *Family Relationships in Later Life.* Rev. ed. Newbury Park, CA: Sage; 1990: 212–228.

Cicirelli V. Siblings as caregivers in middle and late life. In: Dwyer J, Coward R, eds. *Gender, Families and Elder Care.* Newbury Park, CA: Sage; 1992:84–104.

Clarke SDB, Clarke AM. "Sleeper effects" in development. Fact or artifact? *Dev Rev.* 1981;1:344–360.

Clausen J. *American Lives: Looking Back at the Children of the Great Depression.* New York, NY: Free Press; 1993.

Clayton V. Erikson's theory of human development as it applies to the aged: wisdom as contradictive cognition. *Hum Dev.* 1975;18:119–128.

Clayton V. Wisdom and intelligence: the nature and function of knowledge in the later years. *Int J Aging Hum Dev.* 1982;15:315–321.

Clayton V, Birren J. The development of wisdom across the life-span: a reexamination of an ancient topic. In: Baltes P, Brim OG, Jr, eds. *Life-Span Development and Behavior.* Vol. 3. New York, NY: Academic Press; 1980:103–135.

Cockerham WC, Sharp K, Wilcox JA. Aging and perceived health status. *J Gerontol.* 1983;38:349–355.

Cohen-Shalev A. Old age style: developmental changes in creative production from a life-span perspective. *J Aging Stud.* 1989;3:21–37.

Cohler B. Autonomy and interdependence in the family of adulthood: a psychological perspective. *Gerontologist.* 1983;23:33–39.

Cohler B. Resilience and the study of lives. In: Anthony J, Cohler B, eds. *The Invulnerable Child.* New York, NY: Guilford Press; 1987:363–424.

Cohler B. Aging, morale, and meaning: the nexus of narrative. In: Cole T, Achenbaum WA, Jakobi P, Kastenbaum R, eds. *Voices and Visions of Aging: Toward a Critical Gerontology.* New York, NY: Springer; 1993:107–133.

Cohler B, Altergott K. The family of the second half of life: connecting theories and findings. In: Blieszner B, Bedford V, eds. *Handbook of Aging and the Family.* Westport, CT: Greenwood Press; 1995:59–94.

Cohler B, Borden W, Groves L, Lazarus L. Caring for family members with Alzheimer's disease. In: Light E, Lebowitz B, eds. *Alzheimer's Disease, Treatment and Family Stress: Directions for Research.* Washington, DC: US Government Printing Office; 1988:50–105.

Cohler B, Freeman M. Psychoanalysis and the developmental narrative. In: Pollock G, Greenspan S, eds. *The Course of Life.* Vol. 5. Rev. ed. *Early Adulthood.* New York, NY: International Universities Press; 1993:99–177.

Cohler B, Galatzer-Levy R. Self, meaning, and morale across the second half of life. In: Nemiroff R, Colarusso C, eds. *New Dimensions in Adult Development.* New York, NY: Basic Books; 1990:214–259.

Cohler B, Grunebaum H. *Mothers, Grandmothers, and Daughters.* New York, NY: Wiley-Interscience; 1981.

Cohler B, Lieberman M. Personality change across the second half of life: findings from a study of Irish, Italian and Polish-American men and women. In: Gelfand D, Kutznik A, eds. *Ethnicity and Aging*. New York, NY: Springer; 1979:227–245.

Cohler B, Lieberman M. Social relations and mental health: middle-aged and older men and women from three European ethnic groups. *Res Aging*. 1980;2:4454–469.

Cohler B, Stott F, Musick J. Adversity, vulnerability, and resilience: cultural and developmental perspectives. In: Cicchetti D, Cohen D, eds. *Developmental Psychopathology*. Vol. 2. New York, NY: Wiley; 1995:753–800.

Cole TR. *The Journey of Life: A Cultural History of Aging in America*. Cambridge, UK: Cambridge University Press; 1992.

Cole TR, Achenbaum WA, Jakobi P, Kastenbaum R, eds. *Voices and Visions of Aging: Toward a Critical Gerontology*. New York, NY: Springer; 1993.

Colombo J. The critical period concept: research, methodology, and theoretical issues. *Psychol Bull*. 1982;91:260–275.

Cornman JM, Kingson ER. Trends, issues, perspectives, and values for the aging of the baby boom cohorts. *Gerontologist*. 1996;36:15–26.

Costa PT, Jr, McCrae RR. Still stable all these years: personality as a key to some issues in adulthood and old age. In: Baltes PB, Brim OG, eds. *Life-Span Development and Behavior*. Vol. 3. New York, NY: Academic Press; 1980:65–102.

Costa PT, Jr, McCrae RR. Concurrent validation after 20 years: implications of personality stability for its assessment. In: Butcher JT, Spielberger CD, eds. *Advances in Personality Assessment*. Vol. 4. Hillsdale, NJ: Erlbaum; 1985:31–54.

Costa PT, Jr, McCrae RR. Personality continuity and the changes of adult life. In: Storandt M, VandenBos G, eds. *The Adult Years: Continuity and Change*. Washington, DC: American Psychological Association; 1989:54–77.

Costa PT, Jr, McCrae RR. Stability in personality from adolescence through adulthood. In: Halverson CF, Kohnstamm GA, Martin RP, eds. *The Developing Structure of Temperament and Personality From Infancy to Adulthood*. Hillsdale, NJ: Erlbaum; 1994:139–150.

Costa PT, Jr, McCrae RR. Longitudinal stability of adult personality. In: Hogan R, Johnson J, Briggs S, eds. *Handbook of Personality Psychology*. New York, NY: Academic Press; 1997:269–290.

Costa PT, Jr, Yang J, McCrae RR. Aging and personality traits: generalizations and clinical implications. In: Nordhus IH, VandenBos GR, Berg S, Fromholt P, eds. *Clinical Geropsychology*. Washington, DC: American Psychological Association; 1998:33–48.

Cottle T. *Perceiving Time: A Psychological Investigation*. New York, NY: Wiley; 1976.

Cottle T, Klineberg S. *The Present of Things Future*. New York, NY: Free Press; 1974.

Cross S, Markus H. Possible selves across the life span. *Hum Dev*. 1991;34:230–255.

Csikszentmihalyi M. *Creativity*. New York, NY: HarperCollins; 1996.

Csikszentmihalyi M, Larson R. *Being Adolescent: Conflict and Growth in the Teenage Years*. New York, NY: Basic Books; 1984.

Cumming E, Henry W. *Growing Old: The Process of Disengagement*. New York, NY: Basic Books; 1961.

Datan N, Antonovsky A, Maoz B. *A Time to Reap: The Middle Age of Women in Five Israeli Subcultures*. Baltimore, MD: The Johns Hopkins University Press; 1981.

Dean A, Lin N. The stress-buffering role of social support. *J Nerv Ment Dis*. 1977;165:403–417.

Dennis W. Age and achievement: a critique. *J Gerontol.* 1956;11:331–333.

Dennis W. Creative productivity between the ages of 20 and 80 years. *J Gerontol.* 1966; 21:1–8.

Dunkel-Schetter C, Wortman C. Dilemmas of social support: parallels between victimization and aging. In: Kessler SB, Morgan JN, Oppenheimer VK, eds. *Aging: Social Change.* New York, NY: Academic Press; 1981:349–381.

Durkheim E. *The Elementary Forms of the Religious Life.* Swain JW, trans. New York, NY: Free Press/Macmillan; 1963. (Original work published 1912.)

Eckenrode J, Gore S. Stressful events and social supports: the significance of context. In: Gottlieb BH, ed. *Social Networks and Social Support.* New York, NY: Sage; 1981: 43–68.

Ekerdt DJ, Bosse E. Change in self-reported health with retirement. *Int J Aging Hum Dev.* 1982;15:213–223.

Elder G. *Children of the Great Depression.* Chicago, IL: University of Chicago Press; 1974.

Elder G. Historical change in life patterns and personality. In: Baltes P, Brim OG, Jr, eds. *Life-Span Development and Behavior.* New York, NY: Academic Press; 1979: 117–159.

Elder G. Human lives in changing societies: life course and developmental insights. In: Cairns R, Elder GH, Jr, Costello E, eds. *Developmental Science: Multiple Perspectives.* New York, NY: Cambridge University Press; 1996:31–62.

Elder G. The life-course and human development. In: Lerner RM, ed. *Theory.* Damon W, general ed. *Handbook of Child Psychology.* Vol. 1. New York, NY: Wiley; 1997:939–991.

Elder G, Rockwell R. The life-course and human development: an ecological perspective. *Int J Behav Dev.* 1979;2:1–21.

Elwell F, Maltbie-Crannell A. The impact of role loss upon coping resources and life satisfaction of the elderly. *J Gerontol.* 1981;36:223–232.

Elson M. *Self Psychology in Clinical Social Work.* New York, NY: Norton; 1987.

Emde R. Changing the models of infancy and the nature of early development: remodeling the foundation. *J Am Psychoanal Assoc.* 1981;29:179–219.

Emde R. From adolescence to midlife: remodeling the structure of adult development. *J Am Psychoanal Assoc.* 1985;33(suppl):59–112.

Erikson E. *Childhood and Society.* 2nd ed. New York, NY: Norton; 1963. (Original work published 1950.)

Erikson E. Human strength and the cycle of generations. In: Erikson E, ed. *Insight and Responsibility: Lectures on the Ethical Implications of Psychoanalytic Insight.* New York, NY: Norton; 1964:109–158.

Erikson E. *Identity, Youth and Crisis.* New York, NY: Norton.

Erikson E. Reflections on Dr. Borg's life cycle. In: Van Tassel D, ed. *Aging, Death and the Completion of Being.* Philadelphia: University of Pennsylvania Press; 1979; 29–67.

Erikson, E. Elements of a psychoanalytic theory of psychosocial development. In: Greenspan S, Pollock GH, eds. *The Course of Life: Volume 1. Infancy.* Madison, CT: International Universities Press; 1989:15–83. (Original work published 1980.)

Erikson E, Erikson J, Kivnick H. *Vital Involvement in Old Age: The Experience of Old Age in Our Time.* New York, NY: Norton; 1986.

Essex M, Nam S. Marital status and loneliness among older women: the differential importance of close friends and family. *J Marriage Family.* 1987;49:93–106.

The experience of separation-individuation in infancy and its reverberations through the course of life. I: Infancy and childhood. *J Am Psychoanal Assoc.* 1973a;21:135–154.

The experience of separation-individuation in infancy and its reverberations through the course of life. II: Adolescence and maturity. *J Am Psychoanal Assoc.* 1973b;21:155–167.

The experience of separation-individuation in infancy and its reverberations through the course of life. III: Maturity, senescence, and sociological implications. *J Am Psychoanal Assoc.* 1973c;21:633–645.

Ferraro KF. Self-ratings of health among the old and old-old. *J Health Soc Behav.* 1980;21:377–383.

Fillenbaum GG. Social context and self-assessments of health among the elderly. *J Health Soc Behav.* 1979;20:45–51.

Firth R, Hubert J, Forge A. *Families and Their Relatives: Kinship in a Middle-Class Sector of London.* London, England: Humanities Press; 1970.

Fisher B, Specht D. Successful aging and creativity in later life. *J Aging Stud.* 1999;13:457–472.

Fiske M. Tasks and crises of the second half of life: the interrelationship of commitment, coping, and adaptation. In: Birren J, Sloane RB, eds. *Handbook of Mental Health and Aging.* Englewood Cliffs, NJ: Prentice-Hall; 1980:337–373.

Fisseni H-J. Perceived unchangeability of life and some biographical correlates. In: Munnichs J, Mussen P, Olberich E, Coleman P, eds. *Life-span and Change in Gerontological Perspective.* New York, NY: Academic Press; 1985:103–132.

Folkman S, Lazarus R. An analysis of coping in a middle-aged community sample. *J Health Soc Behav.* 1980;21:219–239.

Francis D. Artistic creations from the work years: the New York world of work. In: Calagione J, Francis D, Nugent D, eds. *Workers' Expressions: Beyond Accommodation and Resistance.* Albany: State University of New York Press; 1992:48–67.

Freud A. *The Ego and the Mechanisms of Defense.* Rev. ed. New York, NY: International Universities Press; 1965.

Fung HH, Carstensen LL, Lutz AM. Influence of time on social preferences: implications for life-span development. *Psychol Aging.* 1999;14:595–604.

Galatzer-Levy R, Cohler B. *The Essential Other.* New York, NY: Basic Books; 1993.

George L. *Role Transitions in Later Life.* Belmont, CA: Wadsworth; 1980.

Gergen K. Stability, change and chance in understanding human development. In: Datan N, Reese H, eds. *Life-span Developmental Psychology: Dialectical Perspectives on Experimental Research.* New York, NY: Academic Press; 1977:32–65.

Gergen K. The emerging crisis in life-span development theory. In: Baltes P, Brim OG, Jr, eds. *Life-span Development and Behavior.* Vol. 3. New York, NY: Academic Press; 1980:32–65.

Gergen K. From self to science: what is there to know? In: Suls J, ed. *Psychological Perspectives on the Self.* Vol. 1. Hillsdale, NJ: Erlbaum; 1982:129–149.

Gergen MM, Gergen KJ. The discourse of control and the maintenance of well-being. In: Baltes MM, Baltes PB, eds. *The Psychology of Control and Aging.* Hillsdale, NJ: Erlbaum; 1986:119–138.

Gilligan C. New maps of development: new visions of maturity. *Am J Orthopsychiatry.* 1982;52:199–212.

Glick I, Weiss R, Parkes C. *The First Year of Bereavement.* New York, NY: Wiley; 1974.

Goldberg E, Comstock G. Epidemiology of life events: frequency in general populations. *Am J Epidemiol.* 1980;111:736–752.

Greenblatt M, Becerra R, Serafetinides E. Social networks and mental health: an overview. *Am J Psychiatry.* 1982;139:977–984.

Greene AL. Future time perspective in adolescence: the present of things future revisited. *J Youth Adolesc.* 1986;15:99–113.

Greene AL. Great expectations: constructions of the life-course during adolescence. *J Youth Adolesc.* 1990;19:289–306.

Gutmann D. Parenthood: key to the comparative study of the life-cycle. In: Datan N, Ginsberg L, eds. *Life-span Developmental Psychology: Normative Life-Crises.* New York, NY: Academic Press; 1975:167–184.

Gutmann D. The cross-cultural perspective: notes toward a comparative psychology of aging. In: Birren J, Schaie KW, eds. *Handbook of the Psychology of Aging.* New York, NY: Van Nostrand-Reinhold; 1977:302–326.

Gutmann D. *Reclaimed Powers: Toward a Psychology of Men and Women in Later Life.* New York, NY: Basic Books; 1987.

Gutmann D, Griffin B, Grunes J. Developmental contributions to the late-onset affective disorders. In: Baltes P, Brim OG, Jr, eds. *Life-Span Development and Behavior.* Vol. 2. New York, NY: Academic Press; 1982:244–263.

Haan N, Millsap R, Hartka E. As time goes by: change and stability in personality over fifty years. *Psychol Aging.* 1986;1:220–232.

Hagestad G. *Middle Aged Parents and Their Children* [dissertation]. Minneapolis: University of Minnesota; 1974.

Haight B. Reminiscing: the state of the art as a basis for practice. *Int J Aging Hum Dev.* 1991;33:1–32.

Happé F, Winner E, Brownell H. The getting of wisdom: theory of mind in old age. *Dev Psychol.* 1998;34:358–362.

Harré R. *The Singular Self: An Introduction to the Psychology of Personhood.* Thousand Oaks, CA: Sage; 1998.

Harris L, and Associates. *The Myth and Reality of Aging in America.* Washington, DC: National Council on Aging; 1975.

Hartmann H. *Ego Psychology and the Problem of Adaptation.* Rapaport D, trans. New York, NY: International Universities Press; 1959. (Original work published 1939.)

Hazan H. *The Limbo People: A Study of the Constitution of the Time Universe Among the Aged.* London, England: Routledge & Kegan Paul; 1980.

Heckhausen J, Dixon RA, Baltes PB. Gains and losses in development throughout adulthood as perceived by different adult age groups. *Dev Psychol.* 1989;25:109–121.

Hendricks J. Creativity over the life course. *Int J Aging Hum Dev.* 1999;48:85–111.

Heyman D, Gianturco D. Long term adaptation by the elderly to bereavement. *J Gerontol.* 1973;28:359–362.

Hickson J, Housley W. Creativity in later life. *Educ Gerontol.* 1997;23:539–547.

Hochschild A. Disengagement theory: a critique. *Am Sociol Rev.* 1975;40:553–569.

Holliday S, Chandler M. *Wisdom: Explorations in Adult Competence.* Basel, Switzerland: Karger; 1986.

Hooker K. Possible selves and perceived health in older adults and college students. *J Gerontol.* 1992;47:85–95.

Hooker K, Siegler IC. Separating apples from oranges in health ratings: perceived health includes psychological well-being. *Behav Health Aging.* 1992;2:81–92.

Horton P. *Solace: The Missing Dimension in Psychiatry.* Chicago, IL: University of Chicago Press; 1981.

Horton PC, Gewirtz H, Kreutter KJ. *The Solace Paradigm: An Eclectic Search for Psychological Immunity.* Madison, CT: International Universities Press; 1988.

Hull C. *Principles of Behavior: An Introduction to Behavior Theory.* New York, NY: Appleton-Century; 1943.

Hultsch D, Plemons J. Life-events and life-span development. In: Baltes P, Brim OG, Jr, eds. *Life-Span Development and Behavior.* Vol. 2. New York, NY: Academic Press; 1979:1–37.

Idler EL, Kasl SV. Health perceptions and survival: do global evaluations of health status really predict mortality. *J Gerontol Soc Sci.* 1991;46:S55–S65.

Janis I. *Psychological Stress; Psychoanalytic and Behavioral Studies of Surgical Patients.* New York, NY: Wiley; 1958.

Jaques E. Death and the mid-life crisis. *Int J Psychoanal.* 1965;46:502–514.

Jaques E. The mid-life crisis. In: Greenspan S, Pollock G, eds. *The Course of Life.* Vol. 3: *Adulthood and the Aging Process.* Washington, DC: US Government Printing Office; 1980:1–23.

Jung CG. *Modern Man in Search of a Soul.* New York, NY: Harcourt, Brace & World; 1933.

Kagan J. Perspectives on continuity. In: Brim OG, Jr, Kagan J, eds. *Constancy and Change in Human Development.* Cambridge, MA: Harvard University Press; 1980: 26–74.

Kagan J. *Three Seductive Ideas.* Cambridge, MA: Harvard University Press; 1998.

Kagan J, Kearsley R, Zelazo P. *Infancy: Its Place in Human Development.* Cambridge, MA: Harvard University Press; 1978.

Kahn R. Aging and social support. In: Riley M, ed. *Aging From Birth to Death.* Boulder, CO: Westview Press; 1979:77–91.

Kahn R. Social support: context, causes, and consequences. In: Abeles RA, Gift HC, Ory MG, eds. *Aging and Quality of Life.* New York, NY: Springer; 1994:163–184.

Kahn R, Antonucci T. Convoys over the life course: attachment, roles, and social support. In: Baltes P, Brim OG, Jr, eds. *Life-Span Development and Behavior.* Vol. 3. New York, NY: Academic Press; 1980:253–386.

Kakar S. *The Inner World: A Psychoanalytic Study of Childhood and Society in India.* New Delhi, India: Oxford University Press; 1978.

Kakar S, ed. *Identity and Adulthood.* Delhi, India: Oxford University Press; 1992. (Original work published 1979.)

Kaminsky M. Transfiguring life: images of continuity hidden among the fragments. *J Gerontol Soc Work.* 1984a;7:3–18.

Kaminsky M. The uses of reminiscence: a discussion of the formative literature. *J Gerontol Soc Work.* 1984b;7:137–156.

Kaminsky M. Definitional ceremonies: depoliticizing and reenchanting the culture of age. In: Cole T, Achenbaum WA, Jakobi P, Kastenbaum R, eds. *Voices and Visions of Aging: Toward a Critical Gerontology.* New York, NY: Springer; 1993:1257–1274.

Kaplan G, Barell V, Lusky A. Subjective state of health and survival in elderly adults. *J Gerontol*. 1988;43:114–120.

Kasl S. Stress and health. *Annu Rev Public Health*. 1984;5:319.

Kastenbaum R. The creative impulse: why it won't just quit. *Generations*. 1991;15: 7–12.

Kastenbaum R. The creative process: a life-span approach. In: Cole TR, Van-Tassel D, Kastenbaum R, eds. *Handbook of the Humanities and Aging*. New York, NY: Springer; 1992:285–306.

Kastenbaum R. Encrusted elders: Arizona and the political spirit of modern aging. In: Cole T, Achenbaum WA, Jakobi P, Kastenbaum R, eds. *Voices and Visions of Aging: Toward a Critical Gerontology*. New York, NY: Springer; 1993:160–183.

Kaufman S. *The Ageless Self: Sources of Meaning in Late Life*. Madison: University of Wisconsin Press; 1986.

Kernberg O. Normal narcissism in middle age. In: Kernberg O, ed. *Internal World and External Reality: Object Relations Theory Applied*. New York, NY: Aronson; 1980:121–153.

Killilea M. Interaction of crisis theory, coping strategies, and social support systems. In: Schulberg HC, Killilea M, eds. *The Modern Practice of Community Mental Health*. San Francisco, CA: Jossey-Bass; 1982:163–214.

Kohut H. *The Analysis of the Self*. New York, NY: International Universities Press; 1971.

Kohut H. Remarks about the formation of the self—letter to a student regarding some principles of psychoanalytic research. In: Ornstein P, ed. *The Search for the Self: Selected Writings of Heinz Kohut, 1950–1978*. Vol. 2. New York, NY: International Universities Press; 1978:737–770. (Original work published 1974.)

Kohut H. The self in history. In: Strozier C, ed. *Self Psychology and the Humanities: Reflections on a New Psychoanalytic Approach by Heinz Kohut*. New York, NY: Norton; 1975:161–170.

Kohut H. *The Restoration of the Self*. Madison, CT: International Universities Press; 1977.

Kohut H. Self psychology and the sciences of man. In: Strozier C, ed. *Self Psychology and the Humanities: Reflections on a New Psychoanalytic Approach by Heinz Kohut*. New York, NY: Norton; 1978:73–94.

Kohut H. Introspection, empathy, and the semi-circle of mental health. *Int J Psychoanal*. 1982;63:395–407.

Krantz D. The Santa Fe experience. In: Sarason S, ed. *Work, Aging and Social Change: Professionals and the One Life–One Career Imperative*. New York, NY: Free Press; 1977:123–164.

Krause N. Stress and the devaluation of highly salient roles in late life. *J Gerontol Soc Sci*. 1999;S48:S99–S108.

Lachman ME, Leff R. Beliefs about intellectual efficacy and control in the elderly. *Dev Psychol*. 1989;25:722–728.

Lachman ME, Ziff MA, Spiro A, III. Maintaining a sense of control in later life. In: Abeles RA, Gift HC, Ory MG, eds. *Aging and Quality of Life*. New York, NY: Springer; 1994:216–232.

Lang FR, Featherman DL, Nesselroade JR. Social self-efficacy and short-term variability in social relationships: the MacArthur Successful Aging Studies. *Psychol Aging*. 1997;12:657–666.

Lang FR, Staudinger UM, Carstensen L. Perspectives on socioemotional selectivity in late life: how personality and social context do (and do not) make a difference. *J Gerontol Psychol Sci.* 1998;53B:P21–P30.

Lansford JE, Sherman AM, Antonucci TC. Satisfaction with social networks: an examination of socioemotional selectivity theory across cohorts. *Psychol Aging.* 1998;13: 544–552.

Larson R. Thirty years of research on the subjective well-being of older Americans. *J Gerontol.* 1978;33:109–125.

LaRue A, Bank L, Jarvik LF, Hetland M. Health in old age: how do physicians' ratings and self ratings compare? *J Gerontol.* 1979;34:687–691.

Lazarus R, DeLongis A. Psychological stress and coping in aging. *Am Psychol.* 1983;38: 245–254.

Lazarus R, Folkman S. *Stress, Appraisal and Coping.* New York, NY: Springer; 1984.

Lazarus L, Newton N, Cohler B, Lesser J, Schweon C. Frequency and presentation of depressive symptoms inpatients with primary degenerative dementia. *Am J Psychiatry.* 1987;144:41–45.

Lee G. Children and the elderly: interaction and morale. *Res Aging.* 1979;1:335–359.

Lehman HC. *Age and Achievement.* Princeton, NJ: Princeton University Press; 1953.

Lehman HC. Reply to Dennis' critique of *Age and Achievement. J Gerontol.* 1956;11: 333–337.

Leinberger P, Tucker B. *The New Individualists: The Generation After the Organization Man.* New York, NY: Harper Collins; 1991.

Leon G, Gillum B, Gillum R, Gouze M. Personality stability and change over a 60-year period—middle age to old age. *J Consult Clin Psychol.* 1979;47:517–524.

Lewis M. (*Altering Fate: Why the Past Does Not Predict the Future.* New York, NY: Guilford Press; 1997.

Lichtenstein P, Gatz M, Pedersen NL, Berg S, McClearn G. A co-twin-control study of response to widowhood. *J Gerontol.* 1996;51B:P279–P289.

Lieberman L, Lieberman L. Second careers in art and craft fairs. *Gerontologist.* 1983; 23:266–272.

Lieberman M, Falk J. The remembered past as a source of data for research on the life-cycle. *Hum Dev.* 1971;14:132–141.

Lieberman M, Peskin H. Adult life crises. In: Birren J, Sloane RB, Cohen G, eds. *Handbook of Mental Health Aging.* 2nd ed. New York, NY: Academic Press; 1992: 120–146.

Lieberman M, Tobin S. *The Experience of Old Age: Stress, Coping and Survival.* New York, NY: Basic Books; 1983.

Lindenberger U, Gilberg R, Little TD, Nuthmann R, Pötter U, Baltes PB. Sample selectivity and generalizability of the results of the Berlin Aging Study. In: Baltes PB, Mayer KU, eds. *The Berlin Aging Study: Aging From 70 to 100.* New York, NY: Cambridge University Press; 1999:56–82.

Lorenz K. The nature of instinct. In: Schiller C, ed. *Instinctive Behavior.* New York, NY: International Universities Press; 1957:129–175. (Original work published 1937.)

Lorenzen-Huber L. Self-perceived creativity in the later years: case studies of older Nebraskans. *Educ Gerontol.* 1991;17:379–390.

Lowenthal MF. Social isolation and mental illness in old age. *Am Sociol Rev.* 1964;29: 54–70.

Lowenthal MF, Robinson B. Social networks and isolation. In: Binstock R, Shanas E, eds. *Handbook of Aging and the Social Sciences.* New York, NY: Van Nostrand; 1976:432–456.

Lowenthal MF, Thurnher M, Chiriboga D, et al. *Four Stages of Life.* San Francisco, CA: Jossey-Bass; 1975.

Maas H. The development of adult development: recollections and reflections. In: Munnichs J, Mussen P, Olberich E, Coleman P, eds. *Life-span and Change in Gerontological Perspective.* New York, NY: Academic Press; 1985:161–176.

Mahler M, Pine F, Bergman A. *The Psychological Birth of the Human Infant.* New York, NY: Basic Books; 1975.

Mancini J. Family relationships and morale among people 65 years of age and older. *Am J Orthopsychiatry.* 1979;49:292–300.

Mancini J, Quinn W, Gavigan M, Franklin H. Social network interaction among older adults: implications for life satisfaction. *Hum Relations.* 1980;33:543–554.

Manheimer RJ. Wisdom and method: philosophical contributions to gerontology. In: Cole TR, Van Tassel D, Kastenbaum R, eds. *Handbook of the Humanities and Aging.* New York, NY: Springer; 1992:426–440.

Marris P. *Loss and Change.* Rev. ed. London, England: Routledge & Kegan Paul; 1986. (Original work published 1974.)

Marshall V. Age and awareness of finitude in developmental gerontology. *Omega.* 1975; 6:113–129.

Marshall V. *Last Chapters: A Sociology of Death and Dying.* Belmont, CA: Wordsworth; 1981.

Marshall V. A sociological perspective on aging and dying. In: Marshall V, ed. *Later Life: The Social Psychology of Aging.* Newbury Park, CA: Sage; 1986:125–146.

Martire LM, Schulz R, Mittelmark MB, Newsom JT. Stability and change in older adults' social contact and social support: the Cardiovascular Health Study. *J Gerontol.* 1999;54B:S302–S311.

McCrae R, Arenberg D, Costa PT. Declines in divergent thinking with age: cross-sectional, longitudinal, and cross-sequential analyses. *Psychol Aging.* 1987;2:130–137.

McCrae R, Costa P. *Personality in Adulthood.* New York, NY: Guilford Press; 1990.

McCullough L. Arrested aging: the power of the past to make us aged and old. In: Cole T, Achenbaum WA, Jakobi P, Kastenbaum R, eds. *Voices and Visions of Aging: Toward a Critical Gerontology.* New York, NY: Springer; 1993:184–204.

McMahon A, Rhudick P. Reminiscing: adaptational significance in the aged. *Arch Gen Psychiatry.* 1964;10:292–298.

McMahon A, Rhudick P. Reminiscing in the aged: an adaptational response. In: Levin S, Kahana R, eds. *Psychodynamic Studies on Aging; Creativity, Reminiscing, and Dying.* New York, NY: International Universities Press; 1967:64–78.

Meacham JA. The loss of wisdom. In Sternberg RJ, ed. *Wisdom: Its Nature, Origins, and Development.* Cambridge, UK: Cambridge University Press; 1990:181–211.

Mendes de Leon CF, Kasl SW, Jacobs S. A prospective study of widowhood and changes in symptoms of depression in a community sample of the elderly. *Psychol Med.* 1994;23:613–624.

Miller N, Dollard J. *Social Learning Theory and Imitation.* New Haven, CT: Yale University Press; 1941.

Mischel W. *Personality and Assessment.* New York, NY: Wiley; 1968.

Mischel W, Shoda Y. A cognitive-affective system theory of personality: reconceptualizing situations, dispositions, dynamics and invariance in personality structure. *Psychol Rev.* 1995;102:246–286.

Moody H. A bibliography on reminiscence and life review. *J Gerontol Soc Work.* 1984; 7:231–236.

Moody H. The meaning of life and the meaning of old age. In: Cole TR, Gadow S, eds. *What Does It Mean to Grow Old? Reflections From the Humanities.* Durham, NC: Duke University Press; 1986:11–40.

Moody H. Overview: what is critical gerontology and why is it important. In: Cole T, Achenbaum WA, Jakobi P, Kastenbaum R, eds. *Voices and Visions of Aging: Toward a Critical Gerontology.* New York, NY: Springer; 1993:xv–xli.

Mossey JM, Shapiro E. Self-rated health: a predictor of mortality among the elderly. *Am J Public Health.* 1982;72:800–808.

Munnichs J. *Old Age and Finitude: A Contribution to Psychogerontology.* New York, NY: Karger; 1966.

Murphy G. *Personality: A Biosocial Approach to Organization and Structure.* New York, NY: Basic Books; 1966. (Original work published 1947.)

Myerhoff B. *Number Our Days.* New York, NY: Dutton; 1978.

Myerhoff B. *Remembered Lives: The Work of Ritual, Storytelling, and Growing Older.* Kaminsky M, ed. Ann Arbor: University of Michigan Press; 1992.

Neugarten B. The awareness of middle age. In: Neugarten B, ed. *Middle Age and Aging.* Chicago, IL: University of Chicago Press; 1968:93–98.

Neugarten B. Continuities and discontinuities of psychological issues into adult life. *Hum Dev.* 1969;12:121–130.

Neugarten B. Personality in later life: a developmental perspective. In: Eisdorfer C, Lawton MP, eds. *The Psychology of Adult Development.* Washington, DC: American Psychological Association; 1973:311–338.

Neugarten B. Time, age and the life cycle. *Am J Psychiatry.* 1979;136:887–894.

Neugarten B, Datan N. The middle years. In: Arieti S, ed. *American Handbook of Psychiatry.* Vol. 1. New York, NY: Basic Books; 1974:596–606.

Neugarten B, Hagestad G. Age and the life course. In: Binstock R, Shanas E, eds. *Handbook of Aging and the Social Sciences.* New York, NY: Van Nostrand-Reinhold; 1976:35–55.

Offer D, Offer J. *From Teenage to Young Manhood.* New York, NY: Basic Books; 1975.

Offer D, Sabshin M. Adolescence: empirical perspectives. In: Offer D, Sabshin M, eds. *Normality and the Life Cycle.* New York, NY: Basic Books; 1984: 76–107.

Orwoll L, Achenbaum A. Gender and the development of wisdom. *Hum Dev.* 1993;36: 274–296.

Orwoll L, Perlmutter M. The study of wise persons: integrating a personality perspective. In Sternberg RJ, ed. *Wisdom: Its Nature, Origins, and Development.* Cambridge, UK: Cambridge University Press; 1990:160–177.

Osherson S. *Holding On or Letting Go: Men and Career Change at Midlife.* New York, NY: Free Press; 1980.

Parkes C. *Bereavement: Studies of Grief and Adult Life.* New York, NY: International Universities Press; 1972.

Parkes C, Weiss R. *Recovery From Bereavement.* New York, NY: Basic Books; 1983.

Perlmutter M. Learning and memory through adulthood. In: Riley M, ed. *Aging in Society: Selected Reviews of Recent Research.* Hillsdale, NJ: Erlbaum; 1983:219–241.

Pinquart M, Sörensen S. Influences of socioeconomic status, social network, and competence on subjective well-being in later life: a meta-analysis. *Psychol Aging.* 2000; 15:187–224.

Plath D. Contours of consociation: lessons from a Japanese narrative. In: Baltes P, Brim OG, Jr, eds. *Life-Span Development and Behavior.* Vol. 3. New York, NY: Academic Press; 1980a:287–305.

Plath D. *Long Engagements.* Stanford, CA: Stanford University Press; 1980b.

Pollock G. On time, death and immortality. *Psychoanal Q.* 1971;40:435–446.

Pollock G. Aging or aged: development or pathology. In: Greenspan S, Pollock G, eds. *The Course of Life. Volume 3: Adulthood and the Aging Process.* Washington, DC: US Government Printing Office; 1980:549–585.

Pollock G. Reminiscence and insight. *Psychoanal Study Child.* 1981;36:278–287.

Pruchno R, Blow F, Smyer M. Life events and interdependent lives. *Gerontologist.* 1984; 27:31–41.

Pruyser P. Creativity in aging persons. *Bull Menninger Clin.* 1987;51:425–435.

Rapaport D, Gill M. The points-of-view and assumptions of metapsychology. *Int J Psychoanal.* 1959;40:153–162.

Ricoeur P. *Oneself as Another.* Blaney K, trans. Chicago, IL: University of Chicago Press; 1992.

Riegel K. *Foundations of Dialectical Psychology.* New York, NY: Academic Press; 1979.

Robertson J. Grandparenthood: a study of role conceptions. *J Marriage Family.* 1977; 39:165–174.

Rodin J. Aging and health: effects of the sense of control. *Science.* 1986;233:1271–1276.

Romaniuk JG, Romaniuk M. Creativity across the life span: a measurement perspective. *Hum Dev.* 1981;23:366–381.

Rook K. The negative side of social interaction: the impact of psychological well being. *J Pers Soc Psychol.* 1984;46:1097–1108.

Rook K. Strains in older adults' friendships. In: Adams R, Blieszner R, eds. *Older Adult Friendship: Structure and Process.* Newbury Park, CA: Sage; 1989:108–128.

Rosenmayr L, Kockeis E. Predispositions for a sociological theory of the family. *Int Soc Sci J.* 1963;15:410–426.

Rowe J, Kahn R. Human aging: usual and successful. *Science.* July 10, 1987;237:143–149.

Rowe J, Kahn R. *Successful Aging.* New York, NY: Pantheon Books; 1998.

Ryff C, Heincke S. Subjective organization of personality in adulthood and aging. *J Pers Soc Psychol.* 1983;44:807–816.

Salthouse T. Age-related changes in basic cognitive processes. In: Storandt M, VandenBos G, eds. *The Adult Years: Continuity and Change.* Washington, DC: American Psychological Association; 1989:5–40.

Salthouse T. Cognitive competence and expertise in aging. In: Birren J, Schaie KW, eds. *Handbook of the Psychology of Aging.* 3rd ed. New York, NY: Academic Press; 1990:311–319.

Schaie KW. Psychological changes from midlife to early old age: implications for the maintenance of mental health. *Am J Psychiatry.* 1981;51:199–218.

Schaie KW. The Seattle longitudinal study: a 2-year exploration of the psychometric intelligence of adulthood. In: Schaie KW, ed. *Longitudinal Studies of Personality.* New York, NY: Guilford Press; 1984:64–135.

Schaie KW. Intellectual development in adulthood. In: Birren J, Schaie KW, eds. *Handbook of the Psychology of Aging*. 3rd ed. New York, NY: Academic Press; 1990: 291–310.

Schaie KW. The Seattle longitudinal studies of adult intelligence. *Curr Dir Psychol Sci*. 1993;2:171–175.

Schaie KW. The course of adult intellectual development. *Am Psychologist*. 1994;49: 304–313.

Schaie KW. *Intellectual Development in Adulthood: The Seattle Longitudinal Study*. New York, NY: Cambridge University Press; 1996.

Schaie KW, Labouvie G, Buech B. Generational and cohort-specific differences in adult cognitive behavior: a fourteen-year study of independent samples. *Dev Psychol*. 1973;9:151–166.

Schulz R, Rau MT. Social support through the life course. In: Cohen S, Syme SL, eds. *Social Support and Health*. Orlando, FL: Academic Press; 1985: 129–149.

Seeman T, Unger J, McAvay G, Mendes de Leon C. Self-efficacy beliefs and perceived declines in functional ability: MacArthur studies of successful aging. *J Gerontol*. 1999;54B:P214–P222.

Shanas E, Townsend P, Wedderburn D, Friis H, Milhoj P, Stehouwer J. *Old People in Three Industrial Societies*. London, England: Routledge & Kegan Paul; 1968.

Shweder R. How relevant is an individual difference theory of personality. *J Pers*. 1975; 43:455–484.

Shweder R. Illusory correlation and the MMPI controversy. *J Consult Clin Psychol*. 1977;45:917–924.

Sill J. Disengagement reconsidered: awareness of finitude. *Gerontologist*. 1980;37:587–594.

Silverstone B. Older people of tomorrow: a psychosocial profile. *Gerontologist*. 1996; 36:27–32.

Simonton DK. Creativity in the later years: optimistic prospects for achievement. *Gerontologist*. 1990a;30:626–631.

Simonton D. Creativity and wisdom in aging. In: Birren J, Schaie KW, eds. *Handbook of the Psychology of Aging*. 3rd ed. New York, NY: Academic Press; 1990b:320–329.

Simonton DK. Does creativity decline in the later years? Definition, data, and theory. In: Perlmutter M, ed. *Late Life Potential*. Washington, DC: Gerontological Society of America; 1990c:83–112.

Simonton DK. Career paths and creative lives: a theoretical perspective on late life potential. In: Adams-Price C, ed. *Creativity and Successful Aging*. New York, NY: Springer; 1998:3–18.

Sinnott J. Correlates of sex roles of older adults. *J Gerontol*. 1982;37: 587–594.

Smith J, Baltes PB. Wisdom-related knowledge: age/cohort differences in response to life-planning problems. *Dev Psychol*. 1990;26:494–505.

Smith J, Baltes PB. Trends and profiles in psychological functioning in very old age. In: Baltes PB, Mayer KU, eds. *The Berlin Aging Study: Aging From 70 to 100*. New York, NY: Cambridge University Press; 1999:197–226.

Sorokin P, Merton R. Social time: a methodological and functional analysis. *Am J Sociol*. 1937;42:615–629.

Staudinger UM. Older and wiser? Integrating results on the relationship between age and wisdom-related performance. *Int J Behav Dev*. 1999;23:641–664.

Staudinger UM, Smith J, Baltes PB. Wisdom-related knowledge in a life review task: age differences and the role of professional specialization. *Psychol Aging.* 1992;7: 271–281.

Sternberg RJ, ed. *Wisdom: Its Nature, Origins, and Development.* Cambridge, UK: Cambridge University Press; 1990a.

Sternberg RJ. Wisdom and its relations to intelligence and creativity. In: Sternberg RJ, ed. *Wisdom: Its Nature, Origins, and Development.* Cambridge, UK: Cambridge University Press; 1990b:142–159.

Stevens DP, Truss CV. Stability and change in adult personality over 12 and 20 years. *Dev Psychol.* 1985;21:568–584.

Stolar GE, MacEntee MI, Hill P. Seniors' assessment of their health and life satisfaction: the case for contextual evaluation. *Int J Aging Hum Dev.* 1992;35:305–317.

Strobe W, Strobe MS. *Bereavement and Health: The Psychological and Physical Consequences of Partner Loss.* New York, NY: Cambridge University Press; 1987.

Sulloway F. *Freud, Biologist of the Mind.* New York, NY: Basic Books; 1979.

Szinovacz ME, DeViney S, Atkinson MP. Effects of surrogate parenting on grandparents' well-being. *J Gerontol Soc Sci.* 1999;54B:S376–S388.

Takahashi M, Bordia P. The concept of wisdom: a cross-cultural perspective. *Int J Psychol.* 2000;35:1–9.

Taranto MA. Facets of wisdom: a theoretical synthesis. *Int J Aging Hum Dev.* 1989;29: 1–21.

Thomae H. Stress, satisfaction, competence—findings from the Bonn longitudinal study on aging. In: Bergener M, Finkel S, eds. *Clinical and Scientific Psychogeriatrics. Vol. I. The Holistic Approaches.* New York, NY: Springer; 1990:117–134.

Thomas LL. The grandparent role: a double bind. *Int J Aging Hum Dev.* 1990;32:169–171.

Tinbergen N. *The Study of Instinct.* Oxford, UK: Clarendon Press; 1951.

Tobin S. *Personhood in Advanced Old Age.* New York, NY: Springer; 1991.

Torrance EP. Creativity and the older adult. *Creative Child Adult Q.* 1977;2:136–144.

Townsend P. *The Family Life of Old People.* London, England: Routledge & Kegan Paul; 1957.

Turner J. Social support as a contingency in psychological well-being. *J Health Soc Behav.* 1981;22:357–367.

Uhlenhuth E, Lipman R, Balter M, Stern M. Symptom intensity and life-stress in the city. *Arch Gen Psychiatry.* 1974;31:759–764.

Vaillant G. *The Wisdom of the Ego.* Cambridge, MA: Harvard University Press; 1993.

Vaillant G. *Aging Well.* New York, NY: Little, Brown; 2001.

Wagner M, Schütze Y, Lang FR. Social relationships in old age. In: Baltes PB, Mayer KU, eds. *The Berlin Aging Study: Aging From 70 to 100.* New York, NY: Cambridge University Press; 1999:282–301.

Wan TTH. Health consequences of major role losses in later life: a panel study. *Res Aging.* 1984;6:469–489.

Weiss R. Attachment in adult life. In: Parkes CM, Stevenson-Hinds J, eds. *The Place of Attachment in Human Behavior.* New York, NY: Basic Books; 1982:171–184.

Werner E. Stress and protective factors in children's lives. In: Nicol AR, eds. *Longitudinal Studies in Child Psychology and Psychiatry.* New York, NY: Wiley; 1985:335–355.

Werner E. Protective factors and individual resilience. In: Micelles S, Shonkoff J, eds.

Handbook of Early Childhood Intervention. New York, NY: Cambridge University Press; 1990:97–116.

Werner E, Bierman J, French F. *The Children of Kauai: A Longitudinal Study From the Prenatal Period to Age Ten.* Honolulu: University Press of Hawaii; 1971.

Werner E, Smith R. *Kauai's Children Come of Age.* Honolulu: University Press of Hawaii; 1977.

Werner E, Smith R. *Vulnerable But Invincible: A Study of Resilient Children.* New York, NY: McGraw-Hill; 1982.

Werner E, Smith R. *Overcoming the Odds: High Risk Children From Birth to Adulthood.* Ithaca, NY: Cornell University Press; 1992.

Wertsch J. *Mind as Action.* New York, NY: Oxford University Press; 1998.

Whitbourne S. The psychological construction of the life span. In: Birren J, Schaie KW, eds. *Handbook of the Psychology of Aging.* New York, NY: Van Nostrand-Reinhold; 1985:594–618.

Whitbourne S. Personality development in adulthood and old age: relationships among identity style, health, and well-being. *Annu Rev Gerontol Geriatr.* 1987;7:189–216.

White RW. Motivation reconsidered: the concept of competence. *Psychol Rev.* 1959;66: 297–333.

Wiggins JS, ed. *The Five-Factor Theory of Personality: Theoretical Perspectives.* New York, NY: Guilford Press; 1996.

Wiggins JS. In defense of traits. In: Hogan R, Johnson R, Briggs S, eds. *Handbook of Personality Psychology.* New York, NY: Academic Press; 1997:97–117.

Wiggins J, Trapnell PD. Personality structure and the return of the big five. In: Hogan R, Johnson J, Briggs S, eds. *Handbook of Personality Psychology.* New York, NY: Academic Press; 1997:737–766.

Wood V, Robertson J. Friendship and kinship interaction: differential effect on the morale of the elderly. *J Marriage Family.* 1978;40:367–375.

Wortman C, Silver R. Coping with irrevocable loss. In: VandenBos G, Bryant B, eds. *Cataclysms, Crises and Catastrophes: Psychology in Action.* Washington, DC: American Psychological Association; 1987:189–235.

Wortman C, Silver R. Successful mastery of bereavement and widowhood: a life-course perspective. In: Baltes P, Baltes M, eds. *Successful Aging: Perspectives From the Behavioral Sciences.* Cambridge, UK: Cambridge University Press; 1990:225–264.

Zautra A, Hempel A. Subjective well-being and physical health: a narrative literature review with suggestions for future research. *Int J Aging Hum Dev.* 1984;19:95–110.

Zweibel N, Cassel C. Treatment choices at the end of life: a comparison of decision by older patients and their physician-selected proxies. *Gerontologist.* 1989;29:615–621.

Zweibel N, Lydens L. Incongruent perceptions of older adult/caregiver dyads. *Fam Relations.* 1990;39:63–67.

8

The Role of Religion/Spirituality in the Mental Health of Older Adults

Harold G. Koenig, MD

In this chapter, I examine the role of religion/spirituality in the mental health of older adults, with particular emphasis on coping with stress and disability, prevention of mental illness, and recovery from emotional disorder. I also explore possible mechanisms by which religion has an impact on mental health and discuss clinical applications in geriatric patients. This is a topic that makes many mental health professionals feel uncomfortable; however, there is increasing evidence that avoiding this topic may ignore an important psychological and social resource that could facilitate health and healing. I review some of the research supporting this notion and consider the potentially harmful aspects of religious/spiritual belief and practice. The focus in this chapter is primarily on Western religious traditions, with which I am most familiar; information about Eastern religious traditions (Hinduism, Buddhism, etc.) and mental health is available from other resources (Koenig, 1998a). Some necessary background information is presented next.

DEFINITIONS

The relationship of religion/spirituality to mental health is controversial and complex; thus, it is important to define terms. Religion and spirituality are two concepts defined in a variety of ways; they mean different things to different people. *Religion* is often understood to mean institutional religion, which concerns membership in religious bodies and attendance at religious services. This term has come into disfavor in many academic communities because it is seen as divisive and associated with rules, regulations, and responsibilities. Academicians would much rather talk about *spirituality*, which is more personal and inclusive and not necessarily tied to traditional religion or activities associated with institutional religion. Spirituality has also become a popular term in modern society and is often associated with nonmaterial humanistic qualities that all people possess.

Despite its popularity, however, spirituality has become so broad and diffuse a concept that it is difficult for researchers to define in a way that is distinctive and measurable. Consequently, most studies (perhaps over 90%) measure spirituality by simply assessing religion. Indeed, religious beliefs and activities are much easier to measure, with literally hundreds of instruments developed and used since 1929 (Hill & Hood, 1999). Even the most recent and popular measure of spirituality, the Multidimensional Measure of Religiousness/Spirituality, developed by a consensus panel of experts convened by the National Institute on Aging and Fetzer Institute, asks questions primarily about traditional religious beliefs and activities (Fetzer Institute, 1999).

Furthermore, in many published instruments that profess to measure spirituality as distinct from religion, the concept is usually made operational in terms of positive humanistic traits—a sense of awe and wonder, forgiveness, meaning and purpose, existential well-being, connectedness, and so on. The last are really mental health outcomes of spirituality, not spirituality itself. If spirituality is defined as a positive mental health state, then naturally it will be associated with good mental health, and any research that tries to correlate it with mental health becomes tautological.

In summary, most studies of the religion–mental health relationship have examined traditional religious beliefs and practices. We really do not know much about how broad-based spirituality—unmoored to an established religious tradition—affects the mental or physical health of older adults. The majority of older adults consider themselves both religious and spiritual and seldom distinguish between these concepts (Koenig, 2000a; Zinnbauer et al., 1997). Therefore, I mostly talk about religion in this chapter, including the personal aspects of traditional religious belief and practice (e.g., faith and personal commitment), as well as the social aspects that involve participation in the religious community (e.g., attending religious services, participation in other religious group activity, religious volunteering).

PREVALENCE OF RELIGIOUS BELIEFS AND ACTIVITIES

Traditional religious beliefs and practices are widespread among older adults in the United States. According to Gallup polls, more than 95% of older adults believe in God or a universal spirit, 80% are members of a church or synagogue, and 53% attended religious services in the past week (Princeton Religion Research Center, 1996). Gallup poll results (December 1999 and March 2000) indicated that religious attendance for persons of all ages in the United States is higher than at any time since 1962 (except when measured during Easter week), with 44% to 45% of Americans having attended religious services in the previous 7 days (Princeton Religion Research Center, 2003). The comparable figure for 1939, the first year that religious attendance was measured by the Gallup organization, was 41%. In almost all subsequent years, older adults reported attending religious services more frequently than younger adults. Prayer is also common among Americans in general, with 75% indicating that they pray at least once a day; an additional 15% indicated that they pray at least weekly (Princeton Religion Research Center, 1996).

In an April 2000 Gallup poll release, 61% of Americans of all ages indicated that religion was "very important" in their lives, whereas only 12% said that it was not at all important; women were more likely than men, by a margin of about 14%, to say that religion was important to them. No fewer than 75% of persons aged 65 years or older indicated that religion was very important in their lives (Princeton Religion Research Center, 2003). These findings are consistent with a Gallup poll in 1995, which found 73% of persons over age 65 years reported that religion was very important (Princeton Religion Research Center, 1996).

Approximately 85% of Americans said their religious preference is a form of Christianity, with 59% Protestants and 26% Roman Catholics; 6% of Americans have no religious preference, 4% say that they cannot designate a specific religious affiliation, and 5% indicate a non-Christian religion, of whom 2% are Jewish (Princeton Religion Research Center, 2003). This means that, of those Americans with a religious preference, 97% claim a Judeo-Christian tradition.

To what extent do people become more religious as they age? This is a controversial and much debated topic because few longitudinal studies have tracked people's religious beliefs from childhood through adulthood into old age. Some evidence about changes in religious importance with age can be obtained by comparing rates of religious attendance and importance by age group from 1939 to 2000 (Table 8-1). In virtually every cohort, younger adults have lower religious attendance and lower religious importance than older adults— suggesting that religious involvement may increase with increasing age. Nevertheless, even young adults in the 1950s and early 1960s were more religious than later generations of youths (especially in the 1970s and 1980s), providing support also for a cohort effect.

In a regional study of men aged 65 years or older hospitalized in the Durham Veterans Administration Hospital in North Carolina, 850 consecutively admitted patients were asked if they had ever experienced a significant increase in religious beliefs or commitment at any time. Approximately one quarter to one third of men reported such experiences, and over 40% of them reported the experience occurred after they turned 50 years old (Koenig, 1994). Thus,

TABLE 8-1. **Religious attendance and importance of religion in the United States, percentage**

Year	All ages	18–29 years	30–49 years	50–64 years	65 years or older
Attended religious services in average week					
1939	41	—	—	—	—
1940	37	—	—	—	—
1950	39	—	—	—	—
1955	49	—	—	—	—
1960	47	—	—	—	—
1965	44	—	—	—	—
1970	42	—	—	—	—
1975	40	30	41	46 (≥ 50 years old)	—
1981	41	32	42	45	49
1986	40	33	39	45	49
1989	43	34	40	52 (≥ 50 years old)	—
1995	43	34	40	46	53
2000	44	—	—	—	—
Reported religion "very important"					
1952	75	64	—	—	—
1965	70	57	—	—	—
1975	56	45	58	63 (≥ 50 years old)	—
1981	56	40	—	—	74
1984	56	42	—	66 (≥ 50 years old)	—
1989	55	42	51	68 (≥ 50 years old)	—
1995	58	45	56	61	73
2000	61	50	60	61	75

Source: Data from Princeton Religion Research Center (1976, 1982, 1985, 1990, 1996, 2000).

many adults experience an increase in religiousness during their later years, and this often occurs during a period of physical or emotional stress.

VIEWS OF MENTAL HEALTH PROFESSIONALS TOWARD RELIGION

The views of mental health professionals toward religion have often been negative, with religion seen largely as neurotic and irrational (Ellis, 1980; Freud, 1927/1962). This is not surprising given that many mental health professionals had few or no personal religious beliefs, and few systematic studies were conducted on the religion–mental health relationship in nonpsychiatric samples.

Ragan and colleagues (1980) examined the religious beliefs and practices of a random sample of 555 members of the American Psychological Association. Only 43% believed in God; 27% attended church twice a month or more; and 9% held leadership positions in their congregations. Bergin and Jensen (1990) surveyed a national sample of 425 clinical psychologists, psychiatrists, clinical social workers, and marriage and family therapists. Subjects were asked to respond to the following statement: "My whole approach to life is based on my religion." The category "uncertain/disagree/strongly disagree" was chosen by 67% of psychologists and 61% of psychiatrists (vs. 28% for the general population).

Religious involvement may also vary depending on geographical location. In a survey of 47 randomly sampled psychologists in California, Shafranske and Malony (1990) found that only 26% believed in a personal God in the traditional sense, and 80% had very limited or no involvement in organized religion (51% with no religious affiliation). Religious involvement is even less common among British psychiatrists. In surveying 231 psychiatrists practicing in London, Neeleman and King (1993) found that 73% of psychiatrists reported no religious affiliation, and 78% attended religious services less than once a month. Over 40% of the psychiatrists believed that religiousness can lead to mental illness, and 58% never made referrals to clergy.

PSYCHIATRIC TREATMENT IN EARLY AMERICA

Many psychiatrists today are not aware of the role that religion played in the treatment of mental illness in early America. In fact, the first form of psychiatric care in the United States was called "moral treatment" and arose from the teachings of William Tuke. A devout Quaker, Tuke started the York retreat in England in the late 18th century; patients were treated with a regimen of exercise, work, and recreation—like normal adults expected to behave according to societal norms.

In 1817, Quakers started one of the first psychiatric hospitals (the Friends Asylum) in America in Philadelphia, Pennsylvania; it was modeled after the York retreat. Soon, other mental institutions arose in Hartford, Connecticut, and Worcester, Massachusetts. The early superintendents of these institutions included Samuel Woodward (founder of what was to become the American Psychiatric Association) and Amariah Brigham (Brigham and Woodward were the first coeditors of what was to become the *American Journal of Psychiatry*). These superintendents believed that religious involvement was an important part of psychiatric treatment; in fact, patients were rewarded for good behavior by being allowed to attend chapel services (Taubes, 1998). Furthermore, chaplains lived on the grounds of these institutions and performed an important role in the treatment of patients. All of this was to change with the powerful influence of Freud in the early 1900s.

During the closing decade of the 20th century, there again appeared to be a shift in attitudes of health professionals toward religion. By the year 2000, of 126 US medical schools, 64 offered elective or required courses on religion, spirituality, and medicine. The Accreditation Council on Graduate Medical Education (1994) mandated, in its Special Requirements for Psychiatry Residency Training, that all training programs include didactic training in the "presentation of the biological, psychological, socio-cultural, economic, ethnic, gender, *religious/spiritual*, sexual orientation and family factors that significantly influence physical and psychological development in infancy, childhood, adolescence, and adulthood" (pp. 11–12, emphasis added). Furthermore, it established that

> The residency program should provide its residents with instruction about American culture and subcultures, particularly those found in the patient community associated with the training program. This instruction should include such issues as sex, race, ethnicity, *religion/spirituality*, and sexual orientation. (p. 18, emphasis added)

Thus, psychiatrists are encouraged to ask about and to understand the religious/spiritual beliefs of their patients—and to respect them (American Psychiatric Association, 1995). Why is this especially true for geriatric psychiatrists?

RELIGIOUS COPING AMONG OLDER ADULTS

Aging is associated with a number of losses—loss of youth and vigor, loss of health, loss of independence, loss of role and status in society and family, loss of loved ones and friends, and, ultimately, threat of loss of life. Older adults frequently use religious beliefs and practices to cope with age-related stress. At least 60 studies have examined the prevalence and use of religion in coping by older adults or those with physical illness (Koenig et al., 2001).

The use of religion to cope involves depending on God, prayer, scripture, rituals, religious leaders, or religious communities for support and comfort when encountering psychological or social stress. When medically ill older patients were asked an open-ended question about what enabled them to deal successfully with the stress, between 24% and 42% indicated that religion was the most important factor that enabled them to cope; in some areas of the country, up to 90% of older patients used religion at least moderately when coping with stress (Koenig, 1998b; Koenig et al., 1992). Although religious coping is ubiquitous in the United States, particularly in the South and Midwest, these rates drop to only 1% to 5% of the population in northern European countries like Sweden (Cederblad et al., 1995).

Do older adults adapt more quickly if they use religious coping behaviors? In other words, are religiously active older adults less depressed and less anxious, and do they feel more in control and have a greater sense of well-being than elders not engaged in such practices? In general, the answer to this question is yes, although in particular cases, this is not always so. Religious involvement has been associated with fewer depressive symptoms (Koenig et al., 1992) and faster recovery from depression (Koenig et al., 1998) among older adults—particularly among those with chronic medical illness and physical disability (Idler, 1987; Koenig et al., 1992, 1998; Pressman et al., 1990). Higher self-esteem and greater sense of purpose and meaning in life, as well as greater hope and optimism, help explain these associations.

RELIGIOUS/SPIRITUAL ACTIVITIES AND MENTAL HEALTH

Through a systematic review of the research literature over the past 100 years (the 20th century), my colleagues and I attempted to identify studies that examined the relationship between the religious characteristics of individuals and their mental health (Koenig et al., 2001). Over 850 studies were identified. These studies were conducted in different locations throughout the world, in populations both old and young, and used clinical and population-based community samples. They were carried out at a variety of academic institutions by many scientists, including psychologists, sociologists, epidemiologists, psychiatrists, general medical physicians, nurses, and other health professionals. Mental health outcomes included well-being and life satisfaction, meaning and purpose, hope and optimism, depression, suicide, anxiety, psychosis, personality, marital stability, delinquency, and substance abuse. Between two thirds and three quarters of these studies found religious involvement associated with better mental health. Consider, for example, depression in older adults.

Religion and Depression

COMMUNITY STUDIES   In a random sample of 4,000 persons aged 65 years or older (Established Populations for Epidemiologic Studies in the Elderly, North Carolina site), Koenig and coworkers (1997) examined the relationships among physical health, social support, religious activity, and depression (measured using the Center for Epidemiological Studies–Depression Scale [CES-D]). After controlling for demographic factors and other covariates such as social support and physical health, persons who attended religious services once a week or more were only about half as likely to be depressed as less-frequent attenders (odds ratio [OR] = 0.56; 95% confidence interval [CI], 0.48–0.65); private religious activities like prayer and scripture study were unrelated to depression (OR = 0.88; 95% CI, 0.75–1.04), as was listening to religious radio or viewing religious television programs (OR = 1.11; 95% CI, 0.94–1.31).

Studies of community-dwelling older adults in Connecticut reported similar results. Idler (1987), examining depressive symptoms among 2,811 older adults in the Yale Health and Aging Study, found an interesting pattern of cross-sectional relationships between depressive symptoms and religious activities in 1982. Multivariate analyses revealed that, among older men, public religious activity was unrelated to depression after chronic conditions and disability (along with optimism and fatalism) were controlled. However, the relationship between functional disability and depression weakened at greater degrees of private religiousness, suggesting that private religious activity was particularly effective in shielding from depression those who had severe functional disability. Among women, public religiousness was inversely related to depression (–.08, $P < .01$, after controlling for covariates, including optimism and fatalism); private religiousness, however, was not related to depression after covariates were controlled (and there were no interactions with disability).

A longitudinal study revealed that public and private religiosity had no overall predictive effect on depression, except among men who had become disabled between 1982 and 1985. In the last group, private religiosity in 1982 had an inverse relationship with CES-D depression in 1985 ($\beta = -.50$, $P = .03$). Idler and Kasl (1992) concluded that, "Religious involvement provides some protection against depression for the elderly, especially the vulnerable group of elderly men with deteriorating functional status" (p. 1069). In the last analysis reported for this cohort, Idler and Kasl (1997) found that religious attendance predicted lower levels of disability during 8 to 12 years of follow-up, a finding that largely persisted after controlling for multiple covariates; more important, the effect on religious attendance by impaired physical functioning was much less than the effect of religious attendance on preventing future disability.

Studies in Europe also reported an inverse relationship between religious involvement and depression in community samples (Braam, 1999; Braam, Beekman, van Tilburg, et al., 1997; Braam et al., 2001). In a survey of more than 3,000 persons aged 55 to 85 years living in three different regions of the Netherlands, Braam (1999) hypothesized that religious involvement would cause persons to be more vulnerable to depression than those who had stopped going to church, and that elderly Reformed Christians in particular would be at higher risk for depression. Contrary to expectations, he found that the prevalence of depression varied from 7% to 8% in small villages where most people were Reformed Christians to 20% in Amsterdam, the city with the highest percentage of people who had stopped attending church. The author concluded that church social life and religion itself played an important role in preventing depression. He also indicated that people who had made a conscious decision to leave the church still felt some bitterness as they grew older, experiencing little comfort, forgiveness, or grace.

CLINICAL SAMPLES Studies of clinical samples of medically ill older adults reported similar findings. Pressman and colleagues (1990) examined depressive symptoms (measured by the Geriatric Depression Scale) and religious involvement in a sample of 33 elderly women hospitalized with hip fractures. Religious involvement was inversely related to depressive symptoms and predicted quicker recovery (measured in terms of walking distances at discharge).

Koenig and coworkers (1992) examined the relationship between religious coping (measured by a three-item, 30-point scale) and depressive symptoms in 850 hospitalized men aged 65 years or older. Depressive symptoms (measured by Geriatric Depression Scale and Hamilton Depression Rating Scale) were inversely related to religious coping, a relationship that persisted after controlling for multiple covariates. There was again a significant interaction between physical functioning and religious coping; the relationship between religious coping and depressive symptoms was stronger among those with worse disability.

Interestingly, religious coping was inversely related only to certain types of depressive symptoms (Koenig et al., 1995). Cognitive/emotional symptoms of depression, not somatic symptoms, were less frequent among religious copers. Boredom, loss of interest, social withdrawal, feeling downhearted and blue, restlessness, feeling like a failure, feeling hopeless, or feeling other people were better off were all significantly less common among religious copers; difficulty initiating new activity was the only somatic symptom that was less frequent among religious copers. In contrast, symptoms such as appetite disturbance or weight loss, difficulty sleeping, trouble concentrating, and fatigue were unrelated to religious coping scores. The investigators concluded that religious coping is heavily dependent on cognitive processes and is associated with fewer cognitive, but not somatic, symptoms of depression. Once depression reaches a certain severity (so that it is associated with endogenous symptoms), the patient may be unable to access religious resources for comfort.

In the longitudinal portion of the study by Koenig and coworkers (1992), investigators followed 202 men an average of 6 months after hospital discharge. Religious coping during hospitalization (Time 1) predicted lower depressive symptoms on follow-up. One of only two significant variables in the model, Time 1 religious coping predicted 45% of the explained variance in depressive symptoms at Time 2 after controlling for Time 1 depressive symptoms and other demographic, physical health, and social characteristics.

RECOVERY FROM DEPRESSIVE DISORDER   A few studies have examined the effects of religiousness on recovery from depressive disorder in older adults. Although not examining depressive disorder per se, Braam, Beekman, Deeg, and colleagues (1997) conducted a 12-month prospective study of a community-based sample of 177 persons aged 55 to 89 years living in the Netherlands. Subjects were assessed five times (T1–T5) by mailed questionnaires; change in depression was defined as an increase or decrease of more than 5 points on the CES-D (one-half standard deviation) between measurements, thereby crossing the CES-D threshold of 16. First, for subjects with CES-D less than 16 at T1 ($n = 129$), *incident depression* was determined (there was a 25% incidence). Second, for subjects with CESD higher than 15 at T1 ($n = 48$), those with a chronic course

(CES-D above 15 at all measurements T1–T5, $n = 31$) were compared to those with "clinically relevant improvement of depression" ($n = 17$).

Religiousness was measured by a single variable in the study by Braam, Beekman, Deeg, and coworkers (1997): Subjects were asked to choose the three domains of life they considered most important in their present situation; "a strong faith" was among the eight domains presented to patients. If the subject chose strong faith, religion was considered "salient" (29% of the sample). There was a nonsignificant association between absence of religious salience and incident depression (OR = 2.66; 95% CI, 0.95–7.55); absence of religious salience, however, was associated with chronic depression (OR = 5.91; 95% CI, 1.48–23.6). The effect was stronger among women ($n = 24$); 100% of women for whom religion was not salient had persistent depression compared to 50% of those for whom religion was salient ($P < .01$).

Koenig and coworkers (1998) conducted the first study to diagnose depressive disorder using a structured psychiatric interview (the Diagnostic Interview Schedule); they examined the relationship of depressive disorder to intrinsic religiousness over time. The outcome variable was speed of depression remission (using standard remission criteria). These investigators identified 87 depressed older adults acutely hospitalized for medical illness and followed them for approximately 1 year after discharge. Subjects were contacted every 3 months and assessed for presence or absence of criterion symptoms.

Intrinsic religiousness was measured (Koenig et al., 1998) using a 10-item intrinsic religious motivation scale validated in two prior studies (score range 10–50). After controlling for multiple sociodemographic, medical, and psychosocial covariates using Cox proportional hazards, investigators found that, for every 10-point increase in intrinsic religiosity (approximately one standard deviation), there was a 70% increase in the speed of depression remission. Among subjects whose level of physical disability stayed the same or worsened during the follow-up period, speed of remission from depression increased by over 100% for every 10-point increase on the intrinsic religiosity measure. Again, level of physical disability appeared to influence the inverse relationship between religiousness and depression.

RELIGION AND DEPRESSION IN CAREGIVERS   Religious involvement may also have a protective effect against depression in caregivers of patients with dementia or end-stage cancer (Keilman & Given, 1990; Rabins et al., 1990; Wright et al., 1985; Zunzunegui et al., 1999). Rabins and colleagues (1990) conducted a prospective study of 62 caregivers of persons with either Alzheimer's disease or recurrent metastatic cancer (patients were attending the psychogeriatric clinic at Johns Hopkins). They examined characteristics of caregivers that predicted adaptation 2 years later; adaptation was assessed using the Affect Balance Scale (ABS). Only two characteristics predicted successful adaptation (ABS positive score). Number of social contacts explained 30% of the positive affect score variance, whereas self-reported religious faith explained 13% (F = 15.4,

P < .0001). Strong religious faith, then, and frequency of social contacts were the two most important baseline characteristics predicting caregiver adaptation.

UNDERSTANDING MECHANISMS

How might religious involvement affect mental health and help prevent or facilitate resolution of depression in older adults? Religion provides a package of resources that may help counteract factors involved in late-life depression, particularly in the settings of medical illness and other significant losses. These resources fall into four categories: social support; framework for meaning, purpose, and hope; avoidance of negative coping behaviors; and quality of decision making.

Social Support

Religion provides two kinds of social support that help counteract loneliness and isolation. One form includes support received from other members of the congregation and the clergy. However social support is measured, persons involved in religious communities have more of it. In a systematic review of the literature, 20 studies that examined religion and social support were identified; religious involvement was associated with greater social support in 19 of those 20 studies (Koenig et al., 2001).

The social support obtained in a religious setting appears to be more durable and of higher quality than support obtained in secular group settings (e.g., bridge or bingo clubs, senior centers) (Cutler, 1976; Ellison & George, 1994; Hatch, 1991; Oman & Reed, 1998; Ortega et al., 1983). One reason for this may be that the motivation to provide support to others in religious settings is partly driven by religious belief and commitment. Religious teachings encourage people to love one another and help one another, even when it is not convenient or even desirable (e.g., love thy neighbor, love thy enemy). Religious people provide support because they believe God wants them to and because they will be ultimately rewarded for such acts of kindness (or punished for lack of kindness). In secular settings, on the other hand, the motivation to provide support is based more on the exchange principal—I provide support to you as long as I feel like it, as long as you can provide something for me. Of course, many religious people also provide support based only on the exchange principal, and many secular individuals provide support for altruistic reasons.

Motivation to provide support to others is an important factor, particularly with regard to the elderly, whose ability to engage in social involvement via the exchange principal becomes increasingly threatened as health declines. Disabled older adults may not be able to go out for social activities, requiring friends to come to them or provide the disabled person with assistance in order to participate. This requires work and energy (on both sides), and often, unless powerfully motivated by some independent factor (like religion), social interactions with the disabled or sick elderly often diminish. Furthermore, healthy elderly, unless motivated by strong altruistic drives, may be threatened by elders with declining health because they fear that someday they will have the same problems (and would just as soon not be reminded).

Another form of support that helps reduce loneliness is the relationship with God. No matter where they are or what situation they are in, people can always talk to God—in the middle of the night, in the nursing home or hospital bed, when alone at home, or even in the middle of a crowd. This personal relationship with the Divine can be a powerful source of comfort, support, and self-esteem because the elder feels loved, cared for, and accepted by God. This relationship also provides a perceived link between this world and the next (e.g., the belief that God will not only take care of individuals after death, but also takes care of loved ones who have died and allows for a joyful reunion someday). As mental health professionals, I believe that we have underestimated the supportive power of this real or imagined relationship.

Framework for Meaning, Purpose, and Hope

Freud acknowledged that "only religion can answer the question of the purpose of life. One can hardly be wrong in concluding that the idea of life having a purpose stands and falls with the religious system" (1930/1962, p. 25). Indeed, religion provides a worldview in which even suffering and pain can have meaning and purpose. Viennese psychiatrist Viktor Frankl (1959) said that almost any degree of suffering could be endured if meaning or purpose could be found in it. The older adult with multiple medical problems, hearing or visual problems, chronic pain from arthritis, dependence on others for assistance with basic activities, and loneliness because many other family members have died may have a difficult time determining the meaning and purpose of life. These patients are seen by geriatric psychiatrists all the time because often they are depressed, and their medical doctor does not know what to do with them; consequently, the medical doctor refers the patient to a geriatric psychiatrist. They are placed on antidepressants in the hope that this will help; for many, it does help, but there are many (sometimes, both patient and psychiatrist) who are not completely relieved of a sense of hopelessness and powerlessness.

Religion can help some of these patients. Religion empowers people. In a situation in which the patient feels out of control, religious belief and prayer can give a sense of control. The belief that God is all-powerful, desires good for the person, and responds to prayer gives the patient an indirect form of control over the situation or enables the patient to view the situation in a different light that gives it meaning and purpose. Religious belief also gives the patient hope—hope to make it through, hope that things will turn out okay, hope that if God is in control then the patient does not have to be.

Scripture readings may also be helpful. They provide role models who suffered both physical and mental disease, yet triumphed eventually and were even rewarded (e.g., the Book of Job). These inspiring stories provide a way of understanding pain and suffering and may even help to relieve guilt and receive forgiveness for real or imagined sins believed to be the cause for the suffering. Singing hymns or repeating old, familiar prayers may give the disabled elder a sense of continuity with the past and arouse deeply felt emotions from past experiences. All of this may be therapeutic in one way or another.

Avoidance of Negative Coping Behaviors

Some older adults, when facing pain, disability, declining health, and independence, turn to ways of coping that are ultimately self-destructive. These include heavy alcohol use, dependence on prescription medication, excessive food intake, sometimes even gambling or sexual indiscretions. These behaviors often only plunge the older adult further into isolation, loneliness, and greater pain and suffering. By prohibiting such self-destructive behaviors and offering alternatives to them, religion may help prevent the negative consequences that otherwise follow.

Quality of Decision Making

Religion may influence older adults' decisions that determine level of psychosocial stress. The quality of decisions made both earlier in life and during the present often affect business operations, family relationships, and friendships, contributing to the current level of psychosocial stress in the older adult's life. If such decisions are guided by strong ethical principles, altruistic motives, and concern for others, then stress-producing negative life events are less likely to occur, and supportive resources will be more readily available.

For example, a poor decision in business may result in either the failure of the business or legal difficulties, which ultimately affects the older adult's quality of life, financial state, and reputation in the community. A poor decision concerning family priorities results in divorce and ongoing difficulties with children that reduce the social support and sources of practical assistance available when such support is needed. A decision to ignore others' needs in social and community relationships (through volunteer work, etc.) could adversely affect the social resources available in retirement years. The older adult must decide whether to forgive, to be grateful, to be generous—decisions that will ultimately affect mental health. Religious beliefs can help guide decision making so that negative life stressors are minimized, and quality of life is maximized.

NEGATIVE EFFECTS ON MENTAL HEALTH

There is no doubt that religion can also work in ways the opposite of those described above. Rather than being comforting and freeing, it can be restricting and confining. Religion can be controlling and coercive, particularly when a single powerful religious leader without accountability forms an exclusive group and alienates members from their families and the surrounding community. Religion can arouse excessive guilt, fear, and threat of persecution for past mistakes. Religion can lead to social isolation because a person feels judged by others for not "playing by the rules" and is excluded from religious fellowship because he or she is an alcoholic or a homosexual or she has had an abortion. Religion can be so rule driven that the spirit of religion is lost—the spirit of kindness, patience, forgiveness, compassion, mercy, understanding. A desire for justice, fairness, and truth can be driven by anger or a need for revenge rather than by love.

Gordon Allport, a Harvard psychologist and expert in the area of religious prejudice, wrote about two types of persons in churches that he surveyed: the intrinsically religious and the extrinsically religious. The intrinsically religious person, whom he discovered was relatively low on prejudice against minorities, was motivated to be religious as an end in itself—religious beliefs acted as the primary guide and yardstick for making decisions in life. The extrinsically religious person, who scored relatively high on prejudice, turned to religion as a means to another end, such as social status, prestige, wealth, power, or material gain; it was not religion that was important, but that which could be obtained through use of religion. Succinctly put, "The extrinsic type turns to God, but without turning away from self" (Allport & Ross, 1967, p. 434). A wealth of studies shows that extrinsic religiosity is associated with worse mental health, whereas intrinsic religiosity is correlated with better mental health (Batson & Ventis, 1982; Donahue, 1985).

Religious beliefs and experiences are sometimes confused with psychiatric illness. Many older psychiatric patients experience psychotic symptoms from mania, depression, schizophrenia, or other thought disorder accompanied by religious delusions or hallucinations. In some cases, psychotic symptoms may be difficult to distinguish from culturally sanctioned religious beliefs or experiences. When this occurs, it is important to establish communication with the patient's clergy and sort out with the clergy whether the patient's beliefs are consonant with those of their religious tradition. There is no evidence that religious beliefs or activities will exacerbate psychotic symptoms or "bring them on," even in schizophrenic patients. Rather, traditional beliefs and practices appear to have a stabilizing influence on patients with chronic psychoses (Carson & Huss, 1979; Kehoe, 1999; Verghese et al., 1989).

In some cases, religion may be used to replace necessary psychiatric care. Patients may stop taking a mood stabilizer or antipsychotic drug because they have been "healed" during a prayer service and no longer need medication. Often, these patients did not want to take medication anyway and use religion as an excuse for discontinuing it. Some religious groups view psychiatrists and, especially, psychologists with suspicion; they worry that these mental health professionals do not understand and will not respect their religious faith. Sometimes, religious councilors do not recognize the severity of a mental illness and may not refer patients (suicidal patients, for example) for specialty mental health care in a timely fashion.

Certain extreme religious groups (e.g., Scientologists) in the United States and occasionally even more traditional groups are skeptical about the benefits of antidepressant medication. Taking such medication may be seen as betraying God, with the belief that only God can heal, and God does so through supernatural means in response to prayer or other religious ritual. Sometimes, clergy reinforce these ideas. In general, however, most religious people (even the very devout) take their medication, seek counseling when necessary, and use their religious practices as adjuncts to routine psychiatric care.

APPLICATIONS TO CLINICAL PRACTICE

How does the psychiatrist apply research findings about religion and mental health to the clinical care of the geriatric patient? There is a variety of interventions that the psychiatrist can perform to learn about and utilize the religious resources of patients. Of primary importance, however, is to keep all actions in this sensitive area patient centered, not doctor centered (Koenig, 2000b). I now discuss four areas that address clinical applications: taking a religious/spiritual history, conducting religious interventions, understanding boundaries and limits, and recognizing the role of clergy.

Religious/Spiritual History

Psychiatrists should consider taking a brief religious/spiritual history from all older patients; this can be included as part of the patient's social history in the initial evaluation. The purpose is to learn about the patient's religious background, current practices, religious beliefs relevant to the illness, and the extent to which religion is used as a coping resource. Examples of questions that might be asked include the following:

What is your religious tradition or denomination?

Did you grow up in a religious home, and was this a positive or negative experience?

Have you ever had any notable religious experiences or religious transitions?

Have these experiences had a positive or negative impact on your life?

Are you religious now, and in what kinds of religious activities do you currently engage?

Are you a member of a religious community, and is this religious community supportive?

Is there a particular clergy person that you respect and trust?

Do you think religion is in some way associated with your current medical or psychiatric condition?

Does religion play a role in how you cope with medical or psychiatric illnesses?

How has the physical or mental illness affected your religious beliefs and activities?

If the patient is not religious, then it is important to inquire about what gives that person's life meaning or purpose, particularly in relationship to his or her medical or psychiatric illness. The answers to such questions will reveal a wealth of information about the patient's worldview, thought processes, and level of perceived social support.

A task force of the American College of Physicians (Lo et al., 1999) suggested that medical physicians ask seriously ill or terminally ill patients the following questions: "Is faith (religion, spirituality) important to you in this illness?" "Has faith been important to you at other times in your life?" "Do you have someone to talk to about religious matters?" and "Would you like to explore religious matters with someone?" Although these apply more specifically to medical patients, they may also be useful for geriatric patients with complex medical and psychiatric problems.

Conducting Religious Interventions

Simple interventions include acknowledging and showing respect for the patient's religious beliefs and supporting religious beliefs viewed as generally healthy. If the therapist has the necessary training, he or she may decide to utilize the healthy religious beliefs of the patient to alter dysfunctional cognitions, reframe difficult situations, and bolster the patient's social support network.

Although no studies have been conducted specifically of older adults, a number of clinical trials showed benefit to religious patients receiving religious psychotherapies, whether Christian or Muslim (Azhar et al., 1994; Azhar & Varma, 1995a, 1995b; Propst, 1980; Propst et al., 1992). Furthermore, many older adults who are isolated and lonely may benefit from becoming more involved in a religious community. This is particularly true for those who used to be quite involved, but for health or other reasons cut back or eliminated this activity. Remember that because 80% of older Americans are church members, religious attendance is the most common form of voluntary social activity among older adults in the United States (Cutler, 1976; Princeton Religion Research Center, 1996).

Understanding Boundaries and Limits

Religion is a sensitive area in most people's lives, and there are limits to interventions that psychiatrists should make in this area. First, mental health professionals should probably not prescribe religious beliefs or practices to nonreligious older patients. This does not, however, mean that religious or spiritual topics should be completely avoided with these patients, but rather that the area should be explored respectfully and nonjudgmentally. Second, psychiatrists should be cautious when supporting religious activities even in older patients who are clearly religious; if this is done, the approach should be gentle, nonimposing, and always patient centered. Third, for some patients, any direct religious intervention like prayer will strain their weak ego boundaries and should therefore be avoided. Post and colleagues (2000) provided rational guidelines in this regard, although they were speaking primarily to a medical audience. Transference and countertransference problems that may arise when religion is introduced into the clinical relationship have been discussed elsewhere, and all psychiatrists should be aware of these (Spero, 1981).

Recognizing the Role of Clergy

In the United States, clergy do more counseling with older adults than do mental health professionals. In the Epidemiologic Catchment Area (ECA) study, a higher proportion of patients seen by clergy were elderly than those seen by mental health professionals (9.9% vs. 5.8%, respectively) (Larson et al., 1988). This is not surprising because there are nearly 500,000 churches, synagogues, and mosques with over 300,000 clergy in the United States. Counseling activities by clergy typically take up about 10% to 20% of their time; consequently, religious professionals provide nearly 150 million hours of mental health services per year (not including the activities of nearly 100,000 full-time nuns or chaplains, for whom data are not available) (Weaver, 1995). Older adults with mental health problems are more likely to see clergy for at least two reasons: Clergy usually do not charge for their services, and such visits do not have the stigma associated with mental illness.

Studies have shown that the kinds and severity of mental conditions for which patients see clergy are remarkably similar to those for which they see mental health professionals (Larson et al., 1988). Clergy, however, seldom receive in-depth training on the mental health problems of older adults during seminary training and often feel unprepared to deal with these problems (Koenig & Weaver, 1997). Geriatric psychiatrists should form linkages with community clergy, both as referral sources and as resources to refer patients for community support. Volunteers from religious organizations can often be very helpful in providing respite for stressed, overburdened caregivers of patients with dementia or chronic depression. Psychiatrists can help clergy by educating them concerning how to recognize older members of their church or synagogue with mental disorders that require psychiatric care and when to refer such persons.

On the other hand, psychiatrists should be aware that professional chaplains have extensive training to address the emotional and spiritual needs of persons with complex social, medical, and emotional problems. For clergy to be certified in the Association of Professional Chaplains, 4 years of college, 3 years of divinity school, and between 1 and 4 years of clinical pastoral education are required, and they must take written and oral board exams. Thus, in the hospital setting, chaplains are the true experts in spiritual care and should be included as part of the team caring for older patients with mental disorders.

CONCLUSION

Religious beliefs and practices of older adults in the United States and elsewhere around the world appear to be associated with better mental health, whether mental health is measured as the absence of psychiatric disorder or the presence of well-being, hope, and optimism. This does not mean that all religiously involved older adults are mentally healthier or experience greater quality of life than those who are not religious. Nevertheless, religious involvement is associated with social support and a positive worldview that can provide meaning, purpose, and hope even in the most desperate and difficult of circumstances that many elders with chronic illness and disability face (Koenig, 1999). Sensitive and careful application of this research to clinical practice is warranted.

ACKNOWLEDGMENTS

This work was supported by the National Institute of Mental Health (R01 MH57662-01) and by a grant from the John Templeton Foundation (Radnor, PA).

REFERENCES

Accreditation Council on Graduate Medical Education. *Special Requirements for Residency Training in Psychiatry.* Chicago, IL: Accreditation Council on Graduate Medical Education; 1994.

Allport GW, Ross JM. Personal religious orientation and prejudice. *J Pers Soc Psychol.* 1967;5:432–443.

American Psychiatric Association. American Psychiatric Association practice guidelines for psychiatric evaluation of adults. *Am J Psychiatry.* 1995;152(11 Suppl):64–80.

Azhar MZ, Varma SL. Religious psychotherapy in depressive patients. *Psychother Psychosom.* 1995a;63:165–173.

Azhar MZ, Varma SL. Religious psychotherapy as management of bereavement. *Acta Psychiatr Scand.* 1995b;91:233–235.

Azhar MZ, Varma SL, Dharap AS. Religious psychotherapy in anxiety disorder patients. *Acta Psychiatr Scand.* 1994;90:1–3.

Batson CD, Ventis WL. *The Religious Experience.* New York, NY: Oxford University Press; 1982.

Bergin AE, Jensen JP. Religiosity and psychotherapists: a national survey. *Psychotherapy.* 1990;27:3–7.

Braam A. *Religion and Depression in Later Life: An Empirical Approach* [doctoral dissertation, Vrije University]. Amsterdam, The Netherlands: Thela Thesis; 1999.

Braam AW, Beekman ATF, Deeg DJH, Smith JH, van Tilburg W. Religiosity as a protective or prognostic factor of depression in later life; results from the community survey in the Netherlands. *Acta Psychiatr Scand.* 1997;96:199–205.

Braam AW, Beekman ATF, van Tilburg TG, Deeg DJH, van Tilburg W. Religious involvement and depression in older Dutch citizens. *Soc Psychiatry Psychiatr Epidemiol.* 1997;32:284–291.

Braam AW, Van Den Eeden P, Prince MJ, et al. Religion as a cross-cultural determinant of depression in elderly Europeans: results from the EURODEP collaboration. *Psychological Med.* 2001;31:803–814.

Carson V, Huss K. Prayer: an effective therapeutic and teaching tool. *J Psychiatr Nurs Ment Health Serv.* 1979;17:34–37.

Cederblad M, Dahlin L, Hagnell O, et al. Coping with life span crises in a group at risk of mental and behavioral disorders: from the Lundby study. *Acta Psychiatr Scand.* 1995;91:322–330.

Cutler SJ. Membership in different types of voluntary associations and psychological well-being. *Gerontologist.* 1976;16:335–339.

Donahue MJ. Intrinsic and extrinsic religiousness: review and meta-analysis. *J Pers Soc Psychol.* 1985;48:400–419.

Ellis A. Psychotherapy and atheistic values: a response to A. E. Bergin's "Psychotherapy and religious values." *J Consult Clin Psychol.* 1980;48:635–639.

Ellison CG, George LK. Religious involvement, social ties, and social support in a southeastern community. *J Scientific Study Religion.* 1994;33:46–61.

Fetzer Institute. *Multidimensional Measurement of Religiousness/Spirituality for Use in Health Research: A report of the Fetzer Institute/National Institute on Aging Working Group.* Kalamazoo, MI: Fetzer Institute; October 1999.

Frankl V. *Man's Search for Meaning.* New York, NY: Simon and Schuster; 1959.

Freud, S. Future of an illusion. In: Strachey J, ed-trans. *Standard Edition of the Complete Psychological Works of Sigmund Freud.* London, England: Hogarth Press; 1962: 3–45. (Original work published 1927.)

Freud S. Civilization and its discontents. In: Strachey J, ed-trans. *Standard Edition of the Complete Psychological Works of Sigmund Freud.* London, England: Hogarth Press; 1962. (Original work published 1930.)

Hatch LR. Informal support patterns of older African-American and white women. *Res Aging.* 1991;13:144–170.

Hill PC, Hood R. *Measures of Religiosity.* Chattanooga, TN: Religious Education Press; 1999.

Idler EL. Religious involvement and the health of the elderly: some hypotheses and an initial test. *Soc Forces.* 1987;66:226–238.

Idler EL, Kasl SV. Religion, disability, depression, and the timing of death. Am J Sociol. 1992;97:1052–1079.

Idler EL, Kasl SV. Religion among disabled and nondisabled elderly persons. II. Attendance at religious services as a predictor of the course of disability. *J Gerontol.* 1997;52B:306–316.

Kehoe NC. A therapy group on spiritual issues for patients with chronic mental illness. *Psychiatr Serv.* 1999;50:1081–1083.

Keilman LJ, Given BA. Spirituality: an untapped resource for hope and coping in family caregivers of individuals with cancer. *Oncol Nurs Forum.* 1990;17:159.

Koenig HG. *Aging and God.* Binghamton, NY: Haworth Press; 1994.

Koenig HG, ed. *Handbook of Religion and Mental Health.* San Diego, CA: Academic Press; 1998a.

Koenig HG. Religious beliefs and practices of hospitalized medically ill older adults. *Int J Geriatr Psychiatry.* 1998b;13:213–224.

Koenig HG. *The Healing Power of Faith.* New York, NY: Simon and Schuster; 1999.

Koenig HG. *Impact of Religion and Spirituality on Health Service Use (1998–2002): Preliminary Results.* Durham, NC: Center for the Study of Religion/Spirituality and Health; 2000a.

Koenig HG. Religion, spirituality and medicine: application to clinical practice. *JAMA.* 2000b;284:1708.

Koenig HG, Cohen H, Blazer D, et al. Religious coping and depression in elderly hospitalized medically ill men. *Am J Psychiatry.* 1992;149:1693–1700.

Koenig HG, Cohen HJ, Blazer DG, Kudler HS, Krishnan KRR, Sibert TE. Cognitive symptoms of depression and religious coping in elderly medical patients. *Psychosomatics.* 1995;36:369–375.

Koenig HG, George LK, Peterson BL. Religiosity and remission from depression in medically ill older patients. *Am J Psychiatry.* 1998;155:536–542.

Koenig HG, Hays JC, George LK, Blazer DG, Larson DB, Landerman LR. Modeling the cross-sectional relationships between religion, physical health, social support, and depressive symptoms. *Am J Geriatr Psychiatry.* 1997;5:131–143.

Koenig HG, McCullough M, Larson DB. *Handbook of Religion and Health: A Century of Research Reviewed.* New York, NY: Oxford University Press; 2001.

Koenig HG, Weaver AJ. *Counseling Troubled Older Adults: A Handbook for Pastors and Religious Caregivers.* Nashville, TN: Abingdon Press; 1997.

Larson DB, Hohmann AA, Kessler LG, Meador KG, Boyd JH, McSherry E. The couch and the cloth: the need for linkage. *Hosp Community Psychiatry.* 1988;39:1064–1069.

Lo B, Quill T, Tulsky J. Discussing palliative care with patients. *Ann Intern Med.* 1999; 130:744–749.

Neeleman J, King MB. Psychiatrists' religious attitudes in relation to their clinical practice: a survey of 231 psychiatrists. *Acta Psychiatr Scand.* 1993;88:420–424.

Oman D, Reed D. Religion and mortality among the community-dwelling elderly. *Am J Public Health.* 1998;88:1469–1475.

Ortega ST, Crutchfield RD, Rushing WA. Race differences in elderly personal well-being. *Res Aging.* 1983;5:101–118.

Post SG, Puchalski C, Larson D. Physicians and patient spirituality: professional boundaries, competency, and ethics. *Ann Intern Med.* 2000;132:578–583.

Pressman P, Lyons JS, Larson DB, Strain JJ. Religious belief, depression, and ambulation status in elderly women with broken hips. *Am J Psychiatry.* 1990;147:758–759.

Princeton Religion Research Center. *Religion in America.* Princeton, NJ: Gallup Poll; 1976.

Princeton Religion Research Center. *Religion in America.* Princeton, NJ: Gallup Poll; 1982.

Princeton Religion Research Center. *Religion in America*. Princeton, NJ: Gallup Poll; 1985.

Princeton Religion Research Center. *Religion in America*. Princeton, NJ: Gallup Poll; 1990.

Princeton Religion Research Center. *Religion in America*. Princeton, NJ: Gallup Poll; 1996.

Princeton Religion Research Center. Princeton, NJ: Gallup Organization; 2003. Available at: www.gallup.com/poll/releases/pr010413.asp (accessed June 24, 2003).

Propst LR. The comparative efficacy of religious and nonreligious imagery for the treatment of mild depression in religious individuals. *Cogn Ther Res*. 1980;4:167–178.

Propst LR, Ostrom R, Watkins P, Dean T, Mashburn D. Comparative efficacy of religious and nonreligious cognitive-behavior therapy for the treatment of clinical depression in religious individuals. *J Consult Clin Psychol*. 1992;60:94–103.

Rabins PV, Fitting MD, Eastham J, Zabora J. Emotional adaptation over time in caregivers for chronically ill elderly people. *Age Ageing*. 1990;19:185–190.

Ragan C, Malony HN, Beit-Hallahmi B. Psychologists and religion: professional factors and personal beliefs. *Rev Religious Res*. 1980;21:208–217.

Shafranske EP, Malony HN. California psychologists' religiosity and psychotherapy. *J Religion Health*. 1990;29:219–231.

Spero M. Countertransference in religious therapists of religious patients. *Am J Psychother*. 1981;35:565–575.

Taubes T. "Healthy avenues of the mind": psychological theory building and the influence of religion during the era of moral treatment. *Am J Psychiatry*. 1998;155:1001–1008.

Verghese A, John JK, Rajkumar S, Richard J, Sethi BB, Trivedi JK. Factors associated with the course and outcome of schizophrenia in India: results of a two-year multicentre follow-up study. *Br J Psychiatry*. 1989;154:499–503.

Weaver AJ. Has there been a failure to prepare and support clergy in their role as frontline community mental health workers? A review. *J Pastoral Care*. 1995;49:129–149.

Wright SD, Pratt CC, Schmall VL. Spiritual support for caregivers of dementia patients. *J Religion Health*. 1985;24:31–38.

Zinnbauer B, Pargament KI, Cowell B, et al. Religion and spirituality: unfuzzying the fuzzy. *J Scientific Study Religion*. 1997;36:549–564.

Zunzunegui MV, Beland F, Llacer A, Keller I. Family, religion, and depressive symptoms in caregivers of disabled elderly. *J of Epidemiol Community Health*. 1999;53:364–369.

9

Ethnocultural Aspects of Aging in Mental Health

Kenneth Sakauye, MD

OVERVIEW

A lack of understanding of ethnic differences can be the basis for underdiagnosis, misdiagnosis, insensitivity, or inappropriate or ineffective treatment of psychiatric disorders in minority populations (American Psychiatric Association [APA], 1993). Renewed awareness of the importance of culture to mental health has led to requirements that general psychiatry training must cover cultural psychiatry in the curriculum. Although this has met little opposition, many educators still openly espouse the view that cultural discussions are little more than an attempt to force political correctness.

This chapter focuses on "minorities of color": African Americans, Hispanic Americans, Asian Americans, and Native Americans and Pacific Islanders. However, the chapter is organized around the overriding common issues rather than broad stereotypes of each group because there is such a large variability within these racial divisions, which represents many ethnic groups, intermarriage, assimilation, and distances from immigration. Useful overviews are available in *Mental Health: Culture, Race, and Ethnicity* (US Department of Health and Human Services, 2001) and the *Lexicon of Cross-Cultural Terms in Mental Health* (World Health Organization [WHO], 1997).

Cultural study is not quite a discipline like other fields in psychiatry. There are biological differences between races that may influence different susceptibilities to disease and pharmacokinetic and pharmacodynamic variations. However, the dominant feature of what is commonly seen as "culture" comprises more elusive constructs: institutions that preserve group identification, art and music, food preferences, attitudes, behaviors, and a regulated system of beliefs. Language is often different as well, leading to communication barriers with other cultural groups. Differences in values and beliefs influence the expression of distress, the reason for seeking help, and compliance, which is affected by differing views of the credibility of recommendations from professionals. Strongly hierarchical family and cultural systems may so influence relationships with authority that they inhibit full disclosure or, conversely, lead to excessive attempts to please the professional or blind compliance. The culture of poverty, seen most often in minority populations, creates barriers to access to care and factors that lead to poor compliance.

For practitioners, ethnocentric bias and pseudoscientific racism (such as concepts of racial supremacy) lead to stereotyping, which fosters misdiagnosis, undertreatment, and treatment errors (Table 9-1). Prejudice is often returned by the minority group in the form of oversuspicion of mistreatment by a majority caregiver or even outright hatred (APA, 1993; Gaw, 1993).

Thernstrom and coworkers (1980) catalogued 106 ethnic groups in the *Harvard Encyclopedia of American Ethnic Groups*. Groups were described by

TABLE 9-1. Role of ethnicity in health care

Variable	Clinical relevance
Language	Often a barrier to treatment
	Implies different cultural values and beliefs
Values and beliefs	Credibility of treatment recommendations
	Disease presentation and communication
	Reason for seeking treatment
	Family issues, social networks, habits
Ethnocentric bias (racial stereotyping)	Misdiagnosis
	Undertreatment
	Treatment errors
	Racial pseudoscience
Prejudice (bidirectional)	Distrust
	Overt hostility or mistreatment
	Problems establishing a treatment alliance
Culture of poverty	Barriers to access to care
	Noncompliance and poor health knowledge
	Higher risk factors for illness and mental illness
Biological differences	Risk and prevalence of illness
	Pharmacokinetic and pharmacodynamic differences

socioeconomic status, immigrant status, language, country of origin, religion, way of life, marriage patterns, leisure time activities, food preferences, political attitudes or attitudes for selected issues, and institutions that preserved the culture. However, these objective markers for ethnic identity are usually blurred by intermarriage, assimilation, and progressive American-born generational status. Differences between behaviors due to socioeconomic stratification and those rooted in out-of-awareness cultural identification are not always easy to discern.

The subjective dimension of ethnicity, or social identity, is context bound. That is, its presence and strength vary with the situation. For example, an African American elder may not be aware of race unless interacting with whites. Thus, influences of ethnicity and culture often appear to be a moving target that is better understood for the individual rather than the group. Key issues to consider are developmental influences, motivations, self-esteem, performance, interpersonal relations, and sense of personal control (Liebkind, 1992; Peterson, 1980). The difficult aspect of understanding culture is knowing when to apply group stereotypes and when exceptions would prove the rule.

Since the review "Ethnocultural Aspects" in *The Comprehensive Review of Psychiatry II* (Sakauye, 1996), world events have forced attention to ethnic differences, prejudice, and ethnocentrism on a global scale. Ethnicity and mental health have also received more interest, as reflected in *Mental Health: Culture, Race, and Ethnicity* (US Department of Health and Human Services, 2001). However, ideas about elderly minority individuals are still largely inferred from studies of younger minority group members around the key issues of immigrant status, prejudice, diagnostic differences and prevalence of disease, culture-bound syndromes, family conflicts, and low utilization of resources.

DEMOGRAPHIC PROFILES (65 OR OLDER)

Ethnic minority populations in the United States are growing (Table 9-2). The 2000 census showed 11.6% growth in the general population, from 248,708,873 in 1990 to 281,421,906 in 2000. Meanwhile, the minority population grew

TABLE 9-2. US minority population, change in elderly, 1900–2000

US census	1990	2000	% Change
Total population	248,709,873	281,421,906	+11.6
White, one race	199,686,070	211,460,626	+5.6
Minority (difference)	49,023,803	69,961,280	+29.5
Percent of population	19.7	24.8	+5.1

Source: US Census Bureau (2000). Because mixed races are double counted as white and other races, the calculation for minorities in this table was based on the use of white-only census as the measure of nonminority status and calculated against the total population.

TABLE 9-3.   Minority elderly demographic profile, 2000 census

Cultural group	Number	% Total population
Total population	281,421,906	100
African American	34,658,190	12.3
Hispanic American	35,305,818	12.5
Native American and Alaska Native	2,475,956	0.9
Asian American	10,242,998	3.6
Native Hawaiian and other Pacific Islander	398,835	0.1
Two or more races	6,826,228	2.4

Source: US Census Bureau, Census 2000 Redistricting (Public Law 94-171) Summary File, Tables PL1 and PL2.

29.5%, from 49,023,803 in 1990 to 69,961,280 in 2000, representing an increase in minority percentage from 19.7% of the US population in 1990 to 24.8% in 2000. The melting pot ideal still seems relatively limited, with 97.6% of the population declaring only one racial makeup. Within this context, the nation's median age has grown as the baby boom generation ages and was the highest ever (35.3 years compared to 32.9 years in 1990), while growth in the population 65 years and older seemed to lag with the rise in the middle-aged population. The elderly population showed virtually no percentage change between 1990 (12.6%) and 2000 (12.4%).

When taken as an aggregate of age and two or more races (by intermarriage), of the total population, Hispanic Americans represented 12.5% (35,305,818), African Americans represented 12.3% (34,658,190), Native Americans and Alaska Natives represented 0.9% (2,475,956), Asians represented 3.6% (10,242,998), and Native Hawaiian and other Pacific Islanders represented 0.1% (398,835) (Table 9-3). Although the US Census Bureau special reports on ethnicity, age, and immigrant status usually are not completed until the latter half of the decade, the trends noted since the 1980s in relation to current immigration laws that favor reunification of families under the 1952 immigration law (Gibson & Lennon, 1999; Smith, 1998) show the following patterns (see also Table 9-4):

1. African American elderly are largely American born, although soon a higher proportion of elderly from reunification of African and Caribbean Islander immigrants and individuals of mixed heritage is expected.
2. Approximately 84% of all Asian Americans residing in the United States are of six ethnic groups: Chinese, Filipino, Japanese, Korean, Vietnamese, and Asian Indian. Asian groups with longer and earlier histories of family immigration before the Asian Exclusion Act of 1924 (e.g., Japanese and Filipino) have higher proportions of elderly and American-born natives than other Asian groups.

3. Hispanics are primarily represented by Mexican Americans (60% of Hispanics), Puerto Ricans (12.2% of Hispanics), Cubans (4% of Hispanics), and South and Central Americans.
4. Asian and Hispanic elderly are more likely to be immigrants, posing special risks for mental health and support (APA, 1993; US Census Bureau, 2000).
5. Native American and Alaska Native elders comprise several hundred tribal or cultural groups with different languages and degrees of assimilation. Lower education levels and socioeconomic status characterize minority elderly.

Mental health and well-being are strongly related to physical health status and disability (Stewart et al., 1989). Although there has been a slight reduction in the estimates of excess mortality (shorter life span) for minorities, there are continued health risks for minority elderly, who face many barriers to treatment. In general, minority populations experience more health problems than the white majority population. Over 50% of older blacks and older Mexican Americans report chronic health conditions; this is more than 10% greater than the rate for older whites. Of Native American elders, 50% suffer from adult onset diabetes, and these elders have a 107% higher rate of death from diabetes than the general population. By age 45 years, Native Americans show

TABLE 9-4. Minority elderly demographic profile (1990 census)

Cultural group	Number of elderly (>60 years)	% Elderly (>60 years) within own ethnic group	% Foreign born (elderly 62 years and older only)
African American	2,058,100	8.3	N/A
Hispanic American	1,161,300	5.2	N/A
Mexican		4.4	
Puerto Rican		4.7	
Cuban		14.8	
Central or South American		3.0	
Asian American	454,400	6.2	
Japanese		19.5	37.2
Chinese		12.5	75.9
Korean		7.2	80.1
Filipino		11.3	96.3
Southeast Asian (Vietnamese)		4.6	100
Asian Indian		4.3	19.3
Native American	114,500	5.8	0

Source: US Bureau of the Census (1991) (not revised to estimates of change based on the 1990 census that are published annually). Similar data were not expected to be released until late 2002 from the 2000 census. N/A, not applicable.

the same rate of disabilities as non-Natives at age 65 years, and Native Americans have the shortest life expectancy of any racial group (65 years). They show a 459% higher rate of death from alcoholism and 233% higher rate of death from tuberculosis. The basis for many of these differences lies in socioeconomic disparity, occupations that pose higher risks of injury and disability, poor nutrition, and lack of appropriate illness prevention (health promotion) (American Society on Aging, 1992; APA, 1993). Health concerns must be addressed in the provision of mental health to minority elderly.

DIAGNOSTIC ISSUES

Prevalence of Mental Illness

Differences in rates of mental illness for minority elderly are important to service planners and to inform the direction of clinical research. Many of the well-known risk factors common to mental health problems and mental disorders (US Department of Health and Human Services, 2001), particularly neuropsychological deficits, language disabilities, physical health, social disadvantage, low education, and poverty, are known to be increased in minority elderly (Table 9-5).

A reanalysis of the National Institute of Mental Health (NIMH) epidemiologic catchment area (ECA) data was performed for an American Psychiatric Association task force in 1993 (APA, 1993). The ECA study oversampled Hispanics at the Los Angeles, California, site and African Americans and rural elderly at Piedmont (Duke University, North Carolina), but lacked additional data on Asians or Native Americans, making it statistically unsound to venture prevalence estimates for most minority groups. Nevertheless, unexpected findings were a lower rate of depression in minority groups despite higher mental health risks and a higher rate of phobic disorders for African Americans and Hispanics and cognitive impairment in African Americans (Table 9-6). Another unexpected finding was the lower rate of psychopathology in Mexican American immigrants as opposed to American-born Mexican Americans. Contrary to predictions about increased risk for immigrant elderly, the immigrant group showed only one half the lifetime prevalence for most major psychiatric disorders compared to their US-born counterparts (Escobar, 1993).

This was similar to earlier findings in the Midtown Manhattan Study (another NIMH catchment study), in which immigrants who had been in the United States for over 20 years actually showed fewer mental health problems than recent immigrants or American-born individuals (Srole et al., 1962). A "survivor theory" was proposed, whereby a higher rate of early mortality in minority populations meant that only the individuals with the best mental and physical health survived to old age. To definitively address the questions, it is clear that special sampling procedures are needed to study minority elderly, who are underrepresented in most studies.

TABLE 9-5. Ethnoculturally (racially) determined risk and protective factors in mental disorders

Risk factors common to mental health problems and mental disorders	Protective factors against mental health problems and mental disorders
Individual	Individual
Genetic vulnerability (varies by mental disorder)	Positive temperament
Gender	Above-average intelligence
Neuropsychological deficits	Social competence
Language disabilities	Spirituality or religion
Chronic physical illness	
Dementia/low average intelligence	
Family	Family
Severe marital discord	Smaller family structure
Social disadvantage	Supportive family relationships
Overcrowding or large family size	Good sibling relationships
Paternal criminality	
Elder abuse or neglect	
Community or social	Community or social
Violence	Availability of health and social services
Poverty	Social cohesion
Community disorganization	
Inadequate schools	
Racism and discrimination	

Source: US Department of Health and Human Services (2001).

Suicide rates for African American and Hispanic American elderly have generally been lower than among whites (Group for the Advancement of Psychiatry, 1989). Rates among Japanese, Chinese, and Korean Americans increase with age and seem comparable to those for whites (about 21 per 100,000), with marginally higher rates of suicide in elderly Chinese and Japanese Americans (McIntosh & Santos, 1981). Higher suicide rates might be explainable by anomie, poverty, or other social stressors. The lower rates of suicide in elderly minorities have been explained by stronger family ties and extended family networks (social buffers), stronger social importance in the minority family, and stronger cultural or religious attitudes against suicide.

Japanese Americans have often been assumed to have a higher rate of suicide than whites because of the widely known ritual suicide (seppuku or hara-kiri), related to an old military code of honor (Bushido). However, this ritual was reserved for the noble class, and the actual transmission of such attitudes among Japanese immigrants is doubtful. The incidence of suicides in Japanese Americans is generally equivalent to that for white counterparts, and the pat-

TABLE 9-6. ECA 6-month prevalence by age and race

| | Percentage of psychiatric diagnoses in each race | | | | | |
| | White | | African American | | Hispanic | |
Disorder	18–54 years	55 years and older	18–54 years	55 years and older	18–54 years	55 years and older
Bipolar*	1.1	—	1.3	—	—	—
Major depression	4.4	1.5	3.7	1.6	4.2	—
Dysthymia*	3.7	2.5	2.8	1.8	4.0	—
Alcohol abuse	7.5	2.1	6.3	3.3	8.8	—
Schizophrenia/ schizophreniform illness	1.1	0	1.8	0	—	0
Obsessive-compulsive	2.1	0.9	1.6	1.9	—	0
Phobia	8.9	6.7	15	13.9	8.1	9.1
Somatization	0	0	0	0	0	0
Panic	1.2	—	1.2	—	—	—
Antisocial personality	1.6	—	1.2	—	—	0
Cognitive impairment†	0.3	2.3	1.4	9.2	—	—
Any DIS/DSM-III diagnosis	23.6	14.0	27.3	24.7	23.1	18.5

Source: Adapted from Amerian Psychiatric Association (1993), Tables 2-2 and 2-3. Based on the DIS (Diagnostic Interview Schedule) from the epidemiologic catchment area study, 6-month period, all sites included, weighted. A dash indicates fewer than 20 unweighted positive cases. Asian and Native Americans were not oversampled; there were inadequate numbers for analysis.
*Lifetime diagnosis.
†Determined by MMSE.

tern of suicide does not appear ritualistic (Gaw, 1993; Group for the Advancement of Psychiatry, 1989).

In practice, one must be especially cautious of potential diagnostic errors and minimization of the extent of psychiatric disorders in minority elderly. Similarly, to reduce cultural bias in research, Rogler (1989) summarized his recommendations to (1) include a period of direct immersion in the culture of the study group, (2) look for unexpected findings (as evidence of cultural influences), (3) adapt to the respondent's cultural context (rather than expect the respondent to behave like everyone else), (4) incorporate emic cultural expressions in inquiries, and (5) be aware that cultural factors may influence the psychometric properties of instruments.

Culture-Bound Syndromes and Atypical Presentations

There is a stronger possibility of atypical presentations, culture-bound disorders, and communication barriers in minority elderly. The rates of atypical presentations, culture-bound syndromes, and diagnostic errors are not established, although they are discussed frequently.

From a medical model for psychiatric classification, biology is viewed as the source of pathogenesis with a putative set of nonoverlapping symptoms that characterize disease states. Under this model, psychological and cultural layers of reality are held to be epiphenomenal, exerting a pathoplastic effect on the content of a delusional system or system of thought (Kleinman, 1988).

On the other extreme, diagnosis from a medical anthropology perspective (cultural psychiatry vantage point) views illness behavior, patterns of help seeking, and treatment responses as the distinctive factor rather than symptoms per se. The dichotomy is exemplified by depression experienced entirely as low back pain. The patient might complain that the pain is leading to loss of appetite, inability to go out, weakness, and insomnia. Depressive affect and social disinterest are denied. In the absence of explainable medical causes, this may be conceptualized as a phenomenon similar to existential despair and sadness common to elderly persons.

Although major psychiatric disorders, such as psychosis, major depression, bipolar disorder, or dementia may be less prone to culturally based diagnostic differences, cultural influences seem most evident in diagnosis of personality styles, dysthymia, anxiety, marital or family disorders, and culture-bound syndromes (syndromes that fall outside conventional diagnostic categories) (Littlewood, 1990). It is not difficult to see how a paradigm conflict could cause misdiagnosis of mild psychopathology like dysthymia, make it difficult to engage a patient, or cause a clinician to view some behaviors (like somatic expressions) pejoratively as primitive defense mechanisms.

As possible inclusions as new diagnostic categories, 185 indigenous terms representing culture-bound syndromes (Table 9-7) were investigated in preparation for the *Diagnostic and Statistical Manual of Mental Disorders, Third Edition (DSM-III)* and Fourth Edition (American Psychiatric Association, 1980, 1994) work group (Hughes, 1985; Simons, 1993). These disorders are generally rare even within their cultures of origin, but as local diagnostic entities, have a culturally developed theory of causality and cure (often spiritual or herbal).

The age distribution of these syndromes and their frequency have not yet been defined, but are thought to be greater than a 10% lifetime prevalence rate for some of the anxiety spectrum disorders. In studies from the University of Connecticut (Tolin, Robison, Gatzambide et al., submitted) a survey of Puerto

TABLE 9-7. Culture-bound syndromes

Syndrome	Group and location	Description (estimated incidence if known)	Possible *DSM-III* parallel
Black voodoo	Southern United States	Witchcraft afflictions	Psychosis
Falling out	Southeastern United States Afro-Caribbeans	Sudden collapse, cannot see, but can understand surrounding events	Posttraumatic stress disorder
Indisposition	Bahamians, Haitians		
Wind illness (*p'a-leng*)	Chinese	Morbid fear of the cold, especially of the wind	Specific phobia (300.29)
Neurasthenia	China, Japan	Weakness or exhaustion of the nervous system	Dysthymia (300.40)
Taijinkyofusho	Japan	Embarrassed of being with others due to blushing, unpleasant body order, stuttering	Social phobia Body dysmorphic disorder
Shinkeishitsu	Japanese men	Fear of contact with others (obsessions and phobias)	Agoraphobia (but usually in women in the West)
Latah	Malaysia, Indonesia	Hypersensitivity to sudden fright or startle; hypersuggestibility, echopraxia, echolalia, dissociation	Anxiety or panic disorder
Susto	Central and South America	Tiredness, debility attributed to an antecedent fright or startle	Adjustment disorder/ dysthymia
Espanto	Spain		
Ataque de nervios	Puerto Rico	Out-of-consciousness state caused by malevolent spirits	Psychosis Body dysmorphic disorder
Towatl ye sni	Dakota Sioux	Experience of one's thoughts traveling to the dwelling place of dead relatives, preoccupations with ghosts and spirits, "totally discouraged"	Major depression

TABLE 9-7. *Continued*

Syndrome	Group and location	Description (estimated incidence if known)	Possible *DSM-III* parallel
Ghost sickness	Navajo	Weaknes, loss of appe- tite, dizziness, faint- ing, suffocation, dread caused by witches	Panic attack
Wiacinko	Oglala Sioux	Anger, withdrawal, mutism, immobil- ity, suicide caused by disappointments	Major depression

Source: Selected from Golden (1977), Kleinman (1989), and Simons and Hughes (1993).

Rican adults showed that 16% reported a history of *attaques de nervios* (Tolin, Robison, Fenster et al., submitted), and 75% of these individuals sought medi- cal treatment as a result. Minority elderly seem to be at highest risk to exhibit many culture-bound syndromes because of their foreign-born status, low edu- cation, and low degrees of assimilation.

Insensitivity of existing diagnostic scales (missing a diagnosis when disease is present) as well as poor specificity (failing to distinguish between two somewhat similar disorders, like bipolar disorder and psychosis) are well docu- mented in case examples for minority populations. Examples are as far reach- ing as the Spanish translations of the MMSE (Mini-Mental State Examination), for which linguistic differences even among Hispanic subgroups have required several translation versions (Valle, 1989). Differences in social desirability or response sets have led to artifactually higher depression scores on the CES-D (Center for Epidemiological Studies Depression Scale) (Radloff, 1977) or schiz- oid traits on the MMPI (Minnesota Multiphasic Personality Inventory) in Japanese nationals partly due to cultural (Confucian) values for stoicism and self-sacrifice, which are viewed as part of the depressive continuum in the West (APA, 1993; Robins, 1989).

Considerations in clinical evaluations of minority patients should include potential (1) language barriers, (2) different idioms or concepts of illness, (3) lower socioeconomic status and education, and (4) ethnocentric bias of diag- nosticians. The high proportion of new immigrants for Asian and Hispanic elderly, a generally lower socioeconomic status, and discrimination still persist today and magnify the importance of these factors in evaluations. For physi- cians who deal with non–English-speaking patients, availability of translators is now mandatory. In the absence of translators for non–English-speaking people, non-English brochures and culture-fair non-English tests are necessary. In socially isolated, nonassimilated, American-born groups, like African Americans of lower socioeconomic status, there might be less motivation to change attitudes or behaviors. One might expect greater adherence to traditional cultural values and beliefs in such nonacculturated elderly.

Dementia

Higher rates of poor cognitive performance on screening tests like the MMSE and MSQ (Mental Status Questionnaire) have been noted in studies of ethnic/cultural differences, and estimated incidence rates (new annual cases) of Alzheimer's dementia are often described as being higher in minority patients. However, many cross-cultural studies of Alzheimer's dementia across races and locations showed significantly lower prevalence rates for Alzheimer's dementia in African Americans (Chang et al., 1993), Japanese (with autopsy confirmation) (Homma, 1991), and Cree Native Americans (Hendrie et al., 1993). Rough estimates of the rate of dementia by race are provided in Table 9-8 from pooled sources.

The situation has become very murky given studies presented at a conference sponsored by the NIMH/APA in December 2000 (Genetics Race and Cognitive Enhancers, GRACE), which suggest that incidence rates seem equivalent across races, but survival differences account for different prevalence rates (Jarvik & Mintzer, 2000). Tang and coworkers (1998) found a 4-fold increased incidence rate among African Americans and a 2-fold increased incidence rate among Hispanics without an increased frequency of an APOE ε4 allele.

In reviewing the cross-cultural data, there may be a shift in types of dementia seen over the past two decades. In the 1980s, vascular dementia was reported to be more prevalent than Alzheimer's dementia in Korea, Japan, and China. In the 1990s, reports suggested that Alzheimer's dementia occurs nearly twice as often as vascular dementia in these same countries (Suh & Shah, 2001). As countries "Westernize," perhaps environmental risk factors or diet

TABLE 9-8. Dementia by country

Country	Age in years (N)	Mild (%)	Moderate	Severe (%)
Sweden	60+ (443)	10.8	N/A	5.0
United States (New York)	65+ (1,805)	N/A	N/A	6.8
Denmark	65+ (978)	15.4	N/A	3.1
Scotland	65+ (222)	N/A	N/A	4.5
England	65+ (297)	5.2	N/A	4.9
Japan	65+ (4,716)	1.5	N/A	1.6
China (Beijing)	65+ (1,331)	N/A	N/A	1.82
Nigeria	60+ (not given)	N/A	N/A	0

Source: Homma (1991).
N/A, not applicable.

account for changing risk. Ongoing studies about environmental and genetic risk factors across cultures are in their infancy, and no definitive data are available to report.

Language effects and educational levels have been particularly important in interpreting performance on tests designed to measure cognitive and intellectual function (Loewenstein et al., 1993; Valle, 1989). Tests that seem most vulnerable to language and cultural effects are digit span (possibly due to nonequivalence of phonemes or syllables in particular digits in different languages), verbal comprehension, and verbal fluency (Loewenstein et al., 1993). Low education has been shown to bias even such screening tests as the Folstein MMSE (Chang et al., 1993) due to deficits in fund of knowledge, learning styles, abstraction, and reading abilities. Correction factors are difficult to develop because of the heterogeneity of minority populations (especially in degrees of language competence and self-education). For example, lowering the cutoff score for the MMSE would reduce false-positive results for the poorly educated or those with poor language skills, but would increase false-negative results for others.

An alternative to improve culture-fair tests lies in assessing everyday memory (Cohen, 1989) and IADL abilities through direct observation of performance on familiar tasks or problems or through naturalistic experiments. What is everyday differs for individuals from different cultures. Using this approach will require the establishment and validation of a wide variety of test forms and some method to decide which form to use. For example, rigid gender roles might make household tasks and even household utensils foreign to men in one culture, or memorization of grocery lists might be biased by what is a familiar food to different ethnic populations. In a clinical setting, caution should be exercised when interpreting mild dysfunction or severity from standard tests in minority elderly. Deficits should always be viewed in conjunction with functional correlates and history.

Another approach to enhancing culture-fair testing for dementia is to minimize language dependence in responses. For multiethnic elders, almost half of whom did not use English as their primary language (Asian–Pacific Islanders, African Americans, and Native Americans), the Clock Drawing Test proved more sensitive than the MMSE or Cognitive Abilities Screening Instrument for detection of dementia in poorly educated non-English speakers (Borson et al., 1999, 2000).

PHARMACOLOGY OF ETHNICITY

A growing body of research on the psychobiology of ethnicity suggests important differences between races in isomorphic variations of hepatic enzymes and metabolism of many medications.

Ethnic differences have frequently been noted in response to medications (Table 9-9). Using standardized protocols, a WHO cross-cultural study of anti-

TABLE 9-9. Biological differences

	Pharmacogenetics				Pharmacokinetics				
Group	Cytochrome P$_{450}$ polymorphism	Alcohol and aldehyde dehydrogenase	Acetylation	Conjugation	Neuroleptics	Triclic antidepressants	Benzodiazepines	Lithium	Protein binding
US Caucasian	D 8.7% PM S 2.7% PM	0% PM Reference	52%–68% PM	Reference	Reference	Reference	Reference	Reference	Reference
African American Nigeria Bushman	D 1.9% PM D 0%–10% PM D 18% PM	Not reported	Not reported	Not reported	Not reported	Higher peak plasma concentration (higher delirium rate by age and race)	Increased clearance—higher dose?	Lower membrane counter-transport (higher red blood cell/plasma ratio)—lower therapeutic dose?	N/A
Hispanic Spanish	D 6.6% PM	0% PM	0% PM	N/A	Same as reference	Same as reference	N/A	N/A	N/A

						Higher peak concentrations— lower daily dose?	Higher peak concentrations— lower daily dose?	Slower clearance— lower dose?	Kinetics same— lower therapeutic dose?	TCA, Same as reference
Asian										
Japanese	D 0% PM S 18%–23% PM	44% PM	10%–15% PM	20% Slower rate	Higher COMT activity (faster L-DOPA metabolism; more dyskinesia)					
Chinese	D 0.7% PM	22% PM	22% PM			Chinese, PM				
Filipino	S 5.1 % PM									
Native Americans	N/A	43%–45% PM	N/A			N/A	N/A	N/A	N/A	N/A
Navajo	2% PM									
Sioux	5% PM									
Oklahoma	16% PM									

Source: Mendoza et al. (1991), Lin et al. (1993, 2001). COMT, catechol-*O*-methyltransferase; D, debrisoquine hydroxylase (chytochrome P_{450} IID6) (most tricyclics, propranolol, perphenezine); EM, extensive metabolizers; N/A, not applicable; PM, poor metabolizers; S, S-mephenytoin hydroxylase (cytochrome P_{450} $2C_{mp}$) (diazepam). Alcohol dehydrogenase (ALH) and aldehyde dehydrogenase (ALDH) allelic variations affect ethanol oxidation/acetylation (caffeine, clonazepam, phenylzine, nitrazepam)/conjugation (acetaminophen, amobarbital, L-DOPA).

depressants found minimal differences in effective dose requirements for Asians, blacks, and Caucasians. However, different rates of side effects and early dropouts from intolerable side effects were noted between groups, especially in Japanese (WHO, 1983, 1986). This finding was consistent with the fact that racial groups may have pharmacodynamic differences or enzyme polymorphisms that lead to faster or slower metabolism.

Pharmacodynamic differences have not been studied extensively in minority elderly. However, there is a growing body of published data from the Center for the Psychobiology of Ethnicity (University of California, Los Angeles); the data are mainly for younger minority individuals and suggest differences due to race, dietary differences, body size, and so on (Lin et al., 2001; Ruiz, 2000). One key example is the slow membrane transport of lithium in many African Americans, which leads to higher intracellular lithium levels and explains efficacy at lower blood levels and increased lithium toxicity for many African Americans (Lin et al., 1993). It is unclear if this may be related to the presence of hemoglobin S (sickle cell trait or disease), as suggested in some case reports (APA, 1993).

Genetic polymorphisms of the cytochrome P_{450} system and other enzyme systems help explain pharmacokinetic differences, which lead to marked variation in metabolism of medications (Lin et al., 1993, 2001). Most psychopharmacologically active medications are relatively nonpolar (fat soluble) and require two metabolic steps, oxidative functionalization and conjugation. The rate-limiting step appears to be hepatic oxidation, predominantly through the P_{450} isozyme system, in which a polar group is introduced to increase water solubility. Of greatest interest have been cytochrome 2D6 and cytochrome 3A4, which metabolize many of the major psychotropic medications. The frequency of poor metabolizer variants of cytochrome P_{450} 2D6 seem higher in Caucasians (absent in 7% of Caucasians) than in either African Americans or Asians. Poor metabolizers of mephenytoin hydroxylase (2C19) may exceed 20% in some Asians. Genetic differences, in addition to functional differences, are being increasingly described in younger minority populations, although additional differences for elderly minorities remain unclear.

A sizable proportion of Asians show higher sensitivity and toxicity to older tricyclic antidepressants and neuroleptics. Many African Americans show increased sensitivity to lithium at therapeutic blood levels due to lithium transport differences in affected individuals. Differences in response or dosing for the newer generation psychotropic medications for elderly minorities have not been studied.

It is important to remember that these differences are not universal findings. They represent subtypes that may be more prevalent in different racial groups. In the absence of useful clinical tests to subtype in advance, this is meant to increase caution in dosing.

GENERATIONAL ISSUES

First-Generation Immigrants

The obvious and most widely accepted theme is the problem of culture shock or relocation trauma, which represents adjustment problems for new immigrants (Westermeyer, 1993). This is a major problem for many Asian elderly and Hispanic elderly who move to the United States in late life for family reunification and who are unlikely to work or have language-training opportunities. The problem of isolation is further magnified by the absence of local ethnic neighborhoods given trends to move to the suburbs and away from "ethnic ghettos." In a study of older Mexicans, the first report of differences in the prevalence and risk of depression for US-born and immigrant Mexican American elderly (older than 60 years) showed a higher prevalence of depression in Mexican American elderly compared to non-Hispanic Caucasians. The prevalence rate of severe depression (by CES-D) reached 30%–37% in immigrants older than 70. The rate was about one third greater than in American-born Mexican American elders and higher than reports in other studies of depression rates in either Caucasian or African American elderly (Gonzalez et al., 2001).

However, utilization of professional help is still rare (APA, 1993; US Department of Health and Human Services, 2001). A particular caution must be made here in interpreting reasons for low service utilization information. A recent minority caregiver survey by AARP (formerly known as the American Association of Retired Persons) showed a marked difference by race in the value placed on independence. In response to the statement "My children shouldn't care for me," 72% of Caucasian elderly said "Yes" (my children should not take care of me) as opposed to 68% of African Americans, 60% of Hispanic Americans, and only 49% of Asian Americans (Dessoff, 2001).

When taken as a group, the AARP and similar surveys are often used to explain why formal services are not utilized (minorities take care of their own). However, there are many barriers to care, usually in the areas of finances, language, stigma, referral patterns, and pathways to care (e.g., geographic inaccessibility, alternate health practices). Many minority individuals believe that formal care is fraught with racial or institutional bias, or that the only services available to them are substandard. It is important to think through all possible barriers to care when services are underutilized and not assume that minority families are not interested.

Another unique issue for immigrant elderly is the possibility of heightened isolation from family. The older immigrant may feel irrelevant, and there may actually be a decrease in intergenerational family solidarity for immigrant families (Roberts & Bengston, 1990). American-born children may be ashamed of an immigrant parent and distance themselves affectively despite feeling obligated to help.

A reassuring finding is that, if an immigrant stays in the United States, mental health problems may actually decrease. Immigrants who were in the United States for over 20 years had a lower psychopathology rate than even the national average in an NIMH epidemiological study that focused on immigrants (Srole et al., 1962). The reason proposed is survivor effects, by which only the hardiest stayed or survived.

American-Born Individuals

Much of the minority literature focuses on the special problems of low socioeconomic status in minorities of color. The so-called culture of poverty can exist outside color, but is often highest in minority populations because of biased treatment from individuals and, at times, institutionalized barriers to advancement (poor education, lack of mentors, segregation, inequitable resource distribution). However, it becomes a cultural issue when the disparities become entrenched and are concentrated among the minority populations.

The mental health aspect of prejudice is the question of what impact lifelong experiences of racism and poverty have on self-concept, locus of control (the belief that people control their own lives), and locus of responsibility (who is to blame for shortcomings . . . them or me). Identification with the negative portrayals of violence, being unintelligent, or being incapable of doing anything has been described. Fitting the stereotype will reinforce a nonminority individual's view that minority individuals are hopelessness, apathetic, procrastinating, lazy, depressed, or fearful of trying (Sue & Sue, 1990).

However, negative self-concept among minority individuals is not universal or even normative, despite the privations. Black identity development models have been proposed which speculate that ethnic identity, like other aspects of the self, follows a developmental continuum. Minority individuals progress from identification with the aggressor (with devaluation of self and one's ethnic group), to rejection of the dominant culture (and overvaluation of one's culture), to a balanced and healthy acceptance and tolerance of cultural differences and selective appreciation of attitudes toward the dominant group (Sue & Sue, 1990). This identity model has not been tested empirically across the lifespan (Ponterotto & Wise, 1987), but clinical experience seems to show far less anger and suspiciousness in the majority of minority elderly, as one might expect from developmental progression, and offers promise in trying to involve elderly minorities in a formal care system that had previously excluded them (APA, 1993).

PSYCHOTHERAPY AND FAMILY NEEDS

Sue and Sue (1990, p. 7) suggest: "The reasons why minority-group individuals underutilize and prematurely terminate counseling/therapy lie in the biased nature of the services themselves. The services offered are frequently antagonistic or inappropriate to the life experiences of the culturally different client; they lack sensitivity and understanding, and they are oppressive and discriminating toward minority clients." It is always hoped that this is unconscious on the part of the provider and can be addressed through better training about care for minority individuals.

Specific cultural treatment modalities such as acupuncture (China and Japan), Niakan therapy (self-reflection) or Morita therapy (getting in touch with the outside world rather than self-centeredness, Japan), herbal healing (throughout Asia), or spiritual healing (e.g., *spiritistas* [faith healers], voodoo) are usually unavailable within the formal care system, so many minority patients are known to use local healers simultaneously. These treatments can be geared for treatment of depression and psychiatric problems. The practitioner needs to be aware of any alternative therapy that is being given. From my personal experience, elderly minority patients have occasionally gone to their local healer for permission to follow our advice.

More germane to geriatric psychiatrists, however, is the need to address several generic themes consciously during counseling of minority individuals: (1) culture-bound values (communication patterns; degree of being individually centered, verbally expressive, open, or analytical [i.e., believing in cause and effect]; and how strong a distinction is made between mental and physical illness); (2) class-bound values (time orientation; need for immediate, short-term goals); (3) language; and (4) the stage of racial/cultural identity development, which influences social interactions and self-view (Sue & Sue, 1990).

Attitudes toward authority figures often pose initial problems in establishing a therapeutic alliance with a minority patient. Of course, one must bear in mind that there are different responses to authority figures within the family (parents, grandparents), in the social hierarchy (pastors, community leaders), and regarding outside authorities (doctors, lawyers, etc.). Patients might be overly deferential, inhibited, or ashamed of revealing personal feelings or might alternatively be hostile and suspicious. Strict time consciousness or time pressure may be unimportant if a patient has not worked or is from rural settings. Every ethnic group seems to joke about its "ethnic time," for which 4:00 o'clock actually means 4:15, 4:30, or even later. These factors are general problems that vary within ethnic populations by gender, age, generation level, and other life experience factors. What is important is that awareness of these issues and open discussion of different expectations are often enough to reduce these attitude differences, which are really external to the central therapeutic themes (Sakauye, 1989).

The problems raised also differ for immigrant generations (versus those who are American born) by length of residence in the United States and by degree of assimilation and social class. For new immigrants, the primary issues revolve around adjustment issues and may involve culture-bound presentations and need for bilingual therapists. Established immigrants may have more social and health-related issues. American-born, socioeconomically assimilated elderly may face problems of racial identity and problems of self-concept. Poorly assimilated elderly may face problems related to a culture of poverty and face adjustment issues due to early health disabilities and language barriers. The impact of prejudice, discrimination, and overt racism remain dominant themes for all American-born minority elderly (Fig. 9-1).

Cultural aspects of psychotherapy are also discussed in Chapter 31. Details about specific groups should be reviewed by consulting texts written for each ethnic group, such as Wilkerson's (1986) work for African Americans or that of Sue and Sue (1990) and Gaw (1993) for Asians, which elaborate on these issues. Additional abstracts are available in the APA task force report on minority elderly (1993).

SERVICE UTILIZATION AND ETHNICITY

The American Society on Aging (1992) developed a model for introducing culturally sensitive care within mainstream programs through an Administration on Aging grant (Table 9-10). The major recommendations are inclusion of minority care in the mission statement, involvement of community leaders on the board of directors, hiring of multicultural staff, and development of special multicultural programs and multicultural support staff. A monolingual, English-speaking receptionist, for example, may be the main barrier to service access.

Although there is more attention to minority issues than ever before, racial disparity in service utilization persists. One area of concern in geriatrics is the underutilization of nursing homes by frail minority elderly. In a stratified sample of 59 nursing homes in Maryland, the racial distribution was 78% white, 15% black, and 7% other races. This roughly matches the overall census breakdown of minority status and would suggest a trend toward proportionate utilization. However, cognitively impaired black residents were significantly overrepresented. Of the black residents, 77% were admitted for dementia, as opposed to 57% of white residents. The severity of dementia is often more advanced in African Americans who seek institutionalization (US Department of Health and Human Services, 2001; Weintraub et al., 2000).

Although not specifically dealing with the elderly, a recent analysis of the Veterans Affairs inpatient psychiatric facilities by race and diagnosis showed no significant differences due to race in psychiatric inpatient days or readmission. However, on closer scrutiny, there were significantly fewer visits by African American patients for psychotic disorders and significantly more visits for substance abuse than for their white counterparts (Kales et al., 2000). Hispanics showed no difference from the comparison Caucasian group. The analysis made speculations, but the generalizability from this predominantly male veteran population to the larger universe of minority elderly of both genders was unclear. A commentary followed this study on mental health care by race and diagnosis for elderly and suggested underutilization and possible misdiagnosis

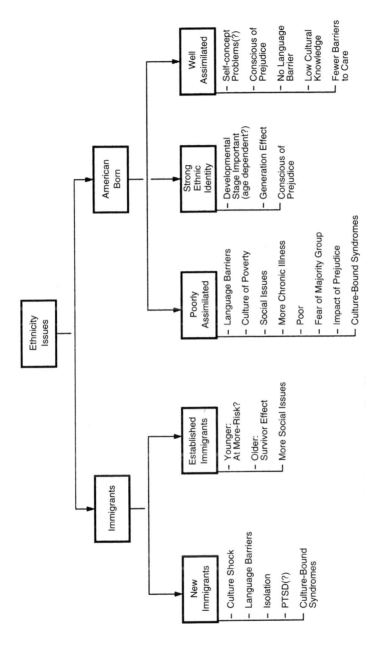

FIGURE 9-1. Impact of ethnicity on mental health care.

245

TABLE 9-10. American Society on Aging: programs for minorities

Commitment and empowerment
Mission: Agencies must have an explicit commitment to serve elders from all racial, ethnic, and cultural groups.
Governance and administration: Seek proportional representation of the communities served on governing bodies and administrative staff. Empower persons of color in decisions and have them serve as spokespeople for the agency.
Service approaches and program: Every effort should be made to make services accessible, understandable, and useful to all sectors of the community.
Targeting: Agencies should understand the prevalence of needs among different populations and know that need may exceed expectations based simply on proportional representation of a group within the community.
Outreach and marketing: The messages and methods of conducting outreach and marketing of services must appreciate cultural diversity and difference.

Considerations for developing a model
1. Understand the cultural traditions, historical experiences, and social and political networks within the community.
2. Identify and involve community leaders, organizations, grant makers, and advocates in planning and organizing efforts (planning committee).
3. The planning group and event participants must decide direction and priorities. Encourage the core group to take ownership of the project by coordinating efforts without imposition of a facilitator's point of view.
4. Define goals based on a realistic time line.
5. Work to develop community leaders (education about aging services and program systems and the skills necessary to effect change).
6. Design interactive sessions that promote discussion and hands-on activities (education to validate the experiences and issues affecting elders and their families and develop the skills necessary to effect change).
7. Be available to provide technical assistance.
8. Conduct monthly follow-up with participants.
9. From relationships between older participants and community professional leadership.
10. Emphasize issues that directly affect elders' lives.

of a greater magnitude than described in the Veterans Affairs study (Baker, 2000).

Caregiver burden and preference for care by minority family members is a necessary area of further investigation. Low utilization of supportive services by minority populations is accompanied by the finding that minority caregivers often complain less about burden (Hinrichsen & Ramirez, 1992; Peifer et al., 2000). What is protective and which attitude differences exist must be studied in more depth. Policy and service planners need data for future decisions.

SUMMARY

The mental health of minority elderly has received little research attention to date, although this appears to be changing. Minority elderly are a growing segment of the population, with a large proportion being poor or foreign born. The reliability of studies on the prevalence of psychiatric disorders in minority elderly has been questioned because of sampling limitations and instrumentation. Viewing problems from the vantage of immigrant versus American-born issues is useful in looking at the psychosocial issues and psychotherapy approaches that emerge. The classical problems of culture shock, language/communication barriers, attitude/value differences, and culture-bound syndromes are greatest for new immigrants and the poorly assimilated American-born groups.

Prejudice and the culture of poverty remain dominant problems for many minority elderly. Biological differences in rates of Alzheimer's dementia in cross-cultural studies have been found, which may lead to greater understanding of genetic and environmental risk factors. Pharmacogenetic and pharmacokinetic differences between races explain observed differences in drug response among racial groups (usually less than 5%–20% are affected).

A major problem in providing service to minority elderly remains a need for sensitization of mental health professionals to the particular ethnic groups that are being seen and developing culturally appropriate services. This requires conscious attention to the generic themes that affect all ethnic minority elderly, involvement of the community in program planning and feedback, and immersion in the culture of the group being served.

REFERENCES

American Psychiatric Association. *Diagnostic and Statistical Manual of Mental Disorders*. 3rd ed. Washington, DC: American Psychiatric Association; 1980.

American Psychiatric Association. *Diagnostic and Statistical Manual of Mental Disorders*. 4th ed. Washington, DC: American Psychiatric Association; 1994.

American Psychiatric Association. *Ethnic Minority Elderly: A Task Force Report of the American Psychiatric Association*. Washington, DC: American Psychiatric Press; 1993.

American Society on Aging. *Serving Elderly of Color: Challenges to Providers and the Aging Network*. San Francisco, CA: American Society on Aging; 1992.

Baker FM. Further reflections on race, psychiatric diagnosis, and mental health care utilization in older persons. *Am J Geriatr Psychiatry*. 2000;8:297–300.

Borson S, Brush M, Gil E, et al. The Clock Drawing Test: utility for dementia detection in multiethnic elders. *J Gerontol*. 1999;54A:M534–M540.

Borson S, Scanlan J, Brush M, Vitaliano P, Dokmak A. The Mini-Cog: a cognitive "vital signs" measure for dementia screening in multi-lingual elderly. *Int J Geriatr Psychiatry*. 2000;15:1021–1027.

Chang L, Miller BL, Lin KM. Clinical and epidemiologic studies of dementia: cross-ethnic perspectives. In: Lin KM, Poland RE, Nakasaki G, eds. *Psychopharmacology and Psychobiology of Ethnicity.* Washington, DC: American Psychiatric Press; 1993:223–252.

Cohen G. *Memory in the Real World.* Hillsdale, NJ: Erlbaum; 1989.

Dessoff A. Caregiving burdens hit low-income and minority boomers the hardest. *AARP Bull.* 2001;42:6.

Escobar JI. Psychiatric epidemiology. In: Gaw AC, ed. *Culture, Ethnicity and Mental Illness.* Washington, DC: American Psychiatric Press; 1993:43–74.

Gaw AC, ed. *Culture, Ethnicity and Mental Illness.* Washington, DC: American Psychiatric Press; 1993.

Gibson CJ, Lennon E. *Historical Census Statistics on the Foreign-Born Population of the United States 1850–1990.* Washington, DC: Population Division US Bureau of the Census; February, 1999. Population Division Working Paper 29.

Golden KM. Voodoo in Africa and the United States. *Am J Psychiatry.* 1977;134:1425–1427.

Gonzalez HM, Haan MN, Hinton L. Acculturation and the prevalence of depression in older Mexican Americans: baseline results of the Sacramento Area Latino Study on Aging. *J Am Geriatr Soc.* 2001;49:948–953.

Group for the Advancement of Psychiatry, Committee on Cultural Psychiatry. *Suicide Among Ethnic Minorities in the United States.* New York, NY: Brunner/Mazel; 1989. Report 128.

Hendrie HC, Hall KS, Pillay N, et al. Alzheimer's disease is rare in Cree. *Int Psychogeriatr.* 1993;5:5–14.

Hinrichsen GA, Ramirez M. Black and white dementia caregivers: a comparison of their adaptation, adjustment, and service utilization. *Gerontologist.* 1992;32:375–381.

Homma A. Gerontopsychiatric surveys on age-associated dementia in Japan: recent findings form epidemiologic view. In: *Proceedings of the 3rd International Symposium on Dementia.* Tokyo, Japan: National Center of Neurology and Psychiatry; 1991: 31–41.

Hughes CC. Culture bound or construct bound? The syndromes of the *DSM-III.* In: Simons RC, Hughes CC, eds. *The Culture Bound Syndromes: Folk Illnesses of Psychiatric and Anthropological Interest.* Dordrecht, Netherlands: Reidel; 1985: 3–24.

Jarvik L, Mintzer J. Expert panel summary. Paper presented at: Genetics, Response, and Cognitive Enhancers: Implications for Alzheimer's Disease (GRACE); December 2–3, 2000; Bethesda, MD.

Kales HC, Blow FC, Bingham CR, Roberts JS, Copeland LA, Mellow AM. Race, psychiatric diagnosis, and mental health care utilization in older patients. *Am J Geriatr Psychiatry.* 2000;8:301–309.

Kleinman A. *Rethinking Psychiatry: From Cultural Category to Personal Experience.* New York, NY: Free Press; 1988.

Liebkind K. Ethnic identity—challenging the boundaries of social psychology. In: Breakwell GM, ed. *Social Psychology of Identity and Self-Concept.* London: Surrey University Press; 1992:147–183.

Lin KM, Poland RE, Nakasaki G, eds. *Psychopharmacology and Psychobiology of Ethnicity.* Washington, DC: American Psychiatric Press; 1993.

Lin KM, Smith MW, Ortiz V. Culture and psychopharmacology. In: Alarcon R, ed. *The Psychiatric Clinics of North America: Cultural Psychiatry: International Perspectives.* Philadelphia, PA: Saunders; 2001:24:523–536.

Littlewood, R. From categories to contexts: a decade of the "new cross-cultural psychiatry." *Br J Psychiatry.* 1990;156:308–327.

Loewenstein DA, Arguelles T, Barker WW, Duara R. A comparative analysis of neuropsychological test performance of Spanish-speaking and English-speaking patients with Alzheimer's disease. *J Gerontol.* 1993;48:P142–P149.

McIntosh JL, Santos JF. Suicide among minority elderly: a preliminary investigation. *Suicide Life Threat Behav.* 1981;11:151–166.

Mendoza R, Smith MW, Poland RE, et al. Ethnic psychopharmacology: the Hispanic and Native American perspective. *Psychopharmacol Bull.* 1991;27:449–461.

Peifer KL, Hu T-W, Vega W. Help seeking by persons of Mexican origin with functional impairments. *Psychiatr Serv.* 2000;51:1293–1298.

Peterson W. Concepts of ethnicity. In: Thernstrom S, Orlov A, Handlin O, eds. *Harvard Encyclopedia of American Ethnic Groups.* Cambridge, MA: Belknap Press/Harvard University Press; 1980:234–242.

Ponterotto JG, Wise SL. Construct validity study of the Racial Identity Attitude Scale. *J Couns Psychol.* 1987;34:218–223.

Radloff LS. The CES-D: a self-report depression scale for research in the general population. *Appl Psychol Meas.* 1977;3:385–401.

Roberts REL, Bengston VL. Is intergenerational solidarity a unidimensional construct? A second test of a formal model. *J Gerontol: Soc Sci.* 1990;45:S12–S20.

Robins LN. Cross cultural differences in psychiatric disorder. *Am J Public Health.* 1989; 79:1479–1480.

Rogler LI I. The meaning of culturally sensitive research in mental health. *Am J Psychiatry.* 1989;146:296–303.

Ruiz P, ed. *Ethnicity and Psychopharmacology: Review of Psychiatry.* Vol. 19. Washington, DC: American Psychiatric Press; 2000.

Sakauye K. Ethnocultural aspects. In: Sadavoy J, Lazarus LW, Jarvik LF, Grossberg GT, eds. *Comprehensive Review of Geriatric Psychiatry.* 2nd ed. Washington, DC: American Psychiatric Press; 1996:197–221.

Sakauye KM. Ethnic variations in family support of the frail elderly. In: Goldstein M, ed. *Family Care of the Frail Elderly.* Washington, DC: American Psychiatric Press; 1989:63–106.

Simons RC, Hughes CC. Culture bound syndromes. In: Gaw AC, editor. *Culture, Ethnicity and Mental Illness.* Washington, DC: American Psychiatric Press; 1993: 75–93.

Smith ML. *Overview of INS History.* Arlington, VA: Bureau of Citizenship and Immigration Services. (Reprinted from Kurian GT, ed. *A Historical Guide to the US Government.* New York, NY: Oxford University Press; 1998.)

Srole I, Langer T, Michael S, Opler M, Rennie T. *Mental Health in the Metropolis: The Midtown Manhattan Study.* New York, NY: McGraw-Hill; 1962.

Stewart AL, Greenfield S, Hays RD, et al. Functional status and well being of patients with chronic conditions: results from the Medical Outcomes Study. *JAMA.* 1989; 262:907–913.

Sue DW, Sue D. *Counseling the Culturally Different: Theory and Practice.* 2nd ed. New York, NY: Wiley; 1990.

Suh GH, Shah A. A review of the epidemiological transition in dementia—cross-national comparisons of the indices related to Alzheimer's disease and vascular dementia. *Acta Psychiatr Scand.* 2001;104:4–11.

Tang MX, Stern Y, Marder K, et al. The APOE-ε4 allele and the risk of Alzheimer disease among African Americans, whites, and Hispanics. *JAMA*. 1998;279:751–755.

Thernstrom S, Orlov A, Handlin O, eds. *Harvard Encyclopedia of American Ethnic Groups*. Cambridge, MA: Belknap Press/Harvard University Press; 1980.

Tolin DF, Robison JT, Fenster J, Gaztambide S, Blank K. *Ataques de nervios* in older Puerto Rican primary care patients: prevalence and phenomenology. Submitted.

Tolin DF, Robison JT, Gaztambide S, Blank K. The prevalence of anxiety disorders among older Puerto Rican primary care patients. Submitted.

US Census Bureau. *1990 Census of Population and Housing Summary*. Washington, DC: US Census Bureau; 1991. Tape File 1C.

US Census Bureau. *Profiles of General Demographic Characteristics and Summary Files*; Washington, DC: US Census Bureau; 2000.

US Department of Health and Human Services. *Mental Health: Culture, Race, and Ethnicity, a Supplement to Mental Health: A Report of the Surgeon General*. Rockville, MD: US Dept of Health and Human Services, Substance Abuse and Mental Health Services Administration, Center for Mental Health Services; 2001.

Valle R. Cultural and ethnic issues in Alzheimer's disease family research. In: Light E, Lebowitz BD, eds. *Alzheimer's Disease Treatment and Family Stress: Directions for Research*. Washington, DC: US Dept of Health and Human Services; 1989:122–154. DHHS Publication (ADM) 89-1569.

Weintraub D, Raskin A, Ruskin PE, et al. Racial differences in the prevalence of dementia among patients admitted to nursing homes. *Psychiatr Serv*. 2000;51:1259–1264.

Westermeyer JJ. Cross-cultural psychiatric assessment. In Gaw AC, ed. *Culture, Ethnicity and Mental Illness*. Washington, DC: American Psychiatric Press; 1993:125–144.

Wilkerson CB. *Ethnic Psychiatry*. New York, NY: Plenum; 1986.

World Health Organization. *Depressive Disorders in Different Cultures: Report on the WHO Collaborative Study on Standardized Assessment of Depressive Disorders*. Geneva, Switzerland: WHO; 1983.

World Health Organization. Dose effects of antidepressant medication in different populations: A World Health Organization collaborative study. *J Affect Disord*. 1986; 10(suppl 2):S1–S67.

World Health Organization. *Lexicon of Cross-Cultural Terms in Mental Health*. Geneva, Switzerland; World Health Organization; 1997.

Principles of Evaluation

10

Comprehensive Psychiatric Evaluation

Ivan L. Silver, MD, MEd, FRCP (C)
Nathan Herrmann, MD, FRCP (C)

The ability of the geriatric psychiatrist to solve clinical problems is related directly to the comprehensiveness and depth of the data obtained from patients and their families. In the past 10 years, more attention has been paid to the psychiatric examination of elderly patients, and comprehensive assessment protocols are now available (Blazer, 1989; Coffey & Cummings, 1994; Lichtenberg, 1999; Zarit & Zarit, 1998). In this chapter, we present a guide for taking the psychiatric history, performing a functional assessment, and examining the mental status of the geriatric patient. More specific details about developmental inquiry, special tests, neuroimaging, and medicolegal issues are found in other relevant sections of this book.

Obtaining a geriatric history and assessing mental status are potentially long and complex tasks because the patient has lived many years and frequently experiences the comorbidity of neurological and medical illness. Emphasis on different aspects of the history will vary depending on the patient's problems. For instance, a corroborative history and a detailed cognitive assessment are priorities in patients with progressive dementing disorders and delirium. The family and past history are important for all patients and are particularly essential in patients with affective or personality disorders.

The goals of the history, functional, and mental status examinations are to (1) establish a provisional diagnosis and differential diagnoses; (2) develop an etiologic formulation that traces the biological, psychological, and social factors that have predisposed, precipitated, and now perpetuate the patient's current mental illness; (3) establish each patient's capacity to function independently; and (4) understand the patient by placing the patient's disorders and problems into a developmental and psychological context.

CHARACTERISTICS OF THE GERIATRIC PSYCHIATRY ASSESSMENT

A geriatric psychiatrist must consider three questions before the assessment begins:

1. Where should the patient be seen? Geriatric assessments may be undertaken in a variety of settings: at the bedside, in an outpatient office, at home, in an institution, in a day hospital, or in a specialized clinic. Where the clinician sees the patient may be critical because it can determine the quantity and quality of the data collected. For example, generally it cannot be expected that completing the assessment in an outpatient office will allow a full assessment of the capacity of a patient with dementia to function at home. This assessment often requires observation and monitoring in the home environment. On the other hand, a medical workup to rule out reversible causes of dementia requires the facilities of a clinic or hospital setting.

2. Who should participate in the assessment? A basis tenet in geriatric assessment is that, whenever possible, a patient's spouse, caregiver, and family are seen for corroborative information, with appropriate regard for issues of consent and confidentiality. This is critically important in the assessment of patients with cognitive impairment and may be equally important in patients who are cognitively intact. When mental disorders interfere with insight into the nature and quality of the illness, especially during an acute illness episode, interviewing family members often will provide a truer picture of the person's history. Historical events are verified and, in many cases, the diagnosis depends on the family members' ability to relate a coherent history. A family member is often the best person to describe the premorbid personality of the patient. This is valuable information because premorbid personality traits may change or become exaggerated in the context of a variety of geriatric mental illnesses, including dementia, affective disorders, and paranoid disorders.

3. How should the interview be conducted? It is important for each assessment to include an opportunity to talk to the patient alone, particularly when suicidal risk, family conflict and abuse, shameful issues, and sexual impairments are present. All psychiatric interviews should allow for a free exchange of information in an atmosphere of mutual trust that leaves patients with the feeling that they are understood. Establishing

rapport by providing appropriate reassurance and encouragement is important. Particular attention should be paid to the capacity of the patient to tolerate a psychiatric interview. Severely disturbed or cognitively impaired patients do not tolerate long, detailed interviews well. Brief interviews with active engagement facilitate the process.

Consideration must be given to the common sensory impairments seen in some geriatric patients. Patients with poor hearing and vision may require special intervention. When dealing with patients with deafness, it may help to ensure the hearing aid is on, to interview in a quiet room, and to speak in a slow, steady, low-pitched voice into the "good ear." A sound-amplifying device may be necessary; if one is unavailable, the "reverse stethoscope" method may be used: Put the stethoscope in the ears of the patient and speak into the diaphragm quietly. For the visually impaired, sitting closer to the patient or ensuring that the patient is wearing corrective lenses is helpful. The appropriate use of touch may reassure the patient and help facilitate the psychiatric interview. Cultural and language issues are also important to consider. The reader is referred to Chapter 9 for a full discussion of these issues.

THE ORGANIZATION OF THE PSYCHIATRIC ASSESSMENT

A schematic for the geriatric psychiatric assessment is presented in Table 10-1. It is meant only as a tool to organize the data and not as a checklist for the examiner.

THE PSYCHIATRIC HISTORY

Several detailed guides to the assessment of younger adults are available (Kaplan & Sadock, 1998; Yates et al., 1998). The following discussion is meant as a guide to adapting the traditional psychiatric history to the needs of the geriatric population.

TABLE 10-1. Schematic for the geriatric psychiatric assessment

Identifying data	Drug and alcohol history
Reliability of informant	Physical examination
Chief complaint	Functional status
History of presenting illness	Mental status
Past psychiatric history	Etiologic formulation
Family history	Provisional diagnosis
Family psychiatric history	Differential diagnoses
Personal history	Investigations
Medical history	Comprehensive management plan
Current medications	

Identifying Data

Identifying data can be amended by adding the name of the primary caregiver, whether in or out of the home. If the patient lives in a residential setting, the type of institution is specified.

History of Presenting Illness

The purpose of the history of presenting illness is to document events and arrange them in the order in which they occurred. It is important to record all recent environmental and physical changes in the patient's life. Environmental events and physical illness may precipitate mental illness in elderly patients. For example, recent losses, separations, moves, and changes in support networks may be associated with the onset of affective and paranoid disorders or the exacerbation of cognitive disability. Cognitively impaired, frail elderly patients are particularly predisposed to superimposed delirium when relatively minor toxic, metabolic, or infectious disease intercedes. Certain physical disorders seem to precipitate specific mental disorders. For example, cerebrovascular accidents have been associated with depression and mania (Cummings, 1997; Starkstein & Robinson, 1989).

To focus the inquiry, the examiner must be familiar with the natural history and symptomatology of the common mental illnesses in elderly patients. This is important because some mental disorders, particularly affective disorders, may present differently in old age. For example, many elderly depressives do not present with the classic sad and tearful demeanor (McCullough, 1991). Common geriatric presentations include the hypochondriacal, agitated depressive who importunes the family in fits of desperation. The patient's frantic pleas for help may look "hysterical" to the observer and feel "manipulative" to the family. Depression may present with negativistic behavior such as refusal to move, eat, or drink. A suicidal gesture may signal the presence of this disorder. The recent onset in advanced age of phobias, obsessions, or compulsive behavior may signal the beginning of depression.

Vegetative symptoms of depression in elderly patients include sleep, appetite, weight, energy, and sexual disturbance and diurnal variation in mood. The clinician distinguishes abrupt changes in sleep, appetite, and energy because the normal aging process can affect these functions. Weight loss may be quantified by changes in dress or belt size.

Interviewing a family member is essential when a cognitive disorder is suspected. The clinician may have to elicit the entire history of the presenting illness from the family. Cognitive disorders affect memory, language, perception, mood, thinking, personality, and the capacity to function independently in the patient's environment. For example, early in the course of Alzheimer's disease, patients will misplace their belongings, have trouble with the names of familiar people, have trouble remembering new information, and show word-finding difficulties. Personality traits may become exaggerated. Apathy, depressive symptoms, or stealing delusions may coexist. The patient may give up usual household activities, have trouble handling finances, and rely more on the primary caregiver. Impaired executive cognitive function may occur because of depression or brain disease; patients may be unable to organize their instrumental activities of daily living (IADLs), although they may remain independent in their activities of daily living (ADLs) (Spector et al., 1987). The primary caregiver is in the best position to provide the clinician with this information.

Past Psychiatric History

The record of past treatment successes and failures can help develop a management plan for the current illness by providing data on the natural history of a patient's mental illness and prognosis.

Family History

Most geriatric patients have deceased parents and may have deceased siblings. The cause of death, age of death, and the health of siblings may give clues about the patient's current problems. Knowing the mental function and living arrangements of the patient's parents or siblings near the end of their lives may be useful. These issues are particularly important with cognitive disorders (Cummings & Benson, 1992). A family psychiatric history provides valuable clues to the patient's diagnosis and may implicate genetic vulnerability, especially with affective and psychotic disorders and the dementias (Zarit & Zarit, 1998).

The past relationship of patients to their parents often determines the quality of family and interpersonal relationships. Because geriatric patients often rely on support for continuous good functioning, it is helpful to know about the quality of their relationships with their spouse or primary caregiver, adult children, grandchildren, and friends. Specific issues that may be important in the geriatric patient include the location of the children and the frequency of their contact with the patient; the health, reliability, and availability of the spouse; the presence of family conflict, especially in immigrant families; and unexpressed disappointments, fears, and resentments.

Personal History

Sometimes it is difficult to decide which events in an elderly patient's past are relevant to current problems and circumstances. Birth, developmental, childhood, and adolescent data are important and may be difficult to verify and corroborate. Knowledge of the patient's past sheds light on the patient's vulnerabilities and strengths and may explain why some patients develop psychiatric symptomatology at particular points in their lives (Vaillant, 2002). A review of the life cycle of an individual establishes the premorbid capacity of each patient to adjust to important life events.

These life cycle events may include starting school, leaving home, establishing a career, getting married, the birth of children, the death of parents, children leaving home, the death of siblings, retirement, and the death of a spouse. It is important to inquire whether the patient has had a history of abuse, neglect, or maltreatment at any time. Immigrants may be especially at risk for earlier trauma and difficulties adapting to a new environment. Holocaust survivors may be especially vulnerable to reliving traumatic events, especially in the context of dementia (Sadavoy, 1997). Patients who have been abused by caregivers may be more likely to show paranoid or agitated behavior in institutional care settings or to mistrust formal caregivers.

The personal history should also include an inquiry into the person's activities, religious affiliation, hobbies, and connections with community resources. This information is useful in assessing each individual's social vulnerabilities and strengths.

Documenting a patient's premorbid personality provides a longitudinal view of the patient's characteristic personality function and helps avoid erroneous diagnostic conclusions based on cross-sectional examination. Although this type of information is elicited from the patient, corroborative history from family or friends is often necessary. Asking about key features of personality such as capacity for empathy and intimacy, regulation of affect in stressful situations, and history of interpersonal relationships can provide a useful context for understanding current behavior.

A sexual history is often omitted in elderly patients. This may be caused by the examiner's lack of knowledge or misconceptions about sexuality in old age. A history of sexual orientation, activities, and practices and how the mental disorder has affected these functions is essential. For example, some elderly patients are very troubled by the sexual side effects of many psychotropic drugs. Developing a comfortable atmosphere for patients to raise these concerns during the assessment can be extremely therapeutic. This can be facilitated by a matter-of-fact manner when taking the history and by expressing empathic concern about any current sexual dysfunction.

Medical History, Medication Use, and Drug and Alcohol History

The clinician should document carefully all past and current medical problems, dates of onset, and treatment. The comorbidity of physical and mental illness, especially depression, is common in elderly patients (Koenig & George, 1998). Several physical illnesses, including Parkinson's disease and cerebrovascular disease, can precipitate a mood disorder or paranoid disorder (Assal & Cummings, 2002; Uekermann et al., 2003).

A variety of medications can precipitate psychiatric disorders such as delirium, affective disorders, and paranoid disorders (Johnson, 1981). A list of all medications, dosages, and date of onset is essential. Over-the-counter medications and so-called herbal remedies (e.g., SAM-e [S-adenosylmethionine] and St. John's wort) need to be included in this survey. Many, such as bromides, aspirin, and antihistamines, are neurotoxic even in moderate doses.

Drug and alcohol abuse often are underestimated in elderly patients (Naranjo et al., 1995). Screening for alcoholism can be assisted by asking questions known by the acronym CAGE (Ewing, 1984):

1. Have you ever felt you ought to Cut down on your drinking?
2. Have people Annoyed you by criticizing your drinking?
3. Have you ever felt bad or Guilty about your drinking?
4. Have you ever had a drink first thing in the morning to steady your nerves or to get rid of a hangover (Eye-opener)?

A careful inquiry into the quantity and frequency of drinking behavior, in addition to the above questions, is essential. A score of 1 or more on the CAGE questionnaire or a history of ingestion of a large quantity of alcohol on a frequent basis should lead the clinician to inquire in more depth. This would include further characterization of the extent of the drinking and the presence of withdrawal symptoms, anxiety, depression, or other comorbid psychiatric or medical illnesses (Schaffer & Naranjo, 1998).

Functional Assessment

Functional status can be defined as the assessment of skills for independent daily living and physical self-care (Loewenstein & Mogosky, 1999). The capacity of an elderly person to remain independent often is jeopardized by the coexistence of physical and mental disability (Lawton, 1988). This is especially relevant in patients who are cognitively impaired and medically frail. The functional assessment quantifies how well the patient performs important tasks and maintains independence. This assessment ideally employs careful observation of the patient's functioning in the patient's residence. If this is not possible, an interview with the primary caregiver is essential.

Lawton and Brody (1969) and Katz and coworkers (1970) divided the functional assessment into two kinds of activities: physical activities of daily living (ADLs) and instrumental activities of daily living (IADLs) (see Table 10-2). This assessment (1) documents each patient's functional strengths and vulnerabilities so that appropriate in-home supports for the caregiver and patient can be organized and (2) monitors a patient's progress over time. The functional assessment can provide clues to potentially remediable and underdiagnosed medical and psychiatric conditions. Linking a mental disorder to an impairment in instrumental function often is a way to bring about acceptance of treatment by the patient and family.

TABLE 10-2. Functional assessment tasks

Activities of daily living	Instrumental activities of daily living
Bathing	Able to use telephone
Ability to transfer	Shopping
Dressing	Food preparation
Going to toilet	Laundry
Grooming	Motor transportation
Ability to feed self	Responsibility for own medication
	Ability to handle finances

Other scales have been developed to quantify activities of daily living: the Barthel Index (Mahony & Barthel, 1965) and the OARS Physical Activities of Daily Living (Pfeiffer, 1975). Instrumental activities of daily living have also been quantified with the OARS Instrumental Activities of Daily Living Scale (Duke University, 1978) and the Direct Assessment of Functional Status Scale (Loewenstein et al., 1989).

The Interview With the Informant

Most geriatric psychiatric assessments require taking a history from a significant other of the patient's problems. If this person is the caregiver, specific attention should be given to assessing the caregiver's health, the caregiver's understanding of the patient's illness, a history of the caregiver's relationship with the patient, the stresses in the relationship with the patient, the degree to which the caregiver is providing practical care, and the degree of burden on the caregiver. This information is intended to provide help to the caregiver. The collaborative history may be influenced by the quality of the informant's relationship with the patient, and it may need to be reinterpreted (Oppenheimer & Jacoby, 1991).

Mental Status

The mental status examination is a cross-sectional assessment of the mental state of the patient at the time of the psychiatric interview. In an office setting, the examination begins as soon as the clinician meets the patient and family in the waiting room. While greeting the patient, the clinician may note the following: How did the patient greet the examiner? Does the patient know the reason for the interview? How did the patient arrive for the assessment? Does the patient defer to the family for explanations? These observations often determine whether the clinician sees the patient or the family first. Much of the mental status examination is completed during the history taking. The skilled clinician uses appropriate moments in an interview to explore the phenomenology associated with the mental disorder. For example, one challenge for the clinician examining an impaired elderly patient is to ask, in words the patient can understand, about phenomena that the patient is experiencing. A schematic for the geriatric mental status examination is presented in Table 10-3.

APPEARANCE AND BEHAVIOR   Geriatric patients' general appearance and behavior often suggest the underlying psychiatric diagnosis. For example, an elderly patient who is sitting quietly; looking vacantly into space; dressed in ill-fitting, stained clothes with buttons missing; and smells of urine suggests the possibility of a cognitive disorder. More specifically, patients with dressing apraxia may button a shirt incorrectly or wear the shirt or pants inside out. Elderly, depressed patients may lose motivation to take care of their appearance. Meeting a patient who greets the clinician with hesitation and furtive glances and who does not want the clinician to see the family suggests paranoid symptomatology.

Posture, facial appearance, and movement can reflect mood and thinking disturbances and can be affected by a variety of neurological conditions and psychotropic drugs. For example, the shuffling, tremulous elderly man who does not look at the examiner when he speaks and who will not get out of bed may reflect a person with both Parkinson's disease and depression. Catatonic behaviors, including mannerisms (goal-directed repetitive movements), stereotypes (repetitive purposeless movements), echopraxia (automatic copying of the examiners' posture or behavior), and waxy flexibility (a patient can be molded into a position that is maintained) can be seen in dementia and mood disorders.

SPEECH   The rate, quantity, and quality of speech and the presence or absence of speech defects may offer clues to the diagnosis. For example, the spontaneity, volume, and quantity of speech often are reduced in geriatric depression.

TABLE 10-3. Schematic for geriatric mental status

Appearance and behavior
Speech
Affect
    • Subjective
    • Objective
Suicide potential
Thought perception: process/content
Obsessive-compulsive/phobic/anxiety symptoms
Insight and judgment
Competencies
Consent
    • Financial
    • Driving
    • Cognitive assessment

Speech sounds are flat and monotonous when depression affects the person's capacity to express emotion (dysprosodia). Loud, insistent, and pressured speech is characteristic of mania.

AFFECT Clinicians elicit and describe the subjective affective disturbance ("the mood") of the patient. These subjective complaints potentially may mislead the examiner. For example, compared to younger depressed patients, the depressed elderly complain less about a depressed mood (Gottfries, 1998). Instead, these patients may express their subjective distress as "bad nerves," "funny feelings all over my body," or just feeling "sick."

The examiner notes the predominant affect expressed during the interview and the range, appropriateness, and control of affect. Disturbance in each of these functions may signal a different underlying etiology. For example, incongruous, unrestricted affect may be associated with multiinfarct dementia, a "pained" facial expression may be associated with melancholia or chronic pain, and a blank or flat affect may be associated with Parkinson's disease.

Each geriatric patient requires a careful review of suicide ideation and intent. The accuracy and depth of the inquiry are aided by first asking about suicide ideation and passive death wishes and then, if appropriate, asking about specific intent, methods, and plans. Additional risk factors in elderly patients include poor physical health, past history of suicide attempts, family history of suicide attempts and completions, chronic pain, concurrent alcoholism, depression and recent losses, the presence of command hallucinations, and social isolation.

THOUGHT The clinician notes the specific preoccupations of the patient and the presence or absence of delusions. For example, preoccupations in depression include somatic and hypochondriacal concerns, especially with the gastrointestinal, musculoskeletal, and nervous systems. Depressed patients may worry that their health is deteriorating, and these worries may replace the subjective complaint of depression.

Delusions that are present are described in detail. The examiner needs to be sensitive to the patient's delusional belief systems. An attitude of concerned interest can help elicit the nature of the delusions, their historical origins, and the patient's response to them. Directly challenging the patient's delusions is generally not helpful. Inquiring about delusions is best accomplished by starting with open-ended questions such as, "Have you noticed anything unusual happening in your neighborhood?" "Are the people around you minding their own business?"

Mood-congruent delusions in severe geriatric depression may include delusions of poverty, sin, guilt, nihilism, and hypochondriasis. Hypochondriacal delusions are common and often center on the functions of the bowel and brain. For example, a patient may believe there is a blockage or tumor in the bowel and may subsequently stop eating.

Delusions associated with dementia are common (Hwang et al., 1999) and include stealing delusions, delusions of persecution, delusional jealousy (involving the spouse), misidentification syndromes (involving the caregiver or spouse), and reincarnation delusions (involving dead relatives). More complex and systematized delusions of persecution may be present in paranoid patients with apparent intact cognition. Themes seen in patients living in the community include fears about drug dealers, criminals, and prostitutes operating in nearby homes. These patients may fear that they are monitored and observed constantly. Ideas of reference often are associated. Schneider's first-rank symptoms are sometimes present in late-onset schizophrenia and in affective psychoses (Howard, 1999). These symptoms can include experiences of influence, thought insertion, thought withdrawal, thought broadcasting, audible thoughts, and specific types of auditory hallucinations.

Thought process abnormalities are less common in elderly schizophrenic patients with intact cognition than in a younger adult psychiatric population (Howard, 1999; Post, 1967). Tangentiality and looseness of associations may be seen in dementia. Flight of ideas is common in mania of old age. Circumstantiality may be associated with an obsessional personality.

PERCEPTION   Perceptual disturbances include illusions, hallucinations, derealization, and depersonalization experiences. Terrifying visual illusions and hallucinations are common in severe delirium in elderly patients. Cerebral lesions, especially of the right posterior cerebral hemisphere, can cause "release" hallucinations that last minutes to hours (Cummings, 1985). Olfactory and auditory hallucinations are seen in a variety of geriatric disorders, including paranoid disorders and affective disorders.

OBSESSIVE-COMPULSIVE, PHOBIC, OR ANXIETY SYMPTOMS   There is considerable evidence that obsessive-compulsive, panic, or phobic symptoms can arise de novo in old age. These symptoms most often appear in the context of a depressive disorder or in the early stages of a dementing disorder. Agoraphobia appears to be the only primary anxiety disorder that appears first in old age to any significant degree (Flint, 1994). Posttraumatic stress disorders may occur in later life, particularly in connection with medicosurgical trauma, or reemerge as a result of earlier trauma, especially in the context of dementia (Mittal et al., 2001). Patients who present with an apparent late-onset anxiety disorder may have had an unrecognized or an untreated anxiety disorder earlier in life. Such individuals often are described by families as always tense, worried, nervous, or controlling (see also Chapter 23).

INSIGHT AND JUDGMENT   Using information obtained in the history, the clinician determines whether the patient's mental illness interferes with judgment to the extent that it could jeopardize personal health and safety or that of others. More subtle alterations in judgment include the inability to make and carry out plans and inappropriate behavior in social situations. Traditional tests of judgment that ask the patient what he or she would do in imaginary situations are not very helpful because they are not sensitive to the subtle alterations in judgment seen in many geriatric disorders.

Insight refers to the degree of awareness and understanding the patient has of his or her illness and the need for treatment. It is important to inquire whether the patient realizes that certain events may have predisposed or precipitated or may be perpetuating his or her illness. Elderly patients' judgment and insight often are affected by dementias, by paranoid disorders, and by affective disorders with delusions.

COMPETENCE   Geriatric psychiatrists often are required to assess a patient's capacity to make decisions. This may involve the patient's ability to make or change a will, give power of attorney, or consent to treatment. The assessment of competence in each area should be tested individually. Competence is best viewed as a task-specific assessment. Therefore, a person might be competent to consent to medical treatment, but might not be competent to manage financial affairs or vice versa.

One of the more common competence assessments involves the capacity of the patient to give consent for medical treatment (Applebaum & Grisso, 1988). The clinician can use the following questions as a guide: Is the patient aware of experiencing a mental illness? Does the patient understand the nature of the proposed treatment? Does the patient understand the need for treatment and the implications of refusing treatment? Does the mental illness sufficiently interfere with judgment and reasoning that it accounts for refusal of treatment?

Geriatric mental illness may interfere with the capacity of a person to manage his or her finances (Lieff et al., 1984). The following questions may be used to complete this assessment: Does the person have knowledge of his or her current assets? Does the person have knowledge of monthly expenses and bills? Does the person know where assets are located and how they are managed? Can the person complete simple calculations? Does the person experience delusions (such as delusions of poverty) that interfere with the capacity to manage his or her finances? Is the person experiencing memory impairment sufficient to interfere with his or her capacity to remember recent and past financial transactions? Is the person's judgment so affected (in a manic episode or in dementia, for example) that personal finances would be jeopardized?

An important area of competency that must be assessed frequently by geriatric psychiatrists is driving ability. Details of mandatory reporting to the Department of Motor Vehicles will vary by locale, but the role of the physician in identifying drivers at risk is almost universally recognized. Concerns about driving ability might be raised by the presence of any late-life mental disorder, but most attention has focused on dementia. There is a strong correlation between cognitive deficits, driving ability, and the risk of motor vehicle accidents, and there is general agreement that patients with moderate dementia should not drive (Johansson & Lundberg, 1997).

What is much more controversial is how to assess driving competence in patients with early, mild dementia. The American Association for Geriatric Psychiatry and others have recommended that patients with mild dementia and a history of motor vehicle accidents or significant impairment of visuospatial or executive functions must be closely monitored (Small et al., 1997). A practice guideline suggested that patients with mild dementia should be warned that they are at increased risk for involvement in motor vehicle accidents and should be considered for referral to a qualified driver examination service. Given the likelihood of progression of cognitive dysfunction, these patients should be reassessed every 6 months (Dubinsky et al., 2000).

At the very least, for every patient assessed by a geriatric psychiatrist, questions should include whether they are driving, if they have been involved in any recent motor vehicle accidents, and if they have received any recent tickets for driving violations. Given corroborative history, findings on mental status examination, and diagnosis, the clinician will then be able to decide what further steps need to be taken.

THE COGNITIVE ASSESSMENT

Purpose. The assessment of cognitive function is a crucial component of the geriatric mental status examination. The purpose of this portion of the comprehensive examination is to allow the clinician to answer the following questions:

1. Is cognitive impairment present or absent? The answer to this question is important for diagnostic purposes. For example, the onset of depressive symptoms for the first time in late life may represent a bona fide major depressive episode, may be secondary to a general medical condition that can also impair cognition (e.g., depression following a cerebrovascular accident), or may be symptoms associated with an underlying neurodegenerative disorder (e.g., Alzheimer's disease). It is important to recognize, however, that geriatric patients may have more than one condition present, and that elderly patients with "functional" illnesses such as major depression and schizophrenia will have cognitive impairment in the absence of other "organic" causes. The presence or absence of cognitive impairment often has an important impact on the treatment of the underlying illness.

2. What is the pattern of the cognitive dysfunction? The pattern of cognitive impairment may reveal important clues about the etiology of the illness. The exact location of a lesion may not be elicited by the screening examination, but the examiner should be able to determine whether

the lesion is diffuse or multifocal (as in Alzheimer's disease) or localized (as in a right parietal lobe tumor).
3. What is the quantity or severity of the cognitive impairment? When cognitive function examinations are performed longitudinally, the answer to this question helps determine the course and prognosis of the illness. A functional assessment and the assessment of the quality and quantity of cognitive impairment are essential to determine how much care or supervision patients require.
4. Is a more elaborate neuropsychological examination necessary? Although much can be learned from a relatively brief screening examination, more detailed testing helps establish a more accurate diagnosis when the findings are extremely subtle or when the clinician suspects an underlying dementia or neurological illness. When the diagnosis of dementia is likely, more detailed testing establishes areas of weakness and strengths in the various cognitive domains for organizing a comprehensive rehabilitation program. The examination should help guide the choice of other investigations, such as electroencephalogram and neuroimaging, required for further diagnosis.

Principles.   The cognitive examination begins immediately with history taking. The examiner should examine attention, concentration, memory, and language by listening to how the patient relates the details of the history. These "passive" observations can be supplemented by subtle "in-context" questioning throughout the history (e.g., asking patients the exact date of a wedding anniversary while talking about their marriage, asking patients to name all their grandchildren, or asking what day of the week they were admitted to the hospital).

The cognitive assessment should be documented carefully. A clinician seeing a patient with Alzheimer's disease 2 years after initial diagnosis will be able to compare findings more meaningfully if the first examiner recorded "could recall three of four objects after 5 minutes" rather than "short-term memory fair."

Another important principle is that the examination must be acceptable to both the patient and the examiner. The examiner should be able to administer the tests easily, with minimal equipment, and in a short period of time. The tests must be nonthreatening to the patient and should not be unduly arduous, particularly if they follow a lengthy history.

The formal assessment always should begin with a short explanation to the patient (e.g., "I would now like to ask you some questions to see how well you can concentrate and remember things"). Elaborate explanations and using of the word *test* only serve to heighten the patient's anxiety; apologies (e.g., "Some of these questions may seem a little silly . . . ") reduce the legitimacy and importance of the exam.

The examination is organized in a hierarchical fashion from basic to more complex functions. For example, attention and concentration need to be assessed before any valid testing of memory is done. The examiner will have to demonstrate a degree of flexibility depending on the clinical situation and the degree of impairment demonstrated during the history (e.g., comprehension will need to be tested early for any patient with a suspected aphasia). This hierarchical approach is extended to assess tasks within a given cognitive domain. For example, a patient with suspected concentration impairment might be asked to count backward by ones from 100 before being asked for serial sevens from 100. The former test is simpler and less threatening; the latter is more likely to demonstrate milder impairment, but it may overwhelm the patient who did not have the opportunity to warm up for the testing procedures. When recording scores on individual tasks, the examiner should note the quality of the responses. "I don't know" responses, confabulations, lack of effort, and perseveration (the pathological repetition of speech or actions) are qualitative comments that provide useful diagnostic information. Table 10-4 outlines an easily administered cognitive assessment that provides the information necessary to answer the questions listed above.

ATTENTION AND CONCENTRATION   Attention traditionally has been tested using the task of repeating a string of digits forward and backward; concentration has been measured with the serial sevens task. Both tests provide useful information, but elderly persons often feel threatened when confronted with tasks involving numbers or arithmetic. The serial sevens subtraction test, in particular, may depend more on a patient's premorbid intellectual capacity, education, and arithmetic ability than on an underlying impairment of concentration. A simple test to assess attention consists of reading a series of random letters to the patient and asking him or her to indicate (tap or say "yes") every time he or she hears the letter A. This task can be scored for errors or omission, com-

TABLE 10-4.   Format of the cognitive assessment

Attention and concentration
Language
   Spontaneous speech
   Comprehension
   Naming
Orientation
Memory
   Recent
   Remote
Constructional ability
Praxis
Frontal systems

mission, or perseveration. Simple tests of concentration include asking a patient to state the days of the week backward, followed by months of the year backward. If these two tasks are performed well, the patient can be asked to do serial sevens from 100.

LANGUAGE The exact characterization of an aphasia may be beyond the scope of a screening examination for cognition, but the examiner can assess some aspects of a patient's expressive and receptive language function during screening for cognition. After taking the patient's history, the examiner should be able to comment on many aspects of spontaneous speech, such as articulation (presence of dysarthria), melody (prosody), the presence of word-finding difficulties, and evidence of specific aphasic errors such as paraphasias. Paraphasias include substituting an incorrect word (referred to as *verbal* or *semantic paraphasia*; for example, "I cut meat with a 'pen'") or substituting a syllable (called a *phonemic* or *literal paraphasia*; for example, "I cut meat with a 'fife").

Comprehension can be tested by asking the patient to point to certain objects in the room. The test can be made more difficult by increasing the number of objects in a single command (e.g., "Point to the ceiling, the wall, and then the door") or by proceeding from the concrete (e.g., "Point to the light") to the abstract (e.g., "Point to the source of illumination"). Alternatively, the examiner may ask a series of questions to which the patient responds yes or no. To detect perseveration, the yes or no responses should vary randomly. This task is made more complex by varying the complexity of the question (e.g., "Is snow white?" versus "Does a stone float on water?" versus "Do you put on your shoes before your socks?"). Comprehension tests that involve asking a patient to perform 1-, 2-, or 3-stage commands may be useful, but difficult to interpret if the patient has a motor problem or apraxia.

Naming difficulties (*anomia*) that occur in aphasic patients may be found in patients with dementia such as Alzheimer's disease, toxic metabolic encephalopathies, and increased intracranial pressure (Cummings, 1985). Naming referred to as *confrontation naming* is tested by pointing to a series of objects and asking the patient to name each one. The objects should include different categories (colors, body parts, clothing), high-frequency words (blue, red, mouth, hand, shirt, tie), and low-frequency words (purple, knuckles, watch crystal).

ORIENTATION Orientation is a function of memory and consists of long-term (orientation to person) and short-term (orientation to place and time) components. Orientation to person, place, and time is tested sequentially. Patients are asked their full name, age, and date of birth. Orientation to place is tested by asking where they are and asking which city, state, and country they are in. Patients may be asked their home address and more details of their present location (hospital floor, ward, or room). Orientation to time includes asking the day, date, month, year, time of day, and season. Patients who respond incorrectly to any of the above can be corrected and retested later in the interview as a test of ability to learn new information.

MEMORY   Testing memory can be extremely complicated if all its dimensions (immediate, recent, remote, recall, recognition, verbal, and visual) are tested individually. Memory can be assessed quickly and simply for cognitive screening purposes to determine whether more elaborate testing is needed. The examiner begins by telling the patient to remember three or four words that the patient will be asked to recall in several minutes. Any unrelated words can be used; the examiner should use the same series of words for every patient to ensure consistency and ease of administration. Immediate recall is tested by asking the patient to repeat the words immediately after the examiner's first recitation. The patient may require several trials to learn all the words; the number of trials should be recorded. Recent memory is examined by asking the patient to recall the words after 5 minutes. The examiner records the number of words recalled spontaneously and those recalled with the use of hints. Two kinds of hints or cues are semantic cues (hints related to the category of the object such as "one word was a kind of animal") and phonemic cues (given by progressively reciting the individual sounds or syllables of the word, "B . . . Bl . . . Bla . . . Black," for example). Patients can also be asked if they can identify the words from a list of related words.

Remote memory is assessed by noting the patient's knowledge of personal history details and by asking several questions about historical or political facts (names of the president and past presidents, dates of World War II, what Sputnik was). The performance on this task depends on the patient's premorbid intelligence, education, and cultural background. This task should be modified to account for sociocultural factors (for example, asking a recent immigrant from England the names of prime ministers instead of presidents).

CONSTRUCTIONAL ABILITY   Constructional ability is assessed by asking the patient to draw or copy two-dimensional and three-dimensional figures. These tasks involve extensive cortical areas and can be quite sensitive to subtle changes in overall cognition; difficulty on these tests may indicate nondominant parietal lobe impairment (Strub & Black, 1999).

For proper evaluation of constructional ability, the clinician must ensure that adequate light, optimum vision (glasses are worn if necessary), and appropriate motor ability (no gross evidence of weakness or incoordination) are present. Paper should be unlined so that it does not produce interference, and the patient should be given a pencil or a pen that writes easily, even at odd angles.

Constructional ability can be tested by asking the patient to draw freehand and to copy figures. The patient can be asked to draw a circle, cross, and a cube (in order of ascending difficulty). If the patient experiences any difficulty, the examiner draws the figure and asks the patient to copy it.

Another simple, useful test of constructional ability is to hand the patient a sheet of paper with a predrawn circle and ask the patient to write in the numbers to make the circle look like the face of a clock. If this is done correctly, the patient can be asked to draw in the hands to make the clock read 3 o'clock (a relatively easy task) or 10 minutes past 11 (a relatively difficult task). Initially conceptualized as a test of visuoconstructive abilities, this task assesses other cognitive domains, including praxis and executive functions. It has also been used as a cognitive screening test. As a single test to detect dementia, clock drawing has a mean sensitivity and specificity of 85%, with excellent reliability, and high correlations with other, lengthier cognitive screening examinations, possibly with less cultural bias (Shulman, 2000). Clock drawing can also be used to document the progression of illness (for example, relative improvement in a resolving delirium or worsening in a dementia). A variety of standardized scoring systems has been described, all with similar psychometric properties (Shulman, 2000).

PRAXIS Ideomotor praxis involves the ability to perform volitional actions on command, in mime, without props (Cummings, 1985). Testing involves limb, whole-body, and buccal-lingual commands. To assess limb commands, the patient can be asked, "Show me how you would comb your hair with your left hand." Other limb commands may include brushing teeth, turning a key, or using a saw. Both hands should be tested separately. Common errors include performing the actions awkwardly, using the hands as the object instead of pretending to hold the object, needing to use both hands, or verbalizing the task first. Whole-body commands include asking the patient to stand like a boxer or to swing a bat like a baseball player. To demonstrate buccal-lingual commands, patients can be asked to pretend to lick crumbs off their lips, blow out a candle, or suck through a straw. Impairment of this kind of praxis (i.e., ideomotor apraxia) usually is related to dominant parietal lobe dysfunction.

FRONTAL SYSTEMS TASKS Frontal systems tasks are used to screen for dysfunction of the frontal lobes and of their interconnected, subcortical structures. These tests are useful for assessing patients with frontal lobe pathology (such as in Pick's disease) and for assessing the cognitive functioning of patients with extrapyramidal disorders (such as Parkinson's disease). In the latter, dysfunction in the basal ganglia, with its multitude of connections to the frontal lobes, may lead to a pattern of cognitive impairment, referred to as *subcortical dementia*, that is quantitatively and qualitatively different from cortical dementias (Cummings & Benson, 1992).

The frontal lobes oversee many cognitive functions, including attention, concentration, verbal fluency, abstraction, insight, and judgment. The following tests have been chosen for use in the cognitive screening because they tend to elicit two important signs associated with frontal lobe dysfunction: perseveration and concrete thinking. (Assessment of attention, concentration, insight, and judgment are described above.)

Perseveration may be obvious from the history and previous testing; it can be assessed further by showing the patient an alternating-sequence diagram or several multiple loops and asking the patient to copy the diagrams exactly and continue the pattern across the page. Perseverative errors include drawing consecutive squares or triangles with the former and adding extra loops to the latter. Alternatively, the patient can be tested with a "go/no-go" sequence. The patient can be asked to tap once when the examiner taps twice and twice when the examiner taps once. The examiner, while tapping randomly once or twice, observes whether the patient can learn the correct response, how many errors are committed, and whether the errors are perseverative (e.g., the patient continues to tap twice every time the examiner taps twice). The task can be made more difficult when the examiner asks the patient to tap twice every time the examiner taps once, but not to tap at all if the examiner taps twice. Particular attention is paid to whether the patient perseverates on the first series of instructions by continuing to tap once when the examiner taps twice.

Tests to elicit concrete thinking involve testing a patient's ability to think abstractly. The results of these tests need to be interpreted cautiously because they are highly dependent on educational level and cultural background. The patient can be asked to interpret metaphorical speech such as "he's blue," "she's yellow," "a heart of gold," or "heavy handed." The patient can be asked to interpret some common proverbs such as "don't cry over spilled milk" (low difficulty) or "a stitch in time saves nine" (higher difficulty).

Concrete thinking can be elicited using a similarities task. The patient is asked to describe how two objects are alike. The task begins with a simple stimulus such as "How are an apple and an orange alike?" The response, They are both round." may indicate concrete thinking, but the patient should be told the examiner was looking for the response, "They are both fruits," before proceeding with the next stimulus. Stimuli are arranged in order of ascending complexity (e.g., orange/apple, shirt/pants, table/chair, airplane/bicycle). Continued responses emphasizing minute individual characteristics (as opposed to the group or category to which the objects belong) are indicative of concrete thinking. This test is less culture biased than interpretation of proverbs.

Another useful test of frontal systems impairment is verbal fluency or word-list generation. The patient is asked to list, in 1-minute trials, as many words as he or she can think of, excluding proper names, beginning with a given letter of the alphabet. Recommended letters have included F, A, and S, and a similar test can be performed by asking the patient to name as many animals as they can in 1 minute. Although age and education can affect performance, most patients should be able to name 10 to 12 words using each letter and 12 to 15 animals in 1-minute trials. Recording the number of perseverative responses adds a qualitative component to this simple test.

STANDARDIZED ASSESSMENT INSTRUMENTS

Standardized assessment instruments are essential tools for clinical investigators, but their utility in everyday clinical practice is often underemphasized.

These instruments are particularly useful in the circumstances listed below, but they never should take the place of the comprehensive biopsychosocial assessment described above.

For Screening Purposes

Standardized assessments can be useful on medical or surgical services as screening instruments. They are particularly useful for identifying diagnoses often missed by nonpsychiatric staff, such as delirium (Elie et al., 2000), depression (Koening & Kuchibhatla, 1998), and alcohol abuse (Johnson, 2000).

For Communicating With Colleagues

Subjective descriptions of symptom severity or degree of impairment can be misleading or unreliable; therefore, scales such as the Mini-Mental State Examination (MMSE) (Folstein et al., 1975) or the Hamilton Depression Rating Scale (HAM-D) (Hamilton, 1967), which are widely recognized, help standardize communication between physicians.

For Medicolegal and Insurance Purposes

Clinicians may argue the validity and reliability of individual scales or diagnostic tools, but many of these have been embraced by the legal system and insurers because they ostensibly provide systemic standardized descriptions of psychopathology.

To Solve Specific Clinical Problems

Certain rating scales can be used to solve specific clinical problems. For example, the Staff Observation Aggression Scale (Palmstierna & Wistedt, 1987) can be used on the ward for documenting antecedents and consequences of aggressive acts. This information is used for designing a behavioral program for aggressive elderly patients.

To Document Change

Recording scores on depression rating scales or cognitive assessment scales effectively can document response to treatment or progression of illness.

For Education Purposes

Standardized assessments often are excellent tools for teaching medical students or allied health professionals. These assessments are taught easily and can elevate awareness of the necessity to consider emotional and cognitive functioning in all elderly patients.

Commonly Used Scales

DEPRESSION RATING SCALES Depression rating scales are divided into interviewer-administered and self-report measures. The former generally are more sensitive and specific, whereas the latter generally are easier and quicker to administer (Thompson et al., 1988). The most commonly used self-report measures in geriatrics are the Geriatric Depression Scale (GDS) (Yesavage & Brink, 1983), the Zung Self-Rating Depression Scale (Zung, 1965), and the Beck Depression Inventory (BDI) (Beck et al., 1961). The GDS, designed specifically for use in elderly patients, is sensitive and specific (Norris et al., 1987). It is easily administered, requiring patients to respond yes or no to a series of 30 statements. A short form (10 items) is available (Sheikh & Yesavage, 1986).

Self-rated scales are not valid when there is significant cognitive impairment, especially when insight is lost. The most widely used interviewer-administered measure is the HAM-D (Hamilton, 1967). Its reliability has been improved by the development of a structured interview guide (Williams, 1988), but its heavy weighting toward somatic symptoms (9 of 17 items) might be problematic for use in an elderly population with a high prevalence of physical illness (Thompson et al., 1988). The Montgomery-Åsberg Depression Rating Scale (MADRS) (Montgomery & Åsberg 1979) places less emphasis on somatic symptoms and may be more suitable in an elderly population (Kearns et al., 1982). This scale is easily administered and very helpful for documenting response to therapy.

COGNITIVE FUNCTION AND DEMENTIA RATING SCALES One of the most widely accepted standardized cognitive screening tests is the MMSE (Folstein et al., 1975). The MMSE provides a measure of cognition that includes tests of orientation, memory, concentration, language, and constructional ability. This examination requires only about 10 minutes and is easy to administer. This tool has been extensively investigated and has stood the test of time with acceptable validity and reliability (Tombaugh & McIntyre, 1992).

The MMSE is not without its weaknesses. Although scores of 23 or less, out of 30, are usually associated with significant cognitive impairment, age, education, race, socioeconomic status, and even hearing impairment may affect scores. Age and education norms have been published to help address some of these problems (Crum et al., 1993). The MMSE is also not sensitive to frontal systems impairment and may lead to false-negative tests in patients with early frontotemporal dementias. It is, therefore, advisable to include some frontal systems tests if using the MMSE exclusively for cognitive screening.

Finally, although the MMSE is not in itself a diagnostic test, it can be used to follow the course of dementing illnesses if performed sequentially. For example, the average decline in scores for patients with Alzheimer's disease has been estimated at 3 points per year (Han et al., 2000). Patients who plateau for lengthy periods, or decline at a slower rate, may not have Alzheimer's disease, although those who decline at a much faster rate may have an intercurrent delirium.

Several longer cognitive screening examinations have been developed, such as the Alzheimer's Disease Assessment Scale (ADAS) (Rosen et al., 1984) and the Mattis Dementia Rating Scale (Mattis, 1976). Although these scales have been used extensively in research, they are probably too lengthy for most clinicians. Another short screening examination, the 7 Minute Neurocognitive Screening Battery (Solomon et al., 1998), appears highly sensitive and specific for Alzheimer's disease; whether this test will experience the same popularity as the MMSE remains to be seen.

Although the assessment of cognition remains critical for the diagnosis of dementia, the assessment of function and behavior are also crucial. A number of scales attempt to rate the stage of dementia or the severity of cognitive and noncognitive dysfunction. Two such scales are the Global Deterioration Scale (Reisberg et al., 1982) and the Clinical Dementia Rating Scale (Hughes et al., 1982). The Disability Assessment for Dementia (DAD) (Gelinas et al., 1998) scale is a clinically useful functional assessment tool that measures basic ADLs, IADLs, and leisure activities by documenting the patient's initiation, planning, and effective performance of 40 items.

With increasing attention to the behavioral and psychological symptoms associated with dementia, a variety of scales has been developed to document these disturbances. The Behavior Pathology in Alzheimer's Disease Rating Scale (Behave AD) (Reisberg et al., 1987), the Cohen-Mansfield Agitation Inventory (CMAI) (Cohen-Mansfield, 1986), and the Neuropsychiatric Inventory (NPI) (Cummings et al., 1994) are three of the more popular scales. The NPI, used frequently for research purposes, is also helpful clinically for documenting the frequency and severity of a variety of disturbances, including delusions, hallucinations, agitation, aggression, irritability, depression, and disinhibition.

MISCELLANEOUS RATING INSTRUMENTS   Scales to measure functional abilities and activities of daily living were discussed above. A number of scales with specific foci can be very useful in clinical practice. The Overt Aggression Scale (OAS) (Yudofsky et al., 1986) and the Staff Observation Aggression Scale (Palmstierna & Wistedt, 1987) are useful for evaluating aggressive behavior. The former scale is much more popular. The latter has the advantage of documenting antecedents, aggressive acts, and consequences of aggression; therefore, it aids in developing behavioral management. Simple systematic observation and documentation with this tool have shown a decrease in aggressive behavior in a group of psychogeriatric inpatients (Nilsson et al., 1988).

Another useful tool is the Abnormal Involuntary Movement Scale (National Institute of Mental Health, 1975). This scale consists of a number of ratings of abnormal movements, including a global measure of severity, a rating of incapacity, and a measure of the patient's awareness of the movements. This scale is particularly helpful for monitoring elderly patients on antipsychotic treatment.

Given the importance and popularity of standardized rating scales in clinical practice and research, readers are encouraged to review texts and review articles on this topic (Burns et al., 1999; Weiner et al., 1996).

PHYSICAL AND NEUROLOGICAL EXAMINATION

All geriatric patients require an appropriate physical examination with special attention directed to the neurological system.

DIAGNOSIS AND FORMULATION

After completing the history and functional, medical, and mental status assessments, the clinician can propose a provisional diagnosis and differential diagnosis, develop an etiologic formulation, and establish the capacity of each patient to function independently. The provisional and differential diagnoses will direct the clinician in planning for an orderly series of investigations and tests that will confirm or refute the provisional diagnosis or the specific diagnoses in the differential.

By reorganizing the salient features of the assessment into an etiologic formulation, the clinician will develop a working hypothesis of the factors that make this patient vulnerable to developing a mental illness at this particular time. Knowledge of the biopsychosocial vulnerability of each patient is necessary for individualizing the case management. Knowledge of the current capacity of a patient to function in his or her environment will aid in determining what specific social supports must be provided to allow a person to continue living there. A comprehensive management plan, including biological, psychological, and social therapies, logically follows from the results of this assessment.

REFERENCES

Applebaum PS, Grisso T. Assessing patients' capacities to consent to treatment. *N Engl J Med.* 1988;319:1635–1638.

Assal F, Cummings JL. Neuropsychiatric symptoms in the dementias. *Curr Opin Neurol.* 2002;15:445–450.

Beck AT, Ward CH, Mendelson M, et al. An inventory for measuring depression. *Arch Gen Psychiatry.* 1961;4:561–571.

Blazer DG. The psychiatric interview of the geriatric patient. In: Busse EW, Blazer DG, eds. *Geriatric Psychiatry.* Washington, DC: American Psychiatric Press; 1989;263–284.

Burns A, Lawlor B, Craig S. *Assessment Scales in Old Age Psychiatry.* London, England: Martin Dunitz; 1999.

Coffey CE, Cummings JL, eds. *Textbook of Geriatric Neuropsychiatry.* Washington, DC: American Psychiatric Press; 1994.

Cohen-Mansfield J. Agitated behaviors in the elderly. II. Preliminary results in the cognitively deteriorated. *Am J Geriatr Soc.* 1986;34:722–727.

Crum RM, Anthony JC, Bassett SS, et al. Population-based norms for the mini-mental state examination by age and education level. *JAMA.* 1993;269:2386–2391.

Cummings JL. *Clinical Neuropsychiatry.* Orlando, FL: Grune and Stratton; 1985:5–16.

Cummings JL. Neuropsychiatric manifestations of right hemisphere lesions. *Brain Lang.* 1997;57:22–37.

Cummings JL, Benson DF. *Dementia: A Clinical Approach.* 2nd ed. Boston, MA: Butterworth-Heinemann; 1992:1–17.

Cummings JL, Mega M, Gray K, et al. The neuropsychiatric inventory: comprehensive assessment of psychopathology in dementia. *Neurology.* 1994;44:2308–2314.

Dubinsky RM, Stein AC, Lyons K. Practice parameter: risk of driving and Alzheimer's disease (an evidence-based review). *Neurology.* 2000;54:2205–2211.

Duke University Centre for Aging and Human Development. *The OARS Methodology.* Durham, NC: Duke University; 1978.

Elie M, Rousseau F, Cole M, et al. Prevalence and detection of delirium in elderly emergency department patients. *CMAJ.* 2000;163:977–981.

Ewing JA. Detecting alcoholism: the CAGE Questionnaire. *JAMA.* 1984;252:1905–1907.

Faber R. Neuropsychiatric assessment. In: Coffey CE, Cummings JL, eds. *Textbook of Geriatric Neuropsychiatry.* Washington, DC: American Psychiatric Press; 1994:99–109.

Flint AJ. Epidemiology and comorbidity of anxiety disorders in the elderly. *Am J Psychiatry.* 1994;151:640–649.

Folstein MF, Folstein SE, McHugh PR. Mini-Mental State: a practical method for grading the cognitive state of patients for the clinician. *J Psychiatr Res.* 1975;12:189–198.

Gelinas I, Gauthier L, McIntyre M, et al. Development of a functional measure for persons with Alzheimer's disease: the disability assessment for dementia. *Am J Occup Ther.* 1998;53:471–481.

Gottfries CG. Is there a difference between elderly and younger patients with regard to the symptomatology and aetiology of depression? *Int Clin Psychopharmacol.* 1998;13(Suppl 5):S13–S18.

Hamilton M. Development of a rating scale for primary depressive illness. *Soc Clin Psychol.* 1967;6:278–296.

Han L, Cole M, Bellavance F, et al. Tracking cognitive decline in Alzheimer's disease using the Mini-Mental State Examination: a meta-analysis. *Int Psychogeriatr.* 2000;12:231–247.

Howard R. Schizophrenia-like psychosis with onset in late life. In: Howard R, Rabins PV, Castle DJ, eds. *Late Onset Schizophrenia.* Philadelphia, PA: Wrightson Biomedical; 1999.

Hughes CP, Berg L, Danziger WL, et al. A new clinical scale for the staging of dementia. *Br J Psychiatry.* 1982;140:566–572.

Hwang JP, Tsai SJ, Yang CH, Liu KM, et al. Persecutory delusions in dementia. *J Clin Psychiatry.* 1999;60:550–553.

Johansson K, Lundberg C. The 1994 International Consensus Conference on Dementia and Driving. *Alzheimers Dis Assoc Disord.* 1997;11(Suppl 1):62–69.

Johnson DAW. Drug-induced psychiatric disorders. *Drugs.* 1981;22:57–69.

Johnson I. Alcohol problems in old age: a review of recent epidemiological research. *Int J Geriatr Psychiatry.* 2000;15:575–581.

Kaplan HI, Sadock BJ. *Synopsis of Psychiatry.* 8th ed. Baltimore, MD: Williams and Wilkins; 1998.

Katz S, Downs TD, Cash HR, et al. Progress in development of the index of ADL. *Gerontologist.* 1970;10:20–30.

Kearns MP, Cruikshank CA, McGuigan KJ, et al. A comparison of depression rating scales. *Br J Psychiatry.* 1982;141:45–49.

Koenig HG, George LK. Depression and physical disability outcomes in depressed medically ill hospitalized older adults. *Am J Geriatr Psychiatry.* 1998;6:230–247.

Koenig HG, Kuchibhatla M. Use of health services by hospitalized medically ill depressed elderly patients. *Am J Psychiatry.* 1998;155:871–877.

Larue A. Geriatric neuropsychology: principles of assessment. In: Lichtenberg PA, ed. *Assessment in Clinical Gerontology.* New York, NY: John Wiley and Sons; 1985.

Lawton MP. Scales to measure competence in everyday activities. *Psychopharmacol Bull.* 1988;24:609–614.

Lawton MP, Brody EM. Assessment of older people: self-maintaining and instrumental activities of daily living. *Gerontologist.* 1969;9:179–186.

Lichtenberg PA. *Handbook of Assessment in Clinical Gerontology.* New York, NY: John Wiley; 1999.

Lieff S, Maindonald K, Shulman K. Issues in determining financial competence in the elderly. *CMAJ.* 1984;130:1293–1296.

Loewenstein DA, Amigo ER, Duara R, et al. A new scale for the assessment of functional status in Alzheimer's disease and related disorders. *J Gerontol.* 1989;44:114–121.

Loewenstein DA, Mogosky BJ. The functional assessment of the older adult patient. In: Lichtenberg PA, ed. *Assessment in Clinical Gerontology.* New York, NY: John Wiley and Sons; 1999.

Mahoney FI, Barthel DW. Functional evaluation: the Barthel Index. *Maryland St Med J.* 1965;14:61–65.

Mattis S. Mental status examination for organic mental syndrome in the elderly patient. In: Bellak L, Karasu T, eds. *Geriatric Psychiatry: A Handbook for Psychiatrists and Primary Care Physicians.* New York, NY: Grune and Stratton; 1976:77–101.

McCullough PK. Geriatric depression: atypical presentations, hidden meanings. *Geriatrics.* 1991;46(10):72–76.

Mittal D, Torres R, Abashidze A, et al. Worsening of post-traumatic stress disorder symptoms with cognitive decline: case series. *J Geriatr Psychiatry Neurol.* 2001;14:17–20.

Montgomery SA, Åsberg MA. A new depression scale designed to be sensitive to change. *Br J Psychiatry.* 1979;134:382–389.

Naranjo CA, Herrmann N, Ozdemir V, Bremner KE. Abuse of prescription and licit psychoactive substances by the elderly. *CNS Drugs.* 1995;4:207–221.

National Institute of Mental Health. *Development of a Dyskinetic Movement Scale.* Rockville, MD: National Institute of Mental Health, Psychopharmacology Research Branch; 1975. Publication 4.

Nilsson K, Palmstierna T, Wistedt B. Aggressive behavior in hospitalized psychogeriatric patients. *Acta Psychiatr Scand.* 1988;78:172–175.

Norris J, Gallagher D, Wilson A, et al. Assessment of depression in geriatric medical outpatients: the validity of two screening measures. *J Am Geriatr Soc.* 1987;35: 989–995.

Oppenheimer C, Jacoby R. Psychiatric assessment of the elderly. In: Jacoby R, Oppenheimer C, eds. *Psychiatry in the Elderly.* Oxford, UK: Oxford University Press; 1991:169–198.

Palmestierna T, Wistedt B. Staff Observation Aggression Scale (SOAS): presentation and evaluation. *Acta Psychiatr Scand.* 1987;76:657–663.

Pfeiffer M. *Multidimensional Functional Assessment: The OARS Methodology.* Durham, NC: Duke University Center for the Study of Aging and Human Development; 1975.

Post F. Aspects of psychiatry in the elderly. *Proc R Soc Med.* 1967;60:249–254.

Reisberg B, Borenstein J, Salob SP, et al. Behavioural symptoms in Alzheimer's disease: phenomenology and treatment. *J Clin Psychiatry.* 1987;48(Suppl 5):9–15.

Reisberg B, Ferris SH, DeLeon J, et al. The global deterioration scale for assessment of primary degenerative dementia. *Am J Psychiatry.* 1982;139:1136–1139.

Rosen WG, Mohs RC, Davis KL. A new rating scale for Alzheimer's disease. *Am J Psychiatry.* 1984;141:1356–1364.

Sadavoy J. A review of the late-life effects of prior psychological trauma. *Am J Geriatr Psychiatry.* 1997;5:287–301.

Schaffer A, Naranjo CA. Recommended drug treatment strategies for the alcoholic patient. *Drugs.* 1998;56:571–585.

Sheikh JI, Yesavage JA. Geriatric depression scale: recent evidence and development of a shorter version. *Clin Gerontol.* 1986;5:165–173.

Shulman KI. Clock-drawing: is it the ideal cognitive screening test? *Int J Geriatr Psychiatry.* 2000;15:548–561.

Small GW, Rabins PV, Barry PP, et al. Diagnosis and treatment of Alzheimer's disease and related disorders. *JAMA.* 1997;278:1363–1371.

Solomon PR, Herschoff A, Kelly B, et al. A 7 minute neurocognitive screening battery highly sensitive to Alzheimer's disease. *Arch Neurol.* 1998;55:349–355.

Spector WD, Katz S, Murphy LB, et al. The hierarchical relationship between activities of daily living and instrumental activities of daily living. *J Chronic Dis.* 1987;40: 481–489.

Starkstein SE, Robinson RG. Affective disorders and cerebrovascular disease. *Br J Psychiatry.* 1989;154:170–182.

Strub RL, Black FW. *The Mental Status Examination in Neurology.* 4th ed. Philadelphia, PA: F. A. Davis; 1999.

Thompson LW, Futterman A, Gallagher D. Assessment of late life depression. *Psychopharmacol Bull.* 1988;24:577–586.

Tombaugh TN, McIntyre NJ. The Mini-Mental State Examination: a comprehensive review. *J Am Geriatr Soc.* 1992;40:922–935.

Uekermann J, Daum I, Peters S, et al. Depressed mood and executive dysfunction in early Parkinson's disease. *Acta Neurol Scand.* 2003;107:341–348.

Vaillant GE. *Aging Well: Surprising Guideposts to a Happier Life From the Landmark Harvard Study of Adult Development.* Boston, MA: Little, Brown; 2002.

Weiner MF, Koss E, Wild KV, et al. Measures of psychiatric symptoms in Alzheimer patients: a review. *Alzheimer Dis Assoc Disord.* 1996;10:20–30.

Williams JBW. A structured interview guide for the Hamilton Depression Rating Scale. *Arch Gen Psychiatry.* 1988;45:742–747.

Yates WR, Kathol RG, Carter JL. Psychiatric assessment, *DSM-IV* and differential diagnosis. In: Stoudamire A, eds. *Clinical Psychiatry for Medical Students.* 3rd ed. Philadelphia, PA: Lippincott-Raven; 1998.

Yesavage J, Brink TL. Development and validation of a geriatric depression screening scale: a preliminary report. *J Psychiatry Res.* 1983;17:37–49.

Yudofsky SC, Silver JM, Jackson W, et al. The overt aggression scale for the objective rating of verbal and physical aggression. *Am J Psychiatry.* 1986;143:35–39.

Zarit SH, Zarit JM. *Mental Disorders in Older Adults.* New York, NY: Guilford Press; 1998.

Zung WWK. A self-rating depression scale. *Arch Gen Psychiatry.* 1965;12:63–70.

11

Medical Evaluation and Common Medical Problems of the Geriatric Psychiatry Patient

Cathy A. Alessi, MD
Christine K. Cassel, MD, MACP

INTRODUCTION

Medical conditions are common among older patients with psychiatric illness. Many medical illnesses may present with psychiatric manifestations. Often, the older psychiatric patient will benefit from a careful medical evaluation to identify physical problems that may contribute to psychiatric disease or that may have an impact on quality of life. Psychiatry services can play a key role in the comprehensive interdisciplinary assessment and management that is felt by many to be the cornerstone of care for the frail and "oldest old" (Blazer, 2000).

Certain medical illnesses and geriatric syndromes are quite common in older people and can be managed by the psychiatrist, with referral when appropriate. In fact, the psychiatrist can play a key role in identifying signs and symptoms that signal physical deterioration or missed diagnoses in the older patient. In addition, several laboratory tests are routinely obtained in older psychiatric patients, and the psychiatrist should be skilled in the initial interpretation and appropriate referral based on these results.

Medical illness may present with subtle or nonspecific findings in the older patient and hence go unrecognized or erroneously ascribed to "normal aging." A large body of literature has attempted to distinguish age-related physiological change versus abnormalities from disease. An awareness of both types of change is important in the care of the older patient. In general, aging-related changes may impair the body's homeostatic mechanisms and may result in decreased ability of the older person to deal with acute insult. Changes from disease are quite common; approximately 80% of people older than 65 years of age have at least one chronic disease or disability (Cohen & Van Nostrand, 1995).

PSYCHIATRIC MANIFESTATIONS OF MEDICAL ILLNESS IN THE OLDER PATIENT

Psychiatric symptoms can occur with practically any physical illness that has systemic involvement, can cause metabolic disturbance, or has direct central nervous system (CNS) effects. In addition, a variety of drugs can cause psychiatric symptoms at toxic doses, at normal therapeutic levels, or during periods of withdrawal (Abramowicz, 1986). In fact, older patients may have several coexisting conditions or be taking several medications that potentially could explain or contribute to their psychiatric symptoms. Drug classes for which there should be a high index of suspicion for causing psychiatric symptoms (particularly in patients with underlying brain disease) include anticholinergics, anticonvulsants, dopaminergic agonists, benzodiazepines and related medications, opioids, certain antidepressants, antipsychotics, corticosteroids, and certain antihypertensives (particularly β-blockers and centrally acting agents).

Physical illness is extremely common in psychiatric patients. In a large study of outpatients and inpatients aged 18 years or older in the California public mental health system, 39% of study patients had an active, important physical disease; 9% had physical disease that was judged to be exacerbating their mental disorders (Koran et al., 1989). Likewise, comorbid psychiatric disorders are extremely common in elderly medical patients. For example, major affective disorder has been identified in up to one third of geriatric medical outpatients and 45% of geriatric medical inpatients (Kitchell et al., 1982; Okineto et al., 1982).

Studies suggest that, among general acute hospital adult inpatients, psychological comorbidity (e.g., depression, anxiety, and organicity) is associated with longer length of stay in the hospital (Saravay et al., 1991). Another study of elderly hospitalized medical inpatients found that 27% of patients had at least one research diagnostic criteria (RDC) psychiatric diagnosis; depression was most common (16% of subjects). One year later, only one third of subjects had received mental health treatment, and 65% of the subjects with depression remained depressed (Rapp et al., 1991).

Physical illness in older patients can present as any of several psychiatric syndromes, such as dementia, delirium, depression (see Table 11-1), or anxiety (see Table 11-2). Each of these syndromes has multiple potential physical etiologies (Alexopoulos et al., 1988; Consensus Conference, 1987; Cummings, 1985; Cummings et al., 1984; Lipowski, 1989; Ouslander, 1982; U'Ren, 1989). Dementia and delirium are discussed in Chapters 16 through 20. Selected phys-

TABLE 11-1. Physical disorders associated with depression in the older patient

Neurological	Endocrine and metabolic
Parkinson's disease	Hyperthyroidism, hypothyroidism
Stroke	Hyperparathyroidism,
Alzheimer's disease	hypoparathyroidism
Temporal lobe epilepsy	Hypercalcemia, hypocalcemia
Amyotrophic lateral sclerosis	Cushing's disease
Multiple sclerosis	Addison's disease
Normal-pressure hydrocephalus	Hyperkalemia, hypokalemia
Subdural hematoma	Hypernatremia, hyponatremia
Malignancy	Hyperglycemia, hypoglycemia
Brain tumor (primary or secondary)	Hypomagnesemia
Leukemia	Hypoxemia
Pancreatic cancer	Vitamin B_{12} deficiency
Lung (particularly oat cell) cancer	Drug related
Bone metastasis with hypercalcemia	Central nervous system drugs (e.g.,
Infections	benzodiazepines, alcohol, levodopa,
Viral illness	major tranquilizers)
Chronic central nervous system infections	Antihypertensives (e.g., β-blockers,
Organ failure	clonidine, reserpine, methyldopa,
Renal failure	prazosin, guanethidine)
Liver failure	Steroids (e.g, prednisone)
Congestive heart disease	Chemotherapy (e.g, with vincristine,
	L-asparaginase, interferon)
	Cimetidine
	Digoxin
	Other
	Chronic pain
	Anemia
	Sleep disorders (e.g, sleep apnea)

ical disorders associated with depression and anxiety are listed in Tables 11-1 and 11-2, respectively.

Several important clinical clues can alert the geriatric psychiatrist to the possibility of an underlying physical disorder in the patient with psychiatric illness (Kaplan et al., 1988; Ouslander, 1982). Some of these clues include

- Abnormal level of consciousness
- Atypical age of onset of symptoms
- Lack of expected family history
- Symptoms more severe than expected
- Coexisting physical illnesses that can cause psychiatric symptoms
- Poor response to psychiatric treatment
- Abrupt personality change followed by psychopathology

TABLE 11-2. Physical disorders associated with anxiety in the older patient

Neurological
  Early dementia
  Transient ischemic attack and stroke
  Seizure disorder
Endocrine
  Hypoglycemia
  Hyperthyroidism
  Hypoparathyroidism
  Pheochromocytoma
  Cushing's disease
Drugs
  Thyroid replacement
  Barbiturates
  Steroids
  Stimulants
  Vasodilators
  Caffeine
  Withdrawal from benzodiazepines,
    alcohol, barbiturates, neuroleptics,
    antidepressants

Cardiac
  Coronary artery disesae
  Cardiac arrhythmias
  Mitral valve prolapse
Pulmonary
  Recurrent pulmonary emboli
  Chronic lung disease
Other
  Chronic pain
  Anemia
  Sleep disorders (e.g,. sleep apnea)

MEDICAL EVALUATION OF THE OLDER
PSYCHIATRIC PATIENT

The medical evaluation of the older psychiatric patient includes a thorough history and physical examination, cognitive screening, mental status examination, functional assessment, and appropriate screening laboratory tests.

The initial history and physical examination of the older patient is usually a lengthy process, particularly for patients with an extensive past medical history, several current physical complaints, or physical limitations that interfere with the examination. In the outpatient setting, this initial evaluation frequently requires more than one visit, particularly for frail patients who fatigue easily from the examination process. For a review of history taking and the initial physical examination, see a geriatric medicine text (e.g., Cassel et al., 2003; Kane, 1999; Osterweil et al., 2000). Psychiatric evaluation of the older patient is essential, and is discussed in Chapter 10.

Screening laboratory tests are commonly ordered (see Table 11-3) for older psychiatric patients to rule out physical illness, particularly for patients with psychiatric symptoms that are of recent onset, severe, or resistant to therapy. This is a different concept from the preventive screening (and preventive interventions) recommended in the routine primary care of older patients; discussion of this concept is beyond the scope of this chapter.

Which screening tests for psychiatric symptoms in the older patient are ordered is determined by the patient's clinical presentation. One study of older

TABLE 11-3. Laboratory screening tests commonly ordered for older psychiatric patients

Complete blood count
Blood glucose
Serum electrolytes
Blood urea nitrogen and creatinine
Liver enzymes
Thyroid function test (thyroxine level, free thyroxine index,
    thyroid-stimulating hormone level)
Syphillis serology
    Vitamin B_{12} and folate assays
    Urinalysis
    Electrocardiogram
Chest x-ray

patients admitted to a psychiatric unit found only the following screening tests useful in the detection and treatment of an illness: midstream urine collection, chest x-ray, vitamin B_{12} assay, electrocardiogram, and blood urea nitrogen (Kolman, 1984). Many clinicians would also screen older psychiatric patients for thyroid disease using an assay of thyroid-stimulating hormone (TSH) level (described in the section on thyroid disease).

COMMON MEDICAL PROBLEMS

The geriatric psychiatrist should be aware of the more common medical conditions of older people. Some aspects of initial diagnosis and therapy of these common conditions can be appropriately managed by the psychiatrist, with referral to the medical care provider when indicated. The psychiatrist can also play a major role in identifying features that signal deterioration or missed diagnoses.

Arthritis

The most common chronic condition among persons aged 65 years and older is arthritis; it affects over 50% (Centers for Disease Control and Prevention, 1994; National Center for Health Statistics, 1990). One study suggested the prevalence is even higher in older inpatients, with over 75% of patients admitted to an acute geriatric unit having evidence of arthritis (Jenkinson et al., 1989).

Painful or stiff joints in older patients are usually because of osteoarthritis, which involves deterioration and abrasion of the articular cartilage. One third of older patients have significant symptoms of joint discomfort, and approximately 10% have significant limitation because of osteoarthritis. The joints usually involved include the hands (proximal and distal interphalangeal joints), hips, knees, feet (first metatarsal-phalangeal joints), and the cervical and lower lumbar spine. The diagnosis is suggested by symptoms in one or more of these joints combined with evidence of degenerative changes on plain x-rays. However, x-ray evidence of degenerative disease does not necessarily correlate with symptom severity. There are no diagnostic blood tests for osteoarthritis. An elevated erythrocyte sedimentation rate, weight loss, or constitutional symptoms suggest another disease process.

Treatment of osteoarthritis is symptomatic; acetaminophen taken on a regular basis several times per day, as well as physical therapy and exercise, can improve comfort and mobility. If these measures are inadequate, aspirin or nonsteroidal antiinflammatory drugs (NSAIDs) can be helpful, but these agents can cause severe gastric mucosal injury and even life-threatening gastric ulceration or renal insufficiency in susceptible patients.

The elderly, particularly women, are at increased risk of major gastrointestinal complications from NSAIDs; the majority are asymptomatic on these drugs prior to the complication. Risk factors for NSAID-induced ulcer include a history of ulcer disease, concurrent therapy with corticosteroids or anticoagulants, serious underlying medical illness, and age older than 70 years. The prostaglandin analog misoprostol is effective in the prevention of NSAID-induced gastric and duodenal ulcers (Jones & Schubert, 1991). Proton pump inhibitors (e.g., omeprazole, lansoprazole, rabeprazole, pantoprazole, esomeprazole) are equivalent or superior to misoprostol for the prevention of recurrent ulcers and are better tolerated than misoprostol, but their impact on NSAID-induced ulcer complications is not firmly established. Additional measures that may decrease gastrointestinal complications include discontinuation of cigarettes and alcohol, use of the lowest effective dose of NSAID, and discontinuation of NSAID when the agent is no longer necessary.

Alternative analgesics, such as nonacetylated salicylates (e.g., salsalate) should be considered. In particular, the use of selective cyclooxygenase-2 (COX-2) inhibitors (e.g., celecoxib, rofecoxib) should be strongly considered when using NSAIDs in older people. Selective COX-2 inhibitors have the important advantage (over nonselective NSAIDs) of less gastrointestinal ulceration. Selective COX-2 inhibitors do not inhibit platelets, but can cause renal dysfunction and may increase the INR (international normalized ratio) in patients taking warfarin; they should be avoided in patients with moderate or severe liver disease.

Small doses of codeine are suggested by some to be useful in patients with severe symptoms who cannot tolerate other agents, but the risk of constipation and sedating side effects are a major concern. Physical therapy can be extremely helpful in many patients with symptoms of osteoarthritis. Joint injection with steroids can be extremely helpful for some and may lessen the need for oral treatment with medications (such as NSAIDs and narcotics) that can have serious side effects. There is some evidence for the effectiveness of glucosamine and chondroitin, and many patients use these preparations. If correction cannot be made through optimal conservative therapy, joint replacement should be considered in older patients with severe limiting symptoms or limitation of an activity that is particularly important or meaningful to the patient.

The other major rheumatologic diseases in older patients with joint discomfort include gout, pseudogout, polymyalgia rheumatica (with or without temporal arteritis), rheumatoid arthritis, and infectious arthritis (Moskowitz, 1987; Sorenson, 1989).

Hypertension

The second most common chronic condition in older people is hypertension. Hypertension affects 40% to 69% of persons aged 65 years and older (Working Group on Hypertension in the Elderly, 1986). Hypertension is defined as systolic blood pressure above 140 and/or diastolic blood pressure above 90. One precaution is the falsely elevated cuff blood pressure that may be seen in some older patients (*pseudohypertension*). This is probably because of calcification of the brachial artery, and it may be accompanied by a positive Osler's sign (a palpable, pulseless brachial or radial artery after blood pressure cuff occlusion) (Messerli et al., 1985).

Secondary causes of hypertension are considered in patients with new onset of hypertension after age 50 years or worsening hypertension in a patient whose hypertension was previously adequately controlled. Refractory hypertension associated with progressive renal insufficiency suggests possible renovascular disease (e.g., renal artery stenosis). Other clinical clues to this surgically correctable lesion include an abdominal bruit or severe retinopathy. A clue to another surgically correctable secondary cause of hypertension, an aldosterone-producing adenoma, is hypokalemia less than 3.6 mEq/L. An extensive workup for secondary causes of hypertension is generally recommended in older patients only when hypertension cannot be controlled medically.

Treatment of hypertension reduces the incidence of stroke and congestive heart failure by up to 50%. Treatment of hypertension in older people is highly efficacious and cost effective (Mulrow et al., 1994). In particular, several trials in older persons with predominantly systolic hypertension have confirmed that antihypertensive therapy prevents fatal and nonfatal myocardial infarction and improves overall cardiovascular survival.

Three major trials of antihypertensive treatment in the elderly (i.e., the American Systolic Hypertension in the Elderly Program [SHEP], the Swedish Trial in Old Patients with Hypertension [STOP-Hypertension], and the British Medical Research Council [MRC] Trial of Treatment of Hypertension in Older Adults) support the treatment of hypertension in older people. These trials all compared diuretic or β-blocking agents with placebo. All three trials showed that treatment of hypertension in the elderly reduces the risk of stroke and cardiovascular events; in the STOP-Hypertension trial, there was also a decrease in total mortality with treatment (Dahlof et al., 1991; Hansson, 1993; MRC Working Party, 1992; SHEP Cooperative Research Group, 1991). In addition, a meta-analysis of systolic hypertension in the elderly strongly supports its treatment, particularly for decreasing mortality and stroke (Staessen et al., 2000).

Authors have varied in their recommendations on how aggressively to treat hypertension in older patients because of concerns about complications of antihypertensive therapy. However, the results of the trials mentioned above have highlighted the importance of antihypertensive treatment in the elderly. Most authors currently recommend that a systolic blood pressure of 160 mm Hg or greater or a diastolic blood pressure of 90 mm Hg or greater in an older person should be treated. Nonpharmacological treatment should include weight reduction in obese patients, smoking cessation, moderate sodium restriction, moderation of alcohol, and regular exercise. It should also be remembered that use of NSAIDs can elevate blood pressure. Antihypertensive drug therapy should be started if nonpharmacological therapy does not reduce blood pressure adequately or if the blood pressure is high enough to mandate immediate drug therapy.

The following guidelines have been suggested when treating older patients with antihypertensive medications: Start with a low dose of one drug, increase the dose slowly, minimize the number of pills and doses, monitor for side effects, encourage home blood pressure monitoring, and choose drugs based on coexisting conditions that may interact with drug treatment. It is useful for the psychiatrist to be familiar with common side effects of various antihypertensive agents to recognize these problems when they occur.

Thiazide diuretics are often used in older patients, but they are generally started at lower doses than for younger patients (e.g., 12.5 mg of hydrochlorothiazide per day). Limiting side effects of diuretics include frequent urination, orthostasis, and dehydration, as well as sodium and potassium depletion and azotemia. Hyperglycemia, hyperuricemia, and increased lipid levels may also occur. The dehydration that diuretics may cause can be a particular problem in patients receiving psychiatric or other medications that can cause orthostatic hypotension. In general, psychiatric symptoms because of diuretic therapy are seen only in patients who develop metabolic abnormalities.

β-Blockers can be used in older patients, but with careful attention to the appearance of bradycardia, heart block, bronchospasm, congestive heart failure, and glucose intolerance. Advantages of β-blockers include antianginal effects, cardioprotective effects in patients with prior myocardial infarction, and low incidence of orthostatic hypotension. Disadvantages include the risk of depression (which may be very significant) and the troublesome side effects of restless sleep and somnolence. These agents may also alter lipid metabolism.

Calcium channel blockers may be used, but important potential side effects include the risk of heart block in susceptible patients; potential decreased cardiac contractility and constipation (with nondihydropyridine calcium antagonists such as diltiazem and verapamil); and ankle edema, flushing, and headache with dihydropyridine calcium antagonists (such as amlodipine, felodipine, and nifedipine). These agents generally do not cause significant orthostatic hypotension or CNS side effects.

Angiotensin-converting enzyme (ACE) inhibitors are generally well tolerated, but potential side effects include hyperkalemia, nonproductive cough, and worsening of renal function in patients with congestive heart failure, hyponatremia, or renal artery stenosis. ACE inhibitors are generally the drugs of choice in hypertensive patients with congestive heart failure because of evidence of increased survival, decreased hospitalization, and other benefits. In patients with diabetes, there is evidence of a renal protective effect and reduced cardiovascular events with ACE inhibitors. CNS side effects are generally not a problem.

Centrally acting agents (such as clonidine) are generally not recommended in older patients because of sedation, but these agents are sometimes used in severe hypertension unresponsive to multiple agents. α-Blockers (e.g., terazosin, doxazosin) can be considered in patients who also have symptoms of prostatism in addition to their hypertension; however, these agents may cause significant orthostasis (Applegate, 1989; Tjoa & Kaplan, 1990; Tuck et al., 1988).

Care should be taken when choosing psychiatric medications in patients who are taking antihypertensives with CNS or orthostatic side effects. It may, at times, be desirable to discuss with the primary care physician a change in antihypertensive medication. The potential side effects of various antihypertensive agents discussed above should not detract from the clear evidence for effectiveness of treating hypertension in older people.

Diabetes Mellitus

Glucose intolerance increases with age; approximately one third of patients older than 65 years have an abnormal glucose tolerance test. However, whether all these patients require therapy is unclear. An abnormal fasting blood sugar is the preferable method of diagnosing diabetes in the older population. Diabetes is identified as a plasma glucose level of 126 mg/dL or higher after an overnight fast on more than one occasion. Of older patients, 10% to 20% have diabetes; it has been estimated that 50% of people with diabetes in the United States are older than 65 years of age. The rates in men and women are virtually equal (Harris, 1990).

The majority of older patients with diabetes have type 2 (non-insulin-dependent diabetes mellitus), although some of these patients may require insulin therapy. Patients are typically overweight and had onset of diabetes after age 40 years. Common symptoms at onset of type 2 diabetes include polyuria and polydipsia; candidal vaginitis in women may be an initial manifestation. Many patients have few or no symptoms.

The required treatment of diabetes varies considerably and may include diet, weight loss, oral hypoglycemic agents, or insulin; some patients will require a combination of these modalities (Edelman, 1998). Doses of oral agents or insulin are started low and increased slowly to avoid hypoglycemia, which is a major risk in older patients. Coexisting hypertension and hyperlipidemia are often associated with type 2 diabetes, and evidence suggests management of these comorbidities is essential in reducing complications of diabetes. Hypoglycemia may present with psychiatric symptoms that range from subtle dullness to coma, and nocturnal hypoglycemia may be a cause of insomnia in treated diabetics.

Serious acute hyperglycemia in older diabetics generally presents not as diabetic ketoacidosis, but as hyperglycemic hyperosmolar nonketotic coma (HHNKC). These patients may present with mental status changes in addition to weakness, polyuria, and polydipsia. Mortality is as high as 25% to 50%. Acute hyperglycemia without HHNKC can also cause psychiatric symptoms ranging from subtle personality changes to delirium and may present with focal neurological signs and symptoms. The mental status changes of hyperglycemia with or without HHNKC may resolve slowly, particularly in those patients with underlying CNS disease (Cooppan, 1987; Riesenberg, 1989).

Complications of chronic diabetes involve multiorgan disease and generally reflect microvascular and macrovascular disease or neurological involvement. Three fourths of deaths in older diabetics are caused by cardiovascular disease, primarily ischemic heart disease and stroke (Harris, 1990). Controlled trials have shown that intensive blood sugar control decreases the risk of complications in both type 1 and type 2 diabetes. Control of hypertension and hyperlipidemia and monitoring of renal function are also important in these patients. Nonspecific complaints such as fatigue may be because of chronic hyperglycemia and may improve with good blood sugar control. Mental efficiency is frequently impaired in older persons with diabetes (U'Ren et al., 1990). In the older patient, attempts at tight control must be balanced with the risks of hypoglycemia. In the management of diabetes, glycohemoglobin (e.g., hemoglobin A1C) levels can help evaluate overall control. Finally, cigarette smoking increases the risk of complications with diabetes, and the psychiatrist can play a key role in assisting their patients to stop smoking, particularly those with diabetes.

Constipation

Most healthy older outpatients have a bowel frequency within the same range as their younger counterparts (three times per day to three times per week), but older patients more often complain of constipation and more often use laxatives (Donald et al., 1985). In one large study, 26% of women and 16% of men older than 65 years reported recurrent constipation; risk factors for constipation were increased age, female gender, use of multiple drugs, pain in the abdomen, and hemorrhoids (Stewart et al., 1992). Additional factors that may contribute to constipation in older patients include decreased fluid and dietary fiber intake, decreased activity, intrinsic bowel lesions, endocrine and metabolic disorders, and constipating drugs. Constipation can be a significant problem in psychiatric patients, particularly those on medications with anticholinergic effects. Common causes of constipation in older patients are listed in Table 11-4.

The older patient with constipation should have a rectal examination to rule out fecal impaction or anorectal disease such as hemorrhoids or rectal fissure. Those who present with new or worsened constipation without obvious etiology should have a study to visualize their colon. Colonoscopy should be considered early in particular patient groups, such as those with a family history of colon cancer and those with weight loss or hemoccult-positive stools. Screening blood tests, particularly a complete blood count and thyroid function tests (TFTs), may aid diagnosis.

The first step in treating constipation is to discontinue unnecessary constipating drugs and treat any contributing diseases. Next, patients should be encouraged to increase physical activity, fluid intake, and dietary fiber. Bulk-forming agents such as methylcellulose or psyllium can be added. Patients with hard stools may benefit from a stool softener such as docusate preparations. Other agents to consider are lactulose or sorbitol, enemas, and suppositories. Lactulose can be given at a starting dose of 15 to 30 cc at bedtime and increased if necessary. Sorbitol is less expensive than lactulose, and evidence suggests it is just as effective (Lederle et al., 1990). Prepackaged enemas are simple and usually safe. Bisacodyl suppositories are usually more effective than glycerin suppositories.

Some agents require special precautions in older patients. Oral mineral oil

TABLE 11-4. Common causes of constipation in the older patient

Intrinsic bowel lesions	Endocrine and metabolic
Colorectal carcinoma	Hypothyroidism
Anorectal disease (e.g., hemorrhoids,	Adrenal and pituitary hypofunction
fissures)	Hypokalemia
Diverticular disease	Hypercalcemia
Inflammatory bowel disease	Uremia
Ischemic bowel disease	Drugs
Irritable bowel disease	Analgesics
Hypomotility disorders (e.g., idiopathic	Antacids (e.g., calcium carbonate,
slow transit, idiopathic megacolon)	aluminum hydroxide)
Neurological	Anticholinergics (e.g., antihistamines,
Dementia	tricyclic antiparkinsonian agents,
Stroke	antidepressants, neuroleptics)
Autonomic neuropathy (e.g., diabetes,	Antihypertensives, diuretics
pernicious anemia)	Laxative abuse
Psychiatric	Other (e.g., iron, phenytoin, barium,
Depression	bismuth)
Chronic psychosis	

is not recommended because of the risks of impaired absorption of fat-soluble vitamins and of aspiration with consequent lipoid pneumonia. Stimulant laxatives (e.g., cascara, senna, bisacodyl, castor oil) are generally recommended for short-term or intermittent use because of cramping and fluid and electrolyte loss, but can be used long term in patients with chronic, predisposing risks for constipation (e.g., narcotic analgesic use). Chronic use of stimulant laxatives can cause colonic smooth muscle changes, resulting in severe, resistant constipation (cathartic colon), but this may be less of a concern in elderly requiring treatment for constipation. Saline laxatives such as magnesium and sodium salts carry a risk of fluid loss with chronic use, but can be used for short-term therapy. Soapsuds or hydrogen peroxide enemas should not be used because of mucosal irritation.

Fecal impaction should be suspected and a rectal examination performed in patients with severe or chronic constipation or in patients who develop fecal incontinence or "paradoxical diarrhea" (which generally presents as oozing of small amounts of liquid stool around the impaction). High fecal impaction beyond the range of digital rectal examination may be visualized on plain x-rays of the abdomen. If enemas are not successful, careful manual disimpaction may be necessary, but can be quite uncomfortable for the patient. A fecal impaction must be removed prior to therapy with stimulant laxatives because of the risk of causing severe cramping or obstruction (Alessi & Henderson, 1988). High fecal impaction may be difficult to relieve, but repeated enemas and suppositories can be successful.

Weight Loss and Malnutrition

Weight loss is a common symptom in older patients with psychiatric or medical illness. Unintentional weight loss of 5% of body weight or more in 6 months or 10% or more in 1 year is significant and should be evaluated for an organic cause. In about one fourth to one third of patients with weight loss, a medical cause is not found. The most common medical causes found are malignancy and gastrointestinal disease. Depression was the most common cause in one study of elderly outpatients with weight loss (Thompson & Morris, 1991). Another study found the best predictor of involuntary weight loss in elderly patients on a geriatric rehabilitation unit was the number of general oral health problems (e.g., poor oral hygiene, inability to chew, etc.); other important predictors were household income, age, smoking, nutritional intake, and education (Sullivan et al., 1993).

The extent of laboratory testing in the older patient with psychiatric symptoms and weight loss depends on clinical clues to an underlying medical illness, degree of weight loss, and overall status of the patient (Morley, 1997). Typical screening tests include complete blood count, electrolytes, blood urea nitrogen, creatinine, liver function tests, glucose, serum protein and albumin, calcium, thyroid function tests, erythrocyte sedimentation rate, stools for occult blood, urinalysis, and chest x-ray. Further testing is guided by the history, physical examination, and results of screening laboratory tests (Morley, 1997).

The prevalence of malnutrition in older patients varies with the population studied. Malnutrition is reported in less than 5% of ambulatory outpatients, but occurs in up to two thirds of hospitalized and institutionalized older persons. The diagnosis is often missed; one study found that physicians did not record malnutrition or weight loss as a problem in nearly 50% of older outpatients with these problems, and the physicians prescribed nutritional supplements in only one fourth of those affected (Manson & Shea, 1991). Malnourished patients can present with weight loss, weakness, skin problems, and changes in mental status.

Unfortunately, it is difficult to assay nutritional status with the laboratory tests that are currently available. Laboratory tests used to identify malnutrition include serum albumin (a value less than 3 to 3.5 g/dL is significant), total lymphocyte count (values less than 1,500/cm^3 are significant), and the presence of anergy on skin testing. However, in older patients albumin may not be reliable, and anergy may occur without malnutrition. Anthropometric measures can also be used, such as age-adjusted weight and height, skinfold thickness, and arm muscle circumference. Another commonly used measure is the body mass index, which is the body weight in kilograms divided by the square of height in meters. Calorie counts can determine if the patient's energy intake is adequate. Treatment of malnutrition includes making food accessible, treating underlying causes, and using nutritional supplements (orally or by tube feedings) when appropriate (Morley, 1997).

Anemia

Although mild anemia is common in older people and frequently no obvious etiology can be found, the anemic older patient should be evaluated for etiology. Healthy older people should maintain a normal hemoglobin value. The World Health Organization criteria for anemia are a hemoglobin less than 13 g/dL for men and 12 g/dL for women. Surveys suggest the incidence of anemia is 6% to 30% for elderly men and 10% to 22% for elderly women (Mansouri & Lipschitz, 1992).

The classic signs of anemia are pallor, weakness, and fatigue. The older anemic patient, however, may present with behavioral changes or confusion. If the anemia is recognized and treated, the symptoms can respond dramatically to relatively small improvements in hemoglobin. Evaluation of the anemic patient should be approached systematically. A coexisting low platelet count and low white blood cell count suggest pancytopenia. An elevated reticulocyte count suggests that the patient's bone marrow is responding appropriately to some insult; such as hemolysis, blood loss, some toxin, or vitamin deficiency. A normal or low reticulocyte count (reticulocyte index less than 2) in the face of anemia suggests that the bone marrow is not responding appropriately.

Traditionally, identification of the anemia is made based on classification of red blood cell size (generally using the mean corpuscular volume) as microcytic, macrocytic, or normocytic. Another classification system for common causes of anemia includes three categories based on etiology; these categories can be identified based on results of the reticulocyte count and mean corpuscular volume (MCV). The categories include (1) hypoproliferative anemia (with low reticulocyte count and normal or low MCV; e.g., iron deficiency anemia); (2) compensatory (hemolytic) states (with elevated reticulocyte count and high, low, or normal MCV; e.g., hemolysis from autoimmune disease, infection, or medication); and (3) ineffective erythropoiesis (with low reticulocyte count and elevated MCV; e.g., from vitamin B_{12} or folate deficiency). It should be remembered that several causes of anemia can coexist in the older patient.

Iron deficiency anemia presents with a low MCV (less than 84 fL). A low serum ferritin is diagnostic of iron deficiency, and serum ferritin is the best predictor of bone marrow iron stores, but ferritin can be falsely increased into the normal range by liver disease or inflammatory disorders (Guyatt et al., 1990). Low serum iron and increased total iron-binding capacity (TIBC) can also be seen in iron deficiency anemia, but these tests may not be reliable in older patients because the presence of a chronic disease can lead to a normal or low TIBC even in the presence of an iron deficiency anemia.

Results from one study suggested that anemic older patients with a serum ferritin greater than 100 µg/L can be treated as not having iron deficiency, patients with serum ferritin less than 18 µg/L can be treated as having iron deficiency, and patients with values between 18 and 100 need additional testing (Guyatt et al., 1990). Some clinicians will use a therapeutic trial of iron replacement to aid in the diagnosis (looking for evidence of bone marrow response to iron supplementation).

However the diagnosis is established, it is essential that the older patient with iron deficiency be evaluated for its etiology, particularly looking for a gastrointestinal lesion. Stool examination for occult blood is important; however, negative stool exams should not preclude bowel studies when an iron deficiency anemia is present. Many geriatricians will avoid barium enema and evaluate the iron-deficient older patient with colonoscopy as the initial test to increase diagnostic accuracy and avoid subjecting the older patient to two bowel preparation procedures.

Anemia of chronic disease is a diagnosis of exclusion made only in patients with anemia who have a documented chronic disease and otherwise normal hematologic evaluation. Iron studies typically show both decreased iron and decreased TIBC.

Macrocytic anemia (defined as an MCV of more than 100 fL) from megaloblastic red blood cell changes in older patients can be because of deficiency of folate or vitamin B_{12} or other etiologies. Red cell folate levels are more reliable than serum folate levels, but are not available in all laboratories. If there is no malabsorption, folate deficiency can be corrected with folic acid (1 mg orally per day).

The most frequent cause of vitamin B_{12} deficiency in the older patient is probably an inability to separate B_{12} from food sources because of low stomach acidity or deficient pancreatic enzymes. Pernicious anemia (i.e., a lack of intrinsic factor) is another important etiology.

The normal lower limit of serum vitamin B_{12} level is uncertain in the older patient, and the necessity for additional testing has been debated. Other measures of vitamin B_{12} deficiency that may help clarify the diagnosis include increased levels of methylmalonic acid in the urine and elevated serum methylmalonic acid or total homocysteine level.

Vitamin B_{12} deficiency has been associated with a variety of neurological symptoms including paresthesias, dysesthesias, abnormal proprioception, and dementia. Psychiatric symptoms have also been described, including delirium, hallucinations, personality changes, delusions, depression, acute psychoses, and mania. Neurological changes of B_{12} deficiency can occur prior to hematologic changes.

Patients with vitamin B_{12} deficiency generally require lifelong monthly intramuscular B_{12} injections, but oral therapy may be effective in patients with mild B_{12} deficiency. Whether folate deficiency alone can cause neurological symptoms has been debated. Correction of folate deficiency in the face of undiagnosed vitamin B_{12} deficiency can precipitate progression of neurological symptoms.

Anemia with an elevated reticulocyte count should be evaluated for evidence of hemolysis. Some recommend testing for iron deficiency anemia and folate and B_{12} deficiency in the older anemic patient with normocytic anemia because of the possibility of early or mixed disease (Cohen & Crawford, 1986; Marcus & Freedman, 1985). Finally, the older patient with unexplained normochromic normocytic anemia should be evaluated (e.g., with serum and urine protein electrophoresis) for multiple myeloma.

Thyroid Disease

Estimates of the prevalence of thyroid disease in the elderly vary from less than 2% to 14%. Higher rates are noted in hospital settings. In one study of hospitalized older patients, only 27% of patients had normal values for all thyroid function studies (Simons et al., 1990). The presentation of thyroid disease in the older patient may be subtle or atypical. Symptoms that are erroneously attributed by some to "old age"—such as fatigue, constipation, and functional decline—may be seen with thyroid disease. Screening for thyroid disease in older patients with psychiatric symptoms is recommended because thyroid disease in older patients is common and the symptoms can mimic or exacerbate psychiatric illness. Abnormalities in thyroid function testing and concerns about thyroid disease are common in older psychiatric patients, so this topic is extensively addressed in this chapter.

The single best test of thyroid function is assay of thyroid-stimulating hormone level. The currently used immunoradiometric methods of TSH assay allow the distinction between normal (euthyroid) and low (hyperthyroid) levels of TSH. Because of this, this supersensitive TSH assay may be used as a single screening test of thyroid function (Caldwell, 1985; Feit 1988). The TSH response to exogenous thyrotropin-releasing hormone (TRH) is less commonly used clinically, but has been studied in older psychiatric patients. For example, patients with major depression have a blunted TSH response; studies have varied as to whether patients with Alzheimer's disease have a blunted TSH response.

Different etiologies have been suggested to explain these findings in terms of the pathophysiology of these psychiatric disorders (Molchan et al., 1991). Older patients with hyperthyroidism may present with the classic signs and symptoms, such as heat intolerance, weight loss, tremor, and palpitations. However, older patients may also present with single-organ-system symptoms (such as atrial fibrillation) or with "apathetic hyperthyroidism" (characterized by anorexia, fatigue, weight loss, and general decline) without the hypermetabolic symptoms of hyperthyroidism.

Laboratory testing in hyperthyroidism reveals a high serum T_4 (levorotatory thyroxine), high FTI (free thyroxine index), and a low, generally undetectable, TSH. An undetectable level of TSH is clear evidence of hyperthyroidism. Detectable, subnormal levels of TSH can occur in medically ill patients. T_3 thyrotoxicosis is a hyperthyroid state with elevated serum T_3 (triiodothyronine) but normal serum T_4. If low, the serum free T_4 index or serum free T_4 concentration should be measured; a high value for either confirms the diagnosis of hyperthyroidism (Woeber, 1992). Free T_3 level should be obtained if TSH is low and T_4 is normal.

Initial therapy of hyperthyroidism in the older patient generally involves a β-blocker such as propranolol and an antithyroid medication such as propylthiouracil. Definitive treatment in older patients is usually accomplished with radioactive iodine therapy, after which up to one third of patients become hypothyroid.

The major symptoms of hypothyroidism in older patients are lassitude, constipation, cold intolerance, fatigue, and decreased mentation. The symptoms may develop slowly and be attributed to aging, depression, or dementia. Patients with myxedema have the features of hypothyroidism along with soft tissue accumulation of mucopolysaccharides. Laboratory testing in hypothyroidism reveals low serum T_4 and FTI with elevated levels of TSH. In frail older patients or those with cardiac disease, thyroid hormone replacement starts at low doses, such as 0.025 mg of L-thyroxine per day, and is gradually increased by 0.025 mg at monthly intervals, with monitoring for side effects and normalization of serum TSH levels. Overreplacement should be avoided, so the thyroid hormone dose should be increased until the TSH level is within, but not below, the normal range.

Myxedema coma is a life-threatening presentation of hypothyroidism that occurs almost exclusively in patients older than 50 years. It generally occurs in patients with chronic myxedema who suffer some additional insult, such as sedating medications or an acute illness. Myxedema coma is a medical emergency that requires intravenous L-thyroxine therapy (Robuschi et al., 1987).

Three additional patterns of TFT abnormality are euthyroid hyperthyroxinemia, euthyroid sick syndrome, and subclinical hypothyroidism. Euthyroid hyperthyroxinemia is characterized by an elevated T_4 with normal TSH. These patients are clinically euthyroid, and the elevated serum T_4 level generally resolves spontaneously. The euthyroid sick syndrome has been described in hospitalized patients with serious systemic illness of various etiologies. In this syndrome, T_4 can be normal or decreased, T_3 is decreased, TSH can be increased or decreased, and the reverse T_3 level is usually increased. It is not appropriate to treat patients with euthyroid sick syndrome with thyroid hormone replacement. Subclinical (compensated) hypothyroidism is a very common pattern of abnormal TFTs in older patients; it is characterized by elevated TSH with normal T_4 and FTI. It may progress to overt hypothyroidism, particularly in patients with TSH values greater than 20 µU/mL or high-titer positive antithyroid antibodies (Rosenthal et al., 1987). In the patient with high TSH, normal T_4,, and depression, if the clinician believes the depression is caused by decreased thyroid function, the hypothyroidism should be treated.

A significant percentage of newly admitted psychiatric patients who are clinically euthyroid have some abnormality in initial TFTs, particularly an elevated T_4 or FTI, which reverts to normal after approximately 2 weeks. In a patient with an acute psychiatric illness, without signs or symptoms of thyroid disease, and with mild or nonspecific abnormalities on initial TFTs, it is reasonable simply to observe the patient and repeat the TFTs after approximately 2 weeks (Feit, 1988).

GERIATRIC SYNDROMES

Certain medical problems are common in older patients, yet may go untreated if not specifically addressed. They are singled out here to alert the psychiatrist to recognize these "geriatric syndromes" and refer patients for evaluation when appropriate.

Hearing and Visual Impairment

Hearing impairment occurs in 25% to 45% of persons older than 65 years and in 90% of those older than 80. The normal ear is most sensitive to frequencies between 500 and 4,000 Hz, the approximate range of human speech (Lavizzo-Mourey & Siegler, 1992). The hearing loss in older people is usually in the high-frequency range, which is important in conversation. Although there are various definitions of hearing impairment, at least one author reported that hearing is abnormal in older people if pure tones softer than 40 dB in more than one frequency are not heard in one or both ears (Lavisso-Mourey & Siegler, 1991).

Hearing impairment can be associated with significant emotional, social, and communication dysfunction, all of which can affect the quality of life of the older person (Mulrow et al., 1990). However, fewer than 20% of those impaired receive any form of hearing aid. Screening guidelines have not been established; however, annual screening of older persons with a handheld audioscope and perhaps a screening questionnaire has been recommended (Mulrow & Lichtenstein, 1991).

When there is a question of hearing impairment, the first step is to examine the ear for cerumen occluding the external ear canal. If the ear is clear of cerumen, patients can be tested with a handheld audioscope or referred to audiology for testing. There are several questionnaires available to evaluate the significance of hearing impairment (American Speech, Language, and Hearing Association, 1989; Lichtenstein et al., 1988; Mader, 1984). Individuals with hearing impairment should be referred to an audiologist for assessment and prescription of an appropriate hearing device. Older patients who are initially reluctant to accept a hearing aid may, with encouragement, markedly benefit from the correction of their hearing impairment.

Visual impairment is present in almost 15% of persons aged 65 and older, and nearly 50% of people older than 75 years have one of the four leading causes of vision impairment. These four common causes of nonrefractive (i.e., excluding presbyopia) visual impairment are cataracts (38% of cases), followed by macular degeneration (14%), diabetic retinopathy (7%), and glaucoma (5%) (Rahmani et al., 1996).

Because of the high prevalence of eye disease in older people, it is generally recommended that routine examination be performed by an eye professional (Straatsma et al., 1985). Treatment of vision impairment in older people has a positive impact on quality of life; one large study found that within 1 year of treatment for vision problems older people had better driving skills, more activities, better mental health, and more life satisfaction (Brenner et al., 1993).

Urinary Incontinence

Urinary incontinence is a problem in up to one third of community-dwelling older patients and in even higher numbers of those acutely hospitalized. The majority of patients with incontinence can have symptom improvement if the incontinence is recognized by the clinician, properly evaluated, and treated. However, the patient may not mention the incontinence unless specifically asked.

Incontinence can be an acute or chronic problem. Common causes of acute incontinence are urinary tract infection, restricted mobility, altered mental status, drugs (particularly those with anticholinergic or sedating properties and diuretics), polyuria, and fecal impaction. Patients who suddenly develop urinary incontinence should have some procedure (by bedside bladder ultrasound or straight catheterization) to rule out urinary retention with overflow incontinence. A postvoid residual of more than 100 mL is considered significant (Ouslander, 1986). A voiding diary, in which the patient records the frequency and severity of continent and incontinent episodes, can be extremely valuable.

There are various classifications of chronic urinary incontinence. One commonly used system classifies chronic incontinence as stress, urge, overflow, or functional incontinence. The initial evaluation of chronic incontinence includes a focused history and physical examination, including pelvic examination in women, a urinalysis, and postvoid residual determination. Literature suggests that asymptomatic bacteriuria (in the absence of urinary incontinence) is common in older people and does not warrant antibiotic treatment. However, in patients undergoing initial evaluation for urinary incontinence who are found to have evidence of a urinary tract infection, a trial of antibiotics may be warranted (Ouslander, 1986).

Symptoms of *stress incontinence* include loss of small amounts of urine with increases in intraabdominal pressure, such as from a cough or laugh. The presence of stress incontinence can be documented by the pad test: The female patient with a full bladder is asked to cough while holding a pad between her legs; involuntary loss of urine establishes the diagnosis. Common treatments of stress incontinence include Kegel exercises or an α-adrenergic agonist or topical estrogen. Kegel exercises with biofeedback in a motivated patient can have a good success rate. Various surgical interventions are also available and have a high success rate.

The patient with *urge incontinence* usually describes an uncontrollable urge to void, with loss of small or large amounts of urine. Voiding at regular intervals and bladder retraining may help relieve the incontinence. Referral for formal cystometry may be indicated. Urge incontinence is commonly treated with a bladder relaxant such as oxybutynin or tolterodine.

Overflow incontinence is the loss of small amounts of urine associated with an overdistended bladder. Patients with overflow incontinence and a significant postvoid residual should have urologic evaluation. *Functional incontinence* is loss of urine associated with an inability to get to the toilet because of immobility or other functional problems. Several measures to improve access to the toilet may improve functional incontinence.

It is essential to realize that a patient may have multiple causes of incontinence. Referral to a specialist is recommended for patients with chronic urinary incontinence that is difficult to diagnose or is present in a patient with other findings, such as severe pelvic prolapse in women, an enlarged prostate in men, or hematuria or prior urologic procedure in either gender.

Falls

Falls occur in one third of community-dwelling persons older than 65 years and more than one half of nursing home residents each year. Falls increase with age and are more common in women until the age of 75 years, after which the frequency is similar in both sexes (Tinetti & Speechley, 1989). Of falls, 5% result in a fracture, and up to 10% result in other serious injury.

There is a wide range of etiologies for falls in older persons, including neurological disorders (such as Parkinson's disease) with gait and postural abnormalities; environmental hazards (such as loose rugs or electric cords); drugs that cause orthostatic hypotension; and mental status changes. There is strong evidence for an association between use of benzodiazepines, other sedative-hypnotics, and antipsychotic medications and falls and hip fracture in older people, and the psychiatrist must be ever vigilant of this potential complication when considering these medications in the elderly. In most cases, falls have multiple causes. The psychiatrist should question the older person about falls, particularly when medications are added or dosage changes are made (Tinetti & Speechley, 1988).

Falls may be a marker for serious underlying illnesses and disabilities that can be identified and potentially treated. The majority of these underlying problems can be identified from a careful history and physical examination (King & Tinetti, 1995; Rubenstein et al., 1990; Tinetti et al., 1995). Interdisciplinary interventions have been shown to reduce fall rates in community-dwelling and institutionalized older people who fall (Ray et al., 1997). Research also suggests that adapted, moderately intensive tai chi may prevent falls (Wolf et al., 1996). Older patients should be screened for falls, and targeted assessments should be performed for those who do present with a history of falls. Strength and endurance training for the prevention of falls are also supported in the literature (American Geriatrics Society, 2001).

Immobility

Immobility of older patients can have serious consequences, such as contractures (which can develop in days to weeks), deep venous thrombosis and embolization, osteopenia, orthostasis, atelectasis and pneumonia, constipation, urinary retention, and pressure sores. Common conditions that lead to immobility in older patients are arthritis, hip fracture, stroke, infection, generalized weakness, and pain. Patients confined to bed should be mobilized as quickly as possible. While bedridden, patients should have range-of-motion exercises to prevent contractures and subcutaneous heparin therapy to prevent thrombosis, and they should be turned frequently to avoid skin breakdown (Harper & Lyles, 1988).

Pressure Sores

The majority of pressure sores occur in older patients, with a prevalence of up to 30% in older hospitalized patients. More than 90% of pressure sores occur over one of the following sites: sacrum, ischial tuberosity, greater trochanter, calcaneus, and lateral malleolus. Factors that can lead to pressure sores include pressure on one area for more than 2 hours, shearing forces, friction on the skin surface, and moisture (Allman, 1989). Methods of preventing (and treating) pressure sores include mobilizing patients, relieving pressure in bedridden patients (by repositioning the body), keeping skin clean and dry, and maintaining adequate nutrition.

Pressure sores that are limited to the dermis (Stage I, nonblanchable erythema with skin intact) are primarily managed with pressure-relieving maneuvers. "Clean" pressure sores that involve skin breakdown (Stage II, generally a superficial ulcer with up to full-thickness skin loss; Stage III, ulcer through the dermis with exposure of subcutaneous fat but limited by the deep fascia) are generally treated with specialized protective dressings. Some Stage III and Stage IV (full-thickness ulcer with exposure of deep structures, not limited by deep fascia) may need surgical repair. Wounds with necrotic tissue should be debrided by mechanical (with a scalpel) or enzymatic means (with specialized enzymatic ointments). The clinician should be wary of closed pressure sores, which are extensive, deep fascia wounds that appear benign on the surface (Shea, 1975).

Many different skin preparations and dressings are available for the treatment of pressure sores. Referral to a wound care specialist is often indicated.

COMMON LABORATORY ABNORMALITIES

Various screening laboratory tests are often obtained in older patients who present with psychiatric symptoms (see Table 11-3). The psychiatrist should be familiar with the initial approach to abnormalities of these tests and obtain referral when appropriate. The approach to anemia, glucose abnormalities, abnormal thyroid function test, and vitamin B_{12} and folate deficiency were addressed separately above.

Serum Electrolytes

Serum sodium level reflects body water balance. Hypernatremia usually is the result of fluid loss (e.g., from diarrhea, osmotic diuresis, insensible losses, and diabetes insipidus from lithium therapy), so these patients (who have increased plasma osmolality) should develop thirst. However, older patients have been shown to have a decrease in thirst sensation (hypodipsia) and are at risk for dehydration. Patients with hypernatremia can present with confusion. Treatment of hypernatremia requires clinical assessment of volume status. This assessment is critical because patients with volume excess and edema and those with the syndrome of inappropriate antidiuretic hormone (SIADH) secretion are treated with water restriction, whereas those with decreased volume status are treated with saline (Narins et al., 1982).

Hyponatremia can result from a variety of etiologies. When hyponatremia is present, it is particularly important to clarify the likely cause because treatment varies drastically with etiology. Measurement of serum (and urine) plasma osmolality can aid in diagnosis. Hyponatremia with increased plasma osmolality can occur with hyperglycemia, in which case management of glucose level and hydration are the typical treatments. Hyponatremia with normal plasma osmolality (i.e., pseudohyponatremia) can occur with severe hyperlipidemia or hyperproteinemia (e.g., multiple myeloma), for which treatment addresses the underlying cause. Hyponatremia with decreased plasma osmolality can be associated with states of excess extracellular fluid (e.g., renal failure, heart failure, and cirrhosis). Hyponatremia with decreased extracellular fluid volume can be caused by renal losses in certain nephropathies, diuretics, vomiting, diarrhea, and other conditions. Hyponatremia with normal extracellular fluid volume can be caused by primary polydipsia, hypothyroidism, adrenal insufficiency, and SIADH.

Many psychiatric medications (e.g., carbamazepine, selective serotonin reuptake inhibitors [SSRIs], and antipsychotics) are associated with hyponatremia. The best approach to drug-induced (and other causes of) SIADH is discontinuation (or tapering off, if indicated) of the offending drug if present, fluid restriction, and liberalizing salt intake.

Symptoms depend on the severity of hyponatremia and how rapidly the change in sodium level has occurred. CNS symptoms such as confusion, lethargy, coma, and seizures (which are generally associated with sodium levels below 120 to 125 mEq/L), or severe hyponatremia (below 120 mEq/L) are an emergency. However, extreme caution is warranted to avoid overrapid correction of sodium levels, which can result in the devastating consequence of central pontine myelinolysis (a.k.a. osmotic demyelination). Referral is indicated for management of moderate-to-severe hyponatremia.

Blood Urea Nitrogen and Creatinine

The glomerular filtration rate declines with age, placing older patients at increased risk for developing acute renal failure when exposed to insults such as nephrotoxic drugs and dyes or episodes of low renal perfusion. Blood urea nitrogen and creatinine may overestimate renal function in older patients because of decreased protein intake and decreased muscle mass. Thus, serum levels of blood urea nitrogen and creatinine may be within normal limits despite decreased renal function, and minor elevations of these tests may represent significant renal impairment. In addition, equations designed to calculate estimated creatinine clearance may be erroneous in older people, by underestimating or overestimating creatinine clearance. Timed collection of urine to estimate creatinine clearance is recommended (Malmrose et al., 1993). Medications with renal excretion (e.g., some antibiotics, aspirin, bronchodilators) should be prescribed initially in low doses in older patients, and drug levels should be monitored if available.

Liver Function Tests

In healthy older people, liver function remains adequate throughout life. However, there is evidence that hepatic metabolism of some drugs decreases with age, and caution should be taken with these agents.

Commonly ordered screening tests that reflect liver disease include those for bilirubin, transaminases, and alkaline phosphatase. These tests may be abnormal in a variety of disorders, such as viral hepatitis, drug-induced hepatitis, cirrhosis, biliary tract obstruction, malignancy, hemolysis, and prolonged fasting. Some psychiatric medications may cause hepatitis. Drug-induced hepatitis can present with a cholestatic, a hepatitic, or a mixed pattern. Phenothiazines can cause a cholestatic-type drug-induced hepatitis with marked bilirubin elevation (primarily direct bilirubin), marked alkaline phosphatase elevation, and only mild-to-moderate transaminase elevations. Monoamine oxidase inhibitors (MAOIs) can cause a predominantly hepatitic picture with marked transaminase elevation and lesser increase in alkaline phosphatase.

Syphilis Serology

There has been a dramatic increase in the number of cases of primary and secondary syphilis reported in the United States. One study suggested an increase in early (recently acquired) syphilis in the elderly (Berinstein & DeHertogh, 1992). There are two basic types of serologic tests for syphilis. The first is nonspecific reagin antibody testing (e.g., VDRL test, rapid plasma reagin [RPR]). The second is specific antitreponemal antibody testing (e.g., fluorescent treponemal antibody absorption [FTA-ABS] test for syphilis, microhemagglutinations *Treponema pallidum* [MHA-TP]).

The VDRL and RPR have a high false-positive rate, so positive results should be followed by an FTA-ABS or MHA-TP. A false-negative VDRL can occur in patients with primary syphilis who have not yet developed reactivity; in one third of patients with latent or tertiary syphilis, the VDRL titer can spontaneously decline over time. One study in an acute care setting found that many older patients with positive syphilis serology did not have adequate evaluation (Naughton & Moran, 1992).

Asymptomatic neurosyphilis develops in approximately one third of patients after 1 year or more of untreated syphilis. Symptomatic neurosyphilis can be meningovascular, parenchymal, or mixed disease. Meningovascular neurosyphilis presents as subacute or chronic meningitis. Parenchymal neurosyphilis may present as general paresis or tabes dorsalis. General paresis is characterized by progressive dementia, alterations in speech, and generalized weakness with hyperreflexia. Irritability, grandiose delusions, and hallucinations may occur. Tabes dorsalis is characterized by progressive ataxia, paresthesias, sharp pains, and sensory dysfunction. The Argyll-Robertson pupil (reacts to accommodation, but not to light) may be seen in both general paresis and tabes dorsalis.

The diagnosis of neurosyphilis is based on cerebrospinal fluid findings of an elevated protein level or mononuclear pleocytosis. A positive cerebrospinal fluid VDRL is diagnostic, but not present in all cases. Older patients with positive serology and neurological symptoms should have a lumbar puncture.

Penicillin is the treatment of choice for all stages of syphilis; alternative agents are used only if the patient has a well-documented allergy to penicillin. However, specific treatment regimen recommendations vary. Early syphilis (less than 1 year's duration) should be treated with 2.4 million units of benzathine penicillin intramuscularly as a single dose. Late syphilis (but not neurosyphilis) is treated with three weekly intramuscular doses. Neurosyphilis is treated with a 10- to 14-day course of intravenous penicillin.

After therapy for syphilis, the VDRL should be followed for evidence of decline in titer or conversion to seronegative status (which may take months). The FTA-ABS may remain positive after successful therapy. Lumbar puncture should be repeated in patients with neurosyphilis to determine adequacy of treatment.

Urinalysis

Urinary tract infection is the most common cause of gram-negative sepsis in older patients. Symptoms of urinary tract infection in older patients can include changes in mental status, functional decline, abdominal pain, or nausea and vomiting in addition to, or instead of, dysuria and urinary frequency. Older patients with serious infection may lack a febrile response. Urinalysis usually reveals bacteriuria, commonly with enteric rods. Some older patients may not have significant pyuria.

Diagnosis of urinary tract infection is made based on urine culture and sensitivity. Mild symptomatic urinary tract infection in older patients should be treated with a 7- to 10-day course of oral antibiotic rather than the single-dose therapy recommended for younger patients. Intravenous antibiotic is recommended for serious infection. Men with urinary tract infections (not related to recent catheterization) and women with recurrent urinary tract infections should have a urologic referral (Zweig, 1987).

Asymptomatic bacteriuria is common in older patients, particularly women, and increases in frequency with age as well as hospitalization and institutionalization. Its significance is unclear. Treatment of asymptomatic bacteriuria has not been shown to affect subsequent morbidity or mortality and probably should not be done (Nordenstam et al., 1986). However, as mentioned, patients with incontinence and asymptomatic bacteriuria probably deserve one trial of antibiotic therapy. Essentially, all patients with chronic indwelling urinary catheters will have bacteriuria and pyuria. These patients should not be treated with antibiotics if asymptomatic (Ouslander, 1986), and "monitoring" urine cultures in asymptomatic catheterized patients is not warranted.

MEDICAL CLEARANCE FOR
ELECTROCONVULSIVE THERAPY

Electroconvulsive therapy (ECT) is an effective and safe form of treatment for depression in the elderly. It is considered by many the treatment of choice in older patients with life-threatening severe depression and medical illness. In addition, patients who fail to respond to chemical antidepressant therapy may respond to ECT at a rate as high as 80% to 85%. However, subjects older than 80 years may have more cardiovascular complications and falls with ECT therapy compared to subjects aged 65 to 80 years (Cattan et al., 1990). Maintenance ECT has been found to be safe and effective for patients older than 75 years, even in the presence of medical disease (Dubin et al., 1992).

Pretreatment evaluation of the older patient prior to ECT should focus on neurological and cardiovascular status. A contraindication to ECT is the presence of increased intracranial pressure. ECT can be safely given in stroke patients after neurological status has stabilized or even in patients with brain tumors who are carefully monitored during treatments.

Cardiac events are the major cause of mortality reported from ECT. Although patients with cardiac disease have a higher rate of cardiac complications during ECT, with close monitoring (for arrhythmias and ischemic episodes), ECT can be given with relative safety even to patients with severe cardiovascular disease (Zielinski et al., 1993). All older patients should have cardiac monitoring during the ECT treatments. ECT causes a diffuse autonomic discharge, which can lead to severe bradycardia or even asystole if patients are not given atropine for cholinergic blockade. If patients are given atropine, however, heart rate, blood pressure, and plasma catecholamines increase immediately after ECT.

Pretreatment evaluation of cardiac status should focus on the presence of hypertension, angina, heart failure, and arrhythmias. If these problems are controlled, the patient may have ECT. Patients with hypertension who develop extreme blood pressure rise after ECT may need to have a prophylactic β-blocker. Calcium channel blockers and nitroprusside have been used to reduce the blood pressure rise after ECT. β-Blockade may also be necessary in patients with angina. Pacemaker patients can receive ECT after pacer function has been documented. Demand pacemakers should be converted to fixed mode with an external magnet immediately prior to ECT, and the patient should be appropriately grounded. ECT is contraindicated in patients with recent myocardial infarction because of an increased risk of cardiac arrhythmias with treatment. However, ECT has been performed in the immediate postmyocardial infarction period in severe cases of depression, generally with a resuscitation team present. However, if possible, it is recommended to wait at least 6 weeks after myocardial infarction to allow cardiac status to stabilize.

There may be increased risk from ECT for patients with respiratory diseases, particularly those with ventilatory compromise or those who retain carbon dioxide and have compromised hypoxic drive, who may not tolerate the brief period of apnea with ECT. Prolonged apnea has been reported in patients taking the drug echothiopate (even in eyedrop form) to prevent glaucoma. This drug should be discontinued before ECT therapy is instituted.

Many of the potential risks of ECT therapy can be prevented with careful technique. In selected patients, pretreatment oxygen therapy may decrease the risk of memory deficits and cardiac arrhythmias. Succinylcholine (or another agent) is given for muscle relaxation to decrease cardiovascular strain and decrease the risk of fractures; it is particularly important in patients with osteoporosis. Cardiac monitoring is required as noted. Atropine can prevent the risk of bradycardia and asystole, but dosage should be decreased or it should be avoided in patients with pacemakers, arrhythmias, or hypertension. Patients with glaucoma should have adequate topical treatment prior to pretreatment atropine (Elliot et al., 1982; Salzman, 1982).

Several psychotropic medications may interact with ECT therapy. Concomitant use of ECT and lithium should be avoided because of the reported risks of developing delirium (sometimes with seizure) and prolongation of neuromuscular blocking drugs used during ECT. Most experts recommend stopping antidepressants prior to ECT, primarily because of concerns over adverse cardiovascular effects. However, there is evidence that the combination of ECT and antidepressant therapy may be beneficial in some cases. In addition, the abrupt discontinuation of certain psychochotropics, especially those with strong anticholinergic effects, can be problematic. There is some evidence that benzodiazepines may reduce the therapeutic effect of ECT. On the other hand, neuroleptics are believed safe with ECT; some data suggest a beneficial effect of the combination of neuroleptics and ECT (Kellner et al., 1991).

Cognitive effects of ECT are another important consideration. Transient memory loss (retrograde and anterograde) is well documented. These cognitive effects may be decreased by attention to electrode placement and stimulus dosage. Animal studies and limited human trials suggest that treatment with drugs with antianmestic properties (e.g., opioid antagonists, vasopressin, adrenocorticotropic hormone, etc.) may decrease cognitive effects; however, usefulness of these agents is not clear (Krueger et al., 1992). There is some evidence that administration of T_3 may attenuate the cognitive effects of ECT. Dementia is not a contraindication to ECT, but demented patients are more prone to memory impairment with treatment.

MEDICAL ASPECTS OF THERAPY
WITH PSYCHIATRIC MEDICATIONS

Specific psychiatric medications, their indications, and their side effects are reviewed in Chapter 30. However, some of the more problematic side effects that can occur using psychiatric medications in older people are reviewed here.

The sedative effects of some antidepressants and other psychiatric medications can pose a major problem in older patients. Nighttime dosing of sedating antidepressants or use of less-sedating drugs can help this problem. In some patients, the sedating side effects are beneficial when the agent is given at night.

Anticholinergic effects can be very problematic in the older patient, and agents with strong anticholinergic effects should be avoided. Anticholinergic effects can occur with nearly all tricyclic and tetracyclic antidepressants. Heterocyclic compounds (e.g., trazodone, fluoxetine) do not cause anticholinergic effects. Typical problematic anticholinergic effects that can occur include delirium, dry mouth, constipation, tachycardia, blurred vision, and urinary retention. An increase in heart rate may not be tolerated in patients with unstable angina, and patients with chronic atrial fibrillation should be carefully observed. Patients should be questioned about these anticholinergic symptoms and about signs of adrenergic hyperactivity, such as tremulousness and sweating. In older patients, it is usually best to manage anticholinergic (and other problematic) side effects by decreasing or eliminating the offending agent rather than adding another drug to treat the side effect.

Clinically significant orthostatic hypotension is another concern with certain antidepressant therapy in older patients and is presumably because of antagonism of peripheral α_1-adrenergic receptors. The best predictor of postural hypotension with antidepressant therapy is preexisting orthostatic hypotension. In addition, orthostatic hypotension is more likely to develop in patients with left ventricular impairment or in patients taking other drugs, like diuretics or vasodilators (Glassman & Preud'homme, 1993). Careful monitoring of orthostatic blood pressure and symptoms of hypotension is required before and during treatment with agents with this side effect. The occurrence of orthostatic hypotension may be reduced by using low doses or divided doses and by slowly increasing the dose to reach a therapeutic effect. Paradoxically, pretreatment orthostatic hypotension has been shown to predict favorable treatment response to antidepressant therapy (Jarvik et al., 1983). Bupropion and SSRIs do not appear to cause orthostatic hypotension. MAOIs, on the other hand, may lead to orthostatic hypotension, supine hypotension, and hypertensive reactions.

Caution is warranted in the use of multiple agents with serotonergic effects. SSRIs should not be used with MAOIs or tryptophan. Caution is also

suggested with many SSRIs when using these agents with lithium, tricyclic antidepressants, phenytoin, warfarin, and other agents.

The major cardiovascular side effect with psychiatric medications that is a
concern in older patients is the cardiac conduction effects of certain agents. A
quinidinelike effect has been demonstrated by reduced frequency of premature
ventricular contractions in patients receiving imipramine, nortriptyline, or maprotiline. In addition, these agents may prolong intracardiac conduction. Caution is recommended in patients with preexisting conduction disturbances and
those receiving class IA antiarrhythmic drugs such as quinidine. If a different
antidepressant cannot be used, then the antiarrhythmic agent may need to be
reduced or discontinued while the patient is receiving such an antidepressant.
In vitro studies have demonstrated that these drugs do not lower cardiac output
even in patients with impaired ventricular function. Agents such as bupropion,
trazodone, and SSRIs appear to be relatively safe in patients with conduction
disease. Bupropion has some antiarrhythmic properties (Glassman & Preud'-
homme, 1993). MAOIs do not seem to have significant cardiac conduction,
rhythm, or left ventricular function effects.

An electrocardiogram should be taken in older patients prior to instituting
an antidepressant with known cardiac conduction effects. It has been suggested
in the past that, if bifascicular block, second-degree heart block, or QT prolongation is present, tricyclic antidepressants should not be started unless the patient is under careful observation in a hospital setting. Simple first-degree AV
block or hemiblock do increase the risk of complications to a small, but probably insignificant, degree. To monitor prolongation of the PR, QT, and QRS
duration (which most patients develop), worsening of AV block, and ventricular arrhythmias, a repeat electrocardiogram after treatment has begun is necessary for all patients with heart disease who are started on one of these medications (Dietch, 1990; Thompson et al., 1983; Veith, 1982). Newer
antidepressants without significant cardiac effects are probably a better choice
for patients with cardiac disease. In addition, ECT is another option in these
patients.

REFERENCES

Abramowicz M. Drugs that can cause psychiatric symptoms. *Med Lett Drugs Ther.*
    1986;28:81–86.
Alessi CA, Henderson CT. Constipation and fecal impaction in the longterm care pa-
    tient. *Clin Geriatr Med.* 1988;4:571–588.
Alexopoulos GS, Young RC, Meyers BS, et al. Late-onset depression. *Psychiatr Clin
    North Am.* 1988;11:101–112.
Allman RM. Pressure ulcers among the elderly. *N Engl J Med.* 1989;320:850–853.
American Geriatrics Society, British Geriatrics Society, and American Academy of Or-
    thopaedic Surgeons Panel on Falls Prevention. Guideline for the prevention of falls
    in older persons. *J Am Geriatr Soc.* 2001;49:664–672.

American Speech, Language, and Hearing Association. Guidelines for the identification of hearing impairment/handicap in adult/elderly persons. *Am Speech Lang Hearing Assoc J.* August 1989:59–63.

Applegate WB. Hypertension in elderly patients. *Ann Intern Med.* 1989;110:901–915.

Berinstein D, DeHertogh D. Recently acquired syphilis in the elderly population. *Arch Intern Med.* 1992;152:330–332.

Blazer DG. Psychiatry and the oldest old. *Am J Psychiatry.* 2000;157:1915–1924.

Brenner MH, Curbow B, Javitt JC, Legro MW, Sommer A. Vision change and quality of life in the elderly. Response to cataract surgery and treatment of other chronic ocular conditions. *Arch Ophthalmol.* 1993;111:680–685.

Caldwell G, Gow SM, Sweeting VM, et al. A new strategy for thyroid function testing. *Lancet.* 1985;1:1117–1119.

Cassel CK, Leipzig RM, Cohen HJ, et al. *Geriatric Medicine: An Evidence-Based Approach.* 4th ed. New York, NY: Springer-Verlag; 2003.

Cattan R, Barry PP, Mead G, Reefe WE, Gay A, Silverman M. Electroconvulsive therapy in octogenarians. *J Am Geriatr Soc.* 1990;38:753–758.

Centers for Disease Control and Prevention. Arthritis prevalence and activity limitations—United States, 1990. *Morb Mortal Wkly Rep.* 1994;43:433–438.

Cohen HJ, Crawford J. Hematologic problems. In: Calkins E, Davis PJ, Ford AB, eds. *The Practice of Geriatrics.* Philadelphia, PA: Saunders; 1986:519–531.

Cohen RA, Van Nostrand JF. Trends in the health of older Americans: United States, 1994, National Center for Health Statistics. *Vital Health Stat.* 1995;3(30).

Consensus Conference. Differential diagnosis of dementing diseases. *JAMA.* 1987;258:3411–3416.

Cooppan R. Determining the most appropriate treatment for patients with non-insulin dependent diabetes mellitus. *Metabolism.* 1987;365:17–21.

Cummings JL. Acute confusional states. In: *Clinical Neuropsychiatry.* New York, NY: Grune and Stratton; 1985:68–74.

Cummings JL, Benson DF. *Dementia: A Clinical Approach.* Boston, MA: Butterworths; 1984.

Dahlof B, Lindholm LH, Hansson L, et al. Morbidity and mortality in the Swedish Trial in old patients with hypertension (STOP-Hypertension). *Lancet.* 1991;338:1281–1285.

Dietch JT, Fine M. The effect of nortriptyline in elderly patients with cardiac conduction disease. *J Clin Psychiatry.* 1990;51:65–67.

Donald IP, Smith RG, Cruikshank JG, et al. A study of constipation in the elderly living at home. *Gerontology.* 1985;31:112.

Dubin WR, Jaffe R, Roemer R, Siegel L, Shoyer B, Venditti ML. The efficacy and safety of maintenance ECT in geriatric patients. *J Am Geriatr Soc.* 1992;40:706–709.

Edelman SV. Type II diabetes mellitus. *Adv Intern Med.* 1998;43:449–500.

Elliot DL, Linz DH, Kane JA. Electroconvulsive therapy: pretreatment medical evaluation. *Arch Intern Med.* 1982;142:979–981.

Feit H. Thyroid function in the elderly. *Clin Geriatr Med.* 1988;4:151–161.

Glassman AH, Preud'homme XA. Review of the cardiovascular effects of heterocyclic antidepressants. *J Clin Psychiatry.* 1993;54(suppl):16–22.

Guyatt GH, Patterson C, Ali M, et al. Diagnosis of iron-deficiency anemia in the elderly. *Am J Med.* 1990;88:205–209.

Hansson L. Future goals for the treatment of hypertension in the elderly with reference to STOP-Hypertension, SHEP, and the MRC trial in older adults. *Am J Hypertens.* 1993;6:405–435.

Harper CM, Lyles YM. Physiology and complications of bedrest. *J Am Geriatr Soc.* 1988;36:1047–1054.

Harris MI. Epidemiology of diabetes mellitus among the elderly in the United States. *Clin Geriatr Med.* 1990;6:703–719.

Jarvik LF, Read SL, Mintz J, et al. Pretreatment orthostatic hypotension in geriatric depression: predictor of response to imipramine and doxepine. *J Clin Psychopharmacol.* 1983;3:368–372.

Jenkinson ML, Bliss MR, Brain AT, Scott DL. Peripheral arthritis in the elderly: a hospital study. *Ann Rheum Dis.* 1989;48:227–231.

Jones MP, Schubert ML. What do you recommend for prophylaxis in an elderly woman with arthritis requiring NSAIDS for control? *Am J Gastroenterol.* 1991;86:264–268.

Kane RL, Ouslander JB, Abrass IB. *Essentials of Clinical Geriatrics.* 4th ed. New York, NY: McGraw-Hill; 1999.

Kaplan C, Lipkin M, Gordon GH. Somatization in primary care. *J Gen Intern Med.* 1988;3:177–190.

Kellner CH, Nixon DW, Bernstein HJ. ECT-drug interaction: a review. *Psychopharm Bull.* 1991;27:595–609.

King MB, Tinetti ME. Falls in community-dwelling older persons. *J Am Geriatr Soc.* 1995;43:1146–1154.

Kitchell MA, Barnes RF, Veith RC, et al. Screening for depression in hospitalized geriatric medical patients. *Am Geriatr Soc.* 1982;30:174.

Kolman PBR. The value of laboratory investigation of elderly psychiatric patients. *J Clin Psychiatry.* 1984;45:112–116.

Koran LM, Sox HC, Marton KI, et al. Medical evaluation of psychiatric patient. I. Results in a state mental health system. *Arch Gen Psychiatry.* 1989;46:733–740.

Krueger RB, Sackeim ITA, Gamzu ER. Pharmacologic treatment of the cognitive side effects of ECT: a review. *Psychopharm Bull.* 1992;28:409–424.

Lavizzo-Mourey RJ, Siegler EL. Hearing impairment in the elderly. *J Gen Intern Med.* 1992;7:191–198.

Lederle FA, Busch DL, Mattox KM, West MJ, Aske DM. Cost-effective treatment of constipation in the elderly: a randomized double-blind comparison of sorbitol and lactulose. *Am J Med.* 1990;89:597–601.

Lichenstein MJ, Bess FH, Logan SA. Validation of screening tools for identifying hearing-impaired elderly in primary care. *JAMA.* 1988;259:2875–2878.

Lipowski ZJ. Delirium in the elderly patient. *N Engl J Med.* 1989;320:578–581.

Mader S. Hearing impairment in elderly persons. *J Am Geriatr Soc.* 1984;32:548–553.

Malmrose LC, Gray SL, Pieper CF, et al. Measured versus estimated creatinine clearance in a high-functioning elderly sample: MacArthur Foundation study of healthy aging. *J Am Geriatr Soc.* 1993;41:715–721.

Manson A, Shea S. Malnutrition in elderly ambulatory medical patients. *Am J Public Health.* 1991;81:1195–1197.

Mansouri A, Lipschitz DA. Anemia in the elderly patient. *Med Clin North Am.* 1992; 76:619–630.

Marcus DL, Freedman ML. Clinical disorders of iron metabolism in the elderly. *Clin Geriatr Med.* 1985;4(1):729–745.

Messerli FH, Ventura HO, Amodea C. Osler's maneuver and pseudohypertension. *N Engl J Med.* 1985;312:1548–1551.

Molchan SE, Lawlor BA, Hill JL, et al. The TRH stimulation test in Alzheimer's disease and major depression: relationship to clinical and CSF measures. *Biol Psychiatry.* 1991;30:567–576.

Morley JE. Anorexia of aging: physiologic and pathologic. *Am J Clin Nutr.* 1997;66:760–773.

Moskowitz RW. Primary osteoarthritis: epidemiology, clinical aspects, and general management. *Am J Med.* 1987;83:5–10.

MRC Working Party. Medical research council trial of treatment of hypertension in older adults: principal results. *BMJ.* 1992;304:405–412.

Mulrow CD, Aguilar C, Endicott JE, et al. Association between hearing impairment and the quality of life of elderly individuals. *J Am Geriatr Soc.* 1990;38:45–50.

Mulrow CD, Cornell JA, Herrera CR, Kadri A, Farnett L, Aguilar C. Hypertension in the elderly: implications and generalizability of randomized trials. *JAMA.* 1994;272:1932.

Mulrow CD, Lichtenstein MJ. Screening for hearing impairment in the elderly: rationale and strategy. *J Gen Intern Med.* 1991;6:249–258.

Narins RG, Jones ER, Stom MC, et al. Diagnostic strategies in disorders of fluid, electrolyte, and acid-base homeostasis. *Am J Med.* 1982;72:496–520.

National Center for Health Statistics. Current estimates from the National Health Interview Survey, 1989. *Vital Health Stat 10.* 1990;176.

Naughton BJ, Moran MB. Patterns of syphilis testing in the elderly. *J Gen Intern Med.* 1992;7:273–275.

Nordenstam GR, Brandenberg CA, Oden AS, et al. Bacteriuria and mortality in an elderly population. *N Engl J Med.* 1986;314:1152–1156.

Okineto JT, Barnes RF, Vieth RC, et al. Screening for depression in geriatric medical patients. *Am J Psychiatry.* 1982;139:799.

Osterweil D, Brummel-Smith K, Beck JC. *Comprehensive Geriatric Assessment.* New York, NY: McGraw-Hill; 2000.

Ouslander JG. Illness and psychopathology in the elderly. *Psychiatr Clin North Am.* 1982;5:145–157.

Ouslander JG. Diagnostic evaluation of geriatric urinary incontinence. *Clin Geriatr Med.* 1986;2(4):715–730.Rahmani B, Tielsch JM, Katz J, et al. The cause-specific prevalence of visual impairment in an urban population. The Baltimore eye survey. *Ophthalmology.* 1996;103:1721–1726.

Rapp SR, Parisi SA, Wallace CE. Comorbid psychiatric disorders in elderly medical patients: a 1-year prospective study. *J Am Geriatr Soc.* 1991;39:124–131.

Ray WA, Taylor RA, Meador KG, et al. A randomized trial of a consultation service to reduce falls in nursing homes. *JAMA.* 1997;278:557–562.

Riesenberg D. Diabetes mellitus. In: Cassel CK, Reisenberg D, Sorenson LB, et al., eds. *Geriatric Medicine.* 2nd ed. New York, NY: Springer-Verlag; 1989:228–238.

Robuschi G, Safran M, Braverman LE, et al. Hypothyroidism in the elderly. *Endocr Rev.* 1987;8:142–153.

Rosenthal MJ, Hunt WC, Garry PJ, et al. Thyroid failure in the elderly: microsomal antibodies as discriminant for therapy. *JAMA.* 1987;258:209–213.

Rubenstein LZ, Josephson KR, Schulman BL, Osterweil D. The value of assessing falls in an elderly population: a randomized clinical trial. *Ann Intern Med.* 1990;113: 308–316.

Salzman C. Electroconvulsive therapy in the elderly patient. *Psychiatr Clin North Am.* 1982;5:191–197.

Saravay SM, Steinberg MD, Weinschel B, Pollack S, Alovis N. Psychological comorbidity and length of stay in the general hospital. *Am J Psychiatry.* 1991;148:324–329.

Shea JD. Pressure sores: classification and management. *Clin Orthop.* 1975;112:89–100.

SHEP Cooperative Research Group. Prevention of stroke by antihypertensive drug treatment in older persons with isolated systolic hypertension. *JAMA.* 1991;265:3255–3264.

Simons RJ, Simon JM, Demers LM, Santen RJ. Thyroid dysfunction in elderly hospitalized patients: effect of age and severity of illness. *Arch Intern Med.* 1990;150:1249–1253.

Smith DM, Winsemius DK, Besdine RW. Pressure sores in the elderly: can this outcome be improved? *J Gen Intern Med.* 1991;6:81–93.

Sorenson LB. Rheumatology. In: Cassel CK, Reisenberg D, Sorenson LB, et al., eds. *Geriatric Medicine.* 2nd ed. New York, NY: Springer-Verlag; 1989:184–211.

Staessen JA, Gasowski J, Wang JG, et al. Risks of untreated and treated isolated systolic hypertension in the elderly: meta-analysis of outcome trials. *Lancet.* 2000;355:865–872.

Stewart RB, Moore MT, Marks RG, Hale WE. Correlates of constipation in an ambulatory elderly population. *Am J Gastroenterol.* 1992;87:859–864.

Straatsma BR, Foos RY, Horwitz J, et al. Aging-related cataract: laboratory investigation and clinical management. *Ann Intern Med.* 1985;102:82–92.

Sullivan DH, Martin W, Flaxman N, Hagen JE. Oral health problems and involuntary weight loss in a population of frail elderly. *J Am Geriatr Soc.* 1993;41:725–731.

Thompson MP, Morris LK. Unexplained weight loss in the ambulatory elderly. *J Am Geriatr Soc.* 1991;39:497–500.

Thompson TL, Moran MG, Nies AS. Psychotropic drug use in the elderly. *N Engl J Med.* 1983;308:194–199.

Tinetti ME, Coucette JT, Claus EB. The contribution of predisposing and situational risk factors to serious fall injuries. *J Am Geriatr Soc.* 1995;43:1207–1213.

Tinetti ME, Speechley M. Prevention of falls among the elderly. *N Engl J Med.* 1989; 320:1055–1059.

Tinetti ME, Speechley M, Ginter SF. Risk factors for falls among elderly persons living in the community. *N Engl J Med.* 1988;319:1701–1707.

Tjoa HI, Kaplan NM. Treatment of hypertension in the elderly. *JAMA.* 1990;264:1015–1018.

Tuck ML, Griffiths RF, Johnson LE, et al. Hypertension in the elderly. *J Am Geriatr Soc.* 1988;36:630–643.

U'Ren RC. Anxiety, paranoia, and personality disorders. In: Cassel CK, Reisenberg D, Sorenson LB, et al., eds. *Geriatric Medicine.* 2nd ed. New York, NY: Springer-Verlag; 1989:491–500.

U'Ren RC, Riddle MC, Lezak MD, Bennington-Davis M. The mental efficiency of the elderly person with type II diabetes mellitus. *J Am Geriatr Soc.* 1990;38:505–510.

Veith RC. Depression in the elderly: pharmacologic considerations in treatment. *J Am Geriatr Soc.* 1982;30:581–586.

Woeber KA. Thyrotoxicosis and the heart. *N Engl J Med.* 1992;327:94–98.

Wolf SL, Barnhart HX, Kutner NG, et al. Reducing frailty and falls in older persons: an investigation of tai chi and computerized balance training. *J Am Geriatr Soc.* 1996; 44:489–497.

Working Group on Hypertension in the Elderly. Statement on hypertension in the elderly. *JAMA.* 1986;256:70–74.

Zielinski RJ, Roose SP, Devanand DP, Woodring S, Sackeim HA. Cardiovascular compliations of ECT in depressed patients with cardiac disease. *Am J Psychiatry.* 1993; 150:904–909.

Zweig S. Urinary tract infections in the elderly. *Am Fam Physician.* 1987;35:123–130.

12

The Neurological Evaluation in Geriatric Psychiatry

Jeff Victoroff, MD

The primary goal of the neurological evaluation in geriatric psychiatry is to identify evidence of nervous system dysfunction that may relate to psychiatric status. Traditionally, this is viewed as the opportunity to discover "organic" causes of psychiatric disturbance. However, our expanding knowledge of the biology of behavior compels us to reconsider this traditional view. Because it is accepted that all behavior is based in brain function, the distinction between organic and nonorganic or functional disturbances represents a false dichotomy. The endeavor is to understand the way in which neurobiological factors interact with environmental/psychological factors to produce behavior.

Therefore, the true goal is to evaluate the role of the nervous system in mediating both the homeostasis of the internal biopsychological milieu and the older patient's responsiveness to his or her environment and to attempt to identify changes in this nervous system/environment interaction that ultimately may be expressed as changes in behavior. In practical terms, the neurological evaluation is used—in concert with the history, mental status examination, medical examination, and selected laboratory tests—as one component of the integrated neurobehavioral approach to the geriatric psychiatric patient. This chapter discusses the neurological evaluation in geriatric psychiatry; it is considered within the framework of some exciting new advances in the understanding of human brain aging.

Perhaps the most passionate—and currently unresolved—debate in the field of geriatric neuropsychiatry is where to draw the lines between normal aging of the brain and aging-related pathology. This debate reflects our slow progress in coming to understand where to draw the line between the intrinsic biology of aging and the extrinsic contribution of aging-related disease (Perry & Kay, 1997). It was not until 1931 that Critchley raised the question of which neurological changes might be expected to occur in the normally aging human (Critchley, 1931), and debates still rage regarding the quality of our knowledge in this area (Drachman, 1997; Fazekas et al., 1998; Katzman, 1997). Debated with equal fervor is the question of where to draw the line between the various forms of late-life brain degeneration, such as what is usually called Alzheimer's disease (AD) and what is usually called Parkinson's disease (PD), and even the boundary between neurodegenerative and vascular forms of dementia (Ball & Murdoch, 1997). While vivid clinical examples of the extremes are encountered—for instance, comparing the highly functional elderly with those suffering with severe dementia or the brain with no pathologically confirmed strokes with the one exhibiting many—it is appreciated that the old paradigms and dichotomies do not adequately capture the shadings across the full spectrum of changes of late human adulthood or the substantial overlaps in the molecular biology of these conditions. The struggle continues to find biologically valid ways to distinguish the many dimensions in which brains tend to change—both for better and for worse—over the years.

These questions cannot be settled definitively yet. However, this chapter offers a clear outline of what is currently known about aging-related changes in the human brain and some practical implications of this knowledge for the diagnosis and management of behavioral distress in the elderly. Thus, the first part of this chapter provides a brief review of the neurology of normal aging. The second describes the neurological disorders of the elderly that are most pertinent to geriatric psychiatry; a third offers a practical guide to the neurological evaluation and its role in the comprehensive assessment of disorders of behavior in geriatric patients.

THE NEUROLOGY OF NORMAL AGING

Aging-related changes in the nervous system are typically regarded as negative and progressive. Yet there are five reasons to reconsider this view. First, as we noted above, it is sometimes extremely difficult to distinguish normal aging from pathological change. Some investigators argue that the role of aging per se has been overemphasized, and that many so-called aging-associated decrements in function can actually be accounted for by a wide array of environmental factors (Rowe & Kahn, 1987).

Second, the pace of decline is neither linear nor exponential for most functions; in fact, there is evidence of a curious leveling off of decline at very advanced ages. Third, although there are clear declines in some nervous system functions, it should not be presumed that all aging-related changes are maladaptive; gerontology theory suggests that some functions improve with age with beneficial effects on fitness (e.g., Partridge, 1997). In fact, changes in the human brain that appear disadvantageous in some ways, such as declining synaptic plasticity, may actually be advantageous in others—for instance, by maintaining our most valued patterns of synaptic connectivity (Victoroff, 1999).

Fourth, there is considerable individual variation, with some individuals exhibiting substantial preservation of function (Griffiths & Meecham, 1990). Fifth, the recent discovery that adult brains may make new neurons overthrows nearly half a century of dogma about aging and neuronal loss. Nonetheless, the average aging nervous system undergoes important changes that may have an impact on behavior, both by directly affecting function and by changing the way in which the older person perceives the environment. Although some of the changes described below are also mentioned in Chapter 5, it may be helpful to review the changes most pertinent to the neurological evaluation.

The peripheral nervous system and the muscular system—the pathway of communication from the central nervous system to the motor system and the final motor effectors themselves—both exhibit a progressive and measurable decline in function with advancing age. In many cases, this represents a combination of aging-related factors, diseases of the nervous system, and systemic diseases, including endocrine, nutritional, and vascular causes (Baker, 1989; Thomas, 1999). Our sensory receptors change in structure and decline in number with aging, and peripheral neurons exhibit (1) demyelination and remyelination, (2) distal greater than proximal axonal degeneration, (3) loss of fast-conducting peripheral axons, and (4) lipofuscin accumulation (Spencer & Ochoa, 1981).

There are age-related declines in the number of anterior horn cells and motor cranial nerve nuclei as well as demyelination and remyelination of motor roots. The result is a progressive decrease in the number of functioning motor units after 60 years of age. Muscle fiber atrophy is common and appears to accelerate after age 50 years, particularly among the type II fibers, such that by 80 years of age roughly half of skeletal muscle has been lost (Booth & Weeden, 1993). Remaining fibers exhibit signs of denervation, with the presence of target cells as well as ragged red fibers, ring fibers, lipofuscin accumulation, and increased interstitial connective tissue and fat (Hubbard & Squier, 1989; Munsat, 1984).

Electrophysiology shows decreased amplitude of sensory action potentials, decline in both sensory and motor nerve conduction velocities, increased duration of motor units, and reduced somatosensory evoked potentials with age (Smith, 1989; Thomas, 1999), which may help to account for increased weakness and sensory impairments with age. There is evidence that exercise may attenuate some of these aging-related changes in skeletal muscle structure and function (Thompson, 1994).

Most pertinent to the neuropsychiatric evaluation, of course, are the aging-related changes in the brain (Mrak et al., 1997). Two findings have revolutionized our understanding of brain aging. The first of these was the discovery that, contrary to popular neurological belief, aging-related neuronal losses might be negligible in many brain regions. Earlier estimates of loss of cortical neurons with aging were as high as 30% to 60% (Anderson et al., 1983; Henderson et al., 1980). It has been assumed that cell loss in the hippocampus was inevitable—an assumption that has been used to explain the commonly observed aging-related decline in short-term memory. It was also long assumed that we could expect a decline in subcortical and brainstem neurons, as well as a relative increase in glial cells (Coleman & Flood, 1987; Riederer & Krusik, 1987). However, this apparent decline in neuronal counts may be due in part to fixation artifacts and to a decline in the average size of neurons (which would deflate any count that is based on neuronal density) rather than to actual disappearance. Newer methods have led to different counts and to the novel idea that cortical and hippocampal neuronal loss with aging may be, to some extent, a myth. For instance, West and colleagues at the University of Aarhus in Denmark, using a quantitative cell-counting method stereology, found aging-related losses in the subiculum and the hilus of the temporal lobe, but reported virtually no loss in the Ammon's horn regions of the hippocampus—the regions most associated with memory (West, 1993). There is also strong evidence to suggest that neocortical neuron loss may be minimal with normal aging (Gomez-Isla et al., 1997; Wickelgren, 1996).

It must be borne in mind that the struggle is to understand human aging as a whole based on results from very few autopsied brains of elderly people whose mental status was assessed just prior to death (Kaye, 1997). Even if we had access to many brains from such people, the neuronal counts and degrees of regional loss might vary significantly from one individual to the next; "normal" comprises a spectrum with boundaries that remain to be defined. Furthermore, even if neurons could be counted with perfect accuracy in thousands of brains and the means and standard deviations of counts could be shown for every age, we would still face a daunting dilemma: If we only count neurons in brains from the subgroup of people with preserved mentation, we cannot know whether to regard those brains as normal or supernormal.

The second discovery is that we are probably not born with our entire lifetime supply of neurons, and that—contrary to long-held dogma—human brains may continue to manufacture new neurons, particularly in the hippocampus, even in later adulthood (Eriksson et al., 1998; Gage, 1998). This discovery constitutes a paradigm shift, providing an exciting new view of the aging brain, which is not to be conceptualized as deteriorating from adolescence, but as a dynamic entity with cells and connections that are likely to be engaged in constant turnover and renewal. Nonetheless, it is not known to what extent adult neurogenesis occurs, in what brain locations, with what individual variability, and with what functional consequence.

Despite the wealth of new findings, much remains unknown about the effects of aging per se on brains. Although it is irresistible to discuss the brain changes that affect behavior in geriatric psychiatry as either intrinsic to aging (as in so-called age-associated memory impairment) or extrinsic (signs of brain disease that lead to organic mental disorder), it is premature to make such distinctions.

The question about aging-related brain change has shifted somewhat from the issue of "how many cells" to that of "how good a brain"; many changes other than decreases in gross numbers of neurons may yield an older brain that is more vulnerable to certain neuropsychiatric conditions. For instance, there seem to be aging-related declines both in synapse density and in reactive synaptogenesis (a marker of plasticity); old brains have fewer synapses, although each remaining synapse is a bit larger—perhaps an adaptive compensatory change. In addition, certain neuronal pools are especially prone to retain the capacity for synaptic sculpting throughout life, another hint of continued adaptability of the older brain (Bertoni-Freddari et al., 1996; Cotman, 1990; Masliah et al., 1993; Perry et al., 1993).

Evidence also suggests that older persons compensate for aging-related changes by recruiting larger cortical regions to support even simple motor tasks (Mattay et al., 2002). As noted in other chapters, there are many changes in the neurochemistry of the aging brain, including declines in the production and metabolism of multiple transmitter systems. Unfortunately, the instability of brain molecules immediately after death has made it challenging to determine typical aging-related changes in neurochemistry, but new technology—such as positron emission tomography (PET) scanning—is making it increasingly practical to measure these aging-related changes in vivo (Meltzer, 1999).

Microvascular changes such as tortuous or "lumpy-bumpy" capillaries are common in brain aging, although it is hard to know the extent to which these are normal changes or signs of subclinical vascular disease (de la Torre, 1997; Moody et al., 1997). These vascular changes are probably responsible, at least in part, for the periventricular white matter changes commonly seen on neuroimaging, which should not be taken as proof of a clinically significant cerebrovascular disorder (Pantoni & Garcia, 1995).

There are also aging-related decreases in cerebral blood flow (CBF) independent of cerebrovascular disease (CVD); it is fairly well accepted that there are global declines in CBF, but there are conflicting data regarding regional declines; again, it is unclear how much CBF decline to regard as normal or excessive for age (Krausz et al., 1998; Takeda et al., 1988). Rather than considering only baseline CBF, it may be important to explore how aging, CBF, and psychiatric disease interact; for example, there may be greater declines in CBF in late-life depression compared with depression seen in younger patients (Nobler et al., 1999). It is less clear whether there is also an aging-related decline in cerebral metabolic rate, with some investigators finding clear aging-related declines using single-photon emission computed tomography (SPECT) or PET scans, particularly in the frontal cortex (e.g., Mielke et al., 1998), and others finding no decline with age (e.g., Rapoport, 1986).

Most important, there seem to be aging-related changes in human function that may relate to the biological changes reviewed above (Timiras, 1994). These changes must be taken into account in the neurological examination of the geriatric psychiatric patient and may be critical to identifying the real cause of behavior changes. While these functional changes are described in more detail below, a brief summary includes the following: Motor performance exhibits an overall decline, more for maximal performance tasks than for habitual tasks (Stones & Kozma, 1985), and both special and general sensory systems suffer a decline in function. Strength, balance, postural reflexes, and hand steadiness all decline with age (Stelmach et al., 1989; Teravainen & Calne, 1983). There is a drop-off in reaction time after the 20s, which is more marked after 50 years of age (Welford, 1988). It should be noted that both endurance and resistive exercise may significantly improve muscle strength and function in the elderly (Rogers & Evans, 1993), suggesting that ongoing physical activity might ameliorate some of these observed age-related deficits.

Normal aging also has an impact on cognition. The most commonly observed declines—even among people who have been carefully screened for brain disease—occur in speed of information processing, fluid intelligence, short-term memory, and executive function (e.g., Keys & White, 2000; Powell, 1994; Rabbitt & Lowe, 2000). These changes may be reflected in functional neuroimaging studies, which perhaps help to visualize how aging effects on brain function result in cognitive compromise (Grady et al., 1998; Rypma & D'Esposito, 2000). Still, it is difficult to determine (and passionately debated) to what degree such cognitive declines represent the inevitable and universal changes of normal aging or the earliest signs of progressive, nonuniversal dementing processes. While a few authorities present evidence that cognition remains stable in the absence of a dementing condition (e.g., Rubin et al., 1998), most find that cognitive decline occurs in normal aging and, indeed, must occur given the universality of aging-related brain changes (Binks, 1989; Celsis, 2000; Gabrieli, 1996; Kirasic & Allen, 1985; Plude & Hoyer, 1985).

In summary, there are almost certainly aging-related declines, both centrally and peripherally, in the structure and the function of the aging nervous system. There is also cognitive decline independent of the pathology of recognized dementing diseases. For both physical and cognitive function, it remains uncertain how much decline is inevitably aging related and how these changes may be modified by lifestyle, environment, or training. A familiarity with these changes may offer perspective to the neurological evaluation of the elderly psychiatric patient by orienting the examination toward vulnerable systems, changes within which may be manifested by abnormal behavior.

NEUROLOGICAL DISORDERS OF THE ELDERLY

Neurological disorders, including dementias, may be the most common cause of geriatric disability, outpacing respiratory, cardiovascular, and orthopedic/

rheumatological disorders (Broe & Creasey, 1989; Drachman & Long, 1983). In addition to their direct impact on function, neurological disorders may interact with other disorders to impair activities of daily living and degrade the quality of life, as for instance when weakness or sensory loss increase the risk of orthopedic injury or interact with restriction of joint motion to impair mobility, a major source of old age disability (Borchelt & Steinhagen-Thiessen, 1992; Jette, 1993). With the aging of the population and the advancement of medical treatment for nonneurological conditions, this disproportionate prevalence of neurological disorders will probably increase in the coming decades. Just as the challenge of determining whether age-related changes in the nervous system are normal or pathological is faced, the challenge of determining whether late-onset neurological disorders represent exaggerations of normal aging or pathophysiologically distinct conditions must be met.

There is also real uncertainty regarding whether the various forms of neurodegeneration currently regarded as clinically distinct disorders (such as Alzheimer's disease versus dementia with Lewy bodies) are in fact biologically distinct diseases. Pending further advances in our knowledge of the biological causes of these disorders, however, it remains important to discriminate between these clinically distinguishable conditions. Nervous system disorders may result from a variety of insults, including trauma, neoplasia, metabolic disorders, infection, demyelinating disease, vascular disease, and neurodegeneration. While the primary dementing conditions are described in other chapters, a brief discussion is offered here to summarize the neurological perspective on clinical features, epidemiology, pathology, and treatment of the most common central nervous system disorders of the elderly.

Neurodegenerative diseases are conditions in which populations of central nervous system neurons die or dysfunction to the point that some changes become clinically apparent, manifested by cognitive loss, psychiatric symptoms, or movement disorders. Several supposedly distinct neurodegenerative conditions are routinely distinguished, although the way in which these conditions perhaps overlap with one another and with normal aging in terms of molecular pathophysiology, environmental precipitants, microscopic pathology, and clinical symptoms are still being investigated, leading to questions about the validity of these conditions as true disease entities. Still, there are practical advantages to distinguishing between conditions (e.g., Parkinson's disease versus Alzheimer's disease) that seem to respond to particular interventions.

The currently popular nosology distinguishes AD, PD, and Parkinson's plus syndromes, which include dementia with Lewy bodies (DLB), frontal lobe dementia (FLD), progressive supranuclear palsy (PSP), and multiple system atrophy (MSA, which encompasses both olivopontocerebellar atrophy [OPCA] and striatonigral degeneration). Other degenerative disorders with perhaps better established biological grounds for consideration as distinct entities include subacute combined degeneration (SCD); the trinucleotide repeat disorders, including myotonic dystrophy and Huntington's disease (HD); the motor neuron diseases, including amyotrophic lateral sclerosis (ALS, also referred to as Lou Gerhig's disease); and the transmissible prion disorders Creutzfeldt-Jakob disease (CJD) and Gerstmann-Sträussler-Scheinker syndrome (GSS). Cerebrovascular disease is typically regarded as biologically distinct from neurodegeneration, although as noted below, CVD shares important features with neurodegenerative conditions and leads to similar clinical problems.

Aging-Related Neurodegeneration of the Alzheimer Type and Alzheimer's Disease

There have been enormous strides in identifying the underlying pathophysiology of Alzheimer-type brain changes in recent years, with the current theory focusing on the interrelated accumulation of two lesions: (1) hyperphosphorylated tau protein that disrupts microtubule assembly to produce neurofibrillary tangles and (2) excessive activity of the β- and γ-secretases that cleave the large amyloid precursor protein (APP) in such a way as to produce the more toxic Aβ42 form of amyloid, forming neuritic plaques and precipitating neuronal apoptosis (programmed cell death). Nonetheless, it remains unclear how these brain changes are provoked in most cases, whether this combination of changes represents a distinct condition or a final common pathway of many types of insults, and how these changes relate to the spectrum of normal brain aging. In addition, while there is an obvious classic presentation of these changes associated with dementia, the underlying biological changes may be developing for many years before a person exhibits the clinical picture that has come to be called Alzheimer's disease or dementia of the Alzheimer's type (*Diagnostic and Statistical Manual of Mental Disorders, Fourth Edition* [*DSM-IV*]; American Psychiatric Association, 1994). For these reasons, it may be more accurate to refer to these brain changes by the more modern term that does not presuppose the presence of dementia, aging-related neurodegeneration of the Alzheimer type (ARNAT) (Victoroff, 2000).

ARNAT may or may not eventually become apparent as a clinical syndrome that meets the criteria for mild cognitive impairment or as full-blown AD. That is, virtually everyone who survives to an advanced age will develop some of the pathological changes of AD, but only a subgroup will exhibit noticeable cognitive impairments. Therapy for AD leans heavily toward the use of cholinergic agents, but advances in primary prevention of ARNAT, as well as the experimental but not yet clinically applicable introduction of agents to block the activity of harmful secretases and vaccines against β-amyloid, may be seen. Indeed, a phase II trial was undertaken to vaccinate AD patients with amyloid peptide aggregates. The trial was halted when some subjects showed signs of a vaccination syndrome involving brain inflammation. However, subsequent work suggests that these vaccinations usually cause a selective antibody response against protein aggregates that may remove fibrillar deposits without provoking inflammation, and this therapeutic approach remains promising (Haass, 2002; Hock et al., 2002).

Classic AD is described in more detail in Chapter 16 and multiinfarct dementia is described in Chapter 17. Other types of dementias and the psychiatric disturbances associated with them are discussed in detail in Chapter 19. The following brief descriptions of several other dementing conditions provide a companion discussion of these issues.

Parkinson's Disease

PD is a progressive, disabling neurological condition. Again, popular thinking sharply distinguishes between PD and AD, although there may in fact be significant overlaps between these conditions. PD should be distinguished from parkinsonism, a constellation of motor and behavioral symptoms described below. While parkinsonism occurs in PD, this syndrome is not diagnostic of PD because it may also occur in other conditions involving damage to the nigrostriatal dopamine system.

PD was first described by James Parkinson in 1817 (Tyler, 1987) and seems to be one of the most common neurodegenerative disorders, although it is difficult to measure the prevalence of PD accurately because of variations in diagnostic threshold and access to expert neurological evaluation. Also, like ARNAT, many cases of PD-type neurodegeneration (probably the majority) will not progress to the point of overt clinical symptoms. It is clear that the prevalence of clinically apparent PD is age related. PD is rare before 40 years of age, with an age-related increase in prevalence that rises rapidly with each decade, affecting roughly 1% of those older than 65 years (Jankovic & Caine, 1987). There may be a slightly higher prevalence among men than among women.

PD is pathologically identified by two brain changes: (1) a massive death of dopaminergic neurons in the substantia nigra (SN) pars compacta, which is the origin of the nigrostriatal dopamine pathway to the basal ganglia; and (2) the presence of Lewy bodies in the brain stem, hypothalamus, basal forebrain, and cortex. The classic brain stem Lewy body is a round, eosinophilic, intracytoplasmic inclusion and contains two key proteins, the presynaptic terminal protein α-synuclein and the neuronal protein-degrading protein ubiquitin. Both proteins are also found in the plaques of Alzheimer's disease.

The cause of most cases of idiopathic PD is unknown; however, three gene mutations that can cause clinical PD have now been identified: (1) a mutation in the α-synuclein gene on chromosome 4 (4q21.3-23); (2) a mutation in the ubiquitin carboxy terminal hydrolase-L1 gene, also on chromosome 4(4p16.3); and (3) a mutation in the *parkin* gene on chromosome 6 (6q25.2-27) associated with autosomal recessive parkinsonism. Four other genetic loci responsible for familial PD have also been identified (2p13, 4p14-15, 1p35-36, and 12p11.2-

q13.1), although the genes involved have not yet been identified (Grimes & Bullman, 2002; Marsden & Olanow, 1998; Olanow & Tatton, 1999). Nonetheless, twin studies have shown little evidence of increased concordance between monozygotic twins than between dizygotic twins, strongly suggesting that the overwhelming majority of PD cases involve an environmental factor (Langston, 1998).

Research into the causes of PD has been advanced by the study of such causes of parkinsonism as the ALS-PD complex that occurs in the Chamorro Indians of Guam and the syndrome produced by the toxic compound 1-methyl-4-phenyl-1,2,5,6-tetrahydropyridine (MPTP). Studies of the latter condition revealed that PD involves dysfunctional energy metabolism, oxidative stress from increased free-radical production, or decreased antioxidant defenses, particularly inhibition of complex I of the mitochondrial respiratory chain. The current hypothesis is that PD usually results from an interaction of environmental neurotoxicants (e.g., pesticides) with genetic vulnerabilities, both acting in the setting of an aging-related reduction in defenses against xenobiotic factors (Le Couteur et al., 2002; Skipper & Farrer, 2002). There is also evidence that those with PD are less likely to have been smokers or coffee drinkers, although it is not clear whether tobacco or caffeine prevent PD or whether those with brains en route to PD will get less of a pleasurable dopamine-mediated boost from these agents (Ross et al., 2000).

Clinically, the core syndrome is marked by an insidious onset of motor slowing associated with a regular rhythmic resting tremor of about 4–7 Hz, most apparent in one or both hands, and a characteristic "cogwheel" rigidity of the limbs that consists of tremulous resistance to passive movement throughout the range of motion around large joints. In patients who have little or no tremor, the rigidity may have a smoother feel than classic cogwheeling. Facial expression is diminished (the masklike facies), and gait is usually abnormal, with a stooped posture, hesitation, shuffling, small steps, and loss of postural righting reflexes that puts the patient at risk for falls.

Behavior change in PD may affect up to 77% of individuals afflicted (Mortimer, 1988); thus, Parkinson's disease may be an important cause of psychiatric disability among the elderly. Identification of even subtle signs of Parkinson's disease on examination is important because there may be a long subclinical prodrome (Ward, 1987) during which the patient may be at risk for behavioral complications such as depression and dementia with little overt evidence of the disease. It is possible that patients with prodromal PD will exhibit increased sensitivity to the extrapyramidal side effects of neuroleptics. Depression in PD appears to be more frequent than can be accounted for by an adjustment reaction to disability, suggesting a specific neurobiological link.

The clinical features of PD may vary considerably among patients, with asymmetrical presentation or with relative predominance of tremor, rigidity, or postural instability. There is also considerable heterogeneity in age of onset, rate of progression, and responsiveness to medications (Koller, 1992).

The differential diagnosis of Parkinsonism includes idiopathic PD, neuro-leptic-induced parkinsonism, PSP, striatonigral degeneration or olivopontocer-ebellar atrophy, and parkinsonism associated with stroke. Certain clinical features may help distinguish Parkinson's disease from the motor slowing of depression and from neuroleptic effects: The bradykinesia of Parkinson's disease, unlike that of depression, will usually be associated with rigidity. Neu-roleptic-induced parkinsonism may present with cogwheel rigidity, but is asso-ciated with resting tremor less often than is idiopathic Parkinson's disease and is less often unilateral.

For many years, the main treatment strategy for idiopathic PD has been to replete the dopamine deficit with the precursor L-dopa (Koller, 2000). To in-crease delivery of L-dopa to the brain, it is usually administered with carbi-dopa, which decreases the peripheral metabolism of L-dopa by inhibiting the enzyme dopa-decarboxylase. Alternate treatment strategies include the use of agents such as pergolide mesylate and bromocriptine mesylate (direct dopa-mine receptor agonists), benztropine mesylate and trihexyphenidyl hydro-chloride (anticholinergics), and the monoamine oxidase B (MAO-B) inhibitor L-deprenyl. These agents have been used alone or in combination with L-dopa/carbidopa. Because L-deprenyl inhibits oxidation, it has been hoped that this treatment might slow disease progression by protecting neurons; it remains un-clear whether this benefit can be expected. Anticholinergic agents may be particularly helpful for ameliorating tremor. There has been expanded use of inhibitors of catechol-O-methyl transferase (COMT), such as entacapone and tolcapone, to increase the "on" time of effective control of PD symptoms (Kie-burtz & Hubble, 2000). While most patients with idiopathic PD will benefit from these anti-Parkinson's treatments, patients with related disorders that cause rigidity, such as stroke-induced parkinsonism, Wilson's disease, or multiple system atrophy, are less likely to respond.

There has been considerable progress in the investigation of treatment op-tions for PD. Experimental strategies for neuroprotection include the use of trophic agents such as GM1 ganglioside and immunomodulators that may spare substantia nigra neurons from damage. Ablative surgical procedures have re-gained favor, the most common of which is *pallidotomy*, lesioning the internal part of the globus pallidus. High-frequency deep brain stimulation of the thala-mus, the subthalamus, the globus pallidus, and the substantia nigra has also been effective in PD and is shifting from the realm of experimental to practical therapy (Jankovic, 1999).

Interest is rapidly increasing regarding the potential benefits of transplant-ing fetal dopamine-producing cells or genetically engineered cells (which pro-duce either dopamine or neurotrophins) into the brain to substitute for the loss of dopaminergic neurons. Although this approach is in the early stages of development, the progress has been rapid (Clarkson & Freed, 1999; Segovia, 2002). There is also an expectation that pigs or other animals will soon become a source of tissue for xenotransplants to treat PD (Barker et al., 2000).

Parkinson's Plus Syndromes

Parkinson's plus syndromes refers to a group of neurodegenerative disorders clinically similar to PD, although each may have distinguishing etiological, pathological, and clinical features. These syndromes include DLB, PSP, MSA, and cortical-basal ganglionic degeneration (CBGD). A debate is under way regarding the classification of these entities, with controversial lumping and splitting that may eventually be resolved by identifying underlying molecular causes (Mark, 2001).

DEMENTIA WITH LEWY BODIES Dementia with Lewy bodies is regarded by some authorities as the second most common form of neurodegenerative dementia (e.g., McKeith et al., 1999). However, because the community involved with neurological diseases began to give more attention to this condition in the 1990s, there has been considerable uncertainty about whether it should be regarded as an entity that is truly distinct from AD, a subtype of AD, or a mixture of AD with features of PD. Pathologically, this condition is supposedly distinguished from AD by the presence of Lewy bodies in the forebrain or the brain stem.

Yet, there is some question as to whether the lesions found in the brain stem are really the same as those found in the cortex: Classic Lewy bodies of the kind seen in Parkinson's disease are brain stem eosinophilic intracytoplasmic inclusions, while the cortical Lewy bodies currently accepted as diagnostic of DLB are less well defined and would be more accurately called Lewylike bodies. Both types of bodies often stain positive for the protein α-synuclein, which may be a useful point of distinction, although this protein is also found in the brains of patients with AD without either of the two types of bodies.

Furthermore, questions have been raised regarding the supposed clinical dichotomy between DLB and AD. According to the DLB International Workshop Consensus Guidelines (McKeith et al., 1996), the clinical diagnosis of probable DLB requires dementia as well as two of the following: fluctuating cognition, recurrent visual hallucinations, or parkinsonism. It has also been claimed that persons with this condition exhibit sensitivity to neuroleptics. However, these symptoms occur in AD without Lewy bodies and in PD; in practice, it has been difficult to assign clear operational criteria for the degree or frequency of these symptoms that would discriminate DLB. As a result, the Quality Standards Subcommittee of the American Academy of Neurology (Knopman et al., 2001) has noted that the clinical diagnosis of DLB has low specificity, sensitivity, and interrater reliability and advised that use of the consensus criteria for DLB is optional in clinical practice.

PROGRESSIVE SUPRANUCLEAR PALSY Progressive supranuclear palsy is another progressive neurodegenerative condition that shares some clinical features with

PD. The precise prevalence is unclear, but PSP is not a rare condition. Onset is typically in the age range of 50 to 70 years, with imbalance, visual complaints, and difficulty swallowing. PSP is frequently misdiagnosed as PD or frontotemporal lobar degeneration (FTLD), especially in the early stages when its special features are ambiguous. As in PD, there is rigidity, most apparent in the trunk, but also in the limbs. Unlike PD, there is a characteristic disorder of extraocular movements; this consists of a supranuclear ophthalmoplegia that first restricts downward gaze, later restricts upward gaze, and later still may paralyze all voluntary eye movements. Reflex eye movements, induced by rapid passive head movement, are preserved, demonstrating that the pathway from the nuclei to the extraocular muscles is intact and that the dysfunction must be superior to these brain stem nuclei (hence, supranuclear). Patients also develop a pseudobulbar palsy that consists of slurred speech, masked facies, and dysphagia. Early falls may help point to the diagnosis. Cognitive deficits are common as the disorder progresses (Rajput & Rajput, 2001).

The etiology of PSP is unknown; however, recent evidence that sporadic PSP is associated with tau gene polymorphisms suggests that this entity belongs to the family of tauopathies. In fact, cerebrospinal fluid levels of tau have been proposed as diagnostic (Pastor & Tolosa, 2002). Pathological degeneration is found in several upper brain stem and diencephalic areas, including the vestibular nuclei, pretectal nuclei, superior colliculi, red nuclei, subthalamic nucleus, and globus pallidus. Treatment with anti-Parkinson agents may be somewhat helpful for the rigidity.

MULTIPLE SYSTEM ATROPHY   Multiple system atrophy refers to a group of primary neurodegenerative conditions that have in common idiopathic neuronal loss in several central sites or systems. These conditions are probably best classified as variations on the theme of combined degeneration. MSA exhibits a predilection for damage to the basal ganglia (especially the posterior putamen and pars externa of the globus pallidus), the brain stem (especially the pontine nuclei and inferior olives), the spinal cord (especially the intermediolateral cell columns), and the cerebellar Purkinje cells. Although the term MSA might well apply to most of the neurodegenerative conditions, including PD, Huntington's disease, Friedreich's ataxia, and progressive supranuclear palsy, it is usually used to refer to (1) degeneration of the pons and cerebellum (OPCA); (2) degeneration of the nigra and striatum (striatonigral degeneration); (3) Shy-Drager syndrome, with degeneration of preganglionic sympathetic neurons, yielding PD symptoms combined with autonomic dysfunction, especially disabling orthostatic hypotension; or (4) combinations of these forms of degeneration (Mark, 2001; Wenning & Braune, 2001).

In general, MSA presents with earlier onset than idiopathic PD, with a variety of neurological symptoms that affect muscle tone, movement, and autonomic function. Distinctive hyperintensities are seen in the base of the pons on magnetic resonance imaging (MRI) scanning in most patients. Survival from diagnosis to death averages 9 years, but new evidence suggests that patients who have both motor and autonomic features at onset have a worse prognosis (Watanabe et al., 2002). A minority of patients derives clinical benefit from dopaminergic agents; ongoing studies of neuroprotective agents (e.g., riluzole) may possibly demonstrate a benefit (Wenning & Braune, 2001).

Olivopontocerebellar Atrophy.   Olivopontocerebellar atrophy is a multiple system atrophy associated with degeneration of the inferior olive and pontine nuclei of the brain stem and cerebellar atrophy most prominent in the middle cerebellar peduncles. The disorder is infrequent, but not rare. It is possible that most cases are inherited dominantly. Cerebellar ataxia is the outstanding clinical feature, but other clinical characteristics include parkinsonism, motor neuron syndrome, spasticity, and autonomic dysfunction with sometimes disabling postural hypotension. OPCA has been shown to be associated with cognitive deficits (Kish et al., 1988) and with depression. The autonomic dysfunction is associated with cell loss in the lateral horns and intermediolateral columns of the spinal cord. The parkinsonism may be associated with a loss of striatal dopamine (Kish et al., 1992). L-dopa therapy is usually ineffective.

Striatonigral Degeneration.   Striatonigral degeneration is a rarely diagnosed multiple system atrophy clinically similar to PD, but with a somewhat different pathological picture. As in PD, there is progressive rigidity, bradykinesia, and postural instability. As in OPCA, postural hypotension may occur in many cases. Pathologically, as in PD, there is major cell loss in the pars compacta of the substantia nigra. What distinguishes striatonigral degeneration from PD is the presence of more severe degeneration in the putamen and caudate nuclei of the basal ganglia. These patients may initially be diagnosed with PD, but tend to respond poorly to anti-Parkinson's agents.

CORTICOBASAL-GANGLIONIC DEGENERATION   CBGD is an unusual PD plus syndrome characterized by striking early apraxia. Patients may have relatively preserved mental status apart from inability to carry out motor commands for which they have intact motor strength and coordination.

Frontotemporal Lobar Degeneration

FTLD is a term that has come to describe a group of degenerative neuropsychiatric disorders marked by disproportionate, or unusually early, degeneration of the frontal and sometimes temporal lobes. It is clear from clinical practice that some patients present with striking loss of social decorum or self-inhibition or a loss of volition out of proportion to memory loss. Structural and functional neuroimaging and neuropathological findings all confirm that some patients experience such disproportionate frontal lobe deterioration.

However, there remains some controversy regarding the degree to which

FTLD truly represents a distinct pathogenetic entity or is instead a manifestation of one part of the ARNAT spectrum. That is, in the most common form of ARNAT, we observe early dysfunction of the temporal and parietal lobes. Yet, ARNAT can definitely strike different lobes—and even different sides of the brain—to varying degrees and at varying paces during its course, leading to the possibility that many cases of so-called FTLD are actually cases of frontally predominant ARNAT.

On the other hand, pathological findings that are highly atypical for ARNAT have been identified in the brain of some patients who present with this pattern of disproportionate frontotemporal dysfunction. Such findings include a pattern of prominent microvacuolar change (most often associated with frontal degeneration) or a pattern of severe gliosis that may or may not also exhibit ballooned cells with inclusion bodies (Pick bodies) (most often associated with combined frontotemporal degeneration). Furthermore, familial forms of FTLD have been linked to mutations on chromosome 17, and other cases were perhaps linked to chromosome 3. While this does not resolve the controversy about the relationship between ARNAT and FTLD, it increases the suspicion that neurons in the frontal lobe may have special biological vulnerabilities (Hutton et al., 1998; Mendez et al., 1996; Miller et al., 1997).

Three clinical subtypes of FTLD have been specified in newly formulated consensus criteria. The first subtype is a frontotemporal dementia, marked by early decline in social conduct, personal conduct, emotional blunting, and loss of insight. The second subtype, a progressive nonfluent aphasia, is marked by agrammatism, phonemic paraphasias (substituting similar sounds for correct words, e.g., *swatch* for *watch*). The third subtype, semantic aphasia with associative agnosia, has fluent but empty speech, loss of word meaning, semantic paraphasias (substituting similar or dissimilar concepts for correct words, e.g., *clock* or *dog* for *watch*), or it is a perceptual disorder characterized by impaired identification of familiar faces or associative agnosia, impaired recognition of objects (Neary et al., 1998).

Again, the extent to which each of these represents a unique clinicopathological entity remains unsettled. It seems most likely that (1) some cases presenting with these features will indeed be due to pathophysiology that is substantially different from that of ARNAT and specific to the clinical syndrome; (2) some cases will be due to pathophysiology that is substantially different from ARNAT, but exhibits pathology that overlaps that seen in other clinical syndromes; and (3) yet others will turn out to be atypical cases of ARNAT—with or without various degrees of cerebrovascular compromise. So, we should hesitate to embrace the new nosology as the truth. But, geriatric psychiatrists encountering atypical forms of progressive dementia may be able to recognize these intriguing syndromes—and await evidence that they may respond to treatments that are different from those we would offer the patient with classic Alzheimer's disease.

Subacute Combined Degeneration

Subacute combined degeneration (SCD) refers to the neurological disorder caused by vitamin B_{12} deficiency, most often related to pernicious anemia. Pathologically, there is loss of both myelin and axons in the white matter of the spinal cord, as well as peripheral neuropathy. This combination of lesions leads to the characteristic mix of upper and lower motor neuron signs, including absent ankle jerks and positive Babinski signs. Patients present with numbness and sometimes tingling of the feet; decreased position sense, which causes sensory ataxia; and spastic paraparesis.

Despite the well-described motor and sensory features of SCD, it remains very unclear exactly how B_{12} deficiency is related to cognitive loss. Although it is known that there is a very rough correlation between low B_{12} levels and dementia, there are two problems: First, it is possible that the lower limit of normal is generally set too high, and that people with modestly low serum B_{12} levels are at elevated risk for cognitive impairment. Second, serum levels may not accurately reflect metabolic deficiency, so even setting a more conservative standard for the normal level may not identify patients with brains at risk (Joosten et al., 1993; Lindenbaum et al., 1994). Furthermore, even if confronted by a patient with dementia and a low B_{12} level, it remains controversial whether the best correlate of cognitive impairment is the B_{12} level, elevated levels of methylmalonic acid, or of transcobolamin II, the carrier protein of B_{12}. For this reason, clinical measurement of methylmalonic acid provides no guidance regarding the likely efficacy of B_{12} supplementation (Hvas et al., 2001).

Cognitive changes and psychiatric symptoms related to B_{12} deficiency are usually attributed to cerebral demyelination. However, there is no good way to detect this pathology in the antemortem setting, which again limits the certainty that, when a patient with low B_{12} and behavioral abnormalities is seen, the two are causally related. In addition, B_{12} deficiency should probably not be regarded as typically acting alone to harm the aging brain. There is evidence that, instead, the combination of low B_{12} and ARNAT may lead to dementia (Levitt & Karlinsky, 1992; Clarke et al., 1998). Finally, when B_{12} deficiency is detected and when the clinician attributes cognitive loss to that deficiency, the extent to which monthly B_{12} injections may restore some function or prevent further deterioration is unclear (Stabler et al., 1997).

It might simply be said that there is persuasive evidence that metabolic deficiencies related to vitamin B_{12} are directly or indirectly related to cognitive loss up to or including clinical dementia. For practical purposes, if the motor and sensory signs of SCD are found, if there is no other obvious cause of these signs, if the B_{12} level is low, and if the patient is demented, then it might be concluded that the dementia is due, at least to some extent, to SCD.

Trinucleotide Repeat Disorders

Huntington's disease is a hereditary neurological condition characterized by movement disorder, dementia, and changes in personality. HD affects about 4 to 8 individuals per 100,000 (Mayeux, 1984; Nance, 1998).

The molecular basis of HD has been discovered, and HD is now considered one form of a larger group of medical problems attributed to abnormal lengthening of consecutively repeating sequences of trinucleotides in the genome. Theoretically, any trinucleotide may repeat, but in practical terms, common repeats are CAG-CAG and so on or CCG-CCG and so on (Margolis et al., 1999). At least 20 diseases seem to be caused by mutations that expand the length of repeating sequences of trinucleotides; these include the relatively common HD, fragile X syndromes, Friedreich's ataxia, and myotonic dystrophy as well as the less common conditions spinocerebellar ataxia type 6 (SCA6) and autosomal dominant cerebellar ataxia (SCA12), oculopharyngeal muscular dystrophy, and dentatorubral-pallidoluysian atrophy (DRPLA) (Wells & Warren, 1998; Yu et al., 1992). Taken together, conditions due to this problem are called the *trinucleotide expansion diseases* (TEDs).

HD is specifically due to an unstable and variable expansion of repeats of the trinucleotide CAG on chromosome 4p (Huntington's Disease Collaborative Research Group, 1993). CAG codes for the amino acid glutamine. When genes containing this repeat are translated, they create toxic forms of proteins that contain excessive glutamines (also known as *polyglutamine repeats*). This abnormal protein leads to early loss of neurons in the striatum, especially the caudate nucleus and putamen, with less damage to the cortex, thalamus, and brain stem.

There is a range of age of onset of HD, and childhood-onset cases occur, but most cases first exhibit symptoms at age 40 to 50 years. Clinically, patients may present with an insidious onset of any of the three cardinal features: (1) a hyperkinetic movement disorder that is usually choreic, with abrupt involuntary jerking or writhing of the muscles of the face, trunk, and limbs; (2) dementia, with progressive deterioration in cognitive function, usually regarded as subcortical dementia due to the relative predominance of slowed speed of information processing (Brandt & Butters, 1986); and (3) psychiatric changes marked by irritability, disinhibition, mood disorder and variably progressing to frank psychosis.

Of HD patients, 70% to 80% exhibit both dementia and some form of psychiatric disorder, and up to 40% of HD patients specifically exhibit a mood disorder (Peyser & Folstein, 1993). On neurological examination, the involuntary limb movements produce a "dancing" type of gait, and patients are unable to hold the tongue protruded.

Neuroleptic therapy may decrease both the dyskinetic motor movements and some of the psychiatric symptoms, while antidepressants may ameliorate depression. Perhaps more important, identification of the genetic basis of this disease, along with genetic counseling and prenatal testing, leads to the hope of a marked decline in incidence of this terrible condition.

Motor Neuron Diseases

Amyotrophic lateral sclerosis, or Lou Gerhig's disease, is a motor neuron disorder with a prevalence of 4 to 6 individuals per 100,000. Onset usually occurs after 40 years of age, with a mean onset at 55 years and a rapid rise in incidence over the subsequent three decades of life. About 10% of cases are familial. Familial ALS is associated with mutations of the gene on chromosome 21q encoding copper/zinc-binding superoxide dismutase, suggesting that the pathophysiology of ALS is related to toxicity by the superoxide anion (Brown, 1997; Rosen et al., 1993).

There is evidence that suggests that the more common sporadic form of ALS may be associated with enterovirus infection of neurons (Berger et al., 2000). In both familial and sporadic ALS, it is possible that excess excitatory neurotransmission is a proximal cause of cell death. The pathology of ALS involves loss of the anterior motor horn cells of the spinal cord and the motor nuclei of the brain stem (sparing the ocular motor nuclei), as well as corticospinal tract degeneration.

The clinical presentation of ALS may reflect the spastic weakness of upper motor neuron damage, the flaccid/atrophic weakness of lower motor neuron involvement, or both. Typically, patients present with weakness of one or more limbs, gait disorder, dysarthria, dysphagia, and muscle atrophy; patients with bulbar onset are possibly distinct from those with limb onset (Subcommittee on Motor Neuron Diseases, 1994). ALS is progressively disabling, ultimately affecting essentially all the major axial muscle groups, including respiratory muscles, with death usually occurring 2 to 5 years after onset. Older patients and those with more respiratory compromise tend to have shorter survival (Stambler et al., 1998).

Although the classic understanding of ALS is that it is a condition confined to motor neurons, there is evidence that some ALS patients—perhaps those with bulbar onset in particular—will also develop precentral cortical cell loss associated with cognitive deficits. These include impairments of working memory and recognition memory, word generation, and visual perception (Strong et al., 1999).

The neurological examination reveals variable degrees of weakness and muscle atrophy with fasciculations, often including characteristic atrophy and fasciculations of the tongue. Deep tendon reflexes may be increased or decreased. Sensation and mentation are typically preserved, unfortunately leaving many patients with clear insight into their inevitable deterioration. The principal differential diagnosis is cervical spondylosis, multiple sclerosis, or less commonly, syrinx, all of which can mimic many features of the clinical syndrome of ALS.

Treatment of ALS is extremely difficult and somewhat controversial. Riluzole was approved by the Food and Drug Administration (FDA) in 1997 and became standard therapy in the late 1990s. The drug acts by inhibiting the release of the excitatory transmitter glutamate and by inhibiting sodium entry (Bensimon et al., 1994; "Practice Advisory on the Treatment of Amyotrophic Lateral Sclerosis," 1997). However, some neurologists and patients have been disappointed with the likelihood and the magnitude of the therapeutic benefit (Ludolph & Riepe, 1999). Hope for the benefit of other treatments, such as recombinant ciliary neurotrophic factor and interferon beta, was largely dashed by controlled trials (ALS CNTF Treatment Study Group, 1996; Beghi et al., 2000). On the other hand, there is preliminary evidence of a treatment benefit with insulinlike growth factor I and perhaps with brain-derived neurotrophic factor ("A Controlled Trial," 1999; Lai et al., 1997). A new category of drugs has been proposed as a treatment for ALS: Caspases are enzymes that turn on apoptosis, essentially becoming neuronal executioners in animal models of ALS; there is now evidence that caspase inhibitors defend the nervous system from this devastating disease (Gurney et al., 2000; Li et al., 2000). Experiments such as this hold out new hope for practical, effective ALS therapy in the reasonably near future.

Transmissible Prion Disorders

CJD and GSS are both rare transmissible degenerative disorders associated with brain accumulation of a protease-resistant prion protein, PrP. Almost all cases of GSS and about 10% to 15% of cases of CJD are familial. CJD garnered international attention due to a statistically significant increase in cases among Europeans who ate beef infected with "mad cow disease" (bovine spongiform encephalopathy), apparently circulating in the food chain because cattle had been fed infected animal protein. Fortunately, new methods have been developed to screen animals rapidly for the presence of this disease.

In the past, it was unclear how the familial and sporadic forms of prion diseases were related. Then, in 1999, it was shown that the common feature of all such diseases is the presence of an excessive amount of a transmembrane version of the prion protein, called ^{Ctm}PrP. Normal prion proteins defend neurons from cell death, while ^{Ctm}PrP fails to do so; excess ^{Ctm}PrP may be responsible for both genetic and transmissible forms of prion diseases (Hedge et al., 1999).

The pathology of CJD is notable for cytoplasmic vacuoles in neurons and glia, giving the brain a characteristic spongiform microscopic appearance. Clinically, CJD manifests with the gradual onset of dementia that becomes accompanied by weakness, spasticity, extrapyramidal-type rigidity, and myoclonic jerks. These jerks are more lightninglike than the choreic jerks of HD and may be evoked by stimuli such as loud noises or tapping the reflexes. CJD is rapidly progressive, with death usually occurring within a year of diagnosis.

GSS is a related transmissible encephalopathy, with the pathological appearance of both amyloid plaques, as in AD, and spongiform change, as in CJD. Clinically, GSS is a rare condition that presents with dementia and ataxia. No treatments are currently available for either CJD or GSS.

Cerebrovascular Disease

CVD is a single term that encompasses a complex, multifaceted disorder. The brain may be injured by acute, subacute, or chronic vascular changes from the intracranial or extracranial circulatory system. In addition, as noted above, certain microvascular changes appear to accompany normal aging. Although CVD may refer to the steady-state condition of abnormal vasculature, in practice it usually refers to a spectrum of clinical events and sequelae related to altered blood flow in the brain: transient ischemic attack (TIA), reversible ischemic neurological deficit (RIND), ischemic and hemorrhagic infarction (stroke), and subarachnoid hemorrhage.

By convention, TIAs refer to sudden focal neurological deficits attributed to cerebral ischemia, with complete clinical resolution within 24 hours, and RINDs refer to deficits persisting beyond 24 hours, but resolving within 2 weeks. However, 35% of RINDs are associated with computed tomographic (CT) changes (Koudstall et al., 1992), suggesting that these categorical distinctions may not represent true pathophysiological differences as much as clinically detectable reference points along a continuum. Stroke is the most common neurological disorder of the elderly and the third leading cause of death in the United States. Stroke rates are age related, doubling with each decade from the fifth through the ninth. After an apparent decline in the rate of stroke during the 1960s and 1970s, attributed to increasingly successful management of hypertension, there is evidence of a leveling off of the rate of decline or possibly even an increase in stroke rate since the early 1980s (Kuller, 1989).

TIAs can occur in the anterior (carotid) or posterior (vertebrobasilar) circulation. Common symptoms of carotid TIAs are transient monocular blindness (or amaurosis fugax) and transient contralateral hemispheric syndromes that often produce motor or sensory changes of a limb. Vertebrobasilar TIAs usually manifest as diplopia, vertigo, dysarthria, or ataxia. Although transient cerebral ischemia may also cause syncope or seizures, these clinical events themselves are not usually referred to as TIAs.

Stroke refers to the syndrome of a lasting change in central function attributed to CVD (Batjer, 1997). The causes of stroke are manifold, but the most common categories include stroke due to thrombosis within the intracranial vessel; stroke due to embolus from the extracranial carotid artery; stroke due to cardiogenic embolus; stroke due to global hypoperfusion; or stroke due to hematological changes such as hypercoagulable states. The symptoms of stroke are extremely variable. Carotid territory hemispheric strokes often present with contralateral motor or sensory deficits, visual field deficits, or impairment of higher cortical functions such as aphasias, apraxias, or confusion. Vertebrobasilar territory strokes often present with dizziness or vertigo, ataxia or staggering gait, diplopia, occipital visual field deficits, or motor or sensory syndromes attributable to ischemia of the brain stem nuclei and tracts.

Intracranial hemorrhage may occur due to primary hypertensive hemorrhage, rupture of aneurysm or arteriovenous malformation, or trauma. Primary hypertensive hemorrhage, usually associated with long-standing chronic hypertension, presents with rapid or sudden onset of focal neurological deficit, often progressing over several hours and sometimes accompanied by impairment of consciousness. The most common sites of primary hypertensive hemorrhage are the putamen and adjacent internal capsule, the thalamus, the cerebellum, and the pons. Subarachnoid hemorrhage, most often due to rupture of a saccular aneurysm, usually presents with the sudden onset of severe headache, often associated with nausea, vomiting, and impairment or loss of consciousness. Focal neurological deficits are less common. The outcome of subarachnoid bleeding is related to the preservation of consciousness after the bleed. Relatively minor head trauma may cause subdural hematoma in the elderly, which may present as headache, focal neurological deficits, lethargy, or simply a change in behavior that is sometimes mistakenly attributed to neurodegenerative dementia or functional psychiatric disorder.

Treatment of stroke can be divided into primary prevention (before the first episode), secondary prevention (after the first episode), acute intervention, and rehabilitation/brain repair. Primary and secondary prevention of stroke focus on control of known risk factors, including hypertension, smoking, alcohol use, obesity, and inactivity (Gorelick et al., 1999). Elevated serum total and low-density lipoprotein (LDL) cholesterol and triglycerides are also risk factors for ischemic stroke, and there is evidence that treatment with HMG-CoA (3-hydroxy-3-methylglutaryl coenzyme A) reductase inhibitors (statins) can reduce this risk (Lewis et al., 1998; Salonen et al., 1995). Elevated serum homocysteine has also gained increased attention as a risk factor for stroke (Bots et al., 1999); in addition, recent evidence suggests that elevated homocysteine levels are associated with increased brain atrophy independent of stroke (Sachdev et al., 2002). Clinical trials are needed to see whether lowering homocysteine with folic acid, vitamin B_{12}, and vitamin B_6 will reduce these risks. There is also intriguing evidence that seropositivity for Chlamydia pneumoniae may be a risk factor for stroke (Fagerberg et al., 1999); again, the appropriate intervention is uncertain.

Chronic antiplatelet therapy with aspirin, ticlopidine, or clopidigrel has been shown to reduce the risk of stroke among patients who have suffered a TIA or stroke, although the use of these agents in primary prevention remains controversial, in part because patients with poorly controlled hypertension treated with antiplatelet agents may actually have an increased risk for hemorrhagic stroke (Antiplatelet Trialists' Collaboration, 1994). After myocardial infarction, warfarin helps prevent stroke in patients who also have atrial fibrillation, decreased left ventricular ejection fraction, or left ventricular thrombus (Gorelick et al., 1999). There is evidence that some patients with symptomatic high-grade carotid stenosis (>60%) will benefit from carotid endarterectomy, although uncertainty remains regarding the best strategy for patient selection and results may depend greatly on the skill of the operative team (Biller at al., 1998).

The management of acute stroke is evolving as new approaches and agents are developed (Fisher & Bogousslavsky, 1998; Marler et al., 1997). By far the major advance in the 1990s was the introduction of the concept of the "brain attack," recognition that—in select patients—intervention within a brief window of opportunity shortly after the stroke might significantly improve outcome.

The primary method of acute intervention consists of thrombolysis via intravenous infusion of tissue plasminogen activator (t-PA). The National Institute of Neurological Disorders and Stroke (NINDS) study showed that patients who underwent t-PA treatment were somewhat more likely to experience intracerebral hemorrhage, but were at least 30% more likely to have minimal or no disability at three months compared with patients treated with placebo (NINDS rt-PA Study Group, 1995); as a result, in 1996, t-PA was approved by the FDA for treatment of stroke within 3 hours of symptom onset. Thrombolytic therapy appears to be especially safe and efficacious when the stroke is small and nonhemorrhagic. Evidence shows that patients treated with t-PA patients maintain their advantage at 1 year (Kwiatkowski et al., 1999).

Other approaches to acute intervention under investigation include several reperfusion strategies, such as hemodilution to reduce viscosity and improve cerebral blood flow and thrombolysis via percutaneous transluminal intracranial angioplasty. Findings regarding the cellular pathophysiological sequence of acute ischemic infarction suggest possible benefits of neuroprotective agents that may interrupt this sequence. Neurotoxicity due to postsynaptic reception of excitatory amino acid (EAA) neurotransmitters such as N-methyl-D-aspartate may be ameliorated by EAA receptor blockers or by agents that prevent EAA release, although receptor blockade may cause unacceptable behavioral side effects. Excessive calcium influx may contribute to cell death and may be inhibited by dihydropyridine calcium channel blockers. Free-radical production may play a role in ischemic cell death, suggesting possible benefits of antioxidants or free-radical scavengers such as the 21 amino steroids (lazaroids). Even high-dose conventional glucocorticosteroids may prove beneficial if introduced early enough. Despite the promise of these new methods, most studies suggest a relatively brief window of opportunity for intervention with neuroprotective agents, perhaps limited to as little as 60 to 120 minutes after a stroke.

Treatment of subarachnoid hemorrhage is focused on limiting further bleeding by management of blood pressure, control of vasospasm with nimodipine, angiography to determine the cause of the bleed, and surgical clipping of aneurysms. Surgery has the best outcome in patients who have retained normal consciousness. Treatment of subdural hematoma depends on the size and the presence of increased intracranial pressure or shift of intracranial structures. Large hematomas require surgical evacuation. CT scanning may be particularly valuable for diagnosing such lesions, because this neuroimaging technique is more sensitive than MRI imaging for identifying hemorrhages.

Improving brain function after acute treatment for stroke is usually regarded as a matter of optimum rehabilitation, and steady progress in this field has led to improved functional outcomes. However, there is already evidence that brain repair—in the form of neuronal transplants—may become a legitimate option in the near future (Zivin, 2000).

It is obvious and well documented that strokes can lead to changes in behavior, many of which are pertinent to geriatric psychiatry. These changes include specific syndromes attributed to the focal impact of strokes, such as aphasias, apraxias, and agnosias, as well as psychiatric disorders such as secondary depression, secondary mania, and psychoses. Some evidence suggests that left-sided and more anterior strokes are more likely to be associated with depression, although a review of 48 reports questioned this claim and demonstrated that the likelihood of poststroke depression is probably not related to the hemisphere affected (Carson et al., 2000; Greenwald et al., 1998; Krishnan et al., 1997).

In contrast, features of aphasia correlate fairly well with the location of the stroke and deserve special mention. Before turning to the brain-behavior correlations of aphasiology, several points bear mentioning: First, the classic aphasias in pure form are rare. This is because few strokes neatly ablate Broca's or Wernicke's areas; many more strokes damage the brain tissue adjacent to or underlying these small classic areas. Aphasias caused by damage to this large swath of tissue near (but not in) the classic language centers are called *transcortical aphasias*. Thus, because strokes are much more likely to strike this large area of language-supporting tissue than to strike the small classic language centers, a clinician is much more likely to encounter a transcortical motor aphasia than a Broca's aphasia and more likely to encounter a transcortical sensory aphasia than a Wernicke's aphasia. Second, lesions in different places can produce identical aphasias. This is because a distributed network of cells rather than a discreet clump of neurons supports each language function. For example, a small stroke in the left anterior thalamus may produce an aphasia that is clinically indistinguishable from that produced by a large stroke in the cortex overlying that part of the thalamus. Third, aphasias evolve with time. This is because the metabolically dramatic initial stage of stroke may produce widespread cortical dysfunction and global aphasia; this resolves to a more circumscribed aphasia after several hours or days, and compensatory recruitment of nearby cortex will reduce the aphasia even more in the following weeks and months.

That said, the anterior language system is located in the dominant frontal lobe in and around Broca's area (a small part of the posterior inferior prefrontal gyrus); it supports fluent production of spoken and written language, so lesions in this region tend to make speech slow, sparse, effortful, or aromatic. The posterior language system is located in the dominant temporal and parietal lobes in and around Wernicke's area (a small part of the posterior superior temporal gyrus); it supports understanding of spoken and written language, so lesions in this region tend to make the patient confused about what has been said and to make their speech confusing to hear (word salad) (Kuest & Karbe, 2002; Saffran, 2000).

One good way to summarize the aphasias—and how to test for them—is to consider the three parts of the language system needed to repeat: (1) Wernicke's area decodes the words that are heard, (2) the arcuate fasciculus carries this information forward, and (3) Broca's area encodes the utterance into speakable form, then sends this information to the motor strip for activation of the cranial nerves serving speech. Because damage to any of these three essential parts will impair repetition, if the patient struggles to repeat a nonsense phrase (e.g., "no ifs, ands, or buts"), there must be damage to one of these parts. However, if repetition is relatively preserved, it suggests that the lesion spared all three parts and is elsewhere in the dominant hemisphere.

Thus, as shown in Table 12-1, the rare-but-classic Wernicke's, Broca's, and conduction aphasias involve impaired repetition, while the more common transcortical motor, transcortical sensory, and mixed transcortical aphasias spare the three-part system and involve relatively preserved repetition. Aphemia can also be explained in terms of this simple three-part system: In *aphemia*, the patient cannot speak fluently, but can write fluently. This is because strokes sometimes selectively damage the tracts that carry language from Broca's area to the sector of the motor strip that controls the muscles of articulation, but spare the tracts going to the hand sector. A geriatric specialist should be familiar with the aphasias listed in Table 12-1.

Perhaps the most important—and controversial—issue regarding CVD and altered behavior in the elderly is the relationship between CVD and dementia. Vascular dementia (VaD; *DSM-IV* 290.4) is typically defined as the presence of the dementia syndrome—a functionally significant decline from the previously established level of cognitive function—that is judged etiologically related to CVD. Yet, there is great uncertainty about the best way to demonstrate that etiological link; as a result, multiple competing criteria for VaD have been developed (Chui et al., 1992; Roman et al., 1993). Furthermore, according to the conventional dichotomy, AD and VaD are substantially different entities: AD is a neurodegenerative disorder marked by a gradual progression and global cognitive changes, while VaD is a vascular disorder marked by stepwise progression and "patchy" cognitive deficits.

Yet, this strict dichotomy oversimplifies the complex relationship between AD and VaD. For one thing, it is clear that CVD increases the expression of

TABLE 12-1. The aphasias

Aphasia type	Lesion location	Fluency (spoken and written)	Comprehension (auditory and writing)	Repetition
Broca's	Posterior inferior dominant frontal lobe	Impaired: limited output with effortful or stereotyped speech	Preserved	Impaired
Wernicke's	Posterior superior dominant temporal gyrus	Often impaired: rate and amount of output preserved, but "word salad"	Impaired	Impaired
Global	Combined frontal plus either temporal or parietal lobe damage	Impaired	Impaired	Impaired
Conduction	Arcuate fasciculus	Relatively preserved	Relatively preserved	Impaired
Transcortical motor aphasia	Dominant frontal lobe near Broca's area	Impaired	Impaired	Relatively preserved
Transcortical sensory aphasia	Dominant posterior temporal or inferior parietal lobe near Wernicke's area	Often impaired: rate and amount of output preserved, but "word salad"	Impaired	Relatively preserved
Mixed transcortical aphasia	Combined frontal plus either temporal or parietal lobe damage*	Impaired	Impaired	Relatively preserved
Aphemia	Base of precentral gyrus	Speaking impaired; writing preserved	Preserved	Spoken impaired; written preserved

*But sparing Broca's area, Wernicke's area, and the arcuate fasciculus.

cognitive deficits in AD, and that, if not for AD-type pathological changes, the relationship between CVD and dementia would be weak (Heyman et al., 1998; Nagy et al., 1997; Wu et al., 2002). For another, AD and VaD overlap in many important ways, including shared risk factors, overlapping microvascular changes, overlapping clinical syndromes, and shared molecular pathways leading to neuronal death (Alavi et al., 1998; Crawford, 1996; de la Torre, 1997). This is not to say that subgroups of demented patients with more or less vascular pathology cannot be distinguished, but instead acknowledges that further research is needed to truly understand the cause-and-effect relationships among CVD, VaD, AD, and dementia.

Temporal arteritis is a perivascular inflammatory condition of the temporal branches of the external carotid artery. The condition occurs almost exclusively in the elderly, most often affecting those in the sixth to eighth decades. The patient presents with unilateral temporal region headache, ipsilateral visual impairment, as well as systemic signs of illness such as fever, anorexia, malaise or depression, increased white count, and elevated sedimentation rate. The involved temporal artery may be tender and prominent. There is an overlap between temporal arteritis and the syndrome of polymyalgia rheumatica, in which diffuse myalgia without focal weakness occurs, sometimes combined with the cranial symptoms and pathological changes of temporal arteritis (DiBartolomeo & Brick, 1992). Because it is possible for temporal arteritis to occur in the presence of a normal sedimentation rate, psychiatrists may conceivably encounter depressed patients in whom this diagnosis has not previously been suspected. Prompt recognition is important because intervention with corticosteroids may preserve vision.

Brain neoplasms present throughout life, with about 40,000 new tumors diagnosed each year and a prevalence of roughly 20 cases per 100,000 adults. Half of these tumors are metastases from other sites (most commonly from the lung, breast, and gastrointestinal tract), and half are primary intracranial tumors. Primary brain tumors exhibit an age-related increase in prevalence. According to the traditional cell-type-based classification scheme, the most common primary brain tumor cell type first diagnosed among the elderly is the glioma, which accounts for nearly 50% of all brain tumors. About half of gliomas are the slower-growing, low-grade astrocytomas, while the other half are the fast-growing glioblastoma multiforme. Meningiomas account for about 15% of adult brain tumors; metastatic tumors, pituitary tumors, and acoustic neuromas each account for about 10% of tumors. It should be noted, however, that advances in molecular oncology have raised the question of a new classification of brain tumors based on underlying genetic pathophysiology (Darling & Warr, 1998; Hill et al., 1999).

The clinical presentation of intracranial tumors depends greatly on both location and rate of growth. Slow-growing tumors may present with focal neurological signs, personality change, or seizures long before there is any symptomatic increase in intracranial pressure. Pituitary tumors may present either with visual field defects related to pressure on the optic chiasm or endocrine dysfunctions related to the changes in the secretion of gonadotropins, prolactin, corticotropin (ACTH), or thyroid-stimulating hormone. Tumors in the cerebellopontine angle, most often acoustic neuromas, may present with unilateral hearing loss and sometimes with facial weakness or numbness. Rapidly growing tumors, either in the cerebellum or the cerebral hemispheres, may present with symptoms of increased intracranial pressure, including headache, lethargy, confusion, ataxia, nausea, and vomiting. Tumors sometimes present suddenly, like a stroke, either because they reach a critical size threshold or because they undergo hemorrhagic change.

The clinical outcome of intracranial tumors also varies significantly depending on cell type, location, and rate of growth. Slow-growing meningiomas may be essentially cured by surgical removal. Fast-growing gliobastomas are notoriously difficult to treat and currently typically lead to death within a year of diagnosis irrespective of therapy.

Treatment of intracranial tumors is directed at decreasing intracranial pressure, unblocking flow of cerebrospinal fluid, removing the bulk of the tumor, and killing neoplastic cells. Depending again on the type and location of the tumor, treatment may involve several modalities, alone or in combination. Corticosteroids are often used to control the vasogenic edema associated with many tumors. Neurosurgery may be used to biopsy the tumor to identify cell type, to remove the entire tumor, to debulk the lesion without complete removal, or to shunt fluid from the ventricles. Conventional chemotherapy has been of limited value in the treatment of gliomas, the most common tumors of adulthood. Radiotherapy has been a mainstay of intracranial tumor treatment, and new techniques make it increasingly possible to deliver focused doses of irradiation via particle beams, high-energy stereotactic radiosurgery, or focused gamma rays.

Brain tumor therapy is undergoing something of a revolution. Exciting new strategies for better treating these difficult neoplasms are being actively developed on multiple fronts, including antiangiogenesis, oncolytic virus therapy, and multiple forms of gene therapy, such as immunogene therapy, the introduction of tumor suppressor genes (such as the p53 gene), cell-cycle modulators, and "suicide" genes that render tumor cells more vulnerable to otherwise nontoxic prodrugs (Fueyo et al., 1999; Shapiro, 1999). Although these therapies are mostly at the stage of animal research, some are already in phase I or II human trials, so significant improvements in outcomes might be seen in the early part of the 21st century. As the possibility of effective treatment increases, so does the need for early diagnosis, meaning that the geriatric psychiatrist will have increased motivation to detect behavioral or neurological changes that might be attributable to a brain tumor.

HIV-1-associated dementia (HAD; sometimes referred to as HIV-1 [human immunodeficiency virus type 1] encephalopathy or the acquired immunodeficiency syndrome [AIDS]–dementia complex) occurs in 15% to 20% of

AIDS patients and is the first AIDS-defining illness in about 7% of cases (Jannsen et al., 1992; McArthur et al., 1993). HAD typically produces a subcortical dementia with significant psychomotor slowing. Other typical mental status changes include short-term memory loss, apathy, depression, and more rarely, psychosis. The neurological exam often reveals psychomotor slowing, tremor, unsteady gait, hyperreflexia, hypertonia, and frontal release signs. Neuroimaging often shows atrophy and white matter changes. The pathological features of HAD include brain atrophy, microglial nodules, multinucleated giant cells, activated macrophages and other signs of inflammatory response, vacuolar myelopathy, pallor of the white matter, and sometimes, frank infarctions (Bouwman et al., 1998; McArthur et al., 1999). Progression and clinical features are variable, depending on whether the patient suffers from a secondary brain infarction causing symptoms. Although the past experience with this condition is that it occurs only in the preterminal phase of AIDS, with survival times averaging 3 to 6 months, new treatments may perhaps prolong the course. As a result, HAD may be seen with increasing frequency in the geriatric neuropsychiatry population, as those infected after 1980 survive for longer periods. The symptoms of HAD may be treated, or even prevented, by antiretroviral therapy with high-dose zidovudine (Sacktor & McArthur, 1997).

NEUROLOGICAL ASSESSMENT IN GERIATRIC PSYCHIATRY: POTENTIAL RELATIONSHIP TO PSYCHOPATHOLOGY

There are a number of ways to regard the relationship between neurological abnormalities and behavioral changes:

1. The neurological condition might be considered the proximate biological cause of the psychiatric condition, such as dementia due to neurosyphilis.
2. The neurological condition and psychiatric condition may be two manifestations of a shared neurobiological change, such as right hemiparesis and depression due to left frontal lobe infarction (Robinson et al., 1984).
3. The neurological condition may represent a psychological stressor that lowers the threshold for appearance of the psychiatric condition, such as an adjustment reaction with depressed mood related to lumbar spondylosis (Love, 1987).
4. A psychiatric condition may serve as a stress under which a previously covert neurological impairment becomes apparent (e.g., the emergence of an underlying dementia during an episode of depression) (Kral, 1983).
5. The treatment for the neurological condition may produce or exacerbate psychopathology, such as psychosis related to L-dopa therapy in Parkinson's disease (Klawans, 1982).
6. Treatment of a psychiatric condition may produce or exacerbate a

neurological problem (e.g., the wide range of neuroleptic-induced extrapyramidal disorders) (Marsden & Jenner, 1980).

7. A somatoform psychiatric disorder may mimic or embellish a neurological disorder, as in hysterical paralysis (Strub & Black, 1988).

8. A psychological factor may lead to elaboration of an underlying neurological disorder; an example would be the co-occurrence of seizures and pseudoseizures.

9. The neurological and psychiatric conditions may be independent but coincident in time.

Determining the causal relationship between co-occurring neurological and psychiatric conditions is valuable, although in many cases, present knowledge does not permit precise determination of causality in behavioral dysfunction. Therefore, in the discussion that follows, the emphasis is on practical strategies to integrate the neurological assessment into the neuropsychiatric evaluation.

The Neurological History in Geriatric Psychiatry

Given the behavioral significance of neurological disease, the geriatric psychiatric evaluation must always include a careful neurological history. In addition, due to the possibilities of denial, somatization, or failing memory, it is important to seek independent confirmation of neurological complaints or experiences, usually from a spouse or other close relative. Further, because even remote or seemingly unrelated neurological events may be important in the genesis of a behavioral problem (e.g., the minor "bump on the head" that led to an undetected subdural hemorrhage and gradual personality change), it is important to press for any neurological experiences or symptoms of possible relevance. The focus and depth of this exploration will depend on individual circumstances; however, a good general neurological review should consider history of the following: cognitive change, personality change, head trauma, acute decline in function, transient or paroxysmal neurological symptoms, dizziness, progressive focal motor or sensory dysfunction, alteration in special senses, new headache, gait disturbance, incontinence, sleep disturbance, or exposure to centrally acting substances.

COGNITIVE CHANGE A neurological disorder may produce both cognitive and noncognitive dysfunction (e.g., dementia and paranoia in Alzheimer's disease). Therefore, the interview should include a careful review of subtle new intellectual deficits, such as forgetfulness, verbal symptoms such as word-finding difficulty, or visuospatial symptoms such as difficulty navigating through town.

PERSONALITY CHANGE Personality is remarkably stable through the life span. When family or friends note a change in a short period of time, it can be an important clue to a new neuropsychiatric condition, including anything from a primary psychiatric condition such as major depression, to an endocrine or metabolic disturbance, to stroke or increased intracranial pressure. New onset of irritability, in particular, can be a tip-off to new cerebral compromise.

HEAD TRAUMA   Of a population of 100,000, 200 to 300 are admitted to hospitals for head trauma each year, and there are probably many more nonhospitalized cases (Jennett & Teasdale, 1981). The chance of persistent behavioral sequelae is probably higher in cases with loss of consciousness lasting more than 24 hours or posttraumatic amnesia lasting more than 1 week. However, even minor head trauma deserves consideration as a possible precipitant of post-concussion syndrome, subdural hematoma, or posttraumatic epilepsy. More-over, injuries without direct trauma to the occiput—such as whiplash—may also produce cognitive or affective changes (Yarnell & Rossie, 1988). The recovery from head trauma is likely to be slower and less complete in older patients (Duffy & Fogel 1994; Wrightson, 1989). Head trauma can definitely be followed by depressive mood disorder, especially after left anterior injury (Ownsworth & Oei, 1998). It is also possible (but not definite) that head trauma is a risk factor for the development of ARNAT and Alzheimer's disease (Launer et al., 1999; Mayeux et al., 1995; Mortimer et al., 1991).

ACUTE DECLINE IN FUNCTION   Any acute change in function raises the question of stroke or transient ischemic attack. Small strokes may escape recognition or medical evaluation until the secondary behavioral problems emerge (e.g., dementia or affective change) because they fail to produce overt focal symptoms or signs. It is also possible for a slowly progressive process to reach a critical stage and then present with acute symptoms suggestive of stroke (e.g., an expanding tumor mass that finally produces observable dysfunction). On the other hand, it is possible for a nonacute process to present in a pseudoacute way when other factors lower the patient's reserve; an example is the appearance of the first signs of primary degenerative dementia during a stressful time such as a move, a loss, or a medical problem.

TRANSIENT OR PAROXYSMAL NEUROLOGICAL SYMPTOMS   Syncopal episodes often suggest a cardiac arrhythmia with increased stroke risk (and possible association with anxiety disorders). However, transient ischemic attacks or partial seizures may go unrecognized due to a vague or atypical history. Inquiring about any faints or "funny turns" may elicit this history.

DIZZINESS   As noted above, peripheral vestibulopathy is common in the elderly and may produce both subjective symptoms and gait unsteadiness. In the patient complaining of "dizziness," it is important to distinguish *light-headed-ness*, a near-fainting sensation that can be due to postural hypotension, vasovagal responses, or presyncopal symptoms of cardiac arrhythmia, from *vertigo*, a sense of movement with respect to the surroundings that may be produced by a wide range of central or peripheral vestibular pathology, including behaviorally relevant conditions such as migraine, vertebrobasilar insufficiency, or posterior fossa tumors (Baloh, 1984).

PROGRESSIVE FOCAL MOTOR OR SENSORY DYSFUNCTION Weakness, numbness, or discoordination of any part of the body requires further neurological evaluation. Although symptoms confined to a single extremity may initially suggest a peripheral process without relevance to behavior, many disorders with potential behavioral associations (for example, multiinfarct dementia [MID], idiopathic PD, ALS) may present with asymmetrical or focal symptoms.

ALTERATION IN SPECIAL SENSES Changes in hearing or vision in particular may relate to psychiatric dysfunction in three ways: Primary sensory disorders may produce sensory deprivation that is associated with hallucinations in the affected sensory modality (Benson, 1989; Cummings, 1985); sensory disorders may create misperceptions of the environment that potentially lead to such problems as the paranoia of the hearing impaired (Cooper & Curry, 1976); sensory disorders may be symptomatic of a central dysfunction (stroke, tumor, demyelinating disease, etc.) that itself may alter behavior.

NEW HEADACHE Although a lifetime history of vascular or muscle tension headaches is probably not relevant to a new behavioral disorder, the recent onset of headaches in an elderly patient or a significant change in previous headache symptoms suggests the possibility of intracranial mass lesion or increased intracranial pressure, chronic meningitis, or temporal arteritis (in addition to more common problems such as hypertension, cervical spondylosis, sinusitis, or glaucoma).

GAIT DISTURBANCE Gait disorders have been reported to produce disability in 13% of the aged, even excluding those gait disturbances caused by specific medical diseases (Larish et al., 1988). Although geriatric gait disorders are often multifactorial, complaints of new dysfunction can be suggestive of behaviorally relevant disorders such as multiinfarct dementia, increased intracranial pressure, normal-pressure hydrocephalus (NPH), or Parkinson's disease.

INCONTINENCE There are, of course, nonneurological causes of new onset incontinence in the aged—especially urinary tract infection or stress incontinence due to bladder neck dependency in women or prostatic hypertrophy in men. However, a history of new-onset incontinence may also be the first sign of normal pressure hydrocephalus or an alert to other neurological problems, such as a recent silent stroke or subdural hematoma.

SLEEP DISTURBANCE Aging is associated with decreased slow-wave sleep and in-creased nocturnal wakefulness. One third of the elderly experience frequent sleep interruptions due to apnea or hypopnea, even in the absence of complaints about sleep. Snoring is increasingly common with age, usually indicates some degree of upper airway obstruction, and is associated with hypertension and cardiovascular disease (Dement et al., 1985). Therefore, nocturnal respiratory status may be compromised not only in patients with sleep complaints such as daytime sleepiness, choking attacks, or morning headache, but also in those who simply snore. A history of snoring or other sleep disturbance may be rele-vant to the presenting psychiatric problem because there is evidence that sleep apnea may be associated with psychopathology or cognitive deficits (Kales et al., 1985; Telakivi et al., 1988).

EXPOSURE TO CENTRALLY ACTING SUBSTANCES Substance use or abuse can result in neurological and psychiatric symptoms, sometimes combined. A history of al-cohol abuse, even if remote, must be taken into account as a possible cause of cognitive decline. Occupational exposure to toxins such as solvents or heavy metals should be queried. Given the evidence that insecticides may precipitate Parkinson's disease, a careful history regarding agricultural or gardening expo-sure is warranted. Because the elderly are both exposed to more prescription medications and may be more sensitive to behavioral side effects than younger patients, it is important to document recent drug use.

Although repetition of the patient encounter and experience are obviously the best ways to acquire expertise, some (myself included) find mnemonic de-vices helpful in the midst of the multitasking intellectual adventure of a busy clinic. A mnemonic that may help physicians ensure a systematic review of key points of the geriatric neurological history and examination can be written as "This is madd!":

T   Trauma recently?
H   Headache?
I   Incontinence?
S   Sleep disturbance?
I   Irritability?
S   Sensory change, including numbness, or special senses such as vision and hearing?
M   Motor changes, such as slowing or tremor?
A   Appetite loss?
D   Delusions?
D   Depression?

The Neurological Examination in Geriatric Psychiatry

The neurological examination requires experience, practice, and sophistication in neuroanatomy to yield the most fruitful results; for this reason, nonneurologists sometimes hesitate to perform a complete examination. However, the elderly psychiatric patient often presents with combined medical, neurological, and psychiatric symptomatology. Proficiency and confidence in the techniques of the neurological examination puts the geriatric psychiatrist in a position to offer a unique synthesis of biological and behavioral knowledge in the assessment of the patient, making the development of these examination skills an extremely valuable asset. Excellent general reviews of the neurological examination are available in specialized references (e.g., Brazis et al., 1985; Gilman, 1999; Haerer, 1992). However, the examination of the elderly patient requires special knowledge of the neurology of aging. The following discussion focuses on both the distinctive features of the geriatric neurological examination and the behavioral significance of neurological signs.

In this examination, there are three goals: (1) to assess physical signs objectively and to distinguish the signs of normal aging from pathological abnormalities; (2) to assess the neurological significance of abnormal signs, both by determining the anatomy of the responsible lesion and by generating testable hypotheses regarding the differential diagnosis of the abnormality; and (3) to assess the potential behavioral significance of abnormal signs. In performing the examination, the geriatric psychiatrist may be faced with a frightened, confused, distracted, uncooperative, or even combative patient. Establishing rapport and maintaining flexibility can mitigate these factors; however, even the most challenging patients can be assessed in some detail by careful observation of their spontaneous activity and responses to events in the environment.

OBSERVATION The neurological examination begins at the first moment the examiner catches sight of the patient. Throughout the historical interview, important information can be gathered regarding the posture; gait; coordination; excesses or deficiencies of movement; the symmetry of facial, truncal, and appendicular activity; attention to or neglect of extrapersonal space; eye movements; and the response to visual, auditory, and somatosensory stimuli in the environment. By the time the formal examination begins, the examiner will have formulated questions about apparent dysfunction that can be tested in depth.

MENTAL STATUS EXAMINATION The mental status examination is described in Chapter 10. As above, the performance of the patient during the course of both the psychiatric interview and mental status examination will provide clues to focus the detailed neurological examination. To take one example, mental slowness may be a sign of subcortical pathology, whether in the white matter, as in the case of severe periventricular white matter changes, or in the subcortical gray matter of the basal ganglia, which produces the mental slowing of parkinson-ism. Therefore, slowing on the mental status examination would heighten the examiner's attention to other physical signs of conditions such as hypertension or diabetes that contribute to white matter changes and to abnormalities of tone, posture, gait, or the presence of resting tremor consistent with parkinson-ism or other basal gangliar pathology. For another example, idiosyncratic speech, paraphasias, or stereotypy (the patient who tends to repeatedly use the same word or phrase) may be subtle signs of aphasia that indicate dominant hemi-sphere dysfunction and may alert the practitioner to look for motor or sensory changes consistent with a left frontal, temporal, or parietal injury.

CRANIAL NERVES   Taste and olfaction both show age-related decline in sensitivity, which is especially pronounced after the age of 50 years, with females exhibit-ing superiority in olfactory abilities throughout the life span. Of those aged 65 to 80 years, 60% show olfactory impairment; nearly a quarter are anosmic (Doty et al., 1984; Verillo & Verillo, 1985); this may be due, in part, to an aging-related slowing in the turnover of olfactory cells (Winkler et al., 1999). Deficiency of the first cranial nerve is most likely to be clinically significant when it is unilateral, suggesting possible basal frontal or mesial-temporal pa-thology on the affected side. In a more general sense, because olfaction is a major component of taste, the decline in olfactory discrimination with aging may contribute to a decrease in the pleasure of eating and a decline in appetite. Olfaction may be tested by exposure to pungent, but nonvolatile, smells such as those of cloves or soap, although the availability of "scratch-and-sniff" cards may improve standardization.

Elderly patients lose visual acuity due to presbyopia and are increasingly vulnerable to ophthalmologic disorders that may be apparent on fundoscopy, including cataracts, glaucoma, age-related macular degeneration, anterior is-chemic optic neuropathy, and retinal vascular disease (Chisholm, 1989; Kasper, 1989). Aging is also associated with some loss of blue-green discrimination and increased sensitivity to glare. Visual acuity can be tested with a handheld Snel-len eye chart at 14 inches, with and without corrective lenses, but presbyopia may make vision at distance the better measure. Visual fields can be roughly assessed by confrontation, testing each eye separately, and overcoming the pa-tient's urge to look directly toward the stimulus by brief, unilateral finger movements. More subtle deficits may be identified in cooperative patients with small test objects such as colored pinheads. Pupils become smaller with aging (senile miosis) and the pupillary light reflex is often diminished or even absent (Chisolm, 1989; Loewenfield, 1979), although asymmetry of response repre-sents an afferent pupillary defect. The presence of papilledema is an important sign of increased intracranial pressure; however, the absence of papilledema cannot be taken as evidence of normalcy because even massive hemispheric tumors may not produce this sign, and papilledema does not usually occur in space-occupying intracranial lesions in the elderly (Caird, 1982; Fetell & Stein, 1989). The loss of previously observed spontaneous venous pulsations in the optic disc may be a more sensitive sign of increased intracranial pressure.

Eye movements change with age; there are increased saccadic latencies (the speed of shifting gaze to fixate on a target) and breakdown of smooth pursuit movements; such disruptions of normal movement may themselves impair vision (Hutton & Morris, 1989). Normal aging is also associated with limitation of upward gaze and less so of downward gaze (Chamberlain, 1971). This normal restriction must be distinguished from two patterns of eye movements with potential relevance to behavioral disorders: (1) the Parinaud syndrome (upgaze paralysis, retraction nystagmus, and pupillary light-near dissociation), which may be associated with pineal region masses; and (2) marked restriction of vertical gaze with preservation of oculocephalic reflexes, which suggests progressive supranuclear palsy. Any other paresis of eye movement, nonconjugate movement, or nystagmus requires further investigation of brain stem, cerebellar, and vestibular function.

Facial asymmetry can be a normal variant or a sign of unilateral facial weakness. Because residual weakness from an old Bell's palsy may be misleading, the examiner should inquire about this past condition and examine the patient's driver's license to determine whether an asymmetry is new. Excessive bucco-oral facial movements are sometimes attributable to ill-fitting dentures or chewing of gum; these confounding variables should be ruled out by examining the patient when the patient's mouth is empty. Dyskinetic lingual-facial-buccal movements are most often encountered in elderly patients with a history of neuroleptic exposure (tardive dyskinesia, TD). However, identical oral dyskinesias can appear spontaneously in never-medicated schizophrenics or in psychiatrically normal, but edentulous, elderly persons (Koller, 1983; McCreadie et al., 2002; Watanabe et al., 1985; Weiner & Klawans, 1973).

Hearing declines with age, primarily due to presbyacusis, a multifactorial condition that can involve (1) sensorineural hearing loss due to a declining population of cochlear ganglion cells, (2) conductive loss, and (3) possible changes in the central auditory pathway (Mackenzie, 1989). The accumulated effect of noise injury, as well as possible effects of toxins, infections, Meniere's disease, and rarely acoustic neuromas can contribute to hearing impairment. The vestibular system declines in function, with up to 40% loss of myelinated fibers in the aged vestibule (Yoder, 1989).

Standard eighth nerve examination should include simple hearing tests, such as assessing the patient's awareness of rubbed fingertips near the ear, a ticking wristwatch, a tuning fork, or whispered words. Because speech perception is probably the most clinically important hearing ability, it is especially useful to document the patient's ability to hear words spoken at conversational level at different distances. The Weber and Rinne tests should supplement these bedside hearing tests to distinguish conductive from sensorineural deficits.

Given the potential for hearing defects to produce emotional distress in the elderly, particularly paranoia, a noticeable deficit on bedside testing justifies formal audiometric evaluation.

Speech may roughen slightly with age, and dysarthria may occur from causes as benign as loose dentures, but progressive hoarseness or nasality may signal more serious problems, such as laryngeal neoplasia, myasthenia, or motor neuron disease. Soft, hypophonic speech can be a sign of pathology in subcortical regions, and patients with Parkinson's disease with dementia will typically have softer speech with impaired melody compared to patients with Alzheimer's disease (Cummings et al., 1988). Excessive movement of the tongue may be a sensitive indicator of tardive dyskinesia, particularly if the patient fails to keep the tongue extended on command. However, fasciculations (a marker of motor neuron disease) can best be observed with the tongue relaxed in the floor of the mouth.

MOTOR EXAMINATION   The initial observation of the patient, as remarked above, is a rich source of information about the function of the motor system. Particular emphasis should be placed on the degree and character of spontaneous movement. Movement disorders in the geriatric psychiatry patient constitute a special diagnostic challenge because they may represent (1) normal aging effects; (2) idiopathic movement disorders, which increase in prevalence among the aged; (3) medication side effects, especially those of neuroleptics; or (4) the consequences of the psychiatric illness. Further, because movement disorders have been associated with depression and dementia (Girotti et al., 1988; Mayeux, 1984), the co-occurrence of movement disorder and psychiatric disturbance raises the question of the degree of interdependence of these diagnoses. To distinguish psychogenic alterations in movement from neurological movement disorders, it is important to supplement observation with examination of resting tone, muscle bulk, power, and deep tendon reflexes.

Resting tone increases with age, both for limbs and axial muscles, with paratonia or *gegenhalten*, the tendency to increase tone in response to rapid displacements of the limb by the examiner, occurring in 10% to 12% of those aged 70 to 79 years and in 21% of those over 80 years old. It remains unclear whether paratonia represents a normal finding or a sign of diffuse cerebral dysfunction (George, 1989; Jenkyn et al., 1985). However, marked rigidity reflects pathology, particularly when accompanied by either a spastic catch, suggestive of upper motor neuron disease, or with cogwheeling, suggestive of basal ganglia disease. Reduction of movement or hypokinesis may represent psychomotor retardation, which can signal depression, but also carries the name *bradykinesia* and is seen in metabolic disorders such as hypothyroidism or especially in basal ganglia disorders, including parkinsonism. The combination of bradykinesia, resting tremor, cogwheel rigidity, and loss of postural reflexes should be familiar as the syndrome of parkinsonism, which can either occur as the result of degenerative nervous system disease such as Parkinson's disease, striatonigral degeneration, and progressive supranuclear palsy or as an extrapyramidal side effect of psychotropic medications, most frequently neuroleptics (Adams & Victor, 1989; Klawans & Tanner, 1984). There is also evidence of an intriguing—and probably centrally mediated—aging-related decline in the induced state of readiness before a spontaneous movement, which may help to explain why older patients sometimes seem slow to respond to commands during the physical examination (Mankovsky et al., 1982).

Excessive movements or *hyperkinesias* may be normal in form (such as the hyperactivity seen in patients with akathisia, agitation, mania, or stimulant intoxication) or abnormal in form (as seen in the neuroleptic-induced dyskinesias or with tremors, tics, and choreoathetosis). Hyperactivity with abnormal form is usually due to basal ganglia pathology; hyperactivity with normal form possibly relates to dysfunction of a limbic-mesencephalic psychomotor activity circuit (Victoroff, 1989). In the presence of generalized hyperactivity with normal form or motor restlessness, clinical features may help distinguish psychogenic hyperactivity from neuroleptic-induced akathisia: Subjective restlessness occurs in both, but patients with akathisia may show more inability to remain still and more shifting from foot to foot and may exhibit a coarse tremor (Braude et al., 1983).

Truncal or appendicular choreic, athetotic, or otherwise dyskinetic movements may be reduced when the patient is seated and so are better examined with the patient standing at rest, walking, and during activating procedures such as touching the thumb with each finger or standing with arms outstretched and eyes closed (Simpson & Singh, 1988). Such dyskinetic movements have a differential diagnosis that includes Huntington's disease, Wilson's disease, acquired hepatocerebral degeneration, senile chorea, and TD (Klawans & Tanner, 1984).

Because the degenerative causes of dyskinesia are rare and because the incidence of tardive dyskinesia is roughly 5% per year among the elderly exposed to neuroleptics (Baldessarini, 1988), it is probable that neuroleptic-induced TD is overwhelmingly the most common pathological cause of dyskinesia in geriatric psychiatric patients. However, as noted above, spontaneous oral dyskinesias also occur in elderly persons not exposed to neuroleptics and with or without a history of schizophrenia, suggesting that the aged nervous system is naturally susceptible to producing these movements (Blowers et al., 1981; McCreadie et al., 2002; Watanabe et al., 1985).

Muscle bulk, as noted above, declines with age. On examination, atrophy of the interosseous muscles of the hands may be particularly evident, and the most common cause of such focal atrophy is probably arthritic joint disease (Baker, 1989). However, focal wasting can also occur with limb disuse from altered activity, trauma, or a cortical insult such as stroke. Neurologically, wasting is important as a sign of lower motor neuron dysfunction, which can be focal, as in spondylosis or spinal mass lesions, or diffuse, as in motor neuron disease. Observation of the resting muscle may reveal fasciculations, which are pathognomonic of lower motor neuron dysfunction, such as occurs in ALS. Measurement of homologous parts on opposite sides of the body will aid in confirming an impression of asymmetry. Diffuse wasting may also signal the anorexia of depression or medical problems, including metabolic, infectious, and neoplastic disorders. The wasting syndrome of human immunodeficiency virus is emerging as another possible diagnosis.

Examination of strength in each major muscle group requires consideration of the patient's willingness to generate maximal effort. Elderly patients may—for good reason—fear excessive exertion, and even their best efforts cannot be compared with those of younger patients. Instead, it is better to use each muscle as the control for the contralateral muscle. For most screening purposes, bedside testing of the upper extremities should include testing of the deltoids, biceps, triceps, flexors and extensors of the wrists and fingers, and intrinsic hand muscles. Testing in the lower extremities should include the iliopsoas, gluteus, quadriceps, hamstrings, anterior tibialis, and soleus/gastrocnemius. Patterns of weakness may have both localizing and diagnostic value. For example, unilateral weakness prompts the search for other localizing signs to discriminate upper from lower motor neuron dysfunction and to delineate the extent of the focal lesion. Disproportionate proximal weakness is common in myopathies or metabolic disorders such as hypothyroidism, while distal weakness may predominate in neuropathies. Disproportionate loss of extensor strength in the arms with relative preservation of flexors is common in upper motor neuron disorders. Diffuse weakness is difficult to interpret and may represent psychogenic enervation or a wide range of medical conditions, including the neuropathic and myopathic disorders.

Tremors are often observed on examinations of elderly persons, and their presence requires diagnosis because pathological and benign tremors are often distinguishable based on a few simple features. In particular, the informal term *senile tremor* should be abandoned because it is does not identify a homogeneous group, and it may obfuscate the important distinction between benign and pathological conditions. A recent consensus statement adopted by the Movement Disorders Society clarifies many of the ambiguities in the classification and differential diagnosis of tremors (Deuschl et al., 1998).

Action tremor is the largest category. It can be defined as tremor seen when the patient is voluntarily holding an extremity in position against gravity. Action tremors include essential tremor, physiological tremor, medication-induced tremor, and parkinsonian tremor.

Classic *essential tremor* is a genetically heterogeneous, usually autosomal dominant, familial tremor of 4 to 10 Hz, which typically is seen in 0.4% to 4% of persons older than 60 years. It is usually bilaterally symmetrical and, although it is classified as an action tremor (seen while holding a position), it is also often seen during willed movement or even at rest. One useful feature of essential tremor that sometimes aids in diagnosis is that about half of patients will report that alcohol helps control the tremor (Koller, 1984; O'Sullivan & Lees, 2000).

Physiological tremor is the universal action tremor; that is, everyone has a fine distal hand tremor of 8–12 Hz on maintaining position against gravity. However, *enhanced physiological tremor* refers to the clinically noticeable version of this tremor that becomes apparent with anxiety, stress, exertion, hypoglycemia, alcohol or benzodiazepine withdrawal, as well as with many medications, including lithium, neuroleptics, antidepressants, and anticonvulsants. Low-dose propranolol often helps control this tremor (Habib-ur-Rehman, 2000; O'Sullivan & Lees, 2000). While parkinsonism is classically associated with resting tremor, it is useful to note that virtually all patients with Parkinson's disease also exhibit some action tremor.

Resting tremor is the second important category and refers to tremors seen when the extremity is immobile and supported against gravity. The most common resting tremor is the classic, slow (4–6 Hz) tremor seen in Parkinson's disease and in many of the Parkinson's plus syndromes. Unlike essential tremor, which most often begins in the hands, Parkinson's tremor often begins in the lower extremities. Thus, the consensus statement recognizes the following: type 1 Parkinson's tremor, which is the classic, slow, resting tremor with or without a slow action tremor; type 2, which is a combined slow resting, faster action tremor; and type 3, which is an uncommon pure action tremor (Deuschl et al., 1998; O'Sullivan & Lees, 2000).

COORDINATION Coordination testing does not assess a single system in isolation, but instead evaluates the orchestration of motor activities due to the harmonious interaction of the pyramidal system, basal ganglia, and cerebellum. Observation of fine finger movements such as rapid, successive opposition of the thumb and other digits may elicit defects of corticospinal tract function. The finger-to-nose test may exhibit abnormalities with dysfunction of different systems: Corticospinal tract pathology may produce smooth, but weak or ineffectual, reaching; basal ganglial pathology may produce bradykinesia and tremor that does not increase with arm extension; cerebellar pathology may produce overshooting, lateral dysmetria, or tremor that increases with arm extension. Some degree of "intention tremor," or dysmetric performance, on the finger-to-nose test may be seen in 20% of normal aged individuals (Howell, 1949).

For this reason, it is sometimes difficult to distinguish between relatively benign age-related incoordination and an important diagnostic clue to cerebellar system pathology. Significant overshoot on attempted rapid movement to a target, whether with saccadic eye movements or limb movements, may distinguish clinically important cerebellar system dysfunction. Cerebellar dysfunction may also produce disorganized or erratic rapid-alternating movements (dysdiadochokinesis, which is often tested by instructing the patient to alternately slap a surface with the pronated or supinated hand), awkward heel-to-shin performance, and failure to check recoil when the examiner suddenly releases the flexed arm.

Disorders that produce these appendicular signs of cerebellar dysfunction may include lesions intrinsic to or compressing the cerebellum, but can also occur with lesions of cerebellar connections, for example, in the vestibular system, red nucleus, inferior olive, ventral lateral thalamus, or even frontal lobe. Causes of this cerebellar type of appendicular incoordination include posterior fossa neoplasm, cerebrovascular disease, demyelinating disease, or less often, one of several degenerative conditions, including OPCA, dentatorubral degeneration, or Azorean disease—a familial condition of cerebellar dysfunction and parkinsonian features in patients of Portuguese-Azorean descent. Alcoholic cerebellar degeneration may also produce these appendicular cerebellar signs, but more often produces truncal ataxia due to midline cerebellar degeneration, with relative preservation of appendicular function.

REFLEXES   Deep tendon reflexes are reduced with age, most often at the ankle, but also, in some studies, at the biceps, triceps, and patella (Howell, 1949; Prakash & Stern, 1973). Because reflexes may be reduced and anxiety may make relaxation difficult for the elderly patient, reinforcing maneuvers are sometimes required to elicit the reflexes, such as asking the patient to clench his or her teeth while testing the upper extremities or using the Jendrassik maneuver (asking patients to hook their hands in front of their chest and pull them in opposite directions as the examiner taps the patellae).

Diffuse hyporeflexia disproportionate to age may commonly be a sign of peripheral neuropathy and less commonly is a sign of myopathy. In hypothyroidism, the reflexes may be slow both to respond and to relax.

Unilateral or focal loss of a reflex may represent peripheral or lower motor neuron damage, commonly as the result of cervical or lumbar spondylosis and less commonly as the result of tabes dorsalis, syringomyelia, or spinal tumor.

Diffuse hyperreflexia occurs in bilateral lesions of the pyramidal system above the midcervical level in states of neuromuscular irritability such as tetany and in hyperthyroidism.

Focally increased reflexes, particularly when combined with pathological signs such as the Babinski or Hoffman, alert the examiner to unilateral pathology affecting the descending pyramidal system; however, it is possible for pathology in cortical regions outside the motor cortex to produce unilateral hyperreflexia (e.g., prefrontal or temporal lesions), possibly by remote effects on the motor strip.

Two patterns of special relevance to behavior are (1) the combination of absent reflexes and positive Babinski signs seen in subacute combined degeneration due to B_{12} deficiency, which is a cause of reversible dementia, and (2) the combination of hyperreflexia and atrophy with fasciculations seen in amyotrophic lateral sclerosis, which may be associated with both depression and dementia (Davis, 1987; Montgomery & Erickson, 1987).

FRONTAL RELEASE SIGNS   A group of reflexes has been referred to as frontal release signs or primitive reflexes. These reflexes represent the exaggeration of normal reflexes or reappearance of reflexes seen in infancy, thereby indicating an impairment of nervous system function. However, it is important to consider the presence of such reflexes in light of their prevalence among the normal aged.

The palmomental reflex (contraction of the mentalis muscle of the face on stroking the palm) has been found in 41% to 60% of the healthy aged, with increasing frequency for each decade from the sixth through the ninth (Jacobs & Gossman, 1980). The snout reflex (puckering or pursing of the lips in response to light pressure above the upper lip) has been found in 26% to 33% of the healthy aged (Jacob & Gossman, 1980; Jenkyn et al., 1985). The glabellar tap response (inability to inhibit blinking during a series of finger taps to the glabellar region) has been found in 37% of healthy aged individuals (Jenkyn et al., 1985).

In addition, Jensen and coworkers (1983) found no difference in the prevalence of the palmomental or glabellar reflexes between normal individuals and patients with cerebral disease, with the exception that patients with basal ganglial disorders more frequently had a positive glabellar tap. Jenkyn et al. (1985) found that 95% of subjects over age 70 years had 5 to 7 "abnormal" signs on examination. Further, patients may have substantial frontal lobe damage, yet have no grasp, snout, suck, rooting, hyperactive jaw jerk, or palmomental reflexes (Benson et al., 1981). Hence, the presence of these reflexes might reveal evidence of nervous system degeneration, but cannot be taken as proof of behaviorally significant frontal lobe pathology, and their absence cannot be used to rule out such pathology.

SENSATION   There is a well-established decline in vibratory sensation beginning by age 50 to 60 years, and there are lesser declines in thermal, touch, and pain discrimination (Olney, 1989; Pearson, 1928). These changes probably relate to combined functional declines of sensory receptors, peripheral nerves, roots, and tracts (Baker, 1989). Although decreased detection of vibratory stimuli may be due to normal aging, marked vibratory insensitivity combined with poor proprioception or a positive Romberg sign (swaying on standing that markedly increases when the eyes are closed) will alert the examiner to peripheral neuropathy or posterior column dysfunction as in subacute combined degeneration. There has also been observed an age-related decline in discrimination of competing tactile stimuli presented to different locations (Kokmen et al., 1977; Levin & Benton, 1973). This insensitivity to double simultaneous stimulation may complicate diagnosis of sensory neglect unless there is a notable asymmetry.

GAIT   Critchley and others noted that the gait of the normal elderly shares many of the features of Parkinson's disease, with short steps, rigidity, and flexion posture (Coffey, 1989; Critchley, 1931). Stoplight photography of walking, healthy, elderly men revealed shortened steps, diminished arm swing, and anteroflexion of the upper torso (Murray et al., 1969). However, these findings are confounded by the fact that elderly patients may walk slowly for a variety of reasons, and a decrease in freely chosen walking rate will naturally produce a decreased length of stride (Larish et al., 1988). Thus, in the aged patient with gait disturbance, it is often difficult to distinguish pathology from normal aging and to sort out the contribution of multiple potential contributory factors, including (1) decreased proprioception; (2) decreased vision; (3) impaired postural reflexes; (4) weakness; (5) rigidity; (6) extrapyramidal dysfunction; (7) vestibulopathy; (8) cerebellar ataxia; (9) diffuse frontal lobe pathology; (10) cervical or lumbar spondylosis; (11) joint restriction; (12) pain; (13) postural hypotension; (14) medication effect; (15) fear of falling based on prior mishaps; and a wide range of focal and diffuse central disorders, including stroke, tumor and hydrocephalus (Adams, 1984; Manchester et al., 1989; Stelmach et al., 1989; Tinetti, 1989).

To best observe gait impairment, the patient should be examined standing in place, walking, walking on heels and toes, and tandem walking (feet in line). The examiner should observe the rate, length and width of stride, stability of turns, arm swing, and foot strike for any atypical features. Postural reflexes can be assessed both on the Romberg test and by observing the response to displacement (lightly pushing the standing patient in different directions). There are several patterns of gait that may have specific diagnostic significance:

Frontal gait "apraxia," with poor initiation, halting steps, and an impression of magnetic attachment to the floor, can be associated with bilateral frontal lobe dysfunction, which may occur due to multiple strokes, Binswanger's disease, or idiopathic frontal lobe degeneration. Normal-pressure hydrocephalus can produce the triad of dementia, incontinence, and a gait disturbance of the frontal type.

Parkinsonian gait will be distinguished from normal aging by the degree of the slowing, rigidity, and shortening of steps; by the presence of festination (acceleration as if chasing the center of gravity); and by the association with resting tremor. Again, depression may produce bradykinesia, but should not produce rigidity or tremor. Parkinsonian gait may occur with idiopathic Parkinson's disease, progressive supranuclear palsy, striatal infarction, or neuroleptic medication exposure.

Broad-based gait occurs with (1) cerebellar or vestibular dysfunction, as in chronic alcoholism that causes midline cerebellar atrophy; (2) loss of proprioception, as in tabes dorsalis due to syphilis or subacute combined degeneration due to vitamin B_{12} deficiency; (3) toxic or metabolic encephalopathy, for example, hepatic encephalopathy; or (4) multiple sensory deficits. Patients with these disorders also often exhibit unsteadiness on the Romberg test.

Spastic gait occurs with myelopathy, most often due to cervical spondylosis. The gait is typically stiff legged, with plantar flexion at the ankle causing the toes to drag.

Hemiparetic gait occurs with any unilateral upper motor neuron disorder, most commonly following a stroke, and typically appears as a limp with unilateral spasticity, foot drop, and circumduction of the affected leg.

Orthopedic gait is a general term for the wide range of alterations in gait occurring in association with focal joint and limb disorders, most often arthritic conditions. In one community study, these disorders were more common than neurological disorders as causes of abnormal gait. (Lundgren-Lindquist et al., 1983)

Table 12-2 summarizes common gait abnormalities seen in a typical neurological referral population.

TABLE 12-2. Causes of gait disorders in a neurological referral practice

Disorder	Frequency, %	Causes
Frontal gait disorder	20	Normal-pressure hydrocephalus Multiple strokes Binswanger's disease
Sensory imbalance	18	Neuropathy Multiple sensory deficits
Myelopathy	16	Cervical spondylosis Vitamin B_{12} deficiency
Parkinsonism	10	Idiopathic Parkinson's disease Drug-induced parkinsonism Progressive supranuclear palsy
Cerebellar degeneration	8	Neurodegenerative disease Alcohol
Toxic or metabolic encephalopathy	6	Hepatic encephalopathy, uremia, hypoglycemia, for instance
Undetermined	14	

Source: Adapted from Sudarsky (1990).

The careful neurological examination of an elderly patient may yield multiple findings that suggest abnormal function. The examiner is sometimes faced with subtle, equivocal findings, findings that do not clearly fit a pattern or even seem contradictory. In part, this may be due to the simultaneous effects of multiple common pathologies, such as cervical or lumbar spondylosis, metabolic or vascular neuropathies, or remote injuries that make it more challenging to identify pertinent new changes. Experience helps in developing a sense for the critical threshold at which a given finding is likely to indicate clinically important dysfunction, and expert examiners may shift their estimate of probability of a certain disorder when certain constellations of signs rise in prominence above the background of softer signs. Nonetheless, the neurological examination can be difficult and somewhat subjective even for experienced clinicians. When the examination yields equivocal positive findings, a reasonable approach may be to err on the side of suspecting meaningful dysfunction and pursue the issue by consultation or appropriate laboratory testing.

The Integrated Neurobehavioral Evaluation

Significant changes occur with age in the structure and function of both the central and the peripheral nervous systems. In addition, the incidence and prevalence of many neurological disorders increase with age. The neurological evaluation should be considered as one component of an integrated neurobehavioral assessment, which includes the psychiatric interview and examination, cognitive testing, neurological examination, and laboratory testing.

Because there is an increased probability of "organicity" with age, there should be a low threshold for supplementing the neurological examination with laboratory tests. Although this is particularly true when the examination suggests a specific central nervous system disorder, we should be modest about the limits of physical diagnosis: Even when no focal or localizing signs are identified, laboratory testing may reveal a specific factor that plays a significant role in the genesis of the behavioral disturbance. While it is often difficult to render a cost-benefit analysis of such testing, the opportunity to discover potentially treatable causes of behavioral disorder is a compelling mandate. As the sophistication in neurobiology grows, so will these opportunities.

The aging of the population will confront the medical community with a large increase in the number of elderly patients who have both psychiatric disturbances and neurological problems. At the same time, the disciplines of neurology and psychiatry are evolving in concert toward an integrated understanding of the neuropsychiatry of behavioral disturbance. The geriatric psychiatrist is in a unique position, drawing on a broad base of knowledge in gerontology, neurology, and psychiatry, to offer a synthesis of disciplinary approaches in the evaluation and treatment of the behavioral distress among the elderly.

ACKNOWLEDGMENTS

This work was supported in part by the State of California Department of Health Services Alzheimer's Research Center (grant 99-86140).

REFERENCES

Adams RD. Aging and human locomotion. In: Albert ML, ed. *Clinical Neurology of Aging*. New York, NY: Oxford University Press; 1984:381–386.

Adams RD, Victor M. *Principles of Neurology*. 4th ed. New York, NY: McGraw-Hill; 1989.

Alavi A, Clark C, Fazekas F. Cerebral ischemia and Alzheimer's disease: critical role of PET and implications for therapeutic intervention. *J Nucl Med*. 1998;39:1363–1365.

ALS CNTF Treatment Study Group. A double-blind placebo-controlled trial of subcutaneous recombinant human ciliary neurotrophic factor (rhCNTF) in amyotrophic lateral sclerosis. *Neurology*. 1996;46:1244–1249.

American Psychiatric Association. *Diagnostic and Statistical Manual of Mental Disorders*. 4th ed. Washington, DC: American Psychiatric Association; 1994.

Anderson JM, Hubbard BM, Coghill GR, Slidders W. The effect of advanced old age on the neuron content of the cerebral cortex. *J Neurol Sci*. 1983;58:235–44.

Antiplatelet Trialists' Collaboration. Collaborative overview of randomized trials of antiplatelet therapy, I: prevention of death, myocardial infarction, and stroke by prolonged antiplatelet therapy in various categories of patients. *BMJ*. 1994;308: 81–106.

Baker PCH. The aging neuromuscular system. *Semin Neurol*. 1989;9:1:50–59.

Baldessarini RJ. A summary of current knowledge of tardive dyskinesia. *Encephale*. 1988;14:263–268.

Ball MJ, Murdoch GH. Neuropathological criteria for the diagnosis of Alzheimer's disease: are we really ready yet? *Neurobiol Aging*. 1997;18(4 suppl):S3–S12.

Baloh RW. *Dizziness, Hearing Loss and Tinnitus: The Essentials of Neurotology*. Philadelphia, PA: F. A. Davis; 1984.

Barker RA, Kendall AL, Widner H. Neural tissue xenotransplantation: what is needed prior to clinical trials in Parkinson's disease? Neural Tissue Xenografting Project. *Cell Transplant*. 2000;9:235–246.

Batjer HH, ed. *Cerebrovascular Disease*. Philadelphia, PA: Lippincott-Raven; 1997.

Beghi E, Chio A, Inghilleri M, et al. A randomized controlled trial of recombinant interferon beta-1a in ALS. Italian Amyotrophic Lateral Sclerosis Study Group. *Neurology*. 2000;54:469–474.

Bensimon G, Lacomblez L, Meininger V, ALS/Riluzole Study Group. A controlled trial of riluzole in amyotrophic lateral sclerosis. *N Engl J Med*. 1994;330:585–591.

Benson DF. Disorders of visual gnosis. In: Brown JW, ed. *Neuropsychology of Visual Perception*. Hillsdale, NJ: Erlbaum; 1989:59–78.

Benson DF, Stuss DT, Naeser MA, et al. The long-term effects of prefrontal leukotomy. *Arch Neurol*. 1981;38:165–189.

Berger MM, Kopp N, Vital C, Redl B, Aymard M, Lina B. Detection and cellular localization of enterovirus RNA sequences in spinal cord of patients with ALS. *Neurology*. 2000;54:20–25.

Bertoni-Freddari C, Fattoretti P, Paoloni R, et al. Synaptic structural dynamics and aging. *Gerontology*. 1996;42:170–180.

Biller J, Feinberg WM, Castaldo JE, et al. Guidelines for carotid endarterectomy: a statement for healthcare professionals from a Special Writing Group of the Stroke Council, American Heart Association. *Circulation*. 1998;97:501–509.

Binks M. Changes in mental functioning associated with normal aging. In: Tallis R, ed. *The Clinical Neurology of Old Age*. Chichester, UK: John Wiley & Sons; 1989: 27–39.

Blowers AJ, Borison RL, Blowers CM, Bicknell DJ. Abnormal involuntary movements in the elderly [letter]. *Br J Psychiatry*. 1981;139:363–364.

Booth FW, Weeden SH. Structural aspects of aging human skeletal muscle. In: Buckwalter JA, Goldberg VM, Woo SLY, eds. *Musculoskeletal Soft-Tissue Aging: Impact on Mobility*. Rosemont, IL: American Academy of Orthopaedic Surgeons; 1993:195–200.

Borchelt MF, Steinhagen-Thiessen E. Physical performance and sensory functions as determinants of independence in activities of daily living in the old and the very old. *Ann N Y Acad Sci*. 1992;673:350–361.

Bots ML, Launer LJ, Lindemans J, et al. Homocysteine and short-term risk of myocardial infarction and stroke in the elderly: the Rotterdam Study. *Arch Intern Med*. 1999;159:38–44.

Bouwman FH, Skolasky R L, Hes D, et al. Variable progression of HIV-associated dementia. *Neurology*. 1998;50:1814–1820.

Brandt J, Butters N. The neuropsychology of Huntington's disease. *Trends Neurosci*. 1986;9:118–120.

Braude WM, Barnes TRE, Gore SM. Clinical characteristics of akathisia, a systematic investigation of acute psychiatric inpatient admissions. *Br J Psychiatry*. 1983;143: 139–150.

Brazis PW, Masdea JC, Biller J. *Localization in Clinical Neurology*. Boston, MA: Little Brown & Company; 1985.

Broe GA, Creasey H. The neuroepidemiology of old age. In: Tallis R, ed. *The Clinical Neurology of Old Age*. Chichester, UK: John Wiley & Sons; 1989:51–65.

Brown RH. Amyotrophic lateral sclerosis: insights from genetics. *Arch Neurol*. 1997; 54:1246–1250.

Caird FI. Examination of the nervous system. In: Caird FI, ed. *Neurological Disorders in the Elderly*. Bristol, UK: Wright PSG; 1982:44–51.

Carson AJ, MacHale S, Allen K, et al. Depression after stroke and lesion location: a systematic review. *Lancet*. 2000;356:122–126.

Celsis P. Age-related cognitive decline, mild cognitive impairment or preclinical Alzheimer's disease? *Ann Med*. 2000;32:6–14.

Chamberlain W. Restriction in upward gaze with advancing age. *Am J Ophthalmol*. 1971;71:341.

Chisolm I. Visual failure. In: Tallis R, ed. *The Clinical Neurology of Old Age*. Chichester, UK: John Wiley & Sons; 1989:335–346.

Chui HC, Victoroff JI, Margolin D, et al. Criteria for the diagnosis of vascular dementia proposed by the State of California Alzheimer's Disease Diagnostic and Treatment Centers. *Neurology*. 1992;42:473–480.

Clarke R, Smith AD, Jobst KA, Refsum H, Sutton L, Ueland PM. Folate, vitamin B12, and serum total homocysteine levels in confirmed Alzheimer disease. *Neurology.* 1998;55:1449–1455.

Clarkson ED, Freed CR. Development of fetal neural transplantation as a treatment for Parkinson's disease. *Life Sci.* 1999;65:2427–2437.

Coffey DJ. Disorders of movement in aging. *Semin Neurol.* 1989;9:1:46–49.

Coleman PD, Flood DG. Neuron numbers and dendritic extent in normal aging and Alzheimer's disease. *Neurobiol Aging.* 1987;8:521–545.

A controlled trial of recombinant methionyl human BDNF in ALS: the BDNF Study Group (phase III). *Neurology.* 1999;52:1427–1433.

Cooper AF, Curry AR. The pathology of deafness in the paranoid and affective psychoses of later life. *J Psychosom Res.* 1976;20:97–105.

Cotman CW. Synaptic plasticity, neurotrophic factors, and transplantation in the aged brain. In: Schneider EL, Rowe JW, eds. *Handbook of the Biology of Aging.* 3rd ed. New York, NY: Academic Press; 1990:255–274.

Crawford JG. Alzheimer's disease risk factors as related to cerebral blood flow. *Med Hypotheses.* 1996;46:367–377.

Critchley M. The neurology of old age. *Lancet.* 1931;1:1221–1230.

Cummings JL. *Clinical Neuropsychiatry.* Orlando, FL: Grune & Stratton; 1985:221–233.

Cummings JL, Darkins A, Mendez M, et al. Alzheimer's disease and Parkinson's disease: comparison of speech and language alterations. *Neurology.* 1988;38:680–684.

Darling JL, Warr TJ. Biology and genetics of malignant brain tumours. *Curr Opin Neurol.* 1998;11:619–625.

Davis AS. Neuropsychological measures in patients with amyotrophic lateral sclerosis [letter]. *Acta Neurol Scand.* 1987;75:284.

de la Torre JC. Cerebromicrovascular pathology in Alzheimer's disease compared to normal aging. *Gerontology.* 1997;43:26–43.

Dement W, Richardson G, Prinz P, et al. Changes of sleep and wakefulness with age. In: Finch CE, Schneider EL, eds. *Handbook of the Biology of Aging.* 2nd ed. New York, NY: Van Nostrand Reinhold; 1985:692–717.

Deuschl G, Bain P, Brin M. Consensus statement of the Movement Disorder Society on Tremor. Ad Hoc Scientific Committee. *Mov Disord.* 1998;13(suppl 3):2–23.

DiBartolomeo AG, Brick JE. Giant cell arteritis and polymyalgia rheumatica. *Postgrad Med.* 1992;91:107–109.

Doty RL, Shaman P, Applebaum SL, Giberson R, Sikorski L, Rosenberg L. Smell identification ability: changes with age. *Science.* 1984;226:1441–1443.

Drachman DA. Aging and the brain: a new frontier. *Ann Neurol.* 1997;42:819–828.

Drachman DA, Long RR. Neurological evaluation of the elderly patient. In: Albert ML, ed. *Clinical Neurology of Aging.* New York, NY: Oxford University Press; 1984: 97–113.

Duffy J, Fogel BS. Elderly patients. In: Silver JM, Yudofsky SC, Hales RE, eds. *Neuropsychiatry of Traumatic Brain Injury.* Washington, DC: American Psychiatric Press; 1994:413–441.

Eriksson PS, Perfilieva E, Bjork-Eriksson T, et al. Neurogenesis in the adult human hippocampus. *Nature Med.* 1998;4:1313–1317.

Fagerberg B, Gnarpe J, Gnarpe H, et al. *Chlamydia pneumoniae* but not cytomegalovirus antibodies are associated with future risk of stroke and cardiovascular disease:

a prospective study in middle-aged to elderly men with treated hypertension. *Stroke.* 1999;30:299–305.

Fazekas F, Schmidt R, Kleinert R, Kapeller P, Roob G, Flooh E. The spectrum of age-associated brain abnormalities: their measurement and histopathological correlates. *J Neural Trans Suppl.* 1998;53:31–39.

Fetell MR, Stein BM. Tumors. In: Rowland LP, ed. *Merritt's Textbook of Neurology.* Philadelphia, PA: Lea & Febiger; 1989:275–285.

Fisher M, Bogousslavsky J. Further evolution toward effective therapy for acute ischemic stroke. *JAMA.* 1998;279:1298–1303.

Fueyo J, Gomez-Manzano C, Yung WK, Kyritsis AP. Targeting in gene therapy for gliomas. *Arch Neurol.* 1999;56:445–448.

Gabrieli JD. Memory systems analyses of mnemonic disorders in aging and age-related diseases. *Proc Natl Acad Sci U S A.* 1996;93:13534–1340.

Gage FH. Stem cells of the central nervous system. *Curr Opin Neurobiol.* 1998;8:671–676.

George J. The neurological examination of the elderly patient. In: Tallis R, ed. *The Clinical Neurology of Old Age.* Chichester, UK: John Wiley & Sons; 1989:67–75.

Gilman S, ed. *Clinical Examination of the Nervous System.* New York, NY: McGraw Hill; 1999.

Girotti F, Soliveri P, Carella F, et al. Dementia and cognitive impairment in Parkinson's disease. *J Neurol Neurosurg Psychiatry.* 1988;51:1498–1502.

Gomez-Isla T, Hollister R, West H, et al. Neuronal loss correlates with but exceeds neurofibrillary tangles in Alzheimer's disease. *Ann Neurol.* 1997;41:17–24.

Gorelick PB, Sacco RL, Smith DB, et al. Prevention of a first stroke. A review of guidelines and a multidisciplinary consensus statement from the National Stroke Association. *JAMA.* 1999;281:1112–1120.

Grady CL, McIntosh AR, Bookstein F, et al. Age-related changes in regional cerebral blood flow during working memory for faces. *Neuroimage.* 1998;8:409–425.

Greenwald BS, Kramer-Ginsberg E, Krishnan KR, et al. Neuroanatomic localization of magnetic resonance imaging signal hyperintensities in geriatric depression. *Stroke.* 1998;29:613–617.

Griffiths TD, Meecham PJ. Biology of aging. In: Ferraro KF, ed. *Gerontology: Perspectives and Issues.* New York, NY: Springer; 1990:45–57.

Grimes DA, Bulman DE. Parkinson's genetics—creating exciting new insights. Parkinsonism Rel Disord. 2002;8:459–464.

Gurney ME, Tomasselli AG, Heinrikson RL. Stay the executioner's hand. *Science.* 2000; 288:283–284.

Haass C. New hope for Alzheimer disease vaccine. *Nature Med.* 2002;8:1195–1196.

Habib-ur-Rehman. Diagnosis and management of tremor. *Arch Intern Med.* 2000;160: 2438–2444.

Haerer A. *Dejong's the Neurologic Examination.* New York, NY: Lippincott Williams & Wilkins; 1992.

Hedge RS, Tremblay P, Groth D, et al. Transmissable and genetic prion diseases share a common pathway of neurodegeneration. *Nature.* 1999;402:822–826.

Henderson G, Tomlinson BE, Gibson PH. Cell counts in human cerebral cortex in normal adults throughout life using an image analyzing computer. *J Neurol Sci.* 1980; 46:113–136.

Heyman A, Fillenbaum G, Welsh-Bohmer K, et al. Clinical and neuropsychological findings in patients with autopsy evidence of Alzheimer's disease with and without cerebral infarction: the CERAD experience. *Neurology.* 1998;50(suppl 4):A408.

Hill JR, Kuriyama N, Kuriyama H, Israel MA. Molecular genetics of brain tumors. *Arch Neurol.* 1999;56:439–441.

Hobson W, Pemberton J. *The Health of the Elderly at Home.* London, England: Butterworth; 1955.

Hock C, Konietzko U, Papassotiropoulos A, et al. Generation of anti-amyloid antibodies by vaccination of patients with Alzheimer's disease. *Nature Med.* 2002;8:1270–1275.

Howell TH. Senile deterioration of the central nervous system. *Br Med J.* 1949;1:56–58.

Hubbard BM, Squier MV. The physical aging of the neuromuscular system. In: Tallis R, ed. *The Clinical Neurology of Old Age.* Chichester, UK: John Wiley & Sons; 1989:3–26.

Huntington's Disease Collaborative Research Group. A novel gene containing a trinucleotide repeat that is expanded and unstable on Huntington's disease chromosomes. *Cell.* 1993;72:971–983.

Hutton JT, Morris JL. Looking and seeing with age related neurologic illness and normal aging. *Semin Neurol.* 1989;9:1:31–38.

Hutton M, Lendon CL, Rizzu P, et al. Association of missense and 5′-splice-site mutations in tau with the inherited dementia FTDP-17. *Nature.* 1998;393:702–705.

Hvas AM, Ellegaard J, Nexo E. Increased plasma methylmalonic acid level does not predict clinical manifestations of vitamin B_{12} deficiency. *Arch Intern Med.* 2001; 161:1534–1541.

Jacobs L, Gossman MD. Three primitive reflexes in normal adults. *Neurology.* 1980;30: 184–188.

Jankovic J. New and emerging therapies for Parkinson disease. *Arch Neurol.* 1999;56: 785–790.

Jankovic J, Caine DB. Parkinson's disease: etiology and treatment. *Curr Neurol.* 1987; 7:193–234.

Janssen RS, Nwanyanwu OC, Selik RM, Stehr-Green JK. Epidemiology of human immunodeficiency virus encephalopathy in the United States. *Neurology.* 1992;42:1472–1476.

Jenkyn LR, Reeves AG, Warren T, et al. Neurologic signs in senescence. *Arch Neurol.* 1985;42:1154–1157.

Jennett B, Teasdale G. Prognosis after severe head injury. In: Jennett B, Teasdale G, eds. *Management of Head Injuries.* Philadelphia, PA: F. A. Davis; 1981:317–332.

Jensen JPA, Gron U, Pakkenberg H. Comparison of three primitive reflexes in neurological patients and in normal individuals. *J Neurol Neurosurg Psychiatry.* 1983;46: 162–167.

Jette AM. Musculoskeletal impairments and associated physical disability in the elderly: insights from epidemiological research. In: Buckwalter JA, Goldberg VM, Woo SLY, eds. *Musculoskeletal Soft-Tissue Aging: Impact on Mobility.* Rosemont, IL: American Academy of Orthopaedic Surgeons; 1993:7–22.

Joosten E, van den Berg A, Riezler R, et al. Metabolic evidence that deficiencies of vitamin B-12 (cobalamin), folate, and vitamin B-6 occur commonly in elderly people. *Am J Clin Nutr.* 1993;58:468–476.

Kales A, Caldwell AB, Cadieux RJ, et al. Severe obstructive sleep apnea—II: associated psychopathology and psychosocial consequences. *J Chronic Dis.* 1985;38:427–434.

Kasper RL. Eye problems of the aged. In: Reichel W, ed. *Clinical Aspects of Aging.* Baltimore, MD: Williams & Wilkins; 1989:445–453.

Katzman R. The aging brain—limitations in our knowledge and future approaches. *Arch Neurol.* 1997;54:1201–1205.

Kaye JA. Oldest-old healthy brain function: the genomic potential. *Arch Neurol.* 1997; 54:1217–1221.

Keys BA, White DA. Exploring the relationship between age, executive abilities, and psychomotor speed. *J Int Neuropsychol Soc.* 2000;6:76–82.

Kieburtz K, Hubble J. Benefits of COMT inhibitors in levodopa-treated parkinsonian patients. *Neurology.* 2000;55(suppl 4):S42–S45.

Kirasic KC, Allen GL. Aging, spatial performance and spatial competence. In: Charness N, ed. *Aging and Human Performance.* Chichester, UK: John Wiley & Sons; 1985: 191–224.

Kish SJ, el-Awar M, Schut L, et al. Cognitive deficits in olivopontocerebellar atrophy: implications for the cholinergic hypothesis of Alzheimer's dementia. *Ann Neurol.* 1988;24:200–206.

Kish SJ, Robitaile Y, El-Awar M, et al. Striatal monoamine neurotransmitters and metabolites in dominantly inherited olivopontocerebellar atrophy. *Neurology.* 1992; 42:1573–1577.

Klawans H. Behavioral alterations and the therapy of parkinsonism. *Clin Neuropharmacol.* 1982;5(suppl 1):S29–S37.

Klawans H, Tanner CM. Movement disorders in the elderly. In: Albert ML, ed. *Clinical Neurology of Aging.* New York, NY: Oxford University Press; 1984:387–403.

Knopman D, Cummings J, DeKosky S, et al. Practice parameter: diagnosis of dementia (an evidence-based review). Report of the Quality Standards Subcommittee of the American Academy of Neurology. *Neurology.* 2001;56:1143–1153.

Kokmen E, Bossemeyer RW, Barney J, et al. Neurological manifestations of aging. *J Gerontol.* 1977;32:411–419.

Koller WC. Edentulous orodyskinesia. *Ann Neurol.* 1983;13:97–99.

Koller WC. Diagnosis and treatment of tremors. *Neurol Clin.* 1984;2:499–514.

Koller WC. How accurately can Parkinson's disease be diagnosed? *Neurology.* 1992; 42(1, suppl 1):6–16.

Koller WC. Levodopa in the treatment of Parkinson's disease. *Neurology.* 2000;55(suppl 4):S2–S7.

Koudstaal PJ, van-Gijn J, Frenken CW, et al. TIA: RIND, minor stroke: a continuum, or different subgroups? *J Neurol Neurosurg Psychiatry.* 1992;55:95–97.

Kral VA. The relationship between senile dementia (Alzheimer type) and depression. *Can J Psychiatry.* 1983;28:304–306.

Krausz Y, Bonne O, Gorfine M, et al. Age-related changes in brain perfusion of normal subjects detected by 99mTc-HMPAO SPECT. *Neuroradiology.* 1998;40:428–434.

Krishnan KR, Hays JC, Blazer DG. MRI-defined vascular depression. *Am J Psychiatry.* 1997;154:497–501.

Kuest J, Karbe H. Cortical activation studies in aphasia. *Curr Neurol Neurosci Rep.* 2002;2:511–515.

Kuller LH. Incidence rates of stroke in the eighties: the end of the decline in stroke? *Stroke.* 1989;20:841–843.

Kwiatkowski TG, Libman RB, Frankel M, et al. Effects of tissue plasminogen activator for acute ischemic stroke at one year. *N Engl J Med.* 1999;340:1781–1787.

Lai EC, Felice KJ, Festoff BW, et al. Effect of recombinant insulin-like growth factor-I on progression of ALS. *Neurology.* 1997;49:1621–1630.

Langston JW. Epidemiology versus genetics in Parkinson's disease: progress in resolving an age-old debate. *Ann Neurol.* 1998;44(suppl 1):S45–S52.

Larish DD, Martin PE, Mungiole M. Characteristic patterns of gait in the healthy old. *Ann N Y Acad Sci.* 1988;515:18–32.

Launer LJ, Andersen K, Dewey ME, et al. Rates and risk factors for dementia and Alzheimer's disease: results from EURODEM pooled analyses. EURODEM Incidence Research Group and Work Groups. European Studies of Dementia. *Neurology.* 1999;52:78–84.

Le Couteur DG, Muller M, Yang MC, Mellick GD, McLean AJ. Age-environment and gene-environment interactions in the pathogenesis of Parkinson's disease. *Rev Environ Health.* 2002;17:51–64.

Levin HS, Benton AL. Age and susceptibility to tactile masking effects. *Geront Clin.* 1973;15:1–9.

Levitt AJ, Karlinsky H. Folate, vitamin B_{12} and cognitive impairment in patients with Alzheimer's disease. *Acta Psychiatr Scand.* 1992;86:301–305.

Lewis SJ, Sacks FM, Mitchell JS, et al. Effect of pravastatin on cardiovascular events in women after myocardial infarction: the cholesterol and recurrent events (CARE) trial. *J Am Coll Cardiol.* 1998;32:140–146.

Li M, Ona VO, Guegan C, et al. Functional role of caspase-1 and caspase-3 in an ALS transgenic mouse model. *Science.* 2000;288:335–339.

Lindenbaum J, Rosenberg IH, Wilson PW, Stabler SP, Allen RH. Prevalence of cobalamin deficiency in the Framingham elderly population. *Am J Clin Nutr.* 1994;60: 2–11.

Loewenfield IE. Pupillary changes related to age. In: Thompson HS, ed. *Topics in Neuroopthalmology.* Baltimore, MD: Williams & Wilkins; 1979.

Love AW. Depression in chronic low back pain patients: diagnostic efficiency of three self-report questionnaires. *J Clin Psychol.* 1987;43:84–89.

Ludolph AC, Riepe MW. Do the benefits of currently available treatments justify early diagnosis and treatment of amyotrophic lateral sclerosis? *Neurology.* 1999; 53(suppl 5):S46–S49.

Lundgren-Lindquist B, Aniansson A, Rundgren A. Functional studies in 79-year-olds. III. Walking performance and climbing capacity. *Scand J Rehab Med.* 1983;15: 125–131.

Mackenzie I. Disturbances of hearing and balance. In: Tallis R, ed. *The Clinical Neurology of Old Age.* Chichester, UK: John Wiley & Sons; 1989:363–375.

Manchester D, Woollacott M, Zederbauer-Hylton N, Marin O. Visual, vestibular and somatosensory contributions to balance control in the older adult. *J Gerontol.* 1989;44:M118–M127.

Mankovsky NB, Mints AY, Lisenyuk VP. Age peculiarities of human motor control in aging. *Gerontology.* 1982;28:314–322.

Margolis RL, McInnis MG, Rosenblatt A, Ross CA. Trinucleotide repeat expansion and neuropsychiatric disease. *Arch Gen Psychiatry.* 1999;56:1019–1031.

Mark MH. Lumping and splitting the Parkinson plus syndromes: dementia with Lewy bodies, multiple system atrophy, progressive supranuclear palsy, and cortical-basal ganglionic degeneration. *Neurol Clin.* 2001;19:607–627.

Marler JR, Jones PW, Emr M, eds. *Rapid Identification and Treatment of Acute Stroke.*

Bethesda, MD: National Institute of Neurological Disorders and Stroke, National Institutes of Health; 1997.

Marsden CD, Jenner P. The pathophysiology of extrapyramidal side-effects of neuroleptic drugs. *Psychol Med.* 1980;10:55–72.

Marsden CD, Olanow CW. The causes of Parkinson's disease are being unraveled and rational neuroprotective therapy is close to reality. *Ann Neurol.* 1998;44(suppl 1): S189–S196.

Masliah E, Mallory M, Hansen L, DeTeresa R, Terry RD. Quantitative synaptic alterations in the human neocortex during normal aging. *Neurology.* 1993;43:192–197.

Mattay VS, Fera F, Tessitore A, et al. Neurophysiological correlates of age-related changes in human motor function. *Neurology.* 2002;58:630–635.

Mayeux R. Behavioral manifestations of movement disorders. *Neurol Clin.* 1984;2:527–540.

Mayeux R, Ottman R, Maestre G, et al. Synergistic effects of traumatic head injury and apolipoprotein-epsilon 4 in patients with Alzheimer's disease. *Neurology.* 1995; 45(3 pt 1):555–557.

McArthur JC, Hoover DR, Bacellar H, et al. Dementia in AIDS patients: incidence and risk factors. *Neurology.* 1993;43:2245–2252.

McArthur JC, Sacktor N, Selnes O. Human immunodeficiency virus-associated dementia. *Semin Neurol.* 1999;19:129–150.

McCreadie RG, Padmavati R, Thara R, Srinivasan TN. Spontaneous dyskinesia and parkinsonism in never-medicated, chronically ill patients with schizophrenia: 18-month follow-up. *Br J Psychiatr.* 2002;181:135–137.

McKeith IG, Galasko D, Kosaka K, et al. Consensus guidelines for the clinical and pathological diagnosis of dementia with Lewy bodies (DLB). *Neurology.* 1996;47: 1113–1124.

McKeith IG, Perry EK, Perry RH, for the Consortium on Dementia with Lewy Bodies. Report of the Second Dementia with Lewy Body International Workshop: diagnosis and treatment. *Neurology.* 1999;53:902–905.

Meltzer CC. Neuropharmacology and receptor studies in the elderly. *J Geriatr Psychiatry Neurol.* 1999;12:137–149.

Mendez MF, Cherrier M, Perryman KM, et al. Frontotemporal dementia versus Alzheimer's disease: differential cognitive features. *Neurology.* 1996;47:1189–1194.

Mielke R, Kessler J, Szelies B, Herholz K, Wienhard K, Heiss WD. Normal and pathological aging—findings of positron-emission-tomography. *J Neural Trans (Budapest).* 1998;105:821–837.

Miller BL, Ikonte C, Ponton M, et al. A study of the Lund-Manchester research criteria for frontotemporal dementia: clinical and single photon emission CT correlations. *Neurology.* 1997;48:937–942.

Montgomery GK, Erickson LM. Neuropsychological perspectives in amyotrophic lateral sclerosis. *Neurol Clin.* 1987;5:61–81.

Moody DM, Brown WR, Challa VR, Ghazi-Birry HS, Reboussin DM. Cerebral microvascular alterations in aging, leukoaraiosis, and Alzheimer's disease. *Ann N Y Acad Sci.* 1997;826:103–116.

Mortimer JA. The dementia of Parkinson's disease. *Clin Geriatr Med.* 1988;4:785–797.

Mortimer JA, van Duijn CM, Chandra V, et al. Head trauma as a risk factor for Alzheimer's disease: a collaborative re-analysis of case-control studies. EURODEM Risk Factors. *Int J Epidemiol.* 1991;20(suppl 2):S28–S35.

Mrak RE, Griffin ST, Graham DI. Aging-associated changes in human brain. *J Neuropathol Exp Neurol.* 1997;56:1269–1275.

Munsat TL. Aging of the neuromuscular system. In: Albert ML, ed. *Clinical Neurology of Aging.* New York, NY: Oxford University Press; 1984:404–423.

Murray MP, Kory RC, Clarkson BH. Walking patterns in healthy old men. *J Gerontol.* 1969;24:169–178.

Nagy Z, Esiri MM, Jobst KA, et al. The effects of additional pathology on the cognitive deficit in Alzheimer disease. *J Neuropathol Exp Neurol.* 1997;56:165–170.

Nance MA. Huntington disease: clinical, genetic, and social aspects. *J Geriatr Psychiatry Neurol.* 1998;11(2):61–70.

National Institute of Neurological Disorders and Stroke rt-PA Stroke Study Group. Tissue plasminogen activator for acute ischemic stroke. *N Engl J Med.* 1995;333:1581–1587.

Neary D, Snowdon JS, Gustafson L, et al. Frontotemporal lobar degeneration. A consensus on clinical diagnostic criteria. *Neurology.* 1998;51:1546–1554.

Nobler MS, Mann JJ, Sackeim HA. Serotonin, cerebral blood flow, and cerebral metabolic rate in geriatric major depression and normal aging. *Brain Res Brain Res Rev.* 1999;30:250–263.

Olanow CW, Tatton WG. Etiology and pathogenesis of Parkinson's disease. *Ann Rev Neurosci.* 1999;22:123–144.

Olney RK. Diseases of peripheral nerves. In: Tallis R, ed. *The Clinical Neurology of Old Age.* Chichester, UK: John Wiley & Sons; 1989:171–189.

O'Sullivan JD, Lees AJ. Nonparkinsonian tremors. *Clin Neuropharmacol.* 2000;23:233–238.

Ownsworth TL, Oei TP. Depression after traumatic brain injury: conceptualization and treatment considerations. *Brain Injury.* 1998;12:735–751.

Pantoni L, Garcia JH. The significance of cerebral white matter abnormalities 100 years after Binswanger's report. A review. *Stroke.* 1995;26:1293–1301.

Partridge L. Evolutionary biology and age-related mortality. In: Wachter KW, Finch CE, eds. *Between Zeus and the Salmon: The Biodemography of Longevity.* Washington, DC: National Academy Press; 1997:78–95.

Pastor P, Tolosa E. Progressive supranuclear palsy: clinical and genetic aspects. *Curr Opin Neurol.* 2002;15:429–437.

Pearson GHJ. Effect of age on vibratory sensibility. *Arch Neurol Psychiatry.* 1928;20:482–496.

Perry E, Kay DW. Some developments in brain ageing and dementia. *Br J Biomed Sci.* 1997;54:201–215.

Perry EK, Piggott MA, Court JA, Johnson M, Perry RH. Transmitters in the developing and senescent human brain. *Ann N Y Acad Sci.* 1993;695:69–72.

Peyser CE, Folstein SE. Depression in Huntington disease. In: Starkstein SE, Robinson RG, eds. *Depression in Neurologic Disease.* Baltimore, MD: Johns Hopkins University Press; 1993:117–138.

Plude DJ, Hoyer WJ. Attention and performance: identifying and localizing age deficits. In: Charness N, ed. *Aging and Human Performance.* Chichester, UK: John Wiley & Sons; 1985:47–99.

Powell DH. *Profiles in Cognitive Aging.* Boston, MA: Harvard University Press; 1994.

Practice advisory on the treatment of amyotrophic lateral sclerosis with riluzole: report of the Quality Standards Subcommittee of the American Academy of Neurology. *Neurology.* 1997;49:657–659.

Prakash C, Stern G. Neurological signs in the elderly. *Age Ageing.* 1973;2:24–27.

Rabbitt P, Lowe C. Patterns of cognitive ageing. *Psychol Res.* 2000;63:308–316.

Rajput A, Rajput AH. Progressive supranuclear palsy: clinical features, pathophysiology and management. *Drugs Aging.* 2001;18:913–925.

Rapoport SI. Positron emission tomography in normal aging and Alzheimer's disease. *Gerontology.* 1986;32(suppl 1):6–13.

Riederer P, Krusik P. Biochemical and morphological changes in the aging brain. *Electroencephalogr Clin Neurophysiol Suppl.* 1987;39:389–395.

Robinson RG, Kubos KL, Starr LB, Rao K, Price TR. Mood disorders in stroke patients: importance of location of lesion. *Brain.* 1984;107:81–93.

Rogers MA, Evans WJ. Changes in skeletal muscle with aging: effects of exercise training. *Exerc Sports Sci Rev.* 1993;21:65–102.

Roman GC, Tatemichi TK, Erkinjutti T, et al. Vascular dementia: diagnostic criteria for research studies. *Neurology.* 1993;43:250–260.

Rosen DR, Siddique T, Patterson D, et al. Mutations in CU/Zn superoxide dismutase gene are associated with familial amyotrophic lateral sclerosis. *Nature.* 1993;362: 59–62.

Ross GW, Abbott RD, Petrovitch H, et al. Association of coffee and caffeine intake with the risk of Parkinson disease. *JAMA.* 2000;283:2674–2679.

Rowe JW, Kahn RL. Human aging: usual and successful. *Science.* 1987;237:143–149.

Rubin EH, Storandt M, Miller JP, et al. A prospective study of cognitive function and onset of dementia in cognitively healthy elders. *Arch Neurol.* 1998;55:395–401.

Rypma B, D'Esposito M. Isolating the neural mechanisms of age-related changes in human working memory. *Nature Neurosci.* 2000;3:509–515.

Sachdev PS, Valenzuela M, Wang XL, Looi JC, Brodaty H. Relationship between plasma homocysteine levels and brain atrophy in healthy elderly individuals. *Neurology.* 2002;58:1539–1541.

Sacktor NC, McArthur JC. Prospects for therapy of HIV-associated neurologic disease. *J Neurovirol.* 1997;3:89–101.

Saffran EM. Aphasia and the relationship of language and brain. *Semin Neurol.* 2000; 20:409–418.

Salonen R, Nyyssonen K, Porkkala E, et al. Kuopio Atherosclerosis Prevention Study (KAPS). A population-based primary preventive trial of the effect of LDL lowering on atherosclerotic progression in carotid and femoral arteries. *Circulation.* 1995; 92:1758–1764.

Segovia J. Gene therapy for Parkinson's disease: current status and future potential. *Am J PharmacoGenomics.* 2002;2:135–146.

Shapiro WR. Current therapy for brain tumors: back to the future. *Arch Neurol.* 1999; 56:429–432.

Simpson GM, Singh H. Tardive dyskinesia rating scales. *Encephale.* 1988;14:175–182.

Skipper L, Farrer M. Parkinson's genetics: molecular insights for the new millennium. *Neurotoxicology.* 2002;23:503–514.

Smith J. Clinical neurophysiology in the elderly. In: Tallis R, ed. *The Clinical Neurology of Old Age.* Chichester, UK: John Wiley & Sons; 1989:89–97.

Spencer PS, Ochoa J. The mammalian peripheral nervous system in old age. In: Johnson J, ed. *Aging and Cell Structure*. New York, NY: Plenum Press; 1981:35–103.

Stabler SP, Lindenbaum J, Allen RH. Vitamin B_{12} deficiency in the elderly: current dilemmas. *Am J Clin Nutr*. 1997;66:741–749.

Stambler N, Charatan M, Cedarbaum JM. Prognostic indicators of survival in ALS. ALS CNTF Treatment Study Group. *Neurology*. 1998;50:66–72.

Stelmach GE, Phillips J, DiFabio RP, Teasdale N. Age, functional postural reflexes and voluntary sway. *J Gerontol*. 1989;44:B100–B106.

Stones MJ, Kozma A. Physical performance. In: Charness N, ed. *Aging and Human Performance*. Chichester, UK: John Wiley & Sons; 1985:261–292.

Strong MJ, Grace GM, Orange JB, et al. A prospective study of cognitive impairment in ALS. *Neurology*. 1999;53:1665–1670.

Strub RL, Black FW. *Neurobehavioral Disorders: A Clinical Approach*. Philadelphia, PA: F. A. Davis; 1988:451–475.

Subcommittee on Motor Neuron Diseases/Amyotrophic Lateral Sclerosis of the World Federation of Neurology Research Group on Neuromuscular Diseases and the El Escorial "Clinical Limits of Amyotrophic Lateral Sclerosis" Workshop Contributors. El Escorial World Federation of Neurology criteria for the diagnosis of amyotrophic lateral sclerosis. *J Neurol Sci*. 1994;124(suppl):96–107.

Sudarsky L. Geriatrics: gait disorders in the elderly. *N Engl J Med*. 1990;322:1441–1446.

Takeda S, Matsuzawa T, Matsui H. Age-related changes in cerebral blood flow and brain volume in healthy subjects. *J Am Geriatr Soc*. 1988;36:293–297.

Telakivi T, Kajaste S, Partinen M, et al. Cognitive function in middle age snorers and controls: role of excessive daytime somnolence and sleep-related hypoxic events. *Sleep*. 1988;11:454–462.

Teravainen H, Calne DB. Motor system in normal aging and Parkinson's disease. In: Katzman R, Terry R, eds. *The Neurology of Aging*. Philadelphia, PA: F. A. Davis; 1983:85–109.

Thomas PK. Electrophysiological and morphological changes in the peripheral nervous system with ageing. *Electroencephalogr Clin Neurophysiol*. 1999(suppl 50):103–108.

Thompson LV. Effects of age and training on skeletal muscle physiology and performance. *Phys Ther*. 1994;74:71–81.

Timiras PS. Aging of the nervous system: functional changes. In: Timiras PS, ed. *Physiological Basis of Aging and Geriatrics*. 2nd ed. Boca Raton, FL: CRC Press; 1994.

Tinetti ME. Instability and falling in elderly patients. *Semin Neurol*. 1989;9:39–45.

Tyler KL. A history of Parkinson's disease. In: Koller WC, ed. *Handbook of Parkinson's Disease*. New York, NY: Marcel Dekker; 1987.

Verillo RT, Verillo V. Sensory and perceptual performance. In: Charness N, ed. *Aging and Human Performance*. Chichester, UK: John Wiley & Sons; 1985:1–46.

Victoroff J. The evolution of aging-related brain change. *Neurobiol Aging*. 1999;20:431–438.

Victoroff J. Central nervous system changes with normal aging. In: Sadock BJ, Sadock VA, eds. *Comprehensive Textbook of Psychiatry*. 7th ed. Philadelphia, PA: Lippincott, Williams & Wilkins; 2000:3101–3020.

Victoroff JI. Hyperactivity syndrome of Alzheimer's disease. *Bull Clin Neurosci*. 1989;54:34–42.

Ward C. The genetics and epidemiology of Parkinson's disease. In: Griffiths RA, McCarthy ST, eds. *Degenerative Neurological Disease in the Elderly*. Bristol, UK: Wright; 1987:20–28.

Watanabe H, Saito Y, Terao S, et al. Progression and prognosis in multiple system atrophy: an analysis of 230 Japanese patients. *Brain*. 2002;125(pt 5):1070–1083.

Watanabe I, Sato M, Yamane H, Nakazawa K. Oral dyskinesia of the aged. I. Clinical aspects. *Gerodontics*. 1985;1:39–43.

Weiner WJ, Klawans HL. Lingual-facial-buccal movements in the elderly. II: Pathogenesis and relationship to senile chorea. *J Am Geriatr Soc*. 1973;21:318–320.

Welford AT. Reaction time, speed of performance, and age. *Ann N Y Acad Sci*. 1988; 515:1–17.

Wells RD, Warren ST. *Genetic Instabilities and Hereditary Neurological Diseases*. San Diego, CA: Academic; 1998.

Wenning GK, Braune S. Multiple system atrophy: pathophysiology and management. *CNS Drugs*. 2001;15:839–852.

West MJ. Regionally specific loss of neurons in the aging human hippocampus. *Neurobiol Aging*. 1993;14:287–293.

Wickelgren I. For cortex, neuron loss may be less than thought. *Science*. 1996;273: 48–50.

Winkler S, Garg AK, Mekayrajjananonth T, et al. Depressed taste and smell in geriatric patients. *J Am Dent Assoc*. 1999;130:1759–1765.

Wrightson P. Management of disability and rehabilitation services after minor head injury. In: Levin HS, Eisenberg HM, Benton AL, eds. *Mild Head Injury*. New York, NY: Oxford University Press; 1989.

Wu CC, Mungas D, Petkov CI, et al. Brain structure and cognition in a community sample of elderly Latinos. *Neurology*. 2002;59:383–391.

Yarnell PR, Rossie GV. Minor whiplash head injury with major debilitation. *Brain Injury*. 1988;2:255–258.

Yoder MG. Geriatric ear nose and throat problems. In: Reichel W, ed. *Clinical Aspects of Aging*. Baltimore, MD: Williams & Wilkins; 1989:454–463.

Yu S, Pritchard M, Kremer E, et al. Fragile X genotype characterized by an unstable region of DNA. *Science*. 1992;252:1179–1181.

Zivin JA. Cell transplant therapy for stroke. Hope or hype. *Neurology*. 2000;55:467.

13

Neuropsychological Testing
of the Older Adult

Clifford A. Smith, PhD
Wilfred G. van Gorp, PhD, ABPP

INTRODUCTION

Significant strides have been made in the field of geriatric neuropsychology in
the past few years. The proliferation of normative data for older adults, the
creation of specialized measures for the assessment of cognitive dysfunction
associated with advanced aging, and the development of neuropsychological
measures and batteries specifically designed for repeated administration over
time are just some of the advances that we discuss.

In this chapter, we focus on key issues pertaining to the role of neuropsychological assessment in evaluating the cognitive functioning of the older adult.
To accomplish this, we review (1) what a neuropsychological assessment is
and when requesting one is most helpful; (2) unique issues associated with the
neuropsychological assessment of the geriatric patient; (3) cognitive domains
that may be evaluated and a selection of tests that should be considered for the
evaluation of the geriatric patient; and (4) the contribution of neuropsychological assessments in assisting with the differential diagnosis of neuropsychiatric
disorders often found in older adults.

THE NEUROPSYCHOLOGICAL EVALUATION

Neuropsychological evaluation is concerned with the psychometric assessment
of cognitive and emotional processes and, as such, can be viewed as being an

in-depth and quantitative extension of the commonly used bedside mental status examination, such as the Mini-Mental State Examination (MMSE).

Ultimately, the goal of every neuropsychological evaluation is to describe and document brain-behavior relationships; however, the specific strategies for conducting a neuropsychological assessment to obtain this information vary widely among clinicians. Broadly speaking, two clinical approaches are currently used in conducting a neuropsychological evaluation. In one approach, neuropsychologists administer a "fixed" or predetermined test battery, such as the Halstead-Reitan Neuropsychological Test Battery (HRNTB; Reitan & Wolfson, 1985), to all patients regardless of the presenting illness or the referral question. While clinicians using this approach may incorporate additional neuropsychological tests in the battery, the core set of tests remains fixed as it is argued that this allows for both clinical utility (i.e., diagnostic specificity) and scientific research.

Pertaining to the evaluation of the elderly, the fixed battery approach has been criticized for being both time and labor intensive, which is particularly relevant in geriatric assessments, and for lacking the flexibility needed given different clinical populations and referral questions. Perhaps more important, Fastenau and Adams (1996) noted that the available normative data for the HRNTB (Heaton et al., 1991) contained serious limitations pertaining to sample size. In addition, several authors have noted that the pattern of cognitive performance for older adults remains poorly defined on the HRNTB (Cullum et al., 1989; Elias et al., 1990; Fastenau, 1998). With this, some have asserted that the use of normative data along with the traditional cutoff scores from the HRNTB may contribute to a high rate of either falsely diagnosing impairment (Cullum et al., 1989) or failing to diagnose actual impairment (Fastenau, 1998).

In contrast to the fixed battery approach, the second general method employed in a neuropsychological assessment incorporates what is often called the "flexible" approach. While a core set of tests (intelligence, memory, language, etc.) is often used, this approach differs from the fixed battery method in that a broad array of tests may be drawn on to design a tailored battery. Advantages of the flexible approach include potentially shorter administration time and the ability to gear the battery specifically to address the referring question and the patient's presenting illness. While this approach is not without potential disadvantages, such as the potential lack of comprehensiveness, many clinicians favor this approach because of its flexibility to the patient and to address the referral question in an economical and focused fashion.

UNIQUE ISSUES IN THE ASSESSMENT OF OLDER ADULTS

The neuropsychological assessment of the older adult presents a number of unique challenges. One of the most significant of these pertains to the concept of "normal" aging, for which a number of definitions have been offered. For example, many researchers have considered normal to constitute optimal aging in which the *super healthy* (individuals free of any comorbid illnesses) are studied (hence, these individuals are often referred to as *supernormals*). However, given that only a very small percentage of older adults remains free of chronic illnesses, such as diabetes and hypertension late in life, many researchers consider truly normal older adults to constitute quite a heterogeneous group in which the effects of illness and medications on neuropsychological function complicate the aging process.

In part, competing notions regarding the cognitive changes associated with normal aging are largely attributable to the problem of defining what is normal. Taking the methodological problems associated with defining normal aging into consideration, a considerable amount of research has demonstrated that cognitive functions are affected differentially in the aging process. For example, increasing age is consistently shown to be associated with psychomotor slowing, decreased mental flexibility and set shifting, and diminished performance on nonverbal tasks (Parkin & Java, 1999; Rinn, 1988; Salthouse, 1998).

In addition, while age-corrected IQ (intelligence quotient) scores do not change with age (these scores are already adjusted for the patient's age), some of the true, underlying intellectual abilities do change with age. A "classic aging pattern" (Albert & Kaplan, 1980) has been demonstrated in a number of studies that evaluated the performance of subjects independent of their age (e.g., Rinn, 1988; Salthouse, 1998). This pattern, demonstrated by relative stability in verbal intellectual abilities (such as vocabulary knowledge) compared to more significant declines in nonverbal intellectual abilities (such as psychomotor speed), highlights the differential sensitivity of timed and novel neuropsychological measures in the assessment of the elderly.

Both verbal and nonverbal memory may also be differentially affected by aging (Craik, 1991; Salthouse, 1998), as cross-sectional (Petersen et al., 1992) and longitudinal studies (Small, 2001; Small et al., 1999) have reported age-related declines on tasks of effortful learning or acquisition, but not on the retention of already learned information.

A second challenge pertains to the use of neuropsychological test results in making a judgment regarding the presence or absence of clinical neuropsychological impairment. To determine if a patient's cognitive functioning is normal or abnormal, the neuropsychologist relies on two general strategies. The first interpretation strategy is to compare the obtained performance to the performance of neurologically intact individuals with similar demographic characteristics (*normative standard*). This method, however, presents a number of limitations, including the failure to take into consideration the level of premorbid ability. To overcome this limitation, neuropsychologists often rely on a second method—that of comparing the observed neuropsychological test performance to the individual's known or estimated premorbid capacity (*individual standard*).

The problems associated with the use of a normative standard have re-

ceived extensive attention (see Lezak, 1995; Spreen & Strauss, 1998). Typically, the normative standard, or *norm*, reflects an average score derived from a
neurologically intact sample. Historically, the normative data that have been
available for comparisons have been limited by small sample sizes, skewed gender distributions, and restricted age and educational ranges (often with few or
no older adults, especially the old-old). With these limitations, the neuropsychological assessment of older adults has often been problematic as these
confounds have potentially contributed to an increase in false diagnosis of impairment (Leckliter & Matarazzo, 1989).

In the past decade, in response to these and other limitations with published normative data, a number of authors published, for a variety of common
neuropsychological measures, extensive normative data based on large sample
sizes with broad age and educational ranges (for a description of the measures,
see Lezak, 1995; Spreen & Strauss, 1998). The Mayo Older Americans Normative Studies (MOANS) represent one of the most systematic efforts to
provide normative data on adults up to the age of 95 years for a variety of
neuropsychological measures. To date, normative data on a variety of measures
have been renormed, including category fluency (Lucas et al., 1998), Controlled Oral Word Association Test (COWAT; Ivnik et al., 1996), the Reading
subtest on the Wide Range Achievement Test–Revised (WRAT-R; Ivnik et al.,
1996), Trail Making Test (TMT; Ivnik et al., 1996), Judgment of Line Orientation (JLO; Ivnik et al., 1996), Stroop Color Word Test (Ivnik et al., 1996),
the Wechsler Memory Scale (WMS; Ivnik et al., 1991), the Wechsler Memory
Scale–Revised (WMS-R; Ivnik et al., 1992b), and the Wechsler Adult Intelligence Scale–Revised (WAIS-R; Ivnik et al., 1992a; Malec et al., 1992).

In addition to extensive normative data, new measures, such as the Repeatable Battery for the Assessment of Neuropsychological Status (RBANS; Randolph, 1998) and revised versions of common neuropsychological measures
such as the California Verbal Learning Test–II (CVLT-II; Delis et al., 2000),
the Wechsler Adult Intelligence Scale–III (WAIS-III; Wechsler, 1997a), and
Wechsler Memory Scale-III (WMS-III; Wechsler, 1997b), now include adults
through the age of 89 years in their standardization samples. In contrast, previous versions (WAIS-R and WMS-R) only included older adults up to 74 years
of age. Perhaps even more important, however, the current version of the WAIS
and WMS were administered and normed on the same standardization sample,
which affords the neuropsychologist the ability simultaneously to compare intellectual functioning with concurrent memory functioning.

COGNITIVE DOMAINS AND AVAILABLE MEASURES

An increasing number of neuropsychological measures are available for the
evaluation of the elderly patient. Below, we review a number of the most common measures, but this review should in no way be considered all-inclusive of

the measures currently available. A number of textbooks describe many of these tests in detail (see Lezak, 1995; Mitrushina et al., 1999; Spreen & Strauss, 1998), but with the proliferation of neuropsychological measures, descriptive information pertaining to additional measures is available predominantly through the specific administration manual available from the test publisher (Table 13-1).

Clinical Interview

The clinical interview is a vital component of the neuropsychological evaluation. Neuropsychological test data should not be interpreted in isolation as a number of factors frequently confound the interpretation of the obtained data. Peripheral sensory impairment, sleep deprivation, psychiatric illness, and suboptimal motivation are just a few of the factors that need to be considered when interpreting neuropsychological data. Although it is time consuming, a complete psychosocial history covering all areas of development, education, vocation, medical, and social functioning should be included in every neuropsychological evaluation (for a complete review, see Strub & Black, 2000). In addition, as the elderly often present with limited or disorganized recall of their personal history, collateral information from a close family member is vital to attain a clear understanding of the onset and course of the presenting illness. Collateral information also serves as corroboration of the patient's recount of personal history.

In addition to the historical information provided by the psychosocial interview, the interview provides a means for gathering behavioral information, which may be critical in differential diagnosis. The careful report of behavior is vital in the diagnosis of acute confusional states (delirium), denial-neglect syndromes, and frontal lobe syndromes, as observations such as abulia, emotional incontinence, or perseverative thoughts and actions can influence both concurrent test performance and the resulting diagnosis.

Premorbid Estimate

To reach a conclusion regarding a patient's current cognitive functioning, knowledge of premorbid intellectual functioning is important. However, as intel-

TABLE 13-1.   Neuropsychological test publishers

The Psychological Corp	www.PsychCorp.com
Psychological Assessment Resources, Inc	www.parinc.com
MHS, Inc	www.mhs.com
Western Psychological Services	www.wpspublish.com
American Guidance Service	www.agsnet.com
Pro-Ed, Inc	www.proedinc.com

lectual functioning is rarely evaluated prior to the event that necessitates a referral, the neuropsychologist must rely on premorbid estimates. However, research has demonstrated that certain cognitive functions, such as reading ability, are less affected by the cognitive changes in neurological illnesses and syndromes, such as dementia (Crawford et al., 1988).

Following this observation, a number of valid and reliable measures of reading ability have been developed for estimating premorbid intellectual functioning in the elderly. Three widely used measures include the WRAT-R, the National Adult Reading Test (NART), and its revision for an American (US) population (AmNART). The first of these measures, the WRAT-R, requires the patient to read a list of 75 increasingly difficult words. While the NART and AmNART also are based on the principle that word recognition (familiarity) reflects attained vocabulary, the NART and AmNART require the reading of a list of phonemically irregular words (e.g., "aisle" and "gouge") in which there must be word familiarity to pronounce the word correctly.

The use of reading tests to establish premorbid IQ functioning has not been without criticism. For example, while the use of reading ability to estimate premorbid IQ in patients with dementia has been criticized (Stebbins et al., 1990), a recent study that looked at a variety of neurological impairments (e.g., dementia, brain injury, and vascular disorders) reported that these measures provided equivalent and accurate IQ estimates (Johnstone et al., 1996). In addition, it has been reported that these measures underestimate the premorbid IQ in higher IQ groups (Wiens et al., 1993), although this assertion remains equivocal (Johnstone et al., 1996).

Like the AmNART, the newer Wechsler Test of Adult Reading (WTAR) consists of 50 irregularly spelled words, but the WTAR offers several advantages over the NART, AmNART, and the WRAT-R. First, the WTAR provides a premorbid estimate for individuals up to the age of 89 years. In addition, the NART and AmNART were developed as measures of reading ability, which was then related to intellectual ability (as assessed by the WAIS-R). In contrast, the WTAR was standardized (normed) on the same sample used in standardizing the WAIS-III and the WMS-III. Because it was conormed on both the WAIS-III and WMS-III standardization sample, the WTAR provides estimates of both premorbid WAIS-III IQ and WMS-III memory abilities.

A final method commonly used to estimate premorbid ability is based on only the use of demographic information that has been shown to be highly correlated with IQ (e.g., education, race, and occupation). A number of regression formulas have been developed (such as the Barona Index; Barona et al., 1984) that have been shown to provide IQ estimates comparable to the WRAT-R (Axelrod et al., 1999; Karaken et al., 1995). However, compared to the WTAR, the Barona Index is limited in that it provides only IQ estimates of the WAIS-R; it does not provide estimates of premorbid memory functioning, and it is also less valid with IQ scores less than 80 and greater than 120.

General Intelligence

The WAIS-III is the most commonly used measure of general intelligence. This measure is composed of a number of subtests designed to assess general knowledge, expressive vocabulary, verbal attention, abstraction, comprehension, and visuospatial construction and perception, which not only provide an overall assessment of the individual's intellectual functioning (Full Scale IQ), but also provide a Verbal IQ score and a Performance IQ score.

In addition, the WAIS-III protocol organizes the subtests into four material-specific indices. The first of these, the Verbal Comprehension Index (VCI), is a measure of acquired verbal knowledge and reasoning and was conceived as a "pure" measure of verbal comprehension as the Digit Span, Arithmetic, and Comprehension subtests are not included in calculating the VCI. Similarly, the Perceptual-Organization Index (POI) was conceived as a purer indicator of nonverbal, fluid reasoning and visuomotor integration, and the subtests related to psychomotor speed (Digit Symbol and Symbol Search) are not included (this index includes the Block Design, Picture Completion, and Matrix Reasoning subtests). Both Digit Symbol and Symbol Search make up the Processing Speed Index (PSI), which represents the individual's ability to process mental information quickly. Finally, the Working Memory Index (WMI) is comprised of the Digit Span, Arithmetic, and Letter-Number Sequencing subtests, which require individuals to attend to information and to hold and briefly manipulate information in immediate memory, somewhat analogous to remembering a telephone number momentarily after hearing it from directory assistance.

Attention

Measures of attention can be composed of simple (e.g., Digit Span Forward from the WAIS-III), complex (e.g., Digit Span Backward from the WAIS-III), and sustained components (e.g., Continuous Performance Test). A visual analog (Spatial Span) to the Digit Span from the WAIS-III is found on WMS-III. In addition, both the WAIS-III and the WMS-III include Letter-Number Sequencing as a component of the Working Memory Index. Other well-validated measures of attention and concentration commonly employed in the assessment of the elderly include the Paced Auditory Serial Addition Test (PASAT), Auditory Consonant Trigrams (ACT), and the Trail Making Test (Part A).

As attention mediates all other cognitive domains, this domain is often examined first. Attention is relatively insensitive to age-associated changes (Berardi et al., 2001), but is highly sensitive to acute disruptions of neural functioning. Determining the etiology of impaired attention and concentration is problematic as performance on measures of attention and concentration can be adversely affected by both diffuse and focal neurological impairment. For example, although digit repetition has been shown to be more vulnerable to left hemisphere damage (Black, 1986), impaired attention is commonly associated with diffuse impairment that is often associated with delirium and toxic exposure (Morrow et al., 1992). Similarly, focalized left and right hemisphere lesions have been associated with impaired performance.

Language

Language disturbances are frequently seen in disorders such as Alzheimer's disease (AD) and vascular dementia (VaD), as well as in focal disease processes of the left hemisphere. The assessment of language includes an evaluation of language comprehension, verbal fluency, repetition, naming, writing, and reading. Standardized language/aphasia batteries, such as the Boston Diagnostic Aphasia Examination (BDAE) and the Multilingual Aphasia Examination (MAE), have been developed and are easily incorporated into a neuropsychological evaluation when suspected language deficits are present. In addition to vocabulary knowledge assessed on the WAIS-III, vocabulary knowledge can be assessed through measures such as the Peabody Picture Vocabulary Test–III (PPVT-III), which requires the individual to select one of four pictures that best represents the meaning of a given word. Finally, tasks of verbal fluency, often divided into category and phonemic components, are typically included in the assessment of language function. On measures of phonemic verbal fluency, such as the COWAT, individuals are asked to generate all the words that they can think of in 1 minute that begin with a certain letter of the alphabet (such as the letter *F*). In contrast, measures of categorical verbal fluency, such as Animal Naming, requires the individual to name different types of animals in a 1-minute period.

While a number of language functions have been shown to be resilient to age-associated changes, language functioning is quite sensitive to left hemisphere damage. While confrontation naming, assessed with measures such as the Boston Naming Test, has been reported to be stable across the life span (Small et al., 1999), other studies have reported that this ability remains stable until individuals are in their 70s, at which point there is a decline in performance (van Gorp et al., 1986). Likewise, verbal fluency, the capacity to generate words in a specific time period, has been shown to change little until around the age of 80 years (Benton et al., 1981; Parkin & Java, 1999; Small et al., 1999).

Visuospatial

As noted above, the Wechsler Adult Intelligence Scale–III contains several visuospatial subtests that focus on construction, attention to visual details, and visual perception. In addition to the WAIS-III subtests, measures such as the Judgment of Line Orientation and Line Bisection are often administered as these measures are sensitive to visual hemineglect. In addition, drawing abilities are particularly sensitive to right hemisphere damage and hemineglect; therefore, elderly patients are often asked to complete increasingly complex drawing tasks ranging from simple designs like a clock and the Necker cube to complex designs such as the Rey Complex Figure Test (RCFT).

While focal lesions in either the left or right hemisphere can produce impaired performance on measures of visuospatial functioning, the parietal region of the right hemisphere has been shown to be especially sensitive to poor performance on these measures (Lezak, 1995). For example, individuals with damage to the left hemisphere tend to lose the details of the figure, producing a poorly copied design (Lezak, 1995). In contrast, right hemisphere damage is commonly associated with piecemeal construction and omitted elements, especially on the left side of the figure (Lezak, 1995).

Functionally, impairment in visuospatial abilities can have a significant impact on the quality of life for the elderly. Spatial neglect seen on drawing and constructional tasks often coincides with problems with dressing and hygiene difficulties. Perhaps the most significant restriction placed on the elderly in regard to their quality of life is the loss of driving privileges because spatial ability is required for successful navigation. A considerable amount of research has demonstrated the association between impaired visuospatial skills and driving ability (Carr, 1993; De Raedt & Ponjaert-Kristoffersen, 2000).

Memory

A variety of measures can be employed to assess memory functioning. The WMS-III is often used in evaluating the elderly patient. The WMS-III incorporates a variety of verbal and visual memory tasks, including prose (Logical Memory I and II) and paired learning (Paired Associates I and II) subtests to assess verbal memory and face recognition (Faces I and II) and character recall (Family Pictures I and II) to assess the visual domain. A number of optional subtests (Word List I and II and Visual Reproduction I and II) are available to supplement the information obtained through the administration of the standard protocol. Each of the WMS-III measures is administered with an immediate recall and delayed recall format, permitting the neuropsychologist to assess immediate and delayed memory and the patient's ability to retain learned information.

In addition to the WMS-III, a variety of list-learning tasks with varying levels of difficulty are available for the elderly patient. One of the most commonly used list-learning measures is the California Verbal Learning Test, now in its second revision. This task of effortful learning presents a series of 16 words over 5 learning trials. Compared to prose learning, list-learning tasks are generally more demanding; as a result, these measures are often more sensitive to subtle memory decline in the elderly and to subtle memory changes associated with depression (Veiel, 1997; Zakzanis et al., 1998).

Executive Function

Executive functioning refers to the cognitive domain consisting of the "higher" cognitive functions, such as abstraction, problem solving, inhibition, and cognitive set shifting, and is anatomically linked to the functioning of the frontal lobes (Miller & Cummings, 1999). Research has demonstrated that, compared to younger adults, older adults demonstrate mild executive decline (Daigneault et al., 1992). A number of validated measures are available to assess executive functioning, including tests of problem solving such as the Wisconsin Card Sorting Test (WCST), tests of verbal fluency such as the COWAT, tests of figure fluency such as the Ruff Figural Fluency Test, and tests of response inhibition such as the Stroop Color Word Test.

Psychomotor Function

Psychomotor speed has been shown to decline with increasing age (van Gorp et al., 1990). In addition to the Processing Speed Index on the WAIS-III, a number of motor tasks are available to assess psychomotor strength (e.g., Hand Dynamometer), speed (e.g., Finger Tapping Test), and manual dexterity (e.g., Grooved Pegboard).

WHEN TO USE A NEUROPSYCHOLOGICAL EVALUATION

There are a number of situations for which a referral for a neuropsychological evaluation may be particularly relevant to the assessment of the geriatric patient. These situations or referral questions may include (1) establishing a baseline of the patient's level of cognitive functioning; (2) using a test-retest paradigm, determining if the patient's current level of cognitive functioning is static or progressive; and (3) determining if a change in medication treatment has produced a corresponding change in neuropsychological functioning.

From these referral objectives, a neuropsychological assessment may be designed specifically to address issues related to the aging process, including the assessment of disorders commonly found among older adults. For example, an evaluation can be requested to determine if neurocognitive difficulties in an older adult are related to normal aging or are more consistent with an acquired neurodegenerative process. In addition, in conjunction with a thorough neurological and psychiatric evaluation, a neuropsychological evaluation is often helpful to assist in the determination whether an individual is capable of living independently, is in need of an assisted-living arrangement, or requires placement in a closed nursing home facility. Finally, by delineating which cognitive domains are differentially affected, neuropsychological assessments may be helpful in assisting with differential diagnosis as part of a comprehensive neuropsychiatric workup.

A thorough neuropsychological evaluation may also be beneficial when a patient scores within normal limits on basic screening measures (such as the MMSE), yet by either self-report or family report, concern remains about cognitive changes. Global screening measures often lack the sensitivity and specificity needed to characterize the mild changes in the patient's cognitive abilities as the results are often skewed by factors such as the patient's educational background. For example, with the MMSE, lower education can contribute to increased false positives, while higher education may mask impairment, leading to an increase in false negatives.

DIFFERENTIAL DIAGNOSIS

Delirium

Cognitively, severely impaired attention is the hallmark feature of delirium and is commonly assessed with the Digit Span subtest from the WAIS-III/WMS-III, serial subtractions (demonstrated on Mental Control on the WMS-III), and spelling a word backward (such as *world* on the MMSE). Impaired speech and language comprehension deficits (demonstrated on measures such as the Token Test) are often seen secondary to the confusion and the clouding of consciousness. Given the impaired attentional abilities, learning and memory are almost always adversely affected; however, delirium can often be distinguished from dementia by the severe inability to encode new information and immediately recall new information (such as demonstrated on the learning trials of the CVLT-II) as opposed to the ability to encode information on the learning trials, but with the rapid loss of the learned information following a long delay.

Alzheimer's Disease

Cognitively, memory dysfunction is the hallmark feature of AD. On memory tasks such as the WAIS-III, CVLT-II, and the Consortium to Establish Registry of Alzheimer's Disease (CERAD) Word List, patterns of rapid forgetting will be demonstrated, especially if the individuals engage in an interference task. In addition, memory performance will not benefit from recognition trials (Lezak, 1995). Beyond incorporating measures that assess the effortful encoding of information and the ability to retain that information across time, it is important to administer measures that assess all other cognitive domains when evaluating cases of probable AD. Notably, early AD will often present with language problems, as seen on measures such as COWAT, Animal Naming, and the Boston Naming Test (Lezak, 1995).

In the past few years, 2 lines of research have been particularly important in increasing our understanding of the cognitive changes associated with AD. First, significant strides have been made in the ability to identify early dementia through the use of neuropsychological measurements (Albert et al., 2002; Morris et al., 2001; Petersen et al., 1999). The use of neuropsychological measures of learning and memory, such as the CVLT-II, Rey Auditory Verbal Learning Test (RAVLT), and WMS-III, identified a transitional period between normality and AD, termed mild cognitive impairment (MCI), which is commonly defined by memory performance at least 1.5 standard deviations below average for age and education. Studies have shown that individuals diagnosed with MCI convert to AD at a rate of 10%–15% each year, which is in stark contrast to normal elderly subjects, who convert at a rate of 1%–2% per year (Petersen, 2000; Petersen et al., 2001).

Second, the role of apolipoprotein E ε4 (APOE ε4) in modulating cognitive decline associated with MCI and AD continues to be delineated. Several studies have reported that, while APOE ε4 is not associated with cognitive decline in normal aging (Dik et al., 2000; Small et al., 2000), the APOE ε4 allele is associated with an earlier decline in memory ability (Caselli et al., 1999). Most important, MCI patients with the APOE ε4 allele have been shown to be especially vulnerable to developing AD (Tierney et al., 1996). In considering the conversion from MCI to AD, the authors reported that algorithms that consider APOE status along with delayed recall and recognition performance demonstrated 83% sensitivity and 96% specificity.

Vascular Dementia

Vascular dementia is one of the leading causes of dementia in the United States (Gorelick et al., 1994; Nyenhuis & Gorelick, 1998) and may be as common or more common than Alzheimer's disease in Asia (Udea et al., 1992).

A number of authors have argued that the current understanding of VaD is limited as the VaD diagnostic criteria for dementia are dominated by criteria for AD (Erkinjuntii & Hachinski, 1993). This is especially true as AD requires the inclusion of memory disturbance (Rockwood et al., 2000); yet, as outlined below, vascular disease may or may not present with memory deficits, and it would exclude persons with vascular cognitive impairment who have not reached the end stage of dementia (Babikian et al., 1990; Rockwood et al., 1999).

Neuropsychological research in VaD has attempted to define the pattern of cognitive impairments in VaD and compare it with the pattern in other dementia syndromes, most often AD (Benthem et al., 1997; Crossley et al., 1997; Fuld, 1984; Starkstein et al., 1996). While VaD often presents with heterogeneous neurocognitive deficits, a guiding clinical heuristic in the assessment of vascular cognitive impairment has been that, in comparison to AD, VaD presents with more deficits in attention, concentration, and executive function and less delayed memory impairment (Kertesz & Clydesdale, 1994; McPherson & Cummings, 1996). Consistent with this, a recent meta-analytic review by Looi and Sachdev (1999) reported that, in contrast to a cortical dementia such as AD, memory loss (assessed by measures such as the CVLT, the RAVLT, and the Hopkins Verbal Learning Test) is often absent in VaD. In contrast, consistent with the propensity for subcortical vascular involvement, Looi and Sachdev reported that the hallmark of VaD is executive dysfunction, as evidenced by fewer attained categories and more perseverative responses on the WCST and poor planning on the Porteus Mazes.

Dementia of the Frontal Lobe Type

There is considerable debate regarding the specific nosologic criteria for dementia of the frontal lobe type (see Grossman, 2002). While the presence of Pick bodies has historically been thought to be a hallmark of the neuropathological changes associated with frontal lobe dementia, it is now recognized that multiple histopathological changes can contribute to a dementia of the frontal lobe type. Based on the presence or absence of certain neuropathological changes, dementia of the frontal lobe type can be described as the classically defined "Pick's disease," dementia lacking distinctive histopathology (i.e., frontotemporal dementia of the non-Alzheimer's type), or corticobasal degeneration.

The core clinical features of dementia of the frontal lobe type are similarly heterogeneous. Neary and colleagues (1998) proposed a classification system composed of three subgroups based on the primary behavioral manifestation. These groups include (1) progressive nonfluent aphasia, (2) semantic aphasia, and (3) frontotemporal degeneration.

Behaviorally, the core features in each clinical subgroup include a progressive aphasia and significant personality change, and the validation of this classification system has been shown to be successful in approximately two thirds of the cases (Davis et al., 2001).

Two key distinguishing features of a dementia of the frontal lobe type can aid in differential diagnosis. First, frontal lobe dementia occurs in patients, on average, a decade earlier than the onset of AD (Brun & Gustafson, 1993). Second, in contrast to the severe memory decline seen in Alzheimer's disease, dementia of the frontal lobe type typically presents with executive dysfunction (evidenced by an increase in perseverative behaviors and a decrease in social manners/conduct) in conjunction with mild-to-moderate memory decline (Grossman, 2002; Neary et al., 1998; Zakzanis, 1998a). Therefore, tests such as the WCST, COWAT, and TMT (Part B) are typically impaired. Performance on measures of memory (such as the CVLT-II and WMS-III) is often poor secondary to the deficits associated with frontal lobe degeneration (Neary et al., 1998).

Huntington's Disease

A common clinical heuristic used for differentiating the cognitive sequelae associated with Huntington's disease (HD) from other forms of dementia, particularly AD, is to characterize the dementia as "cortical" or "subcortical" (Folstein et al., 1990). A recent meta-analytic review of the literature (Zakzanis, 1998b) reported that, like AD, HD typically presents with memory deficits, as seen on the Logical Memory and Visual Reproduction subtests of the WMS-R, and list-learning tasks such as the CVLT. However, unlike AD, memory performance was noted to improve on recognition tasks, suggesting a retrieval deficit as opposed to the rapid forgetting seen in AD. In addition, Zakzanis (1998b) reported that tasks associated with frontal lobe functioning, such as those tested by the WCST, COWAT, and TMT (Part B), are typically impaired due to subcortical-cortical neural dysfunction.

Parkinson's Disease

Parkinson's disease (PD) commonly results in impaired cognitive abilities on measures of attention, memory, and executive function. In regard to the memory deficits, the performance of patients with PD is generally associated with subcortical patterns in that, while the free recall of newly learned information is impaired, both remote memory and recognition are intact. With this, the evaluation of memory performance on measures such as the CVLT-II and the WMS-III may highlight mild-to-moderate impairment of encoding of new material (demonstrated on the learning trials), but with little or no loss of learned information over time. In addition, memory recall will often be enhanced given the recognition trials of these measures (Lezak, 1995).

Beyond the memory patterns associated with PD, researchers have demonstrated that subtle semantic verbal fluency deficits (such as with animals) are present in nondemented patients with PD (Auriacombe et al., 1993), as are deficits in sustained attention, set shifting, and maintaining set (Lezak, 1995). With this cognitive pattern, in addition to measures of memory functioning, measures such as the COWAT, WCST, and TMT (Part B) should be administered as part of the comprehensive neuropsychological assessment.

Dementia Syndrome of Depression

Depression in the elderly often results in a syndrome of dementia (dementia syndrome of depression, DSD) for which reversibility of the cognitive deficits is the hallmark feature. Cognitively, depression in the elderly has been shown to result in memory dysfunction, which is distinct from memory patterns associated with Alzheimer's disease in that the rapid loss of newly learned information is atypical in DSD (Lezak, 1995). In addition, research has demonstrated that the memory deficits are commonly dependent on the difficulty of the measure. For example, Zakzanis and colleagues (1998) reported that depressed patients performed more poorly on the RAVLT compared to the CVLT because the CVLT allows the use of encoding strategies (i.e., grouping the words according to such semantic categories as tools).

In addition to memory decline, deficits in executive function, sustained attention, and psychomotor speed have been reported (Alexopolous et al.,

TABLE 13-2.   Recommended measures for evaluating older adults

Premorbid functioning
  Wechsler Test of Adult Reading
Intelligence
  Wechsler Adult Intelligence Scale–III
  Test of Nonverbal Intelligence–III
Attention
  Digit Span (forward and backward)
  Spatial Span (forward and backward)
  Mental Control from Wechsler Memory Scale–III
Language
  Token Test
  Boston Naming Test
  Controlled Oral Word Association Test
  Peabody Picture Vocabulary Test–III
  Boston Diagnostic Aphasia Examination
  Multilingual Aphasia Examination
Memory
  Wechsler Memory–III
  California Verbal Learning Test–II
  Rey Auditory Verbal Learning Test
  Consortium to Establish Registry of Alzheimer's Disease Word List
Executive functions
  Auditory Consonant Trigrams
  Wisconsin Card Sorting Test
  Category Test
  Trail Making Tests A and B
  Stroop Color-Word Test
Psychomotor
  Digit Symbol
  Symbol Search
  Symbol Digit Modalities Test
  Grooved Pegboard
  Finger Tapping
Repeatable measures
  Repeatable Battery for the Assessment of Neuropsychological Status
  Hopkins Verbal Learning Test–Revised
  Auditory Verbal Learning Test

2000; Lockwood et al., 2000). As with the disorders mentioned above, executive dysfunction will be demonstrated by poor performance on measures of sustained attention (such as the PASAT), sequencing and set shifting (TMT, Part B), and planning and organizing (such as on the WCST). Finally, psychomotor slowing will be evident on measures such as the Processing Speed Index on the WAIS-III and the TMT (Part A).

Although unique cognitive profiles associated with DSD have been suggested, differentiating depressed dementia patients from psychiatrically depressed patients remains problematic. Van Gorp and Cummings (1996) highlighted the importance of multiple (test-retest) neuropsychological evaluations in differentiating DSD from dementia syndromes.

CONCLUSION

Increasing age has been shown to affect cognitive functioning differentially, with speed of information processing the most adversely affected. A number of neurological illnesses associated with aging also present with concurrent psychiatric disturbances. In an effort to provide optimal medical care, clinicians must be familiar with the benign cognitive changes commonly seen with increasing age, as well as the typical cognitive profiles that may suggest the presence of incipient neurocognitive disturbance. Table 13-2 presents a list of measures commonly used in the evaluation of older adults.

REFERENCES

Albert MS, Kaplan E. Organic implications of neuropsychological deficits in the elderly. In: Poon LW, Fozard JL, Cermak LS, Arenberg D, Thompson LW, eds. *New Directions in Memory and Aging: Proceedings of the George A. Talland Memorial Conference.* Hillsdale, NJ: Erlbaum; 1980:403–432.

Albert SM, Tabert MH, Dienstag A, Pelton G, Devanand D. The impact of mild cognitive impairment on functional abilities in the elderly. *Curr Psychiatry Rep.* 2002; 4(1):64–68.

Alexopolous GS, Meyers BS, Young RC, et al. Executive dysfunction and long-term outcomes of geriatric depression. *Arch Gen Psychiatry.* 2000;57:285–290.

Auriacombe S, Grossman M, Carvell S, Gollomp S, Stern MB, Hurtig HI. Verbal fluency deficits in Parkinson's disease. *Neuropsychology.* 1993;7:182–192.

Axelrod BN, Vanderploeg RD, Schinka JA. Comparing methods for estimating premorbid intellectual functioning. *Arch Clin Neuropsychol.* 1999;14:341–346.

Babikian V, Wolfe N, Linn R, Knoefel J, Albert M. Cognitive changes in patients with multiple cerebral infarcts. *Stroke.* 1990;21:1013–1018.

Barona A, Reynolds CR, Chastain R. A demographically based index of pre-morbid intelligence for the WAIS-R. *J Consult Clin Psychology.* 1984;52:885–887.

Benthem PW, Jones S, Hodges JR. A comparison of semantic memory in vascular dementia and dementia of the Alzheimer type. *Int J Geriatr Psychiatry.* 1997;12:575–580.

Benton AL, Eslinger PJ, Damasio AR. Normative observations on neuropsychological tests performance in old age. *J Clin Neuropsychol.* 1981;3:33–42.

Berardi A, Parasurman R, Haxby JV. Overall vigilance and sustained attention decrements in healthy aging. *Exp Aging Res.* 2001;27:19–39.

Black BW. Digit repetition in brain-damaged adults: clinical and theoretical implications. *J Clin Psychol.* 1986;42:770–782.

Brun A, Gustafson L. The Lund longitudinal dementia study: a 25-year perspective on neuropathology, differential diagnosis, and treatment. In: Corain B, Iqbal K, Nicoline M, Winblad B, Wisniewski H, Zatta P, eds. *Alzheimer's Disease: Advances in Clinical and Basic Research.* London, England: Wiley; 1993:3–18.

Carr DB. Assessing older drivers for physical and cognitive impairment. *Geriatrics.* 1993;48(5):46–48, 51.

Caselli RJ, Graff-Radford NR, Reiman EM, et al. Preclinical memory decline in cognitively normal apolipoprotein E-ε4 homozygotes. *Neurology.* 1999;53:201–207.

Craik FIM. Memory functions in normal aging. In: Yanagihara T, Petersen RC, eds. *Memory Disorders: Research and Clinical Practice.* New York, NY: Dekker; 1991: 347–367.

Crawford JR, Parker DM, Besson JAO. Estimation of premorbid intelligence in organic conditions. *Br J Psychiatry.* 1988;153:178–181.

Crossley M, D'Arcy C, Rawson NSB. Letter and category fluency in community-dwelling Canadian seniors: a comparison of normal participants to those with dementia of the Alzheimer or vascular type. *J Clin Exp Neuropsychol.* 1997;19:52–62.

Cullum CM, Thompson LL, Heaton RK. The use of the Halstead-Reitan Test Battery with older adults. In: Pirozzolo FJ, ed. *Clinics in Geriatric Medicine.* Vol. 5, No. 3. Philadelphia, PA: Saunders; 1989:595–610.

Daigneault S, Braun MJ, Whitaker HA. Early effects of normal aging on perseverative and non-perseverative prefrontal measures. *Dev Neuropsychol.* 1992;8:99–114.

Davis KL, Price C, Moore P, Campea S, Grossman M. Evaluating the clinical diagnosis of frontotemporal degeneration: a re-examination of Neary et al., 1998. *Neurology.* 2001;56:A144–A145.

Delis DC, Kramer JH, Kaplan E, Ober BA. *California Verbal Learning Test–II.* San Antonio, TX: Psychological Corp; 2000.

De Raedt R, Ponjaert-Kristoffersen I. The relationship between cognitive/neuropsychological factors and car driving performance in older adults. *J Am Geriatr Soc.* 2000; 48(12):1661–1668.

Dik MG, Jonker C, Bouter LM, Geerlings MI, van Kamp GJ, Deeg DJH. APOE-ε4 is associated with memory decline in cognitively impaired elderly. *Neurology.* 2000; 54:1492–1497.

Elias MF, Podraza AM, Pierce TW, Robbins MA. Determining neuropsychological cut scores for older, healthy adults. *Exp Aging Res.* 1990;16:209–220.

Erkinjuntii T, Hachinski VC. Rethinking vascular dementia. *Cerebrovascular Dis.* 1993; 3:3–23.

Fastenau PS. Validity of regression-based norms: an empirical test of the comprehensive norms with older adults. *J Clin Exp Neuropsychol.* 1998;20:906–916.

Fastenau PS, Adams KM. Heaton, Grant, and Matthews' comprehensive norms: an overzealous attempt. *J Clin Exp Neuropsychol.* 1996;18:444–448.

Folstein SE, Brandt J, Folstein MF. Huntington's disease. In: Cummings JL, ed. *Subcortical Dementia.* New York, NY: Oxford; 1990:87–107.

Fuld PA. Test profile of cholinergic dysfunction and Alzheimer-type dementia. *J Clin Neuropsychol.* 1984;6:380–392.

Heaton RK, Grant I, Matthews CG. *Comprehensive Norms for an Expanded Halstead-Reitan Battery: Demographic Corrections, Research Findings, and Clinical Applications.* Odessa, FL: Psychological Assessment Resources; 1991.

Gorelick PB, Roman G, Mangone CA. Vascular dementia. In: Gorelick PB, Alter MA, eds. *Handbook of Neuroepidemiology.* New York, NY: Dekker; 1994:197–214.

Grossman M. Frontotemporal dementia: a review. *J Int Neuropsychol Soc.* 2002;8:566–583.

Ivnik RJ, Malec JF, Smith GE, Tangalos EG, Petersen RC. Neuropsychological tests' norms above age 55: COWAT, BNT, MAE Token, WRAT-R Reading, AMNART, STROOP, TMT, and JLO. *Clin Neuropsychol.* 1996;10:262–278.

Ivnik RJ, Malec JF, Smith GE, et al. Mayo's older Americans normative studies: WAIS-R norms for age 56 to 97. *Clin Neuropsychol.* 1992a;6(suppl):1–30.

Ivnik RJ, Malec JF, Smith GE, et al. Mayo's older Americans normative studies: WMS-R norms for age 56 to 94. *Clin Neuropsychol.* 1992b;6(suppl):49–82.

Ivnik RJ, Smith GE, Tangalos EG, Petersen RC, Kokmen E, Kurland LT. Wechsler Memory Scale (WMS): IQ dependent norms for persons age 65 to 97. *Psychol Assess.* 1991;3:156–161.

Johnstone B, Callahan CD, Kapila CJ, Bouman DE. The comparability of the WRAT-R reading test and the NAART as estimates of premorbid intelligence in neurologically impaired patients. *Arch Clin Neuropsychol.* 1996;11:513–519.

Karaken DA, Gur RC, Saykin AJ. Reading on the Wide Range Achievement Test–Revised and parental education as predictors of IQ: comparison with the Barona formula. *Arch Clin Neuropsychol.* 1996;10:147–157.

Kertesz A, Clydesdale S. Neuropsychological deficits in vascular dementia versus Alzheimer's disease: frontal lobe deficits prominent in vascular dementia. *Arch Neurol.* 1994;51:1226–1231.

Leckliter IN, Matarazzo JD. The influence of age, education, IQ, gender, and alcohol abuse on Halstead-Reitan Neuropsychological Test Battery performance. *J Clin Psychol.* 1989;45:484–512.

Lezak MD. *Neuropsychological Assessment.* 3rd ed. New York, NY: Oxford University Press; 1995.

Lockwood KA, Alexopoulos GS, Kakuma T, van Gorp WG. Subtypes of cognitive impairment in depressed older adults. *Am J Geriatr Psychiatry.* 2000;8:201–208.

Looi JC, Sachdev PS. Differentiation of vascular dementia from AD on neuropsychological tests. *Neurology.* 1999;53:670–678.

Lucas JA, Ivnik RJ, Smith GE, et al. Mayo's older American normative studies: category fluency norms. *J Clin Exp Neuropsychol.* 1998;20:194–200.

Malec JF, Ivnik RJ, Smith GE, et al. Mayo's older Americans normative studies: utility of corrections for age and education for the WAIS-R. *Clin Neuropsychol.* 1992;6(suppl):31–47.

McPherson SE, Cummings JL. Neuropsychological aspects of vascular dementia. *Brain Cognition.* 1996;31:269–282.

Miller BL, Cummings JL. *The Human Frontal Lobes: Functions and Disorders.* New York, NY: Guilford; 1999.

Mitrushina MN, Boon KB, D'Elia LA. Handbook of Normative Data for Neurpsychological Assessment. New York, NY: Oxford University Press; 1999.

Morris JC, Storandt M, Miller P, et al. Mild cognitive impairment represents early-stage Alzheimer disease. *Arch Neurol.* 2001;58:397–405.

Morrow LA, Robin N, Hodgson MJ, Kamis H. Assessment of attention and memory efficiency in persons with solvent neurotoxicity. *Neuropsychologia.* 1992;30:911–922.

Neary D, Snowden JS, Gustafson L, et al. Frontotemporal lobar degeneration: a consensus on clinical diagnostic criteria. *Neurology.* 1998;51:1546–1554.

Nyenhuis DL, Gorelick PB. Vascular dementia: a contemporary review of epidemiology, diagnosis, prevention, and treatment. *J Am Geriatr Soc.* 1998;46:1437–1448.

Parkin AJ, Java RI. Deterioration of frontal lobe function in normal aging: influences of fluid intelligence versus perceptual speed. *Neuropsychology.* 1999;13:539–545.

Petersen RC. Mild cognitive impairment: transition between aging and Alzheimer's disease. *Neurologia.* 2000;15:93–101.

Petersen RC, Smith G, Kokmen E, Ivnik RJ, Tangalos EG. Memory function in normal aging. *Neurology.* 1992;42:396–401.

Petersen RC, Smith GE, Waring SC, Ivnik RJ, Tangalos EG, Kokmen E. Mild cognitive impairment: clinical characterization and outcome. *Arch Neurol.* 1999;56:303–308.

Randolph C. *Repeatable Battery for the Assessment of Neuropsychological Status (RBANS).* San Antonio, TX: Psychological Corp; 1998.

Reitan RM, Wolfson D. *The Halstead-Reitan Neuropsychological Test Battery.* Tucson, Ariz: Neuropsychology Press; 1985.

Rinn WE. Mental decline in normal aging: a review. *J Geriatr Psychiatry Neurol.* 1988;1:144–158.

Rockwood K, Howard K, MacKnight C, Darvesh S. Spectrum of disease in vascular cognitive impairment. *Neuroepidemiology.* 1999;18:248–254.

Rockwood K, Wentzel C, Hachinski VC, Hogan D, MacKnight C, McDowell I. Prevalence and outcomes of vascular cognitive impairment. *Neurology.* 2000;54:447–451.

Salthouse TA. Independence of age-related influences on cognitive abilities across the life span. *Dev Psychol.* 1998;34:851–864.

Small SA. Age-related memory decline: current concepts and future directions. *Arch Neurol.* 2001;58:360–364.

Small SA, Graves AB, McEvoy CL, Crawford FC, Mullan M, Mortimer J. Is APOE-ε4 a risk factor for cognitive impairment in normal aging? *Neurology.* 2000;54:2082–2088.

Small SA, Stern Y, Tang M, Mayeux R. Selective decline in memory function among healthy elderly. *Neurology.* 1999;52:1392–1396.

Spreen O, Strauss E. *A Compendium of Neuropsychological Tests: Administration, Norms, and Commentary.* 2nd ed. New York, NY: Oxford University Press; 1998.

Starkstein SE, Sabe L, Vazquez S. Neuropsychological, psychiatric, and cerebral blood flow findings in vascular dementia and Alzheimer's disease. *Stroke.* 1996;27:408–414.

Stebbins GT, Wilson RS, Gilley DW, Bernard BA, Fox JH. Use of the National Adult Reading Test to estimate premorbid IQ in dementia. *Clin Neuropsychol.* 1990;4:18–24.

Strub RL, Black FW. *The Mental Status Examination in Neurology.* Philadelphia, PA: FA Davis; 2000.

Tierney MC, Szalai JP, Snow WG, et al. A prospective study of the clinical utility of ApoE genotype in the prediction of outcome in patients with memory impairment. *Neurology.* 1996;46:149–154.

Udea K, Hasuo Y, Fujishima M. Prevalence and etiology of dementia in a Japanese community. *Stroke.* 1992;23:798–803.

van Gorp WG, Cummings JL. Depression and reversible dementia in an HIV-1 seropositive individual: implications for the dementia syndrome of depression. *Neurocase.* 1996;2:455–459.

van Gorp WG, Satz P, Kiersch ME, Henry R. Normative data on the Boston Naming Test for a group of normal older adults. *J Clin Exp Neuropsychol.* 1986;8(6):702–705.

van Gorp WG, Satz P, Mitrushina M. Neuropsychological processes associated with normal aging. *Dev Neuropsychol.* 1990;6:279–290.

Veiel HO. A preliminary profile of neuropsychological deficits associated with major depression. *J Clin Exp Neuropsychol.* 1997;19:587–603.

Wechsler D. *Wechsler Adult Intelligence Scale–III.* San Antonio, TX: Psychological Corp; 1997a.

Wechsler D. *Wechsler Memory Scale–III.* San Antonio, Tex: Psychological Corp; 1997b.

Wiens AN, Bryan JE, Crossen JR. Estimating WAIS-R FSIQ from national adult reading test—revised in normal subjects. *Clin Neuropsychol.* 1993;7:70–84.

Zakzanis KK. Neurocognitive deficit in fronto-temporal dementia. *Neuropsychiatry Neuropsychol Behav Neurol.* 1998a;11:127–135.

Zakzanis KK. The subcortical dementia of Huntington's disease. *J Clin Exp Neuropsychol.* 1998b;20:565–578.

Zakzanis KK, Leach L, Kaplan E. On the nature and pattern of neurocognitive function in major depressive disorder. *Neuropsychiatry Neurobiol Behav Neurol.* 1998;3:111–119.

14

Neuroimaging in Late-Life Mental Disorders

Anand Kumar, MD

Despite recent technical developments and the application of modern neuro-imaging methods to the study of behavioral disorders, their utility in routine clinical psychiatric practice remains circumscribed. The diagnostic utility of these approaches is primarily in the realm of neurodegenerative disorders. The study of regional cerebral glucose metabolism and cerebral blood flow, using positron emission tomography (PET) and single-photon emission computed tomography (SPECT), has revealed physiological patterns that are relatively specific for Alzheimer's disease (AD) (Chase et al., 1984; Duara et al., 1986; Kumar et al., 1991). The metabolic patterns, together with genetic markers, may be helpful in the early detection of AD in selected cases (Small et al., 1995). Outside the neurodegenerative disease spectrum, neuroanatomic approaches are largely used to rule out overt neurological causes of psychiatric/ behavioral disturbances.

Neuroimaging, however, has had greater impact in clinical neuroscience research, in which these techniques have been helpful in testing hypotheses and studying mechanisms that may contribute to the pathophysiology of psychiatric disorders. As neuroimaging techniques become more sophisticated, their relevance to late-life mental disorders from both diagnostic and neurobiological perspectives will also increase (Kumar, 2000a, 2000b).

The focus of this chapter is modern neuroimaging as it relates to the major mental disorders in the elderly. First, some of the principal methodological considerations behind PET and magnetic resonance imaging/magnetic resonance spectroscopy (MRI/MRS) are described (Oldendorf & Oldendorf, 1991; Phelps et al., 1978). This is followed by a description of the major neuroimaging findings in normal aging and specific geriatric mental disorders and a discussion of their clinical and biological significance. Some of the cutting edge approaches in human neuroimaging, such as probabilistic atlases and postmortem MRI, that are being developed in the laboratory and will emerge over the next few years as important probes of brain biology are then discussed.

POSITRON EMISSION TOMOGRAPHY

Positron emission tomography (PET) (Table 14-1) is an imaging technique that helps examine active biological processes, such as regional cerebral glucose utilization and blood flow in the living brain, both in the resting state and during specific pharmacological and behavioral challenge paradigms (the activated state) (Grady et al., 1993; Phelps et al., 1978, 1979; Phelps & Cherry, 1998; Reivich et al., 1979). PET is also used to study neuropharmacological and neurochemical systems in the brain and other organs (Agren et al., 1993; Meltzer et al., 1999).

The fundamental principal of PET involves the intravenous injection of trace amounts of a biologically active substance (such as deoxyglucose or water) that is coupled to a positron-emitting radionuclide (fluorine 18) (Phelps et al., 1978, 1979; Phelps & Cherry, 1998). In the brain, as deoxyglucose participates

TABLE 14-1.   Major in vivo neuroimaging techniques and area of scope in neuroscience research

Technique	Neurobiological domain
MRI	Neuroanatomy: volumes of brain, cerebrospinal fluid and high-intensity lesions
Proton MRS	Neurochemistry: levels of NAA, creatine, choline, myo-inositol, and glutamate/glutamine (GLx)
FDG and H_2O^{15} GLx PET	Neurophysiology: regional cerebral metabolic rate for glucose (rCMR glc) and cerebral blood flow (rCBF)
SPECT	Perfusion: semiquantitative estimate of cerebral blood flow
Xenon Inhalation	Blood flow: quantitative estimate of cortical blood flow
Receptor PET/SPECT	Neuropharmacology: estimate of receptor density (B_{max}) affinity (KD) and composite measures of receptor function; postsynaptic and presynaptic receptors and reuptake sites.
Functional MRI (fMRI)	Physiological activation: regional changes in signal intensity (reflecting deoxyhemoglobin/oxyhemoglobin imbalance) in response to cognitive/sensory challenge

Note: See text for definition of abbreviations.

in metabolic pathways, in a manner similar to endogenous glucose, the radio-nuclide fluorine 18, to which it is coupled, emits positrons. The positrons that are emitted annihilate with an electron and give out two photons at an angle of 180°. The photons are detected by a ring of crystals (detectors) that are part of the external imaging system and surround the head in the scanner.

Using a computerized technique called filtered back projection, it is possi-ble to reconstruct images of brain tissue activity depicting the brain locations where the positrons originated (Phelps et al., 1978; Phelps & Cherry, 1998). With the help of appropriate tracer kinetic modeling (mathematical constants and equations that account for the physiological behavior of deoxyglucose in the bloodstream and the brain) and brain tissue activity images (Figure 14-1), a metabolic map of glucose in the brain can be obtained (Phelps et al., 1979; Reivich et al., 1979). This provides a quantitative estimate of glucose utiliza-tion, both globally and regionally, in the brain. MR segmentation algorithms that separate brain from cerebrospinal fluid (CSF) may then be used to correct for atrophy and tissue heterogeneity (gray versus white matter) in the brain; glucose metabolic values are expressed as milligrams per 100 g of brain per minute.

The same underlying principle is exploited in estimating cerebral blood flow with PET. In this instance, radioactive water H_2O^{15} is injected intrave-nously, and kinetic modeling is integrated with tissue activity maps to obtain quantitative estimates of regional cerebral flow (Grady et al., 1993). The short half-life of the radioisotope O^{15} permits us to obtain multiple scans over a very short period. Prior to the advent of functional magnetic resonance imaging

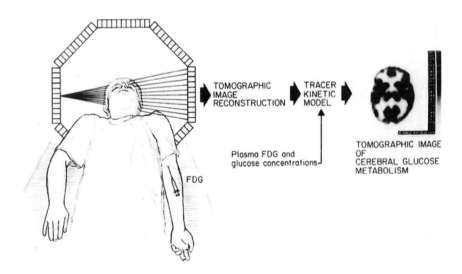

FIGURE 14-1. The steps involved in acquiring a PET image.

(fMRI), H_2O^{15} PET was the principal method of identifying anatomic structures and neural circuits involved in cognitive and sensory processing.

The broad nuclear medicine principle of coupling a positron-emitting radionuclide to a potentially biologically active molecule to track and study physiological/pharmacological phenomena is widely used in clinical neuroimaging. Isotopes such as carbon 11 (^{11}C) and nitrogen 13 (^{13}N) have been used to image and study receptor density, protein synthetic pathways, and neurotransmitter kinetics in humans (Agren et al., 1993; Meltzer et al., 1999). Preliminary testing and development of these approaches in phantom studies and primates increases their validity and facilitates their application in the study of normal controls and patients with specific psychiatric disorders.

MAGNETIC RESONANCE IMAGING

Magnetic resonance imaging uses the magnetic properties of living tissues to produce an image of the organ under study (Oldendorf & Oldendorf, 1991). Because hydrogen makes up two thirds of the atoms in living tissue, it is predominantly the hydrogen in tissue water that is currently imaged using MR. The hydrogen nucleus has only one proton; therefore, imaging of hydrogen is often referred to as proton imaging.

In clinical MR imaging, protons are aligned by placing the subject in a magnetic field. The field strengths of most clinical MR scanners vary from 0.5 Tesla (T) to high-field systems of approximately 4 T. Radio waves are used (as excitation pulses) to perturb hydrogen atoms in the presence of a strong magnetic field. Tissues under study are exposed to single or multiple excitation pulses, which cause the hydrogen atoms to absorb energy and precess (spin) around the common axes. The stimulated protons then release energy and return to their resting orientation.

It is the absorption and release of the energy that forms the fundamental signal of the MR image. Typically, two or more pulses are used for better characterization of tissues. A standard MRI scan provides an image of hydrogen distribution in the organ under study, and it displays a slice of tissue as regions of varying brightness. By varying the time interval between successive pulse cycles (TR) and the interval from a pulse to the measurement of the MR signal (TE), MR images with differing tissue contrasts (i.e., T1, T2 weighting and proton densities) can be obtained.

Each of these images depicts different characteristics of the brain, and they consequently have different applications in clinical geropsychiatry and neurology. In a T1 weighted image, CSF appears black, and tissue discrimination between gray and white matter is sharp. In a T2 weighted image, CSF appears bright, and anatomic detail is less striking. T2 weighted images, however, are useful in detecting certain pathologies that may have special relevance in geriatric psychiatry. This includes high-intensity lesions, areas that appear as bright spots in the parenchyma on T2 weighted images. Proton density images provide tissue contrast with intermediate brightness.

MR has several advantages over computerized tomography (CT) (Hounsfield, 1973; Oldendorf & Oldendorf, 1991). These include the superior spatial resolution of MR, the ability to visualize images in different planes (coronal, sagittal, and axial), better separation of gray and white matter, and the increased sensitivity of MR to different brain pathologies. The confined space of a traditional MR scanner poses a practical problem for patients with claustrophobia. The increasing use of "open" MRI scanners in clinical settings has improved the access of patients to this technology.

MAGNETIC RESONANCE SPECTROSCOPY

Magnetic resonance spectroscopy may be conceptualized as a procedure in which magnetic resonance signals are obtained from nuclei that are components of molecules, other than water, in living tissue. In both MRI and MRS, nuclei are responsible for the signal (Frahm et al., 1989; Kreis et al., 1991; Michaelis et al., 1991; Miller, 1991; Miller et al., 1996; Moore et al., 1999; Thomas & Alger, 1997).

The origin of the signal, however, is different in the two techniques. In MRI, the signal used to create the image originates from hydrogen nuclei in tissue water. In MRS, the signals are generated from nuclei that are parts of other chemicals (metabolites) dissolved in tissue fluid. MRI and MRS scans are routinely performed using the same scanning equipment, and similar biophysical assumptions underlie both approaches. The biological information obtained from these techniques, however, is different (Frahm et al., 1989; Kreis et al., 1991; Michaelis et al., 1991; Miller, 1991; Moore et al., 1999; Thomas & Alger, 1997).

MRS deals with nonradioactive nuclei that are naturally present in tissue and typically involves the detection of either hydrogen (^{1}H) or phosphorus (^{31}P) signals. Signals from different isotopes are distinguishable because they occur at markedly different frequencies (Frahm et al., 1989; Kreis et al., 1991; Michaelis et al., 1991; Miller, 1991). The electronic environment of the different nuclei will determine the frequency at which different nuclei precess. Molecules that are slightly different will precess at different frequencies, thereby producing an MR signal at different chemical shifts. This small effect forms the basis of the ability of MR to distinguish signals from similar nuclei within molecules.

MRS studies of the metabolite signals are generally very weak because the concentration of the molecules that produce them is low (Thomas & Alger, 1997). For example, the concentration of water molecules in human tissue is approximately 100 mol/L (100,000mmol/L). The concentration of several commonly measured metabolites is in the range of 4–10 mmol/L (Thomas & Alger,

1997). Proton spectroscopy is therefore performed by suppressing the MR signal from water.

Obtaining water suppression allows the detection of a number of cerebral metabolites such as N-acetyl aspartate (NAA), creatine/phosphocreatine (Cr), choline (Ch), and myoinositol (MI). Levels of glutamate/glutamine (GLx) and γ-aminobutyric acid (GABA) can also be estimated with MRS. Absolute levels of metabolites and metabolite ratios, such as NAA/Cr and MI/Cr, can be estimated, and both measures are widely reported in the literature (Frahm et al., 1989; Kreis et al., 1991; Michaelis et al., 1991; Miller, 1991). Both single-voxel (where a predetermined region is sampled; Figure 14-2) and multivoxel approaches (commonly called chemical shift imaging, CSI), which permit the concurrent study of multiple regions, have been used in human studies. Each approach has its strengths and limitations.

The precise biological significance and clinical relevance of these metabolites are receiving increasing scrutiny (Bottomley et al., 1992; Cuenod et al., 1995; Thomas & Alger, 1997; Tsai & Coyle, 1995). NAA is widely accepted as a neuronal marker that is absent in mature glia (Tsai & Coyle, 1995). NAA estimates in the gray matter reflect the structural integrity of the cell body, while white matter NAA is a more accurate measure of axonal structure and function (Bottomley et al., 1992). As a putative marker of neuronal viability, it may be more sensitive than volumetric estimates of brain volume (Frahm et al., 1989; Kreis et al., 1991; Michaelis et al., 1991; Miller, 1991; Miller et al., 1996). The choline signal is a composite signal from compounds that contain the choline chemical group and includes phosphocholine, glycerophosphocholine, and phosphotidylcholine (Frahm et al., 1989; Kreis et al., 1991; Michaelis et al., 1991; Miller, 1991).

Many of these compounds are involved in phospholipid and membrane biochemistry. Both creatine and phosphocreatine contribute to the creatine signal (Frahm et al., 1989; Kreis et al., 1991; Michaelis et al., 1991; Miller 1991). This signal is thought to represent a marker of energy metabolism. Myoinositol represents the storage form of the inositol phosphate secondary messenger system and is also a marker of gliosis (Thomas & Alger, 1997). Phosphorous spectra provide important information with respect to phospholipid metabolism, bioenergetics, and pH (Bottomley et al., 1992; Pettegrew et al., 1994). More specifically, phosphorous 31 spectra provide information on metabolically active compounds such as phosphomonoesters, phosphodiesters, and high-energy phosphate bond membrane structure (Bottomley et al., 1992; Cuenod et al., 1995; Pettegrew et al., 1994; Thomas & Alger, 1997).

Within the realm of geriatric psychiatry, proton spectroscopy is used more frequently and provides information on metabolites that is more readily interpretable (Bottomley et al., 1992; Moore et al., 1999; Pfefferbaum et al., 1999). The neurobiological implications of these measures are complex, and the interpretations need to be placed in the context of the overall clinical picture.

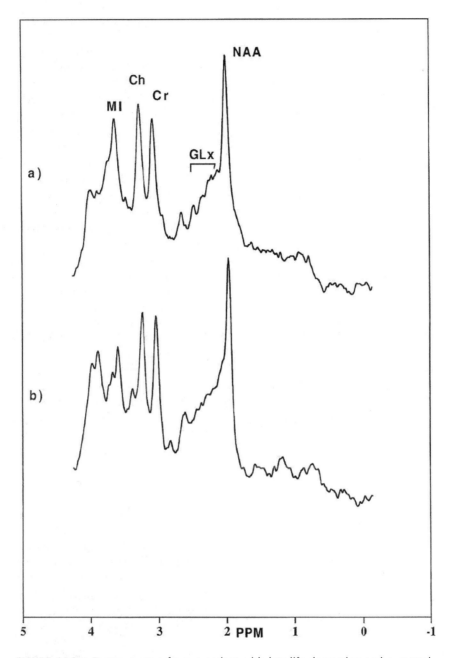

FIGURE 14-2. Proton spectra from a patient with late-life depression and a control. Please note the higher MI and Ch peaks in the patient's spectra.

FUNCTIONAL MAGNETIC RESONANCE IMAGING

Functional magnetic resonance imaging (fMRI) is another MR-based technique that provides information about cerebral perfusion and blood volume in the baseline state and in response to specific cognitive challenges (Cohen & Bookheimer, 1994; Ogawa et al., 1992). The most frequently used fMRI approach is the brain oxygen level dependent (BOLD) contrast technique (Ogawa et al., 1992).

The premise of this approach is that, in the activated state, increased neuronal activity is associated with increased cerebral blood volume and oxygen delivery to specific activated brain areas. This leads to an increased concentration of oxyhemoglobin and a decreased concentration of deoxyhemoglobin (which is a paramagnetic material) in venules and veins. The deoxyhemoglobin/oxyhemoglobin imbalance forms the basis of the fMRI detected in human studies. The areas of activation, which appear red on fMRI images, represent regions with increased neuronal activity.

Differences in signal intensity (brightness) between regions are commonly used as indices of differential activation of regions during performance of a task. Using this approach, it is possible to map regions that are involved in several behavior and cognitive tasks. fMRI provides the opportunity to examine objectively the brain regions and circuits that may be involved in normal information processing in the brain (Cohen & DuBois, 1999; Gabrieli et al., 1997). It further enables a look at psychopathological states for which attenuated circuitry may result in differential activation of brain regions.

Cognitive challenges used in fMRI studies depend on the underlying scientific question. They include working memory tasks and verbal and spatial challenges (Cohen & DuBois, 1999; Gabrieli et al., 1997). These approaches are being widely applied in cognitive neuroscience and brain mapping studies.

DIFFUSION TENSOR IMAGING

Diffusion tensor imaging (DTI) is an MR-related technique that permits noninvasive mapping of the diffusion of proton molecules, a process that is sensitive to the molecular makeup of the surrounding tissue (Alexopoulos et al., 2002; Moseley, 2002; Pfefferbaum et al., 1999). DTI measures the nonrandomness (anisotropy) of water diffusion within tissue, which reflects the degree to which directionally ordered tissues are either maturing or losing their normal integrity. Both anisotropy and the apparent diffusion coefficient (ADC), which is a measure of overall water content, reflect axonal restriction and the myelin content of tissue.

DTI is widely considered to provide important information on the structural integrity of the white matter, including the status of myelin and axons. DTI is being used in neuroscience research to characterize and monitor brain abnormalities associated with normal aging, the dementias, mood disorders, and schizophrenia (Alexopoulos et al., 2002; Moseley, 2002; Pfefferbaum et al., 1999).

Aging has been shown to be associated with a decrease in anisotropy, which may reflect demyelination and loss of myelinated axons. Changes in anisotropy with increasing age may occur in the absence of T2 weighted high-intensity signals. Within the realm of psychiatric disorders, DTI has been used to study dementia of the Alzheimer type (DAT), mood disorders, and schizophrenia. In all these disorders, focal (frontal and temporal) reductions in anisotropy have been identified that have been interpreted as indicating white matter abnormalities in these patient groups when compared with controls (Alexopoulos et al., 2002; Moseley, 2002; Pfefferbaum et al., 1999). While DTI holds much promise, the methodology and its neurobiological underpinnings need to be explored more systematically before its biological relevance to mental disorders can be definitively ascertained.

MAGNETIZATION TRANSFER MAGNETIC
RESONANCE IMAGING

Magnetization transfer MRI (MT-MRI) is a relatively new neuroimaging technique that helps to examine certain biophysical properties of the brain parenchyma using magnetic resonance principals (Eng et al., 1991; Grossman, 1994; Kabani et al., 2002). In MT-MRI, as in any form of MRI, water protons produce the signal that is used to create the images. However, MT-MRI takes advantage of the fact that there are two distinct classes of water within biological tissues: water that is associated with slowly moving macromolecules (bound water) and water that is relatively free to move except for constraints imposed by biological compartmentation (free water). MT-MRI also takes advantage of the fact that individual water molecules exchange back and forth between the bound and free states.

The two forms of tissue water produce remarkably different magnetic resonance signal characteristics. In MT imaging, one of the two image acquisitions (the control acquisition) is performed like any other MRI study. In another image acquisition (the MT acquisition), an "off-resonance" radio-frequency (RF) pulse, which interacts only with the bound water, is used prior to the otherwise-conventional proton density MRI study. This RF pulse nulls (or saturates) the potential for the bound water protons to create signal. This has the effect of reducing the detected free-water MRI signal. In other words, there is signal reduction in the MT acquisition relative to the control acquisition in all tissue regions that have exchanging bound and free water.

A magnetization transfer ratio (MTR) image, which reflects the difference in signal intensity between the two images and provides a semiquantitative estimate of the MT effect, may be obtained by subtracting the off-resonance image from the control acquisition. The extent to which the RF pulse can diminish the transfer of magnetization from the bound-water to the free-water pool depends on the concentration of macromolecules and their chemistry and stoichiometry (Eng et al., 1991; Grossman, 1994; Kabani et al., 2002).

Myelin-related proteins are the primary macromolecules that have been identified as having an important influence on MT imaging in the white matter. The MT ratio is consequently low in disorders characterized by injury to the white matter, such as multiple sclerosis and pontine myelinolysis (Eng et al., 1991; Grossman, 1994; Kabani et al., 2002). In patients with DAT, reductions in the MT ratio have been demonstrated in the gray matter (Kabani et al., 2002). Preliminary evidence in patients with late-life major depressive disorder (MDD) (observations from our laboratory) indicates that the MTR may be lower in normal-appearing white matter regions and subcortical nuclei (the genu and splenium of the corpus callosum, the occipital white matter bilaterally, and the caudate nucleus and the putamen on the right side) in the patient group when compared with controls. Studies using larger clinical samples are needed to confirm this finding. Nonetheless, MT imaging is a technique that permits examination of neurophysiology at another level, thereby providing a better understanding of the biology of mental disorders.

NEUROANATOMIC CHANGES IN AGING

Aging is associated with several neuroanatomic and physiological changes in the central nervous system (CNS) (Coffey et al., 1992; Jernigan et al., 1990, 1991). Anatomically, a decrease in brain volume and an increase in CSF volume occur with increasing age (Coffey et al., 1992). Reductions in the volumes of cerebral hemispheres and frontal and temporal lobes, together with an increase in lateral ventricular volumes, have been reported with increasing age (Coffey et al., 1992; Jernigan et al., 1991). Volumetric reductions have also been demonstrated in the diencephalic, limbic, and subcortical regions (Coffey et al., 1992).

Some groups have reported gender differences in atrophy associated with aging (Cowell et al., 1994). More specifically, these studies suggested that the reduction in frontal lobe volume with increasing age is greater in men compared with women (Cowell et al., 1994).

High-intensity lesions in cortical and subcortical areas also increase with age (Drayer, 1988a, 1988b; Fazekas, 1989; Fazekas et al., 1987, 1988). These findings underscore the need to control for the effects of age when making statements on the neuroanatomic correlates of specific mental disorders in the elderly.

LATE-LIFE DEPRESSION ANATOMIC CHANGES

Estimates of Brain and Cerebrospinal Fluid Volumes

Over the past decade, several groups have reported reductions in brain volumes in critical brain regions in patients with late-life mood disorders when compared with controls (Coffey et al., 1988; Krishnan, 1993a, 1993b; Rabins et al., 1991; Sheline et al., 1996). Anatomic changes in depression fall into two principal categories: reduction in brain volume and increase in volumes of the high-intensity lesions when compared with controls.

Both qualitative and quantitative reports using MRI demonstrated widespread atrophy in neocortical areas and subcortical nuclei in elderly patients with major depressive disorder when compared with controls (Coffey et al., 1988; Sheline et al., 1996). Quantitative studies demonstrated no significant decrease in whole-brain volume in patients with late-life depression when compared with controls. Ventricular and CSF volumes were larger in the patient group when compared with controls (Kumar, Miller, et al., 1997). The broader consensus in the field suggested that reductions in brain volume in patients with late-life depression occur in critical areas such as the frontal lobe, head of the caudate nucleus, and the hippocampus—regions involved in the circuitry and regulation of emotions (Krishnan, 1993b; Kumar, Schweizer, et al., 1997; Sheline et al., 1996). Evidence from my laboratory suggested that patients with late-onset minor depression also present with smaller frontal brain volumes when compared with nondepressed controls (Kumar et al., 1998). These data also indicate that frontal brain volumes in patients with minor depression are between those of patients with major depression and controls (Kumar, Schweizer, et al., 1997). These findings suggest that there may be a common neuroanatomic basis to all clinically significant forms of depression with an onset in late life.

High-Intensity Lesions

Several groups have reported increased severity of high-intensity lesions, principally in the deep white matter and subcortical areas, in patients with late-life major depression when compared with controls (Coffey et al., 1988; Krishnan, 1993b; Rabins et al., 1991). Evidence from community-based epidemiological studies, including the Cardiovascular Health Study, suggested that the clinical correlates of these lesions include increasing age, prior stroke, hypertension, carotid narrowing, and other cerebrovascular risk factors (Kirkpatrick & Hayman, 1987; Manolio et al., 1994; Sullivan et al., 1990; Sze et al., 1981; Yamaji et al., 1997; Zimmerman et al., 1986).

The association between cerebrovascular risk factors and MRI lesions has not been corroborated across all studies and may differ based on underlying sample characteristics (Charletta et al., 1995; Kumar et al., 1992, 2000). Reports from the Cardiovascular Health Study, a large community-based epidemiological study, suggested that the relative role of high-intensity lesions in neocortical, as opposed to subcortical, areas in the pathophysiology of depression remain controversial (Sato et al., 1999; Steffens et al., 1999). Further, one study suggested that the impact of lesions on mood might be mediated through the subjects' activity level and cognitive status (Sato et al., 1999). Despite these caveats, the putative link between MRI high-intensity lesions (Figure 14-3) and vascular disease observed in certain studies forms the basis of the vascular depression concept in late-life mood disorders (Krishnan et al., 1997).

Pathophysiological Significance of Magnetic Resonance Findings in Depression

The increasing use of MRI in psychiatric research has led to several intriguing observations. The precise neurobiological significance of these findings and their relevance to the pathophysiology of depression and other psychiatric disorders, although complex, is now better appreciated (Kumar, 1999). The neuropathological correlates of high-intensity lesions include ischemic changes, demyelination, edema, and perivascular spaces (Bradley et al., 1984; Braffman et al., 1988a, 1988b; Charletta et al., 1995; Chimowitz et al., 1992; Ylikoski et al., 1995).

Data from my laboratory revealed that, in the sample, high-intensity lesions showed a significant correlation to overall medical burden, but not to specific cerebrovascular risk factors (Kumar et al., 2000). The vascular risk factors examined in this study represented the American Heart Association's stroke risk factors (Wolf et al., 1991). Smaller brain volume and larger high-intensity lesion volumes represent complementary, relatively autonomous, pathways to late-life depression (Figure 14-4) (Kumar et al., 2000). These data also indicated that, while age per se had no direct impact on depression, it may indirectly influence depression by contributing to a reduction in brain volume and increase in overall medical burden. Also, while reports focus predominantly on clinical measures of macrovascular disease, microvascular disease may also contribute to mood disorders by compromising brain structure and function (Lyness et al., 1998).

Volumetric decreases ascertained using MRI are commonly interpreted as evidence in support of neuronal atrophy. While the neurobiological basis of smaller brain volumes in depression remain obscure, increased levels of cortisol and a decrease in neurotrophic factors, such as nerve growth factor (NGF) secondary to long-term stress, have been invoked as possible substrates (Duman & Charney, 1999; Gould et al., 1998; Rajkowska et al., 1999; Sapolsky & Pulsinelli, 1985).

It should be emphasized that MR morphometry alone cannot be used to make unequivocal statements regarding the size of the neuronal areas versus that of the glial compartments in the brain. Complementary approaches, such as MRS, are needed before more definitive statements can be made (Lim et al., 1998). The biology of depression in late life is complex, and MRI provides an important approach that, together with other complementary in vivo and in vitro techniques, helps systematic examination of the anatomic and chemical underpinnings of mood disorders. The cumulative findings that result from

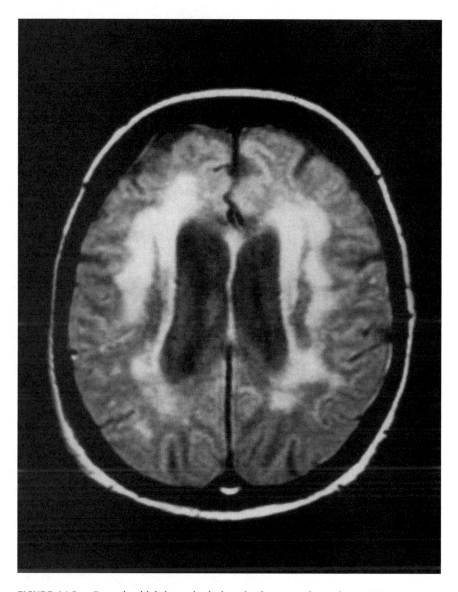

FIGURE 14-3. Extensive high-intensity lesions in the parenchyma in an MRI scan.

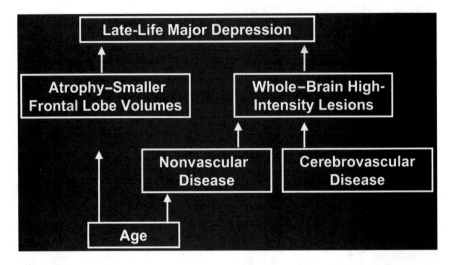

FIGURE 14-4. The pathways to depression in our path analytic model.

these studies will permit development of a more holistic and cohesive model of the neurobiological basis of mood disturbances in the elderly.

NEUROCHEMICAL STUDIES

The use of MRS as a complementary modality to neuroanatomic imaging greatly increases the depth and precision of these approaches in the study of psychiatric disorders. Few studies have focused on neurochemical changes in elderly patients with psychiatric disorders (Charles et al., 1994; Lim & Spielman, 1997; Pfefferbaum et al., 1999). MRS studies of mood disorders have focused on estimating levels of Ch, NAA, and MI in specific brain regions in patients with depression when compared with controls (Charles et al., 1994; Kato et al., 1998). Both metabolite ratios and absolute levels of metabolites have been reported in the literature.

A preliminary report on neurochemical changes in the subcortical/temporal lobe region in elderly patients with depression demonstrated an increase in pretreatment Cho/Cr ratios when compared with controls (Charles et al., 1994). In this study, the choline levels normalized with pharmacological treatment. Data from my laboratory suggested that neurochemical changes in patients with late-life depression include a relative increase in choline and myoinositol (Cho/Cr and MI/Cr) and a decrease in absolute NAA levels when compared with controls (Kumar et al., 2000, 2002) (Figure 14-5). These changes appeared to be more marked in the frontal white matter, thereby suggesting that abnormalities in white matter structure/function may provide important neurobiological substrates to mood disorders in the elderly.

It should be emphasized that the application of MRS to the study of late-

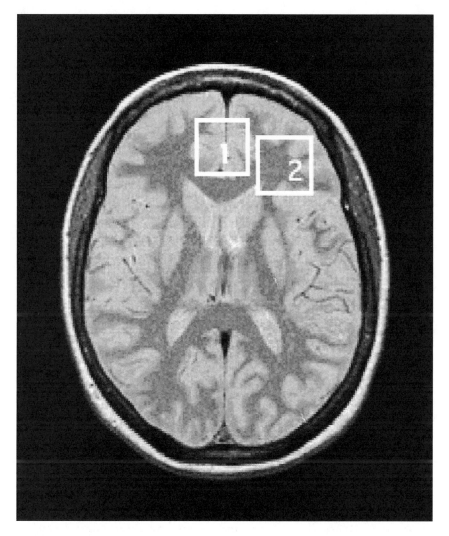

FIGURE 14-5. MRI scan of a healthy comparison subject showing location of magnetic resonance spectroscopy voxels placed in the anterior cingulate gray matter and dorsolateral prefrontal cortex white matter.

life mood disorders, while promising, is still in its preliminary stages. The use of high-field magnets together with cutting edge acquisition methods, such as two-dimensional (2D) acquisitions, will improve the quality of biochemical information obtained using MRS (Thomas et al., 2001). It will also help separate adjacent/overlapping metabolite peaks and improve the quantitation of neurochemical estimates.

The appropriate use of MRS together with MRI can help integrate anatomic and biochemical information in brain areas deemed important in the circuitry of psychiatric diseases. The use of MRS can help the interpretation of the MRI-determined volumetric reductions more precisely (Lim et al., 1998). For example, volumetric reductions, together with a decrease in the regional NAA signal, suggest anatomic compromise in the neurons as opposed to the glial compartment (Table 14-2). NAA reductions in the gray matter suggest compromise in the cell body, while reductions in NAA in the white matter are more indicative of axonal damage (Lim et al., 1998).

PHYSIOLOGICAL CHANGES IN LATE-LIFE DEPRESSION

Xenon inhalation, SPECT, and PET have been used to study the physiological correlates of depression in the elderly (Bonne et al., 1996; Kumar et al., 1993; Lesser et al., 1994; Sackeim et al., 1993; Sackeim & Prohovnik, 1993; Upadhyaya et al., 1990). These studies demonstrated reductions in cerebral blood flow and glucose metabolism (regional cerebral blood flow, rCBF; and regional cerebral metabolic rate for glucose, rCMR glc) in neocortical and subcortical regions, in the resting state, in patients with late-life depression when compared with controls. These findings were demonstrated with absolute glucose metabolic values, relative quantitation of perfusion using SPECT, and a relatively novel statistical approach called the scaled subprofile model, which is used to analyze regional patterns of flow (Kumar et al., 1993; Sackeim & Prohovnik, 1993; Upadhyaya et al., 1990). These findings may be contrasted using fluorodeoxyglucose (FDG) PET with more selective prefrontal metabolic reductions demonstrated in younger patients with both unipolar and bipolar depression (Baxter et al., 1985). The magnitude of the metabolic reductions in patients with late-life MDD may also be comparable to those observed in patients with mild-to-moderate dementia of the Alzheimer type, thereby demonstrating substantial physiological abnormality in the brains of elderly patients with depression (Kumar et al., 1993; Sackeim et al., 1993).

While there is broad agreement on the physiological profile of patients with depression in the pretreatment state, there is more controversy over changes in metabolism and flow after treatment with antidepressants or electroconvulsive therapy (Bonne et al., 1996; Buchsbaum et al., 1997; Kumar, 2000a; Lesser et al., 1994; Nobler et al., 1999). There are reports that demonstrated both increases (normalization) and decreases in cerebral perfusion with successful treatment when compared with the baseline state. The precise relationship between clinical response and physiological changes remains unresolved (Kumar, 2000a). Preclinical studies aimed at elucidating the neurobiological basis of depression and the cellular sites of action of antidepressants are needed to appreciate better the fundamental neuronal changes that occur with clinical response.

TABLE 14-2. Pathophysiological significance of MR findings in late-life MDD and Alzheimer's disease

Measure	Late-life MDD	Alzheimer's disease	Significance
Whole-brain volume	Normal	Reduced	Smaller brain volumes often interpreted as neuronal atrophy
Hippocampal volume	Reduced	Reduced; reduced anterior hippocampus in frontotemporal dementia	
Subcortical nuclei	Reduced*	Reduced	
High-intensity signals	Increased	Variable	
Magnetic resonance spectroscopy			
NAA	Decreased in frontal white matter*	Decreased in cortical and subcortical gray matter	Reliable marker of neuronal structure and function
Cho/Cr	Increased in the frontal and subcortical regions	Increased in the cortex	Reflects increased choline activity and membrane structure
MI/Cr	Increased in the cortical region	Increased in the cortical region	Gliosis and changes in the secondary messenger system
Physiological measure			
rCMR glc, glucose metabolism	Reduced in cortical and subcortical region	Reduced in the neocortex and subcortical regions; relative sparing of primary sensory areas	Reduction in neuronal and synaptic activity
rCBF	Decreased in the frontal, temporal, and parietal lobes	Decreased in the frontal, temporal, and parietal lobes	

Note: See text for definition of abbreviations.
*Compared with controls.

NEUROIMAGING STUDIES IN DEGENERATIVE DISORDERS: DEMENTIA OF THE ALZHEIMER TYPE

Dementias are among the most common mental disorders in the elderly. Dementia of the Alzheimer type (DAT) is the most common form of dementia in the Western Hemisphere. Advances in genetics and protein biochemistry have greatly increased the understanding of the neurobiological correlates of Alzheimer's disease. Neuroimaging in AD has an important role in the early diagnosis of the disorder and in monitoring the impact of pharmacological intervention on physiological and clinical progression of the disease (Chase et al., 1984; Duara et al., 1986; Kumar et al., 1991). FDG PET studies in patients with mild AD demonstrated widespread reductions in glucose metabolism in neocortical and subcortical regions when compared with controls (Kumar et al., 1991).

The metabolic reductions, however, were not uniform across all regions (Chase et al., 1984; Duara et al., 1986; Kumar et al., 1991). The hypometabolism was more striking in the temporal and parietal association neocortices, with relative sparing of the primary sensory regions (sensory motor and calcarine cortex). The in vivo glucose metabolic patterns were consistent with the distribution of plaque and tangles neuropathologically (Kumar et al., 1991). The neuropathological correlates of AD were also predominantly found in the limbic and association neocortices, with relative sparing of the primary sensory areas (Kumar et al., 1991).

NEUROIMAGING AND GENETIC MARKERS IN THE EARLY DETECTION OF ALZHEIMER'S DISEASE

The potential utility of neuroimaging in AD is greatly strengthened by combining neuroimaging approaches with neuropsychological and genetic strategies. Apolipoprotein E (APOE) is a well-recognized risk factor for AD. APOE exists in three forms (alleles) (Corder et al., 1993, 1994): APOE 2, APOE 3, and APOE 4. The presence of the APOE 4 allele increases the risk of developing AD, while APOE 2 may have a protective effect against the disease (Corder et al., 1993, 1994).

In the early stage of the disorder, when mild, subjective memory complaints might be the only symptom (predementia stage), the diagnosis may be difficult to make with any degree of certainty. In this stage, variously called age-associated memory impairment (AAMI) and mild cognitive impairment (MCI), an accurate diagnosis could have enormous clinical and psychosocial implications for patients and their families (Small et al., 1995).

Preliminary FDG PET studies demonstrated that, in patients with mild memory complaints and a family history of AD and an E4 allele, metabolic abnormalities were seen in the parietal and temporal lobes and the posterior cingulated regions in the resting state—a pattern similar to the one described in AD patients (Reiman et al., 1996; Small et al., 1995). A study using func-

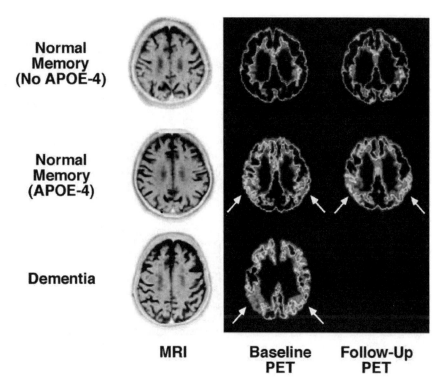

FIGURE 14-6. Displays glucose hypometabolism in the "at risk" APOE 4+ group, when compared with the APOE– group.

tional MRI showed that subjects with normal memory and an APOE 4 allele showed greater physiological activation in the regions typically affected in AD during a verbal memory task when compared with similar subjects with the APOE 3 allele (Bookheimer et al., 2000). Both the magnitude and the extent of the activation were greater in the left hippocampal, parietal, and prefrontal areas in the group positive for APOE 4 (Figure 14-6). Collectively, these findings indicate that the combination of genetic testing and neuroimaging might help in the early detection of AD before all clinical manifestations become evident. Early detection of AD could have substantial practical implications when effective interventions under development become available.

AMYLOID PROTEIN IMAGING

Developments in radioligand synthesis have made it possible to image neurofibrillary tangles and plaques, proteins that are considered central to the pathophysiology of AD (Figure 14-7). In a preliminary report using a small sample of patients with probable/possible Alzheimer's disease, Shoghi-Jadid and co-

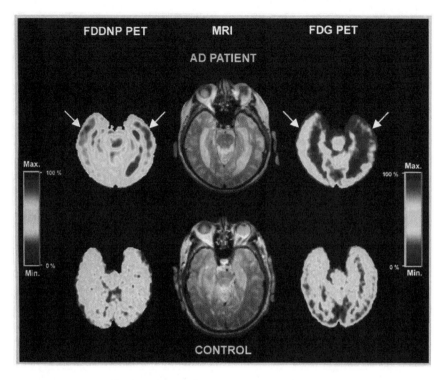

FIGURE 14-7. The [^{18}F]FDDNP and FDG images of each stage are coregistered to their respective MRI images. Areas of FDG hypometabolism are matched with the localization of NFTs and APs resulting from [^{18}F]FDDNP binding (marked arrows). The color bar represents the scaling of the [^{18}F]FDDNP and FDG images.

workers (2002) used 2-(1-{6-[2-[^{18}F]fluoroethyl)(methyl)amino]-2-naphthyl}ethylidene)malononitrile ([^{18}F]FDDNP), a hydrophobic radiofluorinated derivative of 2-{1-[6-(dimethylamino)-2-naphthyl]ethylidene}malononitrile (DDNP), in conjunction with positron emission tomography to characterize pathological deposition, both neurofibrillary tangles and amyloid plaques, in select brain regions. Using PET, the investigators detected greater accumulation and slower clearance of the agent in areas of high plaque and tangle density. Also, these kinetic characteristics correlated with poor performance on memory scores.

Despite the limitations of this preliminary study, it was the first published report of in vivo amyloid imaging in AD and heralded a new era of protein imaging in neuropsychiatric disorders. Studies using larger patient samples are needed to replicate these observations and to investigate further the diagnostic specificity of these findings. The potential of amyloid imaging includes early detection of AD and monitoring the efficacy of interventions over time.

MAGNETIC RESONANCE IMAGING/MAGNETIC RESONANCE SPECTROSCOPY STUDIES IN DEMENTIA

Cross-Sectional Studies

Quantitative neuroanatomic studies using MRI have provided much information both for patients with clinical AD and for patients with isolated memory impairment, the predementia category. AD patients demonstrated reductions in global brain volume and in the volume of focal structures important in memory and cognition (Wahlund, 1996; Xanthakos et al., 1996). These include the temporal lobes, hippocampus, amygdala, entorhinal cortex, and the corpus callosum (Juottonen et al., 1999; Kesslak et al., 1991; Lyoo et al., 1997; Smith, 1996; Wahlund, 1996; Xanthakos et al., 1996).

Cross-sectional studies showed significant reductions in the volume of these structures in patients with AD when compared with controls (Smith, 1996; Wahlund, 1996; Xanthakos et al., 1996). Volumetric reductions in the hippocampus also correlated significantly with clinical measures of cognitive impairment (DeLeon et al., 1997; Jack et al., 1997; Kohler et al., 1998; Laakso et al., 1995). Volumes of the left hippocampus correlated with delayed verbal recall, while the right hippocampal volume correlated with delayed nonverbal memory performance (Peterson et al., 2000). Volumes of the amygdala and the hippocampus may also serve effectively to differentiate AD patients from controls in cross-sectional studies (Lehericy et al., 1994). Despite the biological relevance and potential clinical utility of cross-sectional measures, longitudinal studies provide a more holistic picture of the disease progression over time.

Longitudinal Studies

The hallmark of AD is the progressive nature of the disease, both clinically and neurobiologically. Longitudinal MRI studies corroborated the progressive atrophy that underlies the clinical manifestations of AD (Fox et al., 1999; Jack et al., 1997, 2000; Kaye et al., 1997; Laakso, Lehtovirta, et al., 2000). Progressive volumetric reductions have been demonstrated globally and in more discrete structures (Fox et al., 1999; Jack et al., 2000; Kaye et al., 1997; Laakso, Lehtovirta, et al., 2000). Significant correlations have been found between neuroanatomic measures of atrophy and clinical progression (Jack et al., 2000; Kaye et al., 1997; Laakso, Lehtovirta, et al., 2000). Longitudinal studies have established that volumetric reductions in the hippocampus, per year, are significantly greater in AD patients when compared with age-matched subjects without dementia (Jack et al., 1997).

Other studies suggested that the volume loss in the hippocampus, per year, is greatest in AD patients, followed by subjects with mild cognitive impairment and controls (Jack et al., 2000). Hippocampal atrophy in patients with MCI, which does not meet criteria for dementia, may serve as a predictor of subsequent conversion to AD (Fox et al., 1996; Jack et al., 2000). Also, for patients who meet criteria for MCI, the rate of hippocampal atrophy was greater in those who showed subsequent cognitive decline when compared with patients who remained cognitively stable (Jack et al., 2000). Some studies also suggested that AD patients with the APOE 4 allele showed greater hippocampal atrophy and increased ventricular volume when compared with AD patients without the E4 allele (Yamaguchi et al., 1996).

In summary, both cross-sectional and longitudinal volumetric measures of critical brain structures such as the hippocampus correlated with clinical indices of cognitive compromise. In addition, quantitative morphometry might also serve to predict cognitive decline in patients with mild memory complaints during the initial assessment.

Spectroscopic Studies

Both ^{31}P and ^{1}H spectroscopy have been used to identify biological changes in Alzheimer's disease (Miller et al., 1993; Moats et al., 1994; Shonk et al., 1995; Tedeschi et al., 1996). Most of the studies using proton MRS showed decreases in NAA (in both absolute concentrations and semiquantitative ratios) in several subcortical regions in patients with Alzheimer's disease when compared with controls (Meyerhoff et al., 1994; Rose et al., 1999; Schuff et al., 1998; Tedeschi et al., 1996). The regions examined in these studies include the frontal lobe, temporal regions including the hippocampus, parietal lobe, centrum semoivale, and the subcortical nuclei. AD patients showed an 8% to 50% decline in NAA levels across study samples when compared with controls (Parnetti et al., 1997; Rose et al., 1999).

Combining anatomic and biochemical information, hippocampal NAA levels together with hippocampal volumes are more effective in differentiating AD patients from controls than either measure alone (Schuff et al., 1997). NAA decline in the white matter was less striking in AD patients when compared with changes in the gray matter (Miller et al., 1993; Parnetti et al., 1997). Increases in Cho/Cr and MI/Cr ratios have also been described in AD, although less consistently than the NAA changes (MacKay et al., 1996; Meyerhoff et al., 1994).

Studies using CSI also demonstrated an increase in gray matter NAA after treatment with cholinesterase inhibitors. This suggests that some reversibility in neuronal changes with treatment with a cholinesterase inhibitor. The precise relationship of the modest increase in NAA with treatment to clinical symptoms and disease progression, however, remains to be elucidated (Petrella et al., 2003; Satlin et al., 1997).

Phosphorus MRS provides information on metabolites that reflect the state of cellular energy and membrane lipids (Cousins, 1995; Pettegrew et al., 1997; Ross et al., 1998). The metabolites include phosphomonoesters (PMEs); inorganic orthophosphates (Pi); phosphodiesters (PDE); phosphocreatine (PCr); α-, β-, and γ-phosphates of nucleotide triphosphate (ATP, adenosine triphosphate); and α- and β-phosphates of nucleotide diphosphates (ADP, adenosine diphosphate). PME and PDE reflect the biophysical state of membrane phospholipid, while Pi, PCr, and ATP are indices of energy metabolism (Cousins, 1995; Pettegrew et al., 1997; Ross et al., 1998).

Most phosphorus MRS studies in AD demonstrated elevations in PME and PDE in AD, suggesting accelerated membrane turnover (Klunk et al., 1996; Pettegrew et al., 1988; Smith et al., 1993). Some, although not all, reports also showed an inverse relationship between PME intensity and plaque density in AD (Murphy et al., 1993; Pettegrew et al., 1988). Also, most studies did not show significant changes in ATP, Pi, or PCr in AD patients when compared with controls (Bottomley et al., 1992; Gonzalez et al., 1996; Murphy et al., 1993).

FRONTOTEMPORAL DEMENTIAS

The frontotemporal dementias (FTDs) represent a group of disorders characterized by impairment in memory, executive functions, and behavior together with atrophy largely confined to the frontal lobe and anterior temporal regions (Brun et al., 1994; Kumar & Gottlieb, 1993). FTD is typically associated with an early onset of clinical symptoms, and both familial and sporadic forms of the disorder have been described.

MRI studies revealed a differential pattern of atrophy in patients diagnosed with FTD when compared with AD patients (Duara et al., 1999; Edwards-Lee et al., 1997; Frisoni et al., 1996; Kitagaki et al., 1998; Miller & Gearhart, 1999). FTD patients displayed greater volume loss in the mesial frontal and anterior temporal regions when compared with AD patients (Kitagaki et al., 1998). Also, while hippocampal atrophy was more diffuse in AD, it was localized to the anterior portion of the hippocampus in FTD patients (Laakso, Frisoni, et al., 2000; Laakso, Lehtovirta, et al., 2000). The genu of the corpus callosum was much smaller in FTD patients, although the overall volume of the corpus callosum was comparable in both groups (Kaufer et al., 1997).

Proton MRS studies in FTD revealed a decline in NAA and GLx signal together with an increase in MI in the frontal and temporoparietal gray matter (Ernst et al., 1997). The increase in MI, reflective of gliosis, was significantly greater in the FTD group when compared with the AD group (Ernst et al., 1997).

VASCULAR DEMENTIA

Dementia secondary to vascular pathology is the second most common cause of dementia in the Western Hemisphere (Chui, 1989). Coexisting vascular and AD pathology is also commonly encountered in neuropathological studies of patients with clinical dementia (Chui, 1989; Victoroff et al., 1995). In vascular dementia, the neuronal damage and the consequent atrophy depend in large measure on the location of the vascular injury and its impact on cortico-cortical and cortico-subcortical connections.

Generalized brain atrophy together with loss of cortical gray matter, atrophy of the hippocampus, cerebellum, and the corpus callosum have been reported in patients diagnosed with vascular dementia (Fein et al., 2000; Giubilei et al., 1997; Hershey et al., 1987; Liu et al., 1992; Pantel et al., 1998; Schmidt, 1992). Increased white matter high-intensity lesions on T2 weighted images have been consistently identified in patients with vascular dementia, with some, but not all, studies finding an association between these lesions and cerebrovascular risk factors (Charletta et al., 1995; Corbett et al., 1994; Erkinjuntti et al., 1996; Fukuda et al., 1990; Yamanouchi et al., 1990; Yamauchi et al., 1994).

Proton MRS studies demonstrated a decrease in NAA and increases in the Cho/Cr ratio in neocortical and subcortical regions in patients with vascular dementia (Constans et al., 1995; Kattapong et al., 1996; MacKay et al., 1996). Perfusion and metabolic studies also showed a decline in blood flow and glucose metabolism in specific brain regions in patients with vascular dementia (Sabri et al., 1999; Sultzer et al., 1995). It should be pointed out that the distribution of the anatomic and physiological changes in vascular dementia does not follow a unique, predetermined pattern often encountered in AD. The abnormalities tend to be "patchy" and variable, with the location and extent of the underlying vascular injury primarily determining the neurobiological changes and the resulting neuroimaging findings.

LATE-LIFE PSYCHOTIC DISORDERS

There have been a few studies that have examined the neuroanatomic correlates of psychotic disorders in the elderly (Corey-Bloom et al., 1995; Howard et al., 1994; Kumar, 2000a). Nosological ambiguities and clinical overlap between entities such as late-onset schizophrenia and paraphrenia complicate interpretation of these findings. Increase in ventricular brain ratios and ventricular volumes have been reported in patients with late-onset schizophrenia. Larger thalamic volumes were also identified in this group when compared with controls (Corey-Bloom et al., 1995).

A report indicated that elderly patients with paraphrenia have larger ventricular volumes when compared with elderly patients with schizophrenia and controls. This suggests that the neuroanatomical contributions may be greater in patients diagnosed with paraphrenia when compared with patients with schizophrenia (Howard et al., 1994). Reports also indicated that high-intensity lesions are greater in all patients with late-onset psychoses when compared with controls.

While structural changes have been identified in patients with late-onset psychotic disorders, the specificity of these findings and their pathophysiological significance remain unclear.

NEURORECEPTOR AND NEUROPHARMACOLOGICAL
STUDIES IN THE ELDERLY

The development of ligands specific for receptors and receptor subtypes has broadened the applicability of PET and SPECT imaging in the pursuit of the biochemical basis of mental disorders in all groups, including the elderly (Agren et al., 1993; Biver et al., 1997; Blin et al., 1993; Cohen et al., 1997; Frey et al., 1996; Frost et al., 1993; Gilman et al., 1996; Lee et al., 1996; Meltzer, 1999; Meltzer, Smith, DeKosky, et al., 1998; Meltzer, Smith, Price, et al., 1998; Meltzer & Frost, 1994). Neurotransmitters such as serotonin, acetylcholine, and norepinephrine and neuromodulators such as the opiates have been implicated in the pathophysiology of depression across the age spectrum.

PET provides an opportunity to examine these neurotransmitter systems in the living brain and integrate pharmacological measures with relevant clinical indices. Early PET receptor studies focused largely on examining the density of postsynaptic receptors in specific psychiatric disorders. Efforts in PET imaging have included studies of presynaptic receptors and transporter sites in mood and related CNS disorders (Meltzer et al., 1999). Prime candidate target sites for the investigation include specific receptor subtypes, such as the 5-HT (serotonin) 1-A subtype and 5-HT transporters, which have been implicated in the biology of depression (Meltzer et al., 1999).

Neuroreceptor imaging in the elderly is compounded by additional technical considerations, such as the impact of atrophy and partial volume correction on receptor binding parameters (Meltzer et al., 1999). Additional scientific issues that complicate interpretation of data include the impact of cerebral perfusion and modeling approaches on pharmacokinetics and estimates of receptor density and affinity. Despite the numerous technical challenges, in vivo neurochemical imaging remains a promising approach for characterizing and understanding the biological basis of mental disorders (Meltzer & Frost, 1994).

RESEARCH DIRECTIONS

Probabilistic Anatomic Atlas

While conventional methods of hand tracing of lobar and sublobar regions are widely used in neuroimaging studies, this approach has several limitations (Collins et al., 1994; Dinov et al., 2000; Thompson et al., 1996, 1997). Extreme variations in brain structure across human populations present fundamental challenges in brain-mapping studies. First, wide variations in the gyral patterns of the human cortex make it difficult to integrate data from subjects whose anatomy is different. These difficulties are exacerbated in brain diseases with normal anatomic variation that is compounded by disease-specific atrophic changes. The impact of aging on neuroanatomy introduces an additional source of variance to this already-complex picture.

To distinguish abnormalities from normal variants, a realistically complex mathematical framework to encode information on anatomic variability in homogeneous populations would be very useful. Cortical anatomy is so variable and complex that disease-specific patterns are often hard to identify and characterize consistently. Because there is neither a single representative brain nor a simple method to construct an average anatomy or represent three-dimensional (3D) anatomic variations, the construction of brain atlases to represent large human populations has become the focus of intense research. Probabilistic atlases retain quantitative information on intersubject variation in brain architecture and thus may be more appropriate than a static representation of neuroanatomy for representing particular subpopulations, such as patients with AD and mood disorders.

The principal goal of this approach is to quantify whether an apparent deformity constitutes a clinical abnormality or can be explained by normal variations. It is not automatically assumed that any deviation from the normal or "average" shape is due to the underlying clinical disorder (Collins et al., 1994). Comparisons between subjects, both within and across homogeneous populations, are required to understand the full range of normal variability and to help distinguish genuine structural and functional differences. The approach holds considerable promise and is currently being applied to a broad spectrum of clinical brain disorders.

Antemortem and Postmortem Correlations

While in vivo neuroimaging provides insights into the living brain, correlating in vivo findings with postmortem anatomic information is a potentially more powerful approach to neuroanatomic studies. Correlative imaging—antemortem neuroimaging studies with postmortem neuropathological observations and anatomic image data—provides additional information on the neuropathological substrates of antemortem findings.

For example, this approach makes it possible to study the relationship between areas of hypometabolism determined using FDG PET and the distribution and density of pathological markers such as neurofibrillary tangles and plaques (Mega et al., 1997, 1999). Such approaches have enormous potential in late-life mood and psychotic disorders, for which knowledge about the underlying neurobiological correlates is fragmentary.

Postmortem Magnetic Resonance Imaging

A limitation of studies correlating in vivo neuroimaging with postmortem studies is the time lag between the two studies (Longson et al., 1995). Structural and biochemical changes that occur during the last few weeks of life will not have been captured by earlier neuroimaging studies. Postmortem MRI is an approach that is relatively new to mental disorders in the elderly. Anatomic image data and histology from cryosectioned postmortem tissue provide greater clarity and anatomic data in critical regions when compared with 2-mm MRI slices obtained on a 1.5-T system (Toga et al., 1997). The anatomic details seen in postmortem MRI brain images obtained using a 7-T scanner (MR microscopic imaging) approach those observed in histological preparations (Boyko et al., 1994).

MR scans can be performed after rinsing formalin-fixed preparations of the brain in distilled water (Autti et al., 1997; Cotter et al., 1999; Everall et al., 1997). Brain tissue may be imaged in the plastic bags in which they are wrapped. In certain instances, MRI scans have been performed years after autopsy, although there may be several advantages to rapid postmortem studies. Postmortem MRI also facilitates more precise identification of regions to sample for detailed histopathological examination.

Neuroimaging-neuropathological correlative studies in patients with a history of well-characterized psychiatric disorders are understudied. This important area of research will benefit enormously from the development of brain banks and well-designed clinical-pathological correlative studies.

MicroPET

The microPET is a high-resolution, dedicated small-animal PET system. Its high resolution is realized for a diameter large enough to cover the bodies of mice and rats and the brains of small nonhuman primates (Chatziioannou et al., 1999; Cherry et al., 1997). Developed at the University of California, Los Angeles, it has been tested in complex imaging protocols such as whole-body 18 FDG distribution studies and dynamic studies of receptor ligands in the rat brain. Its high resolution combined with its sensitivity permit it to be applied to study biological changes in laboratory animals such as rats and mice.

It is a powerful noninvasive tool that permits valuable animal studies incorporating both longitudinal and interventional components (Chatziioannou et al., 1999; Cherry et al., 1997). It has potential relevance in behavioral disorders in late life as it permits monitoring of behavioral changes in animal models of disease. Animal models of psychiatric disease, including transgenics, knockouts, and lesion studies, may be scrutinized both physiologically and pharmacologically over time using this approach. It also permits the concurrent study of both behavioral (cognitive and noncognitive) and neurobiological changes in valid animal models as they are developed in the laboratory.

Optical Imaging

Functional activation studies typically depend on perfusion-related signals to localize the source of brain activity. Methods such as PET and fMRI assume close coupling between perfusion and neuronal activity. Most noninvasive brain-mapping techniques are limited by low signal-to-noise ratios, long integration times, and uncertain signal etiology. Optical intrinsic signals (OIS) is a functional neuroimaging technique that measures changes in cortical reflectance with second temporal resolution and micron spatial resolution (Cannestra et al., 1998, 2000; O'Farrell et al., 2000). In vivo optical changes correlate with neuronal activity and are caused by changes in light scattering, blood volume, cellular swelling, and cytochrome activity. Animal studies characterizing optical responses in rodents described temporal profiles in good agreement with more traditional measures of vascular response (Cannestra et al., 1998, 2000; O'Farrell et al., 2000).

OIS is used intraoperatively in patients undergoing neurosurgical procedures. In this context, it is an approach with considerable potential as it allows far greater anatomic and temporal precision than more standard approaches to brain mapping (Cannestra et al., 1998, 2000; O'Farrell et al., 2000). Its application may broaden as technological improvements evolve and increase its relevance to mental disorders in the elderly.

Neuroimaging is a hybrid discipline that encompasses diverse specialties such as physics, chemistry, computer science, and neuroscience. It is a dynamic arena with rapid, ongoing improvements in hardware, software, and acquisition parameters, together with the synthesis of novel ligands to study neurochemical systems. Methods such as magnetization transfer and diffusion tensor imaging already permit close scrutiny of structural and biochemical changes in normal-appearing white matter.

Efforts are also under way to design and build scanners that integrate PET and CT/MRI components. Such advances will introduce a new dimension to clinical neuroimaging as we know it. As more powerful methods are developed and disseminated, their role in diagnosing and understanding psychiatric diseases and their overall clinical relevance are likely to increase.

REFERENCES

Agren H, Reibring L, Hartvig P, et al. Monoamine metabolism in human prefrontal cortex and basal ganglia: PET studies using [b=1−1C]1-5-hydroxytryptophan and [b=1−1C]L-dopa in healthy volunteers and patients with unipolar major depression. *Depression*. 1993;1:71–81.

Alexopoulos GS, Kiosses DN, Choi SJ, et al. Frontal white matter microstructure and treatment response of late-life depression: a preliminary study. *Am J Psychiatry*. 2002;159:1929–1932.

Autti T, Raininko R, Santavuori P, et al. MRI of neuronal ceroid lipofuscinosis. II. Postmortem MRI and histopathological study of the brain in 16 cases of neuronal ceroid lipofuscinosis of juvenile or late infantile type. *Neuroradiology*. 1997;39: 371–377.

Baxter LR, Jr, Phelps ME, Mazziotta JC, et al. Cerebral metabolic rates for glucose in mood disorders. Studies with positron emission tomography and fluorodeoxyglucose F 18. *Arch Gen Psychiatry*. 1985;42:441–447.

Biver F, Wikler D, Lotstra F, et al. Serotonin 5-HT2 receptor imaging in major depression: focal changes in orbito-insular cortex. Br J Psychiatry. 1997;171:444–448.

Blin J, Baron JC, Dubois B, et al. Loss of brain 5-HT2 receptors in Alzheimer's disease. In vivo assessment with positron emission tomography and [^{18}F]setoperone. Brain. 1993;116(pt 3):497–510.

Bonne O, Krausz Y, Shapira B, et al. Increased cerebral blood flow in depressed patients responding to electroconvulsive therapy. J Nucl Med. 1996;37:1075–1080.

Bookheimer SY, Strojwas MH, Cohen MS, et al. Patterns of brain activation in people at risk for Alzheimer's disease. N Engl J Med. 2000;343:450–456.

Bottomley PA, Cousins JP, Pendrey DL, et al. Alzheimer dementia: quantification of energy metabolism and mobile phosphoesters with P-31 NMR spectroscopy. Radiology. 1992;183:695–699.

Boyko OB, Alston SR, Fuller GN, et al. Utility of postmortem magnetic resonance imaging in clinical neuropathology. Arch Pathol Lab Med. 1994;118:219–225.

Bradley WG, Waluch V, Brant-Zawadski M. Patchy, periventricular white matter lesions in the elderly: a common observation during NMR imaging. Noninvasive Med Imaging. 1984;1:41.

Braffman BH, Zimmerman RA, Trojanowski JQ, et al. Brain MR: pathologic correlation with gross and histopathology. 1. Lacunar infarction and Virchow-Robin spaces. AJR Am J Roentgenol. 1988a;151:551–558.

Braffman BH, Zimmerman RA, Trojanowski JQ, et al. Brain MR: pathologic correlation with gross and histopathology. 2. Hyperintense white-matter foci in the elderly. AJR Am J Roentgenol. 1988b;151:559–566.

Brun A, Englund B, Gustafson L, et al. Clinical and neuropathological criteria for frontotemporal dementia. The Lund and Manchester groups. J Neurol Neurosurg Psychiatry. 1994;57:418.

Buchsbaum MS, Wu J, Siegel BV, et al. Effect of sertraline on regional metabolic rate in patients with affective disorder. Biol Psychiatry. 1997;41:15–22.

Cannestra AF, Black KL, Martin NA, et al. Topographical and temporal specificity of human intraoperative optical intrinsic signals. Neuroreport. 1998;9:2557–2563.

Cannestra AF, Bookheimer SY, Pouratian N, et al. Temporal and topographical characterization of language cortices using intraoperative optical intrinsic signals. Neuroimage. 2000;12:41–54.

Charles HC, Lazeyras F, Krishnan KR, et al. Brain choline in depression: in vivo detection of potential pharmacodynamic effects of antidepressant therapy using hydrogen localized spectroscopy. Prog Neuropsychopharmacol Biol Psychiatry. 1994;18:1121–1127.

Charletta D, Gorelick PB, Dollear TJ, et al. CT and MRI findings among African-Americans with Alzheimer's disease, vascular dementia, and stroke without dementia. Neurology. 1995;45:1456–1461.

Chase TN, Foster NL, Fedio P, et al. Regional cortical dysfunction in Alzheimer's disease as determined by positron emission tomography. Ann Neurol. 1984;15(suppl):S170–S174.

Chatziioannou AF, Cherry SR, Shao Y, et al. Performance evaluation of microPET: a high-resolution lutetium oxyorthosilicate PET scanner for animal imaging. J Nucl Med. 1999;40:1164–1175.

Cherry SR, Shao Y, Silverman RW, et al. MicroPET: a high resolution PET scanner for imaging small animals. *IEEE Trans Nucl Sci.* 1997;44:1161–1166.

Chimowitz MI, Estes ML, Furlan AJ, et al. Further observations on the pathology of subcortical lesions identified on magnetic resonance imaging. *Arch Neurol.* 1992; 49:747–752.

Chui HC. Dementia. A review emphasizing clinicopathologic correlation and brain-behavior relationships. *Arch Neurol.* 1989;46:806–814.

Coffey CE, Figiel GS, Djang WT, et al. Leukoencephalopathy in elderly depressed patients referred for ECT. *Biol Psychiatry.* 1988;24:143–161.

Coffey CE, Wilkinson WE, Parashos IA, et al. Quantitative cerebral anatomy of the aging human brain: a cross-sectional study using magnetic resonance imaging. *Neurology.* 1992;42:527–536.

Cohen MS, Bookheimer SY. Localization of brain function using magnetic resonance imaging. *Trends Neurosci.* 1994;17:268–277.

Cohen MS, DuBois RM. Stability, repeatability, and the expression of signal magnitude in functional magnetic resonance imaging. *J Magn Reson Imaging.* 1999;10:33–40.

Cohen RM, Andreason PJ, Doudet DJ, et al. Opiate receptor avidity and cerebral blood flow in Alzheimer's disease. *J Neurol Sci.* 1997;148:171–180.

Collins DL, Peters TM, Evans AC. Automated 3D non-linear image deformation procedure for determination of gross morphometric variability in the human brain. *Proc Vis Biomed Comput.* 1994;3:180–190.

Constans JM, Meyerhoff DJ, Gerson J, et al. H-1 MR spectroscopic imaging of white matter signal hyperintensities: Alzheimer disease and ischemic vascular dementia. *Radiology.* 1995;197:517–523.

Corbett A, Bennett H, Kos S. Cognitive dysfunction following subcortical infarction. *Arch Neurol.* 1994;51:999–1007.

Corder EH, Saunders AM, Risch NJ, et al. Protective effect of apolipoprotein E type 2 allele for late onset Alzheimer disease. *Nat Genet.* 1994;7:180–184.

Corder EH, Saunders AM, Strittmatter WJ, et al. Gene dose of apolipoprotein E type 4 allele and the risk of Alzheimer's disease in late onset families. *Science.* 1993;261: 921–923.

Corey-Bloom J, Jernigan T, Archibald S, et al. Quantitative magnetic resonance imaging of the brain in late-life schizophrenia. *Am J Psychiatry.* 1995;152:447–449.

Cotter D, Miszkiel K, Al Sarraj S, et al. The assessment of postmortem brain volume: a comparison of stereological and planimetric methodologies. *Neuroradiology.* 1999; 41:493–496.

Cousins JP. Clinical MR spectroscopy: fundamentals, current applications, and future potential. *AJR Am J Roentgenol.* 1995;164:1337–1347.

Cowell PE, Turetsky BI, Gur RC, et al. Sex differences in aging of the human frontal and temporal lobes. *J Neurosci.* 1994;14:4748–4755.

Cuenod CA, Kaplan DB, Michot JL, et al. Phospholipid abnormalities in early Alzheimer's disease. In vivo phosphorus 31 magnetic resonance spectroscopy. *Arch Neurol.* 1995;52:89–94.

De Leon MJ, George AE, Golomb J, et al. Frequency of hippocampal formation atrophy in normal aging and Alzheimer's disease. *Neurobiol Aging.* 1997;18:1–11.

Dinov ID, Mega MS, Thompson PM, et al. Analyzing functional brain images in a probabilistic atlas: a validation of subvolume thresholding. *J Comput Assist Tomogr.* 2000;24:128–138.

Drayer BP. Imaging of the aging brain. Part I. Normal findings. *Radiology*. 1988a;166: 785–796.

Drayer BP. Imaging of the aging brain. Part II. Pathologic conditions. *Radiology*. 1988b; 166:797–806.

Duara R, Barker W, Luis CA. Frontotemporal dementia and Alzheimer's disease: differential diagnosis. *Dement Geriatr Cogn Disord*. 1999;10(suppl 1):37–42.

Duara R, Grady C, Haxby J, et al. Positron emission tomography in Alzheimer's disease. *Neurology*. 1986;36:879–887.

Duman RS, Charney DS. Cell atrophy and loss in major depression. *Biol Psychiatry*. 1999;45:1083–1084.

Edwards-Lee T, Miller BL, Benson DF, et al. The temporal variant of frontotemporal dementia. *Brain*. 1997;120(pt 6):1027–1040.

Eng J, Ceckler TL, Balaban RS. Quantitative ^{1}H magnetization transfer imaging in vivo. *Magn Reson Med*. 1991;17:304–314.

Erkinjuntti T, Benavente O, Eliasziw M, et al. Diffuse vacuolization (spongiosis) and arteriolosclerosis in the frontal white matter occurs in vascular dementia. *Arch Neurol*. 1996;53:325–332.

Ernst T, Chang L, Melchor R, et al. Frontotemporal dementia and early Alzheimer disease: differentiation with frontal lobe H-1 MR spectroscopy. *Radiology*. 1997;203: 829–836.

Everall IP, Chong WK, Wilkinson ID, et al. Correlation of MRI and neuropathology in AIDS. *J Neurol Neurosurg Psychiatry*. 1997;62:92–95.

Fazekas F. Magnetic resonance signal abnormalities in asymptomatic individuals: their incidence and functional correlates. *Eur Neurol*. 1989;29:164–168.

Fazekas F, Chawluk JB, Alavi A, et al. MR signal abnormalities at 1.5 T in Alzheimer's dementia and normal aging. *AJR Am J Roentgenol*. 1987;149:351–356.

Fazekas F, Niederkorn K, Schmidt R, et al. White matter signal abnormalities in normal individuals: correlation with carotid ultrasonography, cerebral blood flow measurements, and cerebrovascular risk factors. *Stroke*. 1988;19:1285–1288.

Fein G, Di Sclafani V, Tanabe J, et al. Hippocampal and cortical atrophy predict dementia in subcortical ischemic vascular disease. *Neurology*. 2000;55:1626–1635.

Fox NC, Scahill RI, Crum WR, et al. Correlation between rates of brain atrophy and cognitive decline in AD. *Neurology*. 1999;52:1687–1689.

Fox NC, Warrington EK, Freeborough PA, et al. Presymptomatic hippocampal atrophy in Alzheimer's disease. A longitudinal MRI study. *Brain*. 1996;119(pt 6):2001–2007.

Frahm J, Bruhn H, Gyngell ML, et al. Localized high-resolution proton NMR spectroscopy using stimulated echoes: initial applications to human brain in vivo. *Magn Reson Med*. 1989;9:79–93.

Frey KA, Koeppe RA, Kilbourn MR, et al. Presynaptic monoaminergic vesicles in Parkinson's disease and normal aging. *Ann Neurol*. 1996;40:873–884.

Frisoni GB, Beltramello A, Geroldi C, et al. Brain atrophy in frontotemporal dementia. *J Neurol Neurosurg Psychiatry*. 1996;61:157–165.

Frost JJ, Rosier AJ, Reich SG, et al. Positron emission tomographic imaging of the dopamine transporter with 11C-WIN 35,428 reveals marked declines in mild Parkinson's disease. *Ann Neurol*. 1993;34:423–431.

Fukuda H, Kobayashi S, Okada K, et al. Frontal white matter lesions and dementia in lacunar infarction. *Stroke*. 1990;21:1143–1149.

Gabrieli JD, Brewer JB, Desmond JE, et al. Separate neural bases of two fundamental memory processes in the human medial temporal lobe. *Science.* 1997;276:264–266.

Gilman S, Frey KA, Koeppe RA, et al. Decreased striatal monoaminergic terminals in olivopontocerebellar atrophy and multiple system atrophy demonstrated with positron emission tomography. *Ann Neurol.* 1996;40:885–892.

Giubilei F, Bastianello S, Paolillo A, et al. Quantitative magnetic resonance analysis in vascular dementia. *J Neurol.* 1997;244:246–251.

Gonzalez RG, Guimaraes AR, Moore GJ, et al. Quantitative in vivo ^{31}P magnetic resonance spectroscopy of Alzheimer disease. *Alzheimer Dis Assoc Disord.* 1996;10: 46–52.

Gould E, Tanapat P, McEwen BS, et al. Proliferation of granule cell precursors in the dentate gyrus of adult monkeys is diminished by stress. *Proc Natl Acad Sci U S A.* 1998;95:3168–3171.

Grady CL, Haxby JV, Horwitz B, et al. Activation of cerebral blood flow during a visuoperceptual task in patients with Alzheimer-type dementia. *Neurobiol Aging.* 1993;14:35–44.

Grossman RI. Magnetization transfer in multiple sclerosis. *Ann Neurol.* 1994;36(suppl): S97–S99.

Hershey LA, Modic MT, Greenough PG, et al. Magnetic resonance imaging in vascular dementia. *Neurology.* 1987;37:29–36.

Hounsfield GN. Computerized transverse axial scanning (tomography). 1. Description of system. *Br J Radiol.* 1973;46:1016–1022.

Howard RJ, Almeida O, Levy R, et al. Quantitative magnetic resonance imaging volumetry distinguishes delusional disorder from late-onset schizophrenia. *Br J Psychiatry.* 1994;165:474–480.

Jack CR, Jr, Petersen RC, Xu Y, et al. Rates of hippocampal atrophy correlate with change in clinical status in aging and AD. *Neurology.* 2000;55:484–489.

Jack CR, Jr, Petersen RC, Xu YC, et al. Medial temporal atrophy on MRI in normal aging and very mild Alzheimer's disease. *Neurology.* 1997;49:786–794.

Jernigan TL, Archibald SL, Berhow MT, et al. Cerebral structure on MRI. Part I: Localization of age-related changes. *Biol Psychiatry.* 1991;29:55–67.

Jernigan TL, Press GA, Hesselink JR. Methods for measuring brain morphologic features on magnetic resonance images. Validation and normal aging. *Arch Neurol.* 1990; 47:27–32.

Juottonen K, Laakso MP, Partanen K, et al. Comparative MR analysis of the entorhinal cortex and hippocampus in diagnosing Alzheimer disease. *AJNR Am J Neuroradiol.* 1999;20:139–144.

Kabani NJ, Sled JG, Chertkow H. Magnetization transfer ratio in mild cognitive impairment and dementia of Alzheimer's type. *Neuroimage.* 2002;15:604–610.

Kato T, Inubushi T, Kato N. Magnetic resonance spectroscopy in affective disorders. *J Neuropsychiatry Clin Neurosci.* 1998;10:133–147.

Kattapong VJ, Brooks WM, Wesley MH, et al. Proton magnetic resonance spectroscopy of vascular- and Alzheimer-type dementia. *Arch Neurol.* 1996;53:678–680.

Kaufer DI, Miller BL, Itti L, et al. Midline cerebral morphometry distinguishes frontotemporal dementia and Alzheimer's disease. *Neurology.* 1997;48:978–985.

Kaye JA, Swihart T, Howieson D, et al. Volume loss of the hippocampus and temporal lobe in healthy elderly persons destined to develop dementia. *Neurology.* 1997;48: 1297–1304.

Kesslak JP, Nalcioglu O, Cotman CW. Quantification of magnetic resonance scans for hippocampal and parahippocampal atrophy in Alzheimer's disease. *Neurology.* 1991;41:51–54.

Kirkpatrick JB, Hayman LA. White-matter lesions in MR imaging of clinically healthy brains of elderly subjects: possible pathologic basis. *Radiology.* 1987;162:509–511.

Kitagaki H, Mori E, Yamaji S, et al. Frontotemporal dementia and Alzheimer disease: evaluation of cortical atrophy with automated hemispheric surface display generated with MR images. *Radiology.* 1998;208:431–439.

Klunk WE, Xu C, Panchalingam K, et al. Quantitative ^{1}H and ^{31}P MRS of PCA extracts of postmortem Alzheimer's disease brain. *Neurobiol Aging.* 1996;17:349–357.

Kohler S, Black SE, Sinden M, et al. Memory impairments associated with hippocampal versus parahippocampal-gyrus atrophy: an MR volumetry study in Alzheimer's disease. *Neuropsychologia.* 1998;36:901–914.

Kreis R, Farrow N, Ross BD. Localized ^{1}H NMR spectroscopy in patients with chronic hepatic encephalopathy. Analysis of changes in cerebral glutamine, choline and inositols. *NMR Biomed.* 1991;4:109–116.

Krishnan KR. Magnetic resonance morphometry: image analysis methodology development for affective disorders. *Depression.* 1993a;1:159–171.

Krishnan KR. Neuroanatomic substrates of depression in the elderly. *J Geriatr Psychiatry Neurol.* 1993b;6:39–58.

Krishnan KR, Hays JC, Blazer DG. MRI-defined vascular depression. *Am J Psychiatry.* 1997;154:497–501.

Kumar A. Neuroimaging as a probe of brain function in late-life psychiatric illness: old paradigms, new challenges. *J Geriatr Psychiatry Neurol.* 1999;12:93–94.

Kumar A. Neuroimaging in pursuit of neurobiology: strengths, limitations, and the quest for new paradigms in depression and mood. *Am J Geriatr Psychiatry.* 2000a;8:284–288.

Kumar A. Neuroimaging: special issues. In: Sadock BJ, Sadock VA, eds. *Comprehensive Textbook of Psychiatry.* 7th ed. Philadelphia, PA: Lippincott, Williams & Wilkins; 2000b:3041–3045.

Kumar A, Bilker W, Jin Z, et al. Atrophy and high intensity lesions: complementary neurobiological mechanisms in late-life major depression. *Neuropsychopharmacology.* 2000;22:264–274.

Kumar A, Gottlieb G. Frontotemporal dementias: a new clinical syndrome? *Am J Geriatr Psychiatry.* 1993;1:95–108.

Kumar A, Jin Z, Bilker W, et al. Late-onset minor and major depression: early evidence for common neuroanatomical substrates detected by using MRI. *Proc Natl Acad Sci U S A.* 1998;95:7654–7658.

Kumar A, Miller D, Ewbank D, et al. Quantitative anatomic measures and comorbid medical illness in late-life major depression. *Am J Geriatr Psychiatry.* 1997;5:15–25.

Kumar A, Newberg A, Alavi A, et al. Regional cerebral glucose metabolism in late-life depression and Alzheimer disease: a preliminary positron emission tomography study. *Proc Natl Acad Sci U S A.* 1993;90:7019–7023.

Kumar A, Schapiro MB, Grady C, et al. High-resolution PET studies in Alzheimer's disease. *Neuropsychopharmacology.* 1991;4:35–46.

Kumar A, Schweizer E, Jin Z, et al. Neuroanatomical substrates of late-life minor depression. A quantitative magnetic resonance imaging study. *Arch Neurol.* 1997;54:613–617.

Kumar A, Thomas A, Lavretsky H, et al. Frontal white matter biochemical abnormalities in late-life major depression detected with proton magnetic resonance spectroscopy. *Am J Psychiatry.* 2002;159:630–636.

Kumar A, Yousem D, Souder E, et al. High-intensity signals in Alzheimer's disease without cerebrovascular risk factors: a magnetic resonance imaging evaluation. *Am J Psychiatry.* 1992;149:248–250.

Laakso MP, Frisoni GB, Kononen M, et al. Hippocampus and entorhinal cortex in frontotemporal dementia and Alzheimer's disease: a morphometric MRI study. *Biol Psychiatry.* 2000;47:1056–1063.

Laakso MP, Lehtovirta M, Partanen K, et al. Hippocampus in Alzheimer's disease: a 3-year follow-up MRI study. *Biol Psychiatry.* 2000;47:557–561.

Laakso MP, Soininen H, Partanen K, et al. Volumes of hippocampus, amygdala and frontal lobes in the MRI-based diagnosis of early Alzheimer's disease: correlation with memory functions. *J Neural Transm Park Dis Dement Sect.* 1995;9:73–86.

Lee KS, Frey KA, Koeppe RA, et al. In vivo quantification of cerebral muscarinic receptors in normal human aging using positron emission tomography and [^{11}C]tropanyl benzilate. *J Cereb Blood Flow Metab.* 1996;16:303–310.

Lehericy S, Baulac M, Chiras J, et al. Amygdalohippocampal MR volume measurements in the early stages of Alzheimer disease. *AJNR Am J Neuroradiol.* 1994;15:929–937.

Lesser IM, Mena I, Boone KB, et al. Reduction of cerebral blood flow in older depressed patients. *Arch Gen Psychiatry.* 1994;51:677–686.

Lim KO, Adalsteinsson E, Spielman D, et al. Proton magnetic resonance spectroscopic imaging of cortical gray and white matter in schizophrenia. *Arch Gen Psychiatry.* 1998;55:346–352.

Lim KO, Spielman DM. Estimating NAA in cortical gray matter with applications for measuring changes due to aging. *Magn Reson Med.* 1997;37:372–377.

Liu CK, Miller BL, Cummings JL, et al. A quantitative MRI study of vascular dementia. *Neurology.* 1992;42:138–143.

Longson D, Hutchinson CE, Doyle CA, et al. Use of MRI for measuring structures in frozen postmortem brain. *Brain Res Bull.* 1995;38:457–460.

Lyness JM, Caine ED, Cox C, et al. Cerebrovascular risk factors and later-life major depression. Testing a small-vessel brain disease model. *Am J Geriatr Psychiatry.* 1998;6:5–13.

Lyoo IK, Satlin A, Lee CK, et al. Regional atrophy of the corpus callosum in subjects with Alzheimer's disease and multi-infarct dementia. *Psychiatry Res.* 1997;74:63–72.

MacKay S, Meyerhoff DJ, Constans JM, et al. Regional gray and white matter metabolite differences in subjects with AD, with subcortical ischemic vascular dementia, and elderly controls with ^{1}H magnetic resonance spectroscopic imaging. *Arch Neurol.* 1996;53:167–174.

Manolio TA, Kronmal RA, Burke GL, et al. Magnetic resonance abnormalities and cardiovascular disease in older adults. The Cardiovascular Health Study. *Stroke.* 1994;25:318–327.

Mega MS, Chen SS, Thompson PM, et al. Mapping histology to metabolism: coregistration of stained whole-brain sections to premortem PET in Alzheimer's disease. *Neuroimage.* 1997;5:147–153.

Mega MS, Chu T, Mazziotta JC, et al. Mapping biochemistry to metabolism: FDG-PET and amyloid burden in Alzheimer's disease. *Neuroreport.* 1999;10:2911–2917.

Meltzer CC. Neuropharmacology and receptor studies in the elderly. *J Geriatr Psychiatry Neurol.* 1999;12:137–149.

Meltzer C, Frost J. Partial volume correction in emission computed tomography: focus on Alzheimer disease. In: Thatcher R, Hallet M, Zeffiro T, et al., eds. *Functional Neuroimaging.* St. Louis, MO: Academic Press; 1994:163–170.

Meltzer CC, Price JC, Mathis CA, et al. PET imaging of serotonin type 2A receptors in late-life neuropsychiatric disorders. *Am J Psychiatry.* 1999;156:1871–1878.

Meltzer CC, Smith G, DeKosky ST, et al. Serotonin in aging, late-life depression, and Alzheimer's disease: the emerging role of functional imaging. *Neuropsychopharmacology.* 1998;18:407–430.

Meltzer CC, Smith G, Price JC, et al. Reduced binding of [^{18}F]altanserin to serotonin type 2A receptors in aging: persistence of effect after partial volume correction. *Brain Res.* 1998;813:167–171.

Meyerhoff DJ, MacKay S, Constans JM, et al. Axonal injury and membrane alterations in Alzheimer's disease suggested by in vivo proton magnetic resonance spectroscopic imaging. *Ann Neurol.* 1994;36:40–47.

Michaelis T, Merboldt KD, Hanicke W, et al. On the identification of cerebral metabolites in localized ^{1}H NMR spectra of human brain in vivo. *NMR Biomed.* 1991;4: 90–98.

Miller BL. A review of chemical issues in ^{1}H NMR spectroscopy: N-acetyl-L-aspartate, creatine and choline. *NMR Biomed.* 1991;4:47–52.

Miller BL, Chang L, Booth R, et al. In vivo ^{1}H MRS choline: correlation with in vitro chemistry/histology. *Life Sci.* 1996;58:1929–1935.

Miller BL, Gearhart R. Neuroimaging in the diagnosis of frontotemporal dementia. *Dement Geriatr Cogn Disord.* 1999;10(suppl 1):71–74.

Miller BL, Moats RA, Shonk T, et al. Alzheimer disease: depiction of increased cerebral myo-inositol with proton MR spectroscopy. *Radiology.* 1993;187:433–437.

Moats RA, Ernst T, Shonk TK, et al. Abnormal cerebral metabolite concentrations in patients with probable Alzheimer disease. *Magn Reson Med.* 1994;32:110–115.

Moore CM, Frederick BB, Renshaw PF. Brain biochemistry using magnetic resonance spectroscopy: relevance to psychiatric illness in the elderly. *J Geriatr Psychiatry Neurol.* 1999;12:107–117.

Moseley M. Diffusion tensor imaging and aging—a review. *NMR Biomed.* 2002;15: 553–560.

Murphy DG, Bottomley PA, Salerno JA, et al. An in vivo study of phosphorus and glucose metabolism in Alzheimer's disease using magnetic resonance spectroscopy and PET. *Arch Gen Psychiatry.* 1993;50:341–349.

Nobler MS, Pelton GH, Sackeim HA. Cerebral blood flow and metabolism in late-life depression and dementia. *J Geriatr Psychiatry Neurol.* 1999;12:118–127.

O'Farrell AM, Rex DE, Muthialu A, et al. Characterization of optical intrinsic signals and blood volume during cortical spreading depression. *Neuroreport.* 2000;11: 2121–2125.

Ogawa S, Tank DW, Menon R, et al. Intrinsic signal changes accompanying sensory stimulation: functional brain mapping with magnetic resonance imaging. *Proc Natl Acad Sci U S A.* 1992;89:5951–5955.

Oldendorf W, Oldendorf WH. *MRI Primer.* New York, NY: Raven Press; 1991.

Pantel J, Schroder J, Essig M, et al. In vivo quantification of brain volumes in subcortical vascular dementia and Alzheimer's disease. An MRI-based study. *Dement Geriatr Cogn Disord.* 1998;9:309–316.

Parnetti L, Tarducci R, Presciutti O, et al. Proton magnetic resonance spectroscopy can differentiate Alzheimer's disease from normal aging. *Mech Ageing Dev.* 1997;97: 9–14.

Petersen RC, Jack CR, Jr, Xu YC, et al. Memory and MRI-based hippocampal volumes in aging and AD. *Neurology.* 2000;54:581–587.

Petrella JR, Coleman RE, Doraiswamy PM. Neuroimaging and early diagnosis of Alzheimer disease: a look to the future. *Radiology.* 2003;226:315–336.

Pettegrew JW, Klunk WE, Panchalingam K, et al. Magnetic resonance spectroscopic changes in Alzheimer's disease. *Ann N Y Acad Sci.* 1997;826:282–306.

Pettegrew JW, Moossy J, Withers G, et al. ^{31}P nuclear magnetic resonance study of the brain in Alzheimer's disease. *J Neuropathol Exp Neurol.* 1988;47:235–248.

Pettegrew JW, Panchalingam K, Klunk WE, et al. Alterations of cerebral metabolism in probable Alzheimer's disease: a preliminary study. *Neurobiol Aging.* 1994;15: 117–132.

Pfefferbaum A, Adalsteinsson E, Spielman D, et al. In vivo brain concentrations of N-acetyl compounds, creatine, and choline in Alzheimer disease. *Arch Gen Psychiatry.* 1999;56:185–192.

Phelps ME, Cherry SR. The changing design of positron imaging systems. *Clin Positron Imaging.* 1998;1:31–45.

Phelps ME, Hoffman EJ, Huang SC, et al. ECAT: a new computerized tomographic imaging system for positron-emitting radiopharmaceuticals. *J Nucl Med.* 1978;19: 635–647.

Phelps ME, Huang SC, Hoffman EJ, et al. Tomographic measurement of local cerebral glucose metabolic rate in humans with (F-18)2-fluoro-2-deoxy-D-glucose: validation of method. *Ann Neurol.* 1979;6:371–388.

Rabins PV, Pearlson GD, Aylward E, et al. Cortical magnetic resonance imaging changes in elderly inpatients with major depression. *Am J Psychiatry.* 1991;148:617–620.

Rajkowska G, Miguel-Hidalgo JJ, Wei J, et al. Morphometric evidence for neuronal and glial prefrontal cell pathology in major depression. *Biol Psychiatry.* 1999;45: 1085–1098.

Reiman EM, Caselli RJ, Yun LS, et al. Preclinical evidence of Alzheimer's disease in persons homozygous for the epsilon 4 allele for apolipoprotein E. *N Engl J Med.* 1996;334:752–758.

Reivich M, Kuhl D, Wolf A, et al. The [^{18}F]fluorodeoxyglucose method for the measurement of local cerebral glucose utilization in man. *Circ Res.* 1979;44:127–137.

Rose SE, de Zubicaray GI, Wang D, et al. A ^{1}H MRS study of probable Alzheimer's disease and normal aging: implications for longitudinal monitoring of dementia progression. *Magn Reson Imaging.* 1999;17:291–299.

Ross BD, Bluml S, Cowan R, et al. In vivo MR spectroscopy of human dementia. *Neuroimaging Clin N Am.* 1998;8:809–822.

Sabri O, Ringelstein EB, Hellwig D, et al. Neuropsychological impairment correlates with hypoperfusion and hypometabolism but not with severity of white matter lesions on MRI in patients with cerebral microangiopathy. *Stroke.* 1999;30:556–566.

Sackeim HA, Prohovnik I. Brain imaging studies in depressive disorders. In: Mann J, Kupfer DJ, eds. *Biology of Depression Disorders*. New York, NY: Plenum; 1993: 205–258.

Sackeim HA, Prohovnik I, Moeller JR, et al. Regional cerebral blood flow in mood disorders. II. Comparison of major depression and Alzheimer's disease. *J Nucl Med*. 1993;34:1090–1101.

Sapolsky RM, Pulsinelli WA. Glucocorticoids potentiate ischemic injury to neurons: therapeutic implications. *Science*. 1985;229:1397–1400.

Satlin A, Bodick N, Offen WW, et al. Brain proton magnetic resonance spectroscopy (^{1}H-MRS) in Alzheimer's disease: changes after treatment with xanomeline, an M1 selective cholinergic agonist. *Am J Psychiatry*. 1997;154:1459–1461.

Sato R, Bryan RN, Fried LP. Neuroanatomic and functional correlates of depressed mood: the Cardiovascular Health Study. *Am J Epidemiol*. 1999;150:919–929.

Schmidt R. Comparison of magnetic resonance imaging in Alzheimer's disease, vascular dementia and normal aging. *Eur Neurol*. 1992;32:164–169.

Schuff N, Amend D, Ezekiel F, et al. Changes of hippocampal N-acetyl aspartate and volume in Alzheimer's disease. A proton MR spectroscopic imaging and MRI study. *Neurology*. 1997;49:1513–1521.

Schuff N, Amend DL, Meyerhoff DJ, et al. Alzheimer disease: quantitative H-1 MR spectroscopic imaging of frontoparietal brain. *Radiology*. 1998;207:91–102.

Sheline YI, Wang PW, Gado MH, et al. Hippocampal atrophy in recurrent major depression. *Proc Natl Acad Sci U S A*. 1996;93:3908–3913.

Shoghi-Jadid K, Small GW, Agdeppa ED, et al. Localization of neurofibrillary tangles and beta-amyloid plaques in the brains of living patients with Alzheimer disease. *Am J Geriatr Psychiatry*. 2002;10:24–35.

Shonk TK, Moats RA, Gifford P, et al. Probable Alzheimer disease: diagnosis with proton MR spectroscopy. *Radiology*. 1995;195:65–72.

Small GW, Mazziotta JC, Collins MT, et al. Apolipoprotein E type 4 allele and cerebral glucose metabolism in relatives at risk for familial Alzheimer disease. *JAMA*. 1995; 273:942–947.

Smith CD. Quantitative computed tomography and magnetic resonance imaging in aging and Alzheimer's disease. A review. *J Neuroimaging*. 1996;6:44–53.

Smith CD, Gallenstein LG, Layton WJ, et al. ^{31}P magnetic resonance spectroscopy in Alzheimer's and Pick's disease. *Neurobiol Aging*. 1993;14:85–92.

Steffens DC, Helms MJ, Krishnan KR, et al. Cerebrovascular disease and depression symptoms in the cardiovascular health study. *Stroke*. 1999;30:2159–2166.

Sullivan P, Pary R, Telang F, et al. Risk factors for white matter changes detected by magnetic resonance imaging in the elderly. *Stroke*. 1990;21:1424–1428.

Sultzer DL, Mahler ME, Cummings JL, et al. Cortical abnormalities associated with subcortical lesions in vascular dementia. Clinical and position emission tomographic findings. *Arch Neurol*. 1995;52:773–780.

Sze G, DeArmand SJ, Brant-Zawadski M, et al. Foci of MRI signal anterior to the frontal horns: histologic correlation of a normal finding. *Am J Neuroradiol*. 1981;147: 331–337.

Tedeschi G, Bertolino A, Lundbom N, et al. Cortical and subcortical chemical pathology in Alzheimer's disease as assessed by multislice proton magnetic resonance spectroscopic imaging. *Neurology*. 1996;47:696–704.

Thomas MA, Alger JR. Magnetic resonance spectroscopy of the brain. In: DeSalles AAF, Lufkin R, eds. *Minimal Invasive Therapy of the Brain.* New York, NY: Thieme Medical Publishers; 1997:63–77.

Thomas MA, Yue K, Binesh N, et al. Localized two-dimensional shift correlated MR spectroscopy of human brain. *Magn Reson Med.* 2001;46:58–67.

Thompson PM, MacDonald D, Mega MS, et al. Detection and mapping of abnormal brain structure with a probabilistic atlas of cortical surfaces. *J Comput Assist Tomogr.* 1997;21:567–581.

Thompson PM, Schwartz C, Toga AW. High-resolution random mesh algorithms for creating a probabilistic 3D surface atlas of the human brain. *Neuroimage.* 1996;3: 19–34.

Toga AW, Goldkorn A, Ambach K, et al. Postmortem cryosectioning as an anatomic reference for human brain mapping. *Comput Med Imaging Graph.* 1997;21:131–141.

Tsai G, Coyle JT. N-Acetylaspartate in neuropsychiatric disorders. *Prog Neurobiol.* 1995;46:531–540.

Upadhyaya AK, Abou-Saleh MT, Wilson K, et al. A study of depression in old age using single-photon emission computerised tomography. *Br J Psychiatry.* 1990;Suppl: 76–81.

Victoroff J, Mack WJ, Lyness SA, et al. Multicenter clinicopathological correlation in dementia. *Am J Psychiatry.* 1995;152:1476–1484.

Wahlund LO. Magnetic resonance imaging and computed tomography in Alzheimer's disease. *Acta Neurol Scand.* 1996 Suppl;168:50–53.

Wolf PA, D'Agostino RB, Belanger AJ, et al. Probability of stroke: a risk profile from the Framingham Study. *Stroke.* 1991;22:312–318.

Xanthakos S, Krishnan KR, Kim DM, et al. Magnetic resonance imaging of Alzheimer's disease. *Prog Neuropsychopharmacol Biol Psychiatry.* 1996;20:597–626.

Yamaguchi S, Nakagawa T, Arai H, et al. Temporal progression of hippocampal atrophy and apolipoprotein E gene in Alzheimer's disease. *J Am Geriatr Soc.* 1996;44: 216–217.

Yamaji S, Ishii K, Sasaki M, et al. Changes in cerebral blood flow and oxygen metabolism related to magnetic resonance imaging white matter hyperintensities in Alzheimer's disease. *J Nucl Med.* 1997;38:1471–1474.

Yamanouchi H, Sugiura S, Shimada H. Loss of nerve fibres in the corpus callosum of progressive subcortical vascular encephalopathy. *J Neurol.* 1990;237:39–41.

Yamauchi H, Fukuyama H, Ogawa M, et al. Callosal atrophy in patients with lacunar infarction and extensive leukoaraiosis. An indicator of cognitive impairment. *Stroke.* 1994;25:1788–1793.

Ylikoski A, Erkinjuntti T, Raininko R, et al. White matter hyperintensities on MRI in the neurologically nondiseased elderly. Analysis of cohorts of consecutive subjects aged 55 to 85 years living at home. *Stroke.* 1995;26:1171–1177.

Zimmerman RD, Fleming CA, Lee BC, et al. Periventricular hyperintensity as seen by magnetic resonance: prevalence and significance. *AJR Am J Roentgenol.* 1986;146: 443–450.

15

Electroencephalography

Andrew F. Leuchter, MD
Daniel P. Holschneider, MD

The electroencephalogram (EEG) was developed as a clinical test in the 1930s by a psychiatrist, Dr. Hans Berger. Ironically, in the more than five decades since its introduction into clinical practice, it has become a technique most commonly performed under the supervision of, and interpreted by, neurologists. Neurologists have in fact made the greatest use of this test, using it to help corroborate the diagnosis of seizure disorders.

Since its introduction, however, it has been clear that the EEG has a special role in the assessment of older adults. Berger himself reported that the EEG changes with aging and is abnormal in a high proportion of individuals with dementia (Berger, 1937). To date, the EEG remains the single most cost-effective physiological test to indicate the presence of an encephalopathy. It therefore is incumbent on the geriatric psychiatrist to understand the fundamentals of EEG interpretation.

Despite the frequency with which an EEG is ordered, the specific indications for this test and the guidelines for interpreting its results remain unclear. This chapter reviews the major clinical uses of the EEG, its role in evaluating common clinical syndromes, and the usefulness of EEG results.

INDICATIONS FOR ELECTROENCEPHALOGRAPHY

There are two primary reasons to perform an EEG in geriatric psychiatry: (1) to evaluate the possibility of the presence of an underlying, secondary mental disorder and (2) to evaluate a possible seizure disorder. Although the test is commonly ordered to rule out one of these conditions, normal EEG results cannot rule out brain disease; they simply establish that the presence of such disease is less likely.

An EEG is not indicated whenever brain disease is known or suspected. Rather, in psychiatry, the test is useful primarily in four situations: (1) the presence of brain disease is suspected, but there is no clear etiology or the presentation is unusual; (2) the presence of brain disease is possible, but it is difficult to differentiate from some other psychiatric illness (e.g., depression); (3) the course of a psychiatric illness is unusual, or the illness is refractory to treatment; and (4) a structural imaging study would be advisable, but is unavailable.

ELECTROENCEPHALOGRAM FINDINGS
FOR NORMAL AGING

Any discussion of the application of electroencephalography must consider that the normal EEG in the elderly may differ significantly from that seen in young adults. The EEG cannot fully exclude a diagnosis of brain disease in the elderly because many of the findings of "normal" aging may mimic brain disease.

Although there is considerable variation in the normal EEG at any age, a typical EEG in a young adult (aged 20–60 years) who is awake and resting with eyes closed shows a pattern of moderate-amplitude sinusoidal electrical activity in the back of the head at a frequency of 8 Hz to 12 Hz (the so-called posterior dominant or alpha rhythm), with a mean frequency for young adults of 10 Hz. Visual inspection of the EEG shows negligible slow-wave activity in the range of 0 to 4 Hz (delta) and little detectable activity in the range of 4 to 8 Hz (theta), except when the patient is drowsy. Low-amplitude, fast activity (greater than 12 Hz or beta) predominates in the anterior and central head regions.

In adults older than 60 years, increased slowing occurs as a normal finding. This slowing may be of two types. First, there commonly is slowing of the posterior dominant rhythm. This rhythm remains in the alpha range, but the mean for a group of elderly subjects reportedly slows to 9 Hz by 90 years of age. Some normal elderly subjects have been reported to have alpha rhythms as slow as 8 Hz, but a posterior dominant rhythm below the alpha range in the waking and alert state always is considered pathological (Hubbard et al., 1976; Obrist, 1976; Obrist et al., 1966).

The second type of normal slowing is intermittent theta slowing seen over the temporal regions. This slow activity, which is intermixed with the normal background rhythms, commonly occurs at a frequency of 6 Hz to 8 Hz and may occur in brief runs. It has been reported to occur in up to 40% of normal volunteers (Busse et al., 1954; Torres et al., 1983). Some investigators believe that this pattern of mild, intermixed slowing is indicative of subclinical cerebrovascular disease, and they have shown that, in carefully screened controls, the true prevalence drops 10-fold. For current clinical standards, however, this finding still is considered within normal limits (Van Sweden et al., 1999). When an EEG report mentions "increased slowing" or "increased slow-wave activity," technically it is referring to this second category of slowing.

In clinical practice, the distinction between the two types of EEG slowing frequently is blurred. Slowing of the posterior dominant rhythm and increased intermixed slowing commonly are not specified, and the EEG simply is reported to be slow. Under these circumstances, the key question is whether the electroencephalographer is identifying the presence of pathological slowing (i.e., slow-wave activity that is excessive for age or even under any circumstances). This is a judgment that is made by the electroencephalographer that usually is specified at the end of the report.

Slowing may be accentuated by drowsiness in either young or old, but it is particularly likely to emerge early in drowsiness among elderly subjects. This slowing is most often seen in the frontal regions, where trains of semirhythmic delta activity may be seen. This delta slowing may occasionally be mistaken for frontal intermittent rhythmic delta activity (FIRDA), a pathological rhythm often associated with metabolic encephalopathy and sometimes deep midline lesions (Zurek et al., 1985). Because of sensory losses, the elderly are more likely to become drowsy during EEG recordings, so it is vital that they be alerted often during the procedure and that their state of arousal is noted in the report.

Other EEG changes also are commonly seen with aging. Amplitude of the signal generally decreases, as does the response to photic stimulation (Van Sweden et al., 1999). In some individuals, there is an increase in the amount of sharp-wave activity intermixed with slowing in the temporal regions, but this activity should be readily distinguishable from true epileptiform activity. The changes in beta activity with aging are less clear. The preponderance of evidence suggests modest age-dependent increases, although these are seen mostly when making comparisons across a wide age range (24–90 years), but not across a narrower range (60–90 years) (Holschneider & Leuchter, 1995).

ELECTROENCEPHALOGRAM IN THE EVALUATION
OF SPECIFIC DISORDERS

Many of the various clinical situations that may prompt the geriatric psychiatrist to order an EEG are discussed in the following sections.

Primary Degenerative Dementia
of the Alzheimer's Type

The finding that first generated clinical interest in the EEG was that institutionalized demented patients demonstrated excessive, diffuse slowing of background rhythms and slowing of the posterior dominant rhythm. This finding proved nonspecific, seen primarily in more advanced cases of dementia and in a variety of organic conditions.

Six decades of clinical experience, however, have demonstrated that the EEG has clear uses for patients with possible or definite secondary mental disorders. The most common use is in the initial evaluation of possible dementia of the Alzheimer type (DAT). Experts differ as to the indications for an EEG in the initial evaluation: Some believe it should be ordered in all cases; a National Institutes of Health consensus conference concluded that the test should be ordered when the etiology of the dementia is unclear or the presentation is unusual (Group for the Advancement of Psychiatry, 1988).

When the presentation or course is unusual and the etiology unclear, ordering an EEG may facilitate the diagnostic process. The EEG frequently is not ordered in the initial evaluation of a patient with possible DAT because it is generally believed that the EEG is normal in cases of mild dementia (Cummings & Benson, 1992). Work by our laboratory, however, found that, among 104 patients whose testing showed normal or equivocal mental status and who were to be evaluated for possible dementia, the EEG was abnormal in nearly 50% of cases (Leuchter, Daly, et al., 1993). These findings suggest that the standard EEG is highly sensitive to the presence of even mild encephalopathy. EEG abnormalities are nonspecific, however, and may be seen in patients with depression.

When a baseline tracing from the patient's premorbid state is available, the EEG may be particularly helpful in the evaluation of subsequent dementia. Even when a patient's EEG remains within normal limits overall, it may show slowing that is excessive for the individual. Baseline tracings, however, seldom are available.

Other Causes of Dementia

The EEG does have some utility in the differential diagnosis of dementia, and it may help distinguish DAT from other dementing illnesses. Vascular dementia (VaD) commonly shows focal or lateralizing abnormalities, in contrast to the diffuse and symmetric pattern of slowing seen in DAT (Erkinjuntti et al., 1988; Roberts et al., 1978). Focal abnormalities frequently are absent in cases of vascular dementia, however; cases of diffuse, deep, white-matter ischemic disease (i.e., Binswanger's disease) in which there are no cortical infarcts or lesions "undercutting" the cortex may show a pattern indistinguishable from that of DAT. Structural imaging studies of the brain (computed tomography [CT], magnetic resonance imaging [MRI]) clearly are most useful in corroborating the diagnosis of vascular dementia.

In Creutzfeldt-Jakob disease, an uncommon cause of dementia in the elderly, the EEG reveals frontally predominant triphasic waves, paroxysmal lateralizing epileptiform discharges, or some other pseudoperiodic sharp-wave complex within 12 weeks of onset of clinical symptoms in more than 90% of cases (Spehlmann, 1981). As the disease progresses, these sharp-wave complexes attenuate and disappear into a background of slow-wave activity. Although it is not pathognomonic of the illness, the presence of pseudoperiodic discharges in the presence of a rapidly progressive dementia is highly suggestive of the diagnosis. The absence of these periodic discharges after 10 weeks of clinical symptoms makes the diagnosis suspect (Chiappa & Young, 1978).

Huntington's chorea frequently presents with a progressive loss of amplitude of the EEG, with or without slowing. The dementia accompanying thyroid disease may present with dramatic attenuation of EEG amplitude. Frontotemporal dementias (FTDs) such as Pick's disease may show a well-preserved posterior dominant background rhythm (Groen & Endtz, 1982; Stigsby et al., 1981; Yener et al., 1996). Increases in slow-wave activity appear to be less pronounced in FTD than in DAT and when they occur may be accentuated in anterior regions. Other forms of dementia, such as the dementia accompanying Parkinson's disease or progressive supranuclear palsy, do not have characteristic EEG presentations that help distinguish them from DAT (Brenner, 1999; Spehlmann, 1981). Even in the forms of dementia that do have particular EEG presentations, the EEG usually is primarily a tool for confirming the diagnosis; clinical history and physical examination are likely to be more useful in establishing the diagnosis.

Depression

The EEG may be useful in when there is a suspicion that cognitive impairment is caused by depression. Neuropsychological tests, commonly used in such cases, are liable to be adversely affected by motivational or attention problems. The EEG, however, is a clinically available measure of brain function that can help distinguish between these two illnesses. Abnormal EEG results may be seen in depressed elderly patients (Leuchter, Daly, et al., 1993), but these abnormalities usually are mild. Furthermore, these abnormalities may be caused by subclinical brain disease distinct from dementia (Holschneider & Leuchter, 1999; Oken & Kaye, 1992). Another limitation is that normal EEG results may be seen early in the course of a dementia, so follow-up testing may be necessary to detect an encephalopathy.

Toxic and Metabolic Conditions

The EEG is useful for detecting excess morbidity as a result of reversible toxic or metabolic conditions because it is a sensitive (albeit nonspecific) screen for encephalopathic conditions. For example, a patient with mild cognitive impairment but severe slowing on EEG may have another disease process instead of, or in addition to, DAT (Cummings & Benson, 1983).

A common finding in the elderly is toxic encephalopathy as the result of one or more medications a patient is receiving. Such an encephalopathic process would be expected to present electrographically with increased slow-wave activity and slowing of the posterior dominant rhythm. It may be difficult to determine when medications are causing or contributing to an encephalopathy because, even in therapeutic dosages, many psychoactive and nonpsychoactive drugs may cause EEG changes.

Antidepressants or neuroleptics commonly cause slowing of the posterior dominant rhythm and an increased amount of slow-wave activity (Fink, 1968). Lithium and clozaril similarly may cause increased slowing; at high levels, they may cause focal abnormalities or spike discharges (Freudenreich et al., 1997; Struve, 1987). Benzodiazepines, barbiturates, and other sedative-hypnotics in therapeutic doses usually cause increased 20- to 25-Hz beta activity (Fink, 1968), most commonly in a frontocentral pattern. In high doses, these drugs may cause increased slowing as well.

One of the most common causes of drug-induced cognitive dysfunction in the elderly is drugs with anticholinergic effects. These drugs routinely cause increased amounts of slowing in the EEG (Pfefferbaum et al., 1979). If increased slowing is detected in the EEG of a patient taking a drug known to cause cognitive dysfunction, it may be prudent to discontinue or replace the drug with a nonoffending agent.

The EEG may help detect unsuspected metabolic derangement because blood chemistry panels cannot screen for all possible endocrinopathies, electrolyte imbalances, and toxic substances. Apart from increased slowing, other patterns that may be seen in metabolic encephalopathy include FIRDA, triphasic waves, and sharp waves. Depending on the distribution and the frequency of occurrence of these waveforms, they may suggest a specific etiology of metabolic encephalopathy. For example, the most common cause of frontally predominant triphasic waves that occur two to three times per second is hepatic encephalopathy. Such waveforms also may be seen, however, in patients with chronic renal failure (Hughes, 1982). The clinical history and other laboratory tests clearly are necessary to interpret these nonspecific findings.

Delirium and Changes in Mental Status

Although the EEG is most often ordered in the elderly for evaluating possible dementia, the most justifiable use is in the evaluation of delirium. It first was established in the 1940s that the degree of slowing in the EEG among delirious patients is directly related to the level of confusion, and that improvements in the EEG reflect improvements in mental status (Engel & Romano, 1944; Romano & Engel, 1944). The EEG, therefore, is an important confirmatory tool, and it is difficult to make the diagnosis of delirium in the absence of EEG slowing (Liposwki, 1987). The EEG also may be useful in evaluating the course of delirium. When the mental status exam is equivocal or difficult to perform, as for a patient on a ventilator or one with aphasia, the EEG may be useful for monitoring resolution of the encephalopathy. Interventions to improve the patient's condition should diminish EEG slowing, and persistent severe slowing suggests either that the cause of the delirium has not been corrected or that another illness (i.e., dementia) exists. It is unclear how long EEG slowing may persist after the resolution of a delirium.

When a patient's mental status has declined acutely and a stroke is suspected, the EEG commonly shows focal slowing very early, whereas the CT scan may not show changes for several days (Keilson et al., 1985). When a structural imaging study of the brain is desirable but unavailable, the EEG may be used. It is important to note that there may be a significant mass lesion, particularly in the deep white matter, without any EEG changes.

Finally, the EEG may be useful in following the course of a dementing illness. As a patient's mental status declines, the EEG is marked by concomitant increased slowing, loss of the posterior dominant rhythm, and occasionally, the emergence of spike foci. If the patient has had a baseline EEG and later suffers an abrupt decline in function, a repeat tracing may be useful in determining the cause of the loss in functional status. For example, a significant decline in function with no change in EEG patterns would be unusual and might suggest the development of superimposed depression.

Seizure Disorders

Most patients who develop seizure disorders do so in the first two decades of life. Thereafter, the incidence of new onset seizure disorders drops, only to rise again after 60 years of age. The elderly have been estimated to account for approximately 24% of new-onset cases of epilepsy (Sander et al., 1990). The most common causes of seizures with onset late in life are stroke, trauma, and mass lesions (Ettinger & Shinnar, 1993; Luhdorf et al., 1986; Sung & Chu, 1990). Among these individuals, the EEG is useful to confirm the diagnosis, to help establish the type of seizure, and to define the area of origin of the epileptic discharge. The geriatric psychiatrist generally does not establish the diagnosis of epilepsy or initiate treatment for seizures; these tasks usually are performed by a consulting neurologist. This section therefore focuses primarily on clinical guidelines for ordering and interpretation of EEG in patients with possible seizures.

Seizures in the elderly most commonly present with periodic alterations in level of consciousness or behavior. In most cases, the diagnosis is straightforward, with frank lapses of consciousness that may be associated with loss of motor tone or abnormal movements, incontinence, and postictal confusion. In such cases, the EEG provides confirmatory evidence and may help guide treatment.

In some cases (e.g., patients with possible loss of consciousness, episodic confusion, waxing-and-waning mental status, refractory depression, or panic attacks), a seizure disorder enters the differential diagnosis. The discovery of a seizure focus in these patients may be clinically significant because there are reports in the literature of individuals with seizure foci whose refractory depressions or panic disorders are responsive to anticonvulsants. The index of suspicion for seizures usually is not high in such cases, and the EEG typically is ordered for "atypical" cases, such as for a patient with panic attacks who is briefly unresponsive; it is not routinely recommended for evaluation of patients with panic disorder.

The test usually is requested to rule out seizures. The EEG, however, cannot rule out a seizure disorder; it has been estimated in studies of late-onset epilepsy that 10% to 47% of patients with seizure disorders have normal EEGs (Ahuja & Mohanta, 1982; Carney et al., 1969; Hyllested & Pakkenberg, 1963; Luhdorf et al., 1986; Shigemoto, 1981; Woodcock & Cosgrove, 1964), a rate somewhat lower than that estimated for middle-aged adults. The false-negative rate is dependent in part on the etiology of the seizure, with low false-negative rates reported in patients with brain tumors and higher false-negative rates for seizures of unknown etiology (Carney et al., 1969; Luhdorf et al., 1986).

To perform an adequate electrographic screen for a seizure disorder, a recording at least 30 minutes long should be performed using several different electrode montages. Furthermore, if the patient's physical health and mental state permit, activation procedures such as hyperventilation, photic stimulation, stage II sleep, and sleep deprivation may be useful to activate an underlying seizure focus.

When epileptiform abnormalities (i.e., spikes or spike-and-wave complexes) are detected, a diagnosis of a seizure disorder is not certain. Depending on the location and nature of the abnormality, epileptiform abnormalities predict the existence of a clinical seizure disorder with differing degrees of reliability: Frequent spike-and-wave complexes in the anterior temporal region are correlated with clinical seizures in more than 90% of otherwise healthy adults; isolated occipital spikes have less than a 40% correlation with seizures (Niedermeyer, 1999). The surest method to establish a link between an observed epileptiform abnormality and a possible seizure disorder is to perform prolonged (possibly ambulatory) EEG recording and to observe changes in the state or behavior of the patient that are linked to electrographic changes.

In interpreting the significance of epileptiform abnormalities, the clinical history and condition of the patient must be considered. Some chronic illnesses (such as renal failure) or degenerative diseases of the brain (such as DAT) may lead to the development of generalized sharp waves or spike foci that have a low association with clinical seizures. In the final analysis, seizures are diagnosed on the basis of clinical presentation (Pinkus & Tucker, 1985).

QUANTITATIVE ELECTROENCEPHALOGRAPHY

Several factors limit the application of conventional EEG in psychiatric practice. These include the need for specialized training to interpret an EEG record and problems of interrater reliability. Most difficult perhaps has been the problem of defining a "gold standard" to differentiate normal from abnormal cerebral activity across individuals of different age and gender. In geriatric psychiatry specifically, the value of the EEG (to evaluate a possible encephalopathy) is limited by difficulties in quantitating normal amounts of slowing in the elderly.

Quantitative electroencephalography (QEEG) overcomes several of the limitations of conventional EEG. Using computer-based techniques, QEEG can quantitate the amount of cerebral activity in an individual's EEG and the amount concentrated in slow-wave bands (a measure that may indicate disease) (Figure 15-1). The amount of slowing can be compared to age- and gender-based norms. Statistically significant regional differences are displayed as topographical maps in each frequency band. Quantitative analysis does not eliminate the problem that the EEG changes of normal aging are qualitatively similar to the features of organic brain disease. It yields more reliable and reproducible measurements of brain activity, however, and increases the sensitivity to subtle focal or generalized alterations in brain function (Figure 15-2).

A variety of QEEG parameters, such as absolute power, relative power, and spectral ratios, also provide information not accessible from the visual inspection of the conventional recording. These parameters appear to be com-

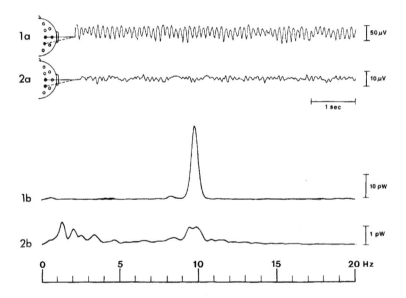

FIGURE 15-1. Samples of (1a) a normal posterior dominant rhythm and (2a) an abnormal rhythm with excessive intermixed slowing such as that seen in patients with dementia. The computer-generated frequency spectra show that (1b) the normal rhythm consists of power concentrated at 10 Hz, whereas (2b) the abnormal rhythm contains considerable power at lower frequencies. (Reproduced from Fisch, 1999.)

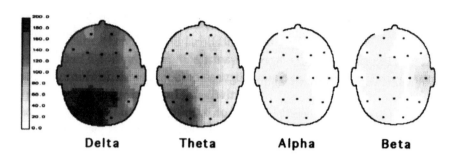

FIGURE 15-2. Quantitative electroencephalographic (EEG) maps of absolute power in the delta, theta, alpha, and beta frequency bands. The maps show excess generalized delta and theta slow-wave power, with maximum focal intensity in the left parietal-occipital region. This patient with vascular dementia had a discrete left parietal infarct. Maps represent the head as viewed from above, with frontal regions at the top of each map. Colors represent the absolute EEG power in each frequency band measured in microvolts squared and displayed according to the color scale on the left.

plementary in that they are additive in the detection of abnormality and yield different regional information regarding abnormality (Leuchter, Cook, et al., 1993).

QEEG is useful for the detection of a dementing illness (Duffy et al., 1984; Nuwer, 1988; Prichep et al., 1983). A number of investigators have demonstrated that patients with dementia have increased delta and theta power, decreased alpha and beta power, as well as decreased mean frequency (Holschneider & Leuchter, 1999), with 90% to 95% correct classification in stages of moderately severe dementia. QEEG measures may reveal normalization of neocortical activity in patients with DAT treated with tacrine (Alhainen et al., 1991). Furthermore, QEEG has been useful in selecting optimal drug dose in patients with DAT with intraventricularly administered bethanechol (a cholinergic agonist), with supraoptimal doses leading to increased slow-wave power (Leuchter et al., 1991).

The issue of how early in the course of a dementia QEEG may be useful as a screening tool remains an active area of research. Different groups have reported sensitivities and specificities in early dementia in the range of 20% to 70% and 70% to 100%, respectively, using differing QEEG measures in a variety of scalp locations (Brenner et al., 1986; Coben et al., 1990; John et al., 1988; Leuchter et al., 1987; Prichep et al., 1983). The highest sensitivity and specificity for any single QEEG variable were reported with percentage theta power (Coben et al., 1990).

Research suggests that patients with early DAT, compared to control subjects, are unable to generate significant amounts of the high-frequency brain electrical activity commonly associated with administration of a barbiturate. Such pharmacological challenge tests may unmask abnormalities in brain function not detected at baseline (Figure 15-3) (Holschneider & Leuchter, 2000) and may distinguish subjects with DAT from those with VaD during later stages of the illness (Holschneider et al., 1997).

New QEEG measures of fiber tract damage have been shown to be useful in the diagnosis and assessment of dementia and its treatment. Coherence, a measure of the synchronization of electrical activity between different regions within an individual, has proved useful in distinguishing subjects with DAT and those with VaD (Leuchter et al., 1992). Subjects with DAT, unlike those with VaD or normal elderly subjects, demonstrate a decrease in coherence between pre-rolandic and post-rolandic areas. This loss in brain electrical synchronization has been hypothesized to reflect the specific deafferentation of long cortico-cortical fiber tracts in DAT, compared to the more diffuse disconnection of cortico-subcortical white matter networks characteristic of VaD.

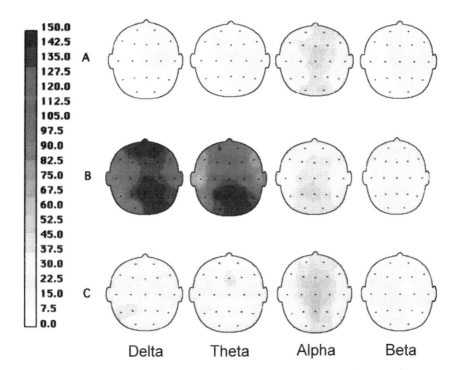

FIGURE 15-3. Quantitative electroencephalographic (EEG) maps of absolute power for a patient (A) at baseline, (B) during acute lithium intoxication, and (C) 2 weeks after the lithium was discontinued. Slow-wave power greatly increased during this episode of delirium and resolved afterward. Each row shows four maps representing (from the left) the delta, theta, alpha, and beta frequency bands. Maps represent the head as viewed from above, with frontal regions at the top of each map. Colors represent the absolute EEG power in each frequency band measured in microvolts squared and displayed according to the color scale on the left.

Low baseline coherence is an indicator of poorer functional status at 2-year follow-up in patients with dementia (Leuchter, Simon, Daly, Rosenberg-Thompson, et al., 1994) and poorer outcome and increased mortality in patients with depression (Leuchter, Simon, Daly, Abrams, et al., 1994). In asymptomatic control subjects, decreases in coherence detect fiber tract dysfunction associated with periventricular white matter changes on MRI. These periventricular fibers are critical components of the networks that subserve higher cortical functions; they contain the projections of the prefrontal cortical neurons and the visual association pathways. The association between white matter disease and the type of disconnection may be a useful model for categorizing cognitive impairment among elderly subjects, even those who do not meet all criteria for dementia (Leuchter et al., 1997).

QEEG has shown distinctive advantages over conventional EEG for assessing the diagnosis, course, and prognosis of subjects with delirium. Grossly excessive slowing in the face of relatively mild cognitive impairment suggests the presence of delirium instead of, or in addition to, dementia (Figure 15-4). This severity of slowing is better estimated by quantitative rather than visual analysis (Brenner, 1991) and may help differentiate delirious from demented subjects (Jacobson et al., 1993a, 1993b; Koponen et al., 1989). Decreases in slow-wave power may actually precede improvements in mental status (Leuchter & Jacobson, 1991).

A new QEEG measure that may prove useful for the study of dementia, depression, and other psychiatric illnesses is called cordance. *Cordance* is a mea-

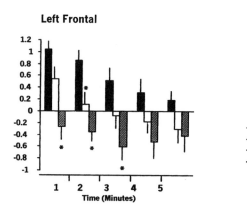 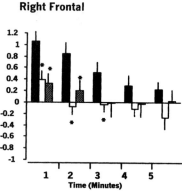

FIGURE 15-4. Changes in $\log_{10}$ (power) (mV^2, 20–28 Hz) over time in the left frontal (F_1–F_3 + F_1–F_7) and right frontal (F_2–F_4 + F_2–F_8) regions after thiopental for normal elderly controls (solid bars), subjects with early DAT (open bars), and subjects with moderately severe DAT (cross-hatched bars). The x axis represents time in minutes after thiopental infusion. Error bars represent 1 standard error. *, a significant difference with respect to control subjects ($P < .05$, Student-Newman-Keuls). (Reproduced with permission of Holschneider and Leuchter, 2000.)

sure of brain electrical activity that is sensitive to damage to afferent fiber tracts supplying the cortex. Cortical deafferentation as might result from a focal lesion produces regional attenuation of perfusion and QEEG power. Although such cortex produces low power, it is concentrated in pathological (i.e., slow-wave) bands. Cordance combines both absolute and relative power (percentage of total power in a given frequency band) to yield a measure that has a stronger association with perfusion than other QEEG measures. Cordance maps have been shown in the research setting to show a striking similarity to positron emission tomographic (PET) or single-photon emission computed tomographic (SPECT) scans (Leuchter, Cook, Mena, et al., 1994; Leuchter, Cook, Lufkin, et al., 1994) and to be as effective as PET in detecting lateralized cerebral activation associated with motor tasks (Leuchter et al., 1999).

The role of QEEG in the assessment of depression remains an area of active research. Pollock and Schneider (1990) reviewed studies performed over the preceding decade that attempted to distinguish depression from dementia and found that no single feature appears to be robust for the diagnosis of depression. Several investigators have used a multivariate statistical approach to the diagnosis of depression (John et al., 1977; Shagass et al., 1984) and have reported overall accuracy in classification of 60% to 90%. The stability of these multivariate methods for diagnosis remains to be verified.

Cordance evaluation of subjects with depression reflects some of the changes in cerebral energy utilization associated with this disorder. Unmedicated depressed patients compared to control subjects demonstrate decreases in global as well as anterior and centrotemporal cordance (Cook et al., 1998). Such differences remit in response to treatment intervention (Figure 15-5). Furthermore, cordance may be useful for patient selection in the early stages of evaluation as it may provide information on the treatment responsiveness to antidepressant medication (Cook et al., 1998, 1999) and assist in identification of placebo responders.

QEEG is useful for a number of routine clinical settings. Quantitative analysis is more sensitive to the proportion of energy in any frequency band and hence may find greater application in the assessment of global brain function or detection of focal brain dysfunction. QEEG is less sensitive in the detection of very fast (milliseconds) transient EEG activity and in the recognition of specific wave morphologies. Thus, conventional EEG remains preferable to QEEG for detecting epileptiform abnormalities.

At present, QEEG remains an adjunct to conventional EEG in the study of psychiatric illnesses (American Psychiatric Association Task Force, 1991), and it should not be considered part of a routine evaluation. Currently, its main usefulness is in selected clinical situations in which mild degrees of encephalopathy may be detected better by QEEG. This includes (1) evaluations of mild head trauma, toxic-metabolic states, and early dementia; (2) serial evaluations of the progression or resolution of a delirium; and (3) evaluations of pseudodementia versus early dementia.

48 hours   2 weeks   8 weeks

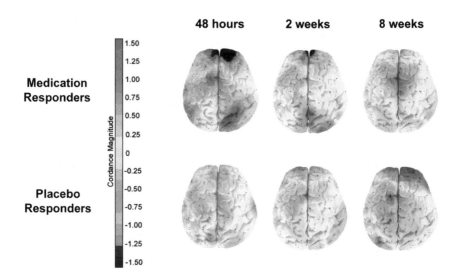

FIGURE 15-5.   These brain maps show changes in brain function measured using quantitative electroencephalography cordance in patients with major depression who responded to treatment either with antidepressants (fluoxetine 20 mg or venlafaxine 150 mg) or a placebo (bottom row). After 48 hours of treatment, the subjects who responded to medication showed decreased cordance in the prefrontal region of the brain indicated by the blue colors (top row, first map on left). This was detected even though the subjects did not show a clinical response until 8 weeks. The subjects who responded to placebo (bottom row) showed no change at 48 hours, but at 2 weeks (middle map) and 8 weeks (far right) showed increased cordance in the prefrontal region (indicated by the red colors). These findings indicate that early changes in prefrontal cordance may be a leading indicator of antidepressant effectiveness and may help distinguish patients with a lasting medication response from those with a a placebo response. (Adapted from Cook et al., 2002; Leuchter et al., 2002.)

CONCLUSION

The EEG plays a prominent role in the evaluation of brain disease among geriatric psychiatry patients, and it generally is quite sensitive to the presence of encephalopathic conditions and seizure disorders. The EEG tracing generally does not yield results diagnostic for any illness; rather, its findings are either consistent with (e.g., slowing in DAT), supportive of (e.g., triphasic waves in Creutzfeldt-Jakob disease), or highly suggestive of the presence of a particular illness (e.g., anterior temporal spike-and-wave foci in a seizure disorder).

EEG is a noninvasive, inexpensive, and portable technology. Its cost effectiveness is likely to be increased further by computer analysis, which will require less physician time. With the decline of computer prices, QEEG systems are increasingly becoming more available for imaging pathophysiological changes in brain function. Stress tests that examine brain electrical function during cognitive or pharmacological activation and the development of new QEEG measures such as coherence and cordance hold great promise for improving not only diagnostic accuracy, but also the monitoring and prediction of treatment response.

REFERENCES

Ahuja GK, Mohanta A. Late onset epilepsy: a prospective study. *Acta Neurol Scand.* 1982;66:216–226.

Alhainen K, Partanen J, Reinikainen K, Laulumaa V, Airaksinen M. Riekkinen P. Discrimination of tetrahydroaminoacridine responders by a single dose pharmaco-EEG in patients with Alzheimer's disease. *Neurosci Lett.* 1991;127:113–116.

American Psychiatric Association Task Force on Quantitative Electrophysiologic Assessment. Quantitative electroencephalography: a report on the present state of computerized EEG techniques. *Am J Psychiatry.* 1991;148:961–964.

Berger H. On the electroencephalogram of man: twelfth report. *Arch Psychiatr Nervenkr.* 1937;106:165–187.

Brenner RP. Utility of EEG in delirium: past views and current practice. *Int Psychogeriatr.* 1991;3:211–229.

Brenner RP. EEG and dementia. In: Niedermeyer E, Da Silva FL, eds. *Electroencephalography: Basic Principles, Clinical Applications, and Related Fields.* Baltimore, MD: Williams and Wilkins; 1999:349–359.

Brenner RP, Ulrich RF, Spiker DG, et al. Computerized EEG spectral analysis in elderly normal, demented and depressed subjects. *Electroenceph Clin Neurophysiol.* 1986; 64:483–492.

Busse EW, Barnes RH, Silverman AJ, et al. Studies of the process of aging: factors that influence the psyche of elderly persons. *Am J Psychiatry.* 1954;110:897–903.

Carney LR, Hudgins RL, Espinosa RE, Klass DW. Seizures beginning after the age of 60. *Arch Int Med.* 1969;124:707–709.

Chiappa K, Young R. The EEG as a definitive diagnostic tool early in the course of Creutzfeldt-Jacob disease. *Electroenceph Clin Neurophysiol.* 1978;45:26.

Coben LA, Chi D, Snyder AZ, Storandt M. Replication of a study of frequency analysis of the resting awake EEG in mild probable Alzheimer's disease. *Electroenceph Clin Neurophysiol.* 1990;75:148–154.

Cook IA, Leuchter AF, Uijtdehaage SH, et al. Altered cerebral energy utilization in late life depression. *J Affect. Disord.* 1998;49:89–99.

Cook IA, Leuchter AF, Witte E, et al. Neurophysiologic predictors of treatment response to fluoxetine in major depression. *Psychiatr Res.* 1999;85:263–273.

Cummings J, Benson F. *Dementia. A Clinical Approach.* 1st ed. London: Butterworths; 1983.

Cummings J, Benson D. *Dementia: A Clinical Approach.* 2nd ed. Boston, MA: Butterworths; 1992.

Duffy FH, Albert MS, McAnulty G. Brain electrical activity in patients with presenile and senile dementia of the Alzheimer type. *Ann Neurol.* 1984;16:439–448.

Engel G, Romano J. Delirium II: reversibility of the electroencephalogram with experimental procedures. *Arch Neurol Psychiatry.* 1944;51:378–392.

Erkinjuntti T, Larsen T, Sulkava R, Ketonen L, Laaksonen R, Palo J. EEG in the differential diagnosis between Alzheimer's disease and vascular dementia. *Acta Neurol Scand.* 1988;77:36–43.

Ettinger AB, Shinnar S. New-onset seizures in an elderly hospitalized population. *Neurology.* 1993;43:489–492.

Fink M. EEG classification of psychoactive compounds in man: a review and theory of behavioral associations. In: Effron DH, ed. *Psychopharmacology: A Review of Progress 1957–1967.* Washington, DC: US Government Printing Office; 1968:497–507.

Fisch B. *Fisch and Spehlmann's EEG Primer: Basic Principles of Digital and Analog EEG.* 3rd ed. New York, NY: Elsevier Science; 1999.

Freudenreich O, Weiner RD, McEvoy JP. Clozapine-induced electroencephalogram changes as a function of clozapine serum levels. *Biol Psychiatry.* 1997;42:132–137.

Groen JJ, Endtz LJ. Hereditary Pick's disease, second re-examination of a large family and discussion of other hereditary cases with particular reference to electroencephalography and computerized tomography. *Brain.* 1982;105:443–459.

Group for the Advancement of Psychiatry. *The Psychiatric Treatment of Alzheimer's Disease.* New York, NY: Brunner/Mazel; 1988.

Holschneider DP, Leuchter AF. Beta activity in aging and dementia. *Brain Topogr.* 1995; 8:169–180.

Holschneider DP, Leuchter AF. Clinical neurophysiology using electroencephalography in geriatric psychiatry: neurobiological implications and clinical utility. *J Geriatr Psychiatry Neurol.* 1999;12:150–164.

Holschneider DP, Leuchter AF. Attenuation of brain high frequency electrocortical response after thiopental in early stages of Alzheimer's dementia. *Psychopharmacology.* 2000;149:6–11.

Holschneider DP, Leuchter AF, Uijtdehaage SH, Abrams M, Rosenberg-Thompson S. Loss of high-frequency brain electrical response to thiopental administration in Alzheimer's-type dementia. *Neuropsychopharmacology.* 1997;16:269–275.

Hubbard O, Sunde D, Goldensohn ES. The EEG in centenarians. *EEG Clin Neurophysiol.* 1976;40:407–417.

Hughes JR. *EEG in Clinical Practice.* Boston, MA: Butterworths; 1982.

Hyllested K, Pakkenberg H. Prognosis in epilepsy of late onset *Neurology.* 1963;13:651–654.

Jacobson SA, Leuchter AF, Walter DO. Conventional and quantitative EEG in the diagnosis of delirium among the elderly. *J Neurol Neurosurg Psychiatry.* 1993a;56:153–158.

Jacobson SA, Leuchter AF, Walter DO, Weiner H. Serial quantitative EEG among elderly subjects with delirium. *Biol Psychiatry.* 1993b;34:135–140.

John ER, Karmel BZ, Corning WC, et al. Neurometrics. *Science.* 1977;196:1393–1410.

John ER, Prichep LS, Fridman J, Easton P. Neurometrics: computer-assisted differential diagnosis of brain dysfunctions. *Science.* 1988;239:162–169.

Keilson MJ, Miller AE, Drexler ED. Early EEG and CTT scanning in stroke—a comparative study [abstract]. *Electroenceph Clin Neurophysiol.* 1985;61:21P.

Koponen H, Partanen J, Paakkonen A, Mattila E, Riekkinen PJ. EEG spectral analysis in delirium. *J Neurol Neurosurg Psychiatry.* 1989;52:980–985.

Leuchter A, Spar J, Walter D, Weiner H. Electroencephalographic spectra and coherence in the diagnosis of Alzheimer's-type and multi-infarct dementia. *Arch Gen Psychiatry.* 1987;44:993–998.

Leuchter AF, Cook IA, Lufkin RB, et al. Cordance: a new method for assessment of cerebral perfusion and metabolism using quantitative electroencephalography. *Neuroimage* 1994;1:208–219.

Leuchter AF, Cook IA, Mena I, et al. Assessment of cerebral perfusion using quantitative EEG cordance. *Psychiatry Res.* 1994;55:141–152.

Leuchter AF, Cook IA, Newton TF, et al. Regional differences in brain electrical activity in dementia: use of spectral power and spectral ratio measures. *Electroenceph Clin Neurophysiol.* 1993;87:385–393.

Leuchter AF, Cook IA, Uijtdehaage SHJ, et al. Brain structure and function and the outcomes of treatment for depression. *J Clin Psychiatry.* 1997;58:22–31.

Leuchter AF, Daly KA, Rosenberg-Thompson S, Abrams M. Prevalence and significance of electroencephalographic abnormalities in patients with suspected organic mental syndromes. *J Am Geriatr Soc.* 1993;41:605–611.

Leuchter AF, Jacobson SA. Quantitative measurement of brain electrical activity in delirium. *Int Psychogeriatr.* 1991;3:231–247.

Leuchter AF, Newton TF, Cook IA, Walter DO, Rosenberg-Thompson S, Lachenbruch PA. Changes in brain functional connectivity in Alzheimer-type and multi-infarct dementia. *Brain.* 1992;115:1543–1561.

Leuchter AF, Read SL, Shapira J, Walter DO, Smith C. Stable bimodal response to cholinomimetic drugs in Alzheimer's disease. Brain mapping correlates. *Neuropsychopharmacology.* 1991;4:165–173.

Leuchter AF, Simon SL, Daly KA, et al. Quantitative EEG correlates of outcome in older psychiatric patients, Part II: 2-year follow-up of patients with depression. *Am J Geriatr Psychiatry.* 1994;2:290–299.

Leuchter AF, Simon SL, Daly KA, et al. Quantitative EEG correlates of outcome in older psychiatric patients, Part I: cross-sectional and longitudinal assessment of patients with dementia. *Am J Geriatr Psychiatry.* 1994;2:200–209.

Leuchter AF, Uijtdehaage SHJ, Cook IA, O'Hara R, Mandelkern M. Relationship between brain electrical activity and cortical perfusion in normal subjects. *Psychiatr Res.* 1999;90:125–140.

Lipowski ZJ. Delirium (acute confusional states). *JAMA.* 1987;258:1789–1792.

Luhdorf K, Jensen LK, Plesner AM. Etiology of seizures in the elderly. *Epilepsia.* 1986;27:458–463.

Niedermeyer E. Epileptic seizure disorders. In: Niedermeyer E, Da Silva FL, eds. *Electroencephalography: Basic Principles, Clinical Applications, and Related Fields.* Baltimore, MD: Williams and Wilkins; 1999:476–585.

Nuwer MR. Quantitative EEG. II. Frequency analysis and topographic mapping in clinical settings. *J Clin Neurophys.* 1988;5:45–85.

Obrist WD. Problems of aging. In: Rémond A, ed. *Handbook of Electroencephalography and Clinical Neurophysiology.* Vol. 6, Part A. Amsterdam, The Netherlands: Elsevier; 1976:207–229.

Obrist WD, Henry CE, Justiss WA. Longitudinal changes in the senescent EEG: a 15-year study. In: *Proceedings of the Seventh International Congress of Gerontology.* Vienna, Austria: International Association of Gerontology; 1966.

Oken BS, Kaye JA. Electrophysiologic function in the healthy, extremely old. *Neurology.* 1992;42:519–526.

Pfefferbaum A, Davis KL, Coulter CL, Mohs RC, Tinklenberg JR, Kopell BS. EEG effects of physostigmine and choline chloride in humans. *Psychopharmacology.* 1979;62:225–233.

Pinkus J, Tucker G. *Behavioral Neurology*. New York, NY: Oxford University Press; 1985.

Pollock VE, Schneider LS. Quantitative, waking EEG research on depression. *Biol Psychiatry*. 1990;27:757–780.

Prichep L, Gomez MF, Johns ER, et al. Neurometric electroencephalographic characteristics of dementia. In: Reisberg B, ed. *Alzheimer's Disease: The Standard Reference*. New York, NY: Macmillan; 1983:252–257.

Roberts M A, Mcgeorge AP, Caird FI. Electroencephalography and computerized tomography in vascular and nonvascular dementia in old age. *J Neurol Neurosurg Psychiatry*. 1978;41:903–906.

Romano J, Engel G. Delirium I: electroencephalographic data. *Arch Neurol Psychiatry*. 1944;51:356–377.

Sander JW, Hart YM, Johnson AL, Shorvon SD. National General Practice Study of Epilepsy: newly diagnosed epileptic seizures in a general population. *Lancet*. 1990; 336:1267–1271.

Shagass C, Roemer RA, Straumanis JJ, Josiassen RC. Psychiatric diagnostic discriminations with combinations of quantitative EEG variables. *Br J Psychiatry*. 1984;144: 581–592.

Shigemoto T. Epilepsy in middle or advanced age. *Folia Psychiatr Neurol Jpn*. 1981;35: 287–294.

Spehlmann R. *EEG Primer*. New York, NY: Elsevier Biomedical Press; 1981.

Stigsby B, Johannesson G, Ingvar DH. Regional EEG analysis and regional cerebral blood flow in Alzheimer's and Pick's diseases. *Electroenceph Clin Neurophysiol*. 1981;51:537–547.

Struve FA. Lithium-specific pathological electroencephalographic changes: a successful replication of earlier investigative results. *Clin Electroenceph*. 1987;18:46–53.

Sung CY, Chu NS. Epileptic seizures in elderly people: aetiology and seizure type. *Age Ageing*. 1990;19:25–30.

Torres F, Faoro A, Loewenson R, Johnson E. The electroencephalogram of elderly subjects revisited. *EEG Clin Neurophysiol*. 1983;56:391–398.

Van Sweden V, Wauquier A, Niedermeyer E. Normal aging and transient cognitive disorders in the elderly. In: Niedermeyer E, Da Silva FL, eds. *Electroencephalography: Basic Principles, Clinical Applications, and Related Fields*. Baltimore, MD: Williams and Wilkins; 1999:340–348.

Woodcock S, Cosgrove J. Epilepsy after the age of 50. *Neurology*. 1964;14:34–40.

Yener GG, Leuchter AF, Jenden D, Read SL, Cummings JL, Miller BL. Quantitative EEG in frontotemporal dementia. *Clin Electroenceph*. 1996;27:61–68.

Zurek R, Schiemann Delgado J, Froescher W, Niedermeyer E. Frontal intermittent rhythmical delta activity and anterior bradyrhythmia. *Clin Electroenceph*. 1985;16: 1–10.

Psychiatric Disorders of the Elderly

16

Alzheimer's Disease

Barry Reisberg, MD
Muhammad Usman Saeed, MD

Alzheimer's disease (AD) is one of the major illness entities of the modern era. Prevalence varies in part with the age of the population; however, as a rule approximately 1% of the population of most modern industrialized nations is probably afflicted by overt manifestations of the illness. Findings in prevalence studies differ depending in part on the definitions and methodologies used and whether institutionalized populations are surveyed, subjects with mild cognitive impairment are included, and other factors in case ascertainment.

EPIDEMIOLOGY

In the United States, community population surveys have indicated that up to 10% to 15% of elderly community residents have AD or closely related dementias of late life (Evans et al., 1989; Katzman, 1986). Because there are presently more than 30 million persons in the United States older than 65 years, it is frequently estimated that as many as 4 million persons in the United States suffer from AD (Small et al., 1997).

Because AD is an illness with a marked association with age and because the prevalence of AD is greater in women, prevalence rates vary markedly with age and gender. For example, the US General Accounting Office estimates that the prevalence of AD doubles with every 5 years of age from 65 to 85 years (US General Accounting Office, 1998).

AD is the major cause of institutionalization in the United States. At present, more than 1.5 million persons in the United States reside in nursing homes.

It should be noted by comparison that well under 1 million persons are institutionalized in US hospital settings at any particular time. An absolute majority of the more than 1.5 million US nursing home residents, approximately three quarters in some surveys (Chandler & Chandler, 1988; Rovner et al., 1986), suffer from dementia. The majority of these nursing home residents with dementia suffer from AD as a major underlying cause or contributor to their cognitive disturbance. Consequently, AD is estimated to be a significant source of morbidity and reason for institutionalization of 800,000 to 900,000 US nursing home residents—approximately the same number of persons as in all US hospitals at any given time.

AD is also a major cause of death, particularly in industrialized nations with aged populations. Dementia in general, and AD in particular, has long been known to be a source of increased mortality in comparison with comparably aged cohort populations (Barclay et al., 1985; Go et al., 1978; Goldfarb, 1969; Jarvik & Falek, 1963; Kaszniak et al., 1978; Kral, 1962; Molsa et al., 1986; Reding et al., 1984; Reimanis & Green, 1971; Roth, 1955; Thompson & Eastwood, 1981). The dimensions of AD and the morbidity and mortality associated with AD are such that this single major illness entity is frequently calculated to be the fourth leading cause of death in the United States and other industrialized nations after all forms of heart disease combined, all forms of cancer combined, and all forms of stroke (Eagles et al., 1990; Weiler, 1987). These mortality statistics are likely to become increasingly disturbing because the incidence and mortality associated with stroke have been steadily decreasing for many years, and the incidence of AD has been steadily increasing with the increasing age of the population. Consequently, AD is likely soon to replace stroke as the third leading cause of death in the United States and many other industrialized nations.

DIAGNOSIS AND SYMPTOMATOLOGY

The diagnosis of AD is presently made based on clinical observations of the onset, course, and characteristic symptomatology of this common condition (American Psychiatric Association, 1994). The presence of dementia is generally established initially. This may be accomplished by documenting deterioration in both cognitive and functional symptomatic domains. A mental status screening instrument such as the Mini-Mental State Examination (MMSE) (Folstein et al., 1975) can be useful in documenting the magnitude of cognitive capacity. However, the clinician must be aware of the limitations of such screening instruments.

Lack of education is one well-known cause of lower scores on mental status assessment (Crum et al., 1993; Murden et al., 1991; Uhlmann & Larson, 1991). Other illnesses and conditions will also produce lower scores on various mental status assessments. These include conditions that interfere with the ability to write (e.g., severe arthritis, severe Parkinson's disease [PD], paralysis secondary to a stroke), conditions that interfere with concentration (e.g., mania and maniform states, depression, acute intoxication, delirium associated with any of numerous medical disorders), conditions that interfere with speech (e.g., severe depression or a stroke), and sensory disturbances such as marked impairment of vision or audition.

Once the presence of dementia is suspected, a dementia workup should be performed. This includes (1) a comprehensive metabolic screen with serum glucose, electrolytes, renal function, serum protein, and serum enzyme studies; (2) corpuscular blood counts and differentials; (3) urinalysis; (4) serum B_{12} and serum folate studies; (5) thyroid studies; and (6) a magnetic resonance imaging (MRI) or computerized tomographic (CT) brain scan. Salient conditions that may produce or contribute to the dementia process and are revealed by these studies include electrolyte disturbances, hypoglycemia, severe hepatic or renal disease, anemia, B_{12} or folate deficiency, thyroid disease, space-occupying brain lesions, and hydrocephalus. If considered appropriate, other studies, such as serum homocysteine testing for evidence of "chemical" cobalamin (B_{12}) deficiency, a rapid plasma reagin (RPR) or VDRL screen for syphilis, and human immunodeficiency virus (HIV) testing should also be performed.

Having established the suspected presence of dementia and the possible primary or secondary role of identifiable contributory factors, the clinician should then examine the evidence for a decline in cognitive and functional capacities and determine whether the nature of the decline and the clinical presentation are consistent with that of dementia of the Alzheimer's type (AD). Because the presentation and history of decline in AD vary markedly depending on the stage of the illness process and other factors, diagnosis ultimately is dependent on knowledge of the symptomatology of AD.

Clearly, differential diagnosis is ultimately dependent not only on an adequate knowledge of AD symptomatology, but also on knowledge of the symptomatology of other similar and related conditions. Consensus conferences have concluded that the diagnosis of AD should be considered a diagnosis of inclusion based on recognition of the characteristic clinical features of the illness and adequate consideration of related disorders and complicating factors (Reisberg, Burns, et al., 1997; Small et al., 1997).

Symptoms and Signs of Alzheimer's Disease: An Overview

The clinical symptomatology of AD consists most notably of cognitive, functional, and behavioral concomitants. Each of these symptomatic domains can be described on a continuum with the corresponding symptoms in normal aging, including age-associated memory impairment (AAMI), mild cognitive impairment (MCI), and the progressive dementia of AD as presented in Table

16-1. Tables 16-2 and 16-3 provide more specific and detailed descriptions of the losses that occur in association with aging and AD, and their approximate relationship to the seven Global Deterioration Scale (GDS) stages (Reisberg et al., 1982) and the stages of functional loss of capacity (Reisberg, 1988). Table 16-4 outlines the major behavioral changes that occur commonly in AD and that appear amenable to neurotransmitter psychopharmacological intervention. Figure 16-1 provides a general outline of the frequency of these behavioral and psychological symptoms of dementia (BPSD) as AD advances.

NORMAL BRAIN AGING   It should be noted that many aged persons are free of both subjective complaints of cognitive decrement and objective clinically manifest evidence of cognitive or functional decline (Lane & Snowdon, 1989; Lowenthal et al., 1967; Reinikainen et al., 1990; Sluss et al., 1980). The prognosis for continued robust mental health for these normal aged persons is excellent (de Leon et al., 2001, including unpublished data; Geerlings et al., 1999; Kluger et al., 1999).

AGE-ASSOCIATED MEMORY IMPAIRMENT   Many aged persons, when queried, maintain the conviction that they can no longer remember such things as personal names as well as they could 5 or 10 years previously (Table 16-2). Persons with these subjectively perceived deficits, in the absence of overt clinically manifest deficit or deterioration, fall into the category of those with age-associated memory impairment (AAMI) (Crook et al., 1986; Reisberg, Ferris, et al., 1986).

It should be noted that these subjective complaints of cognitive decrement are very troubling to many aged persons. They are sufficiently troubling such that many persons throughout the world take medications for these symptoms. In the United States, these substances include multivitamins, vitamin E, hormones such as estrogen, lecithin, choline preparations, and various nonprescription mixtures of these and other substances.

The prognosis for persons with these symptoms remains controversial (Bolla et al., 1991; Christensen, 1991; Geerlings et al., 1999; Jorm et al., 1997; Tobiansky et al., 1995). The etiology of these subjective deficits is also uncertain. However, some current studies indicate that these subjective complaints presage a greater likelihood of subsequent decline in comparison with persons who are free of these complaints (e.g., de Leon et al., 2001; Geerlings et al., 1999; Hänninen et al., 1995). About 12% per year of these subjects appear to progress to an MCI diagnosis; in 4 years, 10% to 15% progress to a dementia diagnosis in some studies (Table 16-1) (de Leon et al., 2001; Hänninen et al., 1995; Kluger et al., 1999).

Predictions of which of these ostensibly "normal aged" persons will, years later, manifest overt symptoms of AD are not sufficiently reliable for clinical purposes. However, ongoing research in this area indicates that, although elderly persons with these subjective complaints do perform well within the normal range on many neuropsychological tests, those who subsequently dete-

Table 16-1. Typical time course of normal brain aging and Alzheimer's disease

Clinical diagnosis	Normal adult	Age-associated memory impairment	Mild cognitive impairment	Mild AD	Moderate AD	Moderately severe AD	Severe AD
CDR stage*	0	0	0.5	1	2	3	4, 5
GDS and FAST stage*	1	2	3	4	5	6	7
FAST substage						a b c d e	a b c d e f
Years†	Many decades	Approximately 15 years	0	7	9	10.5	13 19
MMSE score	29	29	25	19	14	5	0

Usual point of death

Source: Adapted from Reisberg et al. (1994).

AD, Alzheimer's disease; CDR, Clinical Dementia Rating; FAST, Functional Assessment Staging; GDS, Global Deterioration Scale; MMSE, Mini-Mental State Examination.

*Stage range comparisons shown between the CDR and GDS/FAST stages were based on published functioning and selfcare descriptors.

†Numerical values represent time from the earliest clinically manifest symptoms of Alzheimer's disease (i.e., the beginning of GDS and FAST stage 3).

TABLE 16-2. Stages of normal brain aging, mild cognitive impairment, and Alzheimer's disease and corresponding care needs

GDS stage*	Clinical characteristics*	Diagnosis	Approximate mean MMSE†,‡	Equivalent CDR stage§,‖	Dominant emotional impact on the patient¶	Impact on the family¶	Care needs¶	Care recommendations¶
1	No subjective complaints of memory deficit: No memory deficit evident on clinical interview.	Normal	29–30	0	None	None	None	None
2	Subjective complaints of memory deficit, most frequently in following areas: (a) Forgetting where one has placed familiar objects (b) Forgetting names one formerly knew well. No objective evidence of memory deficit on clinical interview. No objective deficit in employment or social situations. Appropriate concern with respect to symptomatology.	Age-associated memory impairment (AAMI)	29	0	Subjective discomfort; no overt emotional symptoms	Family less concerned than the subject with AAMI about subjective deficits.	None	Reassurance with respect to relatively benign prognosis.

454

| 3 | Earliest subtle deficits: Manifestations in more than one of the following areas: (a) Patient may have gotten lost when traveling to an unfamiliar location. (b) Coworkers become aware of patient's relatively poor performance. (c) Word- or name-finding deficit becomes evident to intimates. (d) Patient may read a passage or book and retain relatively little material. (e) Patient may demonstrate decreased facility remembering names on introduction to new people. (f) Patient may have lost or misplaced an object of value. (g) Concentration deficit may be evident on clinical testing. | Mild cognitive impairment | 25 | 0.5 | Anxiety may be manifest | Retirement and the subject's withdrawal from demanding tasks are considered by the subject and the family unit | None | "Tactical" withdrawal from situations that have become, by virtue of their complexity, anxiety provoking |

(continued)

TABLE 16-2. *Continued*

GDS stage*	Clinical characteristics*	Diagnosis	Approximate mean MMSE†,‡	Equivalent CDR stage§,‖	Dominant emotional impact on the patient¶	Impact on the family¶	Care needs¶	Care recommendations¶
	Decreased performance in demanding employment and social settings. Denial begins to become manifest in patient. Mild-to-moderate anxiety frequently accompanies symptoms.							
4	Clear-cut deficit on careful clinical interview: Deficit manifest in following areas: (a) Decreased knowledge of current and recent events. (b) May exhibit some deficit in memory of personal history.	Mild AD	20	0.5	Denial and emotional withdrawal	Family takes over finances and associated responsibilities; begins to supervise the patient	Independent survival still attainable	Assistance toward goal of maximum independence with financial supervision; structured or supervised travel; identification bracelets and labels may be useful Cholinesterase inhibitors have been useful in the treatment of symptoms at this stage

			(c) Concentration deficit elicited on serial subtractions. (d) Decrease ability to travel, handle finances, etc. Frequently no deficit in following areas: (a) Orientation to time and place. (b) Recognition of familiar persons and faces. (c) Ability to travel to familiar places. Inability to perform complex tasks. Denial is dominant defense mechanism. Flattening of affect and withdrawal from challenging situations.				
5	Moderate AD	15	Patient can no longer survive without some assistance. Patient is unable during interview to recall major relevant aspect of their current life, such as: (a) Their address or telephone number of many years. (b) The names of close members of their family (such as grandchildren).	1	Denial and emotional withdrawal with occasional tearfulness and anger	Family begins to take on the emotional burden of the patient's illness; supervision of the patient begins to become a necessity	Patient can no longer survive in the community without assistance; needs supervision with respect to travel and social behavior.	Part-time home health care assistance can be very useful in assisting the patient's caregiver. Driving becomes hazardous and should be discontinued at some point over the course of this stage. Family may require guidance in handling patient's emotional outbursts.

(continued)

TABLE 16-2. *Continued*

GDS stage*	Clinical characteristics*	Diagnosis	Approximate mean MMSE†,‡	Equivalent CDR stage§,‖	Dominant emotional impact on the patient¶	Impact on the family¶	Care needs¶	Care recommendations¶
	(c) The names of the high school or college from which they graduated. Frequently some disorientation to time (date, day of the week, season, etc.) or to place. An educated person may have difficulty counting back from 40 by 4s or from 20 by 2s. Persons at this stage retain knowledge of many major facts regarding themselves and others. They invariably know their own names and generally know spouse's and children's names. They require no assistance with toileting or eating, but may have difficulty choosing the proper clothing to wear.							Cholinesterase inhibitors have been useful in the treatment of symptoms at this stage.

| 6 | Moderately severe AD | 5 | May occasionally forget the name of the spouse, on whom they are entirely dependent for survival. Will be largely unaware of all recent events and experiences in their lives. Retains some knowledge of their surroundings; the year, the season, etc. May have difficulty counting by 1's from 10, both backward and sometimes forward. Will require some assistance with activities of daily living: (a) Will become incontinent as this stage progresses. (b) Will require travel assistance, but occasionally will be able to travel to familiar locations. Diurnal rhythm frequently disturbed. Almost always recalls own name. Frequently continues to be able to distinguish familiar from unfamiliar persons in their environment. | 2 to 3 | Personality and emotional changes occur. This is frequently referred to as agitation. These symptoms peak in magnitude in this stage and include verbal or physical aggressivity and activity disturbances such as wandering, pacing, and storing or hiding objects in inappropriate places. Denial somewhat protects against the emotional impact of the illness on the patient. | The spouse or other caregiver is frequently forced to devote his or her life to the care of the patient, who in return frequently cannot verbally recall the kindness shown to them and may occasionally even forget the spouse's identity. Emotional burden frequently becomes unbearable. Institutionalization considered. | Patient requires assistance with basic ADL. Early in this stage, assistance with dressing and bathing is required. Subsequently, assistance with continence becomes necessary as well. | Full-time home health care assistance is frequently very useful in assisting the patient's caregiver. Strategies for assistance with bathing, toileting, and in the management of incontinence should be discussed with the family. Psychopharmacological intervention based on neurotransmitter modulation is generally useful and indicated to control the behavioral and psychological symptoms (BPSD) in the patient and associated agitation. Emotional stress in the caregiver should be minimized with supportive techniques. |

(continued)

TABLE 16-2. *Continued*

GDS stage*	Clinical characteristics*	Diagnosis	Approximate mean MMSE†,‡	Equivalent CDR stage§,‖	Dominant emotional impact on the patient¶	Impact on the family¶	Care needs¶	Care recommendations¶
	Personality and emotional changes occur. These are quite variable and include (a) Delusional behavior (e.g., patients may accuse their spouse of being an imposter; may talk to imaginary figures in the environment or to their own reflection in the mirror). (b) Obsessive symptoms (e.g., person may continually repeat simple cleaning activities). (c) Anxiety symptoms, agitation, and even previously nonexistent violent behavior may occur. (d) Cognitive abulia, that is, loss of will power because an individual cannot carry a thought long enough to							

determine a pur-
poseful course of
action.

| 7 | All verbal abilities are lost over the course of this stage. Early in this stage, words and phrases are spoken but speech is very circumscribed. Later, there is no serviceable speech, only unintelligible utterances and infrequent emergence of seemingly forgotten words and phrases. Incontinent; requires assistance toileting and feeding. Basic psychomotor skills (e.g., ability to walk) are lost with the progression of this stage. The brain appears to no longer be able to tell the body what to do. Generalized rigidity and developmental neurological reflexes are usually present. | Severe AD | 0 | 4 to 5 (rules for assigning these CDR stages have not yet been established) | Screams and other verbal outbursts, as well as babbling, become a means of communication and must be distinguished from true distress. Pathologic passivity also develops. If proper care is provided, patients can experience happiness and contentment. | Acceptance and coping mechanisms begin to mitigate the emotional trauma and distress. Most families institutionalize their beloved spouses and parents early in the evolution of this stage. | Early in this stage, assistance with feeding as well as dressing, bathing, and toileting is required. Subsequently, assistance with ambulation and purposeful movement becomes necessary. Prevention of decubiti, aspiration, and contractures is a major issue in care. | Full-time assistance in the community home residence or institutional setting is a necessity. Strategies for maintaining locomotion should be explored. The need for psychopharmacological intervention for BPSD decreases. Soft food or liquid diet is generally tolerated. Patients must be fed and instructed/encouraged to maintain chewing and basic eating skills. |

TABLE 16-3. Functional capacities and losses in normal brain aging, mild cognitive impairment, and progressive Alzheimer's disease* and time course of functional loss† (choose highest consecutive level of disability)

Functional (FAST) stage	Clinical characteristics	Level of functional incapacity	Clinical diagnosis	Estimated duration of FAST stage or substage in AD‡
1	No difficulty, either subjectively or objectively.	No deficit	Normal adult	
2	Complains of forgetting location of objects. Subjective work difficulties.	Subjective forgetting	Age-associated memory impairment	
3	Decreased job functioning evident to coworkers. Difficulty in traveling to new locations. Decreased organizational capacity§	Complex occupational performance	Mild cognitive impairment	7 years
4	Decreased ability to perform complex tasks (e.g., planning dinner for guests), handling personal finances (e.g., forgetting to pay bills), difficulty marketing, etc.§	Instrumental activities of daily life (IADL)	Mild AD	2 years
5	Requires assistance in choosing proper clothing to wear for the day, season, or occasion (e.g., patient may wear the same clothing repeatedly, unless supervised)§	Incipient activities of daily life (ADL)	Moderate AD	18 months
6	(a) Improperly putting on clothes without assistance or cuing (e.g., may put street clothes on over night clothes, or put shoes on wrong feet, or have difficulty buttoning clothing) occasionally or more frequently over the past weeks.§	Deficient ADL	Moderately severe AD	5 months

	(b) Unable to bathe properly (e.g., difficulty adjusting bathwater temperature), occasionally or more frequently over the past weeks.§		Deficient ADL	5 months
	(c) Inability to handle mechanics of toileting (e.g., forgets to flush, does not wipe properly or properly dispose of toilet tissue) occasionally or more frequently over the past weeks.§		Deficient ADL	5 months
	(d) Urinary incontinence (occasionally or more frequently over the past weeks)§		Incipient incontinence	4 months
	(e) Fecal incontinence (occasionally or more frequently over the past weeks).§		Incipient incontinence	10 months
7	(a) Ability to speak limited to approximately half a dozen intelligible different words or fewer, in the course of an average day or in response to queries in the course of an interview.	Severe AD	Semiverbal	12 months
	(b) Speech ability limited to the use of a single intelligible word in an average day or in response to queries in the course of an interview (the person may repeat the word over and over).		Semiverbal	18 months
	(c) Ambulatory ability lost (cannot walk without personal assistance).		Nonambulatory	12 months

(continued)

TABLE 16-3. *Continued*

Functional (FAST) stage	Clinical characteristics	Level of functional incapacity	Clinical diagnosis	Estimated duration of FAST stage or substage in AD‡
	(d) Cannot sit up without assistance (e.g., the individual will fall over if there are no lateral rests on the chair).	Immobile		12 months
	(e) Loss of ability to smile.	Immobile		18 months
	(f) Loss of ability to hold up head independently.	Immobile		12 months

*Reisberg (1988).

†Adapted from Reisberg (1986). Copyright © 1984 by Barry Reisberg, MD.

‡In subjects without other complicating illnesses who survive and progress to the subsequent deterioration stage.

§Scored primarily on the basis of information obtained from a knowledgeable informant or caregiver.

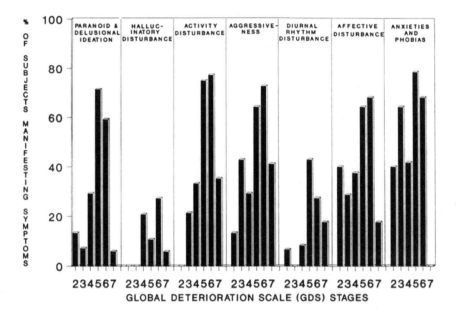

FIGURE 16-1. Prevalence of behavioral and psychological symptoms of dementia (BPSD). The stages correspond to the following diagnoses: Global Deterioration Scale (GDS) stage 2 = age-associated memory impairment (AAMI); GDS stage 3 = mild cognitive impairment (MCI); GDS stages 4 to 7 = mild, moderate, moderately severe, and severe AD, respectively. (Data from Reisberg et al., 1989.)

riorate perform relatively poorly on certain kinds of test measures that involve relatively greater complexity of cognitive processing, multimodality cognitive processing, or a delayed recall element (Flicker et al., 1993; Grober et al., 2000; Hänninen et al., 1995; Kluger et al., 1999).

Examples of tests that appear to be useful in discriminating subjects who subsequently deteriorate from those who do not (from Flicker et al., 1993) include the digit symbol substitution test from the Wechsler Adult Intelligence Scale (WAIS; Wechsler, 1955); a selective reminding-and-recall test (Buschke & Fuld, 1974; Grober et al., 2000); a delayed spatial-and-paragraph recall task (Flicker et al., 1984; Kluger et al., 1999); a facial recognition memory task (Ferris, Crook et al., 1980); and a remote memory questionnaire (Squire, 1974). Other measures, such as neuroimaging of hippocampal atrophy (Golomb et al., 1996) and more generalized brain atrophy (Fox et al., 2001) have also been useful as discriminators of benign from deteriorating outcomes in these and more broadly defined, ostensibly normal, aged subjects.

Possibly the most robust potential predictor of subsequent impairment in subjects with subjective complaints of impairment and other at risk, cognitively intact subjects is neurometabolic activity (de Leon et al., 2001; Small et al., 2000). For example, one study found that neurometabolic activity in the ento-

TABLE 16-4.   Behavioral symptomatology in Alzheimer's disease*

A. Paranoid and Delusional Ideation
  1. *The "people are stealing things" delusion.* Alzheimer's patients can no longer re-
     call the precise whereabouts of household objects. This is probably the psycho-
     logical explanation for what apparently is the most common delusion of pa-
     tients with AD—that someone is hiding or stealing objects. More severe
     manifestations of this delusion include the belief that persons are actually speak-
     ing with or listening to the intruders.
  2. *The "house is not one's home" delusion.* As a result of their cognitive deficits, pa-
     tients with AD may no longer recognize their home. This appears to account, in
     part, for the common conviction of the patient that the place in which they are re-
     siding is not their home. Consequently, while actually at home, patients commonly
     request that their caregiver "take me home." They may also pack their bags for
     their return home. More disturbing to the caregiver, and of great potential danger
     to the patient, are actual attempts to leave the house to go home. Occasionally, at-
     tempts to prevent the patient's departure may result in anger or even violence to-
     ward the caregiver, which is extremely upsetting to the spouse caregiver.
  3. *The "spouse (or other caregiver) is an imposter" delusion.* As cognitive deficit pro-
     gresses, patients with AD recognize their caregivers less well. Perhaps in part for
     this reason, a frequent delusion of the patients is that persons are imposters. In
     some instances, anger and even violence may result from this conviction.
  4. *The delusion of "abandonment."* With the progression of intellectual deficit in
     AD, patients retain a degree of insight into their condition. Although patients
     with AD are largely aware of their cognitive deficits, denial protects them from
     their awareness. Similarly, they may be aware of the burden they have become.
     These insights are probably related to common delusions of abandonment, insti-
     tutionalization, or conspiracy or a plot to institutionalize the patient.
  5. *The "delusion of infidelity."* The insecurities described above are also related to the
     occasional conviction of the patient with AD that the spouse is unfaithful, sexually
     or otherwise. This conviction of infidelity may also apply to other caregivers.
  6. *Other suspicions, paranoid ideation, or delusions.* Although the above specific de-
     lusions are the most commonly observed in AD, others may also be present
     (e.g., phantom boarder [the false belief that strangers are living in the home]);
     delusions that one still carries on activities in which one actually no longer par-
     ticipates (e.g., working, traveling); delusions about former family members or
     the present status of family members (e.g., father is still alive; daughter is still a
     child); delusions of doubles (e.g., there are two of the same person). Suspicion
     and paranoid ideation may occur regarding strangers—people staring, people
     plotting to do harm, and so forth.
B. Hallucinations
  1. *Visual hallucinations.* These can be vague or clearly defined. Commonly, patients
     with AD see intruders or dead relatives at home or have similar hallucinatory ex-
     periences.
  2. *Auditory hallucinations.* Occasionally, in the presence or absence of visual halluci-
     nations, patients with AD may hear dead relatives, intruders, or others whisper-
     ing or speaking to them; sometimes, voices are only heard when caregivers are
     not present.

TABLE 16-4. *Continued*

3. *Other hallucinations.* Less commonly, other form of hallucinations may be observed in patients with AD (e.g., smelling a fire or something burning; perceiving imaginary objects, such as piece of paper, which they offer the caregiver).

C. Activity disturbances

The decreased cognitive capacity of patients with AD renders them less capable of channeling their energies in socially productive ways. Since motor abilities are not severely compromised until the final stage of illness, the patient may develop various psychological/motoric solutions for the need to channel their energies. A few of the most common examples follow:

1. *Wandering.* For a variety of reasons, including inability to channel energies, anxieties, delusions such as those described above, and the decreased cognitive abilities per se, patients with AD frequently wander away from the home or caregiver. Restraints may be necessary; this in turn may provoke anger or violence in the patient.

2. *Purposeless activity (cognitive abulia).* As the condition advances, the patient with AD loses the ability to complete or to carry out many of the activities in which they formerly engaged. This may be the basis in part of a variety of purposeless, frequently repetitive, activities, including opening and closing a purse or pocketbook; packing and unpacking clothing; repeatedly putting on and removing clothing; opening and closing drawers; incessant repetition of demands or questions; or simply pacing. In the absence of more productive, structured activities, these purposeless activities provide a means for the patient to channel energy and their need for movement. Among the most severe manifestations of this syndrome is repetitive self-abrading.

3. *Inappropriate activities.* These occur primarily as a result of decreased cognitive capacities, increased anxieties and suspiciousness, and excess physical energies. They include storing and hiding objects in inappropriate places (e.g., throwing clothing in the wastebasket, putting empty plates in the oven). Attempts by the caregiver to prevent these inappropriate activities may be met by anger or even violence.

D. Aggressivity

1. *Verbal outbursts.* As noted, these may occur in association with many of the behavioral symptoms already described. They can also occur as isolated phenomena. For example, a patient with AD may begin to use unaccustomed foul and abrasive language with intimates or with strangers.

2. *Physical outbursts.* These also may occur as a part of aforementioned syndromes or as an isolated manifestation. The patient with AD may, in response to frustration or seemingly without cause, strike out at the spouse or caregiver.

3. *Other agitation.* This includes anger expressed nonverbally, for example, the patient's "stewing." Also common is negativity manifested by the patient's resistance to bathing, dressing, toileting, walking, or participating in other activities. Agitation may also be expressed as continuous and seemingly incessant talking (i.e., pressured speech), by panting (hyperventilation), by banging, or in other ways.

E. Diurnal rhythm disturbance

Sleep problems are a frequent and significant part of the behavioral syndrome of AD. They may, in part, be the result of decreased cognition (which upsets habitual and other diurnal cues), the energy and motoric changes that occur in the illness, and the neurochemical processes that predispose to agitation and false beliefs.

(continued)

TABLE 16-4. *Continued*

1. *Day/night disturbance.* The most common sleep problem in patients with AD is multiple awakenings in the course of the evening. These can occur in the context of an overall decrease in sleep or in association with increased daytime napping.

F. Affective disturbance

The depressive syndrome of AD is primarily reactive in nature; it frequently tends to become manifest somewhat earlier in the course of AD than many of the other symptoms described above and may be related to the pattern of insight and denial in the patient.

1. *Tearfulness.* This predominant depressive manifestation generally occurs in brief periods. If queried regarding the reason for tearfulness, the patient might respond that he or she is crying because "the person I once was is gone," "because of what is happening to me," or "I forgot the reason." This tearfulness frequently may be a precursor of more severe behavioral symptomatology.

2. *Other depressive manifestations.* A depressive syndrome may coexist with early AD just as other illnesses may coexist with AD. The most common affective symptom in AD is the patient saying "I wish I were dead" or uttering a similar phrase, frequently in a repetitive and manneristic fashion. These pessimistic commentaries of the patient are not accompanied by any more overt suicidal ideation or gestures.

G. Anxieties and phobias

These may be related to the previously described behavioral manifestations of AD or may occur independently.

1. *Anxiety regarding upcoming events (Godot syndrome).* This common symptom appears to result from decreased cognition and, more specifically, anxiety regarding memory disabilities in patients with AD. Consequently, the patient will repeatedly query with respect to an upcoming event. These queries may be so incessant and so persistent as to become intolerable to the family or the patient's caregiver.

2. *Other anxieties.* Patients commonly express previously nonmanifest anxieties regarding their finances, their future, and their health (including their memory) and regarding previously nonstressful activities, such as being away from home.

3. *Fear of being left alone.* This is the most commonly observed phobia in AD, but as a phobic phenomenon, it is out of proportion to any real danger. For example, the anxieties may become apparent as soon as a spouse goes into another room. Less dramatically, the patient may simply request of the spouse or caregiver, "don't leave me alone."

4. *Other phobias.* Patients with AD sometimes develop a fear of crowds, of travel, of the dark, or of activities such as bathing.

Source: Reisberg, Borenstein, et al. (1986). Copyright © 1986 by Barry Reisberg, MD. All rights reserved.
*Adapted from Reisberg et al. (1987).

rhinal cortex, a brain region with very early involvement of AD pathology (Braak & Braak, 1991), predicted subsequent clinical decline at 3-year follow-up with about 85% accuracy (de Leon et al., 2001).

MILD COGNITIVE IMPAIRMENT   The MCI category is presently reserved for persons whose deficits become manifest, only subtly, in the context of a detailed clinical interview (Flicker et al., 1991; Petersen, 2000; Petersen et al., 2001; Sherwin, 2000). Persons at this stage can generally carry out all activities of daily life in which they formerly engaged (Tables 16-2 and 16-3).

Clinical examination at this stage may reveal evidence of decreased capacities in various areas. For example, concentration and calculation deficits may be noted on serial subtractions of 7s from 100. Memory deficits may be suspected on detailed questioning or when the patient repeats queries or phrases in the course of a conversation. Decreased performance on queries related to the patient's orientation may or may not be evident or suspected. Clinicians may also detect seeming deficits in performance on a variety of cognitive tasks that reflect the ability to copy designs, to perform simple arithmetic calculations, or to perform in other areas. However, at this stage the deficits are subtle and evident only to the clinician who is very familiar either with the patient's previous capacities or with the performance of elderly patients on the particular task more generally (Reisberg et al., 1988). Occasionally, clinicians will encounter patients at this stage who score perfectly on the MMSE, but show overt deficits such as repeating themselves or demonstrate major recall deficits.

Longitudinal studies indicate that many of these subjects manifest deterioration when followed over intervals of a few to several years (Bowen et al., 1997; Daly et al., 2000; Devanand et al., 1997; Flicker et al., 1991; Kluger et al., 1999; Morris et al., 2001; Petersen et al., 1999; Tierney et al., 1996). However, a substantial minority of these patients do not manifest deterioration even when followed over a decade or longer. Their deficits may be associated with subtle brain trauma (which may not be clearly evident from neuroimaging or other investigations) or undetected medical or psychiatric conditions (e.g., anxiety, mild depression, hypomania). Most of these patients will subsequently (perhaps as long as 7 years later) manifest AD (Reisberg et al., 2000). Alternatively, these symptoms might not be clinically notable even in retrospect, particularly in elderly persons who are not called on to perform complex occupational or social tasks.

It is important to recognize that, apart from clinically manifest deficits, deficits in psychometric test performance, executive functions, and other clinically relevant domains may occur in this MCI stage. Methodologies for identifying subjects who will subsequently deteriorate are in development (De Santi et al., 2001; Kluger et al., 1999; Touchon & Ritchie, 1999).

MILD ALZHEIMER'S DISEASE Functionally, persons at the mild AD stage (Tables 16-2 and 16-3) frequently manifest deficits in such complex activities of daily life as managing their personal finances or in complex meal preparation or complex marketing skills. For example, they may come to professional attention because they fail to pay their rent properly, or family members may note that the mother or grandmother no longer prepares the holiday meal with accustomed facility. Sometimes, patients will avoid tasks that have become difficult, saying, for example, that they are now "too old for that" or "no longer have the energy they used to," thereby forestalling exposure of their decreased capacities. Nonetheless, persons at this stage generally still perform all basic activities of daily life, including independent dressing and bathing.

Overt deficits in recent memory are frequently apparent. For example, patients may forget where they were or whom they visited on a recent holiday. Other changes also become evident at this stage. For example, family members may note that the patient seems quieter, more withdrawn, or walks more slowly than formerly. Family members frequently interpret these symptoms as signs of depression, and physicians frequently treat these patients with antidepressants. However, in most cases, the psychiatrist notes the absence of overtly dysphoric mood, feelings of guilt, suicidal ideation, initial or terminal insomnia, and appetite disturbance, symptoms commonly seen in depressive disorders.

Longitudinal studies indicate that, in most cases, a diagnosis of AD can reliably be made at this stage, provided other causes of cognitive and functional decrements have been excluded or taken into consideration (McKhann et al., 1984; Reisberg, Burns, et al., 1997; Small et al., 1997). The mean duration of this stage has been estimated as 2 years (Reisberg et al., 1996).

MODERATE ALZHEIMER'S DISEASE   At the moderate AD stage, deficits are of sufficient magnitude to preclude independent survival in the community (Tables 16-2 and 16-3). Recent memory deficits characteristically are such that, for example, patients may not recall their current address, the weather conditions, or the name of the current US president. Generally, patients will recall some of these major aspects of current life and not others. Remote memory deficits are not overt unless the clinician queries in detail. Mood disturbances in this stage are most overtly an exaggeration of those manifest in the previous stage. Specifically, slowing of gait and withdrawal frequently become more evident. Other symptoms such as tearfulness, delusions, and agitation may become increasingly evident, although the magnitude of these symptoms, collectively, is greatest in the next disease stage. The mean duration of this fifth global deterioration and functional stage is 1.5 years (Reisberg et al., 1996).

MODERATELY SEVERE ALZHEIMER'S DISEASE   In moderately severe AD, patients begin to require increasing assistance with basic activities of daily life (Table 16-3). Urinary incontinence generally precedes fecal incontinence. Ambulation is frequently compromised to the extent that the patient takes small steps while walking. Medication or concomitant medical illness may further compromise ambulatory abilities, and there may be a tendency to fall, further increasing the burden of care.

At the end of this stage, speech ability begins to break down. This may be manifested in the patient repeating words or phrases (verbigeration), interspersing genuine words with neologisms, or simply becoming quieter with increasing paucity of speech. The total duration of this moderately severe stage of AD is approximately 2.5 years.

SEVERE ALZHEIMER'S DISEASE   At the severe stage of AD, which may last for many years, patients require continuous assistance with basic activities of daily life, including dressing, bathing, and toileting (Tables 16-2 and 16-3). One third of the total US nursing home population, approximately half a million Americans, appear to be in this stage (German et al., 1985; Gurland et al., 1992; Mayeux et al., 1992; Teresi et al., 1994).

Late in this stage, patients lose ambulatory ability, but they may still be able to walk with personal assistance. Generally, they are not able to use a walker or to manipulate a wheelchair in a purposeful direction. Eventually, patients lose the ability to sit independently in a chair.

Many patients with AD succumb at about the point when they lose the ability to walk or to sit up. Common sources of morbidity and mortality include decubiti (pressure ulcerations), which may become infected, and pneumonia, frequently associated with aspiration. Patients with AD who survive go on to lose the ability to smile. Facial expressions become limited to grimaces. Subsequently, patients lose the ability to move their head or to hold up their head without assistance. A few patients with AD survive for years even beyond this point. The most striking observation in such patients is increasing contractures of all four extremities.

Even early in this final stage, some behavioral problems generally begin to decrease, and they continue to decrease as this final stage evolves (Table 16-3). Consequently, patients may require less and less medication for control of behavioral problems. An exception is screaming, which, although uncommon, is a dramatic symptom of the early seventh stage (Tables 16-2 and 16-3). A few "screamers" can be severely disruptive in chronic care or other settings.

Patients with AD generally succumb approximately 2 years after the onset of this final stage, although some survive for 7 years or longer. Even early in this final stage, AD patients generally achieve only zero or bottom scores on traditional cognitive, mental status, and psychometric tests (Mohs et al., 1986; Wilson & Kaszniak, 1986). Consequently, it was not clear whether the continuing functional decline seen in AD patients was accompanied by continuing cognitive decrements. Tests have been developed for these patients with severe AD; these tests in fact demonstrate continual loss of cognition as AD evolves in this final stage (Auer et al., 1994).

Symptomatology: Behavioral and Psychological Symptoms of Dementia

Behavioral and psychological symptoms (BPSD) are characteristic concomitants of AD (Alzheimer, 1907; American Psychiatric Association, 1994; Burns et al., 1990a, 1990b; Cummings et al., 1987; Drevets & Rubin, 1989; Finkel, 1996; Finkel & Burns, 2000; Lyketsos et al., 2000; Merriam et al., 1988; Reisberg et al., 1987; Reisberg et al., 1989; Rubin et al., 1987; Steele et al., 1990; Teri et al, 1992; Wragg & Jeste, 1989). Seven major categories of potentially remediable BPSD symptoms in AD are readily identified: (A) paranoid and delusional ideation, (B) hallucinatory disturbances, (C) activity disturbances, (D) aggressivity, (E) sleep disturbances, (F) affective disturbances, and (G) anxieties and phobias. Although these general categories are not specific for AD, certain symptomatic manifestations in each of these categories are characteristic of AD and related dementias (Table 16-4). The general occurrence of symptoms in each of the major categories with the advance of AD can be seen in Figure 16-1.

OTHER SYMPTOMS SOMETIMES CLASSIFIED WITH BEHAVIORAL AND PSYCHOLOGICAL SYMPTOMS OF DEMENTIA Other symptoms have occasionally been classified with BPSD that either are not related to the AD illness process or are generally not related to neurobehavioral disturbances in AD. One example of a symptom not related to AD is elation and euphoria (Lyketsos et al., 2000). If symptoms of this nature occur, then superimposed delirium secondary to possibly remediable factors should be suspected and appropriate medical investigations conducted.

Another example of a non-BPSD symptom in AD is weight loss. As AD advances in the moderately severe and severe stages, patients commonly lose weight. This weight loss becomes increasingly dramatic as AD advances in the final stage and particularly in the immobile patient.

Apathy is a symptom psychiatrists understand as emotional withdrawal. This apathetic emotional withdrawal is most clearly and frequently observed in the mild AD stage. Apathy in the AD patient has frequently been misdefined as decreased involvement in activities. When wrongly defined in this manner, apathy becomes synonymous with the increasing functional incapacity seen in the AD patient. However, emotional withdrawal, apathy in the true and therapeutically meaningful sense of the term, does not increase with the continued clinical progression of AD.

NEUROLOGICAL SIGNS Subtle increments in activity of the deep tendon reflexes are detectable even in patients with mild cognitive impairment (Franssen et al., 1991). An increased frequency of nociceptive reflexes (e.g., the glabellar, snout, and palmomental reflexes) may also be noted in patients with mild cognitive impairment or mild AD. Other reflexes, the so-called primitive, developmental, or infantile reflexes (grasp, sucking, rooting, and an abnormal plantar response) (Basavaraju et al., 1981; Franssen et al., 1991, 1993, 1997; Huff et al., 1987; Paulson & Gottlieb, 1968), become clearly manifest only with the advent of severe AD. Because the patient with AD is so much larger and stronger than infants are, the grasp reflex in the patient with severe AD can be very tenacious, and clinicians should be prepared to counsel caregivers on strategies for releasing the patient's grasp (e.g., by gently stroking the dorsal aspect of the hand and removing the hand) (Souren et al., 1997).

Perhaps the most striking neurological concomitant of AD in the later stages is an increase in rigidity (Franssen et al., 1991, 1993; Huff & Growdon,

1986). This appears associated with a stooped posture prior to the loss of ambulation and with the development of contractures in the nonambulatory and increasingly immobile AD patient.

Other Findings in Alzheimer's Disease

NEURORADIOLOGICAL FINDINGS   Cortical brain atrophy and cerebral ventricular dilatation have long been recognized as concomitants of aging in general and as occurring more prominently in AD (Baillie, 1795/1977; de Leon et al., 1979; Huckman et al., 1975; Roberts et al., 1976; Wilks, 1864). The advent of CT scanning has permitted the clear visualization of these changes; however, there is considerable overlap between cognitively normal aged subjects and patients with AD (only a 0.3 Pearson correlation coefficient between global dementia severity in AD and cerebral ventricular dilation magnitude) (Reisberg et al., 1988). Similar results have been obtained in MRI studies of the relationship between cerebral ventricular dilatation and mental status scores or other cognitive severity measures (Kumar et al., 1994; Murphy et al., 1993).

The essential clinical message emerging from these studies is that atrophic changes on neuroimaging alone are not adequate for a diagnosis of dementia. Such changes may, however, be a cause for a comprehensive clinical assessment. It is also important for clinicians to recognize that generalized atrophic changes seen on neuroimaging may be associated not only with aging and AD, but also with various non-AD-related neuropsychiatric and medical conditions, such as chronic ethanol usage and schizophrenia (Burns, 1994; Rabins et al., 1987).

Another neuroimaging change commonly seen, particularly using MRI, in patients with AD is cerebral white matter disease, also known as leukoariosis or Binswanger's changes. These commonly observed findings have been associated with hypertension, age, and cerebral infarctions. They also may have some association with the magnitude of dementia; however, this association is not strong, and white matter changes clinically are clearly not diagnostic either of dementia or of cerebral infarction (Besson, 1994; Erkinjuntti et al., 1994).

The magnitude of hippocampal atrophy visualized with MRI or similar techniques can be useful in distinguishing normal aged patients from patient groups with early AD if special procedures are followed (de Leon et al., 1993a, 1993b; Golomb et al., 1996). However, these techniques have not come into general clinical use either for the early diagnosis of AD or for tracking the course of the disease (De Toledo-Morrell et al., 2000; Fox et al., 2001; Hampel et al., 2002; Killany et al., 2000; Smith, 2002).

Most frequently, neuroimaging is used to detect the presence of a space-occupying lesion that might account for, or add to, the patient's clinical symptomatology. Ventricular dilatation out of proportion to the magnitude of cortical atrophy, indicative of normal-pressure hydrocephalus, is another possible and not infrequent finding on neuroimaging that can influence the clinical dementia presentation. For clinical diagnostic purposes, a noncontrast CT or MRI scan is an appropriate part of the workup. For patients with cardiac pacemakers or other metallic devices that interfere with magnetic-based imaging, a CT scan, with or without contrast dye, is generally obtained.

ELECTROPHYSIOLOGICAL FINDINGS Progressive increments in slow-wave activity have long been recognized as concomitants of progressive dementia in AD (Hughes et al., 1989; Kaszniak et al., 1979; McAdam & Robinson, 1957). Studies using quantitative electroencephalographic (EEG) analysis (Breslau et al., 1989; Coben et al., 1990; Prichep et al., 1994; Sterletz et al., 1990; Williamson et al., 1990) have demonstrated a progressive increase in theta wave activity that appears to accompany even the earliest cognitive changes in AD. With increasing cognitive impairment, increments in delta wave EEG activity also become evident. The magnitude of these relationships between cognitive and other aspects of deterioration in AD and the progressive EEG slowing does not exceed approximately a 0.5 Pearson correlation coefficient (Prichep et al., 1994).

These and related findings (see Chapter 15) may have potential value in early diagnosis (Jelic et al., 2000); however, they remain controversial, and further data are needed. Because EEG slowing is seen in non-AD dementias as well as in other physiological states, EEG changes can be indicative of AD, however, they are not diagnostic unless utilized in conjunction with other clinical procedures.

EEG assessment is not recommended as a necessary part of the standard workup of dementia. However, the EEG can be useful in cases of suspected delirium, seizure, or Creutzfeld-Jakob disease. Other electrophysiological parameters (e.g., evoked potentials) have also been studied in patients with AD, but have not been convincingly demonstrated to be important in diagnostic or symptomatologic assessment in AD.

NEUROMETABOLIC FINDINGS Cerebral blood flow has long been recognized as diminished in normal aging (Kety & Schmidt, 1948) and, to a greater extent, in dementia (Obrist et al., 1970). The advent of positron emission tomography (PET) in the 1980s permitted an examination of cerebral metabolism in AD. Initial studies showed decreased cerebral metabolism in AD (Ferris, de Leon et al., 1980), and these generalized cerebral metabolic decrements have been confirmed in numerous studies (Silverman et al., 2001). The decrements are greatest in the parietotemporal regions and frontal cortex, but are less notable in the motor cortical regions, occipital regions, and cerebellum. PET has also shown considerable promise as an early marker of preclinical AD (de Leon et al., 2001; Haxby et al., 1986). In part because of availability limitations, PET has not as yet come into general clinical use.

Single-photon emission computerized tomography (SPECT) provides information (using a technicium tracer) on cerebral blood flow. Results of studies to date indicate blood flow decrements in AD (Gemmell et al., 1987; Hurwitz et al., 1991; Neary et al., 1987; Neugroschl & Davis, 2002; Podreka et al., 1987). Clinical correlation is an absolute necessity in interpreting these SPECT findings.

CEREBROSPINAL FLUID   Studies have indicated that cerebrospinal fluid (CSF) examinations may become useful in the early diagnosis and in the differential diagnosis of AD (Buerger, Teipel, et al., 2002; Buerger, Zinkowski, et al., 2002; de Leon et al., 2002; Riemenschneider et al., 2002). CSF levels of tau and particular tau moieties (tau is the most important protein constituent of the neurofibrillary degeneration characteristic of AD) and amyloid β subtypes are being explored for potential clinical usefulness.

PATHOLOGY, PATHOGENESIS, AND ETIOLOGY

The salient pathological brain changes of AD are the presence of senile plaques and neurofibrillary tangles (Alzheimer, 1907; Blessed et al., 1968; Braak & Braak, 1991; Khachaturian, 1985; Mirra et al., 1991; Redlich, 1898). Studies have elucidated the nature of these pathological features of AD and their possible relationship to etiopathogenesis. However, the primary versus secondary roles of these pathological features in late-life AD continue to require elucidation.

Classical neuritic senile plaques are composed of a central core of homogeneous-appearing material, termed *amyloid*, surrounded by cellular debris, referred to as the *neurite*. The amyloid consists of the amyloid β-peptide (Aβ), a peptide with 42 to 43 amino acids. The Aβ is a heterogeneous peptide that exists in various forms; Aβ1-42 and Aβ1-40 are the most common. The longer moiety, Aβ1-42, is believed more prone to aggregation and possibly more pathogenic than the Aβ1-40 (Näslund et al., 2000).

The Aβ peptide is derived from the amyloid precursor protein (APP), which has been shown to be encoded in the long arm of chromosome 21 (Goldgaber et al., 1987; Kang et al., 1987; Tanzi et al., 1987). At least two naturally occurring cleavage mechanisms for the breakdown of APP have been demonstrated; one results in amyloid-β deposition (Esch et al., 1990; Golde et al., 1992; Haass et al., 1992; Sisodia et al., 1990). These alternative APP proteolytic pathways are known as α-secretase cleavage and β-secretase cleavage. The latter cleavage is followed by γ-secretase cleavage and the generation of amyloid β. There is evidence that the amyloid β peptide is widely distributed in the body and is present in increased quantities in the brain in aged individuals and, especially, in patients with AD (Näslund et al., 2000; Seubert et al., 1992).

The neurofibrillary tangles are composed of paired helical filaments (Kidd, 1963). The major constituent of these paired helical filaments is the tau protein (Kondo et al., 1988; Wischik, Novak, Thogersen, et al., 1988; Wischik, Novak,

Edwards, et al., 1988). Other constituents have been identified, including ubiquitin, a very widely distributed protein (Mori et al., 1987; Perry et al., 1987).

In normal human infancy, the tau protein is hyperphosphorylated (i.e., there are multiple phosphorylation sites on the tau protein). This hyperphosphorylated tau state is believed to provide necessary flexibility for the microtubular cytoskeleton, for which tau protein provides some of the scaffolding. In the normal adult, tau is in a nonhyperphosphorylated state, with resultant loss of flexibility.

Although patients with AD have hyperphosphorylated tau, the precise sites of hyperphosphorylation in AD differ somewhat from those in infancy. The loss of rigidity of the microtubules in AD resulting from the tau hyperphosphorylation is believed similar to that occurring in the course of normal development and is believed responsible for the neurofibrillary tangle formation (pairs of intraneuronal 20-nm filaments twisted with a periodicity of 80 nm) seen in brains of patients with AD.

It should be emphasized that these hallmark neuropathological features of AD, the amyloid-containing senile plaques and the neurofibrillary tangles containing paired helical filaments, are also found in normal aged subjects and are age-associated phenomena. There is variable evidence that amyloid plaque burden in the cortex correlates with cognitive loss and stronger evidence that tangle burden in various hippocampal regions does so. These neuropathological hallmarks of AD are also found in non-AD pathological conditions. For example, amyloid deposits in the brain have been noted as a feature of hereditary cerebral hemorrhage with amyloidosis–Dutch type (HCHWA-DA) (Levy et al., 1990), and neurofibrillary tangles similar or identical to those in AD may be seen in such diverse conditions as myotonic dystrophy and progressive supranuclear palsy (Bancher et al., 1987; Kiuchi et al., 1991).

The possible role of these neuropathological features of AD in the etiopathogenesis of the disease has been strengthened most notably by two groups of observations. One is that persons with Down syndrome (i.e., trisomy of chromosome 21) develop the neuropathological features of AD relatively early in life and are also prone to the development of dementia in midlife. Another stems from the finding that some families with early onset of AD have mutations in the APP gene (Goate et al., 1991; Mullan et al., 1992).

However, it should be noted that APP mutations have not been shown to occur in the common, late-life form of AD and do not occur in many familial forms of AD. In addition, mutations have been found on chromosome 14 associated with familial, early-onset AD (Schellenberg et al., 1992) and mutations on chromosome 19 are associated with familial, late-onset AD (Pericak-Vance et al., 1991).

A possible role for a very different kind of genetic factor in AD etiopathogenesis has been suggested by findings that persons with a certain kind of genetic marker that codes for an apolipoprotein (apolipoprotein E, apoE), a molecule primarily responsible for lipid transport in various organs, are prone to the development of AD. Three different apoE alleles are inherited: *apoE-2,* *apoE-3,* and *apoE-4.* Persons who are homozygous for the *apoE-4* allele have as much as an eightfold increase in the risk of developing AD (Corder et al., 1993; Poirier et al., 1993). Persons with *apoE-4* in heterozygous form also are at increased risk for the development of AD. The precise role of the apolipo-protein genes in AD etiopathogenesis is currently a subject of considerable speculation and investigation (see Chapter 2).

Many other factors, apart from those noted in the discussion above, have been implicated or considered in AD etiopathogenesis. Stress is known to be associated with brain damage through corticosteroid-related mechanisms that have been considered possibly relevant in AD. For example, oxidative damage and a possible role for antioxidants have long been considered as possibly fundamental in pathogenesis, and there is clear evidence for neurometabolic and mitochondrial changes in AD (Beal, 1994). Also, neuronal damage in AD has been associated with an inflammatory cascade that may be of primary or secondary relevance in terms of continuing neurodegeneration.

Many of the major risk factors for cerebrovascular disease, stroke, and cardiovascular disease are demonstrated risk factors for AD as well (Hofman et al., 1997; O'Brien et al., 2003; Seshadri et al., 2002). Vascular amyloid angiopathy is present in virtually all AD cases and has been independently associated with cognitive impairment (Natte et al., 2001; O' Brien et al., 2003; Premkumar et al., 1996). The association between cerebrovascular disease and AD is sufficiently strong to implicate possible common mechanisms in etio-pathogenesis.

Current knowledge regarding AD etiology can be summarized briefly as follows: (1) The etiology is unknown; and (2) age, genetic mutations, chromosome 21 trisomy, and the presence of an apolipoprotein E4 allele have been convincingly implicated as major risk factors and cerebrovascular disease as an associated factor.

RELATIONSHIP BETWEEN ETIOPATHOGENESIS AND CLINICAL SYMPTOMATOLOGY

Although the etiology of AD remains unknown, research has clarified the relationship between the pathogenic basis of AD and the nature of AD clinical symptomatology. Neuronal stressors, including amyloid β and neuroinflammation (Wu et al., 2000), produce a mitogenic response in the neurons, as evidenced by the appearance of various cell cycle markers (Arendt, 2001). In the terminally differentiated neurons of the adult brain, the mitogenic response is toxic and results in tau hyperphosphorylation and the development of neurofibrillary changes (Kobayashi et al., 1993; Ledesma et al., 1992) and, ultimately, neuronal cell death (Liu & Greene, 2001; Qin et al., 1994). The most metabolically active brain regions, subsuming the most recently acquired information and skills, appear to be the most vulnerable to this process. Consequently, when skills are lost in the AD patient, they appear to be lost in reverse order of their acquisition in normal development. Cognitively, AD changes also reverse those of normal development (Shimada et al., 2001). For example, the MMSE score shows the same correlation with the mental age of children as it does with neuropathological changes of AD (Ouvrier et al., 1993). Because of this functional and cognitive reversal of normal development, a process that has been termed *retrogenesis*, the stages of AD can be usefully translated into developmental ages (Reisberg et al., 1999, 2002).

Using the developmental age of the patient with AD, it has been demonstrated that neurodevelopmental reflexes emerge at the point in AD that corresponds to the developmental age at which they disappear in late infancy (Franssen et al., 1997). Also, recognition of the developmental age of the patient with AD provides an explanation of the general management needs of the AD patient and the nature and causes of many BPSD symptoms.

For example, AD delusions are not constant or firmly held as in schizophrenic patients, and seem similar in many ways to childhood fantasies. Also, a patient with AD who is not provided with activities will pace back and forth in much the same way that a child at the corresponding developmental age who is not provided with activities will run back and forth. Aggressivity in patients with AD is also similar in many ways to that of children at the corresponding developmental age.

DIFFERENTIAL DIAGNOSIS

AD remains a clinical diagnosis. Consequently, the differential diagnosis of AD is based on a recognition of the characteristic clinical features and course. Laboratory procedures, neuroimaging, and—in selected cases—electrophysiological studies and other investigations may assist the clinician in arriving at a proper diagnosis. Differential diagnosis in AD encompasses two kinds of decisions: (1) establishing the primary etiology of cognitive impairment and (2) establishing the nature and relevance of excess morbidity in the patient with AD. A complete discussion of differential diagnostic issues is potentially very broad and requires detailed knowledge of diverse relevant diagnostic entities. However, some salient elements particularly relevant for the geriatric psychiatrist are reviewed here.

Geriatric Depression

The presentation of early AD has certain clinical features very similar to those that occur in depressive disorder, such as flattening of affect, decreased verbalization (i.e., paucity of speech), slowing of gait, and, to a lesser extent, generalized psychomotor slowing (Table 16-5). Consequently, family members of

TABLE 16-5.   Symptomatology associated with Alzheimer's disease (AD) and depressive disorder: Similarities and differences

Symptoms shared by patients with AD and depressive disorder and secondary mainly to the cognitive and dementia-related (not mood) disturbance in AD	Symptoms occurring in those with AD and depressive disorder that are superficially similar*	Symptoms primarily associated with depressive disorder
Flattened affect	Paranoid and delusional ideation	Pervasive dysphoria
Paucity of speech	Hallucinations	Feeling of guilt
Slowed gait	Aggressivity	True suicidal ideation
Generalized psychomotor slowing	Diurnal rhythm disturbance (i.e., sleep disturbance)	
	Affective disturbance	
	Anxiety and phobias	

Source: Adapted from Reisberg (1992).
*Although categorically similar, the specific symptoms in these broad categories of behavioral disturbance differ in AD and depressive affective disorder. The nature and incidence of specific symptoms in the behavioral pathology syndrome of AD are outlined in Table 16-4 and Figure 16-1.

patients with AD presenting for the first time to the clinician commonly bring the patient with such a complaint as "My spouse is depressed."

In mild and moderate AD, the observed emotional withdrawal appears in part a response to the patients' decreased cognitive capacities. Similarly, the decrease in verbalizations in AD appears to be associated in part with the patient's decreased cognitive capacity to respond appropriately. Patients in these early stages remain socially intelligent and aware. A wise person, or, in this case, the wise patient, keeps quiet when not certain what to say. It is clear that the slowed gait and generalized motoric slowing of the patient with AD are on a continuum that begins early in the course of the disease and ultimately results in complete loss of ambulatory and other motor capacities (Kluger et al., 1997; Reisberg et al., 2000; Souren et al., 1995).

The etiology of these overlapping clinical symptoms of AD and depressive disorder is sometimes clarified by cognitive assessment. In depressive disorder, the above symptoms occur frequently in the absence of coexisting manifest cognitive disturbance; in AD, these symptoms are almost invariably manifest at a point in the evolution of the disease at which cognitive disturbances are overtly manifest. However, differential diagnosis is complicated by the frequent presentation of cognitive disturbance as a manifestation of geriatric depression and by the occasional inability to observe clearly manifest cognitive losses in mild AD. For these reasons, the clinician must be aware of additional differentiating and potentially overlapping clinical features as well as the outcome of cognitive disturbance when this occurs in the context of depressive disorder. The clinician must bear in mind the possibility that the two disorders may coexist.

Delusional ideation may occur both in AD and in depressive disorder. However, in AD common delusions are that people are stealing things, that the spouse is an imposter, and other delusions noted in Table 16-4. In depressive disorder, the nature of observed delusional ideation is generally different; commonly, delusions are self-deprecating. Another example is that both AD and depressive disorder are characterized by sleep disturbance. However, in AD the sleep disturbance is primarily manifested as fragmented sleep. In depressive disorder, sleep disturbance is classically manifested as initial or terminal insomnia.

At times, the cognitive disturbance is subjective only; that is, the patient complains of cognitive impairment. However, objective assessment does not reveal evidence of impairment; consequently, the complaints of disturbance seem out of proportion to the actual magnitude of cognitive deficit. In these cases, when sufficient affective symptomatology is present, a diagnosis of "pure" affective disturbance may be made, and treatment plans and prognosis are formulated accordingly.

At other times, the cognitive impairment accompanying geriatric depression is objectively and subjectively manifest (LaRue et al., 1986). In some of these cases, the cognitive disturbance does not return. However, follow-up studies have shown that, in a substantial fraction of these cases, cognitive disturbance may become manifest over the subsequent 2 to 4 years, and the depressive disorder will, in retrospect, be identifiable as a harbinger of subsequently manifest AD (Agbayewa, 1986; Baker et al., 1991; Kral, 1982).

For example, in a study of 44 subjects whose mean age was older than 75 years at baseline, who were assessed as having "depressive pseudodementia" (i.e., both depression and cognitive disturbance) at baseline, and whose cognitive disturbances remitted initially, 39 patients (89%) developed dementia consistent with AD at follow-up (Kral & Emery, 1989). In this study, follow-up occurred at intervals of 4 to 18 years. However, the proportion of patients who advance to dementia varies in different studies, probably depending on the population studied, follow-up interval, criteria for dementia, and other factors. For example, a study of 11 patients found only 1 who manifested overt dementia after a 2-year follow-up interval (Pearlson et al., 1989).

Another possibility is that the depression remits, but the cognitive disturbance continues after successful treatment of the affective symptoms. It is important for the clinician to recognize that the cognitive disturbance may nevertheless remit in the subsequent interval of weeks to months after the affective symptoms have been successfully treated. If the cognitive disturbance does remit, it may or may not return in succeeding months and years.

Another possible clinical scenario is that the affective symptoms are successfully treated, but the cognitive disturbance persists. In retrospect, it will be clear in these cases that the depressive symptoms occurred in the context of an underlying dementia, most commonly AD.

It is clear that depression and AD have many areas of similarity and overlap in terms of symptomatology. This is not surprising because many of the neurotransmitter changes that occur in depressive disorder and in AD are also similar and, to some extent, overlapping (Forstl et al., 1992; Whitehouse, 1987; Zubenko et al., 1990). For example, noradrenergic deficits (Bondareff et al., 1982), dopaminergic decrements (Cross, Crow, Johnson, et al., 1984), and serotonergic changes (Bowen et al., 1983; Cross, Crow, Ferrier, et al., 1984) have been reported in both disorders, although all of these changes appear to be more consistently reported in depressive disorder.

Strokes and Cerebrovascular Dementia

Classical neuropathological studies indicated that cerebrovascular factors, more specifically, loose soft tissue and blood, also termed *cerebral softening* (presumably resulting from cerebral ischemia), appeared to be the major contributor to dementia etiopathogenesis in approximately 10% to 15% of patients autopsied (Tomlinson et al., 1970). An additional quarter of patients autopsied in these classic studies manifested marked cerebrovascular changes in association with Alzheimer's neuropathological brain changes (i.e., senile plaques and neurofibrillary tangles) (see also Chapters 12 and 17).

STROKES Building on the above-noted findings, Hachinski and associates (1974) coined the term *multiinfarct dementia* to encompass those cases for which cerebrovascular factors are primary features in dementia etiopathogenesis. As conceptualized by Hachinski, multiinfarct dementia was characterized by an abrupt onset; a stepwise course; evidence of strokes, including focal neurological signs and symptoms; and associated stroke risk factors, such as hypertension (Hachinski, 1983).

A modified version of a scale designed by Hachinski for the assessment of infarct risk has come into wide usage (Rosen et al., 1980). In clinical practice, this classically conceptualized picture of a dementia with both an abrupt onset and a stepwise course is infrequently observed. On those occasions when a fluctuating stepwise course is seen in association with dementia, the clinician will frequently trace the source of fluctuation to a low serum B_{12} level, severe arteriosclerotic narrowing, or some other, non–multiple infarct, pathological origin.

Current understanding of the role of cerebrovascular factors in dementia etiology includes the salient observation that strokes clinically or radiologically manifest can produce pathology that may include cognitive impairment. The likelihood of dementia depends on the extent to which the lesions are bilateral and/or damage relevant brain regions such as the hippocampi and particular cortical regions. However, as focal neurological lesions, strokes can also produce a variety of signs and symptoms not seen in AD, such as unilateral deficits in motoric function, cranial nerve findings, and so on.

Strokes can also produce other pathology seen in the course of AD, but out of sequence with the temporal and ordinal emergence of pathology in the course of AD. For example, strokes can produce urinary incontinence with or without the cognitive changes typical in AD (Table 16-2). Also, strokes can produce urinary incontinence out of sequence from the characteristic pattern of functional loss in AD (Table 16-3). To cite another example, a cerebral infarction can produce a loss of ambulatory capacity. This ambulatory loss may or may not be accompanied by associated cognitive and functional disturbances secondary to the stroke. Even if the stroke does produce associated cognitive and functional losses, these will not necessarily follow or mimic the patterns of disturbance seen in AD and summarized in Tables 16-2 and 16-3. In general, the pervasiveness of the damage produced by the stroke and the extent to which the infarct lesions produce bilateral deficits determine the extent to which the clinical picture of the dementia secondary to the infarction mimics or resembles that seen in AD.

Although the stepwise pattern of loss described by Hachinski is rarely observed, infarct-related dementia is frequently accompanied by an abrupt onset or a temporal pattern of deficit and loss that is distinct from that observed in AD. Functionally, the temporal pattern of loss in AD can be retrospectively reconstructed. The approximate temporal sequence of functional loss in AD is shown in Table 16-3.

For example, in a study of patients with probable AD free of non-AD-related central nervous system (CNS) pathology, approximately 90% of patients followed the ordinal sequence of deficit shown in Table 16-3 precisely. For the remaining 10%, the order of functional loss differed only slightly (Sclan & Reisberg, 1992). Consequently, the ordinal and temporal patterns of functional losses shown in Table 16-3 can assist clinicians in making judgments of the extent to which the etiology of deficits observed is inconsistent with those anticipated in AD and therefore possibly attributable to infarction-related pathology. Aids in differential diagnosis such as provided in Table 16-3 are particularly important for the clinician because, in many cases, AD and cerebral infarction coexist, and the relevant contributory pathological conditions to the observed clinical symptomatology must be assessed by the geropsychiatric specialist.

For example, a patient may abruptly present with urinary incontinence, ambulatory loss, or loss of speech or one or more of the other functional changes shown in Table 16-3. This abrupt presentation may be attributable after appropriate pathological studies to an infarction. Another patient may have a gradual onset of cognitive and functional losses (e.g., inability to handle complex activities and to pick out clothing without the spouse's assistance).

This patient may suddenly stop speaking and walking. A workup might reveal a cerebral infarction of uncertain age. The clinician might conclude that the patient has a mixed dementia with AD and infarction-related cerebrovascular dementia. The clinician would attribute the gradually appearing ordinal functional losses to AD and and further conclude that an infarction resulted in excess morbidity, including the loss of speech and ambulation.

CEREBROVASCULAR DEMENTIA AND VASCULAR COGNITIVE IMPAIRMENT The incidence and prevalence of cerebrovascular dementia remains controversial, with widely divergent estimates from different studies. These differences are due in part to competing diagnostic criteria. There is an emerging consensus that (1) multiinfarct dementia (cognitive loss because of strokes) may represent only one form of vascular dementia (VaD), and that small-vessel disease may be an equally or even more common cause of cognitive loss with aging; and (2) the diagnosis of a dementia that is entirely due to vascular changes is extremely difficult because the pathological evidence suggests that aging-related neurodegenerative changes of the Alzheimer's type are present to some degree in most patients previously diagnosed with vascular dementia.

All of the well-known risk factors for stroke and heart disease are also believed to be risk factors for small-vessel VaD, including hypertension, diabetes, smoking, and hypercholesterolemia (Jick et al., 2000; Launer et al., 2000; Ott et al., 1998, 1999; Skoog et al., 1996). The terminology *vascular cognitive impairment* (VCI) has been proposed for the entity resulting from this small-vessel disease VaD, which may result in an MCI diagnosis as well as a dementia diagnosis. It appears clear that the pathology associated with VCI adds to that of AD pathology when the conditions occur together, as is commonly the case (Snowdon et al., 1997).

Although risk factors for VCI are known, the etiology is not precisely known in most cases. However, there is an entity known as CADASIL (cerebral autosomal dominant arteriopathy with subcortical infarcts and leukoencephalopathy), which is dominantly inherited and which produces VCI as well as other pathology, in middle-aged persons (Dichgans et al., 1998). In the great majority of late-life cases, the etiology of the small-vessel cerebrovascular disease appears to be multifactorial. This vascular change is now believed to result in incomplete infarctions as well as small infarcts (lacunes) (Chui, 2001). These changes are believed associated with the commonly observed white matter changes seen on MRI imaging.

Although there is agreement on the risk factors for VCI, on its prevalence, and on associated pathological features, there is also agreement that this entity exists on a continuum with AD, and that both conditions pertain to some extent in most cases. Consequently, for differential diagnosis, clinicians should currently recognize and be aware of this continuum and its possible impact on prognosis and therapy.

Lewy Body Dementia

Lewy bodies are spherical, intracytoplasmic inclusions that characteristically contain a protein known as α-synuclein. They were first described by the German neurologist Frederic Lewy in 1912 in association with Parkinson's disease. Since the 1980s, the postmortem neuropathological presence of Lewy bodies has been associated with dementia (Kosaka et al., 1984). Lewy bodies were more readily recognized with the advent of new staining techniques in the 1990s, and they are now believed to be present in the brain stem or cortex in approximately 15% to 25% of dementia patients at the time of death (McKeith et al., 1996).

These pathologically observed Lewy bodies on postmortem examination of the brain frequently occur in association with common dementing disorders, including AD and vascular dementia. When this pathological dementia with Lewy bodies (DLB) occurs in association with AD or vascular dementia, the clinical features are generally not distinctive. For example, one study found that the only clinical features that differentiated patients with neuropathological AD and Lewy bodies from patients with AD without Lewy bodies were more rapid onset and fluctuating evolution (Del Ser et al., 2001).

The relationship among DLB, AD, and PD remains unclear, with some advocating that these are distinct entities, and others pointing to evidence of clinical and pathogenetic overlap. As a result, the criteria first proposed to diagnose DLB as a clinically distinct disorder are not sensitive for the purposes of case detection. In particular, although interrater reliability for visual hallucinations and parkinsonism is acceptable, fluctuating cognition cannot be reliably detected according to the Consortium on Dementia with Lewy Bodies (McKeith et al., 1999).

Nonetheless, the diagnosis of DLB is important for clinicians. For example, according to one study (Ballard et al., 1998), sensitivity to neuroleptics with increased frequency of the neuroleptic malignant syndrome has occurred, as has a threefold increase in mortality. These adverse events have been reported mainly for traditional neuroleptics, but also to some extent for the newer atypical agents, such as risperidone.

Despite these possible adverse events, behavioral disturbances in patients with DLB have been treated successfully with risperidone (Allen et al., 1995). Consequently, clinicians may conclude that they need to proceed with neuroleptic treatment in patients with DLB, but if possible they should avoid so-called typical, traditional neuroleptics and neuroleptics with extrapyramidal side effects. Haloperidol particularly should be avoided.

Finally, it has been found that patients with Lewy body dementia may be particularly responsive to cholinestrase inhibitor treatment. The course of DLB appears to be more rapid than that of AD, and urinary incontinence appears earlier in the course of the dementia (Del Ser et al., 2001).

Frontotemporal Lobar Dementia

Frontotemporal lobar dementia is a clinically and neuropathologically diverse group of dementias. Collectively, they are believed to represent the fourth most common group of progressive dementias after AD, vascular dementia, and DLB. The characteristic feature of these dementias is that there is prominent pathological involvement of the frontal or temporal cortex. In general, they tend to occur at a younger age than AD.

Neuropathologically, two major distinct forms appear to occur: those with microvascular pathology and a laminar spongiosis and those with intraneuronal Pick bodies (Pick's disease) (Mann et al., 2000). Pick bodies are intracytoplasmic inclusions consisting of accumulations of filaments in a granulovacuolar matrix (Rewcastle & Ball, 1968; Wisniewski & Coblentz, 1972). The Pick bodies are approximately the same size as the nucleus. They are strongly immunoreactive for the tau protein. In one pathological series, approximately a quarter of cases of frontotemporal lobar dementia contained Pick bodies (Mann et al., 2000).

In addition to a neuropathological classification of the frontotemporal lobar dementias, it is now possible to classify these entities molecularly. Some of these dementias are "tauopathies" in that tau immunoreactivity is prominent. These tauopathies include Pick's disease and an entity known to be associated with mutations in the tau gene, frontotemporal dementia with Parkinsonism linked to chromosome 17 (FTDP-17). In the series of Mann and colleagues (2000), about 10% of the frontotemporal lobar dementias were patients with FTDP-17.

For clinicians, the clinicopathological classification of the frontotemporal lobar dementias is probably most relevant (Neary et al., 1998). In general, these are entities in which changes in personality and social behavioral disturbance are more prominent features than the memory disturbance. Early disturbance in decision making or executive function is sometimes emphasized (Grafman & Litvan, 1999; Neary et al., 1998). Three clinicopathological subtypes have been identified based on the regions of brain involvement and the nature of prominent clinical symptomatology. In frontotemporal dementia, there is prominent bilateral involvement of the frontal lobes. In progressive aphasia, there is mainly left frontotemporal atrophy and difficulty in reading and writing. In semantic dementia, there is bilateral atrophy, especially in the anterior temporal cortex. In this syndrome, there is a severe naming and comprehension deficit, but speech output is fluent and grammatical.

Other Dementia Etiologies

A broad variety of conditions that have an impact on cerebral function can produce generalized cognitive disturbances and either dementia or a clinical syndrome very similar to dementia. These diverse conditions include head trauma; cerebral primary or secondary neoplasms; encephalitis because of infectious agents, fungal agents, or other organisms producing diffuse cerebral trauma; prions (replicating misfolded proteins) such as Creutzfeldt-Jacob disease; metabolic or electrolyte disturbances; endocrine disturbances; nutritional disturbances including B_{12} and folate deficiencies; hereditary conditions such as Huntington's disease; cerebral toxins such as heavy metal poisoning; various pharmacological agents; normal-pressure hydrocephalus; and progressive supranuclear palsy in addition to AD and the other conditions already described in some detail, including depression, cerebral infarction, cerebrovascular disease, DLB, and frontotemporal lobar dementia.

A standard clinical workup will assist in determining the relevance of these diverse pathological possible etiologies. This workup should include the procedures described in the beginning of this chapter as well as medical, psychiatric, and neurological evaluations and, very importantly, a history of the onset and course of the condition, concomitant medications, and an environmental, social, and family history. The clinician should treat any elucidated remediable pathology.

Knowledge of the clinical symptomatology and course of AD will also assist in the differential diagnosis of these diverse conditions. For example, normal-pressure hydrocephalus commonly presents with gait disturbance. This is generally followed by urinary incontinence and subsequently by cognitive and cognition-related functional disturbances, such as decreased ability to manage instrumental activities of daily life. In AD, the temporal order of cognitive and functional losses is very different, as noted in Tables 16-2 and 16-3.

Excess Morbidity

Physical pathology, apart from CNS pathology, may also have an impact on morbidity in the patient with AD. For example, arthritis, a history of hip fracture, scoliosis associated with osteoporosis, peripheral vascular disease, and loss of vision associated with cataracts or other ocular pathology all commonly occur in elderly persons and may interfere with ambulation in the patient with AD. When AD and these sources of comorbidity coexist, they frequently increase specific morbidity in a synergistic manner (i.e., the resulting disability may be greater than the sum of its parts).

The clinician must assess the relevance of any such additional pathology for the patient with AD. The temporal and ordinal sequence of functional losses in AD as outlined in Table 16-3 can be very useful to the clinician in these assessments. For example, if a clinician is treating a patient with GDS and Functional Assessment Staging (FAST) stage 6 with haloperidol and the patient loses ambulatory capacity, the clinician must determine whether this ambulatory loss is the result of an extrapyramidal side effect from the haloperidol treatment or the result of the progression of AD. If the patient with AD is still capable of speaking in sentences, then the ambulatory loss is likely associated with excess morbidity, such as an extrapyramidal side effect of the haloperidol treatment. The clinician will need to adjust pharmacological treatment accordingly.

TREATMENT

The treatment of AD consists of proper clinical management and pharmacological intervention. Although no treatment has convincingly been demonstrated to halt or even retard the fundamental pathological process of AD, appropriate management and pharmacological intervention can decrease stress and burden for the patient and the caregiver, postpone institutionalization, mitigate clinical symptomatology, and minimize excess morbidity.

Management

Management needs in aging and AD vary enormously, depending on the stage (severity) of the condition (Table 16-2). Special management strategies that should be considered in the patient with AD apart from those outlined in Table 16-2 include support groups and day care centers. Support groups are sometimes available for patients in the incipient and early stages (mainly mild cognitive impairment and mild AD) and appear to be useful. Spouse and family member support groups have long been available and are an important and frequently used and useful resource. Day care centers are particularly useful for patients with moderate AD and less-agitated patients with moderately severe AD.

The Alzheimer's Association based in Chicago, Illinois, is an important resource and can assist families in many ways. Local chapters of the Alzheimer's Association can be found throughout the United States. Internationally, Alzheimer's Disease International (ADI) has affiliate national organizations in more than 50 nations. These organizations and others can assist family members in locating resources, such as obtaining appropriate legal advice, appropriate financial planning, and the like.

Pharmacological Treatment

There are presently two major forms of pharmacological treatment of AD. The first are treatments that remediate the cognitive and global symptomatology in the context of its continued decline in AD. The second are treatments that more specifically alleviate the BPSD and affective symptoms that occur in the context of the disease.

For treatment of the cognitive and global symptoms of AD, the first class of agents that has been approved in the United States and elsewhere is the cholinesterase inhibitors. These agents inhibit the breakdown of acetylcholine by the enzyme acetlycholinesterase at the synapse and thereby enhance cholinergic neurotransmitter activity. Activity of the cholinergic neurotransmitter system. especially the activity of choline acetyltransferase, the enzyme responsible for acetylcholine synthesis, has long been believed to be decreased in the brains of patients with AD (Bartus et al., 1982; Coyle et al., 1983; Davies & Maloney, 1976; Perry et al., 1977; Spillane et al., 1977; Whitehouse et al., 1981). Consequently, these treatments are believed to alleviate this prominent deficit in AD.

Four cholinesterase inhibitors have been approved in the United States: tacrine, donepezil, rivastigmine, and galantamine. Tacrine was the first cholinesterase inhibitor to be introduced. Approved in 1995, the use of tacrine has long been limited by its potential hepatic toxicity, which requires frequent monitoring of hepatic enzymes. Consequently, tacrine is rarely used now, and it is not recommended for new patients.

The cholinesterase inhibitors have all been approved for the treatment of mild-to-moderate AD (Tables 16-1, 16-2, and 16-3; GDS and FAST stages 4 and 5). Evidence for the efficacy of these agents in the treatment of mild cognitive impairment is not available. Also, there is very limited evidence for the efficacy of the cholinesterase inhibitors in treating more severe stages of AD (Farlow et al., 2000; Feldman et al., 2001). A notable exception is a study by Feldman et al. of the efficacy of donepezil; the study included patients with deficits in basic activities of daily life (a FAST score of 6) and an MMSE as low as 5. This study did indicate that donepezil might be useful in patients with this magnitude of dementia severity (i.e., for some patients with moderately severe AD). However, there is no good evidence at this time that the cholinesterase inhibitors are useful either for the full spectrum of moderately severe AD or for severe AD.

In terms of efficacy in the treatment of mild-to-moderate AD, patients treated with the cholinesterase inhibitors showed statistically significantly less deterioration than placebo-treated patients in randomized controlled trials generally extending over a 6-month period. The cognitive assessment sensitive in this range is known as the ADAS-Cog (Alzheimer's Disease Assessment Scale, Cognitive subscale) (Rosen et al., 1984). They also demonstrated statistically significant improvement on an overall assessment of change known as the CIBIC (Clinician's Interview Based Impression of Change) (Reisberg, Schneider, et al., 1997).

However, clinicians should recognize that the magnitude of these effects is not large. For example, in controlled trials, efficacy is demonstrable with sample sizes larger than 100 subjects per group. Smaller sample sizes would not necessarily show statistical significance. Also, the MMSE is optimally sensitive in this mild-to-moderate dementia range. Nevertheless, MMSE scores do not necessarily show statistically significant effects, and the overall magnitude of change on the MMSE with these agents is slightly more than 1 point. What this means for clinicians in part is that the magnitude of the effects of the cholinesterase inhibitors is clearly much too small for clinicians to see or make judgments for individual patients.

The three currently utilized cholinesterase inhibitors differ to some extent in their duration of action and in their side effect profiles. As cholinesterase inhibitors, all can produce cholinergic side effects. These include nausea; increased secretions, including salivation and a tendency to cough; loose stools; and in some cases, emesis. Donepezil is relatively long acting and can be administered on a once-daily schedule. It can cause nightmares and insomnia and is therefore preferentially administered in the morning rather than at night. It tends to be relatively well tolerated, particularly when administered in a 5 mg dosage in the morning.

Rivastigmine differs from donepezil in that it is particularly important to start at the low dosage strength (i.e., 1.5 mg twice daily). Cholinergic side effects are common at the higher dosage, so many patients may be treated with less than the maximum dose. It can be argued that these procedures are associated with treatment utilizing the maximum tolerated cholinesterase inhibition.

Like rivastigmine, galantamine is administered on a twice-daily basis. The recommended starting dose is 4 mg twice daily, and a maximum of either 8 mg twice daily or 12 mg twice daily can be given over a titration period of several weeks (4 weeks minimum between dosage increments). It is recommended that rivastigmine and galantamine be given with meals; however, donepezil can be administered with or without food.

Studies have indicated that cholinesterase inhibitors may be particularly efficacious in patients with DLB. A study has indicated that galantamine was efficacious in patients with vascular dementia (Erkinjuntti et al., 2002). Consequently, the role of cholinesterase inhibitors appears to be extending to dementing disorders in addition to AD.

More recently, an entirely different neurochemical approach to the treatment of AD has been approved in the United States and in Europe (specifically by the Committee for Proprietary and Medicinal Products [CPMP] of the European Union). This treatment approach works on the glutaminergic/NMDA (N-methyl-D-aspartate) chemical messenger/receptor system.

Glutamate is the major excitatory neurotransmitter in the brain (Orrego & Villanueva, 1993). Under conditions of neurodegeneration, there is an excess of glutaminergic neurotransmission presynaptically. This excess results in overstimulation of the postsynaptic neuron (Lipton & Rosenberg, 1994). One major glutaminergic receptor on the postsynaptic neuron is the NMDA receptor. This receptor mediates a process known as long-term potentiation, a process associated with the postsynaptic formation of a "memory trace" (Shimizu et al., 2000). The compound memantine is believed to block the NMDA receptor in a reversible manner (i.e., it is an uncompetitive NMDA receptor antagonist) and thereby mitigate glutamate-induced excitotoxicity (Danysz et al., 2000) induced by neurodegenerative conditions such as AD.

Although memantine was marketed in Germany for many years, until recently there were no studies that demonstrated its utility using current diagnostic and assessment standards. Two such studies have now been completed and formed the basis for European Union and US Food and Drug Administration (FDA) approval (Reisberg et al., 2003; Winblad & Poritis, 1999).

The first study was conducted in a mixed dementia population with AD and vascular dementia, GDS stages 5 to 7, in several nursing homes in Latvia (Winblad & Poritis, 1999). The other study was a US multicenter trial with outpatients with a GDS stage of 5 or above, a FAST stage of 6a or above, and an MMSE range of 14 to 3 (Reisberg et al., 2003). These studies resulted in the European approval of memantine for severe AD, a condition for which no treatments were previously approved. The effects of this treatment approach on less-severe stages of AD are currently under investigation.

The second major form of pharmacological treatment in AD is the remediation of the commonly occurring BPSD manifestations shown in Table 16-4 (Reisberg et al., 1987). A general rule is that these BPSD symptoms should only be treated if they are troubling or burdensome for the caregiver(s) of the AD patient or a source of distress or danger for the AD patient. This rule is particularly important because many of these symptoms are a logical or therapeutic response to the patient's changed level of cognition and capacity.

For example, patients with moderate and moderately severe AD commonly develop a fear of being left alone (Reisberg, Franssen, et al., 1989). This fear and anxiety are expressed concomitantly with the patient's decreased capacity to care for themselves independently. Consequently, treating this appropriate anxiety pharmacologically may not be in the best interest of the patient because the pharmacological treatment might mask the patient's genuine need for assistance.

Another common example of a BPSD symptom for which pharmacological treatment might be deleterious for the patient is pacing. This symptom commonly occurs in patients with moderately severe impairment from AD (Reisberg, Franssen, et al., 1989). Pharmacological treatment that simply reduces the level of mobility and activity may be deleterious to the patient's physical health and well-being because it decreases the patient's movement and increases the tendency toward increased joint rigidity that occurs in these stages and appears to eventuate in contractures and very severe physical disabilities that are very seriously detrimental to the patient's comfort and health (Franssen et al., 1991, 1993; Souren et al., 1995).

In terms of pharmacological treatment of BPSD, experience and research (Reisberg et al., 1987) indicate that the BPSD symptoms generally respond particularly well to a low dosage of neuroleptic treatment when the symptoms occur in the patient who is mildly or moderately impaired by AD (i.e., GDS stages 4 and 5). BPSD symptoms peak in terms of magnitude of disturbance in moderately severe AD (GDS stage 6). Treatment of these symptoms in this stage also becomes particularly difficult.

The advent of the newer, so-called atypical, neuroleptics represents a major advance pharmacologically in the treatment of these symptoms. Evidence for efficacy with pharmacological treatment is particularly compelling for risperidone (De Deyn et al., 1999; Katz et al., 1999). In the study of Katz and colleagues (1999), the magnitude of severity of the "paranoid and delusional ideation" and "aggressivity" symptomatic categories on the Behavioral Pathology in Alzheimer's Disease Rating Scale (BEHAVE-AD) (Reisberg et al., 1987) decreased by approximately 50% with the optimal dosage of risperidone treatment (1 mg per day in this 12-week trial). However, the placebo-treated patients in this study of Katz and colleagues and in other BPSD studies improved at approximately 50% of the extent of the pharmacologically treated patients, emphasizing the importance of nonpharmacological approaches as well as pharmacological treatments.

In terms of pharmacological treatment of BPSD symptomatology, the clinical adage "start low, go slow" applies. For risperidone treatment, this rule translates into an optimal starting dose of 0.25 mg daily. Although clinical circumstances dictate the schedule of dosage titration, an optimal clinical response is not achieved for many weeks on any particular dosage of medication. Also, extrapyramidal side effects may not peak until a patient has been on a particular dosage of medication for as long as 6 months (Stephen & Williamson, 1984). Therefore, ideally, the clinician should endeavor to leave a patient on a particular dosage of medication for many weeks before further dosage adjustments. The exigencies of particular situations, of course, will frequently not permit this time luxury in dose adjustments, and clinicians will frequently need to make rapid dosage adjustments. However, the clinician should also be prepared to adjust medication dosage downward as well as upward in response to particular patient needs and the emergence of side effects. After some months of treatment, a steady-state dosage of approximately 0.25 to 1 mg of risperidone daily is frequently effective in controlling BPSD symptoms.

Pharmacological treatment should always be given in conjunction with nonpharmacological treatment approaches. Also, the emergence of extrapryamidal symptoms, including rigidity and akathasia, is a continuing concern with risperidone treatment of BPSD. Other atypical neuroleptics, such as olanzapine, have less tendency to produce extrapyramidal side effects than risperidone. A study of nursing home patients found an optimal response with 5 mg of olanzapine daily (Street et al., 2000). The most frequent side effects were somnolence and gait disturbance.

Treatment of BPSD symptomatology in the patients with AD with traditional, so-called typical, neuroleptic agents such as haloperidol can cause severe problems. With acute or intramuscular dosing, falling is a major problem (Caligiuri et al., 1991). The more severely the patient is affected by AD, the greater the gait and balance disturbance of the patient (Franssen et al., 1991, 1993, 1999) and the greater the likelihood of falling. Extrapyramidal symptoms are a great concern with haloperidol usage. Resulting rigidity can cause loss of ambulation and even a decreased capacity to eat or swallow (Rohrbaugh & Siegal, 1989). In a milder form, the rigidity can result in decreased participation in activities. The emergence of akathasia with haloperidol usage can result in an increase in agitation and a consequent increase in the same symptoms the clinician is treating with the medication. It is often impossible to distinguish akathasia as a medication side effect from the activity disturbances resulting from AD. Under these circumstances, the clinician frequently increases the medication dosage and thereby worsens the condition of the patient.

Depressive symptoms are also common in patients with mild to moderate AD (GDS stages 4 and 5), and a fully manifest major depressive disorder may occur. Depressive symptoms such as dysphoric mood with associated anxieties or sleep disturbance may respond to antidepressant pharmacological treatment. Many clinicians treat sleep disturbances of patients with AD with sedating antidepressant medications. One commonly used medication for this purpose is trazodone. Another useful medication is a low dose of doxepin (i.e., approximately 10 mg to 25 mg), which generally produces sedation with very few anticholinergic side effects.

Behavioral problems and agitation continue to wax and wane throughout the course of moderately severe AD (GDS stage 6), a stage that lasts, as noted, an average of 2.5 years. Control of these symptoms is a major problem at this point in the illness.

In severe AD (GDS stage 7), behavioral symptoms abate and continue to decline as this stage advances over the course of years. A symptom that sometimes becomes dramatically manifest at this point in the illness is screaming (Teri et al., 1992). This symptom is actually quite infrequent. However, when it occurs, it is dramatic and can be a major problem. Screaming generally occurs in patients who have excess physical disability in addition to their severe AD, such as patients with AD who can still speak some words but have lost the ability to ambulate or patients with severe sensory disturbances in addition to their severe dementia. Above all, it is the clinician's responsibility to investigate whether the patient has been injured or developed a new, painful medical condition. Only after ruling out such remediable causes should other treatment decisions be made. Screaming generally does not respond to pharmacological intervention, and nonpharmacological management and treatment should be the primary modality. Treatment of other BPSD symptoms in this final stage is similar to the previous stage; however, in general the dosages of medication can be gradually reduced as this final stage progresses.

Nonpharmacological Treatment of Behavioral Disturbances

It is important for the clinician to recognize that pharmacological approaches alone are inadequate for the treatment of behavioral disturbances in AD. These disturbances are related to various factors, notably including (1) the patient's inability to channel his or her energies in useful directions; (2) the patient's anger and fear regarding reduced capacities; (3) the spouse's anger at the disastrous turn of events the illness has imposed on him or her and the patient's response to the spouse's anger; (4) the patient's anxieties and discomfort regarding being bathed and dressed and the advent of incontinence; and (5) in institutional settings, the understandable patient reaction to institutionalization needs and constraints. The clinician should be prepared to arrange for the mitigation of all of these psychological aspects of AD treatment (Jarvik & Small, 1988; Mace & Rabins, 1981; Rabins et al., 1982; Teri et al., 1992).

For example, in terms of the patient's inability to channel his or her energies in useful directions, an activity planning approach has been advocated for patients cared for in community settings (Tanner & Shaw, 1985). In addition, day care centers for patients with Alzheimer's disease are available in most communities; they provide various kinds of structured activities for patients and simultaneously provide a respite for spouses. When patients with AD are institutionalized, nursing homes provide a full day of structured activities for their residents.

Another treatment approach has been developed for mitigating the cycle of anger and resultant behavioral disturbance that frequently occurs between patients with AD and their caregivers. This cycle of anger and disturbance may be particularly severe between the spouse, who is understandably frustrated and disturbed by the patient's illness, and the patient, who is also frustrated and disturbed by cognitive and other difficulties and losses. The psychological treatment entails a behavioral approach that examines the antecedents of the disturbing behaviors, the nature of the disturbing behaviors themselves, and the consequences of the behavioral disturbance. Having identified these ABCs (antecedents, behaviors, and consequences), efforts are devoted to breaking the cycle of disturbance by appropriate interventions (Teri & Logsdon, 1990).

A "science of AD management" has been suggested based upon recognition of the developmental ages (DAs) corresponding to the AD patient stages (Reisberg et al., 1999, 2002). This approach emphasizes observations that the DA of the AD patient can provide a guide to the overall management and care needs of the patient. This DA can also inform the activities required for AD patient care, the basis of BPSD symptoms, and other aspects pertaining to care needs in AD.

The clinician should also be prepared to intervene to mitigate disturbances associated with the functional losses that occur with the progression of AD. For example, incontinence can be mitigated by a schedule of regular toileting. Nighttime incontinence may be relatively less avoidable. If this occurs, the clinician should be prepared to suggest absorbent bedding and proper procedures for maintaining optimal cleanliness and skin care.

With the progression of AD, patients become less steady on their feet and more fearful regarding the basic mechanisms of activities of daily life, which they no longer fully comprehend. The clinician can assist by suggesting bath rails, bath mats, handheld showers, toilet railings, and the like. When patients become relatively immobile, the clinician should recommend appropriate frequent movement schedules to prevent the occurrence and development of pressure ulcers. Ulcerated skin or soiled clothing from incontinence may result in increased agitation in the patient. The clinician must counsel appropriately regarding the prevention and treatment of these conditions as part of a comprehensive program of treatment of agitation.

PROGNOSIS AND OUTCOME

Table 16-1 provides a synopsis of current understanding regarding the prognosis of AD. A few salient features of the course of AD should be noted:

1. The "border stage" of mild cognitive impairment is frequently not noted clinically or noted only retrospectively. However, when detected at the earliest possible point, generally in a patient who is called on to perform complex occupational tasks, fully a third of the potential clinically manifest time course of AD may be in this stage.
2. Clinicians can generally reliably diagnose degenerative AD from the beginning of GDS stage 4, corresponding to a MMSE score of about 23. The mean duration of AD to a MMSE score of 0, corresponding to the end of GDS stage 6, is about 6 years. Therefore, patients lose approximately an average of 3 to 4 points on the MMSE per year.
3. Most patients succumb after they have become nonverbal, at approximately the point when ambulatory ability and the ability to sit up are lost. Consequently, patients generally survive about 2 to 3 years after the bottoming out of traditional mental status assessments, such as the MMSE. However, some patients survive for 6 or more years in this final stage of severe AD (stage 7 on the GDS and FAST).

The total duration of AD naturally depends on how soon it is detected and how quickly the patient dies, among other factors. The mean time from diagnosis to death is presently approximately 6 to 8 years; however, as shown in Table 16-1, the potential duration of AD from the earliest clinical manifestations to death is about 20 years. Age and gender have not been shown to influence the course of AD. Excess morbidity, such as the occurrence of cerebral infarctions (mixed dementia), appears to result in a more rapid clinical deterioration. The influence of most AD risk factors, such as APOE genotype, on AD course appears to be negligible or is presently unknown. However, some familial, early-onset, genetically based forms of AD appear to manifest a more rapid deteriorating course than the common, later-life onset forms of AD.

The most common cause of death in AD is pneumonia, generally associated with aspiration. Patients with severe AD have decreased capacity to masticate and swallow food. Consequently, a soft food or liquid diet becomes necessary, and proper time must be devoted to feeding. Even with proper care, aspiration may occur. Psychotropic medication may further interfere with swallowing and increase the tendency to aspiration as a result of extrapyramidal and other side effects. Progressive immobility also predisposes to pneumonia.

A second major cause of morbidity and death in the final stage of AD is decubital ulceration. Proper motility and nursing care is necessary to prevent this common complication. Proper management of incontinence is also essential in preventing ulcerations. If not prevented, ulcerations can serve as a locus of infection, with resultant sepsis, fever, and frequently death.

Patients with AD are also prone to death from stroke, cancer, and other common causes of death in the elderly. For some patients, no specific cause of death is found other than the AD illness process.

ACKNOWLEDGMENTS

This work was supported in part by the US Department of Health and Human Services (DHHS), grants AG03051, AG08051, and AG09127 from the National Institute on Aging of the US National Institutes of Health; by grants 90AR2160 and 90AM2552 from the US DHHS Administration on Aging; by grant M01 RR00096 from the General Clinical Research Center Program of the National Center for Research Resources of the US National Institutes of Health; by the Fisher Center for Alzheimer's Disease Research Foundation; and by a grant from William Silberstein.

REFERENCES

Agbayewa O. Earlier psychiatric morbidity in patients with Alzheimer's disease. *J Am Geriatr Soc.* 1986;34:561–564.

Allen RL, Walker Z, D'Ath PJ, Katona CLE. Risperidone for psychotic and behavioral symptoms in Lewy body dementia. *Lancet.* 1995;346:185.

Alzheimer A. Uber eine eigenartige Erkrankung der Hirnrinde. *Allgemeine Z Psychiatr Psychisch-Gerichtlich Med.* 1907;64:146–148.

American Psychiatric Association. *Diagnostic and Statistical Manual of Mental Disorders.* 4th ed. Washington, DC: American Psychiatric Association; 1994.

Arendt T. Alzheimer's disease as a disorder of mechanisms underlying structural brain self-organization. *Neuroscience.* 2001;102:723–765.

Auer SR, Sclan SG, Yaffee RA, Reisberg B. The neglected half of Alzheimer disease: cognitive and functional concomitants of severe dementia. *J Am Geriatr Soc.* 1994; 42:1266–1272.

Baillie M. *The Morbid Anatomy of Some of the Most Important Parts of the Human Body (1795).* Oceanside, NY: Dabo; 1977.

Baker FM, Kokmen E, Chandra V, Schoenberg BS. Psychiatric symptoms in cases of clinically diagnosed Alzheimer's disease. *J Geriatr Psychiatry Neurol.* 1991;4: 71–78.

Ballard C, Grace J, McKeith I, Holmes C. Neuroleptic sensitivity in dementia with Lewy bodies and Alzheimer's disease. *Lancet.* 1998;351:1032–1033.

Bancher C, Lassmann H, Budka H, et al. Neurofibrillary tangles in Alzheimer's disease and progressive supranuclear palsy: antigenic similarities and differences. *Acta Neuropathol.* 1987;74:39–46.

Barclay LL, Zemcov A, Blass JP, McDowell FH. Factors associated with duration of survival in Alzheimer's disease. *Biol Psychiatry.* 1985;20:86–93.

Bartus RT, Dean RL, Beer B, Lippa AS. The cholinergic hypothesis of geriatric memory dysfunction. *Science.* 1982;217:408–417.

Basavaraju NG, Silverstone F, Libow L, Paraskeros K. Primitive reflexes and perceptual sensory tests in the elderly—their usefulness in dementia. *J Chronic Dis.* 1981;34: 367–377.

Beal MF. Energy, oxidative damage, and Alzheimer's disease: clues to the underlying puzzle. *Neurobiol Aging.* 1994;15:S171–S174.

Berg L. Clinical Dementia Rating. *Br J Psychiatry.* 1984;145:339.

Berg L. Clinical Dementia Rating (CDR). *Psychopharmacol Bull.* 1988;24:637–639.

Besson JAO. Magnetic resonance imaging and spectroscopy in dementia. In: Burns A, Levy R, eds. *Dementia.* London, England: Chapman and Hall; 1994:427–436.

Billig N, Cohen-Mansfield J, Lipson S. Pharmacological treatment of agitation in a nursing home. *J Am Geriatr Soc.* 1991;39:1002–1005.

Blessed G, Tomlinson BE, Roth M. The association between quantitative measures of dementia and senile change in the cerebral gray matter of elderly subjects. *Br J Psychiatry.* 1968;114:797–811.

Bolla KI, Lindgren KN, Bonaccorsy C, Bleecker ML. Memory complaints in older adults: fact or fiction? *Arch Neurol.* 1991;48:61–64.

Bondareff W, Mountjoy CQ, Roth M. Loss of neurons of origin of the adrenergic projection to cerebral cortex (nucleus locus ceruleus) in senile dementia. *Neurology (NY).* 1982;32:164–168.

Bowen DM, Allen SJ, Benton JS, et al. Biochemical assessment of serotonergic and cholinergic dysfunction and cerebral atrophy in Alzheimer's disease. *J Neurochem.* 1983;41:266–272.

Bowen J, Teri L, Kukull W, McCormick W, McCurry SM, Larson EB. Progression to dementia in patients with isolated memory loss. *Lancet.* 1997;349:763–765.

Braak H, Braak E. Neuropathological staging of Alzheimer related changes. *Acta Neuropathol (Berlin).* 1991;82:239–259.

Breslau J, Starr A, Sicotte N, Higa J, Buchsbaum MS. Topographic EEG changes with normal aging and SDAT. *Electroencephalogr Clin Neurophysiol.* 1989;72:281–289.

Buerger K, Teipel SJ, Zinkowski R, et al. CSF tau protein phosphorylated at threonine 231 correlates with cognitive decline in MCI subjects. *Neurology.* 2002;59:627–629.

Buerger K, Zinkowski R, Teipel SJ, et al. Differential diagnosis of Alzheimer disease with cerebrospinal fluid levels of tau protein phosphorylated at threonine 231. *Arch Neurol.* 2002;59:1267–1272.

Burns A. Computed tomography. In: Copeland JRM, Abou-Saleh MT, Blazer DG, eds. *Principles and Practice of Geriatric Psychiatry.* Chichester, UK: John Wiley and Sons; 1994:467–471.

Burns A, Jacoby R, Levy R. Psychiatric phenomena in Alzheimer's disease. 1. Disorders of thought content. *Br J Psychiatry.* 1990a;157:72–76.

Burns A, Jacoby R, Levy R. Psychiatric phenomena in Alzheimer's disease. 2. Disorders of perception. *Br J Psychiatry* 1990b;157:76–81.

Buschke H, Fuld PA. Evaluating storage, retention and retrieval in disordered memory and learning. *Neurology.* 1974;11:1019–1025.

Caligiuri MP, Lohr JB, Jeste DV. Instrumental evidence that age increases motor instability in neuroleptic-treated patients. *J Gerontol.* 1991;46:B197–B200.

Chandler JD, Chandler JE. The prevalence of neuropsychiatric disorder in a nursing home population. *J Geriatr Psychiatry Neurol.* 1988;1:71–76.

Christensen H. The validity of memory complaints by elderly persons. *Int J Geriatr Psychiatry.* 1991;6:307–312.

Chui HC. Vascular dementia, a new beginning. Shifting focus from clinical phenotype to ischemic brain injury. *Neurol Clin.* 2001;18:951–977.

Coben LA, Chi D, Snyder AZ, Storandt M. Replication of a study of frequency of the resting awake EEG in mild probable Alzheimer's disease. *Electroencephalogr Clin Neurophysiol.* 1990;75:148–154.

Corder EH, Saunders AM, Strittmatter WJ, et al. Gene dose of apolipoprotein E type 4 allele and the risk of Alzheimer's disease in late onset families. *Science.* 1993;261: 921–923.

Coyle JT, Price DL, DeLong MR. Alzheimer's disease: a disorder of cortical cholinergic innervation. *Science.* 1983;219:1184–1190.

Crook T, Bartus RT, Ferris SH, Whitehouse P, Cohen GD, Gershon S. Age-associated memory impairment: proposed diagnostic criteria and measures of clinical change—report of a NIMH Work Group. *Dev Neuropsychol.* 1986;2:261–276.

Cross AJ, Crow TJ, Ferrier IN, Johnson JA, Bloom SR, Corsellis JAN. Serotonin receptor changes in dementia of the Alzheimer type. *J Neurochem.* 1984;43:1574–1581.

Cross AJ, Crow TJ, Johnson JA, et al. Studies on neurotransmitter receptor systems in neocortex and hippocampus in senile dementia of the Alzheimer-type. *J Neurol Sci.* 1984;64:109–117.

Crum RM, Anthony JC, Bassett SS, Folstein MF. Population-based norms for the Mini-Mental State Examination by age and educational level. *JAMA.* 1993;269:2386–2391.

Cummings JL, Miller B, Hill M, Neshkes R. Neuropsychiatric aspects of multi-infarct dementia and dementia of the Alzheimer type. *Arch Neurol.* 1987;44:389–393.

Daly E, Zaitchik D, Copeland M, Schmahmann J, Gunther J, Albert M. Predicting conversion to Alzheimer disease using standardized clinical information. *Arch Neurol.* 2000;57:675–680.

Danysz W, Parsons CG, Möbius HJ, Stöffler A, Quack G. Neuroprotective and symptomatological action of memantine relevant for Alzheimer's disease—a unified glutamatergic hypothesis on the mechanism of action. *Neurotox Res.* 2000;2:85–98.

Davies P, Maloney AJF. Selective loss of central cholinergic neurons in Alzheimer's disease. *Lancet.* 1976;2:1403.

De Deyn PP, Rabheru K, Rasmussen A, et al. A randomized trial of risperidone, placebo, and haloperidol for behavioral symptoms of dementia. *Neurology.* 1999;53:946–955.

de Leon MJ, Convit A, Wolf OT, et al. Prediction of cognitive decline in normal elderly subjects with 2-[18F]fluoro-2-deoxy-D-glucose/positron-emission tomography (FDG/ PET). *Proc Natl Acad Sci U S A.* 2001;98:10966–10971.

de Leon MJ, Ferris SH, Blau I, et al. Correlations between CT changes and behavioral deficits in senile dementia. *Lancet.* October 20, 1979:859–860.

de Leon MJ, Golomb J, George AE, et al. Hippocampal formation atrophy: prognostic significance for Alzheimer's disease. In: Corain B, Iqbal K, Nicolini M, Wisniewski H, Zatta P, eds. *Alzheimer's Disease: Advances in Clinical and Basic Research.* Chichester, UK: John Wiley and Sons; 1993a:35–46.

de Leon MJ, Golomb J, George AE, et al. The radiologic prediction of Alzheimer's disease: the atrophic hippocampal formation. *Am J Neuroradiol.* 1993b:14:897–906.

de Leon MJ, Segal S, Tarshish CY, et al. Longitudinal cerebrospinal fluid tau load increases in mild cognitive impairment in humans. *Neurosci Lett.* 2002;333:183–186.

Del Ser T, Hachinski V, Merskey H, Munoz DG. Clinical and pathologic features of two groups of patients with dementia with Lewy bodies: effect of coexisting Alzheimer-type lesion load. *Alzheimer Dis Assoc Disord.* 2001;15:31–44.

De Santi S, de Leon MJ, Rusinek H, et al. Hippocampal formation glucose metabolism and volume losses in MCI and AD. *Neurobiol Aging.* 2001;22:529–539.

De Toledo-Morrell L, Goncharova I, Dickerson B, Wilson RS, Bennett DA. From healthy aging to early Alzheimer's disease: in vivo detection of entorhinal cortex atrophy. *Ann N Y Acad Sci.* 2000;911:240–253.

Devanand DP, Folz M, Gorlyn M, Moesller JR, Stern Y. Questionable dementia: clinical course and predictors of outcome. *J Am Geriatr Soc.* 1997;45:321–328.

Dichgans M, Mayer M, Uttner I, et al. The phenotypic spectrum of CADASIL: clinical findings in 102 cases. *Ann Neurol.,* 1998;44:731–739.

Drevets W, Rubin E. Psychotic symptoms and the longitudinal course of senile dementia of the Alzheimer type. *Biol Psychiatry.* 1989;25:39–48.

Eagles JM, Beattie JAG, Restall DB, Rawlinson F, Hagen S, Ashcroft GW. Relation between cognitive impairment and early death in the elderly. *BMJ.* 1990;300:239–240.

Erkinjuntti T, Gao F, Lee DH, Eliasziw M, Merskey H, Hachinski VC. Lack of difference in brain hyperintensities between patients with early Alzheimer's disease and control subjects. *Arch Neurol.* 1994;51:260–268.

Erkinjuntti T, Kurz A, Gauthier S, Bullock R, Lilienfeld S, Damaraju CV. Efficacy of galantamine in probable vascular dementia and Alzheimer's disease combined with cerebrovascular disease: a randomized trial. *Lancet.* 2002;359:1283–1290.

Esch FS, Keim PS, Beattie EC, et al. Cleavage of amyloid beta peptide during constitutive processing of its precursor. *Science.* 1990;248:1122–1124.

Evans DA, Funkenstein HH, Albert MS, et al. Prevalence of Alzheimer's disease in a community population of older persons: higher than previously reported. *JAMA.* 1989;262:2551–2556.

Farlow M, Anand R, Messina J, Hartman R, Veach J. A 52-week study of the efficacy of rivastigmine in patients with mild to moderately severe Alzheimer's disease. *Eur Neurol.* 2000;44:236–241.

Feldman H, Gauthier S, Hecker J, et al. A 24-week, randomized, double-blind study of donepezil in moderate to severe Alzheimer's disease. *Neurology.* 2001;57:613–620.

Ferris SH, Crook T, Clark E, McCarthy M, Rae D. Facial recognition memory deficits in normal aging and senile dementia. *J Gerontol.* 1980;35:707–714.

Ferris SH, de Leon MJ, Wolf AP, et al. Positron emission tomography in the study of aging and senile dementia. *Neurobiol Aging*. 1980;1:127–131.

Finkel SI, guest ed. Behavioral and psychological signs and symptoms of dementia: implications for research and treatment. *Int Psychogeriatr*. 1996;8(Suppl 3).

Finkel SI, Burns A, guest eds. Behavioral and psychological symptoms of dementia: a clinical and research update. *Int Psychogeriatr*. 2000;12(Suppl 1).

Flicker C, Bartus RT, Crook T, Ferris SH. Effects of aging and dementia upon recent visuospatial memory. *Neurobiol Aging*. 1984;5:275–283.

Flicker C, Ferris SH, Reisberg B. Mild cognitive impairment in the elderly: predictors of dementia. *Neurology*. 1991;41:1006–1009.

Flicker C, Ferris SH, Reisberg B. A two-year longitudinal study of cognitive function in normal aging and Alzheimer's disease. *J Geriatr Psychiatry Neurol*. 1993;6:84–96.

Folstein MF, Folstein SE, McHugh PR. Mini-Mental State: a practical method for grading the cognitive state of patients for the clinician. *J Psychiatry Res*. 1975;12:189–198.

Forstl H, Burns A, Luthert P, Cairns N, Lantos P, Levy R. Clinical and neuropathological correlates of depression in Alzheimer's disease. *Psychol Med*. 1992;22:877–884.

Fox NC, Crum WR, Scahill RI, Stevens JM, Janssen JC, Rossor MN. Imaging of onset and progression of Alzheimer's disease with voxel-compression mapping of serial magnetic resonance images. *Lancet*. 2001;358:201–205.

Franssen EH, Kluger A, Torossian CL, Reisberg B. The neurologic syndrome of severe Alzheimer's disease: relationship to functional decline. *Arch Neurol*. 1993;50:1029–1039.

Franssen EH, Reisberg B, Kluger A, Sinaiko E, Boja C. Cognition-independent neurologic symptoms in normal aging and probable Alzheimer's disease. *Arch Neurol*. 1991;48:148–154.

Franssen EH, Souren LEM, Torossian CL, Reisberg B. Utility of developmental reflexes in the differential diagnosis and prognosis of incontinence in Alzheimer's disease. *J Geriatr Psychiatry Neurol*. 1997;10:22–28.

Franssen EH, Souren LEM, Torossian CL, Reisberg B. Equilibrium and limb coordination in mild cognitive impairment and mild Alzheimer's disease. *J Am Geriatr Soc*. 1999;47:463–499.

Geerlings MI, Jonker C, Bouter LM, Ader HJ, Schmand B. Association between memory complaints and incident Alzheimer's disease in elderly people with normal baseline cognition. *Am J Psychiatry*. 1999;156:531–537.

Gemmell HG, Sharp PF, Besson JA, et al. Differential diagnosis in dementia using the cerebral blood flow agent 99m-Tc-HMPAO: a SPECT study. *J Comput Assist Tomogr*. 1987;11:398–402.

German PS, Shapiro S, Kramer M. Nursing home study of the eastern Baltimore epidemiological catchment area study. In: Harper MS, Lebowitz B, eds. *Mental Illness in Nursing Homes: Agenda for Research*. Washington. DC: National Institute of Mental Health; 1985.

Gershon S, Ferris SH, Kennedy JS, et al. Methods for the evaluation of pharmacologic agents in the treatment of cognitive and other deficits in dementia. In: Prien RF, Robinson DS, eds. *Clinical Evaluation of Psychotropic Drugs: Principles and Guidelines*. New York, NY: Raven Press; 1994:467–499.

Go RCP, Todorov AB, Elston RC, Constantinidis J. The malignancy of dementias. *Ann Neurol*. 1978;3:559–561.

Goate A, Chartier-Harlin M-C, Mullan M, et al. Segregation of a missense mutation in the amyloid precursor protein gene with familial Alzheimer's disease. *Nature*. 1991; 349:704–706.

Golde TE, Estus S, Younkin LH, Selkoe DJ, Younking SG. Processing of the amyloid protein precursor to potentially amyloidogenic fragments. *Science*. 1992;255:728–730.

Goldfarb A. Predicting mortality in the institutionalized aged. *Arch Gen Psychiatry*. 1969;21:172–176.

Goldgaber D, Lerman MI, McBride OW, Saffiotti U, Gajdusek DC. Characterization and chromosomal localization of a cDNA encoding brain amyloid of Alzheimer's disease. *Science*. 1987;235:877–880.

Golomb J, Kluger A, de Leon MJ, et al. Hippocampal formation size predicts declining memory performance in normal aging. *Neurology*. 1996;47:810–813.

Grafman J, Litvan I. Importance of deficits in executive function. *Lancet*. 1999;354: 1921–1923.

Grober E, Lipton RB, Hall C, Crystal H. Memory impairment on free and cued selective reminding predicts dementia. *Neurology*. 2000;54:827–832.

Gurland BJ, Wilder DE, Cross P, Teresi JA, Barrett VW. Screening scales for dementia: toward a reconciliation of conflicting cross-cultural findings. *Int J Geriatr Psychiatry*. 1992;7:105–113.

Haass C, Koo E, Mellon A, Hung A, Selkoe D. Targeting of cell-surface beta-amyloid precursor protein to lysosomes: alternative processing into amyloid-bearing fragments. *Nature*. 1992;357:500–503.

Hachinski VC. Differential diagnosis of Alzheimer's dementia: multi-infarct dementia. In: Reisberg B, ed. *Alzheimer's Disease*. New York, NY: Free Press; 1983:188–192.

Hachinski VC, Lassen NA, Marshall J. Multi-infarct dementia, a cause of mental deterioration in the elderly. *Lancet*. 1974;2:207–210.

Hampel H, Teipel SJ, Alexander GE, Pogarell O, Rapoport SI, Moller H-J. In vivo imaging of region and cell type specific neocortical neurodegeneration in Alzheimer's disease. *J Neural Transm*. 2002;109:837–855.

Hänninen T, Hallikainen M, Koivisto K, et al. A follow-up study of age-associated memory impairment: neuropsychological predictors of dementia. *J Am Geriatr Soc*. 1995;43:1007–1015.

Haxby JV, Grady CL, Duara R, Schlageter N, Berg G, Rapoport SI. Neocortical metabolic abnormalities precede nonmemory cognitive defects in early Alzheimer's-type dementia. *Arch Neurol*. 1986;43:882–885.

Hofman A, Ott A, Breteler MMB, et al. Atherosclerosis, apolipoprotein E, and prevalence of dementia and Alzheimer's disease in the Rotterdam Study. *Lancet*. 1997; 349:151–154.

Huckman MS, Fox J, Topel J. The validity of criteria for the evaluation of cerebral atrophy by computed tomography. *Radiology*. 1975;116:85–92.

Huff FJ, Boller F, Luchelli F, Querriera R, Beyer J, Belle S. The neurologic examination in patient's with probable Alzheimer's disease. *Arch Neurol*. 1987;44:929–932.

Huff FJ, Growdon JH. Neurological abnormalities associated with severity of dementia in Alzheimer's disease. *Can J Neurol Sci*. 1986;13:403–405.

Hughes CP, Berg L, Danziger WL, Coben LA, Martin RL. A new clinical scale for the staging of dementia. *Br J Psychiatry*. 1982;140:566–572.

Hughes CP, Berg L, Danziger WL, Coben LA, Martin RL. Clinical Dementia Rating

(CDR) scale. In: Task Force for the Handbook of Psychiatric Measures, eds. *Handbook of Psychiatric Measures*. Washington, DC: American Psychiatric Association; 2000:446–450.

Hughes JR, Shanmugham S, Wetzel LC, Bellur S, Hughes CA. The relationship between EEG changes and cognitive functions in dementia: a study in a VA population. *Clin Electroencephalogr.* 1989;202:77–85.

Hurwitz T, Ammann W, Chu D, Clark C, Holden J, Brownstone R. Single photon emission computed tomography using 99m-Tc-HM-PAO in the routine evaluation of Alzheimer's disease. *Can J Neurol Sci.* 1991;18:59–62.

Jarvik L, Small G. *Parentcare: A Commonsense Guide for Adult Children.* New York, NY: Crown; 1988.

Jarvik LF, Falek A. Intellectual stability and survival in the aged. *J Gerontol.* 1963;18: 173–176.

Jelic V, Johansson SE, Almkvist O, et al. Quantitative electroencephalography in mild cognitive impairment longitudinal changes and possible prediction of Alzheimer's disease. *Neurobiol Aging.* 2000;21:533–540.

Jick H, Zornberg GL, Jick SS, Seshadri S, Drachman DA. Statins and the risk of dementia. *Lancet.* 2000;356:1627–1631.

Jorm AF, Christensen H, Korten AE, Henderson AS, Jacomb PA, Mackinnon A. Do cognitive complaints either predict future cognitive decline or reflect past cognitive decline? A longitudinal study of an elderly community sample. *Psychol Med.* 1997; 27:91–98.

Kang J, Lemaire HG, Unterbeck A, et al. The precursor of Alzheimer's disease amyloid βA4 protein resembles a cell-surface receptor. *Nature.* 1987;325:733–736.

Kaszniak AW, Fox J, Gandell DL, Garron DC, Huckman MS, Ramsey RG. Predictors of mortality in presenile and senile dementia. *Ann Neurol.* 1978;3:246–252.

Kaszniak AW, Garron DC, Fox JC, Bergen D, Huckman M. Cerebral atrophy, EEG slowing, age, education and cognitive functioning in suspected dementia. *Neurology.* 1979;29:1273–1279.

Katz IR, Jeste DV, Mintzer JE, Clyde C, Napolitano J, Brecher M for the Risperidone Study Group. Comparison of risperidone and placebo for psychosis and behavioral disturbances associated with dementia: a randomized, double-blind trial. *J Clin Psychiatry.* 1999;60:107–115.

Katzman R. Alzheimer's disease. *N Engl J Med.* 1986;314:964–973.

Kety S, Schmidt C. The nitrous oxide method for quantitative determination of cerebral blood flow in man: theory, procedure and normal values. *J Clin Invest.* 1948;27: 475–483.

Khachaturian ZS. (1985). Diagnosis of Alzheimer's disease. *Arch Neurol.* 1985;42: 1097–1105.

Kidd M. Paired helical filaments in electron microscopy in Alzheimer's disease. *Nature.* 1963;197:192–193.

Killiany RJ, Gomez-Isla T, Moss M, et al. Use of structural magnetic resonance imaging to predict who will get Alzheimer's disease. *Ann Neurol.* 2000;47:430–439.

Kiuchi A, Otsuka N, Namba Y, Nakano I, Tomonaga H. Presenile appearance of abundant Alzheimer's neurofibrillary tangles without senile plaques in the brain in myotonic dystrophy. *Acta Neuropathol.* 1991;82:1–5.

Kluger A, Ferris SH, Golomb J, Mittelman MS, Reisberg B. Neuropsychological prediction of decline to dementia in nondemented elderly. *J Geriatr Psychiatry Neurol.* 1999;12:168–179.

Kluger A, Gianutsos J, Golomb J, Ferris SH, Reisberg B. Motor/psychomotor dysfunction in normal aging, mild cognitive decline and early Alzheimer's disease: diagnostic and differential diagnostic features. *Int Psychogeriatr.* 1997;9(Suppl 1):307–316.

Kobayashi S, Ishiguro K, Omori A, et al. A cdc2-related kinase PSSALRE/cdk5 is homologous with the 30kDa subunit of tau protein kinase II, a proline-directed protein kinase associated with microtubule. *Fed Eur Biochem Soc Lett.* 1993;335:171–175.

Kondo J, Honda T, Mori H, et al. The carboxyl third of tau is tightly bound to paired helical filaments. *Neuron.* 1988;1:827–834.

Kosaka K, Yoshimura M, Ikeda K, Budka H. Diffuse type of Lewy body disease: progressive dementia with abundant cortical Lewy bodies and senile changes of varying degree—a new disease? *Clin Neuropathol.* 1984;3:185–192.

Kral VA. Senescent forgetfulness: benign and malignant. *Can Med Assoc J.* 1962;86:257–260.

Kral VA. Depressiv pseudodemenz und senile demenz von Alzheimer-type: eine pilot-studie. *Nervenarzt.* 1982;53:284–288.

Kral VA, Emery OB. Long-term follow-up of depressive pseudodementia of the aged. *Can J Psychiatry.* 1989;34:445–446.

Kumar A, Newberg A, Alavi A, et al. MRI volumetric studies in Alzheimer's disease. *Am J Geriatr Psychiatry.* 1994;2:21–31.

Lane R, Snowdon J. Memory and dementia: a longitudinal survey of suburban elderly. In: Lovibond P, Wilson P, eds. *Clinical and Abnormal Psychology.* Amsterdam, The Netherlands: North-Holland; 1989:365–376.

LaRue A, D'Elia LF, Clark EO, Spar JE, Jarvik LF. Clinical tests of memory in dementia, depression, and healthy aging. *J Psychol Aging.* 1986;1:69–77.

Launer LJ, Ross GW, Petrovik H, et al. Midlife blood pressure and dementia: the Honolulu-Asia aging study. *Neurobiol Aging.* 2000;21:49–55.

Ledesma MD, Correas I, Avila J, Diaznido J. Implication of brain Cdc2 and Map2 kinases in the phosphorylation of tau protein in Alzheimer's disease. *Fed Eur Biochem Soc Lett.* 1992;308:218–224.

Levy E, Carman MD, Fernandez-Madrid IJ, et al. Mutation of the Alzheimer's disease amyloid gene in hereditary cerebral haemorrhage, Dutch type. *Science.* 1990;248:1124–1126.

Lewy FH. Paralysis agitans. I. Pathologische anatomie. In: Lewandowski M, ed. *Handbuch der Neurologie.* Vol. 3/II. Berlin, Germany: Julius Springer; 1912:920–933.

Lipton SA, Rosenberg PA. Excitatory amino acids as a final common pathway for neurologic disorders. *N Engl J Med.* 1994;330:613–622.

Liu DX, Greene LA. Neuronal apoptosis at the G1/S cell cycle checkpoint. *Cell Tissue Res.* 2001;305:217–228.

Lowenthal PM, Berkman PL, Buehler JA, Pierce RC, Robinson BC, Trier ML. *Aging and Mental Disorder in San Francisco: A Social Psychiatric Study.* San Francisco, CA: Jossey Bass; 1967.

Lyketsos CG, Steinberg M, Tschanz JT, Norton MC, Steffens DC, Breitner JCS. Mental and behavioral disturbances in dementia: findings from the Cache County Study on Memory and Aging. *Am J Psychiatry.* 2000;157:708–714.

Mace N, Rabins PV. *The 36-Hour Day*. Baltimore, MD: Johns Hopkins University Press; 1981.

Mann DMA, McDonagh AM, Snowden J, Neary D, Pickering-Brown SM. Molecular classification of the dementias. *Lancet*. 2000;355:626.

Mayeux R, Denaro J, Hemenegildo N, et al. A population-based investigation of Parkinson's disease with and without dementia: relationship to age and gender. *Arch Neurol*. 1992;49:492–497.

McAdam W, Robinson RA. Prognosis in senile deterioration. *J Ment Sci*. 1957;103: 821–823.

McKeith IG, Galasko D, Kosaka K, et al. Consensus guidelines for the clinical and pathologic diagnosis of dementia with Lewy bodies (DLB): report of the consortium on DLB international workshop. *Neurology*. 1996;47:1113–1124.

McKeith IG, Perry EK, Perry RH. For the Consortium on Dementia With Lewy Bodies: Report of the Second Dementia With Lewy Body International Workshop: diagnosis and treatment. *Neurology*. 1999;53:902–905.

McKhann G, Drachman D, Folstein M, Katzman R, Price D, Stadlan EM. Clinical diagnosis of Alzheimer's disease: report of the NINCDS-ADRDA work group under the auspices of Department of Health Human Services Task Force on Alzheimer's Disease. *Neurology*. 1984;34:939–944.

Merriam AE, Aronson M, Gaston P, Wey S, Katz I. The psychiatric symptoms of Alzheimer's disease. *J Am Geriatr Soc*. 1988;36:7–12.

Mirra SS, Heyman A, McKeel D, et al. The consortium to establish a registry for Alzheimer's disease (CERAD). Part II. Standardization of the neuropathologic assessment of Alzheimer's disease. *Neurology*. 1991;41:479–486.

Mohs R, Kim G, Johns C, Dunn D, Davis K. Assessing changes in Alzheimer's disease: memory and language. In: Poon LW, ed. *Handbook for Clinical Memory Assessment*. Washington, DC: American Psychological Association; 1986:149–155.

Molsa PK, Marttila RJ, Rinne UK. Survival and cause of death in Alzheimer's disease and multi-infarct dementia. *Acta Neurol Scand*. 1986;74:103–107.

Mori H, Kondo J, Ihara Y. Ubiquitin is a component of paired helical filaments in Alzheimer's disease. *Science*. 1987;235:1641–1644.

Morris JC. The Clinical Dementia Rating (CDR): current version and scoring rules. *Neurology*. 1993;43:2412–2414.

Morris JC, Storandt M, Miller P, et al. Mild cognitive impairment represents early-stage Alzheimer disease. *Neurology*. 2001;58:397–405.

Mullan M, Crawford F, Axelman K, et al. A pathogenic mutation for probable Alzheimer's disease in the APP gene at the N-terminus of B-amyloid. *Nat Genet*. 1992;1: 345–347.

Murden RA, McRae TD, Kaner S, Bucknam ME. Mini-Mental State Exam scores vary with education in blacks and whites. *J Am Geriatr Soc*. 1991;39:149–155.

Murphy DGM, DeCarli CD, Daly E, et al. Volumetric magnetic resonance imaging in men with dementia of the Alzheimer type: correlations with disease severity. *Biol Psychiatry*. 1993;34:612–621.

Näslund J, Haroutunian V, Mohs R, et al. Correlation between elevated levels of amyloid β-peptide in the brain and cognitive decline. *JAMA*. 2000;283:1571–1577.

Natte R, Maat-Schieman LC, Haan J, Bornebroek RRAC, van Duinen G. Dementia in hereditary cerebral hemorrhage with amyloidosis-Dutch type is associated with cerebral amyloid angiopathy, but is independent of plaques and neurofibrillary tangles. *Ann Neurol.* 2001;50:765–772.

Neary D, Snowden JS, Gustafson L, et al. Frontotemporal lobar degeneration: a consensus on clinical diagnostic criteria. *Neurology.* 1998;51:1546–1554.

Neary D, Snowden JS, Shields RA, et al. Single photon emission tomography using 99m-Tc-HMPAO in the investigation of dementia. *J Neurol Neurosurg Psychiatry.* 1987; 50:1101–1109.

Neugroschl J, Davis KL. Biological markers in Alzheimer's disease. *Am J Geriatr Psychiatry.* 2002;10:660–677.

O'Brien JT, Erkinjuntti T, Reisberg B, et al. Vascular cognitive impairment. *Lancet Neurol.* 2003;2:89–98.

Obrist WD, Chivian E, Cronquist S, Ingvar DH. Regional cerebral blood flow in senile and presenile dementia. *Neurology.* 1970;20:315–322.

Orrego F, Villanueva S. The chemical nature of the main excitatory transmitter: a critical appraisal based upon release studies and synaptic vesicle localization. *Neuroscience.* 1993;56:539–555.

Ott A, Slooter AJ, Hofman A, et al. Smoking and risk of dementia and Alzheimer's disease in a population-based cohort study: the Rotterdam Study. *Lancet.* 1998; 351:1840–1843.

Ott A, Stolk RP, van Harskamp F, Pols HA, Hofman A, Breteler MM. Diabetes mellitus and the risk of dementia: the Rotterdam Study. *Neurology.* 1999;53:1937–1942.

Ouvrier RA, Goldsmith RF, Ouvrier S, Williams IC. The value of the Mini-Mental State Examination in childhood. A preliminary study. *J Child Neurol.* 1993;8:145–148.

Paulson G, Gottlieb G. Developmental reflexes: the reappearance of foetal and neonatal reflexes in aged patients. *Brain.* 1968;91:37–52.

Pearlson GD, Rabins PV, Kim WS, et al. Structural brain CT changes and cognitive deficits in elderly depressives with and without reversible dementia ("pseudodementia"). *Psychol Med.* 1989;19:573–584.

Pericak-Vance MA, Bebout JL, Gaskell PC Jr, et al. Linkage studies in familial Alzheimer's disease: evidence for chromosome 19 linkage. *Am J Hum Genet.* 1991;48: 1034–1050.

Perry EK, Perry RH, Blessed G, Tomlinson BE. Necropsy evidence of central cholinergic deficits in senile dementia. *Lancet.* 1977;1:189.

Perry G, Friedman R, Shaw G, Chau V. Ubiquitin is detected in neurofibrillary tangles and senile plaque neurites of Alzheimer disease brains. *Proc Natl Acad Sci U S A.* 1987;84:3033–3036.

Petersen RC. Mild cognitive impairment: transition between aging and Alzheimer's disease. *Neurologia.* 2000;15:93–101.

Petersen RC, Smith GE, Waring SC, Ivnik RJ, Tangalos EG, Kokmen E. Mild cognitive impairment: clinical characterization and outcome. *Arch Neurol.* 1999;56:303–308.

Petersen RC, Stevens JC, Ganguli M, Tangalos EG, Cummings JL, DeKosky ST. Practice parameter: early detection of dementia: mild cognitive impairment (an evidence-based review). Report of the Quality Standards Subcommittee of the American Academy of Neurology. *Neurology.* 2001;56:1133–1142.

Pfeffer RI, Kurosaki TT, Harrah CH, Chance JM, Files S. Measurement of functional activities in older adults in the community. *J Gerontol.* 1982;37:323–329.

Podreka I, Suess E, Goldenberg G, et al. Initial experience with technetium-99m HM-PAO brain SPECT. *J Nucl Med.* 1987;28:1657–1666.

Poirier J, Davignon J, Bouthillier D, Kogan S, Bertrand P, Gauthier S. Apolipoprotein E polymorphism and Alzheimer's disease. *Lancet.* 1993;342:697–699.

Premkumar DRD, Cohen DL, Hedera P, Friedland RP, Kalaria RN. Apolipoprotein E-ε4 alleles in cerebral amyloid angiopathy and cerebrovascular pathology in Alzheimer's disease. *Am J Pathol.* 1996;148:2083–2095.

Prichep LS, John ER, Ferris SH, et al. Quantitative EEG correlates of cognitive deterioration in the elderly. *Neurobiol Aging.* 1994;15:85–90.

Qin X, Livingston DM, Kaelin WG, Adams GP. Deregulated transcription factor E2F-1 expression leads to S-phase entry and p53-mediated apoptosis. *Proc Natl Acad Sci U S A.* 1994;91:10918–10922.

Rabins P, Mace N, Lucas M. The impact of dementia on the family. *J Am Med Assoc.* 1982;248:333–335.

Rabins PV, Pearlson GD, Jayaram G, Steele C, Tune L. Elevated ventricle-to-brain ratio in late-onset schizophrenia. *Am J Psychiatry.* 1987;144:1216–1218.

Reding AJ, Haycox J, Wigforss K, Brush D, Blass JP. Follow-up of patients referred to a dementia service. *J Am Geriat Soc.* 1984;32:265–268.

Redlich E. Ueber miliare sklerose der Hirnrinde bei seniler Atrophie. *Jahrbucher F Psych Neurol.* 1898;17:208–216.

Reimanis G, Green RF. Imminence of death and intellectual decrement in the aging. *Dev Psychol.* 1971;5:270–272.

Reinikainen KJ, Koivisto K, Mykkänen L, et al. Age-associated memory impairment in aged population: an epidemiologic study. *Neurology.* 1990;40(Suppl 1):177.

Reisberg B. Functional assessment staging (FAST). *Psychopharmacol Bull.* 1988;24:653–659.

Reisberg B. Memory dysfunction and dementia: diagnostic considerations. In: Salzman C, ed. *Clinical Geriatric Psychopharmacology.* 2nd ed. Baltimore, MD: Williams and Wilkins; 1992:255–276.

Reisberg B, Borenstein J, Franssen E, Shulman E, Steinberg G, Ferris SH. Potentially remediable behavioral symptomatology in Alzheimer's disease. *Hosp Community Psychiatry.* 1986;37:1199–1201.

Reisberg B, Borenstein J, Salob SP, Ferris SH, Franssen E, Georgotas A. Behavioral symptoms in Alzheimer's disease: phenomenology and treatment. *J Clin Psychiatry.* 1987;48(Suppl):9–15.

Reisberg B, Burns A, Brodaty H, et al. Diagnosis of Alzheimer's disease: report of an International Psychogeriatric Association Special Meeting Work Group under the cosponsorship of Alzheimer's Disease International, the European Federation of Neurological Societies, the World Health Organization, and the World Psychiatric Association. *Int Psychogeriatr.* 1997;9(Suppl 1):11–38.

Reisberg B, Doody R, Stöffler A, Schmitt F, Ferris S, Möbius H-J for the Memantine Study Group. Memantine in moderate to severe Alzheimer's disease. *N Engl J Med.* 2003;348:1333–1341.

Reisberg B, Ferris SH. Emergency issues in the assessment and management of Alzheimer's disease. In: O'Neill ES, ed. *The Psychiatric Emergency.* New York, NY: Haworth Press; 1986:55–76.

Reisberg B, Ferris SH, de Leon MJ, Crook T. The global deterioration scale for assessment of primary degenerative dementia. *Am J Psychiatry.* 1982;139:1136–1139.

Reisberg B, Ferris SH, de Leon MJ, et al. Stage-specific behavioral, cognitive, and in vivo changes in community residing subjects with age-associated memory impairment (AAMI) and primary degenerative dementia of the Alzheimer type. *Drug Dev Res.* 1988;15:101–114.

Reisberg B, Ferris SH, Franssen E, Kluger A, Borenstein J. Age-associated memory impairment: the clinical syndrome. *Dev Neuropsychol.* 1986;2:401–412.

Reisberg B, Ferris SH, Franssen E, et al. Mortality and temporal course of probable Alzheimer's disease: a five-year prospective study. *Int Psychogeriatr.* 1996;8:291–311.

Reisberg B, Franssen E, Sclan SG, Kluger A, Ferris SH. Stage specific incidence of potentially remediable behavioral symptoms in aging and Alzheimer's disease: a study of 120 patients using the BEHAVE-AD. *Bull Clin Neurosci.* 1989;54:95–112.

Reisberg B, Franssen E, Shah MA, Weigel J, Bobinski M, Wisniewski HM. Clinical diagnosis of dementia. In: Maj M, Sartorius N, eds. *World Psychiatric Association Series: Evidence and Experience in Psychiatry, Vol. 3, Dementia.* Chichester, UK: John Wiley and Sons; 2000:69–115. Commentaries by Larson EB, O'Brien J, Sachdev PS, Heun R, Ransmayr G, Roth Sir M, Finkel SI, Gold G, Kloszewska I, Gifford DR, and Wibisono S, pp. 116–141.

Reisberg B, Franssen EH, Souren LEM, Auer SR, Akram I, Kenowsky S. Evidence and mechanisms of retrogenesis in Alzheimer's and other dementias: management and treatment import. *Am J Alzheimer's Dis.* 2002;17:202–212.

Reisberg B, Kenowsky S, Franssen EH, Auer SR, Souren LEM. President's report: towards a science of Alzheimer's disease management: a model based upon current knowledge of retrogenesis. *Int Psychogeriatr.* 1999;11:7–23.

Reisberg B, Schneider L, Doody R, et al. Clinical global measures of dementia: position paper from the International Working Group on Harmonization of Dementia Drug Guidelines. *Alzheimer Dis Assoc Disord.* 1997;11(Suppl 3):8–18.

Reisberg B, Sclan SG, Franssen E, Kluger A, Ferris S. Dementia staging in chronic care populations. *Alzheimer Dis Assoc Disord.* 1994;8(Suppl 1):S188–S205.

Rewcastle NB, Ball MJ. Electron microscopic structure of the "inclusion bodies" in Pick's disease. *Neurology* 1968;18:1205–1213.

Riemenschneider M, Lautenschlager N, Wagenpfeil S, Diehl J, Drzezga A, Kurz A. Cerebrospinal fluid tau and β-amyloid 42 proteins identify Alzheimer disease in subjects with mild cognitive impairment. *Arch Neurol.* 2002;59:1729–1734.

Roberts MA, Caird FI, Grossart KW, Steven JL. Computerized tomography in the diagnosis of cerebral atrophy. *J Neurol Neurosurg Psychiatry.* 1976;39:905–915.

Rohrbaugh RM, Siegal AP. Reversible anorexia and rapid weight loss associated with neuroleptic administration in Alzheimer's disease. *J Geriatr Psychiatry Neurol.* 1989;2:45–47.

Rosen WG, Mohs RC, Davis KL. A new rating scale for Alzheimer's disease. *Am J Psychiatry.* 1984;141:1356–1364.

Rosen WG, Terry RD, Fuld PA, Katzman R, Peck A. Pathological verification of ischemia score in differentiation of dementias. *Ann Neurol.* 1980;7:486–488.

Roth M. The natural history of mental disorders arising in the senium. *J Ment Sci.* 1955;101:218.

Rovner BW, Kafonek S, Filipp L, Lucas MJ, Folstein MF. Prevalence of mental illness in a community nursing home. *Am J Psychiatry.* 1986;143:1446–1449.

Rubin E, Morris J, Storandt M, Berg L. Behavioral changes in patients with mild senile dementia of the Alzheimer's type. *Psychiatry Res.* 1987;21:55–61.

Schellenberg GD, Bird TD, Wijsman EM, et al. Genetic linkage evidence for a familial Alzheimer's disease locus on chromosome 14. *Science*. 1992;258:668–671.

Sclan SG, Reisberg B. Functional assessment staging (FAST) in Alzheimer's disease: reliability, validity and ordinality. *Int Psychogeriatr*. 1992;4(Suppl 1):55–69.

Seshadri S, Beiser A, Selhub J, et al. Plasma homocysteine as a risk factor for dementia and Alzheimer's disease. *N Engl J Med*. 2002;346:476–483.

Seubert P, Vigo-Pelfrey C, Esch F, et al. Isolation and quantification of soluble Alzheimer's B-peptide from biological fluids. *Nature*. 1992;359:325.

Sherwin BB. Mild cognitive impairment: potential pharmacological treatment options. *J Am Geriatr Soc*. 2000;48:431–441.

Shimada M, Meguro K, Inagaki H, Ishizaki J, Yamadori A. Global intellectual deterioration in Alzheimer's disease and a reverse model of intellectual development: an applicability of the Binet Scale. *Psychiatry Clin Neurosci*. 2001;55:559–563.

Shimizu E, Tang YP, Rampon C, Tsien JZ. NMDA receptor-dependent synaptic reinforcement is a crucial process for memory consolidation. *Science*. 2000;290:1170–1174.

Silverman DHS, Small GW, Chang CY, et al. Positron emission tomography in evaluation of dementia: regional brain metabolism and long-term outcome. *JAMA*. 2001; 286:2120–2127.

Sisodia S, Koo E, Beyreuther K, Unterbeck A, Price D. Evidence that beta-amyloid protein in Alzheimer's disease is not derived by normal processing. *Science*. 1990;248: 492–495.

Skoog I, Lernfelt B, Landahl S. 15-year longitudinal study of blood pressure and dementia. *Lancet*. 1996;347:1141–1145.

Sluss TK, Rabins P, Gruenberg EM. Memory complaints in community residing men [abstract]. *Gerontologist*. 1980;20:201.

Small GW, Ercoli LM, Silverman DHS, et al. Cerebral metabolic and cognitive decline in persons at genetic risk for Alzheimer's disease. *Proc Natl Acad Sci U S A*. 2000; 97:6037–6042.

Small GW, Rabins PV, Barry PP, et al. Diagnosis and treatment of Alzheimer's disease and related disorders: consensus statement of the American Association for Geriatric Psychiatry, the Alzheimer's Association, and the American Geriatrics Society. *JAMA*. 1997;278:1363–1371.

Smith AD. Imaging the progression of Alzheimer's pathology through the brain. *Proc Natl Acad Sci U S A*. 2002;99:4135–4137.

Snowdon DA, Greiner LH, Mortimer JA, Riley KP, Greiner PA, Markesbery WR. Brain infarction and the clinical expression of Alzheimer's disease: the Nun Study. *JAMA*. 1997;277:813–817.

Souren LEM, Franssen EH, Reisberg B. Contractures and loss of function in patients with Alzheimer's disease. *J Am Geriatr Soc*. 1995;43:650–655.

Souren LEM, Franssen EH, Reisberg B. Neuromotor changes in Alzheimer's disease: implications for patient care. *J Geriatr Psychiatry Neurol*. 1997;10:93–98.

Spillane JA, White P, Goodhardt MJ, Flack RH, Bowen DM, Davison AN. Selective vulnerability of neurons in organic dementia. *Nature*. 1977;266:558–559.

Squire LR. Remote memory as affected by aging. *Neuropsychologia* 1977;12:429–435.

Steele C, Rovner B, Chase GA, Folstein M. Psychiatric symptoms and nursing home placement of patients with Alzheimer's disease. *Am J Psychiatry*. 1990;147:1049–1051.

Stephen PJ, Williamson J. Drug-induced parkinsonism in the elderly. *Lancet.* 1984;2: 1082–1083.

Sterletz LJ, Reyes PF, Zolewska M, Katz L, Fariello RG. Computer analysis of EEG activity in dementia of the Alzheimer type and Huntington's disease. *Neurobiol Aging.* 1990;11:15–20.

Street JS, Clark WS, Gannon KS, et al. Olanzapine treatment of psychotic and behavioral symptoms in patients with Alzheimer disease in nursing care facilities: a double-blind, randomized, placebo-controlled trial. The HGEU Study Group. *Arch Gen Psychiatry.* 2000;57:968–976.

Tanner F, Shaw S. *Caring: A Family Guide to Managing the Alzheimer's Patient at Home.* East Hanover, NJ: Sandoz Pharmaceuticals; 1985.

Tanzi RE, Gusella JF, Watkins PC, et al. Amyloid beta protein gene: cDNA, mRNA distribution, and genetic linkage near the Alzheimer locus. *Science.* 1987;235:880.

Teresi J, Lawton MP, Ory M, Holmes D. Measurement issues in chronic care populations: dementia special care. *Alzheimer Dis Assoc Disord.* 1994;8(Suppl 1):S144–S183.

Teri L, Logsdon R. Assessment and management of behavioral disturbances in Alzheimer's disease. *Compr Ther.* 1990;6:36–42.

Teri L, Rabins P, Whitehouse P, et al. Management of behavior disturbance in Alzheimer's disease: current knowledge and future directions. *Alzheimer Dis Assoc Disord.* 1992;6:77–88.

Thompson EG, Eastwood MR. Survivorship and senile dementia. *Age Aging.* 1981;10: 29–32.

Tierney MC, Szalai JP, Snow WG, et al. Prediction of probable Alzheimer's disease in memory-impaired patients: a prospective longitudinal study. *Neurology.* 1996;46: 661–665.

Tobiansky R, Blizard R, Livingston G, Mann A. The Gospel Oak Study, stage IV: the clinical relevance of subjective memory impairment in older people. *Psychol Med (England).* 1995;25:779–786.

Tomlinson BE, Blessed G, Roth M. Observations on the brains of demented old people. *J Neurol Sci.* 1970;11:205–242.

Touchon J, Ritchie K. Prodromal cognitive disorder in Alzheimer's disease. *Int J Geriatr Psychiatry.* 1999;14:556–563.

Uhlmann RF, Larson EB. Effect of education on the Mini-Mental State Examination as a screening test for dementia. *J Am Geriatr Soc.* 1991;39:876–880.

US General Accounting Office. *Alzheimer's Disease: Estimates of Prevalence in the United States.* Washington, DC: US General Accounting Office; 1998.

Wechsler D. *Wechsler Adult Intelligence Scale.* New York, NY: Psychological Corporation; 1955.

Weiler P. The public health impact of Alzheimer's disease. *Am J Public Health.* 1987; 77:1157–1158.

Whitehouse PJ. Neurotransmitter receptor alterations in Alzheimer disease: a review. *Alzheimer Dis Assoc Disord.* 1987;1:9–18.

Whitehouse PJ, Price DL, Clark AW, Coyle JT, DeLong MR. Alzheimer's disease: evidence for selective loss of cholinergic neurons in the nucleus basalis. *Ann Neurol.* 1981;10:122–126.

Wilks S. Clinical notes on atrophy of the brain. *J Ment Sci.* 1864;10:383.

Williamson PC, Merskey H, Morrison S, et al. Quantitative electrophysiologic correlates of cognitive decline in normal elderly subjects. *Arch Neurol.* 1990;47:1185–1188.

Wilson R, Kaszniak A. Longitudinal changes: progressive idiopathic dementia. In: Poon LW, ed. *Handbook for Clinical Memory Assessment*. Washington, DC: American Psychological Association; 1986:285–293.

Winblad B, Poritis N. Memantine in severe dementia: results of the 9M-BEST Study (benefit and efficacy in severely demented patients during treatment with memantine). Int J Geriatr Psychiatry. 1999;14:135–146.

Wischik CM, Novak M, Edwards PC, Klug A, Tichelaar W, Crowther RA. Structural characterization of the core of the paired helical filament of Alzheimer disease. *Proc Natl Acad Sci U S A*. 1988;85:4884–4888.

Wischik CM, Novak M, Thogersen HC, et al. Isolation of a fragment of tau derived from the core of the paired helical filament of Alzheimer disease. *Proc Natl Acad Sci U S A*. 1988;85:4506–4510.

Wisniewski HM, Coblentz JM. Pick's disease: a clinical and ultrastructural study. *Arch Neurol*. 1972;26:97–108.

Wragg R, Jeste D. Overview of depression and psychosis in Alzheimer's disease. *Am J Psychiatry*. 1989;146:577–587.

Wu Q, Combs C, Cannady SB, Geldmacher DS, Herrup K. Beta amyloid activated microglia induce cell cycling and cell death in cultured cortical neurons. *Neurobiol Aging*. 2000;21:797–806.

Zubenko GS, Mossy J, Koop U. Neurochemical correlates of major depression in primary dementia. *Arch Neurol*. 1990;47:209–214.

17

Vascular Dementias

Stephen Read, MD

Dementia associated with cerebrovascular disease is one of the defining syndromes of geriatric psychiatry. The term *multiinfarct dementia* in the *Diagnostic and Statistical Manual of Mental Disorders, Third Edition* (*DSM-III*; American Psychiatric Association [APA], 1987) has been supplanted by the term *vascular dementia* (VaD) in the fourth edition of the manual (*DSM-IV*; APA, 1994) and its text revision (*DSM-IV-TR*; APA, 2000). Diagnosis depends on comprehensive geropsychiatric evaluation with multiaxial diagnosis, as covered in Chapter 10 of this book, plus evaluation as covered in additional topics in Chapters 11 through 15.

Careful consideration must be paid to the relationship between clinical findings and general medical conditions (Axis III) and to complicating psychiatric syndromes—especially depression, paranoia, and hallucinations—which can be of overriding importance in the course, care, and management of the patient with VaD. In addition, deficits because of stroke have provided one of the most fruitful sources of brain-localization concepts clinically, dating to Broca's claim, derived from examination of a stroke patient in 1861, that speech and language production depended on left prefrontal brain function. Cardiovascular and cerebrovascular diseases and related medical conditions are highly prevalent in the elderly. The geriatric psychiatrist, therefore, can expect to encounter a variety of cerebrovascular-related neuropsychiatric syndromes in practice; successful diagnosis and effective treatment can be crucial to optimal recovery of these patients.

DIAGNOSIS AND SYMPTOMATOLOGY

Diagnostic Criteria

Although the *DSM-IV-TR* (APA, 2000) Criteria A and B are the same for vascular dementia (see Table 17-1) as for other dementias, the clinical presentation of the patient with VaD often can be distinguished from the presentations of other dementing illnesses. For example, the requisite cognitive deficits (Criterion A) can be expected to vary more in a cohort of patients with VaD than in a cohort of patients with Alzheimer's disease (AD) or frontal lobe dementia. In particular, memory impairment will not be severe in some patients who have other severe cognitive deficits because of cerebrovascular injury that cause severe impairment, such as the patient with a fluent (Wernicke-type) aphasia or with Balint's syndrome of "cortical blindness." Pending response to suggestions that memory impairment be individually specified for diagnosing dementia (Knopman et al., 2001; Royall, 2003), an alternative diagnosis, such as cognitive disorder not otherwise specified (294.9), may then be technically indicated, although the distinction is of uncertain significance in practice.

TABLE 17-1. *DSM-IV* criteria for vascular dementia

A. The development of multiple cognitive deficits manifested by both
   (1) memory impairment (impaired ability to learn new information or to recall previously learned information)
   (2) one or more of the following cognitive disturbances:
      (a) aphasia (language disturbance)
      (b) apraxia (impaired ability to carry out motor activities despite intact motor function)
      (c) agnosia (failure to recognize or identify objects despite intact sensory function)
      (d) disturbance in executive functioning (i.e., planning, organizing, sequencing, abstracting)
B. The cognitive deficits in criteria A1 and A2 each cause significant impairment in social or occupational functioning and represent a significant decline from a previous level of functioning.
C. Focal neurological signs and symptoms (e.g., exaggeration of deep tendon reflexes, extensor plantar response, pseudobulbar palsy, gait abnormalities, weakness of an extremity) or laboratory evidence indicative of cerebrovascular disease (e.g., multiple infarctions involving cortex and underlying white matter) that are judged to be etiologically related to the disturbance.
D. The deficits do not occur exclusively during the course of a delirium.
Code based on predominant features:
   290.41 with delirium
   290.42 with delusions
   290.43 with depressed mood
   290.40 uncomplicated
Specify if (can be applied to any of the above subtypes): with behavioral disturbance

---

For VaD, the patient's history is crucial not only for the delineation of symptoms and functional deficits, but also for supporting the etiologic distinction of Criterion C, which requires positive present evidence of cerebrovascular disease "judged to be etiologically related to the disturbance" (APA, 2000, p. 161), either in the form of residual neurological signs or laboratory evidence (including neuroimaging). The causative inference is strongest when it is supported by a history of impairment that has developed concomitant with cerebrovascular insults for which there are corresponding residual clinical signs or imaging evidence. Most important, the circumstances of any acute change in the course of a patient's dementia should be examined for evidence of possible cerebrovascular disease. Familiarity with the features of stroke syndromes will increase the clinician's confidence in evaluating the likelihood of cerebrovascular insult. Acute episodes of motor, sensory, or mental status changes, especially if transient, may go unmentioned by the patient or caregiver, who is focused on a condition that is "obviously" (but mistakenly) thought to be AD. On the other hand, stroke may be overemphasized in an otherwise progressive course in a patient with underlying degenerative disease.

While eliciting this history, it is also important to have in mind the many disorders that predispose to cerebrovascular disease (see Table 17-2). A rating-scale approach has been used, mostly derived from the Ischemia Scale (IS) originally developed by Hachinski and colleagues (1975). Scores on the IS distinguished patients with multiinfarct and degenerative dementia. Items scored include features of mental status (depression, relative preservation of personality, somatization), the presence of historical or signs and symptoms of stroke, and a history suggestive of vascular events, although other risk factors for VaD (e.g., diabetes mellitus and atrial fibrillation) are not represented in the IS.

TABLE 17-2.   Risk factors for cerebrovascular disease

Hypertension: Major predisposing factor for arteriosclerosis, atherosclerosis, and ischemic heart disease as well as for stroke

Arrhythmia: Frequent in patients with vascular dementia, especially atrial fibrillation and sick sinus syndrome with bradycardia

Hypoxic/ischemic events: Multiple causes related to hypoperfusion episodes; related to vascular dementia independent of stroke (Moroney et al., 1996)

Diabetes mellitus: Significantly elevated risk for stroke (between 2:1 and 3:1) and for myocardial infarction (between 2:1 and 5:1) (Nathan, 1993) and, independently, direct risk for cognitive impairment (Perlmuter et al., 1984) and vascular dementia (Curb et al., 1999)

Coagulopathy, hyperviscosity, and vasculitis (especially temporal arteritis)

Pulmonary disease: Cognitive deficits due to chronic hypoxemia (Grant et al., 1987)

Substance abuse: Tobacco, especially cigarette smoking, and alcohol predispose to hypertension and vascular disease

Hyperlipidemia

Source: Wolf (1985).

Criteria sets other than the *DSM-IV* (APA, 1994) have also been proposed for vascular dementia, but there is a substantial lack of concordance among them. For example, Verhey and coworkers (1996) found that only 8 of 124 patients with dementia were diagnosed by all of seven different criteria sets, with a range of VaD diagnosis varying from 6% to 32% in that sample. In any event, the presence of these factors is not diagnostic per se, but can appropriately guide the search for further information during the history and examination of the patient.

Examination

Comprehensive evaluation of the patient with VaD requires an examination that elicits performance in cognitive domains, functional capacities, neurological findings, and neuropsychiatric problems. Classically, the cognitive deficits of vascular dementia have been described as "patchy" (Slater & Roth, 1963); that is, there is relative sparing of some mental functions compared to devastation in others. When specific deficits can be correlated with identified vascular injury, it clearly strengthens the case for cerebrovascular etiology. Familiarity with focal stroke syndromes will improve the clinician's skill in this analysis; see Chapters 10 and 12; other rich sources include Absher and Benson (1993), Chui (1989), and Fisher (1982).

In addition to documenting a detailed and thorough mental status examination, the diagnostician must consider neurological signs and symptoms, choosing to rely on other physicians' examinations or to incorporate elements of the neurological examination (especially gait and posture, reflexes, facial and eye movements) as a part of a comprehensive geropsychiatric evaluation. Analysis of functional deficits, required for Criterion B, can also be expected to identify problems related to specific motor or sensory lesions from the vascular injury.

Neuropsychiatric Phenomena Associated with Vascular Dementia

The expertise of the geriatric psychiatrist caring for the patient with VaD is likely to focus on the noncognitive difficulties of these patients. These problems may, indeed, have prompted the original consultation, or the psychiatrist's detection may prove to be an important contribution to the care of the patient with VaD. Because psychiatric and behavioral symptoms are so critical in patient safety and caregiver burden (Rabins et al., 1982) and significantly shorten the time to nursing home placement (Phillips & Diwan, 2003), the geriatric psychiatrist can be the pivotal professional in sustaining the VaD patient's capacity to stay in the community or at home.

The paucity of data on psychiatric syndromes in VaD abets the continuing lack of clarity of the specificity of these phenomena. Differing interpretations of some issues (e.g., whether apathy should be considered a symptom of depression or as a separate matter) confound some assessments. Sultzer and coworkers (1993) found that patients with VaD had significantly higher rates of depression and associated symptoms, but not psychosis, compared to patients with AD. Specifically, they found that over one third of the patients with VaD had blunted affect, depressed mood, emotional withdrawal, motor retardation, low motivation, anxiety, unusual thoughts, and somatic concerns, symptoms that were much less frequent in the patients with AD. Leroi and coworkers (2003) also found high rates of psychosis in patients with both AD and VaD and presented a detailed description of the psychotic phenomena cataloged in the 9 of 59 patients with VaD in their sample.

Laboratory Studies

As in the evaluation of any dementia, physiological sources of brain dysfunction (i.e., delirium, per Criterion D) must be considered, either as causative or as an exacerbation of the cognitive impairment; in addition, some studies may be of specific diagnostic import in VaD (National Institutes of Health Consensus Development Conference, 1987). Items of special relevance to the diagnosis of VaD include anemia (complete blood count), evidence of blood sugar dysregulation (fasting and postprandial blood glucose, glycosylated hemoglobin), and sedimentation rate for possible inflammatory vasculitis. Electrocardiogram (EKG) may reveal arrhythmia or evidence of ischemic cardiac disease, and ambulatory EKG monitoring or other, more invasive, testing may be indicated for other conditions that can predispose the patient to emboli, syncope, or ischemic events. Some patients may have had x-ray contrast or ultrasound studies of the vasculature. Pulmonary impairment can exacerbate the effects of vascular disease by limiting oxygenation directly.

Neuroimaging

Neuroimaging is reviewed in Chapter 14; note that findings suggestive of vascular disease are commonly found in studies of patients with dementia because of other causes and in nondemented individuals. However, delineation of focal areas of brain infarction by magnetic resonance imaging (MRI) or x-ray computed tomography (CT), especially when supported by temporal and clinical correlation to the patient's findings, provides strong support for a diagnosis of VaD.

Controversy continues about the significance of multiple small or confluent abnormalities in the subcortical white matter (WM), which may be referred to as subcortical arteriosclerotic encephalopathy, unidentified bright objects, or leukoaraiosis (Hachinski et al., 1987). Although presumed vascular in origin, these features provide less-specific support for a diagnosis of VaD because they have been reported in patients with AD and other diseases. Some degree of these findings may be compatible with normal mental function, although more detailed investigation supports the opinion that they are indeed associated with deficits. For example, Boone and coworkers (1992) found that attention and frontal lobe function correlated with the amount of WM tissue involvement, and Ylikoski and associates (1993) found that leukoaraiosis correlated with decreased speed of mental processing.

Functional brain imaging techniques, including positron emission tomography (PET), single-photon emission computed tomography (SPECT), functional magnetic resonance imaging (fMRI), MR spectroscopy, and quantitative electroencephalography (QEEG) can assist in determining the significance of cerebrovascular lesions. For example, Sultzer and colleagues. (1995) showed that presumptively vascular subcortical lesions seen on MRI scan were linked to areas of hypometabolism in structurally normal cortex; diagnostic utility and specificity of functional brain imaging is also supported by clinical-pathological case series (e.g., Read et al., 1995).

In summary, the role of neuroimaging in the assessment of VaD is important, but firm guidelines remain elusive. Despite its utility, functional imaging should continue to be done selectively (Talbot et al., 1998). Some question routine CT or MRI in dementia assessment on the basis of yield and cost. The frequency of vascular abnormalities, however, and their undoubted contribution to dementia, degree of disability, and overall prognosis (Snowdon et al., 1997) argue strongly for continued use of MRI or CT, particularly in the evaluation of VaD (Cummings, 2000).

Neuropsychology

Gainotti and coworkers (1989) found that patients with VaD had relative preservation of a primacy effect on memory testing compared to patients with AD, and patients with VaD may also have impaired motor function in relation to cognitive deficits compared with patients with AD (Storrie & Doerr, 1981). Neuropsychological evaluation may be valuable for characterizing the patient's deficits more fully in anticipation of repeat evaluation in the future. Testing can be seen as "objective" evidence of deficits that may prove to be persuasive for patients or family members in denial. In patients with deficits after a vascular event that has been termed transient, neuropsychological testing instead may confirm a clinical impression of persisting deficits despite normal structural neuroimaging and absence of physical neurological signs (Delaney et al., 1980; Russell & Polakoff, 1993).

PATHOLOGY

Brain tissue is intimately associated with vascular structures down to a microscopic level. Neurons cannot utilize energy resources other than glucose and oxygen and are therefore dependent on the steady supply of oxygenated blood with sufficient glucose. The early appreciation of these phenomena and the recognition that cerebrovascular disease was ubiquitous with aging underlay the assumption until well past the middle of the 20th century that senile dementia was caused by cerebral arteriosclerosis. The explosion of knowledge of microcellular anatomy and molecular signaling has begun to delineate the details of the factors regulating and coordinating brain blood flow and function, including the substantial and early increase in blood flow that anticipates regional brain activation. Potential factors include products of neuronal activity (such as K+ and adenosine), neuronal afferents (monoamines, acetylcholine, peptides), and NMDA (N-methyl-D-aspartate) receptor activation resulting in the production of nitrous oxide (NO) (Parri & Crunelli, 2003). Zonta and associates (2003) have proposed that astrocytes provide the critical anatomical link between neuronal cell activity and vasodilation.

The landmark finding in dementia pathology was that of Tomlinson, Blessed, and Roth (1970), who determined that the most common pathological finding in elderly patients with dementia was indistinguishable from that of AD and not related to cerebrovascular disease. Still, cerebral infarction, usually multiple, was the second most common pathological condition identified. These data led to the definition of multiinfarct dementia because they correlated the degree of dementia with the total amount of infarcted brain tissue; subsequent workers have delineated a more complex picture of multiple vascular and ischemic lesions (Roman et al., 1993, Wallin & Blennow, 1993).

Pathological variability has been confirmed in recent studies (Garcia & Brown, 1992; Hulette et al., 1997; Munoz, 1991; Vinters et al., 2000), and Table 17-3 presents a list of different pathological features. The variability of clinical presentation and the fact that similar pathology is found in autopsies of subjects judged cognitively normal prevent a confident assignment of dementia to any specific cerebrovascular pathology. Rather, findings are "associated with" the clinical syndrome of dementia. Because detailed review of the complexity of these findings and their combinations is beyond the scope of this review, I summarize the following key conclusions of these reports:

1. Is it the *location* of cerebrovascular lesions that is critical for the evolution of dementia? "Strategic" injury, such as to the hippocampus (memory) or dominant angular gyrus (Gerstmann syndrome), can result in symptom complexes that substantially fulfill the criteria for dementia. For example, Vinters and coworkers (2000) found hippocampal injury (of various types) in 11 of their 20 cases of vascular dementia. Isolated hippocampal lesions are rare, however, and cannot account for most cases of VaD.

2. Is it the *type* of cerebrovascular lesion that is critical? For example, large cystic infarctions versus lacunar versus microinfarcts versus laminar necrosis (from ischemic/hypoxic injury, e.g., postcardiac arrest). In

TABLE 17-3.   Pathological findings in vascular dementia

A. Focal, "strategic" infarction or ischemic lesions
   1. Hippocampal/mesial temporal structures
   2. Angular gyrus (Gerstmann syndrome in dominant hemisphere)
   3. Frontal/cingulate infarcts (anterior cerebral artery)
   4. Caudate and thalamic infarcts
B. Multifocal and/or diffuse ischemic disease
   1. "Border zone" infarcts
   2. Ischemia with antiphospholipid antibodies
   3. Multiple cortical microinfarcts ("granular atrophy")
   4. Multiple lacunar infarcts
   5. Multifocal subcortical leukoencephalopathy (Binswanger's disease)
   6. Cerebral autosomal dominant arteriopathy with subcortical infarcts and leu-kencephalopathy (CADASIL)
   7. Vasculitis and angiopathies
   8. Cortical laminar necrosis (occurring post–cardiac arrest, posthypotensive)
   9. Cerebral amyloid angiopathy (CAA; note familial forms and link to Alzheimer's disease/pathology)
Caveat: It is the exception for these findings to occur in isolation, but rather the rule that tissue from an individual will reveal more than one cerebrovascular process.

Source: From Vinters et al. (2000); Wallin and Blennow (1993).

brief, the answer is no. None of the lesions in Table 17-3 has been found in all cases of vascular dementia. Most common is more than one type of lesion, further complicating the problem of attribution.

3. Are lesions caused by cerebrovascular disease only *incidental* to dementia because of another underlying disorder (e.g., AD)? Again, briefly, the answer is no; some patients with dementia have only vascular brain injury at autopsy. However, vascular damage may also be significant in addition to a degenerative disorder: Snowdon and colleagues (1997) found that nuns who met neuropathological criteria for AD and who also had brain infarcts were more demented than those without infarcts.

4. Are the pathological lesions of cerebrovascular disease simply markers for some additional pathological process that is present, or perhaps precipitated by cerebrovascular insult, and possibly in some rather than others? This question cannot be answered with certainty at this time, but molecular responses may prove to be the "missing link" between identified cerebrovascular events and cognitive impairment, perhaps especially in those with a slowly progressing vascular dementia. For example, β-amyloid protein may be overexpressed in brain ischemia (Popa-Wagner et al., 1998; Suenaga et al., 1994), and other molecules may be secreted in response to vascular or metabolic insults. Other

findings suggest the possibility of a more unitary view of dementia etiology at the molecular level; for instance, the ε4 allele of apolipoprotein E (APOE) is associated both with AD and VaD (Marin et al., 1998), as are certain measures of cerebral oxidative states (Berr et al., 2000).

EPIDEMIOLOGY

The "true" incidence of vascular dementia remains uncertain, with the extremes of the range of reported estimates 4.5% to 39%. Considerations of sample selection play some role in the variance of these estimates: Relevant factors include age structure of the sample, stage of dementia, and case-finding biases (contrast mild dementia cases in an outpatient evaluation clinic and patients dying of prolonged dementia in a nursing home). The incidence of dementia with cerebral infarcts increases with age; rates per 100,000 below age 60 years are 1.0, rising to 20.7, 105.2, and 213.2 in each succeeding decade cohort. There is also evidence for declining prevalence of vascular dementia coinciding with the declining incidence of stroke in general (Kokmen et al., 1988). Kase (1991) suggests that less that 10% of a community sample of patients with dementia will have vascular dementia, although cerebrovascular pathology complicates another dementing condition in another 10% to 20%.

CARE AND TREATMENT

Care for patients with VaD includes treatment for the primary cognitive impairment syndrome as well as accompanying psychiatric syndromes and medical care issues; support and therapy for the patient, family, and caregivers; overseeing and coordinating care at home, in day care, and in assisted-living and nursing facilities. The medical management of the patient with VaD is the quintessential interdisciplinary challenge, requiring continual consideration and coordination of the interactions and effects on both Axis I and Axis III conditions. In addition, patients with VaD are subject to unpredictable changes in mental status that can be troubling in and of themselves as well as requiring assessment for the presence of delirium because of potential adverse physiological events, drug interactions, or renewed cerebrovascular events. Continuity of care, regularity of contact, and clear lines of communication are valuable for allowing optimal response and adaptation to such episodes.

Although reversal of cerebrovascular damage is not yet possible, evidence is beginning to emerge for the direct treatment of cognitive deficits in VaD: Deficits in brain cholinergic function have been defined in VaD, and cholinesterase inhibitors benefit patients with VaD with or without concomitant AD (Kaufer, 2002). Memantine is a reversible NMDA receptor antagonist that has been available in Germany since 1989, although it is not approved in the United States. Memantine has been reported as significantly better than placebo on measures of global function, care dependence, and motor, social, and cognitive function in patients with severe VaD (Winblad & Poritis, 1999) as well as those with mild-to-moderate VaD (Orgogozo et al., 2002).

The frequency and burden of neuropsychiatric complications of VaD are addressed above. Although the management and care of specific psychiatric syndromes—depression, anxiety, paranoia and psychosis, delirium, sleep, and other behavioral issues—are covered elsewhere in this volume, several factors deserve extra consideration in the patient with VaD.

First, the medical regimen may already confer a substantial burden of anticholinergic activity that threatens to compromise neuropsychiatric function (Mulsant et al., 2003). The geriatric psychiatrist must be aware that any addition from psychotropic or other medications may add to this confound in the condition of the patient with VaD.

Second, patients with VaD can be expected to be especially sensitive to individual and combined vascular effects and pharmacological and pharmacokinetic interactions of prescribed medications; for instance, a high percentage of patients will be taking coumadin or medications to regulate blood sugar.

The geriatric psychiatrist's involvement with the care of the patient with dementia may be limited to a single consultation as an ongoing member of the treatment team. Exceptionally, the geriatric psychiatrist may function as the primary care provider and coordinator (e.g., Tan, 2001), particularly when behavioral issues predominate. Recommendations are most effective when they derive from the comprehensive specifics of the patient's situation, taking into account not only psychiatric symptoms and behaviors, but also basic capacities such as gait stability, hygiene, and nutrition. Safety considerations include the potential for wandering, household security, managing appliances, use of drugs and alcohol, smoking, driving, and access to weapons. Referral for advice on legal and financial matters may be indicated. Cultural and individual values must be weighed to balance dignity, autonomy, safety, and supervision.

Caring for patients with dementia can be stressful and may provide the potential for physical or emotional abuse of the patient. Emotional and practical support for the caregiver may be vital. Ascertaining the patient's values in terms of intensity of care may alleviate later decision-making difficulties for the caregivers; physician assessment of condition and prognosis facilitates realistic discussion of advanced directives. The optimal treatment setting depends on community options, family resources, and the patient's condition (Read, 1990):

- Mild dementia usually is compatible with the patient remaining at home. In-home support and successful management of psychiatric syndromes can be critical in sustaining the family's ability to care for the patient at home.
- Moderate dementia requires closer supervision. Programs such as adult day care can provide critical support, but the possibility of assisted living may also arise.

- Severe dementia mandates full-time care. With sufficient support and resources, this may be provided successfully in a home environment, but for many patients, an institutional setting will be required. Such settings may be favored by financial considerations as the patient's needs increase.

Support and advocacy groups may be identified through the local chapter of the Alzheimer's Association or stroke support programs. The geriatric psychiatrist can be a most valuable resource for patients, family members, and care teams trying to reach decisions about these complex and often emotionally conflicted choices; selective use of specific psychotherapeutic approaches may be helpful.

Rehabilitation efforts for the patient with VaD may be attempted on an empiric, case-by-case basis. Identification of relatively "spared" mental functions may suggest ways to compensate for those areas of impairment. Documentation of deficits may be needed to support evaluations for capacity or disability. There may be prognostic value for these assessments. Sotaniemi and associates (1981), for instance, found that impaired performance on the Stroop preoperatively predicted postcardiac surgery impairment. Note, however, that poorer outcomes are associated with reduced intensity of rehabilitation, and because access to rehabilitation services varies according to managed care practices (Kramer et al., 2000), the assiduous clinician's documentation of deficits perversely risks becoming the basis for denial of access to rehabilitation services that may benefit the patient.

PROGNOSIS

Mortality in patients with VaD is increased compared to age- and sex-matched control subjects. For example, Molsa and coworkers (1986) found a relative mortality of 1.6 : 1 for patients with VaD compared to patients with AD. Skoog and colleagues (1993) reported that 3-year mortality of 85-year-olds in Sweden was 23% for those without dementia, 42% for those with AD, and 66.7% for those with VaD. It would also be plausible that a more precise prognosis would derive from the status of the patient's underlying medical (Axis III) condition. On the other hand, as the incidence of stroke declines and the treatment of other vascular risk factors improve, VaD is the most potentially preventable form of dementia.

CONCLUSION

Controversy persists about the clinical and pathological aspects of vascular dementia, and effective treatment remains elusive. Stroke and related conditions continue to be significant public health problems, however, and are a fruitful and valuable area of expertise for the geriatric psychiatrist.

REFERENCES

Absher JR, Benson DF. Disconnection syndromes: an overview of Geschwind's contributions. *Neurology.* 1993;43:862–867.

American Psychiatric Association. *Diagnostic and Statistical Manual of Mental Disorders.* 3rd ed., rev. Washington, DC: American Psychiatric Association; 1987.

American Psychiatric Association. *Diagnostic and Statistical Manual of Mental Disorders.* 4th ed. Washington, DC: American Psychiatric Association; 1994.

American Psychiatric Association. *Diagnostic and Statistical Manual of Mental Disorders.* 4th ed., text revision. Washington, DC: American Psychiatric Association; 2000.

Berr C, Balansard B, Arnaud J, et al. Cognitive decline is associated with systemic oxidative stress: the EVA study. *J Am Geriatr Soc.* 2000;48:1285–1291.

Boone KB, Miller BL, Lesser IM, et al. Neuropsychological correlates of white-matter lesions in healthy elderly subjects. *Arch Neurol.* 1992;49:549–554.

Chui HC. Dementia: a review emphasizing clinicopathologic correlation and brain-behavior relationships. *Arch Neurol.* 1989;46:806–814.

Cummings JL. Neuroimaging in the assessment of dementia: is it necessary? *J Am Geriatr Soc.* 2000;48:1345–1346.

Curb JD, Rodriguez BL, Abbott RD, et al. Longitudinal association of vascular and Alzheimer's dementias, diabetes, and glucose tolerance. *Neurology.* 1999;52:971–975.

Delaney RC, Wallace JD, Egelko S. Transient cerebral ischemic attacks and neuropsychological deficit. *J Clin Neuropsychol.* 1980;2:107–114.

Fisher CM. Lacunar strokes and infarcts: a review. *Neurology.* 1982;32:871–876.

Gainotti G, Monteleone D, Parlato E, et al. Verbal memory disorders in Alzheimer's disease and multi-infarct dementia. *J Neurolinguistics.* 1989;4:327–345.

Garcia JH, Brown GG. Vascular dementia: neuropathologic alterations and metabolic brain changes. *J Neurol Sci.* 1992; 109:121–131.

Grant I, Prigatano GP, Heaton RK, et al. Progressive neuropsychologic impairment and hypoxemia. *Arch Gen Psychiatry.* 1987;44:999–1006.

Hachinski VC, Iliff LD, Zilhka E, et al. Cerebral blood flow in dementia. *Arch Neurol.* 1975;32:632–637.

Hachinski VC, Potter P, Merskey H. Leuko-araiosis. *Arch Neurol.* 1987;44:21–23.

Hulette C, Nochlin D, McKeel D, et al. Clinical-neuropathologic findings in multi-infarct dementia: a report of six autopsied cases. *Neurology.* 1997;48:668–672.

Kase CS. Epidemiology of multi-infarct dementia. *Alzheimers Dis Assoc Disord.* 1991; 5:71–76.

Kaufer DI. Cholinesterase-inhibitor therapy for dementia: novel clinical substrates and mechanisms for treatment response. *CNS Spectrums.* 2002;7:742–750.

Knopman DS, DeKosky ST, Cummings JL, et al. Practice parameter: diagnosis of dementia (an evidence-based review). Report of the Quality Standards Subcommittee of the American Academy of Neurology. *Neurology.* 2001;56:1143–1153.

Kokmen E, Chandra VJ, Schoenberg BS. Trends in incidence of dementing illness in Rochester, Minnesota, in three quinquennial periods, 1960–1974. *Neurology.* 1988;38:975–980.

Kramer AM, Kowalsky, Lin M, Grigsby J, Hughes R, Steiner JF. Outcome and utilization differences for older persons with stroke in HMO and fee-for-service systems. *J Am Geriatr Soc.* 2000;48:726–734.

Leroi I, Voulgari A, Breitner JCS, Lyketsos CG. The epidemiology of psychosis in dementia. *Am J Geriatr Psychiatry.* 2003;11:83–91.

Marin DB, Breuer B, Marin ML, et al. The relationship between apolipoprotein E, dementia, and vascular illness. *Atherosclerosis.* 1998;140:173–180.

Molsa PK, Marttilla RJ, Rinne UK. Survival and cause of death in Alzheimer's disease and multi-infarct dementia. *Acta Neurol Scand.* 1986;74:103–107.

Moroney JT, Bagiella E, Desmond DW, et al. Risk factors for incident dementia after stroke: role of hypoxic-ischemic events. *Stroke.* 1996;27:1283–1289.

Mulsant BH, Pollock BG, Kirshner M, Shen C, Dodge H, Ganguli M. Serum anticholinergic activity in a community-based sample of older adults: relationship with cognitive performance. *Arch Gen Psychiatry.* 2003;60:198–203.

Munoz DG. The pathological basis of multi-infarct dementia. *Alzheimers Dis Assoc Disord.* 1991;5:77–90.

Nathan DM. Long-term complications of diabetes mellitus. *N Engl J Med.* 1993;328: 1676–1685.

National Institutes of Health. *Consensus. Development Conference Statement—Differential Diagnosis of Dementing Diseases.* Bethesda, MD: US Dept of Health and Human Services; July 6–8, 1987;6(11):1–27.

Orgogozo J-M, Rigaud A-S, Stoffler A, Mobius H-J, Forette F. Efficacy and safety of memantine in patients with mild to moderate vascular dementia. *Stroke.* 2002;33: 1834–1839.

Parri R, Crunelli V. An astrocyte bridge from synapse to blood flow. *Nat Neurosci.* 2003;6:5–6.

Perlmuter LC, Hakami MK, Hodgson-Harrington C, et al. Decreased cognitive function in aging non-insulin-dependent diabetic patients. *Am J Med.* 1984;77:1043–1048.

Phillips VL, Diwan S. The incremental effect of dementia-related problem behaviors on the time to nursing home placement in poor, frail, demented older people. *J Am Geriatr Soc.* 2003;51:188–193.

Popa-Wagner A, Schroder E, Walker LC, Kessler C. Beta-amyloid precursor protein and beta-amyloid peptide immunoreactivity in the rat brain after middle cerebral artery occlusion. Effect of age. *Stroke.* 1998; 29:2196–2202.

Rabins PV, Mace NL, Lucas MJ. The impact of dementia on the family. *JAMA.* 1982; 248:333–335.

Read S. Community resources. In: Cummings JL, Miller BL, eds. *Alzheimer's Disease: Treatment and Long-Term Management.* New York, NY: Marcel Dekker; 1990: 235–244.

Read SL, Miller B, Mena I, Kim R, Itabashi H, Darby A. SPECT in dementia: clinical and pathological correlation. *J Am Geriatr Soc.* 1995;43:1243–1247.

Roman GC, Tetemichi TK, Erkinjuntti T, et al. Vascular dementia: diagnostic criteria for research studies (Report of the NINDS-AIREN International Workshop). *Neurology.* 1993;43:250–260.

Royall D. The "Alzheimerization" of dementia research. *J Am Geriatr Soc.* 2003;51: 277–278.

Russell EW, Polakoff D. Neuropsychological test patterns in men for Alzheimer's and multi-infarct dementia. *Arch Clin Neuropsychol.* 1993;8:327–343.

Skoog I, Nilsson L, Palmertz B, et al. A population-based study of dementia in 85-year-olds. *N Engl J Med.* 1993;328:153–158.

Slater E, Roth M. *Clinical Psychiatry*. 3rd ed. Baltimore, MD: Williams and Wilkins; 1963:593–596.

Snowdon DA, Greiner LH, Mortimer JA, Riley KP, Greiner PA, Markesbery WR. Brain infarction and the clinical expression of Alzheimer disease: the Nun study. *JAMA*. 1997;277:813–817.

Sotaniemi KA, Juolasmaa A, Hokkanen ET. Neuropsychologic outcome after open-heart surgery. *Arch Neurol*. 1981;38:2–8.

Storrie M, Doerr H. Characterization of Alzheimer type dementia utilizing an abbreviated Halstead-Reitan Battery. *Clin Neuropsychol*. 1981;2:78–82.

Suenaga T, Ohnishi K, Nishimura M, Nakamura S, Akiguchi I, Kimura J. Bundles of amyloid precursor protein-immunoreactive axons in human cerebrovascular white matter lesions. *Acta Neuropathol*. 1994;87:450–455.

Sultzer DL, Levin HS, Mahler ME, High WM, Cummings JL. A comparison of psychiatric symptoms in vascular dementia and Alzheimer's disease. *Am J Psychiatry*. 1993; 150:1806–1812.

Sultzer DL, Mahler ME, Cummings JL, Van Gorp WG, Hinkin CH, Brown C. Cortical abnormalities associated with subcortical lesions in vascular dementia. *Arch Neurol*. 1995;52:773–780.

Talbot PR, Lloyd JJ, Snowden JS, Neary D, Testa HJ. A clinical role for 99mTc-HMPAO SPECT in the investigation of dementia? *J Neurol Neurosurg Psychiatry*. 1998;64:306–313.

Tan A. *The Bonesetter's Daughter*. New York, NY: G. P. Putnam's Sons; 2001.

Tomlinson BE, Blessed G, Roth M. Observations on the brains of demented old people. *J Neurol Sci*. 1970;11:205–242.

Verhey FR, Lodder J, Rozendaal N, Jolles J. Comparison of seven sets of criteria used for the diagnosis of vascular dementia. *Neuroepidemiology*. 1996;15:166–172.

Vinters HV, Ellis WG, Zarow C, et al. Neuropathologic substrates of ischemic vascular dementia. *J Neuropathol Exp Neurol*. 2000;59:931–945.

Wallin A, Blennow K. Heterogeneity of vascular dementia: mechanisms and subgroups. *J Geriatr Psychiatry Neurol*. 1993;6:177–188.

Winblad B, Poritis N. Memantine in severe dementia: results of the 9M-Best study (benefit and efficacy in severely demented patients during treatment with memantine). *Int J Geriatr Psychiatry*. 1999;14:135–146.

Wolf PA. Risk factors for stroke. *Stroke*. 1985;16:359–360.

Ylikoski R, Ylikoski A, Erkinjuntti T, et al. White matter changes in healthy elderly persons with attention and speed of mental processing. *Arch Neurol*. 1993 50:818–824.

Zonta M, Angulo MC, Gobbo S, et al. Neuron-to-astrocyte signaling is central to the dynamic control of brain microcirculation. *Nat Neurosci*. 2003;6:43–50.

18

Delirium

Benjamin Liptzin, MD

D elirium has been recognized as a global disturbance of brain function for several thousand years (Lipowski, 1990). Geriatric psychiatrists need to be knowledgeable about delirium because it is common (particularly in elderly patients in general hospitals); it is frequently overlooked (up to 67% of cases according to one study); it may be associated with high morbidity (e.g., institutionalization, pressure sores, or aspiration pneumonia) or mortality; and it is often caused by medical or surgical interventions. Recognition of delirium is important because it may be the only sign of an underlying medical illness or a toxic effect from medication. Significant attention has been paid to the diagnostic criteria that define delirium; the epidemiology, course, and outcomes of patients diagnosed with delirium; the differential diagnosis; etiologies; underlying pathophysiology; and assessment and management of patients with delirium. This review summarizes the current state of knowledge of these areas. More complete information is available in a monograph on delirium (Carlson et al., 1999). The "Practice Guideline for the Treatment of Patients with Delirium" was published by the American Psychiatric Association (APA; 1999).

DIAGNOSIS AND SYMPTOMATOLOGY

In the last 50 years, the diagnostic manual published by the American Psychiatric Association has evolved from a volume with vague terms with no specific criteria or definitions (such as "acute" versus "chronic brain disorders") to more specific terms that use explicit criteria that have been empirically tested and validated. In the *DSM-IV* (APA, 1994), the symptoms of delirium are as follows:

> A disturbance of consciousness (i.e. reduced clarity of awareness of the environment) with reduced ability to focus, sustain or shift attention; a change in cognition (such as memory deficit, disorientation, language disturbance) or the development of a perceptual disturbance that is not better accounted for by a pre-existing, established, or evolving dementia; and the disturbance develops over a short period of time (usually hours to days) and tends to fluctuate during the course of the day. (p. 129)

The condition is further specified as due to a general medical condition, substance intoxication, substance withdrawal, or multiple etiologies if there is evidence from the history, physical examination, or laboratory findings that suggests specific etiologies. If no specific etiology is confirmed, the delirium is classified as "not otherwise specified" (NOS). In addition to the core symptoms, many patients show other associated features, such as a disturbance in the sleep-wake cycle with daytime sleepiness or nighttime agitation. In some cases, there may be a complete reversal of the night-day sleep-wake cycle.

Several subtypes of delirium have been described and studied based on associated features (Liptzin & Levkoff, 1992; Sandberg et al., 1999). The *hyperactive* type is characterized by increased psychomotor activity, hypervigilance, hyperalertness, hallucinations, delusions, fast or loud speech, irritability, combativeness, impatience, swearing, singing, laughing, uncooperativeness, euphoria, anger, wandering, easy startling, distractibility, tangentiality, nightmares, or restlessness. These patients are usually recognized in general hospitals because they may be at risk of falling, pulling out catheters or intravenous lines, or trying to leave the hospital. In contrast, the *hypoactive* type of delirium is characterized by decreased activity, unawareness, decreased alertness, somnolence, lethargy, staring into space, apathy, and sparse, slow, or decreased speech. These patients are often undiagnosed, but may be at increased risk of developing pressure skin ulcerations or aspiration pneumonia or may be at risk of not taking medication properly at home. The majority of patients exhibit features of hyperactive and hypoactive delirium at different times, and their delirium is considered *mixed* type. Some patients fit none of these subtypes.

O'Keeffe (1999) also discussed subtypes of delirium based on psychomotor activity. He suggested that different subtypes may be associated with specific etiologic factors and neurotransmitter pathways and may require different treatment approaches, including specific pharmacological treatments. Furthermore, patients with hyperactive delirium may have a better outcome than those with hypoactive delirium (Camus et al., 2000; Meagher & Trzepacz, 2000; O'Keeffe & Lavan, 1999).

EPIDEMIOLOGY

Reviews by Bucht et al. (1999) and Fann (2000) highlighted the methodological difficulties encountered in studying the epidemiology of delirium. Nevertheless, it is clear that delirium is very common in general hospitals, but there is a wide range of prevalence estimates depending on the population studied (Levkoff et al., 1991). In medical inpatients, the prevalence of delirium has been reported as 11% to 16%, and the incidence of new cases that develop while the patient is in the hospital ranged from 4% to 10%. A review of postoperative delirium cited rates of 0% to 73.5% (van der Mast, 1999). Although cognitive dysfunction is common in elderly persons 1 to 3 days after surgery, this is usually transient and thought to be related directly to the surgery and anesthesia (Goldstein & Fogel, 1993; Ritchie et al., 1997).

Massie and coworkers (1983) found that up to 80% of patients with terminal illness developed delirium near death, although one study found that even when present in patients with advanced cancer, delirium was reversible in 50% of episodes (Lawlor et al., 2000). Hospitalized patients with acquired immunodeficiency syndrome (AIDS) have a 30%–40% incidence of delirium (Breitbart et al., 1996). One study found an association between a decline in cognitive performance after cardiac bypass surgery and the presence of the *apo-E4* allele (Newman et al., 1995).

Most of the studies have been done with hospitalized populations because patients who develop delirium usually have a serious medical illness that requires the services provided by a hospital. In a community survey, Folstein and colleagues (1991) estimated the prevalence of delirium in persons over 55 years of age as 1.1%. In the last 10 years that percentage may have risen as the population over 55 increased in age and as patients were discharged more quickly after hospitalization and before they were fully recovered because of managed care pressures. Lerner and coworkers (1997) found that 22% of community-dwelling patients with Alzheimer's disease had episodes of delirium during the course of their illness.

Table 18-1 summarizes the risk factors that have been associated with de-

TABLE 18-1.   Risk factors for delirium

Cognitive impairment
Older age
Psychoactive drug use
Severe illness/comorbidity
Azotemia/dehydration
Male gender
Alcohol abuse
Infection/fever
Metabolic abnormality

Source: Adapted from Inouye (1999).

lirium. Most of the risk factors for delirium (e.g., older age) cannot be modified. However, they can alert clinicians to the need for careful monitoring to
detect and treat early symptoms of delirium.

Inouye and colleagues (1993) studied predisposing factors that could help
predict which patients were likely to develop delirium during hospitalization.
They found that a simple predictive model based on 4 predisposing factors
(vision impairment, severe illness, cognitive impairment, and serum urea nitrogen [BUN]/creatinine ratio greater than 18) could identify, at hospital admission, older persons at greatest risk for delirium and enable investigators to
target high-risk patients for future studies of interventions.

In a later study, Inouye and Charpentier (1996) identified 5 precipitating factors associated with the development of delirium during hospitalization:
use of physical restraints, malnutrition, more than 3 medications added, use
of a bladder catheter, and any iatrogenic event. Inouye (1999) suggested that
precipitating and predisposing factors are highly interrelated and contribute to
delirium in independent, substantive, and cumulative ways. Taken together,
these factors can help target at-risk patients and develop interventions to prevent delirium in hospitalized older patients.

Martin and coworkers (2000) also identified as potentially modifiable risk
factors the number of medications and number of procedures. Inouye, Schlesinger, and colleagues (1999) have suggested that in-hospital delirium may be
a marker of ways to improve the quality of hospital care for older persons.

As an example of such an intervention study, Inouye, Bogardus, and colleagues (1999) studied 852 patients 70 years of age or older admitted to the
general medicine service at a teaching hospital. Patients on the intervention unit
benefited from standardized protocols for the management of 6 risk factors for
delirium: cognitive impairment, sleep deprivation, immobility, visual impairment, hearing impairment, and dehydration. Delirium developed in only 9.9%
of the intervention group compared with 15.0% of the usual care group. The
total number of days with delirium and the total number of episodes were significantly lower in the intervention group. However, the severity of delirium
and recurrence rates were not significantly different. Intervention led to significant improvement in the degree of cognitive impairment among patients with
cognitive impairment at admission and to a significant reduction in the use of
sleep medications. There were trends toward improvement in immobility, visual impairment, and hearing impairment. Prevention techniques may be specific to delirium in special populations. For example, Hammon and coworkers
(1997) suggested that microemboli may be the cause of neurobehavioral changes
after coronary artery bypass grafting (CABG) procedures and recommended
techniques for reducing manipulation of the ascending aorta.

CLINICAL COURSE AND OUTCOMES

The course of delirium varies widely in individual patients. Delirium generally
presents on admission or early in a hospitalization. Bowman (1992) found that

the highest incidence of delirium in patients undergoing surgery occurred on the third postoperative day. Although delirium is generally thought to have an acute onset, many patients experience a prodromal period with some symptoms of delirium prior to the onset of the full syndrome.

Levkoff and colleagues (1992) found that of all patients who met *DSM-III* (APA, 1980) criteria for delirium, 50% met it the same day that they experienced the onset of a new individual symptom; 86% met criteria within 2 days of the appearance of their first new symptom.

Rudberg and colleagues (1997) studied a group of elderly medical and surgical inpatients and found that 44 of the 64 patients (69%) who developed delirium experienced it for only a single day. They also noted that there was considerable variation in the presentation and time course of the delirium.

Although delirium is usually thought of as acute and transient, for some patients, the course is often prolonged. Koponen and colleagues (1989c) found a range of 3 to 81 days for resolution of delirium, with a mean of 20 days. Levkoff and coworkers (1992) found that only 4% of delirious patients experienced resolution of all new symptoms of delirium before hospital discharge. At 3- and 6-month follow-up after hospital discharge, this had risen to 20.8% and 17.7%, respectively, but the majority had persistent or recurrent symptoms. Levkoff and colleagues (1996) also reported that many patients have some symptoms of delirium without the full blown syndrome, and that this subsyndromal group has outcomes that are intermediate between patients with fully evolved delirium and those with no delirium.

Delirium is associated with significant morbidity and mortality. Thomas and coworkers (1988) found that the mean length of hospitalization was significantly longer in delirious than in nondelirious hospitalized patients, and the mortality rate was also much higher. Patients who developed delirium after elective orthopedic surgery were more likely to have postoperative complications, longer recuperation periods, longer hospital stays, and long-term disability (Rogers et al., 1989). Murray and coworkers (1993) found that over half the patients who had in-hospital delirium had worsening physical function 6 months after discharge. This was twice the rate of decline seen in nondelirious patients. O'Keeffe and Lavan (1997) found that delirium in patients admitted due to an emergency to an acute geriatric unit in a university teaching hospital was independently associated with prolonged hospital stay (versus nondelirious emergency geriatric admissions; 21 vs. 11 days), functional decline during hospitalization, and increased admission to long-term care (36% vs. 13%). Delirious, compared to nondelirious, patients were more likely to develop urinary incontinence, falls, pressure sores, and other complications during hospitalization. Rockwood and coworkers (1999) found that an episode of delirium was associated with much higher rates of subsequent dementia. Studies have found that delirium was independently associated with poor functional recovery 1 month (Marcantonio et al., 2000) or 2 years (Dolan et al., 2000) after hip fracture. It has been suggested that occult hypoxia may be the cause of delirium after femoral neck fracture and elective hip surgery (Clayer & Bruckner, 2000).

The effects of delirium on mortality are less clear-cut. Francis and colleagues (1990) found that delirious patients stayed in the hospital longer and were more likely to die or be institutionalized than patients who did not develop delirium. At 2-year follow-up (Francis & Kapoor, 1992), patients with a history of delirium had a higher mortality rate and a higher rate of loss of independent community living. Patients with "quiet" presentations of acute confusion, who often were not recognized by physicians as having delirium, also had a poor prognosis. Francis (1996) cited a meta-analysis that found a 1-month mortality of 14% and a 6-month mortality of 22% following a diagnosis of delirium; this contrasted with rates of 5% and 10%, respectively, in controls without delirium.

However, when adjustments are made for illness severity, delirium appears to have only a modest impact on mortality. In fact, Levkoff and coworkers. (1992) reported that delirium was not associated with an increased risk of mortality in 6 months of follow-up when controlling for age, sex, preexisting cognitive impairment, and illness severity. Delirium was, however, associated with a prolonged hospital stay and an increased risk of institutional placement among elderly people admitted from home.

In summary, the presence of delirium during a hospitalization places the patient at higher risk for intrahospital complications, a longer stay, and a generally poorer long-term prognosis.

DIFFERENTIAL DIAGNOSIS

The differential diagnosis of delirium includes a number of other psychiatric conditions, as discussed in *DSM-IV* (APA, 1994). Given the high prevalence of concurrent dementia in patients with delirium, the first question is whether the patient has dementia rather than delirium or has both disorders. That question is usually resolved by taking a careful history of the patient's prior symptoms to determine if dementia was present before the acute change and by following the patient's subsequent course to see how completely the symptoms clear. Patients with delirium generally fluctuate more over the course of a day or from day to day than patients with dementia.

Most critically, the sine qua non of delirium is an alteration in the level of consciousness that fluctuates. As noted in *DSM-IV* (APA, 1994), memory impairment is common to both delirium and dementia, but the person with dementia alone is usually alert. The person's alert state in the hospital is generally stable under normal conditions. Dementia patients do not have the acute fluctuating disturbance in consciousness that is characteristic of delirium. In the majority of hospitalized elderly patients who develop delirium, the symptoms are superimposed on preexisting dementia.

Intoxicated patients or patients in substance withdrawal may show some of the features of delirium without the complete syndrome. Other psychiatric syndromes may also present with symptoms suggestive of delirium. Manic patients who are restless, irritable, pressured, agitated, delusional, and hallucinating can be difficult to differentiate from hyperactive delirious patients. Manic patients are generally younger than delirious patients and have a history of prior affective episodes, usually depression. On follow-up, they are also more likely to have subsequent affective episodes.

Patients with hypoactive delirium may also be diagnosed as having major depression, particularly if they are anhedonic, apathetic, dysphoric, and unable to concentrate and show other depressionlike cognitive impairments (Nicholas & Lindsey, 1995). Delirious patients who present with delusions or hallucinations need to be distinguished from those with a brief psychotic disorder, schizophrenia, schizophreniform disorder, or other psychotic disorders. In delirium, the psychotic symptoms occur in the context of fluctuating consciousness and reduced ability to maintain and shift attention. There is also usually evidence of an underlying acute general medical condition, substance intoxication, or substance withdrawal. The psychotic symptoms tend to be fragmented and unsystematized. In rare cases, patients may have atypical presentations of symptoms of delirium due to malingering, a factitious disorder, or a conversion disorder.

ETIOLOGIES

Case reports and systematic studies suggest that delirium can be caused by almost any serious medical illness or drug intoxication in a vulnerable individual. Table 18-2 lists the common causes of delirium. These possible etiologies should be considered in the evaluation of delirious patients (see the section on evaluation). The search for etiologies is essential so that the underlying illness can be treated.

However, in many cases, no single cause can be identified (Brauer et al., 2000). For example, Francis and colleagues (1990) reported the most common etiologies of delirium in their study population as fluid and electrolyte disturbances, infection, drug toxicity, metabolic disturbances, and sensory or environmental disturbances. Drugs associated with delirium included narcotics, benzodiazepines, anticholinergic medications, methyldopa, and nonsteroidal antiinflammatory agents. An intracerebral process was implicated in only 2 cases. Alcohol or sedative drug withdrawal was a possible cause or comorbid condition in 5 cases. In only 36% of the cases could a single definite etiology be established. In another 20%, a single medical condition was believed to be a probable cause of delirium. For the remainder of the patients, multiple possible etiologies were assigned.

Medication-induced side effects, substance intoxication, and substance withdrawal are common causes of delirium and are often easily reversible. Older patients have changes in the pharmacokinetics of drugs due to changes in metabolism and excretion. This can result in a higher blood level than for a younger patient given the same oral dose. In addition, changes in pharmacody-

TABLE 18-2. Frequent causes of delirium

Medication-induced side effects
Substance intoxication
Substance withdrawal
Infections
Postanesthesia or postoperative states
Metabolic disorders
  Electrolye imbalances, dehydration, hypoglycemia or hyperglycemia, kidney failure,
    hepatic failure, anemia, vitamin deficiencies, endocrinopathies
Cardiovascular disorders
  Congestive heart failure, myocardial infarction, cardiac arrhythmia, shock, pulmonary
    emboli
Central nervous system
  Head trauma, seizures, stroke, brain injury, meningitis, encephalitis, space-occupying
    lesions (tumor, subdural hematoma, abscess)
Fracture or other trauma
Hypoxia or hypercapnia
Obstructive sleep apnea
Sleep deprivation
Sensory deprivation

namics make older persons more sensitive to the effects of drugs so that even
at a "therapeutic" blood level, an older patient may develop delirium. A good
example of this is delirium from lithium toxicity even at therapeutic or very
low blood levels in the elderly. Older patients may also be on multiple drugs
that interact and potentiate each other's effects.

With respect to substance-related delirium, the symptoms are characteristic
of delirium and in excess of those usually associated with intoxication from or
the withdrawal syndrome associated with the particular substance. The history
of substance use is the key factor in determining whether the delirium is due
to active intoxication or withdrawal. Even in individuals who appear to be
intoxicated, it is critical to assess for other possible causes of delirium, such as
head injury from a fall or from a fight. Reisner (1979) found that 13 of 27
patients referred to a psychiatric clinic in a delirious state after prolonged intoxication had chronic subdural hematomas.

Delirium due to withdrawal from alcohol or sedative, hypnotic, or anxiolytic drugs is accompanied by anxiety, sleep disturbance, and signs of autonomic hyperactivity, such as tremor, hyperreflexia, tachycardia, elevated blood
pressure, diaphoresis, flushed face, and sensory hyperacuity. In severe and untreated cases, this can progress to grand mal seizures. There are often vivid
visual hallucinations, although auditory hallucinations can also occur. The time
of onset for alcohol withdrawal is less than 24 hours, in contrast to sedative-
hypnotic withdrawal of longer-acting benzodiazepines, which tends to begin 1

or 2 days after stopping the drug. Severe alcohol withdrawal syndrome (delirium tremens) can begin as late as 7 to 10 days after alcohol has been discontinued. This latency in onset may be longer if the patient has been taking benzodiazepines.

In general, the cause of the delirium does not have much effect on the presentation of specific symptoms, although a patient in alcohol withdrawal who is hypoactive may well have an occult subdural hematoma or pneumonia. Delirium appears to be a final common pathway for conditions that interfere with higher cortical functions.

From a research point of view, a number of investigators have studied or hypothesized about the underlying mechanisms involved in the development of delirium. Brown (2000) suggested that delirium

> as a reversible dysregulation of neuronal membrane function: 1. is initiated by a functional lesion of the brain structures most sensitive to the insult in question— this is the principle of "selective vulnerability"; 2. is intimately linked to the specific functions and properties of a few neurotransmitters; 3. is a progression of characteristic signs and symptoms as structures more resistant to deliriogenic impairment are progressively affected—the principle of "progressive vulnerability." (p. 571)

He suggests that a number of neurotransmitters may be involved in the development of delirium. Excess dopamine, which can be produced under conditions of hypoxia, can facilitate the excitotoxic effects of glutamate. He also noted that acetylcholine is an important neuromodulator of cortical and hippocampal neuronal function and can disrupt higher cognitive function if its release is altered or if its effects are pharmacologically blocked.

Flacker and Lipsitz (1999b) found that serum anticholinergic activity levels were elevated in elderly patients with a febrile illness. In a review, they hypothesized that specific disruptions of neurological pathways and neurotransmitter systems may lead to delirium (Flacker & Lipsitz 1999a). Trzepacz (2000) also emphasized the importance of acetylcholine and dopamine.

Other neurotransmitters have also been studied, including somatostatin and β-endorphin (Koponen et al., 1989a, 1989b; Koponen & Riekkinen, 1990). Reduced plasma tryptophan levels, and hence serotonergic function, have been suggested as a cause of postcardiotomy delirium (van der Mast 2000). Ross (1991) hypothesized that the GABAergic, histaminergic, and serotonergic systems may also be important in different aspects of delirium. Another study found an increase in the plasma free MHPG (3-methoxy-4-hydroxyphenylglycol) concentration in the delirious state, suggesting involvement of the noradrenergic system (Nakamura et al., 1997). At present, no specific clinically useful tests to measure dysfunction in any of these neurotransmitter systems are available or used in patients with delirium.

ASSESSMENT

In community-dwelling elderly, the prevalence of delirium is low. However, older patients may be referred to a geriatric psychiatrist because of an acute change in mental status, particularly after a new medication has been started. As noted, delirium is much more common in the hospital setting, and a change in mental status may be a significant factor in the decision to hospitalize a patient. Patients may present with delirium or may develop delirium while in the hospital.

Elderly patients admitted to a hospital are at high risk for delirium; therefore, the admission history and physical should include a basic mental status exam with observations of the patient's orientation, memory, and attention. The Mini-Mental State Examination (MMSE) (Folstein et al., 1975) is recommended to screen patients for delirium (Malloy et al., 1997). The MMSE tests orientation, memory, attention, and other cognitive functions and is useful for distinguishing patients with delirium or dementia from those who are not impaired. However, the MMSE cannot distinguish delirium from dementia based on the rating alone. Furthermore, as a result of low intelligence, little schooling, or trouble understanding the questions, patients may score low even though they do not have delirium or dementia (Anthony et al., 1982).

Once an initial screening has detected some cognitive impairment, a more specific instrument should be used to diagnose delirium. The Confusion Assessment Method (CAM) was developed by Inouye and coworkers (1990) as a screening instrument for use by nonpsychiatrically trained clinicians or trained lay interviewers, and it can be completed in 10–15 minutes. A structured screening interview using the CAM for elective surgical patients was developed (Marcantonio et al., 1994) The instrument has been shown to have high sensitivity and specificity for delirium and high negative predictive accuracy, which makes it useful for screening populations at high risk for delirium. However, the false-positive rate is as high as 10%; therefore, it is recommended that all patients identified as delirious by the CAM have a complete clinical evaluation to confirm the diagnosis.

Even patients who have symptoms of delirium but who do not meet the full criteria should be carefully assessed. They may be in a prodromal stage that will progress to full-blown delirium. Even if the symptoms do not progress, Levkoff and colleagues (1996) have shown that patients with subsyndromal delirium have outcomes that are worse than patients with no symptoms of delirium, although the outcomes are not as severe as for patients with the full-blown syndrome.

EVALUATION

The clinical history is key to the evaluation of patients suspected of delirium. The first step is the recognition that symptoms of delirium are present. Any abnormalities in cognition, perception, or behavior should be checked with family members or caretakers or by examination of previous medical records to determine if they were present before the acute illness that led to the hospitalization. Prior history will identify patients whose symptoms may be due to dementia or some other psychiatric disorder. The history should also focus on any recent new medications or changes in medication dosage, use of alcohol or illicit drugs, or changes in the patient's physical condition. Prescription and nonprescription medications can cause delirium in an older person who has reduced metabolism of the drug or increased sensitivity to its effects because of age or drug-disease or drug-drug interactions. Brown and Stoudemire (1998) wrote an entire book on prescription and over-the-counter medications that cause delirium.

Medications with anticholinergic activity have been of particular interest because it has been known for many years that they can cause delirium (Golinger et al., 1987). Elderly patients appear to be particularly vulnerable to the effects of these medications because of age-related declines in cholinergic neurotransmission, which are accentuated by subclinical or clinically overt Alzheimer's disease. Significant correlations have been reported between elevated serum concentrations of anticholinergics measured by a radioreceptor assay and the development of cognitive impairment, including delirium. Mach and colleagues (1995) found that delirious patients whose syndrome resolved with discontinuation of medications had higher initial serum anticholinergic levels compared with those whose symptoms persisted. In addition, all patients in their sample in whom delirium resolved had a decrease in serum anticholinergic activity.

Mussi and colleagues (1999) found significantly higher levels of serum anticholinergic activity in delirious patients. The assay is not yet commercially available, however, and the usual approach when faced with a delirious patient is to reduce any medication with anticholinergic activity. Tune and colleagues (1992) measured the anticholinergic activity of commonly used drugs and found that many drugs have anticholinergic activity that they did not suspect as having such properties. These include furosemide, digoxin, theophylline, prednisolone, and cimetidine.

Following the history, during the clinical examination, the patient should be observed for behavioral symptoms of delirium, including restlessness, suspiciousness, somnolence, hyperalertness, unstable mood, belligerence, or distractibility. Even if a patient seems completely unaffected, it is important to review any notes written in the medical record over the past 48 hours and to ask the nursing staff on the unit about any abnormal behavior. It is not unusual for patients to seem pleasant and cooperative on rounds in the morning, but agitated and disoriented at night.

As noted, delirium can be caused by many different disorders. In addition to the history described above, these possibilities also need to be investigated systematically with a thorough physical examination and laboratory evaluation. The physical examination should include careful attention to the patient's vital signs and evaluation of the patient's neurological, cardiac, and pulmonary systems. The standard laboratory assessment includes a complete blood count with differential and platelet count; serum chemistries, including albumin, BUN, calcium, creatinine, electrolytes, sedimentation rate; thyroid and liver function tests; a urinalysis; electrocardiogram; and chest X ray. Serum drug levels are very important in identifying high or potentially toxic levels of certain drugs (e.g., lithium, digoxin, tricyclic antidepressants, anticonvulsants, cyclosporine, or quinidine). The clinical history or physical examination may suggest other possible etiologies that require more specific workup (e.g., if the patient is febrile or had occupational exposure to toxins). In alcoholics, vitamin B_{12} and folate levels are usually routine.

One of the challenges in determining etiology is that often multiple laboratory abnormalities turn up as part of the workup. Furthermore, the abnormality may be "borderline abnormal" (e.g., a serum sodium of 132 mmol/L, with 136–142 mmol/L the reference range), which is unlikely to be the direct cause of delirium. Similarly, in a recently drinking alcoholic who presents with a hypoactive delirium, the patient's alcoholism is unlikely to be the cause, and a second diagnosis should be suspected, such as head trauma, subdural hematoma, pneumonia, or liver failure. It is very important that a consulting psychiatrist work closely with the other physicians caring for the patient to identify and correct any conditions that may be contributing to the delirium. A judgment that some condition is etiologically related to the delirium may also depend on the time course of symptoms. An abnormality that is likely to be etiologic should precede the onset of delirium and should return to normal when the delirium clears.

If a specific central nervous system disorder is suspected, a computed tomographic (CT) or magnetic resonance imaging (MRI) scan, a lumbar puncture, and an electroencephalogram (EEG) should be considered. The EEG has been used for over 50 years in the study of delirium, although a routine EEG or 24-hour ambulatory monitoring are primarily indicated for a patient who is suspected of having seizures. From a research point of view, Romano and Engel (1944) found that decreased background EEG frequency and disorganization of the EEG correlated with reduced arousal. Brenner (1991) reviewed the usefulness of EEGs in the evaluation of delirium and noted that, in most patients with delirium, the EEG shows diffuse slowing, and the degree of the EEG changes correlates with the severity of the encephalopathy. If the delirium is due to withdrawal from alcohol or sedative-hypnotic drugs, the EEG may show a paroxysmal burst of high-voltage, slow-frequency activity, which precedes the development of seizures. Leuchter and coworkers (1993) suggested that the EEG is a moderately sensitive, but nonspecific, indicator of brain dysfunction in elderly people. Jacobson and colleagues (1993) used quantitative EEG techniques to assist in the differential diagnosis of encephalopathy in elderly subjects with delirium, dementia, and delirium with dementia. At present, quantitative EEGs are infrequently used as part of the routine workup for delirium, although it may be advantageous (Jacobson & Jerrier, 2000).

Similarly, brain-imaging techniques, including single-photon emission computed tomography (SPECT) scans, have been used in the study of delirium (Lerner & Rosenstein, 2000), but are not routinely used unless structural brain disease or space-occupying lesions are suspected. Hall and associates (1999) found that impaired cerebral perfusion on SPECT scans may identify patients at risk for cognitive deficits after cardiac surgery. Many, if not most, agitated delirious patients will not be able to tolerate the noise, immobility, and confinement of an MRI scan unless sedated.

Koponen, Hurri, and coworkers (1989) found that patients with delirium had significantly more ventricular dilatation and cortical atrophy on CT scans than control subjects. Focal changes were also more common in the delirious patients, and these changes tended to concentrate in the high-order association areas of the right hemisphere. They indicated that structural brain disease plays a marked predisposing role in the development of delirium in elderly patients.

MANAGEMENT

The approach to the management of delirium involves screening patients at high risk of developing delirium, preventing the disorder when possible, recognizing it as soon as it appears, evaluating the patient to determine the underlying cause, reversing the primary cause if possible, providing supportive care while the patient is delirious, and if necessary, treating behavioral symptoms such as agitation, delusions, or hallucinations.

Prevention involves a variety of approaches. The study by Inouye, Bogardus, and colleagues (1999) is the best clinical trial of a multifactorial prevention strategy. In geriatric medical practice, it is always preferable to minimize the number and dosages of medications, particularly those that may cause confusion. Sometimes, the substitution of different drugs within therapeutic class (e.g., using a selective serotonin reuptake inhibitor [SSRI] instead of a tricyclic antidepressant or an angiotensin-converting enzyme [ACE] inhibitor instead of a beta-blocker) can eliminate symptoms of delirium. On the other hand, it is critical to treat and stabilize a patient's underlying medical conditions so that the patients are better able to withstand acute events such as elective surgery.

Studies of risk factors discussed above also suggest preventive measures. For example, Gustafson and colleagues (1991), using several interventions, reduced the incidence and severity of postoperative delirium in elderly patients with hip fracture from 61.3% to 47.6%. These interventions included operating as soon as possible, having a specialist in geriatric medicine do careful preoperative assessments, giving extra doses of diuretic to patients with clinical signs of heart failure, giving heparin for thrombosis prophylaxis in patients with heart failure, measurement of blood gases and use of nasal oxygen to ensure adequate oxygenation, and anesthetic techniques to manage perioperative hypotension aggressively. In addition, patients were carefully assessed and treated postoperatively for complications such as anemia, heart failure, urinary tract infections, urinary retention, pneumonia, and the like.

Aakerlund and Rosenberg (1994) showed that supplemental oxygen was effective in treating delirium in patients who underwent thoracotomy for pulmonary malignancy. It is also important to ensure that patients are getting adequate hydration and nutrition.

Psychological support may also be helpful, such as carefully explaining to patients and family members what to expect in the postoperative period. This can reduce anxiety and improve the detection of symptoms of delirium so that proper treatment can be instituted.

If a patient becomes delirious, it is very helpful to have the family stay (even around the clock) with the patient to provide reassurance and orientation. Maintaining the patient's sleep-wake cycle is important, and patients with exposure to sunlight in rooms with windows (properly secured) are less likely to become confused.

Recognition, evaluation, and treatment of the specific cause have been described above. In addition, supportive measures are often helpful. Nursing interventions have been described for general medical patients (Morency, 1990), postoperative patients (Neelon, 1990), cancer patients (Rando, 1990), and hip fracture patients (Brannstrom et al., 1989; Williams et al., 1985). Table 18-3 lists some of the approaches used to manage confused patients. The decision whether a delirious patient can be better managed on a medical floor or on a psychiatric inpatient unit is usually made on the basis of the severity of the patient's medical illness and behavioral problems, the intensity of the treatment interventions needed, and the sophistication of the nursing staff in both units.

TABLE 18-3.   Nursing interventions for the patient with delirium

Keep the patient in a quiet room with lights on in the daytime and a night-light after bedtime.

Avoid excessive sensory stimulation, but provide some gentle music or television.

Have orientation cues such as a calendar or clock clearly visible to the patient.

Correct sensory impairments with eyeglasses or a hearing aid.

Keep the patient near the nursing station for regular checks and staff interaction.

Encourage family presence for reassurance and orientation.

Have available familiar objects from home such as family pictures.

Explain staff interventions in a clear, firm, but caring manner.

Use physical restraints only if the patient is unsupervised and at risk of falling or pulling out intravenous lines, urinary catheters, or other tubes. Adequate documentation, frequent nursing checks, and proper and rotating positioning are absolutely essential. Follow hospital policy guidelines.

Carefully monitor intake of fluids and food and ensure adequate intake.

PHARMACOLOGICAL MANAGEMENT

The quietly confused patient can generally be managed safely using the above interventions, including careful monitoring. Patients who are highly agitated or psychotic will often need pharmacological intervention to help manage their behavioral disturbance, particularly on a medical or surgical unit.

If the delirium is due to withdrawal from alcohol, an evidence-based practice guideline for pharmacological management is available (Mayo-Smith, 1997). This guideline was largely developed for younger patients and needs to be adapted to the geriatric patient. Benzodiazepines reduce withdrawal severity, the incidence of delirium, and seizures. The American Society of Addiction Medicine Working Group on Pharmacological Management of Alcohol Withdrawal (Mayo-Smith, 1997) recommended benzodiazepines over most other sedative-hypnotics because of their documented efficacy, greater margin of safety, and low abuse potential. All benzodiazepines appear to have similar efficacy in reducing signs and symptoms of withdrawal. In general, shorter acting benzodiazepines such as lorazepam or oxazepam are preferred for older patients. Other medications, such as beta-blockers, clonidine, and carbamazepine, can be used adjunctively because they reduce the severity of withdrawal, but their effect on delirium and seizures is unclear.

If the delirium does not appear to be associated with substance abuse but the patient is agitated, several treatment options are available. If the patient is clearly psychotic, the first choice is generally to use a neuroleptic drug, perhaps because of their dopamine-blocking activity. In general, butyrophenones (e.g., haloperidol) or atypical neuroleptics (e.g., risperidone or olanzapine) are preferable to phenothiazines because the phenothiazines have anticholinergic effects that can cause or worsen delirium and α-adrenergic blocking effects that can cause hypotension. Haloperidol, in doses from 0.5 to 5 mg, can be given orally, intramuscularly, or intravenously every 4 hours up to a maximum of 20 mg per day and can be titrated to the patient's response. High doses of haloperidol may be associated with fatal cardiac arrhythmias (Hunt & Stern, 1995), and cardiac monitoring is advisable if high doses of haloperidol are used. In an attempt to avoid the side effects associated with haloperidol or other typical neuroleptics, atypical neuroleptics such as risperidone, olanzapine, or quetiapine have been used, although there is little systematic study of their use in delirium or in medically ill geriatric patients.

As an alternative to neuroleptics for patients who are not psychotic and primarily require sedation, a short-acting benzodiazepine can be used. Lorazepam 0.25 to 2 mg can be given at bedtime or every 4 hours orally, intramuscularly, or intravenously up to a maximum of 6 mg per day. There is extensive clinical experience using lorazepam in delirium, but data from controlled clinical trials are limited. Breitbart and coworkers (1996) compared lorazepam with haloperidol or chlorpromazine for the treatment of delirium in hospitalized AIDS patients. They found that both neuroleptics were effective and caused few side effects. However, all 6 patients who received lorazepam developed treatment-limiting side effects, including oversedation, disinhibition, ataxia, and increasing confusion, leading to refusal to take the drug or requiring discontinuation of the drug. Although this study was done in a highly specialized population, it does raise some serious concerns about the use of lorazepam as an alternative to haloperidol.

Given the association of high-serum anticholinergic levels in patients with delirium, there has been some interest in the use of cholinesterase inhibitors for delirium. For patients whose delirium is most likely due to an overdose of an anticholinergic drug such as benztropine, parenteral physostigmine has been successfully used to reverse the symptoms (Burns et al., 2000; Stern, 1983). This is often done more for diagnostic than therapeutic purposes. Given the risks involved with physostigmine, its administration should be done under cardiac monitoring by an internist or anesthesiologist. Longer acting oral cholinesterase inhibitors such as tacrine, donepezil, rivastigmine, or galantamine have been used in the treatment of Alzheimer's disease because of the evidence for a cholinergic deficit in such patients. Cummings (2000) suggests these agents may contribute to the management of other neuropsychiatric disorders with cholinergic abnormalities. To date, there are no published controlled studies of their use in delirium in patients with or without Alzheimer's disease, but case reports have suggested that symptoms of delirium caused by anticholinergic medication can be reversed by cholinesterase inhibitors (Itil & Fink, 1966; Wengel et al., 1998). The newer cholinesterase inhibitors (i.e., rivastigmine and galantamine) may have fewer drug-drug interactions.

REFERENCES

Aakerlund LP, Rosenberg J. Postoperative delirium: treatment with supplementary oxygen. *Br J Anaesth*. 1994;72:286–290.

American Psychiatric Association. *Diagnostic and Statistical Manual of Mental Disorders*. 3rd ed. Washington, DC: American Psychiatric Press; 1980.

American Psychiatric Association. *Diagnostic and Statistical Manual of Mental Disorders*. 4th ed. Washington, DC: American Psychiatric Press; 1994.

American Psychiatric Association. Practice guideline for the treatment of patients with delirium. *Am J Psychiatry*. 1999;156(5 suppl):1–20.

Anthony JC, LeResche L, Niaz U, et al. Limits of the "Mini-Mental State" as a screening test for dementia and delirium among hospital patients. *Psychol Med*. 1982;12:397–408.

Bowman AM. The relationship of anxiety to development of postoperative delirium. *J Gerontol Nurs*. 1992;1:24–30.

Brannstrom B, Gustafson Y, Norberg A, et al. Problems of basic nursing care in acutely confused and non-confused hip-fracture patients. *Scand J Caring Sci*. 1989;1:27–34.

Brauer C, Morrison RS, Silberzweig SB, et al. The cause of delirium in patients with hip fracture. *Arch Intern Med*. 2000;160:1856–1860.

Breitbart W, Marotta R, Platt MM, et al. A double-blind trial of haloperidol, chlorpromazine, and lorazepam in the treatment of delirium in hospitalized AIDS patients. *Am J Psychiatry.* 1996;153:231–237.

Brenner RP. Utility of EEG in delirium: past views and current practice. *Int Psychogeriatr.* 1991;3:211–229.

Brown TM. Basic mechanisms in the pathogenesis of delirium. In: Stoudemire A, Fogel BS, Greenberg DB, eds. *Psychiatric Care of the Medical Patient.* 2nd ed. Washington, DC: American Psychiatric Press; 2000:571–580.

Brown TM, Stoudemire A. *Psychiatric Side Effects of Prescription and Over the Counter Medications.* Washington, DC: American Psychiatric Press; 1998.

Bucht G, Gustafson Y, Sandberg O. Epidemiology of delirium. *Dement Geriatr Cogn Disord.* 1999;10:315–318.

Burns MJ, Linden CH, Gravdins A, et al. A comparison of physostigmine and benzodiazepines for the treatment of anticholinergic poisoning. *Ann Emerg Med.* 2000;35:374–381.

Camus V, Gonthier R, Dubos G, et al. Etiologic and outcome profiles in hypoactive and hyperactive subtypes of delirium. *J Geriatr Psychiatry Neurol.* 2000;13:38–42.

Carlson LA, Gottfries CG, Winblad B, et al. Delirium in the elderly. *Dement Geriatr Cogn Disord.* 1999;10:305–430.

Clayer M, Bruckner J. Occult hypoxia after femoral neck fracture and elective hip surgery. *Clin Orthop.* 2000;370:265–271.

Cummings JL. Cholinesterase inhibitors: a new class of psychotropic compounds. *Am J Psychiatry.* 2000;157:4–15.

Dolan MM, Hawkes WG, Zimmerman SI, et al. Delirium on hospital admission in aged hip fracture patients: prediction of mortality and 2-year functional outcomes. *J Gerontol.* 2000;55A:M527–M534.

Fann JR. The epidemiology of delirium: a review of studies and methodological issues. *Semin Clin Neuropsychiatry.* 2000;5:64–74.

Flacker JM, Lipsitz LA. Neural mechanisms of delirium: current hypotheses and evolving concepts. *J Gerontol.* 1999a;54A:B239–B246.

Flacker JM, Lipsitz LA. Serum anticholinergic activity changes with acute illness in elderly medical patients. *J Gerontol.* 1999b;54A:M12–M16.

Folstein MF, Bassett SS, Romanoski AJ, et al. The epidemiology of delirium in the community: the Eastern Baltimore Mental Health Survey. *Int Psychogeriatr.* 1991;3:169–176.

Folstein MF, Folstein SE, McHugh PR. Mini-Mental State: a practical method for grading the cognitive state of patients for the clinician. *J Psychiatr Res.* 1975;12:189–198.

Francis J. Delirium. In: Reuben DB, Yoshikawa TT, Besdine RW, eds. *Geriatrics Review Syllabus: A Core Curriculum in Geriatric Medicine.* 3rd ed. Dubuque, IA: Kendall-Hunt Publishing Company for the American Geriatrics Society; 1996:120–123.

Francis J, Kapoor WN. Prognosis after hospital discharge of older medical patients with delirium. *J Am Geriatr Soc.* 1992;40:601–606.

Francis J, Martin D, Kapoor WN. A prospective study of delirium in hospitalized elderly. *JAMA.* 1990;8:1097–1101.

Goldstein MZ, Fogel BS. Cognitive change after elective surgery in nondemented older adults. *Am J Geriatr Psychiatry.* 1993;1:118–125.

Golinger R, Peet T, Tune L. Association of elevated plasma anticholinergic levels with delirium in surgical patients. *Am J Psychiatry.* 1987;144:1218–1220.

Gustafson Y, Brannstrom B, Norberg A, et al. Underdiagnosis and poor documentation of acute confusional states in elderly hip fracture patients. *J Am Geriatr Soc.* 1991; 39:760–765.

Hall RA, Fordyce DJ, Lee ME, et al. Brain SPECT imaging and neuropsychological testing in coronary artery bypass patients. *Ann Thorac Surg.* 1999;68:2082–2088.

Hammon JW, Stump DA, Kon ND, et al. Risk factors and solutions for the development of neurobehavioral changes after coronary artery bypass grafting. *Ann Thorac Surg.* 1997;63:1613–1618.

Hunt N, Stern T. The association between intravenous haloperidol and torsades de pointes. Three cases and a literature review. *Psychosomatics.* 1995;36:541–549.

Inouye SK. Predisposing and precipitating factors for delirium in hospitalized older patients. *Dement Geriatr Cogn Disord.* 1999;10:393–400.

Inouye SK, Bogardus ST, Charpentier PA, et al. A multicomponent intervention to prevent delirium in hospitalized older patients. *N Engl J Med.* 1999;340:669–676.

Inouye SK, Charpentier PA. Precipitating factors for delirium in hospitalized elderly persons predictive model and interrelationship with baseline vulnerability. *JAMA.* 1996;275:852–857.

Inouye SK, Schlesinger MJ, Lydon TJ. Delirium: a symptom of how hospital care is failing older persons and a window to improve quality of hospital care. *Am J Med.* 1999;106:565–573.

Inouye SK, VanDyck CH, Alessi CA, et al. Clarifying confusion: the confusion assessment method: a new method for detection of delirium. *Ann Intern Med.* 1990;113: 941–948.

Inouye SK, Viscoli CM, Horwitz RI, et al. A predictive model for delirium in hospitalized elderly medical patients based on admission characteristics. *Ann Intern Med.* 1993;119:474–481.

Itil T, Fink M. Anticholinergic drug-induced delirium: experimental modification, quantitative EEG and behavioral correlations. *J Nerv Ment Dis.* 1966;6:492–507.

Jacobson SA, Jerrier H. EEG in delirium. *Semin Clin Neuropsychiatry.* 2000;5:86–92.

Jacobson SA, Leuchter AF, Walter DO. Conventional and quantitative EEG in the diagnosis of delirium among the elderly. *J Neurol Neurosurg Psychiatry.* 1993;56:153–158.

Koponen H, Hurri L, Stenback U, et al. Computed tomography findings in delirium. *J Nerv Ment Dis.* 1989;4:226–231.

Koponen H, Riekkinen P. A longitudinal study of cerebrospinal fluid beta-endorphin-like immunoreactivity in delirium: changes at the acute stage and at one-year follow-up. *Acta Psychiatr Scand.* 1990;82:323–326.

Koponen H, Stenback U, Mattila E, et al. Cerebrospinal fluid somatostatin in delirium. *Psychol Med.* 1989a;19:605–609.

Koponen H, Stenback U, Mattila E, et al. CSF beta-endorphin-like immunoreactivity in delirium. *Biol Psychiatry.* 1989b;25:938–944.

Koponen H, Stenback U, Mattila E, et al. Delirium among elderly persons admitted to a psychiatric hospital: clinical course during the acute stage and 1-year follow-up. *Acta Psychiatr Scand.* 1989c;79:579–585.

Lawlor PG, Gagnon B, Mancini IL, et al. Occurrence, causes, and outcome of delirium in patients with advanced cancer. *Arch Intern Med.* 2000;160:786–794.

Lerner AJ, Hedera P, Koss E, et al. Delirium in Alzheimer disease. *Alzheimer Dis Assoc Disord.* 1997;11:16–20.

Lerner DM, Rosenstein DI. Neuroimaging in delirium and related conditions. *Semin Clin Neuropsychiatry.* 2000;5:98–112.

Leuchter AF, Daly KA, Rosenberg-Thompson S, et al. Prevalence and significance of electroencephalographic abnormalities in patients with suspected organic mental syndromes. *J Am Geriatr Soc.* 1993;41:605–611.

Levkoff S, Cleary P, Liptzin B, et al. Epidemiology of delirium: an overview of research issues and findings. *Int Psychogeriatr.* 1991;3:149–167.

Levkoff SE, Evans DA, Liptzin B, et al. Delirium: the occurrence and persistence of symptoms among elderly hospitalized patients. *Arch Intern Med.* 1992;152:334–340.

Levkoff SE, Liptzin B, Cleary PD, et al. Subsyndromal delirium. *Am J Geriatr Psychiatry.* 1996;4:320–329.

Lipowski ZJ. *Delirium: Acute Confusional States.* New York, NY: Oxford University Press; 1990.

Liptzin B, Levkoff SE. An empirical study of delirium subtypes. *Br J Psychiatry.* 1992; 161:843–845.

Mach JR, Dysken MW, Kuskowski M. Serum anticholinergic activity in hospitalized older persons with delirium: a preliminary study. *J Am Geriatr Soc.* 1995;43:491–495.

Malloy PF, Cummings JL, Coffey CE, et al. Cognitive screening instruments in neuropsychiatry: a report of the committee on research of the American Neuropsychiatric Association. *J Neuropsychiatry Clin Neurosci.* 1997;9:189–197.

Marcantonio ER, Flacker JM, Michaels M, et al. Delirium is independently associated with poor functional recovery after hip fracture. *J Am Geriatr Soc.* 2000;48:618–624.

Marcantonio ER, Goldman L, Mangione CM, et al. A clinical prediction rule for delirium after elective non-cardiac surgery. *JAMA.* 1994;271:134–139.

Martin NJ, Stones MJ, Young JE, et al. Development of delirium: a prospective cohort study in a community hospital. *Int Psychogeriatr.* 2000;12:117–127.

Massie MJ, Holland JC, Glass E. Delirium in terminally ill cancer patients. *Am J Psychiatry.* 1983;140:1048–1050.

Mayo-Smith MF. Pharmacological management of alcohol withdrawal: a meta-analysis and evidence-based practice guideline. *JAMA.* 1997;278:144–151.

Meagher DJ, Trzepacz PT. Motoric subtypes of delirium. *Semin Clin Neuropsychiatry.* 2000;5:75–85.

Morency CR. Mental status change in the elderly: recognizing and treating delirium. *J Prof Nurs.* 1990;6:356–365.

Murray AM, Levkoff SE, Wetle TT, et al. Acute delirium and functional decline in the hospitalized elderly patient. *J Gerontol.* 1993;48:M181–M186.

Mussi C, Ferrari R, Ascari S, et al. Importance of serum anticholinergic activity in the assessment of elderly patients with delirium. *J Geriatr Psychiatry Neurol.* 1999;12: 82–86.

Nakamura J, Uchimura N, Yamada S, et al. Does plasma free-3-methoxy-4-hydroxyphenyl (ethylene) glycol increase in the delirious state? A comparison of the effects of mianserin and haloperidol on delirium. *Int Clin Psychopharmacol.* 1997;12:147–152.

Neelon VJ. Postoperative confusion. *Crit Care Nurs Clin North Am.* 1990;4:579–587.

Newman MF, Croughwell ND, Blumenthal JA, et al. Predictors of cognitive decline after cardiac operation. *Ann Thorac Surg.* 1995;59:1326–1330.

Nicholas LM, Lindsey BA. Delirium presenting with symptoms of depression. *Psychosomatics.* 1995;36:471–479.

O'Keeffe ST. Clinical subtypes of delirium in the elderly. *Dement Geriatr Cogn Disord.* 1999;10:380–385.

O'Keeffe ST, Lavan JN. The prognostic significance of delirium in older hospital patients. *J Am Geriatr Soc.* 1997;45:174–178.

O'Keeffe ST, Lavan JN. Clinical significance of delirium subtypes in older people. *Age Ageing.* 1999;28:115–119.

Rando EV. Delirium in elderly cancer patients: nursing management. *Dimensions Oncol Nurs.* 1990;2:5–8.

Reisner H. Das chronische subdurale Hamatom-Pachymeningeosis haemorrhagica interna. *Nervenarzt.* 1979;50:74–78.

Ritchie K, Polge C, deRoquefeuil G, et al. Impact of anesthesia on the cognitive functioning of the elderly. *Int Psychogeriatr.* 1997;9:309–329.

Rockwood K, Cosway S, Carver D, et al. The risk of dementia and death after delirium. *Age Ageing.* 1999;28:551–556.

Rogers MP, Liang MH, Daltroy LH, et al. Delirium after elective orthopedic surgery: risk factors and natural history. *Int J Psychiatry Med.* 1989;19:109–121.

Romano J, Engel GL. Studies of delirium I: electroencephalographic data. *Arch Neurol Psychiatry.* 1944;51:356–377.

Ross CA. CNS arousal systems: possible role in delirium. *Int Psychogeriatr.* 1991;3:353–371.

Rudberg MA, Pompei P, Foreman MD, et al. The natural history of delirium in older hospitalized patients: a syndrome of heterogeneity. *Age Ageing.* 1997;26:169–174.

Sandberg O, Gustafson Y, Brannstrom B, et al. Clinical profile of delirium in older patients. *J Am Geriatr Soc.* 1999;47:1300–1306.

Stern T. Continuous infusion of physostigmine in anticholinergic delirium: a case report. *J Clin Psychiatry.* 1983;44:463–464.

Thomas RI, Cameron DJ, Fahs MC. A prospective study of delirium and prolonged hospital stay. *Arch Gen Psychiatry.* 1988;45:937–940.

Trzepacz PT. Is there a final common neural pathway in delirium? Focus on acetylcholine and dopamine. *Semin Clin Neuropsychiatry.* 2000;5:132–148.

Tune L, Carr S, Hoag E, et al. Anticholinergic effects of drugs commonly prescribed for the elderly: potential means for assessing risk of delirium. *Am J Psychiatry.* 1992;149:1393–1394.

van der Mast RC. Postoperative delirium. *Dement Geriatr Cogn Disord.* 1999;10:401–405.

van der Mast RC. Is delirium after cardiac surgery related to plasma amino acids and physical condition? *J Neuropsychiatry Clin Neurosci.* 2000;12:57–63.

Wengel SP, Roccaforte WH, Burke WJ. Donepezil improves symptoms of delirium in dementia: implications for future research. *J Geriatr Psychiatry Neurol.* 1998;11:159–161.

Williams MA, Campbell EB, Raynor WJ, et al. Reducing acute confusional states in elderly patients with hip fractures. *Nurs Health.* 1985;8:329–337.

19

Other Dementias and Mental Disorders Due to General Medical Conditions

David K. Conn, MB, BCh, BAO, FRCP (C)

The most frequently diagnosed forms of dementia are Alzheimer's disease (AD) and the vascular dementias. The first half of this chapter focuses on the other forms of dementia that should always be considered in the differential diagnosis of progressive cognitive impairment. The second half of this chapter describes the secondary mental disorders that were referred to as "organic mental disorders" in the *Diagnostic and Statistical Manual of Mental Disorders, Third Edition, Revised* (*DSM-III-R*; American Psychiatric Association [APA], 1987). In the fourth edition of the *DSM* (*DSM-IV*; APA, 1994) the term *organic* was deleted; instead, the actual physical disorder or responsible substance must be specified (e.g., mood disorder due to stroke).

OTHER DEMENTIAS

In *DSM-IV* (APA, 1994), the requirement for a diagnosis of dementia includes the development of multiple cognitive deficits manifested by both (1) memory impairment and (2) at least one of aphasia, apraxia, agnosia, or a disturbance in executive functioning. In addition, the deficits must cause significant impairment in social or occupational functioning and represent a significant decline from a previous level of functioning. Many disorders are known to cause dementia. Katzman (1991) lists approximately 70 diseases; an abbreviated list of the more important causes can be found in Table 19-1.

TABLE 19-1.   Diseases that may present as dementia

Alzheimer's disease	Multiple sclerosis
Other degenerative diseases	Vasculitis
Frontotemporal dementia	Toxic dementia
Huntington's disease	Alcoholic dementia
Parkinson's disease	Metallic poisons
Dementia with Lewy bodies	Organic poisons (e.g., solvents)
Amyotrophic lateral sclerosis	Dementia following head injury
Progressive supranuclear palsy	Dementia syndrome of depression
Wilson's disease	Nutritional disorders
Vascular dementias	Vitamin B_{12} deficiency
Multiinfarct dementia	Folate deficiency
Lacunar dementia	Pellagra (vitamin B_6 deficiency)
Binswanger's disease	Thiamine deficiency
Infections	Metabolic/endocrine disorders
Creutzfeldt-Jakob disease	Hyperthyroidism
AIDS	Hypothyroidism
Postencephalitic dementia	Hypercalcemia
Neurosyphilis	Renal failure
Normal-pressure hydrocephalus	Hepatic encephalopathy
Space-occupying lesions	Cushing's syndrome
Subdural hematoma	Addison's disease
Brain tumor	

In a review of nine published studies, Katzman (1991) found that 65.9% of patients had Alzheimer's disease; 17.1% had other progressive dementias, most commonly multiinfarct dementia; 10.5% had dementias for which specific treatment was indicated (most commonly hydrocephalus or dementias associated with alcohol dependence or tumors); 4.7% had dementias suitable for specific interventions (most commonly caused by drug toxicity or metabolic disturbances); and 1.8% had dementias of uncertain etiology. However, neuropathological autopsy studies have found that between 15% and 25% of elderly patients with dementia have Lewy bodies in their brain stem and cortex (McKeith et al., 1996). Although dementia with Lewy bodies (DLB) is considered a type of dementia distinct from Alzheimer's disease, criteria for this diagnosis are evolving and remain the subject of much debate.

Clarfield (1988), in a review of 42 published studies of 2,889 subjects, investigated the "reversibility" of dementia. Of the subjects, 56.8% had Alzheimer's disease, 13.3% had multiinfarct dementia, and depression accounted for 4.5%, alcohol abuse for 4.2%, and drug abuse for 1.5%. Follow-up was described in 11 studies and revealed that 8% of the patients improved, at least partially; 3% fully returned to premorbid levels of functioning. These etiologies most commonly included depression (26%), drugs (28%), and metabolic conditions (15.5%). Maletta (1990) criticized the use of the term *reversible* dementia and noted that the concept creates misunderstanding. Maletta suggested that an alternative would be to label those dementias with a continuing decline that responds to treatment as remediable, remittable, or arrestable. Regardless of terminology, the effective treatment of many conditions that cause patients to meet contemporary criteria for dementia can lead to full recovery of cognitive functioning.

Frontotemporal Dementia

The onset of frontotemporal dementia (FTD) occurs most commonly between the ages of 45 and 65 years, although it can present earlier or in the elderly (Snowden et al., 2002). The mean duration of the illness is 8 years, with a range from 2 to 20 years. Dementia affecting the frontal and temporal lobes was first reported by Pick in 1892, who described a 71-year-old man with a 3-year history of dementia. For many years, almost all frontal dementias were termed Pick's disease.

A variety of classification systems has been proposed for dementias that primarily affect these regions. The Lund and Manchester groups first used the term frontotemporal dementia and developed consensus criteria for diagnosis (Lund and Manchester Groups, 1994). The criteria were subsequently revised (Neary et al., 1998) as outlined in Table 19-2. FTD can be subclassified on the basis of clinical presentation (see below) or according to histological findings. About 20% of FTD cases demonstrate a distinct neuropathology that includes Pick bodies, inflated cells, white matter gliosis, and the loss of dendritic spines (Pick type). A Pick body is an intracytoplasmic mass composed of neurofilaments and neurotubules. These distinctive histological features are not seen in other FTDs. The most common histological finding in FTD is spongiform degeneration or microvacuolation of the superficial neuropil with minimal gliosis (microvacuolar type).

Clinically, there are several different presentations in FTD, with the earliest changes usually related to personality. Disinhibited and socially inappropriate behaviors are associated with pathological changes in the orbitomedial frontal and anterior temporal regions. However, some patients present primarily with apathy and lack of motivation and others with stereotyped, ritualistic behavior. These different clinical presentations appear to be related to the location of brain damage rather than to the underlying histological findings. Speech language disturbances may include slow deliberate speech with long pauses, anomia, echolalia, perseveration, and subsequent mutism (Jung & Solomon, 1993).

During the early course of the illness, the Kluver-Bucy syndrome may occur, but there is sparing of memory, visuospatial abilities, and the ability to calculate. The potential features of Kluver-Bucy syndrome in patients with FTD include hyperphagia, gluttony, hypermetamorphosis, emotional blunting, hypersexuality, and visual or auditory agnosia. Increased food intake with weight gain and affective changes are especially common (Cummings & Duchen, 1981).

TABLE 19-2.   Clinical diagnostic features of frontotemporal dementia (FTD)

I. Core diagnostic features
  A. Insidious onset and gradual progression
  B. Early decline in social interpersonal conduct
  C. Early impairment in regulation of personal conduct
  D. Early emotional blunting
  E. Early loss of insight
II. Supportive diagnostic features
  A. Behavioral disorder
    1. Decline in personal hygiene and grooming
    2. Mental rigidity and inflexibility
    3. Distractibility and impersistence
    4. Hyperorality and dietary changes
    5. Preservative and stereotyped behavior
    6. Utilization behavior
  B. Speech and language
    1. Altered speech output
      a. Aspontaneity and economy of speech
      b. Press of speech
    2. Stereotypy of speech
    3. Echolalia
    4. Preservation
    5. Mutism
  C. Physical signs
    1. Primitive reflexes
    2. Incontinence
    3. Akinesia, rigidity, and tremor
    4. Low and labile blood pressure
  D. Investigations
    1. Neuropsychology: significant impairment on frontal lobe tests in the absence
       of severe amnesia, aphasia, or perceptuospatial disorder
    2. Electroencephalography: normal or conventional electroencephalogram de-
       spite clinically evident dementia
    3. Brain imaging (structural or functional): predominant frontal or anterior tem-
       poral abnormality

Source: From Neary et al. (1998).

A study of the Lund-Manchester criteria showed that loss of personal awareness, hyperorality, stereotyped and perseverative behavior, progressive reduction of speech, and preserved spatial orientation differentiated 100% of
subjects with FTD and AD (Miller et al., 1997).

  Some individuals with FTD have a family history of dementia with autosomal dominant inheritance. In some families, linkage to chromosome 17 has
been demonstrated, and mutations in the tau gene have also been identified
(Hutton et al., 1998).

In addition to delineating criteria for FTD, Neary and coworkers (1998) developed clinical criteria for two related clinical syndromes: progressive nonfluent aphasia (PA) and semantic dementia (SD). PA is characterized by a disorder of expressive language with relative preservation of other aspects of cognition. Core diagnostic features include nonfluent spontaneous speech with at least one of the following: agrammatism, phonemic paraphasias, and anomia. The initial dominant feature of SD is impaired understanding of word meaning or object identity with relative preservation of other cognitive functioning. Patients develop progressive, fluent, empty spontaneous speech with impaired word naming and comprehension and semantic paraphasias. They may develop impaired recognition of faces (prosopagnosia) or impaired recognition of object identity (associative agnosia). Amyotrophic lateral sclerosis can be associated with FTD, the features of which may pre-date the motor neuron findings. This variant has shown linkage to chromosome 9 (Hosler et al., 2000).

The computed tomography (CT) scan may be normal during the early stages of FTD; subsequently, focal atrophy of the frontal or temporal lobes is often seen. The magnetic resonance imaging (MRI) scan may also reveal lobar atrophy, and the positron emission tomographic (PET) scan reveals diminished glucose metabolism in the frontal and temporal lobes (Kamo et al., 1987). Similarly, single-photon emission computed tomography (SPECT) studies have shown hypoperfusion of the frontal lobes.

The etiology of FTD is unknown. As a result, no specific treatment is available; management consists primarily of supportive and symptomatic treatment. The behavioral symptoms of FTD may improve with serotonin reuptake inhibitors (Moretti et al., 2003; Swartz et al., 1997).

Other Dementias With Frontal Lobe Involvement

Several other degenerative disorders can affect frontal lobe function. Frontotemporal dementia with features of parkinsonism, linked to chromosome 17, has been reported. These patients develop atrophy of the frontal and temporal cortex and the basal ganglia and substantia nigra (Foster et al., 1997). Progressive subcortical gliosis can also affect frontal and temporal lobes. Other disorders that can lead to a frontal lobe syndrome with dementia include stroke, particularly involving the anterior cerebral artery; multiple sclerosis; hydrocephalus; and syphilis. In addition, depression may be associated with features of a dementia of the frontal lobe type (dementia syndrome of depression) with evidence of reduced frontal lobe metabolic activity.

Dementia With Lewy Bodies

It is possible that DLB is the second most frequent cause of dementia after AD. Neuropathological studies have suggested that cases of DLB represent 7.7% to 19% of all patients with dementia (Lindboe & Hansen, 1998; McKeith et al.,

1992). Lewy bodies are intracytoplasmic eosinophilic neuronal inclusions that were once considered characteristic of Parkinson's disease.

The Consortium on Dementia with Lewy Bodies recommended DLB as an inclusive term for all patients with significant numbers of Lewy bodies. This includes patients with the presence of diffuse Lewy bodies and those with Lewy bodies predominantly in the brain stem. The criteria established by the consortium are outlined in Table 19-3 (McKeith et al., 1996).

Mega and coworkers (1996) studied the reliability and validity of these criteria and found that the sensitivity and specificity for probable DLB criteria were 75% and 79%, respectively. Another study by Lopez and colleagues (1999) found high specificity for DLB (94%), but much lower sensitivity (34%). The authors suggested that the heterogeneity of the clinical presentation of DLB significantly affected interrater agreement and accuracy.

The relationship between DLB and other forms of dementia remains controversial. Some researchers believe that DLB constitutes a variant of Alzheimer's disease or Parkinson's disease, and others believe that it is an independent disease process (Cercy & Bylsma, 1997). There appear to be cases with pure DLB, cases with limited or no concurrent Alzheimer's disease pathology and other cases with mixed DLB and Alzheimer's pathology. Features that dis-

---

TABLE 19-3.   Dementia with Lewy bodies (DLB)

Both A and B should be present to make a diagnosis of probable or possible dementia with Lewy bodies.
A. Central feature a progressive cognitive decline of sufficient magnitude to interfere with normal social or occupational function.
   Memory impairment may not necessarily occur in the early stages, but is usually evident with progression; prominent deficits on tests of attention, frontal-subcortical skills, and visuospatial ability
B. Two of the following (probable DLB) or one of the following (possible DLB):
   1. Fluctuating cognition with pronounced variations in attention and alertness
   2. Recurrent visual hallucinations (typically well formed and detailed)
   3. Spontaneous motor features of parkinsonism
C. Features supportive of the diagnosis are
   1. Repeated falls
   2. Syncope
   3. Transient loss of consciousness
   4. Neuroleptic sensitivity
   5. Systemized delusions
   6. Hallucinations in other modalities
D. A diagnosis of DLB is less likely in the presence of
   1. Stroke disease (focal neurological signs or brain imaging)
   2. Evidence of any physical illness or other brain disorder sufficient to account for the clinical picture

---

Source: From Consortium Criteria (McKeith et al., 1996).

tinguish between DLB and Parkinson's disease include myoclonus, absence of resting tremor, lack of response to levodopa, and lack of perceived need to treat with levodopa (Louis et al., 1997).

Simard and coworkers (2000) carried out a detailed review of the cognitive and behavioral symptoms in DLB. Longitudinal studies demonstrated significantly faster cognitive and functional decline in patients with DLB compared to those with AD (Ballard et al., 1996; Olichney et al., 1998). The most consistent cognitive deficit in DLB compared to AD was impairment of spatial working memory (Simard et al., 2000).

Patients with DLB also seem to have more visuospatial dysfunction compared to those with AD. The most frequently reported psychotic symptoms in DLB are visual hallucinations; hallucinations in general have been found significantly more frequently in DLB than in AD (Galasko et al., 1996). Some, but not all, studies reported significantly more delusions and major depression in DLB than in AD.

With regard to treatment, patients with DLB are extremely sensitive to the extrapyramidal side effects of antipsychotic medications. Some reports have suggested that atypical antipsychotic medications can be tolerated by these patients (Allen et al., 1995; Conn & Simard, 1999). Preliminary data suggest that patients with DLB may respond well to cholinesterase inhibitors (Levy et al., 1994); in a case series of nine patients, donepezil appeared to result in fewer hallucinations and an improvement of overall function (Shea et al., 1998). In a randomized placebo-controlled study of rivastigmine in DLB, patients receiving the active medication were less apathetic and anxious and had fewer psychotic symptoms than those on placebo (McKeith et al., 2000).

Subcortical Dementias

The concept of subcortical dementia was first described by Albert and colleagues in 1974. In describing the cognitive deficits of progressive supranuclear palsy (PSP), four cardinal features were proposed as characteristic of subcortical dementia. These included forgetfulness, slowness of mental processes, affective changes—particularly depression—and intellectual deficits, characterized by an impaired ability to manipulate acquired knowledge. In contrast, aphasia, agnosia, and apraxia, which are common in cortical dementia, are absent in patients with pure subcortical dementia.

HUNTINGTON'S DISEASE Huntington's disease is an idiopathic degenerative disease characterized by dementia and chorea; it was first described by George Huntington in 1872. The disease is inherited as an autosomal dominant trait, with approximately 50% of the children affected; the gene for the illness is located on chromosome 4. Isolation of the gene will permit more accurate presymptomatic testing (Huntington's Disease Collaborative Research Group, 1993). When requested by family members, such testing must take place within a carefully designed genetic counseling program. The average length of time from onset to death is 14 years. The average age of onset is 35 to 40 years, although more than 20% develop the illness after 50 years of age.

Dementia is a consistent component of the disorder. In addition, affective illness occurs in more than 50% of patients, and many also develop psychotic features or a schizophrenialike disorder (Caine & Shoulson, 1983; Lieberman et al., 1979). Evidence suggests that suicide accounts for the death of as many as 7% of sufferers (Reed et al., 1958).

The first mental status changes are usually irritability, untidiness, loss of interest, and other personality changes. Dewhurst and colleagues (1969) reported that 57 of 102 patients presented with psychiatric disturbances. The dementia is primarily subcortical and consists of slowed cognition and memory disturbance, which become apparent soon after the chorea begins. Language problems include mild word-finding difficulties, impaired verbal fluency, and dysarthria. The memory disturbance, which is prominent, is characterized by equal difficulty in recalling remote and recently learned information. Subjects perform poorly on frontal systems tasks, and concentration and judgment are impaired.

The CT scan often shows atrophy of the caudate nuclei. The PET scan may show decreased metabolic activity before caudate atrophy is visible on the CT scan (Hayden et al., 1986), and the cerebrospinal fluid (CSF) may show decreased levels of γ-aminobutyric acid (GABA; Bala Manyam et al., 1978). Levels of GABA and glutamic acid decarboxylase are reduced by up to 90% in the basal ganglia.

There is no specific treatment for the illness. However, the associated psychiatric disorders often respond to treatment. The depression may improve with antidepressants, lithium, or electroconvulsive therapy (ECT) (Leonard et al., 1974; McHugh & Folstein, 1975), and psychosis or severe irritability may improve with neuroleptic medication. During the early course of the illness, chorea can also be treated with low-dose neuroleptics or tetrabenazine, a monoamine-depleting agent (Gimenez-Roldan & Mateo, 1989). Patients on tetrabenazine must be carefully monitored as it can cause severe depression.

DEMENTIA IN PARKINSON'S DISEASE   Most studies of large numbers of patients with Parkinson's disease estimated that dementia is present in 35% to 55% (Cummings & Benson, 1992). The age-specific prevalence of dementia in Parkinson's disease ranged from 12.4% in a group with individuals 50 to 59 years old to 68.7% in the group older than 80 years (Mayeux et al., 1992). In a study of the combined effect of age and severity on the risk of dementia in Parkinson's disease, Levy and colleagues (2002) found that the group with older age and higher severity of extrapyramidal signs had a significantly increased risk of incident dementia (relative risk of 9.7). Even in the absence of dementia or depression, patients with advanced Parkinson's disease are likely to show evidence of clinically significant impairments on neuropsychological measures of frontal lobe function (Green et al., 2002).

Dementia in Parkinson's disease may be related to a mixture of cortical and subcortical syndromes caused by a variety of underlying pathologies and neurochemical deficits (McKeith, 2000). Neuropsychological testing tends to demonstrate preservation of recognition memory, but impairment of spontaneous recall and of temporal ordering of learned information. Abnormalities are also present on tests of frontal-subcortical systems. Although some individuals may suffer from both Alzheimer's disease and Parkinson's disease, the dementia of Parkinson's disease does not appear to derive generally from associated Alzheimer's disease. A number of studies demonstrated that Parkinson patients with dementia have severe neuronal loss in subcortical nuclei, but many do not have the characteristic pathology of Alzheimer's disease.

Lewy bodies (hyaline inclusion bodies) may accompany neuronal loss in involved nuclei (e.g., nucleus basalis of Meynert and brain stem nuclei). The relationship between Parkinson's disease and DLB remains unclear. Cummings (1988) suggested that marked dopamine deficiency may result in cognitive deterioration, and that cholinergic deficiency also contributes.

There is evidence of significant degeneration of the nucleus basalis of Meynert in Parkinson patients with dementia (Whitehouse et al., 1983). Many patients receiving dopaminergic agents develop psychotic symptoms. These patients create a clinical dilemma because reduction of the dopaminergic agent may increase the severity of neuromuscular symptoms, and addition of antipsychotic medications might worsen the Parkinson's symptoms. Atypical antipsychotics such as olanzapine, quetiapine, or clozapine may be useful in this situation (Friedman & Factor, 2000; Friedman & Lannon, 1989). Clinicians must be aware that Parkinson's disease is commonly associated with autonomic nervous system dysfunction, making these patients particularly sensitive to developing side effects such as orthostatic hypotension and constipation from concomitant psychiatric medications.

It is always important to consider a diagnosis of depression in patients with Parkinson's disease because depression may worsen cognitive performance and often responds well to treatment. A review of the literature suggested that depression occurs in approximately 40% of patients with Parkinson's disease (Cummings, 1992). The relationship between Parkinson's disease and depression is discussed more fully in the section, "Mood Disorders Due to General Medical Conditions."

PROGRESSIVE SUPRANUCLEAR PALSY The PSP disorder was described by Steele and coworkers (1964). It is an extrapyramidal syndrome characterized by pseudobulbar palsy, axial rigidity, supranuclear gaze paresis, and dementia. The onset of the illness is most common in the sixth or seventh decade, and the average length of time until death is 5 to 10 years. The illness is more common in males than females.

Apathy and slowness are often part of the initial presentation of PSP. Memory consolidation and retrieval of information are impaired; in addition, performance of frontal system tasks is abnormal. The clinical characteristics include more rigidity of midline structures than in the limbs. In contrast to individuals with Parkinson's disease, patients with PSP have an erect posture, often with extension of the neck. The associated ophthalmoplegia is manifested by an initial loss of downward gaze. Subsequently, upward gaze is also impaired. Sleep disturbance and depression occur frequently (Aldrich et al., 1989).

The areas most affected include the subthalamic nucleus, red nucleus, globus pallidus, substantia nigra, and dentate nucleus. The pathology consists of cell loss, neurofibrillary tangles, and granulovacuolar degeneration.

A variety of treatments, including dopaminergic agents, has been tried. Akinesia may improve with levodopa (Mendell et al., 1970), although response is usually disappointing. Some improvement has also been noted with amantadine, and other reports indicated that benztropine and amitriptyline have been helpful for some patients (Haldeman et al., 1981; Newman, 1985). Aggressive behavior in PSP has been effectively treated with trazodone (Schneider et al., 1989). A pilot study of the efficacy of electroconvulsive therapy found a dramatic response in one of five patients (Barclay et al., 1996). A double-blind, placebo-controlled trial of cholinergic stimulation with physostigmine failed to show improvement of swallowing or oral motor functions (Frattali et al., 1999).

Normal-Pressure Hydrocephalus

The syndrome of normal-pressure hydrocephalus (NPH) was first described by Adams and colleagues (1965). The clinical presentation includes a triad of dementia, gait disturbance, and urinary incontinence. These features are associated with evidence of ventricular dilatation in the absence of significantly elevated intracranial pressure. These patients may present to a psychiatrist with symptoms of memory loss and apathy or depression. The presence of an apraxic gait disturbance and urinary incontinence assist in making the correct diagnosis. The etiology of NPH is generally idiopathic, although about one third of patients have a history of subarachnoid bleeding, most commonly because of a ruptured aneurysm (Katzman, 1977). Depressive symptoms and apathy are common (Price & Tucker, 1977), but psychosis is rare (Dewan & Bick, 1985).

Common radiologic findings include enlarged ventricles with a ballooned appearance on CT scan and with disproportionate enlargement of frontal and temporal—compared to posterior—horns of the lateral ventricles. Isotope cisternography can be helpful, although the results do not reliably predict treatment outcome. In NPH, following the injection of an isotope into the lumbar region, there is rapid diffusion into the ventricles and a subsequent failure of the isotope to rise into the sagittal region over the next 48–72 hours.

There is some evidence that CSF drainage tests may predict response to treatment. The possibility that a progressively dementing illness can be reversed by a surgical procedure remains very appealing. Initially, the surgical shunt may have been excessively used, but with careful selection of appropriate patients, it appears that about 50% to 60% of those who receive surgery improve to some degree. In a PET study of 14 patients, those with temporoparietal hypometabolism were less likely to improve than those with a diffuse pattern (Junck et al., 1997). A study by Thomsen et al. (1986), in which 40% of 40 patients improved cognitively following ventricular atrial shunt, suggested that a better postoperative outcome was associated with a known cause of NPH, a short history, and absence of gyral atrophy. Nevertheless, some serious complications can occur, including infection, hemorrhage, or blockage of the shunt. It is noteworthy that the literature on surgery for NPH consists primarily of case series rather than controlled trials. Patients with significant depression may respond to antidepressants, and there is one report of a patient with a shunt who was treated with ECT (Tsuang et al., 1979).

Creutzfeldt-Jakob Disease

Prions are infectious pathogens that cause a group of lethal neurodegenerative disorders presenting as sporadic, familial, or transmissible. They arise from abnormal protein folding of a normal cellular prion protein (PrP^c) to create a pathological isoform (PrP^{sc}). The classical form of dementia from Creutzfeldt-Jakob disease (CJD) was first described by Creutzfeldt in 1920 and by Jakob in 1921. It is a rapidly dementing illness that is extremely rare (incidence of about 1 per 1 million). Onset of the illness is usually in the sixth or seventh decade of life.

The disease is rapidly progressive, with 50% of patients dying in 6 to 9 months. Three disease stages have been identified. Initially, the person presents with vague symptoms, which may include fatigue, insomnia, depression, anxiety, mental slowness, or unpredictable behavior. Subsequently, in the second stage, there is evidence of widespread disease of the central nervous system, with the development of dementia and numerous neurological disturbances, including cerebellar ataxia, aphasia, blindness, brain stem involvement, and myoclonic jerks. In the final stage of the illness, the person enters a vegetative state and coma, which leads to death. This illness is believed to be caused by spontaneous conversion of normal to pathogenic prion protein.

Isolation of patients who are suspected to be suffering from this illness is not required. Special care must be taken with blood or cerebrospinal fluid. Objects contaminated by infected tissue should be autoclaved. Tissues and disposable equipment should be incinerated. Decontamination techniques were reviewed by Ozanne (1994). It is not believed that stool, urine, saliva, or other secretions are infectious (Cummings & Benson, 1992).

The CT scan may show cortical atrophy or no significant change. The electroencephalogram (EEG) may show slowing or synchronous triphasic sharp-wave complexes. Neuropathological findings include neuronal degeneration and proliferation of astrocytes, and the gray matter becomes spongy. Neuronal loss is found throughout the cortex, thalamus, brain stem, and spinal cord. As there is no recognized specific treatment, patients primarily require supportive care.

Iatrogenic CJD involving human-to-human transmission has occurred following corneal transplantation, the use of depth electrodes, and the use of human growth hormone from pituitary glands.

Additional transmissible forms of the disease include variant CJD, believed to be transmitted from cattle suffering from bovine spongiform encephalopathy (BSE) (Fishbein, 1998; Painter, 2000). It has been seen primarily in the United Kingdom, although cases have been reported in France. It generally affects younger adults (20–40 years). Initial symptoms include paresthesia, behavioral changes, and ataxia. Expected survival is about 2 years. Zeidler and colleagues (1997) reviewed the psychiatric features in a series of new variant CJD and reported that depression and psychotic symptoms occurred in the majority of cases.

Human Immunodeficiency Virus Encephalopathy

Although most individuals who suffer from acquired immunodeficiency syndrome (AIDS) are in the younger age groups, a French study suggested that 5% of cases occur in individuals over the age of 60 years (Nguyen et al., 1989). When the human immunodeficiency virus (HIV) produces dementia, the disorder is referred to as HIV encephalopathy or AIDS dementia complex. It is believed that HIV invades the brain shortly after systemic infection and subsequently remains latent for long periods (Resnick et al., 1988).

The HIV virus tends to affect subcortical structures with relative sparing of the cortex (Navia et al., 1986). Early complaints include forgetfulness and poor concentration with slowed thinking. Apathy and social withdrawal may occur, with psychotic symptoms present occasionally. Patients do not develop disturbances of language ability. The term *AIDS dementia complex* refers to a combination of advanced intellectual deficits plus a complex of motor and behavioral abnormalities. The term has been criticized because not all components of the complex are always present.

A study of 132 patients with equivocal or subclinical AIDS reported that about 25% developed clinically significant dementia within 9 months, and another 25% developed it within 1 year (Sidtis et al., 1989). However, a longitudinal study found no decline in neuropsychological profile among 238 patients with Centers for Disease Control and Prevention (CDC) Stages 2 and 3 for 1 year (Selnes et al., 1990). Fifty subjects who developed AIDS during the study were excluded. It is also important to consider that individuals with AIDS may have systemic illness, infections, or CNS malignancies, which could account for their cognitive impairment.

Antiretroviral treatment may lead to improved cognitive functioning of individuals with HIV encephalopathy (Brouwers et al., 1997; McGuire &

Marder, 2000; Yarchoan et al., 1987). One study suggested that zidovudine had a positive impact, as measured by event-related potentials, on AIDS dementia (Evers et al., 1998). It has also been reported that apathy, poor motivation, and attentional deficits may respond to methylphenidate or dextroamphetamine (Fernandez et al., 1988).

Dementia Associated With Metabolic and Endocrine Disorders

Metabolic disorders and toxic states often result in a disturbance of cognitive and intellectual functioning. When this occurs in association with an altered state of consciousness, whether heightened or depressed, a diagnosis of delirium is made. In delirium, the onset is abrupt, and the course is usually limited, provided the underlying disorder is successfully treated. When the onset is gradual and the course progresses insidiously, the disorder may evolve into dementia. Because of the high rates of chronic illness and the relatively high rates of drug consumption in the elderly, those older than 65 years are more likely to suffer from toxic or metabolic dementias (Warshaw et al., 1982). Recognition of these causes of dementia is vital as they are often reversible.

The causes of dementia include endocrine disorders (e.g., thyroid, adrenal, and parathyroid disorders), hypoxia, hepatic encephalopathy, renal failure, vitamin deficiencies, and electrolyte disturbances.

Hypothyroidism can lead to dementia with or without psychosis. Hyperthyroidism may present as a dementia without classical features of an overactive thyroid. Both Cushing's and Addison's diseases may lead to features of dementia, and if serum calcium levels are elevated in a patient with dementia, hyperparathyroidism should be suspected. The most common cause of basal ganglia calcification with dementia is hypoparathyroidism.

Dementia Following Head Injury

Approximately 500,000 individuals per year in the United States suffer from a head injury that is serious enough to warrant hospitalization. It has been estimated that between 70,000 and 90,000 of these individuals will develop a lifelong disability (Goldstein, 1990). The majority of these injuries result from motor vehicle accidents. It has been shown that significant posttraumatic amnesia and residual cognitive impairment may follow head injuries in which there was no obvious loss of consciousness (Cummings & Benson, 1992).

Dementia following head trauma may result from three different forms of neuropathological injury: (1) diffuse axonal injury as a result of shearing forces; (2) focal contusions, hemorrhages, and lacerations; and (3) hypoxic ischemic insults. Diffuse axonal injury primarily affects subcortical white matter, the mesencephalon, and the diencephalon. Brain injury may occur at the point of injury (coup injury) or on the opposite side of the brain (contracoup). Traumatic contusions are especially common in the anterior temporal and inferior frontal lobes.

Cognitive difficulties include retrograde and anterograde amnesia, with deficits in both encoding and retrieval of new information, disorganized thinking, and poor concentration. Language disturbances, especially fluent aphasias, occur in about 30% of individuals with severe head injury. The post–head injury syndrome may include symptoms of depression, apathy, withdrawal, or anxiety, and the full syndrome of posttraumatic stress disorder may coexist. Additional features may be related to damage in specific brain regions. Patients with permanent frontal lobe damage from a head injury are likely to demonstrate the features of frontal lobe syndrome described in this chapter.

Following severe injuries, the CT scan may show contusions and subsequent atrophy. In addition, the MRI scan may reveal white matter abnormalities. However, in some patients with permanent disability, the CT and MRI scans may be normal, although SPECT and PET studies may demonstrate abnormalities.

Dementia pugilistica is a syndrome of dementia and ataxia that may develop as a result of repeated head trauma. This is epitomized by the study of former boxers. Neuropathological findings have included diffuse brain atrophy, ventricular dilatation, and deep pigmentation of the substantia nigra.

Patients require intensive neurorehabilitation programs as continued recovery often occurs over several years. In addition, treatment of depression is often necessary.

Dementia Associated With Toxic Substances

It appears that consistently heavy alcohol intake for a prolonged period (10–20 years) can result in dementia. Individuals who abuse alcohol are also vulnerable to the development of deficiency syndromes such as Korsakoff's psychosis or pellagra. In addition, there is a high risk of subdural hematoma or hepatic encephalopathy, which can further complicate the presentation. Alcoholic dementia itself is generally mild and slowly progressive. Many chronic alcoholics show enlarged lateral ventricles and widening of the cortical sulci, but remarkably, these abnormalities may reverse if the individual refrains from further alcohol intake (Carlen et al., 1978). There is some evidence that alcohol primarily causes white matter atrophy because of its toxic effect on myelin (de la Monte, 1988). A study suggested that it might be possible to differentiate the cognitive deficits of alcohol-related dementia from typical Alzheimer's disease. Alcoholic dementia subjects were more impaired than controls on initial letter fluency, fine motor control, and free recall (Saxton et al., 2000).

Exposure to a number of metals can also result in dementia. These metals include lead, arsenic, mercury, manganese, nickel, bismuth, and tin. In addition, exposure to a variety of industrial compounds, such as organic solvents and insecticides, can result in the development of dementia. Aluminum has been implicated as a cause of dialysis dementia and may have a role in the development of Alzheimer's disease. Dialysis dementia is a serious, often fatal, syndrome that occurs primarily in patients receiving long-term hemodialysis (Mach et al., 1988). The development of this dementia appears to be related to the amount, source, and duration of aluminum exposure, although yet-undefined cofactors also appear to exist. The development of dialysis dementia is not related to the age, sex, or race of the patient. Clinical features include personality change, myoclonus, and seizures. Management includes reduction of aluminum exposure and use of the chelating agent deferoxamine.

Dementia Associated With Brain Tumors

The symptoms and signs resulting from brain tumors depend on the location and speed of growth of the tumor and the presence or absence of increased intracranial pressure or local edema. The onset is often insidious, although persistent headache is not uncommon. Some patients may develop localizing signs such as focal weakness, sensory disturbance, or visual field defects. It is important for the clinician to be aware that some tumors (most likely frontal, temporal, or midline) may present with only cognitive difficulties or personality changes. Dementia occurs in up to 70% of patients with frontal lobe tumors, most commonly meningiomas, gliomas, or metastatic tumors (Avery, 1971; Cummings & Benson, 1992).

Dementia or delirium can also occur with tumors of other brain regions. Tumors that invade the hypothalamus can cause somnolence, hyperphagia, and rage attacks. Basal ganglia tumors can present with memory impairment, poor concentration, depression, and personality changes. Tumors of the brain stem can result in lethargy, personality changes, and mutism. The possibility that a tumor can present with features similar to those of Alzheimer's disease or vascular dementia supports the practice of obtaining neuroimaging if the course or features of a dementing illness are atypical. Psychiatrists should be aware that gradually increasing intracranial pressure because of a brain tumor may cause apathy and withdrawal that can be mistaken for depression. This possibility must be considered in patients who present with a recent change in level of arousal, associated with withdrawal, without other evidence suggestive of depression.

MENTAL DISORDERS DUE TO GENERAL MEDICAL CONDITIONS

In *DSM-IV*, the secondary organic mental disorders were renamed "mental disorders due to a general medical condition" (APA, 1994). When judged etiologically related to the mental disorder, the medical condition should be listed both on Axis I and Axis III.

The new classification of "organic" mental disorders in *DSM-III* represented a radical departure from previous classification systems (APA, 1980). In discussing the approach of *DSM-III*, Lipowski (1984) noted that the essential feature of the newly described syndromes was no longer cognitive impairment, but "psychological or behavioral abnormality associated with transient or permanent dysfunction of the brain" (p. 542). The concept of organicity was no longer synonymous with the presence of cognitive impairment. The division of organic syndromes into acute and chronic subtypes was abandoned in *DSM-III* because it forced the clinician to classify, on the basis of a purely cross-sectional assessment, the patient's condition as either reversible or not.

A number of criticisms were leveled against the new classification system (Spitzer et al., 1983). It was accused of being overinclusive and overcomplex, possibly hindering case finding for epidemiological studies, imposing premature closure on the issue of cause, and in general leaving too much to the clinician's judgment. It is certainly noteworthy that the organic mental syndromes and disorders constituted the only section in *DSM-III-R* (APA, 1987) in which the clinician must make an etiologic diagnosis.

The clinician using the *DSM-III-R* diagnostic system may have encountered difficulties. Using history, physical examination, or laboratory tests, the clinician had to judge whether a specific factor was etiologically relevant to particular psychopathology. It should be noted that the same challenge exists with *DSM-IV*. Indeed, in *DSM-IV* the clinician must determine that the disturbance is the direct physiological consequence of a particular medical condition. When a patient has a past psychiatric history or strong family psychiatric history plus significant medical disease, it may be virtually impossible to determine which of these factors is most relevant. Patients often have features of several organic syndromes, and according to *DSM-III-R* it was necessary to use the residual category of organic mixed syndrome. Patients with mild symptoms of depression, an organic labile (pseudobulbar) affect, or localized cognitive impairment did not always fulfill diagnostic criteria and therefore were difficult to classify. A similar residual category (cognitive disorder not otherwise specified) is available in *DSM-IV*, with examples such as postconcussional disorder noted as appropriate (APA, 1994).

One particular clinical concern relates to the consequences of establishing a definitive biological etiology. For example, if a patient's depression is attributed entirely to his or her stroke, then other etiological factors such as early life experiences, family history of depression, medications, and other recent losses may be overlooked. It is vitally important, therefore, that the clinician, in spite of establishing an etiological factor, continue to search for other contributing factors and thereby consider the full array of potential interventions (Conn, 1989).

Spitzer and colleagues (1992) noted that the term organic implies functional/structural, psychological/biological, and mind/body dualisms. They suggested that, in *DSM-IV*, the term *organic mental disorders* should be renamed either *secondary disorders* (if they are due to physical disorders) or *substance induced disorders*. Although acknowledging that the original dichotomies may have been valuable when there was little understanding of how the CNS functions, they argued that these terms are at variance with the growing body of evidence of the importance of biological factors in the etiology of major "nonorganic" mental disorders.

There were several criticisms of this proposal. Lipowski (1990, 1991) argued that the term organic still served a useful function, and that its abolition would create confusion, impede communication, and be at odds with the *International Classification of Diseases, 10th Revision* (ICD-10). Goldman (1991) argued that loss of the term would have a negative impact on consultation-liaison psychiatry. Whether the terms organic mental disorder or secondary mental disorder or simply naming the specific related medical condition is preferred, it is clear that the disorders remain the same.

Amnestic Disorder

In the text revision to *DSM-IV* (*DSM-IV-TR*; APA, 2000), the first criterion for amnestic syndrome is "the development of memory impairment as manifested by the inability to learn new information *or* the inability to recall previously learned information." Clinically, three types of memory are recognized: (1) immediate memory, as measured, for example, by digit span, which is highly dependent on capacity for attention; (2) short-term memory, for example, recall after a short period of distraction (there are differences of opinion as to how long this period should be, but most clinicians use a period of 2 to 5 minutes); and (3) long-term memory, measured, for example, by recall of early life events or historical figures.

The central feature of the amnestic syndrome is the inability to store, retain, and reproduce new information, leading to anterograde amnesia (i.e., an impairment in the ability to lay down new memories during the period following the onset of an illness). In contrast, the ability to recall information immediately is preserved. Although less severe than the loss of short-term memory, defects in long-term memory are usually present. The result is retrograde amnesia: impaired ability to recall information that existed prior to the onset of an illness.

Neuropsychologists divide the deficits in anterograde amnesia into (1) faulty encoding, (2) faulty consolidation, (3) accelerated forgetting, and (4) faulty retrieval (Kopelman, 1987). Confabulation (the production of inaccurate, erroneous answers to straightforward questions) may occur in the amnestic patient. Patients may provide incorrect answers based on personal or past experiences, in which case the responses are coherent and reasonable, or they may give impossible, inappropriate, adventurous, or even gruesome responses ("fantastic" confabulation).

The most common cause of amnestic syndrome is Wernicke's encephalopathy, which is believed caused by thiamine deficiency (Adams & Victor, 1985). It is most often seen in chronic alcoholics, but it may also occur in malnourished elderly who have a primary psychiatric diagnosis, such as depression or delusional disorder, that has led to social isolation and decreased intake.

Prompt treatment with parenteral thiamine is critical. The majority of patients subsequently develop Korsakoff's syndrome (Reuler et al., 1985), which is chronic and characterized by severe anterograde and moderate retrograde amnesia. Patients with Korsakoff's syndrome often have severely compromised insight, and only 25% of patients make a full recovery (Victor et al., 1971).

Disease processes that affect the diencephalic and medial temporal structures (i.e., mamillary bodies, fornix, and hippocampus) can cause the amnestic syndrome. In patients with thiamine deficiency, the symptoms appear to be related to bilateral sclerosis of the mamillary bodies and degenerative changes in the dorsal medial nucleus of the thalamus (Stoudemire, 1987).

DIFFERENTIAL DIAGNOSIS *Transient global amnesia* is a syndrome characterized by the development of anterograde amnesia, which may persist for several hours, and a short period of retrograde amnesia. Patients are bewildered, but have no other clinical or neurological deficits. The syndrome appears related to hypoperfusion in mesial temporal lobe structures (Jovin et al., 2000). Transient global amnesia can be precipitated by emotional stressors, and Merriam (1988) has suggested that this disorder may result from a disturbance in the brain's intrinsic benzodiazepine ligand system.

Psychogenic amnesia is characterized by inability to recall vital personal information, for example, one's name. There may be a loss of specific emotionally charged information, such as memory of a recent loss. Postictal states should also be considered in the differential diagnosis.

TREATMENT Medical treatment of the primary etiologic factor is the first consideration. Subsequently, rehabilitation may involve specific therapies (both cognitive and behavioral) to maximize the individual's level of functioning. Strategies useful at any age to help patients increase memory function include reorientation therapy; the programmed use of diaries, notebooks, or other aids; and specific memory training programs.

Mood Disorder Due to a General Medical Condition

In *DSM-IV*, the category "mood disorder due to a general medical condition" replaced organic mood syndrome (APA, 1994). Subtypes include those "with depressive features," "with major depressive-like episode," and "with manic features." Mood disorders are also listed in the substance-related disorders category.

Psychiatrists are frequently consulted to rule out depression in the medically ill, and a number of diagnostic difficulties may emerge. Many physical illnesses and drugs may cause symptoms that are also associated with depression (e.g., fatigue, decreased energy, insomnia, weakness, poor concentration, and anorexia). It is at times difficult for the clinician to decide whether to attribute these symptoms to depression. The rate of depression in medical populations appears to be between 12% and 32% (Stoudemire, 1988). Approximately 20% of nursing home residents and 35% of elderly patients in chronic care hospitals have symptoms that suggest the presence of major depression (Katz et al., 1989; Sadavoy et al., 1990).

Many patients with neurological disease display evidence of aprosodia or organic emotional lability. Prosody is the affective and inflectional coloring of speech, including syllable and word stress, rhythm, cadence, and pitch. Along with gesture and mimicry, prosody provides the emotional element to speech. Prosody can be disturbed by right hemisphere lesions and by disorders of the basal ganglia, cerebellum, and brain stem. As a result, the patient may present with a flat, rather monotonous voice, which can lead to either underestimation or overestimation of the severity of an emotional disorder, such as depression. The flat, emotionless voice may be mistaken for depression; conversely, genuine feelings of sadness and distress may be unconvincingly presented. Patients with brain disease may have organic emotional lability; that is, they cry (or occasionally laugh) frequently and intensely with decreased control, often in response to a question or other interaction that produces emotional change. This behavior may also give the clinician the false impression of depression. However, affective lability may occur in association with depression (Ross & Rush, 1981) and may improve with antidepressants (Schiffer et al., 1985).

Many illnesses and drugs are said to cause depression. However, it would be more accurate to state that many of these conditions are associated with specific depressive symptoms. Stoudemire (1987) cautioned that the attribution of "medication or disease as the cause of depression should be approached with some degree of caution and skepticism and case reports and lists of such should be approached and evaluated critically."

In the elderly, both stroke and Parkinson's disease are associated with depression. At least 25% of stroke victims appear to develop a major depression, and depressive symptoms may occur in more than one half of all patients following stroke (Robinson et al., 1984). However, House and colleagues (1991), in a study of all strokes occurring in an English health district, found much lower rates of depression. In the study by House and coworkers, only 9% of patients had a major depression 6 months poststroke, with an additional 11% diagnosed as having dysthymic disorder or adjustment disorder with depressed mood. Follow-up studies reported that the high-risk period for poststroke depression lasted for approximately 2 years (Robinson & Price, 1982).

According to Robinson and colleagues (1983), patients with left hemisphere strokes are more vulnerable to depressive symptoms, particularly when the lesion is close to the frontal pole. Other studies, however, have failed to show a consistent association between site of lesion and presence of depression

(House, 1987). A systematic review offered no support for the hypothesis that the risk of depression after stroke is affected by the location of the brain lesion (Carson et al., 2000).

There is evidence from animal studies that poststroke depression may be related to widespread depletion of norepinephrine following a localized lesion of the cortex. In addition, Mayberg and colleagues (1988) reported concerning a PET study that showed alterations in serotonin receptor binding following stroke, which correlated with the severity of depression.

Studies of the frequency of depression in Parkinson's disease vary considerably. They suggest that 25% to 70% of patients with Parkinson's disease suffer from depression (Cummings, 1992). Cummings (1992) suggested that this depression may be mediated by dysfunction in mesocortical and prefrontal reward, motivational, and stress response systems. Depressed patients with Parkinson's disease have lower levels of the serotonin metabolite 5-hydroxyindoleacetic acid in their cerebrospinal fluid than do nondepressed patients with Parkinson's disease (Mayeux et al., 1984). The degree of physical disability and the duration of the disease do not seem to correlate with the severity of the depression. Parkinson's disease can present with depression (Kearney, 1964), but this relation has not been well studied.

Other disorders that are clearly associated with depression include endocrine disorders, particularly hypothyroidism, Addison's disease, and Cushing's syndrome. Hyperthyroidism also may present with depressive symptoms in the elderly (apathetic hyperthyroidism). Other important conditions include occult carcinomas (particularly of the pancreas), viral illnesses, pernicious anemia, and collagen-vascular diseases.

Medications associated with depression include antihypertensives, especially reserpine and methyldopa. The evidence that other antihypertensives (such as propranolol) cause depression is much weaker (Paykel et al., 1982). Some clinicians believe that β-blockers such as atenolol, which are less likely to cross the blood–brain barrier than others (e.g., propranolol), are consequently less likely to cause depressive symptoms. Steroids appear to have effects on mood, including depression, mood lability, and features of euphoria and anxiety. Factors that alter the major neurotransmitter systems implicated in primary mood disorders (norepinephrine and serotonin) or limbic-hypothalamic functions probably precipitate the development of secondary mood disorders (Cummings, 1985a).

In comparison with depressive symptoms, which are very common in the elderly medically ill population, manic states occur less often. The presentation includes pressure of speech, flight of ideas, hyperactivity, insomnia, distractibility, grandiosity, and poor judgment. A variety of conditions can mimic mania, such as agitated delirium or the disinhibited subtype of frontal lobe syndrome, which might account for some of the conditions that are said to be associated with secondary mania. Table 19-4 lists the more common diseases and drugs associated with secondary mania in the elderly. In elderly patients who develop

TABLE 19-4. Important causes of "secondary" mood disorder (mania) in the elderly

Medical illnesses
    Central nervous system
        Stroke
        Cerebral neoplasms (especially right hemisphere)
        Multiple sclerosis
        Encephalitis
    Syphilis
    Head injury
    Hyperthyroidism
    Uremia
    Hemodialysis
Medications
    Corticosteroids
    Thyroxin
    Levodopa
    Bromocriptine
    Sympathomimetics
    Amphetamines
    Cimetidine

mania for the first time at 60 years of age or older, there appears to be a preponderance of cerebral organic disorders, particularly among men (Shulman & Post, 1980). Cummings (1985a) suggested that the localized neurological conditions linked to mania appear to include right hemisphere lesions or lesions close to the third ventricle and hypothalamus.

There is evidence that both antidepressants and electroconvulsive therapy can be effective in the treatment of mood disorder accompanying stroke or Parkinson's disease (Andersen et al., 1994; Murray et al., 1986; Robinson et al., 2000; Tom & Cummings, 1998). There is also evidence that psychostimulants (e.g., methylphenidate) can be effective in treatment of poststroke depression and depression associated with other medical illnesses (Grade et al., 1998; Emtage & Semla, 1996). However, whether psychostimulants actually treat the syndrome of major depression rather than improve depressive symptoms such as fatigue and apathy has not been demonstrated.

Treatment of the acute manic state generally requires antipsychotic or anticonvulsant medication. Lithium has been shown effective in treating secondary mania occurring in conjunction with brain disease, although these patients are more sensitive to developing neurological side effects during lithium treatment (Rosenbaum & Barry, 1975; Young et al., 1977).

In the same way that patients with a primary mood disorder may benefit from a combination of psychopharmacological agents and psychotherapy, patients with secondary depression may also benefit from a variety of psychiatric treatments. Individual supportive therapy and group therapy may be beneficial. The families of elderly patients who are suffering from physical illness and an associated mood disturbance often require a great deal of support.

Anxiety Disorder Due to a General Medical Condition

In *DSM-IV*, the term "anxiety disorder due to a general medical condition" replaced organic anxiety syndrome (APA, 1994). Anxiety disorders are also listed in the substance-related disorders category. Common symptoms include feelings of apprehension, tension, dread, or panic; autonomic and visceral symptoms also occur, including tachycardia, hyperventilation, increased sweating, dizziness, numbness and tingling, dilatation of the pupils, diarrhea, and urinary frequency. Other symptoms include decreased concentration, tremor, restlessness, and occasionally perceptual changes such as derealization, depersonalization, or even hallucinations.

Anxiety may be a learned response or may reflect a neurotransmitter abnormality. Factors predisposing an individual to anxiety (e.g., genetic and psychodynamic factors) probably also play a role in the development of anxiety as a result of medical conditions. The most common etiologies of this disorder include hyperthyroidism, hypercortisolism, hypoglycemia, and some potentially toxic agents such as amphetamines and other psychostimulants, caffeine, and sympathomimetic agents (Cummings, 1985a; Stoudemire, 1987). Rare etiologies include pheochromocytoma, carcinoid syndrome, brain tumors, and epilepsy, particularly complex partial seizures. Any condition that causes hypoxia, particularly chronic obstructive pulmonary disease, is likely to cause anxiety. Alcohol and drug withdrawal syndromes produce an anxiety syndrome, but are separately classified.

Management should focus on identifying and treating the primary cause. While this process is under way, benzodiazepines or buspirone may be helpful in controlling the symptoms of anxiety. The β-blockers are also said to have a role in the management of anxiety, especially somatic symptoms such as tremor and tachycardia, but their use in this capacity has not been well studied in the elderly. Psychotherapy, relaxation techniques, and hypnosis may also help the patient.

Psychotic Disorder Due to a General Medical Condition, With Delusions

In *DSM-IV*, the term "psychotic disorder due to a general medical condition with delusions" replaced organic delusional syndrome (APA, 1994). Psychotic disorders are also listed in the substance-related disorders category. The delusions may be simple and persecutory in nature, or they may be complex, systematized beliefs. The delusions may be related to specific neurological deficits such as anosagnosia, denial of blindness (Anton's syndrome), or reduplicative paramnesia (in which a patient claims to be present simultaneously in two locations). Specific delusions, such as Capgras syndrome (the delusion that significant people have been replaced by identically appearing imposters), delusional jealousy, delusions of infestation, and De Clerambault's syndrome (erotomania) have all been linked to specific organic causes, as discussed in Cummings' (1985b) extensive review of organic delusions.

Cummings documented approximately 70 medical causes, drugs, and toxic agents that have been implicated in the production of delusions. However, he noted that many of these occur in the context of confusional states, such as delirium, and would not qualify for a diagnosis of organic delusional syndrome. Table 19-5 lists some of the possible causes of secondary delusional syndrome in the elderly (Cummings, 1985b; Stoudemire, 1987).

Certain conditions and medications have been clearly linked to the development of delusions. They include central nervous system disorders such as Huntington's disease, Parkinson's disease, idiopathic calcification of the basal ganglia, and spinocerebellar degenerations. Disorders affecting the temporal-limbic regions (e.g., epilepsy and herpes encephalitis) and tumors or strokes involving the temporal lobe or subcortical regions are all implicated. Among the medications and toxic agents linked to the development of psychosis, certain medications such as levodopa and corticosteroids appear to be frequent culprits. Lo and coworkers (1997) compared inpatients with organic delusional disorder to those with delusional disorder. The patients with an organic disorder had a family history less often and had an older age of onset of psychiatric disorder, longer hospital stays, and lower treatment dosage of antipsychotic medication.

Cummings (1985b) suggested the following relationship among organic delusional syndrome, cortical function, and the limbic system. He proposed that limbic or basal ganglia dysfunction predisposes to abnormal emotional experiences, which are subsequently interpreted by the intact cortex and lead

TABLE 19-5. Important causes of "secondary" psychotic disorder with delusions in the elderly

Medical illnesses	Drugs and toxins
Central nervous system	Levodopa
Stroke	Bromocriptine
Parkinson's disease	Amantadine
Epilepsy	Isoniazid
Idiopathic basal ganglia calcification	Corticosteroids
Spinocerebellar degeneration	Digitalis
Herpes encephalitis	Amphetamines
Huntington's disease	Methylphenidate
Thyroid and adrenal disorders	Lidocaine
Vitamin B_{12} deficiency	Procainamide
Folate deficiency	Ephedrine
Systemic lupus erythematosus	Phenytoin

to complex, intricately structured delusions. Subcortical and limbic lesions may disrupt ascending dopaminergic pathways, which have been implicated in schizophrenia. He cited genetic constitution, early life experiences, personality characteristics, the location and extent of lesions, and the age of onset of the primary illness as possible predisposing factors.

In conjunction with treatment of the primary condition, neuroleptics may be indicated in the treatment of organic delusional syndrome. Cummings's (1985b) prospective study of 20 consecutive patients with organic delusions suggested that the response to treatment was variable. Simple delusions, which are more common in patients with dementia, responded best to neuroleptic treatment, whereas complex delusions were more resistant. It should be noted, of course, that simple delusions tend to have a better prognosis even without treatment. Goldman (1992) reported a positive response to haloperidol in a small series of patients with organic delusional disorder on a consultation-liaison psychiatry service.

The delusions, particularly complex delusions, can lead to misguided actions, which may be highly disruptive to family or nursing home routines. As a result, staff or families may need a considerable degree of support and education with regard to the management of patients with persisting delusions. Because paranoid thinking may be linked to cognitive impairment and misinterpretation of the environment, the gradual development of a trusting relationship with staff and ongoing reorientation and reassurance may be particularly beneficial. Although the mainstay of treatment is psychopharmacological, other approaches (e.g., behavioral management and psychotherapy) may play an important role (Proulx, 1989; Sadavoy & Robinson, 1989).

Psychotic Disorders Due to a General Medical Condition, With Hallucinations

In *DSM-IV*, the term "psychotic disorder due to a general medical condition with hallucinations" replaced organic hallucinations (APA, 1994). Hallucinations can occur in any sensory modality (auditory, visual, tactile, olfactory, or gustatory) and can vary from simple and unformed to highly complex and organized. The individual may be aware that the hallucinations are imaginary or may be convinced of their reality.

Sensory deprivation related to loss of vision or hearing is a frequent cause of hallucinations in the elderly. In a study of visual hallucinations in the elderly, 29% of 150 successive referrals to a geriatric psychiatrist reported visual perceptual disturbances. There was a significant correlation between the presence of hallucinations and eye pathology (Berrios & Brook, 1984).

Visual hallucinations have been subdivided into "release" and "irritable" types (Brust & Behrens, 1977). Release hallucinations are usually formed images and tend to occur in the area of a field deficit. They are associated with any focal lesion in the visual pathway. Irritable (ictal) hallucinations are brief, stereotyped visual experiences. With primary eye disease, the hallucinations may be simple or complex, for example, following eye surgery (especially if the eyes are patched).

Other causes of hallucinations include alcoholic hallucinosis (auditory), delirium tremens (visual and tactile), complex partial seizures, and lesions, especially of temporal-limbic structures. The differential diagnosis includes schizophrenia, especially when auditory hallucinations occur.

Medications and toxic agents responsible for hallucinations include hallucinogens, amphetamines, antiparkinsonian agents, thyroxin, steroids, antibiotics (especially intravenous penicillin), digoxin, sympathomimetics, cimetidine, narcotics, and heavy metals.

Tactile hallucinations are said to occur most commonly in toxic and metabolic disturbances or drug withdrawal states (Berrios, 1982). Olfactory and gustatory hallucinations are most commonly caused by complex partial seizures.

Mechanisms suggested in the pathophysiology of hallucinations include a perceptual release theory (i.e., decreased sensory input results in the release of spontaneous central nervous system activity); the intrusion of dreams into the waking state (narcolepsy, hypnogogic hallucinations); serotonin antagonism (hallucinogens); synaptic elimination; and the role of hemispheric specialization (more commonly, right hemisphere lesions or seizure foci) (Cummings, 1985a; Hoffman & McGlashan, 1997).

Management includes ensuring maximum sensory input through treatment of underlying disorders or through improved hearing or visual aids. Anticonvulsants used for temporal lobe epilepsy are indicated for the treatment of seizures. The use of antipsychotics may be helpful, but has not been well studied. As mentioned, there is preliminary evidence to suggest that cholinesterase inhibitors may reduce visual hallucinations in patients with DLB (Shea et al., 1998).

Personality Change Due to a General Medical Condition

The cardinal feature of personality change due to a general medical condition, which was previously termed organic personality syndrome, is a personality disturbance due to a specific medical condition. The personality disturbance represents a change from the individual's previous characteristic personality pattern. Exclusion criteria include delirium and dementia. The subtypes in DSM-IV-TR include labile, disinhibited, aggressive, apathetic, and paranoid types (APA, 2000).

Any disease that damages frontal lobes may lead to a frontal lobe personality syndrome. Neoplasms, head trauma, cerebrovascular accidents, multiple sclerosis, and Huntington's disease are all associated with this syndrome. An insidious presentation of personality change may herald the onset of a more global dementia, particularly in patients with FTD, which primarily affects the frontal lobes; the same can also be true of other dementias, such as Alzheimer's disease.

Cummings (1985a) described three separate frontal lobe syndromes, although in practice they tend to overlap. The syndromes described are (1) orbitofrontal syndrome, characterized by disinhibition and impulsive behavior ("pseudopsychopathic"); (2) frontal convexity syndrome, in which apathy predominates; and (3) medial-frontal syndrome, which is associated with akinesia. Disinhibited behavior may cause dramatic behavioral change, and there may be totally uncharacteristic behavior incorporating loss of social tact; rude, tasteless, or inappropriate language; and antisocial behavior. The emotions may be labile with episodic euphoria, as well as inappropriate jocularity and hyperactivity. There may be inappropriate sexual behavior. Individuals are often highly distractible and lack the ability to monitor and evaluate their behavior and performance. Insight and judgment are often significantly impaired. On examination, patients may display some of these behaviors or, conversely, be quite apathetic. Inability to program new motor tasks (e.g., the fist-cut-slap test) may lead to motor perseveration or impersistence. There may be decreased word fluency, impaired abstraction and categorization skills, and difficulty shifting set (switching concepts) on tests of executive functioning.

Another personality syndrome is described in some patients with long-standing seizure disorders, particularly complex partial seizures. The essential features consist of emotional "viscosity" (pedantic and overinclusive thinking), hyperreligiosity, hypergraphia, intense emotional reactions, humorlessness, hypermoralism, and changes in sexual behavior, most frequently hyposexuality (Bear & Fedio, 1977). There are no specific data for the elderly.

Frontal lobe syndrome may cause dramatic problems for the patient and the family. Behavior may be frightening to others; at times, the police or outside agencies are called. Because of decreased insight, it may be difficult to involve the individual in a treatment program. Patients with disinhibited behavior may require a combined behavioral and pharmacological approach. Various medications have been used to control disinhibited and aggressive behavior. The first line of treatment is generally a neuroleptic. Other drugs reported anecdotally to improve this behavior include propranolol, lithium, trazodone, and carbamazepine. Behavior management programs may be beneficial, but require the cooperation of families or caregivers living with the patient (Haley, 1983; Proulx, 1989).

CONCLUSION

There is clearly a need for further research if the complex relationships between behavior and neuropsychiatric disorders are to be understood. Although the emphasis from an etiologic standpoint is on organic factors, it is also important to consider psychosocial factors that predispose to the development of these disorders. Understanding these predisposing factors—such as premorbid personality style, previous life experiences, family psychodynamics, and environmental-cultural influences—may be helpful in managing a patient's symptoms.

Optimal care of these patients, whether in the institution or in the community, requires an integrated and multidisciplinary approach. The primary interventions often involve treating the underlying organic factors and using psychopharmacological agents. However, other interventions, such as individual and family psychotherapy, behavioral management programs, and environmental manipulations, may be important adjuncts.

REFERENCES

Adams RD, Fisher CM, Hakim S, et al. Symptomatic occult hydrocephalus with "normal" cerebrospinal fluid pressure: a treatable syndrome. *N Engl J Med.* 1965;273: 117–126.

Adams RD, Victor M. *Principles of Neurology.* 3rd ed. New York, NY: McGraw-Hill; 1985.

Albert M, Feldman RG, Wills AL. The "subcortical dementia" of progressive supranuclear palsy. *J Neurol Neurosurg Psychiatry.* 1974;37:121–130.

Aldrich MS, Foster NL, White RF, et al. Sleep abnormalities in progressive supranuclear palsy. *Ann Neurol.* 1989;25:577–581.

Allen RL, Walker Z, J D'ath P, et al. Risperidone for psychotic and behavioral symptoms in Lewy body dementia. *Lancet.* 1995;346:185.

American Psychiatric Association. *Diagnostic and Statistical Manual of Mental Disorders.* 3rd ed. Washington, DC: American Psychiatric Association; 1980.

American Psychiatric Association. *Diagnostic and Statistical Manual of Mental Disorders,* 3rd ed., rev. Washington, DC: American Psychiatric Association; 1987.

American Psychiatric Association. *Diagnostic and Statistical Manual of Mental Disorders.* 4th ed. Washington, DC: American Psychiatric Association; 1994.

American Psychiatric Association. *Diagnostic and Statistical Manual of Mental Disorders.* 4th ed., text revision. Washington, DC: American Psychiatric Association; 2000.

Andersen G, Vestergaard K, Lauritzen L. Effective treatment of poststroke depression with the selective serotonin reuptake inhibitor citalopram. *Stroke.* 1994;25:1099–1104.

Avery TL. Seven cases of frontal tumour with psychiatric presentation. *Br J Psychiatry.* 1971;119:19–23.

Bala Manyam NV, Hare TA, Katz L, et al. Huntington's disease: cerebrospinal fluid GABA levels in at-risk individuals. *Arch Neurol.* 1978;35:728–730.

Ballard C, Pagel A, Oyebode F, et al. Cognitive decline in patients with Alzheimer's disease, vascular dementia and senile dementia of Lewy body type. *Age Ageing.* 1996;25:209–213.

Barclay CL, Duff J, Sandor P, Lang AE. Limited usefulness of electroconvulsive therapy in progressive supranuclear palsy. *Neurology.* 1996;46:1284–1286.

Bear DM, Fedio P. Quantitative analysis of interictal behavior in temporal lobe epilepsy. *Arch Neurol.* 1977;34:454–467.

Berrios GE. Tactile hallucinations: conceptual and historical aspects. *J Neurol Neurosurg Psychiatry.* 1982;45:285–293.

Berrios GE, Brook P. Visual hallucinations and sensory delusions in the elderly. *Br J Psychiatry*. 1984;144:662–664.

Brouwers P, Hendricks M, Lietzau JA, et al. Effect of combination therapy with zidovudine and didanosine on neuropsychological functioning in patients with symptomatic HIV disease: a comparison of simultaneous and alternating regiments. *AIDS*. 1997;1:59–66.

Brust JCH, Behrens MM. "Release hallucinations" as the major symptom of posterior cerebral artery occlusion: a report of 2 cases. *Ann Neurol*. 1977;2:432–436.

Caine ED, Shoulson I. Psychiatric syndromes in Huntington's disease. *Am J Psychiatry*. 1983;140:728–733.

Carlen PL, Wortzman G, Holgate RC, et al. Reversible atrophy in recently abstinent chronic alcoholics measured by computed tomography scans. *Science*. 1978;200:1076–1078.

Carson AJ, MacHale S, Allen K, et al. Depression after stroke and lesion locations: a systematic review. *Lancet*. 356:122–126.

Cercy SP, Bylsma FW. Lewy bodies and progressive dementia: a critical review and meta-analysis. *J Int Neuropsychol Soc*. 1997;3:179–194.

Clarfield AM. The reversible dementias: do they reverse? *Ann Intern Med*. 1988;109:476–486.

Conn DK. Neuropsychiatric syndromes in the elderly: an overview. In: Conn DK, Grek A, Sadavoy J, eds. *Psychiatric Consequences of Brain Disease in the Elderly—A Focus on Management*. New York, NY: Plenum; 1989:1–50.

Conn DK, Simard M. Case report: successful treatment of psychosis with olanzapine in a case of early dementia with Lewy bodies. *Int J Geriatr Psychopharmacol*. 1999;2:47–49.

Cummings JL. *Clinical Neuropsychiatry*. New York, NY: Grune and Stratton; 1985a.

Cummings JL. Organic delusions: phenomenology, anatomical correlations, and review. *Br J Psychiatry*. 1985b;146:184–197.

Cummings JL. Intellectual impairment in Parkinson's disease: clinical, pathologic, and biochemical correlates. *J Geriatr Psychiatry Neurol*. 1988;1:24–36.

Cummings JL. Depression and Parkinson's disease: a review. *Am J Psychiatry*. 1992;149:443–454.

Cummings JL, Benson DF. *Dementia—a clinical approach*. Boston, MA: Butterworth-Heinemann; 1992.

Cummings JL, Duchen LW. The Kluver-Bucy syndrome in Pick disease. *Neurology*. 1981;31:1415–1422.

de la Monte SM. Disproportionate atrophy of cerebral white matter in chronic alcoholics. *Arch Neurol*. 1988;45:990–992.

Dewan MJ, Bick A. Normal pressure hydrocephalus and psychiatric patients. *Biol Psychiatry*. 1985;20:1127–1131.

Dewhurst K, Oliver J, Trick KLK, et al. Neuro-psychiatric aspects of Huntington's disease. *Confin Neurol*. 1969;31:258–268.

Emtage RE, Semla TP. Depression in the medically ill elderly: a focus on methylphenidate. *Ann Pharmacother*. 1996;30:151–157.

Evers S, Grotemeyer KH, Reichelt D, Luttmann S, Husstedt IW. Impact of antiretroviral treatment on AIDS dementia: a longitudinal prospective event-related potential study. *J Acquir Immune Defic Syndr Hum Retrovirol*. 1998;17:143–148.

Fernandez F, Adams F, Levy JK, et al. Cognitive impairment due to AIDS-related complex and its response to psychostimulants. *Psychosomatics*. 1988;29:38–46.

Fishbein L. Transmissible spongiform encephalopathies, hypotheses and food safety: an overview. *Sci Total Environ*. 1998;217:71–82.

Foster NL, Wilhelmsen K, Sima AA, Jones MZ, D'Amato CJ, Gilman S. Frontotemporal dementia and parkinsonism linked to chromosome 17: a consensus conference. Conference Participants. *Ann Neurol*. 1997;41:706–715.

Frattali CM, Sonies BC, Chi-Fishman G, Litvan I. Effects of physostigmine on swallowing and oral motor functions in patients with progressive supranuclear palsy: a pilot study. *Dysphagia*. 1999;14:165–168.

Friedman JH, Factor SA. Atypical antipsychotics in the treatment of drug-induced psychosis in Parkinson's disease. *Mov Disord*. 2000;15:201–211.

Friedman JH, Lannon MC. Clozapine in the treatment of psychosis in Parkinson's disease. *Neurology*. 1989;39:1219–1221.

Galasko D, Katzman R, Salmon DP, et al. Clinical and neuropathological findings in Lewy body dementias. *Brain Cogn*. 1996;31:166–175.

Gimenez-Roldan S, Mateo D. Huntington disease: tetrabenazine compared to haloperidol in reduction of involuntary movements. *Neurologia*. 1989;4(8):282–287.

Goldman SA. Concerns and issues of the diagnostic category of organic mental disorders in the *DSM-IV* [letter]. *Psychosomatics*. 1991;32:112.

Goldman SA. Organic delusional disorder on a consultation-liaison psychiatry service. *Psychosomatics*. 1992;33:343–352.

Goldstein M. Traumatic brain injury: a silent epidemic. *Ann Neurol*. 1990;27:327.

Grade C, Redford B, Chrostowski J, Toussaint L, Blackwell B. Methylphenidate in early poststroke recovery: a double-blind, placebo-controlled study. *Arch Phys Med Rehabil*. 1998;79:1047–1050.

Green J, McDonald WM, Vitek JL, et al. Cognitive impairments in advanced PD without dementia. *Neurology*. 2002;59:1320–1324.

Haldeman S, Goldman JW, Hyde J, et al. Progressive supranuclear palsy, computed tomography, and response to antiparkinsonian drugs. *Neurology*. 1981;31:442–445.

Haley WE. A family-behavioral approach to the treatment of the cognitively impaired elderly. *Gerontologist*. 1983;23:18–20.

Hayden MR, Martin AJ, Stoessl AJ, et al. Positron emission tomography in the early diagnosis of Huntington's disease. *Neurology*. 1986;36:888–894.

Hoffman RE, McGlashan TH. Synaptic elimination, neurodevelopment, and the mechanism of hallucinated "voices" in schizophrenia. *Am J Psychiatry*. 1997;154:1683–1689.

Hosler BA, Siddique T, Sapp PC, et al. Linkage of familial amyotrophic lateral sclerosis with frontotemporal dementia to chromosome 9q21-q22. *JAMA*. 2000;284:1664–1669.

House A. Mood disorders after stroke: review of the evidence. *Int J Geriatr Psychiatry*. 1987;2:211–221.

House A, Dennis M, Mogridge L, et al. Mood disorders in the year after first stroke. *Br J Psychiatry*. 1991;158:83–92.

Huntington's Disease Collaborative Research Group. A novel gene containing a trinucleotide repeat that is expanded and unstable on Huntington's Disease chromosomes. *Cell*. 1993;72:971–983.

Hutton M, Lendon CL, Rizzu P, et al. Association of missense and 5'-splice-site mutations in tau with the inherited dementia FTDP-17. *Nature*. 1998; 393:702–705.

Jovin TG, Vitti RA, McCluskey LF. Evolution of temporal lobe hypoperfusion in transient global amnesia: a serial single photon emission computed tomography study. *J Neuroimaging*. 2000;10:238–241.

Junck L, Minoshima S, Kuhl DE, Frey KA. Normal pressure hydrocephalus: use of PET FDG scans in the prediction of shunt response. *J Cereb Blood Flow Metab*. 1997; 17(Suppl 1):S225.

Jung R, Solomon K. Psychiatric manifestations of Pick's disease. *Int Psychogeriatr*. 1993; 5:187–202.

Kamo H, McGeer PL, Harrop R, et al. Positron emission tomography and histopathology in Pick's disease. *Neurology*. 1987;37:439–445.

Katz IR, Lesher E, Kleban M, et al. Clinical features of depression in the nursing home. *Int Psychogeriatr*. 1989;1:5–15.

Katzman R. Normal pressure hydrocephalus. In: Wells CE, ed. *Dementia*. 2nd ed. Philadelphia, PA: Davis; 1977:69–92.

Katzman R. Diagnosis and management of dementia. In: Katzman R, Rowe JW, eds. *Principles of Geriatric Neurology*. Philadelphia, PA: Davis; 1991.

Kearney TR. Parkinson's disease presenting as a depressive illness. *J Irish Med Assoc*. 1964;54:117–119.

Kopelman MD. Amnesia: organic and psychogenic. *Br J Psychiatry*. 1987;150:428–442.

Leonard DP, Kidson MA, Shaunon PJ, et al. Double-blind trial of lithium carbonate and haloperidol in Huntington's chorea. *Lancet*. 1974;2:1208–1209.

Levy G, Schupf N, Tang M, et al. Combined effect of age and severity on the risk of dementia and Parkinson's disease. *Ann Neurol*. 2002;51:722–729.

Levy R, Eagger S, Griffiths M, et al. Lewy bodies and response to tacrine in Alzheimer's disease. *Lancet*. 1994;343:176.

Lieberman A, Dziatolowski M, Neophytides A, et al. Dementias of Huntington's and Parkinson's disease. *Adv Neurol*. 1979;23:273–280.

Lindboe CF, Hansen HB. The frequency of Lewy bodies in a consecutive autopsy series. *Clin Neuropathol*. 1998;17:204–209.

Lipowski ZJ. Organic mental disorders—an American perspective. *Br J Psychiatry*. 1984;144:542–546.

Lipowski ZJ. Is "organic" obsolete? *Psychosomatics*. 1990;31:342–344.

Lipowski ZJ. Reply to R. L. Spitzer, M. First, G. Tucker. Organic mental disorders and *DSM-IV* [letter]. *Am J Psychiatry*. 1991;148:396.

Lo Y, Tsai SJ, Chang CH, Hwant JP, Sim CB. Organic delusional disorder in psychiatric in-patients: comparison with delusional disorder. *Acta Psychiatr Scand*. 1997;95:161–163.

Lopez OL, Litvan I, Catt KE, et al. Accuracy of four clinical diagnostic criteria for the diagnosis of neurodegenerative dementias. *Neurology*. 1999;53:1292–1299.

Louis ED, Klatka LA, Liu Y, et al. Comparison of extrapyramidal features in 31 pathologically confirmed cases of diffuse Lewy body disease and 34 pathologically confirmed cases of Parkinson's disease. *Neurology*. 1997;48:376–380.

The Lund and Manchester Groups. Clinical and neuropathological criteria for frontotemporal dementia. *J Neurol Neurosurg Psychiatry*. 1994;57:416–418.

Mach J, Korchik W, Mahowald M. Dialysis dementia. In: Maletta G, ed. *Treatment Considerations for Alzheimer's Disease and Related Dementing Illnesses. Clinics in Geriatric Medicine.* Philadelphia, PA: Saunders; 1988:853–868.

Maletta GJ. The concept of "reversible" dementia: how nonreliable terminology may impair effective treatment. *J Am Geriatr Soc.* 1990;38:136–140.

Mayberg HS, Robinson RG, Wond DF, et al. PET imaging of cortical S_2 serotonin receptors after stroke—lateralised changes and relationship to depression. *Am J Psychiatry.* 1988;145:937–943.

Mayeux R, Denaro J, Hemenegildo N, et al. A population-based investigation of Parkinson's disease with and without dementia: relationship to age and gender. *Arch Neurol.* 1992;49:492–497.

Mayeux R, Stern Y, Cote L, et al. Altered serotonin metabolism in depressed patients with Parkinson's disease. *Neurology.* 1984;34:642–646.

McGuire D, Marder K. Pharmacological frontiers in the treatment of AIDS in dementia. *J Psychopharmacol.* 2000;14:251–257.

McHugh PR, Folstein MF. Psychiatric syndromes of Huntington's chorea: a clinical and phenomenologic study. In: Benson DF, Blumer D, eds. *Psychiatric Aspects of Neurologic Disease.* New York, NY: Grune and Stratton; 1975:267–285.

McKeith I, Del Ser T, Spano P, et al. Efficacy of rivastigmine in dementia with Lewy bodies: a randomised, double-blind, placebo-controlled international study. *Lancet.* 2000;356:2031–2036.

McKeith IG. Spectrum of Parkinson's disease, Parkinson's dementia, and Lewy body dementia. *Neurol Clin.* 2000;18:865 902.

McKeith IG, Fairbairn A, Perry R, et al. Neuroleptic sensitivity in patients with senile dementia of Lewy body type. *BMJ.* 1992;305:673–678.

McKeith IG, Galasko D, Kosaka K, et al. Consensus guidelines for the clinical and pathologic diagnosis of dementia with Lewy bodies (DLB): report of the consortium on DLB international workshop. *Neurology.* 1996;47:1113–1124.

Mega MS, Masterman DL, Benson F, et al. Dementia with Lewy bodies: reliability and validity of clinical and pathologic criteria. *Neurology.* 1996;47:1403–1409.

Mendell JR, Chase TN, Engel WK. Modification by L-dopa of a case of progressive supranuclear palsy. *Lancet.* 1970;1:593–594.

Merriam AE. Emotional arousal-induced transient global amnesia: case report, differentiation from hysterical amnesia, and an etiologic hypothesis. *Neuropsychiatry Neuropsychol Behav Neurol.* 1988;1:73–78.

Miller BL, Ikonte C, Ponton M, et al. A study of the Lund-Manchester research criteria for frontotemporal dementia: clinical and single-photon emission CT correlations. *Neurology.* 1997;48:937–942.

Moretti R, Torre P, Antonello R, et al. Frontotemporal dementia: paroxetine as a possible treatment of behavior symptoms. *Eur Neurol.* 2003;49:13–19.

Murray GB, Shea VA, Conn DK. Electroconvulsive therapy for post-stroke depression. *J Clin Psychiatry.* 1986;47:258–260.

Navia BA, Jordan BD, Price RW. The AIDS dementia complex. I. Clinical features. *Ann Neurol.* 1986;19:517–524.

Neary D, Snowden JS, Gustafson L, et al. Frontotemporal lobar degeneration: a consensus on clinical diagnostic criteria. *Neurology.* 1998;51:1546–1554.

Newman GC. Treatment of progressive supranuclear palsy with tricyclic antidepressants. *Neurology.* 1985;35:1189–1193.

Nguyen Q, Laurent M, Bouchon JP, et al. AIDS in elderly patients. Apropos of 22 cases observed in the Paris region. *Ann Med Interne (Paris)*. 1989;140:299–403.

Olichney JM, Galasko D, Salmon DP, et al. Cognitive decline is faster in Lewy body variant than in Alzheimer's disease. *Neurology*. 1998;51:351–357.

Ozanne WG. Creutzfeldt-Jacob disease decontamination of tissues and contaminated materials. *Can J Med Technol*. 1994;56:35–38.

Painter MJ. Variant Creutzfeldt-Jakob disease. *J Infect*. 2000;41:117–124.

Paykel ES, Fleminger R, Watson JP. Psychiatric side effects of antihypertensive drugs other than reserpine. *J Clin Pharmacol*. 1982;2:14–39.

Price TRP, Tucker GJ. Psychiatric and behavioral manifestations of normal pressure hydrocephalus. *J Nerv Ment Dis*. 1977;164:51–55.

Proulx GB. Management of disruptive behaviors in the cognitively impaired elderly: integrating neuropsychological and behavioral approaches. In: Conn DK, Grek A, Sadavoy J, eds. *Psychiatric Consequences of Brain Disease in the Elderly: A Focus on Management*. New York, NY: Plenum; 1989:147–162.

Reed TE, Chandler JH, Hughes EM, et al. Huntington's chorea in Michigan. I. Demography and genetics. *Am J Hum Genet*. 1958;10:201–225.

Resnick L, Berger JR, Shapshak P, et al. Early penetration of the blood-brain barrier by HIV. *Neurology*. 1988;38:9–14.

Reuler JB, Girard DE, Cooney TG. Wernicke's encephalopathy. *N Engl J Med*. 1985; 312:1035–1039.

Robinson RG, Kubos KL, Starr LB, et al. Mood changes in stroke patients: relationship to lesion location. *Compr Psychiatry*. 1983;24:555–566.

Robinson RG, Price TR. Post-stroke depressive disorders: a follow-up study of 103 patients. *Stroke*. 1982;13:635–641.

Robinson RG, Schultz SK, Castillo C, et al. Nortriptyline versus fluoxetine in the treatment of depression and in short-term recovery after stroke: a placebo-controlled, double-blind study. *Am J Psychiatry*. 2000;157:351–359.

Robinson RG, Starr LB, Price TR. A two-year longitudinal study of mood disorders following stroke: prevalence and duration at six months follow-up. *Br J Psychiatry*. 1984;144:256–262.

Rosenbaum AH, Barry MJ Jr. Positive therapeutic response to lithium in hypomania secondary to organic brain syndrome. *Am J Psychiatry*. 1975;132:1072–1073.

Ross ED, Rush J. Diagnosis and neuroanatomical correlates of depression in brain-damaged patients. *Arch Gen Psychiatry*. 1981;38:1344–1354.

Sadavoy J, Robinson A. Psychotherapy and the cognitively impaired elderly. In: Conn DK, Grek A, Sadavoy J, eds. *Psychiatric Consequences of Brain Disease in the Elderly*. New York, NY: Plenum; 1989:101–136.

Sadavoy J, Smith I, Conn DK, et al. Depression in geriatric patients with chronic medical illness. *Int J Geriatr Psychiatry*. 1990;5:187–192.

Saxton J, Munro CA, Butters MA, Schramke C, McNeil MA. Alcohol, dementia, and Alzheimer's disease: comparison of neuropsychological profiles. *J Geriatr Psychiatry Neurol*. 2000;13:141–149.

Schiffer RB, Herndon RM, Rudick RA. Treatment of pathological laughing and weeping with amitriptyline. *N Engl J Med*. 1985;312:1480–1482.

Schneider LS, Gleason RP, Chui HC. Progressive supranuclear palsy with agitation: response to trazodone but not to thiothixine or carbamazepine. *J Geriatr Psychiatry Neurol*. 1989;2:109–112.

Selnes OA, Miller E, McArthur J, et al. HIV-1 infection: no evidence of cognitive decline during the asymptomatic stages. *Neurology.* 1990;40:204–208.

Shea C, MacKnight C, Rockwood K. Aspects of dementia: donepezil for treatment of dementia with Lewy bodies: a case series of nine patients. *Int Psychogeriatr.* 1998; 10:229–238.

Shulman K, Post F. Bipolar affective disorder in old age. *Br J Psychiatry.* 1980;136: 26–32.

Sidtis JJ, Thaler H, Brew BJ, et al. The interval between equivocal and definite neurological signs and symptoms in the AIDS dementia complex. In: *Abstracts of the Fifth International Conference on AIDS.* Montreal, Quebec, Canada: International Development Research Centre; 1989.

Simard M, van Reekum R, Cohen T. A review of the cognitive and behavioral symptoms in dementia with Lewy bodies. *J Neuropsychiatry Clin Neurosci.* 2000;12:425–450.

Snowden JS, Neary D, Mann DMA. Frontotemporal dementia. *Br J Psychiatry.* 2002; 180:140–143.

Spitzer RL, First MB, Williams JBW, et al. Now is the time to retire the term "organic mental disorders." *Am J Psychiatry.* 1992;149:240–244.

Spitzer RL, Williams JBW, Skodol AE. *International Perspectives on DSM-III.* Washington, DC: American Psychiatric Press; 1983.

Steele JC, Richardson JC, Olszewski J. Progressive supranuclear palsy. *Arch Neurol.* 1964;10:333–359.

Stoudemire A. Depression in the medically ill. In: Michels R, Cooper AM, Guze SB, et al., eds. *Psychiatry.* Rev. ed. Philadelphia, PA: Lippincott; 1988.

Stoudemire GA. Selected organic mental disorders. In: Hales RE, Yudofsky SC, eds. *Textbook of Neuropsychiatry.* Washington, DC: American Psychiatric Press; 1987: 125–139.

Swartz JR, Miller BL, Lesser IM, Darby AL. Frontotemporal dementia: treatment response to serotonin selective reuptake inhibitors. *J Clin Psychiatry.* 1997;58:212–216.

Thomsen AM, Borgeson SE, Bruhn P, et al. Prognosis of dementia in normal pressure hydrocephalus after a shunt operation. *Ann Neurol.* 1986;20:304–310.

Tom T, Cummings JL. Depression in Parkinson's disease: pharmacological characteristics and treatment. *Drugs Aging.* 1998;12:55–74.

Tsuang MT, Tidball JS, Geller D. ECT in a depressed patient with shunt in place for normal pressure hydrocephalus. *Am J Psychiatry.* 1979;136:1205–1206.

Victor M, Adams RD, Collins GH. *The Wernicke-Korsakoff Syndrome.* Oxford, UK: Blackwell Scientific; 1971.

Warshaw GA, Moore JT, Friedman SW, et al. Functional disability in the hospitalized elderly. *JAMA.* 1982;248:847–850.

Whitehouse PJ, Hedreen SC, White CL, Price DL. Basal forebrain neurons in the nucleus of Meynert in dementia of Parkinson's disease. *Ann Neurol.* 1983;13:243–248.

Yarchoan R, Berg G, Brouwers P, et al. Response of human immunodeficiency-virus-associated neurological disease to 3-azido-3-deoxythymidine. *Lancet.* 1987;1:132–135.

Young LD, Taylor I, Holmstrom V. Lithium treatment of patients with affective illness associated with organic brain symptoms. *Am J Psychiatry.* 1977;134:1405–1407.

Zeidler M, Johnstone EC, Bamber RW, et al. New variant Creutzfeld-Jakob disease: psychiatric features. *Lancet.* 1997;350:908–910.

20

Grief and Bereavement

Sidney Zisook, MD
Stephen R. Shuchter, MD
Laura B. Dunn, MD

As testimony to the adaptive capacities of elderly persons, most bereaved individuals ultimately are able to grieve for their loss, to reengage, and to function adequately in their daily lives. Yet, other challenges associated with aging—declining health, mobility, cognitive abilities, income, and function; loss of social and occupational roles; diminished personal independence; and loss of friends and relatives—may compound the distress associated with bereavement. A minority of bereaved persons recovers only marginally or not at all. These individuals may continue to suffer for years from limitations in physical, psychological, or social functioning. Informed by comprehensive knowledge of normal grief, common complications, and risk factors, health practitioners who work with elderly patients can better understand the experiences that bereaved individuals encounter, avert complications that may be preventable, and manage most effectively those that are not.

Although elderly persons are vulnerable to myriad losses (e.g., of spouse, siblings, adult children, grandchildren, friends, and pets), this chapter focuses primarily on spousal bereavement. The death of a spouse is by far the most studied form of bereavement in late life. In the United States, there are more than 900,000 new widows and widowers each year. Most of these men and women are elderly: among people aged 65 years or older, almost 50% of all women and more than 10% of men have been widowed at least once (US Bureau of the Census, 1997).

Spousal bereavement, often considered the prototypical severe life stressor

(Holmes & Rahe, 1967), is associated with prolonged personal suffering, declining mental and physical health (Klerman & Izen, 1977; Osterweis et al., 1984; M. S. Stroebe & W. Stroebe, 1993), an elevated risk for suicide (Duberstein et al., 1998; MacMahon & Pugh, 1965), and an increased risk of death from causes other than suicide (Kaprio et al., 1987; Martikainen & Valkonen, 1996; Schaefer et al., 1995). The mean duration of widowed life is 4 years for widowers and 7 years for widows. The fact that widowed persons, especially women, have much of their lives before them adds to the burden as many widows face living alone on a reduced income into old age. They must confront the tasks of establishing a life independent of their deceased spouses, dealing with evolving family relationships and support networks, and meeting emotional, health, and practical needs over the long term (Hansson et al., 1993).

NORMAL GRIEF

The Duration of Grief

There is little agreement about the time course of normal grief and bereavement. Several investigators have found that depressive symptoms often continue for as long as 1 year (Bornstein et al., 1973; Zisook & Shuchter, 1991a) or 2 years (Harlow et al. 1991; Lund et al., 1985; Zisook & Shuchter, 1993a) after the death of a loved one. Parkes (1971) found that only a minority of widows could recall the past with pleasure or anticipate the future with optimism 13 months after the death of their husbands. Most widows described themselves as being sad, adjusting poorly, feeling depressed, thinking often of their deceased husbands, having clear visual memories of them, and still grieving a great deal of the time. Parkes concluded that the process of grieving often continued for more than 13 months, and that the question of how long grief lasts was still unanswered. Other findings (Zisook, 1987) are in agreement with those of Goin and coworkers (1979), who suggested that "you don't get over it—you get used to it." For a significant proportion of otherwise normally bereaved individuals, some aspects of the grieving process may never end.

Stages of Grief

Proposed models of stages of emotional response through which bereaved individuals pass generally include an initial period of shock, disbelief, and denial; an intermediate mourning period of acute somatic and emotional discomfort and social withdrawal; and a culminating period of reorganization and recovery (Bowlby, 1980; DeVaul et al., 1979; Horowitz, 1986). The existing data on bereavement suggest, however, that individuals vary considerably in the types, intensity, and sequence of emotions experienced (Lund, 1989; Silver & Wortman, 1980). Grief is a composite of overlapping, fluid phases that differ from person to person (Shuchter & Zisook, 1993). Thus, such "stages" of grief should be viewed not literally, but as general guideposts describing, not pre-scribing, where an individual may be in the normal grieving process.

Multidimensional Assessment of Grief

A multidimensional approach seems best suited to understanding the highly individualized process of grief. Table 20-1 presents six overlapping dimensions of grief, including emotional and cognitive experiences, coping strategies, con-tinuing relationship with the deceased, functioning, new relationships, and an evolving new identity (Shuchter, 1986).

DIMENSION 1: EMOTIONAL AND COGNITIVE EXPERIENCES Most people experience some form of initial shock and denial on learning that a loved one is dead; varying degrees of numbness and detachment often are present during this time. The emotional pangs and anguish of grief soon emerge. These are painful, often total body, experiences: a wrenching of the gut, shortness of breath, chest pain, lightheadedness, weakness, rapid welling up of tears, and uncontrollable cry-ing. These responses often erupt suddenly and unexpectedly in the first days and weeks. Over time, such reactions are more apt to be precipitated by re-minders of the deceased. For some bereaved persons, everything is a reminder of their loss, and their pain remains unremitting for an extended period. The frequency and intensity of such pain generally subsides as time passes, although it may reemerge in response to reminders of the loss.

Closely associated with the emotional pain is a sense of loss, yearning, pining, and searching behaviors (Bowlby, 1973). The sense of loss is not limited to the deceased person: also gone are intimacy, companionship, security, life-style, roles, a sense of meaning, and visions of the future. In the wake of these fundamental losses, bereaved individuals may experience disruption of attach-ment bonds, intense insecurity, fear, and anxiety. The anxiety may be felt as free-floating waves or time-limited panic. Vivid and detailed intrusive images of the deceased often arise, particularly at times when the individual's mind is not actively engaged, such as when home alone or before falling sleep. These intrusive images may be more common when the death was sudden and unex-pected (Horowitz, 1986; Jacobs, 1993; Rynearson, 1990).

Clinical experience shows that feelings such as anger, guilt, or regret may

TABLE 20-1. Dimensions of grief

- Emotional and cognitive experiences
- Coping strategies
- Continuing relationship with the deceased
- Health, occupational, and social functioning
- Relationships
- Identity, self-esteem, and worldview

plague the bereaved person intermittently. After the loss of a loved one, be-reaved persons normally, although not universally, experience feelings of anger that may be felt as irritability, hatred, resentment, envy, or a sense of unfair-ness. The anger may be directed at the deceased, family, friends, God, physi-cians, or self. Guilt is common, yet variable. Intense and lasting forms of guilt often may be experienced by bereaved persons, who feel they may have con-tributed to the death or suffering of the deceased through improper nutrition, inadequate support, failure to prevent unhealthy attitudes or lifestyles, or fail-ure to push physicians hard enough to detect the disorder. Survivor guilt may be particularly intense and tenacious when the bereaved person may, in fact, have been in some way responsible for the loss (e.g., having been the driver in a fatal vehicular accident). Often, after a long life together, the bereaved person is disturbed by a sense of unfinished business or unfulfilled wishes. The ultimate regret, however, is that the loved one was not able to continue to live a healthy and happy life.

Mental disorganization may manifest as distractibility, poor concentration, confusion, forgetfulness, and lack of clarity, particularly in the early weeks of bereavement. The cumulative effects of upheavals in the mental, emotional, and cognitive lives of the bereaved person often lead to a sense of being over-whelmed. Bereaved individuals describe feeling out of control, helpless, and powerless. The prospect of facing daily living and survival alone, of dealing with recurrent pain, and of being cognitively impaired may be perceived as a set of unmanageable challenges. Even individuals who previously considered themselves emotionally strong may feel unable to cope.

Loneliness often becomes more severe after the first several months of be-reavement when family and friends begin to pull back and levels of support decrease. Loneliness can be one of the most painful, persistent aspects of be-reavement for older bereaved spouses and is often felt even when the bereaved person is with others (Lund et al., 1986a).

Not all of a bereaved person's affective experiences are negative and pain-ful. Relief may be felt, occasionally leading to increased feelings of guilt, espe-cially if the deceased person suffered a protracted illness. Bereaved persons often are surprised at their capacity to feel joy, peace, or happiness at the same time as sorrow.

DIMENSION 2: COPING   Facing reality initiates pain, which sets off a variety of pro-tective mechanisms. Ideally, bereaved persons are able to regulate the amount of pain they can bear at one time and divert the rest, using the most adaptive coping strategies possible. Coping strategies to protect against the pain of grief include numbness and disbelief; emotional control and suppression; altered per-spectives, such as intellectualization, rationalization, and humor; faith; avoid-ance or exposure; activity; involvement with others; passive distraction, such as listening to the radio or watching television; and indulgence in food or drink. Individuals generally use coping strategies to help them through bereavement similar to those they use to manage other stress in their lives. It is possible, however, that frail, elderly patients—who often are limited by fewer supports, resources, and coping capacities—may be at a disadvantage for making use of coping skills. We have found that no one coping strategy fits all bereaved individuals under all circumstances; rather, the capacity to utilize many different coping skills over time appears most adaptive.

DIMENSION 3: THE CONTINUING RELATIONSHIP WITH THE DECEASED The fundamental dilemma facing the bereaved person may be that reality demands they accept life without their loved one at the same time that (equally important) inner psychological forces dictate that they maintain their attachment and that they retrieve what has been lost (Bowlby, 1969). Freud (1917/1957) originally conceptualized the work of grief as the gradual detachment of the libido from the deceased: "Reality-testing has shown that the loved object no longer exists, and it proceeds to demand that all libido shall be withdrawn from its attachment to it" (p. 243). In modifying Freud's original libidinal theory, contemporary theorists postulate that the task of grief is to realign, rather than give up, attachment bonds (Bowlby, 1961; Glick et al., 1974; Parkes, 1972; Rubin, 1990; Shuchter & Zisook, 1987; Worden, 1991). In one sense, the person is dead, and a major aspect of a living and breathing relationship has been lost; in another sense, the deceased person lives on indefinitely.

Bereaved individuals may maintain important aspects of the relationship with the deceased in many ways. Many bereaved persons perceive that the deceased continues to have an existence either in a spiritual form, such as in heaven, or in a material form, such as being at the burial site or where ashes have been scattered (Klass & Goss, 1999). The bereaved person frequently maintains contact during the early weeks and months by an intermittent sense of anticipation that the deceased will suddenly appear: the bereaved searches in crowds, hears approaching footsteps or voices, sees an image of the deceased, and feels the deceased hovering and protecting the bereaved person. Bereaved individuals often communicate with the deceased, asking for advice or summarizing the day's events. All these "unusual" experiences occur in the context of normal reality testing.

Other ways of maintaining contact with the deceased include symbolic representations, such as maintaining the deceased's clothing, writings, favored possessions, jewelry, or pets, and through living legacies such as identification phenomena (e.g., identifying with the illness, mannerisms, or goals of the deceased), carrying out the deceased's mission, making memorial donations, or seeing the deceased live on in descendants (Field et al., 1999; Klass & Goss, 1999; Shuchter, 1986). Bereaved individuals often dream of the deceased, sometimes experiencing vivid visions of the individual returning or explaining why they have been away. Periodic visitations to the cemetery or lighting candles at a place of worship may keep memories alive. Ultimately, memories become the most powerful means of continuing the relationship with the de-

ceased, yet these memories often are bittersweet, providing comfort by bringing
the spouse back to life, yet stimulating pain as a reminder of loss.

DIMENSION 4: FUNCTIONING   Bereavement has an impact on health, occupational
functioning, and social functioning. Health may be compromised after the
death of a loved one (Caserta et al., 1990); bereaved persons are also at risk
for increased drinking, abuse of drugs, major depression, anxiety disorders, and
disorders similar to posttraumatic stress disorder (PTSD) (Zisook & Downs,
1998). The section of this chapter on the complications of grief discusses this
in greater detail. Other forms of dysfunction include impaired work performance, social inhibition, and isolation. The challenges of new roles or new
demands, such as filing insurance claims or obtaining social security benefits,
may appear overwhelming to bereaved persons. Older men may have to learn
to take care of themselves for the first time, including cooking, shopping, and
keeping house. Women may be challenged by the requirements of home repairs, servicing the car, or maintaining legal and financial records (Lund et al.,
1986a). Help with some of these mundane, but troublesome, difficulties may
obviate turmoil and complications.

DIMENSION 5: RELATIONSHIPS   Bereavement alters the dynamics of many relationships (Lund et al., 1990). There may be changes in needs, in levels of closeness
or support, or in the nature of roles. Some relationships may end, and others
may begin, but all are affected. Complex changes occur within the family. For
example, there may be conflicts in the expectations of the children and surviving parent over issues of emotional support, finances, decision making, and
future directions in a family in which a spouse dies and there are grown children. The survivor may have to contend with the grief of surviving parents,
children, in-laws, and siblings. While there are opportunities for achieving greater
intimacy, repairing old wounds, and sharing grief, conflict and disruption may
be exacerbated.
      Friends may be a major source of support for the bereaved person, espe-
cially when friends can provide empathy and sympathy freely and are accepting
of the enormous fluctuations of feelings, moods, and needs of the bereaved
individual. This may be true especially for elderly people, whose friends may
have had similar experiences and can form an informal support group. Enduring and supportive friendships may evolve with those people whose life experiences are similar to the survivor's. Generally, people who have experienced
grief can offer greater acceptance and comfort to bereaved persons. Nevertheless, there are times when friends may feel threatened or overwhelmed by the
intensity of a bereaved person's neediness and suffering.
      Eventually, most widows and widowers must deal with the intricacies of
single life. When they attempt to begin a new romance, they may be challenged
by continued devotion to the spouse, societal sanctions, fears of recurring loss,
and children's perception of disloyalty (Lund et al., 1993). This transition may

be particularly difficult for older individuals who have not dated for many years; contemporary social and dating customs may be frightening or perplexing. Yet, many widows, and even more widowers, do ultimately develop new intimate relationships and remarry. In the San Diego Project, more than half of all widowers were remarried or in a new intimate relationship by the end of the second year after their wife's death (Schneider et al., 1996).

DIMENSION 6: NEW IDENTITY Persons living through the profoundly disruptive experience of bereavement experience dramatic changes in the way they view themselves and their world. Bereaved individuals initially feel helpless and overwhelmed; these feelings eventually give way to more positive self-images as bereaved individuals find themselves able to tolerate their grief, carry out tasks, and learn new ways of dealing with the world. There is an evolving sense of strength, autonomy, independence, assertiveness, and maturity (Pollock, 1987). Bereaved individuals frequently become more appreciative of daily living and (perhaps) more patient, accepting, and giving; people unable to meet these challenges stagnate and do not experience personal growth. Therapy or support groups may be necessary in such cases to facilitate growth and to help the bereaved person achieve an integrated, healthy self-concept and a stable worldview.

COMPLICATIONS OF GRIEF

Grief is a complex, multidimensional process involving physical, psychological, and sociological reactions. Although the majority of people do not become seriously ill or die immediately following a significant loss, prevailing evidence suggests that bereaved persons are at high risk for a number of complications. Sanders (1993) pointed out that "grief affects everyone, but unequally" (p. 267). Some bereaved individuals have relatively uncomplicated grief reactions, painfully acknowledging the loss while managing to go on with their lives (Cleiren, 1991). Others experience multiple complications. Some people are affected so severely that they die. The two major categories of complications are (1) those that arise from the process of grief itself (too little, too much, or too long) and (2) medical and psychiatric disorders that often occur or worsen following a significant loss.

Risk Factors

There is no one-to-one correlation between known risk factors and specific complications of grief. Several risk factors, however, can potentially lead to a number of possible complications (Table 20-2). These may be categorized as factors related to the type of death (Osterweis et al., 1984; Parkes, 1993; Rynearson & McCreery, 1993; Sanders, 1980), factors related to psychological and psychiatric characteristics of the bereaved individual (Gallagher et al.,

TABLE 20-2.   Risk factors for complications of grief

A. Death-related factors
    Sudden, multiple, or unexpected deaths; suicide; murder; stigmatized deaths; death
    of a child
B. Personality and social factors of the bereaved
    Insecurity, low self-esteem, dependence, coping, difficulties, poor health, depression,
    prior substance abuse, multiple concurrent life stresses, perceived lack of social sup-
    port
C. Relationship with the deceased
    Marked by ambivalence or undue dependency
D. Factors for which the literature is unclear
    Gender (men at greater risk versus women)
    Age (greater risk in younger versus older individuals)
E. Factors for which there are few data
    Cognitive impairment, decline in general medical health
    Grief reactions in the oldest old and frail elderly

1981; Hays et al., 1994; Parkes, 1971, 1990; Raphael, 1983; Vachon, 1982; Zisook & Shuchter, 1993a), and factors associated with the relationship to the deceased person (Parkes, 1975).

Other variables, such as gender and age, remain controversial as substantial risk factors (Jacobs, 1993; Osterweis et al., 1984; Sanders, 1993; W. Stroebe & M. S. Stroebe, 1993; Turvey et al., 1999). While younger age may be a relative risk factor, this may be related more to the effects of age on the pacing of grief rather than on the occurrence of complications. Zisook and colleagues (1994) and Sanders (1981) found that the observed increased intensities of grief and depression found in young compared with old individuals during the first year of bereavement diminish or even reverse during the second year.

Predictors of better adjustment to widowhood have also been investigated. Lund and coworkers (1993) found that those widows and widowers who remarried, who had supportive relationships with others, or who were active in their religion were somewhat more likely to be doing well at follow-up than were individuals with more problematic social relationships. The strongest predictors of adjustment to bereavement, however, were the personal resources unique to each person: positive self-esteem and personal competencies in managing the tasks of daily life.

Complications in the Process of Grief

The grief process itself may become complicated in the amount (too little or too much) or duration of symptoms (Table 20-3).

ABSENT, DELAYED, OR INHIBITED GRIEF (TOO LITTLE GRIEF)   Absent or inhibited grief has led some to speculate about the reasons for and effects of this phenomenon.

TABLE 20-3.   Complications of grief related to the grief process

A. Too little: absent, delayed, or inhibited grief
   Common in elderly
   Most likely when relationship unduly dependent or ambivalent or lacked a deep
   quality of attachment
   Detrimental effects not supported by empirical studies of grief outcomes
B. Too much: hypertrophic grief
   Less common in older than in younger individuals
   May predict long-term functional impairment and heightened risk of physical and
   psychological morbidity
   Consider evolving major depression, anxiety disorder, posttraumatic stress disorder
C. Too long: chronic grief
   May be the most common type of complication
   Risk factors include loss of a child, a dependent relationship with the deceased, or
   an unnatural death
   Characteristics: unrelenting sorrow, overwhelmed by yearning and despair, unable
   to relinquish intense preoccupation with the deceased
   Consider underlying depression, posttraumatic stress disorder, or substance use dis-
   order

Deutsch (1937) wrote that this was a pathological state. Stern and coworkers (1951) speculated that grief was channeled into somatic symptoms by older people. Others wrote that after 65 years of age, a process of "disengagement" occurred; thus, the loss of a spouse was less traumatic in older than in younger people (Cumming & Henry, 1961). The quality of attachment to the deceased person appears to represent a risk factor for inhibited grief (Parkes & Weiss, 1983; Raphael et al., 1993). The empirical evidence, however, does not support an argument for the pathological nature or detrimental effects of "too little" grief (Parkes, 1965; Wortman & Silver, 1989). Nevertheless, we are often consulted by concerned friends or relatives of bereaved individuals (particularly elderly ones) who appear to be displaying too little grief. While these family or friends are concerned that the bereaved person is keeping everything inside and will ultimately "burst," it is clear that individuals do not burst, but rather grieve in their own way and in their own time.

HYPERTROPHIC GRIEF (TOO MUCH GRIEF)   Overly intense grief has not been described fully or studied comprehensively. Grief is one of the most painful emotions; therefore, it is difficult to state when its intensity might be considered extreme. The syndrome appears to be uncommon, particularly in older individuals (Parkes & Weiss, 1983; Zisook, Mulvihill, et al., 1990), although no specific risk factors have been identified. Usually, the frequency and intensity of the acute pangs of grief begin to lessen by the third to fourth month after the loss. The syndrome of *traumatic grief* (formerly *complicated grief reaction*), character-ized by searching, yearning, preoccupation to the point of distraction, disbelief, and lack of acceptance (Prigerson et al., 1995, 1997), appears to be a variant of hypertrophic grief. A grief reaction and preoccupation so intense as to interfere with function—and that does not substantially abate within the first few months—should raise the question of whether a major depression, anxiety disorder, or a posttraumatic stress disorder has emerged, complicating the bereavement and impeding its progress.

CHRONIC GRIEF (GRIEF FOR TOO LONG)   Chronic grief frequently affects young and middle-aged adults, most commonly women, as well as adolescents; it appears to be the most common type of grief complication (Parkes, 1965). There is no consensus, however, regarding the duration of grief that would be considered chronic. Unmodulated, intense preoccupation with the deceased and interference with other relationships or functioning, rather than the length of grieving, define pathological grief. Most investigators would not consider periodic preoccupation with the deceased (such as on or around holidays or anniversaries) to be evidence of chronic grief. However, the existence of persistent and pervasive preoccupation accompanied by dysphoria or other complications of grief beyond the first year after the loss is considered too long and requires clinical attention.

Specific risk factors that have been identified include loss of a child (Raphael, 1983), a dependent relationship with the deceased (Parkes & Weiss, 1983), or an unnatural death (Rynearson, 1987). Treatment often is protracted and difficult. In our experience, an underlying undiagnosed depression, posttraumatic stress disorder, or substance use disorder often underpins what appears to be chronic grief. Effective treatment of the underlying condition may allow normal grief resolution to unfold.

High-Risk Medical and Psychiatric Complications

MEDICAL MORBIDITY   The effects of bereavement on medical health (Table 20-4) are somewhat controversial. Some investigators have found minimal deleterious effects on the health of survivors (Clayton, 1979; Murrell et al., 1988; Norris & Murrell, 1990), particularly in individuals who were healthy before the death. Other investigators have reported an association between bereavement and complaints of somatic symptoms or declining health status, especially in those experiencing symptoms of complicated or traumatic bereavement (Bierhals et al., 1996; Clayton, 1990; Maddison & Viola, 1968; Parkes, 1972; Pasternak et al., 1997; Raphael, 1983; Thompson et al., 1984; Zisook & Shuchter, 1991a, 1993b).

In addition, elderly widows and widowers have been shown to use increased levels of medical services compared to married men and women (McHorney & Mor, 1988; Mor et al., 1986; Parkes, 1964; Shuchter & Zisook, 1993). Evidence regarding an increased incidence of specific medical disorders after loss

TABLE 20-4.   Complications of grief: medical manifestations

A. Morbidity
   Increased somatic complaints
   Increased risk of worsening preexisting illnesses
   Risk greater in widows versus widowers, particularly in early months
   Increased use of medical services
B. Mortality
   Excess mortality compared to nonbereaved individuals
   Widowers: highest mortality risk in first 6 months after loss
   Widows: period of risk delayed 1 or 2 years
   Risk factors:
      Moving into a chronic care facility
      Social isolation, living alone, or not remarrying (for widowers)
      Sudden deaths (for widows/widowers younger than 50 years)

is meager (Jacobs & Douglas, 1979; Klerman & Izen, 1977; Osterweis et al., 1984; Stroebe et al., 1981, 1982), although cardiovascular disease is the most frequently mentioned disorder with putative links to bereavement (Bierhals et al., 1996; Engel, 1961; Parkes, 1972; Prigerson et al., 1997).

Widows may be particularly vulnerable to both worsening of existing illnesses and development of new ones, especially in the months immediately following the death (Gallagher-Thompson et al., 1983; Thompson et al., 1984). Some have speculated that the increased risk of medical problems in widows immediately after the death may be related to the higher burden often assumed by wives (Chentsova-Dutton et al., 2000; Hutchin, 1993; Moss et al., 1993). These widows may have neglected personal health while focusing on the needs of their dying husbands.

MORTALITY   Most studies on medical mortality are limited by design flaws and small sample sizes (Osterweis et al., 1984). Nevertheless, a comprehensive review (M. S. Stroebe & W. Stroebe, 1993) and several large-scale studies have demonstrated higher mortality rates for widows and widowers compared to their married counterparts (Cox & Ford, 1964; Helsing & Szklo, 1981; Kaprio et al., 1987; Kraus & Lilienfeld, 1959; Levav et al., 1988; Rees & Lutkins, 1967). Death rates appear lowest for married individuals, followed by (in order) single, widowed, and divorced persons. The highest period of risk for widowers appears to be during the first 6 months after the loss (Helsing & Szklo, 1981; Rees & Lutkins, 1967; Young et al., 1963); for widows, the risk period may be delayed 1 or 2 years (Cox & Ford, 1964; Helsing & Szklo, 1981). Other risk factors for mortality after bereavement are listed in Table 20-4 (Bowling & Charlton, 1987; Gallagher-Thompson et al., 1993; Helsing & Szklo, 1981; M. S. Stroebe & W. Stroebe, 1993).

Although elderly persons have more chronic illnesses than younger people, younger widows are at greatest risk of dying (relative to their peers) following the death of a loved one (Helsing & Szklo, 1981; Jones, 1987; Kaprio et al., 1987; Mellstrom et al., 1982). One study reported that the oldest old may also be at relatively higher risk compared to controls (Bowling & Charlton, 1987). One well-known study of survivors of Israeli soldiers killed in war did not reveal an overall increase in mortality, but found that widowed or divorced parents who lost a son had an increased mortality rate that was statistically significant in the mothers (Levav et al., 1988).

No consistent pattern emerges for the causes of excess mortality during bereavement (M. S. Stroebe & W. Stroebe, 1993). The most compelling data implicate death from suicide (Kaprio et al., 1987; MacMahon & Pugh, 1965), accidents (Helsing & Szklo, 1981; Jones, 1987; Mellstrom et al., 1982), and heart disease (Jones, 1987; Kaprio et al., 1987; Mellstrom et al., 1982; Parkes et al., 1969). Impaired immunologic function, observed in a high proportion of recently bereaved individuals, especially in those with substantial depressive symptomatology, could theoretically be a mechanism for the increased morbidity and mortality noted in bereavement (Zisook et al., 1994). The increase in smoking and drug abuse observed in some bereaved individuals could also play a role (Zisook, Schuchter, et al., 1990).

PSYCHIATRIC MORBIDITY   The loss of a spouse is a severe life stress event that has been linked to the onset, exacerbation, and continuance of a variety of psychiatric disorders (see Table 20-5).

Substance Use.   Widows and widowers have been found to be at high risk for increased use of alcohol, tobacco, and other substances (Blankfield, 1983; Clayton, 1979; Klerman & Izen, 1977; Maddison & Viola, 1968; Osterweis et al., 1984; Valanis et al., 1987). Several investigators have reported that increased alcohol consumption occurs primarily in those with preexisting alcohol problems (Clayton, 1979; Valanis et al., 1987). Depressed women and those with fewer economic resources appear to be more vulnerable to increased use. Zisook, Mulvihill, et al. (1990) found approximately equal numbers of middle-aged and elderly widows and widowers (mean age 61 years) who increased (30%) versus decreased (26%) the number of days per month they drank, although more people increased (34%) than decreased (10%) the quantity of alcohol consumed per drinking day.

Anxiety Symptoms and Syndromes.   Anxiety related to bereavement has received little attention in the literature. Anxiety is not listed as one of the morbid complications of bereavement, yet Lindemann (1944) described symptoms of somatic anxiety (tightness in throat, choking sensation, sighing) and intense subjective anxiety (tension, mental pain, restlessness, feelings of unreality, and depersonalization) as part of "normal" grief. The "waves of grief" Lindemann described resemble the "pangs of pining and yearning" that Bowlby (1969) ascribed to separation anxiety and that he conceptualized as the characteristic features of grief. Lending some biological support to the close relationship of separation anxiety to bereavement, Shuchter and colleagues (1986)

TABLE 20-5.   Complications of grief: psychiatric manifestations

A. Substance use

Increased use in those with preexisting problems

Risk factors: male, past or bereavement-related depression, poor social/emotional support

B. Anxiety syndromes

Higher than expected rates of both anxiety symptoms and disorders

Risk for panic/generalized anxiety disorder highest with past history of anxiety disorder

Risk factors for continued high anxiety months after the death:

    Female, lower income, younger age

    Increased depression and anxiety symptom intensity soon after the loss

    Nonresolution of grief

    Less environmental support

C. Posttraumatic stress

Bereavement qualifies as a DSM-IV A criterion for posttraumatic stress disorder

Some overlap with traumatic grief

Common after unexpected death of a loved one

Incidence greater when loved one died from unnatural causes

Risk factors:

    Perceived unanticipated death or lack of opportunity to say goodbye

    Not associated with duration of the deceased spouse's terminal illness

D. Depression

Same clinical characteristics, course, and morbidity as nonbereavement depressions

May last 2 years or longer; episodic course probably common

Subsyndromal depressive syndromes probably most common variant in elderly

Risk factors:

    Not associated clearly with gender

    Unnatural, sudden, or unexpected death

    Preexisting physical or mental health problems, including depression/dysphoria

    Early intense or depressive reactions after the loss

    Poor physical health at the time of the loss

    Increased alcohol consumption soon after the loss

    Family history of major depression

    Poor social supports

reported that dexamethasone nonsuppression was related more to anxiety levels than to depressive symptoms in a group of recently bereaved widows.

During the first year of spousal bereavement, anxiety symptoms such as restlessness, tension, insomnia, headaches, weight loss, fatigue, decreased concentration, poor memory, shortness of breath, palpitations, and blurred vision and irritability are common; panic attacks are also common in the first months to the first year (Clayton, 1974; Clayton et al., 1968; Jacobs et al., 1990; Parkes, 1964). Elevated levels of somatization, interpersonal sensitivity, and obsessions, as well as an increased use of prescribed antianxiety medications, hypnotics, and over-the-counter "nerve pills" in older widows and widowers compared to community norms have also been reported (Zisook, Schuchter, et al., 1990; Zisook et al., 1993).

While most of the studies noted above emphasized anxiety symptoms rather than syndromes or disorders, Jacobs and coworkers (1990), using the modified Structured Clinical Interview for *DSM-III* (American Psychiatric Association [APA], 1980), found that more than 40% of bereaved spouses (mean age 55 years) had at least one type of anxiety disorder during the first year of spousal bereavement.

Posttraumatic Stress. The association between bereavement and trauma has been noted since Lindemann's (1944) landmark study of survivors and family members of victims of the infamous Coconut Grove fire. Given the horrific nature of the event, it is not surprising that Lindemann's description of ordinary grief overlaps considerably with symptoms now considered core components of PTSD: bursts of somatic and psychic distress, a sense of unreality, numbness, avoidance, preoccupation, guilt, and hostility. More recent investigators have found that people bereaved by a homicidal event experience intrusive, vivid, and repetitive images of the death; impaired cognitive processes; nightmares; heightened arousal; hypervigilance; and avoidance (Parkes, 1993; Rynearson, 1990).

The features of PTSD-complicated bereavement and traumatic grief overlap. Intrusive phenomena that often reflect the scene of the death or other traumatic images, anxiety, hyperarousal, nightmares, and other ongoing re-experiencing or avoidance phenomena characterize bereavement complicated by PTSD (Middleton et al., 1993). Traumatic grief is described as intense and prolonged preoccupation with thoughts of the deceased, yearning and searching behavior, disbelief, and avoidance (Prigerson et al., 1996, 1999). Prigerson and colleagues (1997) conceptualized traumatic grief, however, as related more to attachment disturbances than to the traumatic nature of the loss.

Until the publication of the fourth edition of the *Diagnostic and Statistical Manual of Mental Disorders (DSM-IV)* by the APA in 1994, bereavement did not qualify as an "A" criterion (i.e., the traumatic stressor criterion) for the diagnosis of PTSD. When the *DSM-IV* broadened the scope of the A, or stress, criteria, it opened the door for bereavement leading to PTSD. In the first published epidemiological study of PTSD using *DSM-IV* criteria, the sudden unexpected death of a loved one was the most common trauma found (Breslau et al., 1998). The prevalence of PTSD-like phenomena in the elderly is yet to be determined. Zisook et al. (1998) retrospectively applied *DMS-IV* criteria to their San Diego Widowhood data and found that 10% of the widows and widowers experienced PTSD 2 months after the spouse's death; a higher rate (36%) of PTSD was observed in those whose spouses died from unnatural causes (e.g., accident or suicide). These findings are consistent with the report of Schut and coworkers (1991) of high rates of PTSD-like phenomena in widows and widowers.

Preliminary studies looking at various approaches to treating these syndromes, pharmacologically or psychotherapeutically, appear promising (Shear et al., 2001; Zygmont et al., 1998).

Depression. Symptoms of depression, which are experienced intermittently by most widows and widowers as part of their grief (Clayton, 1990; Gallagher-Thompson et al., 1983; Nuss & Zubenko, 1992), are frequently persistent and pervasive enough to meet criteria for a major depressive syndrome. These episodes are common, occurring in 29% to 58% of widows and widowers 1 month after their spouse's death (Clayton et al., 1972; Gilewski et al., 1991; Harlow et al., 1991); 2 months after the death, it occurs in 24% to 30% (Futterman et al., 1990; Zisook & Shuchter, 1991a), and 4 months after the death, it occurs in approximately 25% (Clayton et al., 1972; McHorney & Mor, 1988).

Prevailing clinical wisdom suggests these depressive syndromes are aspects of bereavement, not major depression. According to *DSM-IV*, if a major depressive syndrome occurs within 2 months of the death of a loved one, the depression generally should not be considered major depression, but should be considered uncomplicated bereavement (APA, 1994). It is not at all clear, however, that such early depressive syndromes are as self-limiting or benign as the V-Code diagnosis (i.e., no psychiatric diagnosis) of bereavement might imply. Zisook and Shuchter (1991a) and Gilewski and colleagues (1991) independently found that these early depressive syndromes strongly predicted continued depression over longer term follow-up. Even those bereaved persons experiencing so-called uncomplicated bereavement showed increased rates of medical service utilization, poor self-perceived health status, and increased use of substances, including alcohol and psychotropic medications (Zisook & Shuchter, 1993b).

Although many studies on widowhood contain large percentages of elderly subjects, few bereavement studies have focused on elderly persons until recently. In the late 1970s, the National Institute on Aging established bereavement and aging as research funding priorities and funded three controlled, prospective, longitudinal studies to examine depression and its risk factors after late-life bereavement (Lund et al., 1993). The first of these studies took place in California (Breckenridge et al., 1986; Futterman et al., 1990; Gallagher-Thompson et al., 1982, 1983; Gilewski et al., 1991; Thompson et al., 1984), the second in Utah (Caserta et al., 1989; Caserta & Lund, 1992; Dimond et al., 1987; Lund, 1989; Lund et al., 1985, 1986a, 1986b, 1990, 1993), and the third in Florida (Faletti et al., 1989). They were followed by a number of other investigations that examined depressive reactions in late-life bereavement (Bruce et al., 1990; Goldberg et al., 1988; Harlow et al., 1991; McHorney & Mor, 1988; Norris & Murrell, 1990; Zisook & Shuchter, 1991a, 1991b).

These studies and others found that the risk for depressive symptoms and syndromes after bereavement is substantial in late life (Breckenridge et al., 1986; Bruce et al., 1990; Gallagher-Thompson et al., 1983; Harlow et al., 1991).

In perhaps the largest study on spousal bereavement and depression in persons 70 years and older, Turvey and coworkers (1999) reported a rate of syndromal depression in the newly bereaved nearly 9-fold higher than that for married individuals. The risk for both depressive symptoms and syndromes remains greater than the risk for married controls for at least 2 years after the death of a loved one (Harlow et al., 1991; Turvey et al., 1999; Zisook & Shuchter, 1993b). Age (range 70 to 103 years), gender, prior psychiatric history, or the expectation of the death did not differentiate between depressed and non-depressed newly bereaved subjects in the study of Turvey and colleagues (1999).

In general, the depressive reactions experienced by older versus younger individuals appear to be more similar than different. On the other hand, several investigators have found that the frequency and intensity of depressive symptoms and syndromes after late-life bereavement may be less than in younger individuals (Faletti et al., 1989; McHorney & Mor, 1988; VanZandt et al., 1989), particularly in the first year (Zisook & Shuchter, 1993a). This observed delay may indicate not that older widows and widowers are less distressed or depressed than younger ones, but rather that it takes older individuals somewhat longer to experience the full impact of bereavement.

Major depressive syndromes associated with bereavement in late life are similar to nonbereavement-related depression in most ways, although there may be subtle distinguishing characteristics. Various investigators have observed that the depressions experienced by late-life widows and widowers tend to be milder than other major depressive syndromes, with a lower prevalence of self-depreciation, guilt, and feelings of worthlessness (Breckenridge et al., 1986; Bruce et al., 1990; Gallagher-Thompson et al., 1982). Abnormal sleep architecture in depressed elderly widows also supports the similarity of bereavement-related major depressive syndrome to other forms of major depression (Reynolds et al., 1992). More studies using structured diagnostic interviews and carefully selected ambulatory depressed controls are needed to verify or revise these observations.

Subsyndromal depressions (painful symptoms of depression that do not quite meet full criteria for major depression) are gaining increased attention from clinicians and investigators (Judd et al., 1996, 1997). These depressions—frequent in both bereaved and nonbereaved elderly persons and associated with substantial suffering and morbidity—appear to go largely unrecognized in elderly bereaved individuals (Blazer, 1994; Blazer & George, 1987; Broadhead et al., 1990; Pasternak et al., 1994; Zisook et al., 1994, 1997). Subsyndromal depressions may represent early preclinical major depression, may be the aftermath of partially remitted major depression, or may be a form of attenuated major depression important in its own right. Much more investigation is needed on the frequency, course, burden, and treatment of subsyndromal depressions.

The course of depressive symptoms and syndromes associated with bereavement is quite variable. Most investigators have found a decreasing frequency of depressive symptoms and major depressive syndromes during the first year of widowhood (Bornstein et al., 1973; Futterman et al., 1990; Gilewski et al., 1991; Harlow et al., 1991; Zisook & Shuchter, 1991a). However, two studies that continued to track depressive syndromes during the second year of bereavement found little evidence of further decrease in their frequency. In one of the studies, the frequency of depressive syndromes was 16%, compared with 10% in married control subjects at the end of 2 years of bereavement (Harlow et al., 1991); in the other study, the respective frequencies were 14% versus 4% (Zisook & Shuchter, 1993a). Murrell and colleagues (1988) initially reported that the depressive symptoms in elderly bereaved individuals are intense, but temporary. The same group later reported that spousal bereavement (but not loss of a parent or child) in elderly persons is associated with an increased risk for depression that is not transient (i.e., lasting at least 9 months) (Norris & Murrell, 1990). The course of major depressive syndrome for many widows and widowers may be much more episodic than previously thought (Zisook & Shuchter, 1993a, 1993b).

Not all bereaved individuals experience major depressive syndromes. The adaptive capacities of individuals undergoing severe life stressors are impressive (McCrae & Costa, 1993; Pollock, 1987; Shuchter & Zisook, 1993; Silverman, 1972; Tedeschi et al., 1998). Nevertheless, because the risk for developing a major depressive syndrome after bereavement is substantial and the morbidity of untreated depression so great, it is important to identify risk factors.

The data on gender as a risk factor for bereavement-related depression are conflicting (Bruce et al., 1990; Gallagher-Thompson et al., 1983; Richards & McCallum, 1979); most studies have not found substantial differences between bereaved men and women (Clayton, 1990; Feinson, 1986; Zisook & Shuchter, 1991a). Other risk factors include loss of a spouse (vs. most other types of losses) (Norris & Murrell, 1990) and poor prior physical and mental health, including pre-bereavement depression or dysphoria (Bruce et al., 1990; McHorney & Mor, 1988; Norris & Murrell, 1990; Nuss & Zubenko, 1992). Unnatural deaths (e.g., suicide) may be especially likely to result in persistent depressive syndromes (Gilewski et al., 1991).

Others have identified early intense reactions soon after the loss (Farberow et al., 1987; Lund et al., 1985; Parkes & Weiss, 1983; Zisook & Shuchter, 1991a) and early depressive reactions (Dimond et al., 1987; Gilewski et al., 1991; Zisook & Shuchter, 1991a) as powerful predictors of later depression. Additional risk factors include financial problems and global stress (Norris & Murrell, 1990), recent disability (Goldberg et al., 1988), and subsequent losses in widowers (Siegel & Kuykendall, 1990).

Using a stepwise logistic regression procedure, Zisook and Shuchter (1993a) were able to identify a six-variable model that explained 27% of the variance and correctly classified 91% of widows and widowers in terms of major depressive syndrome 2 years after loss. The six variables are (1) presence of a major depressive syndrome soon after the loss, (2) intense symptoms of depression soon after the death, (3) family history of major depression, (4) increased alcohol consumption soon after the loss, (5) poor physical health around the time of the death, and (6) a sudden and unexpected death.

Several investigators have emphasized the protective role of social supports in attenuating the risks for depression associated with late-life bereavement (Dimond et al., 1987; Goldberg et al., 1988; Norris & Murrell, 1990; Nuss & Zubenko, 1992).

TREATMENT

Most bereaved individuals grieve, adapt to their loss, and get on with their lives without requiring any professional intervention (Chentsova-Dutton et al., 2002; McCrae & Costa, 1993; Pollock, 1987; Shuchter & Zisook, 1993). Time is the great healer for the majority of persons who are not at high risk for complications. People do not necessarily "get over it," but they do "get used to it" and "get on with it" over time (Goin et al., 1979). Healthy and secure people whose life experiences have led to a reasonable trust in themselves and others can be expected to cope effectively in adjusting to the death of a loved one.

In circumstances, however, in which a variety of factors place the bereaved individual at heightened risk for complications (see Table 20-2), preventive interventions may help ward off the development of full-blown complications. Once complications develop, prompt and focused treatment may help reverse symptoms or minimize long-term disability.

Prebereavement Counseling

The first level of primary prevention may happen before the death occurs. Most late-life bereavement occurs in the context of chronic illness and provides the possibility of "anticipatory" mourning (Schoenberg et al., 1974). Although data concerning the benefits of anticipatory grief are sparse, there is some support for the value of counseling families and loved ones before the death of a terminally ill family member (Cameron & Parkes, 1983). It is important that this counseling not encourage a sense of helplessness in the bereaved person or premature withdrawal from the dying person. Honest and open communication builds trust and allows the family to address unresolved conflicts, repair miscommunications, and begin to prepare for inevitable changes. Ideally, information is provided in a straightforward way so that it is heard but does not provoke an overwhelmingly traumatic confrontation with the impending loss (Parkes & Weiss, 1983).

Before the death of a loved one, bereaved persons may neglect personal medical needs, especially when involved in a substantial caregiving role. Such neglect may add to the already heightened risks of medical and psychiatric complications both during the caregiving period (Chentsova-Dutton et al., 2000) and after the death of the loved one (Chentsova-Dutton et al., 2002). Sound preventive principles ensure that caregivers take care of their medical needs, eat and sleep well, and visit their physician for routine care (Shuchter & Zisook, 1993). If they have a past history of major depression or anxiety disorders, their families and health providers should be alert to the heightened risk of exacerbation.

HOSPICE   Hospice offers comprehensive care to dying patients and their families during the terminal stage of illness and is committed to continued bereavement care for the bereaved person. In one small study of a hospice treatment program in Britain, Parkes (1981) randomly assigned high-risk survivors to no special treatment or to a brief supportive intervention 10 to 14 days after the death. After a 20-month follow-up, the supported group had better health scores and lower use of drugs, alcohol, and tobacco. Hospice programs offer great opportunities for prebereavement and postbereavement intervention studies, although few such studies have been completed.

MUTUAL SUPPORT   Since the development of Silverman's (1972, 1986) Widows-to-Widows Program, self-help interventions have played an important role in bereavement outcome (Lieberman, 1993). Barrett (1978) was unable to demonstrate benefits for self-help groups, but several studies have suggested their effectiveness, especially for high-risk individuals. For example, in a controlled study of relatively young widows (mean age 52 years), Vachon and colleagues (1980) found that the emotional support and practical assistance from a "widow contact" accelerated the rate of achieving landmark stages, especially for widows who were most distressed initially.

Constantino (1988) reported lower depression scores and better social adjustment in widows treated with self-help groups than in a nontreatment control group; Lieberman and Videka-Sherman (1986) found that self-help groups significantly decreased depression scores and psychotropic medication use compared to no such treatment. Marmar and colleagues (1988) found self-help groups were approximately as effective as brief, dynamic psychotherapy in bereaved women who were experiencing adjustment disorder, posttraumatic stress disorder, or major depression. Referral to self-help groups may provide needed support and "protection" for elderly bereaved individuals, especially for those with high-risk indicators or weak social supports.

GROUP PSYCHOTHERAPY   Yalom and Vinogradov (1982) argued that bereavement groups constitute a particularly efficient preventive intervention for a large at-risk population and represent excellent preventive mental health practice. In a controlled study of brief group therapy for widows and widowers, Lieberman and Yalom (1992) found that group participants showed modest improvements in role functioning and positive psychological states compared with untreated controls. Both groups, however, showed improvement during the year; overall, the adjustments of those in the two groups to their losses were more alike than different. Group therapy clearly is a form of treatment that requires further study.

INDIVIDUAL PSYCHOTHERAPY   Surprisingly few controlled studies have evaluated the efficacy of individual psychotherapy for preventing or lessening the impact of bereavement complications. Two studies were unable to provide strong support for the efficacy of brief therapy for preventing long-term complications. Polak and coworkers (1975) found no differences between bereaved individuals who received immediate crisis intervention after the sudden death of a family member and those who did not receive treatment. Gerber and colleagues (1975) also found no differences in outcome between elderly widows and widowers assigned either to brief supportive psychotherapy or to no active treatment.

In contrast to these two negative studies, Raphael (1977, 1978) found that high-risk widows benefited from early supportive psychotherapy. In widows who were at risk because of perceived lack of support from their social networks, such psychotherapy led to a reduction in health care use; those at risk because of ambivalent relationships with their husbands benefited from an attenuation of the severity of depressive symptoms. Raphael's study did not include elderly widows; therefore, it is important to replicate these important findings in older widows and widowers.

There are several published treatment studies, in addition to the preventive studies reviewed above, that support the usefulness of prompt treatment once complications arise. For example, Horowitz and coworkers (1984) found dynamic psychotherapy to be effective for adults with postbereavement adjustment disorders following the death of a parent or spouse. Interpersonal psychotherapy using grief as its primary paradigm may be suited for dealing with chronic grief, depression, or anxiety disorders associated with bereavement (Klerman, 1989). A small case report series suggested the potential effectiveness of interpersonal psychotherapy for bereavement-related depression following loss of a spouse in late life (Miller et al., 1994).

Another randomized controlled study found nortriptyline, but not interpersonal psychotherapy, to be more effective than placebo treatment. In that same study, however, the combination of medication plus psychotherapy was associated with the highest rates of treatment completion (Reynolds et al., 1999).

Other forms of psychotherapy that have been described include "guided mourning" (Mawson et al., 1981), "re-grief work" (Volkan, 1975), "grief resolution therapy" (Melges & DeMaso, 1980), and conjoint family therapy (Paul & Grosser, 1965). Lazare (1979) advocated an individualized approach for treating unresolved grief; Worden (1991) and Shuchter and Zisook (1987) described individualized, task-specific forms of treatment that may involve multiple modalities of care. These modes of treatment have not yet been sys-

tematically compared to each other in bereaved individuals; it is therefore difficult for clinicians to know when one form of treatment may be preferable to
others. These psychotherapies may have more similarities than differences.
Most of these therapies include some degree of education, support, attention
to the relationship with the deceased as it developed before the death and as it
has changed since, provocative techniques for those whose expression of grief
is blocked, and assurances of "normality" for bereaved individuals who need
to be reminded that their wide-ranging feelings and experiences are not deviant, abnormal, or fixed (Raphael et al., 1993; Zisook & Shuchter, 2001).

MEDICATIONS Although many clinicians have strong opinions about the use of
medications in grief reactions, there are few controlled studies on any medications for prevention or treatment of grief complications. Sleep is a frequent and
persistent bereavement-related problem (Clayton, 1979, 1990). Hypnotics may
therefore be helpful on an as-needed basis because persistent lack of sleep can
adversely affect anyone's health or well-being. There are few data on pharmacological approaches to anxiety disorders associated with bereavement, but
there is no reason to think that treatment should not be similar to that given
to nonbereaved individuals with anxiety syndromes.

Depression is perhaps the best-documented complication of bereavement.
One small, noncontrolled study of mostly middle-aged individuals with traumatic bereavement (mean age 57 ± 10.1 years) found paroxetine had positive
effects on both depressive and traumatic grief symptoms (Zygmont et al.,
1998). Two open studies supported the safety and efficacy of tricyclic antidepressants for bereavement-related major depressive syndromes (Jacobs et al.,
1987; Pasternak et al., 1991). Another study found nortriptyline, but not interpersonal psychotherapy, effective for major depressive syndromes following bereavement (Reynolds et al., 1999). Another open study found bupropion SR
effective in reducing symptoms of depression and grief in widows and widowers with major depressive syndromes within 2 months of a spouse's death
(Zisook et al., 2001). It is possible that treatment of the early depressive syndromes often seen within months of the death of a loved one may help prevent
some of the prolonged suffering, morbidity, and even mortality associated with
bereavement. Longitudinal controlled trials are needed, however.

SPECIAL CONCERNS

Most information on late-life bereavement comes from studies on widows and
widowers. More information is needed on the natural history and epidemiology
of other losses—such as loss of children, siblings, friends, and nondeath losses—
faced in late life. In addition, little is known about the influence of cultural
differences on the course and outcome of bereavement. The oldest old persons
have also not been well described in the bereavement literature, and the particular characteristics and needs of bereaved persons with cognitive difficulties

are unknown. There are few treatment studies specifically of late-life bereavement.

Should subsyndromal depressions be treated? If so, how? How soon after the death should a major depressive syndrome be considered pathological and be treated? Under what circumstances are particular psychotherapeutic approaches, antidepressant medications, or combinations indicated? How long should treatment continue? These and other unanswered questions require further inquiry.

REFERENCES

American Psychiatric Association. *Diagnostic and Statistical Manual of Mental Disorders.* 3rd ed. Washington, DC: American Psychiatric Association; 1980.

American Psychiatric Association. *Diagnostic and Statistical Manual of Mental Disorders.* 4th ed. Washington, DC: American Psychiatric Association; 1994.

Barrett CJ. Effectiveness of widow's groups in facilitating change. *J Consult Clin Psychol.* 1978;46:20.

Bierhals AJ, Prigerson HG, Fasiczka AL. Gender differences in complicated grief among the elderly. *Omega J Death Dying.* 1996;32:303–317.

Blankfield A. Grief and alcohol. *Am J Drug Alcohol Abuse.* 1983;9:435–446.

Blazer DG. Epidemiology of depressive disorders in late life. In: Schneider LS, Reynolds CF, Leibowitz BD, eds. *Diagnosis and Treatment of Depression in Late Life: Results of the NIMH Consensus and Development Conference.* Washington, DC: American Psychiatry Press; 1994:9–20.

Blazer DG, George LK. The epidemiology of depression in an elderly community population. *Gerontologist.* 1987;27:281–287.

Bornstein PE, Clayton PJ, Halikas JA, et al. The depression of widowhood after 13 months. *Br J Psychiatry.* 1973;122:561–566.

Bowlby J. *Attachment and Loss: Attachment.* Vol. 1. New York, NY: Basic Books; 1969.

Bowlby J. *Attachment and Loss. Separation, Anxiety and Anger.* Vol. 2. New York, NY: Basic Books; 1973.

Bowlby J. *Attachment and Loss: Loss, Sadness and Depression.* Vol. 3. New York, NY: Basic Books; 1980.

Bowlby J. Processes of mourning. *Int J Psychoanal.* 1961;42:317–340.

Bowling A, Charlton J. Risk factors for mortality after bereavement: a logistic regression analysis. *J R Coll Gen Pract.* 1997;37:551–554.

Breckenridge JN, Gallagher D, Thompson LW, et al. Characteristic depressive symptoms of bereaved elders. *J Gerontol.* 1986;41:163–168.

Breslau N, Kessler RC, Chilcoat HD, et al. Trauma and posttraumatic stress disorder in the community: the 1996 Detroit area survey of trauma. *Arch Gen Psychiatry.* 1998;55:626–632.

Broadhead WE, Blazer DG, George LK, et al. Depression, disability days, and days lost from work in a prospective epidemiologic survey. *JAMA.* 1990;264:2524–2528.

Bruce M, Kim K, Leaf P, et al. Depressive episodes and dysphoria resulting from conjugal bereavement in a prospective community sample. *Am J Psychiatry.* 1990;147:608–611.

Cameron J, Parkes CM. Terminal care: evaluation of effects on surviving family of care before and after bereavement. *Postgrad Med.* 1983;59:73–78.

Caserta MS, Lund DA. Bereaved older adults who seek early professional help. *Death Stud.* 1992;16:17–30.

Caserta MS, Lund DA, Dimond MF. Understanding the context of perceived health ratings: the case of spousal bereavement in later life. *J Aging Stud.* 1990;4:231–243.

Caserta MS, Van Pelt J, Lund DA. Advice on the adjustment to loss from bereaved older adults: an examination of resources and outcomes. In: Lund DA, ed. *Older Bereaved Spouses: Research with Practical Applications.* New York, NY: Taylor and Francis/Hemisphere; 1989:123–133.

Chentsova-Dutton Y, Shuchter S, Hutchin S, et al. Depression of grief reactions in hospice caregivers: from pre-death to 1 year afterwards. *J Affective Disorders.* 2002; 69:53–60.

Chentsova-Dutton Y, Shuchter S, Hutchin S, et al. The psychological and physical health of hospice caregivers. *Ann Clin Psychiatry.* 2000;12:19–27.

Clayton PJ. Bereavement and depression. *J Clin Psychiatry.* 1990;51:34–40.

Clayton PJ. Mortality and morbidity in the first year of bereavement. *Arch Gen Psychiatry.* 1974;30:747–750.

Clayton PJ. The sequelae and nonsequelae of conjugal bereavement. *Am J Psychiatry.* 1979;136:1530–1534.

Clayton PJ, Desmarais L, Winokur G. A study of normal bereavement. *Am J Psychiatry.* 1968;125:168–178.

Clayton PJ, Halikas JA, Maurice WL. The depression of widowhood. *Br J Psychiatry.* 1972;120:71–76.

Cleirin MPHD. *Adaptation After Bereavement.* Leiden, Netherlands: Leiden University, DSWO Press; 1991.

Constantino RE. Comparison of two group interventions for the bereaved. *Image.* 1988; 20:83–87.

Cox PR, Ford JR. The mortality of widows shortly after widowhood. *Lancet.* 1964;1: 163–164.

Cumming E, Henry WR. *Growing Old.* New York, NY: Basic Books; 1961.

Deutsch H. Absence of grief. *Psychoanal Q.* 1937;6:12–22.

DeVaul RA, Zisook S, Faschingbauer TR. Clinical aspects of grief and bereavement. *Prim Care Clin Office Pract.* 1979;6:391–402.

Dimond MF, Lund DA, Caserta MS. The role of social support in the first 2 years of bereavement in an elderly sample. *Gerontologist.* 1987;27:599–604.

Duberstein PR, Conwell Y, Cox C. Suicide in widowed persons. A psychological autopsy comparison of recently and remotely bereaved older subjects. *Am J Psychiatry.* 1998;6:328–334.

Engel GL. Is grief a disease? *Psychosom Med.* 1961;23:18–22.

Faletti MV, Gibbs JM, Clark C. Longitudinal course of bereavement in older adults. In: Lund DA, ed. *Older Bereaved Spouses: Research With Practical Applications.* New York, NY: Taylor & Francis/Hemisphere; 1989:37–51.

Farberow NL, Gallagher DE, Gilewski MJ, et al. An examination of the early impact of bereavement on psychological distress in survivors of suicide. *Gerontologist.* 1987; 27:592–598.

Feinson MC. Aging widows and widowers: are there mental health differences? *Int J Aging Hum Dev.* 1986;23:241–255.

Field NP, Nichols C, Holen A, et al. The relation of continuing attachment to adjustment in conjugal bereavement. *J Consult Clin Psychol.* 1999;67:212–218.

Freud S. Mourning and melancholia. In: Strachey J, ed. *The Standard Edition of the Complete Psychological Works of Sigmund Freud.* Vol. 14. London, England: Hogarth Press; 1957:239–269. (Originally published 1917.)

Futterman A, Gallagher D, Thompson LW, et al. Retrospective assessment of marital adjustment and depression during the first two years of spousal bereavement. *Psychol Aging.* 1990;5:277–283.

Gallagher DE, Thompson LW, Peterson JA. Psychosocial factors affecting adaptation to bereavement in the elderly. *Int J Aging Hum Dev.* 1981;14:79–95.

Gallagher-Thompson DE, Breckenridge J, Thompson LW, et al. Effects of bereavement on indicators of mental health in elderly widows and widowers. *J Gerontol.* 1983; 38:565–571.

Gallagher-Thompson DE, Breckenridge JN, Thompson LW. Similarities and differences between normal grief and depression in older adults. *Essence.* 1982;5:127–140.

Gallagher-Thompson D, Futterman A, Farberow N, et al. The impact of spousal bereavement on older widows and widowers. In: Stroebe MS, Stroebe W, Hansson RO, eds. *Handbook of Bereavement: Theory, Research and Intervention.* Cambridge, UK: Cambridge University Press; 1993:227–239.

Gerber I, Weiner A, Battin D, et al. Brief therapy to the aged bereaved. In: Schoenberg B, Gerber I, eds. *Bereavement: Its Psychosocial Aspects.* New York, NY: Columbia University Press; 1975:310–313.

Gilewski MJ, Farberow NL, Gallagher DE, et al. Interaction of depression and bereavement on mental health in the elderly. *Psychol Aging.* 1991;6:67–75.

Glick IO, Weiss RS, Parkes CM. *The First Year of Bereavement.* New York, NY: Wiley; 1974.

Goin MK, Burgoyne RW, Goin JM. Timeless attachment to a dead relative. *Am J Psychiatry.* 1979;136:988–989.

Goldberg EL, Comstock GW, Harlow SD. Emotional problems and widowhood. *J Gerontol.* 1988;3:5206–5208.

Hansson RO, Carpenter BN, Fairchild SK. Measurement issues in bereavement. In: Stroebe MS, Stroebe W, Hansson RO, eds. *Handbook of Bereavement.* Cambridge, UK: Cambridge University Press; 1993:62–74.

Harlow SD, Goldberg EL, Comstock GW. A longitudinal study of the prevalence of depressive symptomatology in elderly widowed and married women. *Arch Gen Psychiatry.* 1991;48:1065–1068.

Hays JC, Kasl S, Jacobs S. Past personal history of dysphoria, social support, and psychological distress following conjugal bereavement. *J Am Geriatr Soc.* 1994;42: 712–718.

Helsing KJ, Szklo M. Mortality after bereavement. *A J Epidemiol.* 1981;114:41–52.

Holmes T, Rahe R. The social readjustment rating scale. *J Psychosom Res.* 1967;11: 213–218.

Horowitz MJ. *Stress Response Syndromes.* Northvale, NJ: Aronson; 1986.

Horowitz MJ, Marmar C, Weiss DS, et al. Brief psychotherapy of bereavement reactions. *Arch Gen Psychiatry.* 1984;41:438–448.

Hutchin S. The distress of care giving. Paper presented at: 146th Annual Meeting of the American Psychiatric Association; May 22–27, 1993; San Francisco, CA.

Jacobs S. *Pathologic Grief.* Washington, DC: American Psychiatric Press; 1993.

Jacobs SC, Douglas L. Grief: a mediating process between a loss and illness. *Compr Psychiatry.* 1979;20:165–175.

Jacobs SC, Hansen F, Kasl S, et al. Anxiety disorders in acute bereavement: risk and risk factors. *J Clin Psychiatry.* 1990;51:267–274.

Jacobs SC, Nelson JC, Zisook S. Treating depression of bereavement with antidepressants: a pilot study. *Psychiatr Clin North Am.* 1987;10:501–510.

Jones DR. Heart disease mortality following widowhood: some results from the OPCS longitudinal study. *J Psychosom Res.* 1987;31:325–333.

Judd LL, Akiskal HS, Paulus MP. The role and clinical significance of subsyndromal depressive symptoms (SSD) in unipolar major depressive disorder. *J Affect Disord.* 1997;45:5–17.

Judd LL, Paulus MP, Wells KB, et al. Socioeconomic burden of subsyndromal depressive symptoms and major depression in a sample of the general population. *Am J Psychiatry.* 1996;153:1411–1417.

Kaprio J, Koskenvuo M, Rita H. Mortality after bereavement: a prospective study of 95,647 widowed persons. *Am J Public Health.* 1987;77:283–287.

Klass D, Goss R. Spiritual bonds to the dead in cross-cultural and historical perspective: comparative religion and modern grief. *Death Stud.* 1999;23:547–567.

Klerman GL. Depressive disorders: further evidence for increased medical morbidity and impairment of social functioning. *Arch Gen Psychiatry.* 1989;46:856–858.

Klerman GL, Izen J. The effects of bereavement and grief on physical health and general well being. *Adv Psychosom Med.* 1977;9:63–104.

Kraus AS, Lilienfeld AM. Some epidemiological aspects of the high mortality rate in the young widowed group. *J Chronic Dis.* 1959;10:207–217.

Lazare A. Unresolved grief. In: Lazare A, ed. *Outpatient Psychiatry.* Baltimore, MD: Williams & Wilkins; 1979:498–512.

Levav I, Friedlander Y, Kark J, et al. An epidemiologic study of mortality among bereaved parents. *N Engl J Med.* 1988;319:457–461.

Lieberman MA. Bereavement self-help groups: a review of conceptual and methodological issues. In: Stroebe MS, Stroebe W, Hansson RO, eds. *Handbook of Bereavement: Theory, Research and Intervention.* Cambridge, UK: Cambridge University Press; 1993:411–426.

Lieberman MA, Videka-Sherman L. The impact of self-help groups on the mental health of widows and widowers. *Am J Orthopsychiatry.* 1986;56:435–449.

Lieberman MA, Yalom I. Brief group psychotherapy for the spousally bereaved: a controlled study. *Int J Group Psychother.* 1992;42:117–132.

Lindemann E. Symptomatology and management of acute grief. *Am J Psychiatry.* 1944;101:141–148.

Lund DA. *Older Bereaved Spouses: Research with Practical Applications.* New York, NY: Taylor & Francis/Hemisphere; 1989.

Lund DA, Caserta MS, Dimond MF. The course of spousal bereavement in later life. In: Stroebe MS, Stroebe W, Hansson RO, eds. *Handbook of Bereavement: Theory, Research and Intervention.* Cambridge, UK: Cambridge University Press; 1993:240–254.

Lund DA, Caserta MS, Dimond MF. Gender differences through two years of bereavement among the elderly. *Gerontologist.* 1986a;26:314–320.

Lund DA, Caserta MS, Dimond MF, et al. Impact of bereavement on self-conceptions of older surviving spouses. *Symbolic Interact.* 1986b;9:235–244.

Lund DA, Caserta MS, Van Pelt J, et al. Stability of social support networks after late life spousal bereavement. *Death Stud.* 1990;14:53–73.

Lund DA, Dimond MF, Caserta MS, et al. Identifying elderly with coping difficulties after two years of bereavement. *Omega.* 1985;16:213–223.

MacMahon B, Pugh TF. Suicide in the widowed. *Am J Epidemiol.* 1965;81:23–31.

Maddison D, Viola A. The health of widows in the year following bereavement. *J Psychosom Res.* 1968;12:297–306.

Marmar CR, Horowitz MJ, Weiss DS, et al. A controlled trial of brief psychotherapy and mutual-help group treatment of conjugal bereavement. *Am J Psychiatry.* 1988; 145:203–209.

Martikainen P, Valkonen T. Mortality after the death of a spouse: rates and causes of death in a large Finnish cohort. *Am J Public Health.* 1996;86:1087–1093.

Mawson D, Marks IM, Ramm L, et al. Guided mourning for morbid grief: a controlled study. *Br J Psychiatry.* 1981;138:185–193.

McCrae RR, Costa PT. Psychological resilience among widowed men and women: a 10-year follow-up of a national sample. In: Stroebe MS, Stroebe W, Hansson RO, eds. *Handbook of Bereavement.* Cambridge, UK: Cambridge University Press; 1993: 196–207.

McHorney CA, Mor V. Predictors of bereavement depression and its health services consequences. *Med Care.* 1988;26:882–893.

Melges FT, DeMaso DR. Grief resolution therapy: reliving, revising and revisiting. *Am J Psychother.* 1980;34:51–61.

Mellstrom D, Nilsson A, Oden A, et al. Mortality among the widowed in Sweden. *Scand J Soc Med.* 1982;10:33–41.

Middleton W, Raphael B, Martinek N, et al. Pathological grief reactions. In: Stroebe MS, Stroebe W, Hansson RO, eds. *Handbook of Bereavement: Theory, Research and Intervention.* Cambridge, UK: Cambridge University Press; 1993:44–61.

Miller MD, Frank E, Cornes C, et al. Applying interpersonal psychotherapy to bereavement-related depression following loss of a spouse in late-life. *J Psychother Pract Res.* 1994;3:149–162.

Mor V, McHorney C, Sherwood S. Secondary morbidity among the recently bereaved. *Am J Psychiatry.* 1986;143:158–163.

Moss MS, Moss SZ, Rubinstein R, et al. Impact of elderly mother's death on middle age daughters. *Int J Aging Hum Dev.* 1993;37:1–22.

Murrell SA, Himmelfarb S, Phifer JF. Effects of bereavement/loss and pre-event status on subsequent physical health in older adults. *Int J Aging Hum Dev.* 1988;27: 89–107.

Norris FH, Murrell SA. Social support, life events, and stress as modifiers of adjustment to bereavement by older adults. *Psychol Aging.* 1990;5:429–436.

Nuss WS, Zubenko GS. Correlates of persistent depressive symptoms in widows. *Am J Psychiatry.* 1992;149:346–351.

Osterweis M, Solomon F, Green ME, eds. *Bereavement: Reactions, Consequences, and Care.* Washington, DC: National Academy Press; 1984.

Parkes CM. The effects of bereavement on physical and mental health: a study of the medical records of widows. *Br Med J.* 1964;2:274–279.

Parkes CM. *Bereavement: Studies of Grief in Adult Life.* 2nd ed. New York, NY: International Universities Press; 1972.

Parkes CM. Determination of outcome following bereavement. *Omega.* 1975;6:303–323.

Parkes CM. Bereavement and mental illness. *Br J Med Psychol.* 1965;38:388–397.

Parkes CM. Evaluation of a bereavement service. *J Prev Psychiatry.* 1981;1:179–188.

Parkes CM. Psychiatric problems following bereavement by murder or manslaughter. *Br J Psychiatry.* 1993;162:49–54.

Parkes CM. Risk factors in bereavement: implications for the prevention and treatment of pathologic grief. *Psychiatr Ann.* 1990;20:308–313.

Parkes CM. Psycho-social transitions: a field for study. *Soc Sci Med.* 1971;5:101–115.

Parkes CM, Benjamin B, Fitzgerald RG. Broken heart: a statistical study of increased mortality among widowers. *Br Med J.* 1969;1:740–743.

Parkes CM, Weiss RS. *Recovery From Bereavement.* New York, NY: Basic Books; 1983.

Pasternak RE, Prigerson H, Hall M, et al. The posttreatment illness course of depression in bereaved elders. High relapse/recurrence rates. *Am J Geriatr Psychiatry.* 1997;5: 54–59.

Pasternak RE, Reynolds CF III, Miller MD, et al. The symptom profile and two-year course of subsyndromal depression in spousally bereaved elders. *Am J Geriatr Psychiatry.* 1994;2:210–219.

Pasternak RE, Reynolds CF III, Schlernitzauer M, et al. Acute open-trial nortriptyline therapy of bereavement-related depression in late life. *J Clin Psychiatry.* 1991;52: 307–310.

Paul N, Grosser G. Operational mourning and its role in conjoint family therapy. *Community Ment Health J.* 1965;1:339–345.

Polak PR, Egan D, Vandenburgh R, et al. Prevention in mental health: a controlled study. *Am J Psychiatry.* 1975;132:146–149.

Pollock GH. The mourning-liberation process in health and disease. *Psychiatr Clin North Am.* 1987;10:345–354.

Prigerson HG, Bierhals AJ, Kasl SV, et al. Complicated grief as a disorder distinct from bereavement-related depression and anxiety: a replication study. *Am J Psychiatry.* 1996;153:1484–1486.

Prigerson HG, Bierhals AJ, Kasl SV, et al. Traumatic grief as a risk factor for mental and physical morbidity. *Am J Psychiatry.* 1997;154:616–623.

Prigerson HG, Maciejewski PK, Reynolds CF III, et al. Inventory of Complicated Grief: a scale to measure maladaptive symptoms of loss. *Psychiatry Res.* 1995;59:65–79.

Prigerson HG, Shear MK, Jacobs SC, et al. Consensus criteria for traumatic grief: a preliminary empirical test. *Br J Psychiatry.* 1999;174:67–73.

Raphael B. *The Anatomy of Bereavement.* New York, NY: Basic Books; 1983.

Raphael B. Mourning and the prevention of melancholia. *Br J Med Psychol.* 1978;41: 303–310.

Raphael B. Preventive intervention with the recently bereaved. *Arch Gen Psychiatry.* 1977;34:1450–1454.

Raphael B, Middleton W, Martinek N, et al. Counseling and therapy of the bereaved. In: Stroebe MS, Stroebe W, Hansson RO, eds. *Handbook of Bereavement: Theory, Research, and Intervention.* Cambridge, UK: Cambridge University Press; 1993: 427–453.

Rees W, Lutkins S. Mortality of bereavement. *Br Med J.* 1967;4:13–16.

Reynolds CF III, Hoch CC, Buysse DJ, et al. Electroencephalographic sleep in spousal bereavement and bereavement-related depression of late life. *Biol Psychiatry*. 1992; 31:69–82.

Reynolds CF III, Miller MD, Pasternak RE, et al. Treatment of bereavement-related major depressive episodes in later life: a controlled study of acute and continuation treatment with nortriptyline and interpersonal psychotherapy. *Am J Psychiatry*. 1999;156:202–208.

Richards JG, McCallum J. Bereavement in the elderly. *N Z Med J*. 1979;89:201–204.

Rubin S. Treating the bereaved spouse: a focus on the loss process, the self and the other. *Psychother Patient*. 1990;6:189–205.

Rynearson EK. Pathologic grief: the queen's croquet ground. *Psychiatr Ann*. 1990;20: 295–303.

Rynearson EK. Psychological adjustment to unnatural dying. In: Zisook S, ed. *Biopsychosocial Aspects of Bereavement*. Washington, DC: American Psychiatric Association; 1987:75–93.

Rynearson EK, McCreery JM. Bereavement after homicide: a synergism of trauma and loss. *Am J Psychiatry*. 1993;150:250–261.

Sanders CM. A comparison of adult bereavement in the death of a spouse, child and parent. *Omega*. 1980;10:303–322.

Sanders CM. Comparison of younger and older spouses in bereavement outcome. *Omega*. 1981;11:217–232.

Sanders CM. Risk factors in bereavement outcome. In: Stroebe MS, Stroebe W, Hansson RO, eds. *Handbook of Bereavement: Theory, Research, and Intervention*. Cambridge, UK: Cambridge University Press; 1993:255–267.

Schaefer C, Quesenberry CPJ, Wi S. Mortality following conjugal bereavement and the effects of a shared environment. *Am J Epidemiol*. 1995;141:1142–1152.

Schneider DS, Sledge PA, Shuchter SR, et al. Dating and remarriage over the first 2 years of widowhood. *Ann Clin Psychiatry*. 1996;8:51–57.

Schoenberg B, Carr AC, Kutscher AH, et al. *Anticipatory Grief*. New York, NY: Columbia University Press; 1974.

Schut HA, de Keijser J, Van den Bout J, Dijkhuis JH. Posttraumatic stress symptoms in the first years of conjugal bereavement. *Anxiety Res*. 1991;4:225–234.

Shear MK, Frank E, Foa E, et al. Traumatic grief management in primary care: a pilot study. *Am J Psychiatry*. 2001;158:1506–1508.

Shuchter SR. *Dimensions of Grief: Adjusting to the Death of a Spouse*. San Francisco, CA: Jossey-Bass; 1986.

Shuchter SR, Zisook S. The course of normal grief. In: Stroebe MS, Stroebe W, Hansson RO, eds. *Handbook of Bereavement*. Cambridge, UK: Cambridge University Press; 1993:23–43.

Shuchter SR, Zisook S. A multidimensional model of spousal bereavement. In: Zisook S, ed. *Biopsychosocial Aspects of Bereavement*. Washington, DC: American Psychiatric Association; 1987:35–47.

Shuchter SR, Zisook S, Kirkorowicz C, et al. The dexamethasone test in acute grief. *Am J Psychiatry*. 1986;143:879–881.

Siegel JM, Kuykendall DH. Loss, widowhood, and psychological distress among the elderly. *J Consult Clin Psychol*. 1990;58:519–524.

Silver RL, Wortman CB. Coping with undesirable life events. In: Gabor J, Seligman MEP, eds. *Human Helplessness: Theory and Applications*. New York, NY: Academic Press; 1980:279–340.

Silverman PR. Widowhood and prevention intervention. *Family Coordinator*. 1972;21: 95–102.

Silverman PR. *Widow-to-Widow*. New York, NY: Springer; 1986.

Stern K, Williams GM, Prados M. Grief reactions in later life. *Am J Psychiatry*. 1951; 108:289–294.

Stroebe MS, Stroebe W. The mortality of bereavement: a review. In: Stroebe MS, Stroebe W, Hansson RO, eds. *Handbook of Bereavement: Theory, Research, and Intervention*. Cambridge, UK: Cambridge University Press; 1993:175–195.

Stroebe MS, Stroebe W, Gergen KJ, et al. The broken heart: Reality or myth? *Omega*. 1981;12:87–105.

Stroebe W, Stroebe MS. Determinants of adjustment to bereavement in younger widows and widowers. In: Stroebe MS, Stroebe W, Hansson RO, eds. *Handbook of Bereavement: Theory, Research and Intervention*. Cambridge, UK: Cambridge University Press; 1993:208–226.

Stroebe W, Stroebe MS, Gergen K, et al. The effects of bereavement on mortality: a social psychological analysis. In: Eiser JR, ed. *Social Psychology and Behavioral Medicine*. Chichester, UK: Wiley; 1982:527–560.

Tedeschi RG, Park CL, Calhoun LG. *Posttraumatic Growth: Positive Changes in the Aftermath of Crisis*. Mahwah, NJ: Erlbaum; 1998:258.

Thompson LW, Breckenridge JN, Gallagher D. Effects of bereavement on self-perception of physical health in elderly widows and widowers. *J Gerontol*. 1984;39:309–314.

Turvey CL, Carney C, Arndt S, et al. Conjugal loss and syndromal depression in a sample of elders aged 70 years or older. *Am J Psychiatry*. 1999;156:1596–1601.

US Bureau of the Census. *Statistical Abstract of the United States*. 117 ed. Washington, DC: US Government Printing Office; 1997.

Vachon MLS. Predictors and correlates of adaptation in conjugal bereavement. *Am J Psychiatry*. 1982;139:998–1002.

Vachon MLS, Sheldon AR, Lancee WJ, et al. A controlled study of self-help intervention for widows. *Am J Psychiatry*. 1980;137:1380–1384.

Valanis B, Yeaworth RC, Mullis MR. Alcohol use among bereaved and non-bereaved older persons. *J Gerontol Nurs*. 1987;13:26–32.

VanZandt S, Mou R, Abbott R. Mental and physical health of rural bereaved and non-bereaved elders: a longitudinal study. In: Lund DA, ed. *Older Bereaved Spouses: Research With Practical Applications*. New York, NY: Taylor & Francis/Hemisphere; 1989:25–36.

Volkan VD. "Regrief" therapy. In: Schoenberg B, Kutscher AH, Carr AC, eds. *Bereavement: Its Psychosocial Aspects*. New York, NY: Columbia University Press; 1975: 334–350.

Worden JW. *Grief Counseling and Grief Therapy: A Handbook for the Mental Health Practitioner*. New York, NY: Springer; 1991.

Wortman CB, Silver RC. The myths of coping with loss. *J Consult Clin Psychol*. 1989; 57:349–357.

Yalom ID, Vinogradov S. Bereavement groups: techniques and themes. *Int J Group Psychother*. 1982;34:419–430.

Young M, Benjamin B, Wallis C. Mortality of widowers. *Lancet*. 1963;2:254–256.

Zisook S. Unresolved grief. In: Zisook S, ed. *Biopsychosocial Aspects of Bereavement*. Washington, DC: American Psychiatric Association; 1987:23–34.

Zisook S, Chentsova-Dutton Y, Shuchter SR. PTSD following bereavement. *Ann Clin Psychiatry.* 1998;10:157–163.

Zisook S, Downs NS. Diagnosis and treatment of depression in late life. *J Clin Psychiatry.* 1998;59:80–91.

Zisook S, Mulvihill M, Shuchter SR. Widowhood and anxiety. *Psychiatr Med.* 1990;8: 99–116.

Zisook S, Paulus M, Shuchter SR, et al. The many faces of depression following spousal bereavement. *J Affect Disord.* 1997;45:85–94.

Zisook S, Shuchter SR. Depression through the first year after the death of a spouse. *Am J Psychiatry.* 1991a;148:1346–1352.

Zisook S, Shuchter SR. Early psychological reaction to the stress of widowhood. *Psychiatry.* 1991b;54:320–333.

Zisook S, Shuchter SR. Major depression associated with widowhood. *Am J Geriatr Psychiatry.* 1993a;1:316–326.

Zisook S, Shuchter SR. Treatment of the depressions of bereavement. *Am Behav Scientist.* 2001;44:782–797.

Zisook S, Shuchter SR. Uncomplicated bereavement. *J Clin Psychiatry.* 1993b;54:365–372.

Zisook S, Shuchter SR, Mulvihill M. Alcohol, cigarette, and medication use during the first year of widowhood. *Psychiatr Ann.* 1990;20:318–326.

Zisook S, Shuchter SR, Pedrelli P, et al. Acute, open-trial of bupropion SR therapy of bereavement. *J Clin Psychiatry.* 2001;62:227–230.

Zisook S, Shuchter SR, Sledge P, et al. Diagnostic and treatment considerations in depression associated with late-life bereavement. In: Schneider LS, Reynolds CF, Leibowitz BD, et al., eds. *Diagnosis and Treatment of Depression in Late Life: Results of the NIMH Consensus and Development Conference.* Washington, DC: American Psychiatric Press; 1994:419–435.

Zisook S, Shuchter SR, Sledge P, et al. Aging and bereavement. *J Geriatr Psychiatry Neurol.* 1993;6:137–143.

Zygmont M, Prigerson HG, Houck PR, et al. A post hoc comparison of paroxetine and nortriptyline for symptoms of traumatic grief. *J Clin Psychiatry.* 1998;59:241–245.

21

Late-Life Mood Disorders

George S. Alexopoulos, MD

THE MAGNITUDE OF THE PROBLEM

Epidemiological studies show that major depression occurs in 1% of the general elderly population; 3% of community-residing elderly individuals suffer from dysthymia, and 8% to 15% have clinically significant depressive symptomatology (NIH consensus conference, 1992). Reanalysis of epidemiological data suggests that the lower prevalence of depression in older compared to younger adults may result from the tendency of elders to underreport depressed mood (Gallo et al., 1999). Underreporting of depressed mood by elders has also been documented in clinical populations (Gallo & Rabins 1999). Finally, epidemiological findings that suggest that older persons have lower lifetime prevalence of depression than younger adults may result from the documented tendency of elders to "forget" previous episodes (Gallo et al., 1999).

Several studies have shown that the prevalence of geriatric depression is much higher in medical settings than in the community (Schneider et al., 1994). In mixed-age patients treated in primary care settings, clinically significant depressive symptoms and signs were identified in 17% to 37% of patients (Alexopoulos, 1996a). Approximately 30% of these patients have major depression; the remainder have a variety of depressive syndromes that could benefit from medical attention (Koenig et al., 1988). In medically hospitalized patients, major depression occurs in 11%, and less severe, yet clinically significant, depressive symptomatology is identified in 25% of the population (NIH consensus conference, 1992).

Elders who reside in long-term care settings suffer higher rates of depression than those living in the community, and half of those relocated to nursing homes are at increased risk for depression (Parmelee et al., 1989). Depression estimates for nursing home residents range from 12% to 22.4% for major depression and an additional 17% to 30% for minor depression (Burrows et al., 1995; Katz et al., 1995). About 13% of residents develop new episodes of major depression in a 1-year period, and another 18% develop new depressive symptoms (NIH consensus conference, 1992).

DEPRESSIVE SYNDROMES

Several syndromes of geriatric depression have been identified and are included in the current classification system of the *Diagnostic and Statistical Manual of Mental Disorders, Fourth Edition* (*DSM-IV*; American Psychiatric Association [APA], 1994): major depression, dysthymia, psychotic depression, adjustment disorder with depressed mood, and other syndromes of late-life depression.

Major Depression

The diagnosis of major depression requires five of the following nine symptoms for at least 2 weeks: depressed mood, diminished interest or pleasure in all or almost all activities, weight loss or gain (more than 5% of body weight), insomnia or hypersomnia, psychomotor agitation or retardation, fatigue, feelings of worthlessness or inappropriate guilt, reduced ability to concentrate, recurrent thoughts of death or suicide. Depressed mood or loss of interest or pleasure are necessary to meet criteria for major depression and must be one of the five required symptoms.

Although not part of the diagnostic criteria, nondemented elderly individuals often have cognitive impairment when they develop depression (Alexopoulos, 1990), including disturbances in attention, speed of mental processing, and executive function, even when they are not demented (Kindermann et al., 2000; Lockwood et al., 2000). Processing speed and working memory deficits persist after remission of geriatric depression and may be a trait marker of this disorder (Butters et al., 2000; Nebes, 2000).

Dysthymia

The *DSM-IV* defines *dysthymia* as a chronic depression (more than 2 years) of mild or moderate severity. Depressed mood is the cardinal symptom of dysthymia and should not be absent for longer than 2 months. The *DSM-IV* criteria require that at least two of the following symptoms: poor appetite or overeating, insomnia or hypersomnia, fatigue, low self-esteem, poor concentration or difficulty in making decisions, and hopelessness. In elderly patients, major depression, dysthymia, and even clinically significant depressive symptomatology that does not meet criteria for a distinct depressive syndrome occur frequently in the context of neurological and medical disorders and pose diagnostic difficulties.

Psychotic Depression

Patients with psychotic depression, as a rule, have delusions; hallucinations are less frequent. The usual themes of depressive delusions are guilt, hypochondriasis, nihilism, persecution, and sometimes jealousy. Depressive delusions can be distinguished from delusions of demented patients in that the latter are less systematized and less congruent to the affective disturbance. Psychotic depression occurs in 20% to 45% of hospitalized elderly depressives (Meyers, 1995).

Adjustment Disorder With Depressed Mood

Negative life events are associated with increased depressive symptoms in the elderly (Hays et al., 1998). Financial problems, socioeconomic deprivation (Wilson et al., 1999), poor physical health, disability, and social isolation are significant contributors to depressive symptomatology in late life (West et al., 1998). Among older women, the effects of aging, mood, and chronic life stress are interactive and may affect regulation of interleukin-6, a cytokine that is implicated in both the aging process and health problems such as osteoporosis (Lutgendorf et al., 1999).

Other causes of adjustment disorders in the elderly are relocation to a long-term care facility and bereavement because of loss of a spouse. Marked increases in the risk for medical morbidity and mortality occur following involuntary relocation. However, when elderly persons have control over such decisions and when they move to a high-quality institution, relocation may have a neutral or even a beneficial effect (Armer, 1993).

Approximately 10% to 20% of persons who lose a spouse develop clinically significant depressive symptoms in the first year of bereavement. If left untreated, the depression frequently persists (Zisook et al., 1994). Older persons appear to be at lower risk for developing depressive symptoms or syndromes than younger adults during the first months of widowhood. However, by the end of the second year, older and younger individuals have same rates of major depression. In fact, the prevalence of major depression continues to increase during the second year of bereavement (Zisook et al., 1994). At the end of the second year after loss, 14% of the bereaved individuals have major depression, a percentage much higher than the prevalence of major depression in the elderly community population (1%). Bereaved elderly individuals who do not meet criteria for major depression often have significant depressive symptomatology that can contribute to compromised function, disability, and impaired quality of life.

Other Syndromes of Late-Life Depression

Several syndromes of geriatric depression have been described. Research on these syndromes has facilitated the development of pathogenetic hypotheses and stimulated research on brain mechanisms in geriatric depression. Some clinically useful information was derived from the description of these syndromes, but their main contribution to the field has been heuristic.

LATE-ONSET DEPRESSION   It has been suggested that depression with the onset of the first episode in late life includes a large subgroup of patients with neurological brain disorders that may or may not be evident when the depression first appears (Alexopoulos, 1990). This assertion is supported by differences observed between late-onset and early-onset geriatric depression. Compared to those with early-onset geriatric depression, patients with late-onset depression appear to have less-frequent family history of mood disorders, higher prevalence of dementing disorders, more impairment in neuropsychological tests, higher rate of dementia development on follow-up, more neurosensory hearing impairment, greater enlargement in lateral brain ventricles, and more white matter hyperintensities.

The late-onset syndrome has served as the basis of pathogenetic hypotheses that link neurological brain abnormalities to development of late-life depression and has stimulated research on specific brain abnormalities that underlie geriatric depressive disorders. However, there have been significant limitations in using age of onset as a distinguishing clinical characteristic. On a clinical level, onset of depression is difficult to identify, especially in patients whose early episodes are mild (Wiener et al., 1997). On a theoretical level, an episode that occurs in late life may be contributed by neurological brain changes regardless of whether the patient did or did not have other depressive episodes in early life. Moreover, early-onset depression may predispose to brain abnormalities by increasing secretion of stress-related hormones, which reduce neurotrophic factor secretion and ultimately decrease neurogenesis (Duman et al., 1997).

DEPRESSION WITH REVERSIBLE DEMENTIA   Some elderly depressed patients develop a reversible dementia syndrome that improves or completely subsides after remission of depression. This syndrome has been termed *pseudodementia, depression with reversible dementia,* and *dementia of depression* and mainly occurs in patients with late-onset depression (Alexopoulos, Young, et al., 1993). Depressed elderly patients who remain with some cognitive impairment even after improvement of depression usually have an early-stage dementing disorder with cognitive manifestations that are exaggerated when the depressive syndrome is superimposed. It appears that even patients with more or less complete cognitive recovery have high rates of irreversible dementia (about 40% within 3 years) on follow-up. Most of these patients do not meet criteria for dementia for 1 to 2 years after the initial episode of depression with reversible dementia (Alexopoulos, Meyers, et al., 1993). Therefore, identification of a reversible dementia syndrome in elderly depressives constitutes an indication for thorough diagnostic workup aimed at the identification of treatable dementing disorders and frequent follow-up.

VASCULAR DEPRESSION   It has been proposed that cerebrovascular disease may predispose, precipitate, or perpetuate some geriatric depressive syndromes (Alexopoulos et al., 1997b; Alexopoulos, Bruce, Silbersweig, et al., 1999). The vascular depression hypothesis is supported by the comorbidity of depression and vascular disease and risk factors and the association of ischemic lesions to distinctive behavioral symptomatology. Elderly patients with vascular depression have greater overall cognitive impairment and disability than those in the nonvascular depression group (Alexopoulos et al., 1997a; Krishnan et al., 1997). Fluency and naming are most impaired in vascular depression. Patients with vascular depression have more apathy and retardation and less agitation as well as less guilt and greater lack of insight. Disruption of prefrontal systems or their modulating pathways by single lesions or by an accumulation of lesions exceeding a threshold have been hypothesized as the central mechanisms in vascular depression.

DEPRESSION–EXECUTIVE DYSFUNCTION SYNDROME   Clinical, structural, and functional neuroimaging and neuropathology studies suggest that frontostriatal dysfunction contributes to the pathogenesis of at least some late-life depressive syndromes. Based on these findings, the depression–executive dysfunction syndrome has been described and conceptualized as an entity with pronounced frontostriatal-limbic dysfunction (Alexopoulos, 2001a). On a clinical level, the syndrome is characterized by psychomotor retardation, reduced interest in activities, suspiciousness, impaired instrumental activities of daily living (IADL), and limited vegetative symptoms. The clinical significance of identifying the depression–executive dysfunction syndrome of late life is that emerging evidence suggests that the syndrome has poor or slow and unstable response to classical antidepressants and selective serotonin reuptake inhibitors (SSRIs) (Alexopoulos et al., 2000; Alexopoulos, Kiosses, Choi, et al., 2002; Kalayam & Alexopoulos, 1999). In contrast, a preliminary study showed that the depression–executive dysfunction syndrome responds well to problem-solving therapy (Alexopoulos et al., 2003).

DEPRESSION OF ALZHEIMER'S DISEASE   Depressive symptoms and syndromes are common in Alzheimer's patients. The "National Institute of Mental Health—Provisional Diagnostic Criteria for Depression of Alzheimer's Disease" (Olin et al., 2002) have been developed to assist clinicians in making the diagnosis and to promote research on the mechanisms and treatment of these disorders. The criteria require (1) establishing the diagnosis of dementia of the Alzheimer's type and (2) identifying clinically significant depressive symptoms. Clinical assessment should focus on the temporal associations between the onset and course of the depression and the dementia to establish that the depression is not better accounted for by an idiopathic depression, other mental disorders, other medical conditions, or adverse effects of medication.

The criteria require that three (or more) depressive symptoms have been present during the same 2-week period and represent a change from previous functioning; at least one of the symptoms must be either depressed mood or decreased positive affect or pleasure. Depressive symptoms, part of the criteria, are as follows:

1. Clinically significant depressed mood (e.g., depressed, sad, hopeless, discouraged, tearful)
2. Decreased positive affect or pleasure in response to social contacts and usual activities
3. Social isolation or withdrawal
4. Disruption in appetite
5. Disruption in sleep
6. Psychomotor changes (e.g., agitation or retardation)
7. Irritability
8. Fatigue or loss of energy
9. Feelings of worthlessness, hopelessness, or excessive or inappropriate guilt
10. Recurrent thoughts of death or suicidal ideation, plan, or attempt

Symptoms that, in the clinician's judgment, are clearly because of a medical condition other than Alzheimer's disease or are a direct result of non-mood-related dementia symptoms (e.g., loss of weight because of difficulties with food intake) should not be used in making the diagnosis of depression of Alzheimer's disease.

CAREGIVERS' DEPRESSION   Individuals caring for disabled family members often develop depressive symptoms or syndromes (Gallant & Connell, 1997). Depressive symptoms are twice as common among caregivers than noncaregivers (Baumgarten et al., 1992). Depression is most likely to occur during long-term caregiving (Collins et al., 1994). Behavioral problems by the care recipient and limited help from family and friends contribute significantly to caregiver burden and predispose to symptoms of depression (Clyburn et al., 2000). About 25% of caregivers develop significant symptoms of depression following nursing home placement of the care recipient. Male caregivers underreport depression compared to female caregivers. Similarly, African American caregivers report less depression and role strain than their white counterparts, although there was no interaction between race and caregiver distress (Farran et al., 1997).

Once identified, depression remains relatively unchanged over time in female caregivers, but worsens in male caregivers (Schulz & Williamson, 1991).

COMORBIDITY AND COMPLICATIONS
OF LATE-LIFE DEPRESSION

Medical Burden

The relationship of geriatric depression to medical illnesses is complex. There is evidence that depression often occurs in elders with significant medical burden and itself promotes medical morbidity, worsens the outcome of medical illnesses, and increases mortality (Alexopoulos, Buckwalter, et al., 2002).

Geriatric depression as a rule occurs in the context of multiple medical illnesses. A study showed that patients with any medical diagnosis were twice as likely to have depression than patients without a medical diagnosis (Luber et al., 2000). The total mean number of medical diagnoses in depressed patients was 7.9, compared to 3.0 medical diagnoses in nondepressed patients. These differences persisted when the elderly group was examined separately.

There is evidence that depression increases mortality (National Center for Health Statistics, 1991). Depressed hospitalized patients have increased mortality even when the severity of medical illnesses and disability is controlled (Covinsky et al., 1998). Depression has been associated with increased mortality in institutionalized elders (Parmelee et al., 1992; Samuels et al., 1996). It has been reported that presence of major depression on admission to a nursing home increases the likelihood of death by 59% a year later (Rovner, 1993). The effect of depression on mortality was independent of other medical health parameters.

Depression may increase medical morbidity. Depressive symptoms, especially chronic symptoms, are associated with more medical morbidity than other psychiatric disorders of late life (Lacro & Jeste, 1994). In older community residents, long-term, but not short-term, depressive symptoms had an adverse impact on health. In contrast, medical burden contributed only to short-lived depressive symptoms (Meeks et al., 2000). In elderly medical inpatients, those with six depressive symptoms had greater comorbid illness, cognitive impairment, and functional impairment (Covinsky et al., 1999). Depression may adversely affect the prognosis of comorbid disease, as suggested by evidence of prolonged recovery from illness, long hospital stays, increased medical complications, and earlier mortality in depressed patients (Cooper et al., 1994). Increased mortality risk has been reported in depressed compared to nondepressed medical and psychiatric patients (Jorm, Henderson, et al., 1991; Murphy et al., 1988; Shamash et al., 1992).

Depression worsens the outcomes of medical disorders. Depression after surgery has been associated with poorer recovery in both functional and psychosocial status (Mossey et al., 1989). Among patients hospitalized after hip fractures, those with chronic or acute cognitive and depressive symptoms had poorer functional recovery 1 year after discharge than those who did not. Similarly, patients who had more contact with family and friends after leaving the hospital had better recovery than those who had less contact (Magaziner et al., 1990). Depressed medical patients stay in bed more days compared to patients with chronic diseases, such as chronic lung disease, diabetes, arthritis, and hypertension (Wells et al., 1989).

Depression increases the perception of poor health (Wells et al., 1989) and utilization of medical services. In primary care clinic populations, 75% of distressed overutilizers were found to have clinically significant depressive symptomatology. Depressed primary care patients had almost twice the number of appointments per year compared to nondepressed patients (5.3 vs. 2.9) (Luber et al., 2001). Depressed patients had more than twice the number of hospital days over the expected length of stay compared to nondepressed patients. Finally, 65% of depressed patients received more than five medications compared to 35.6% of nondepressed patients.

Depression increases the economic burden on the health care system. Data from a large health maintenance organization population suggest that the health care cost of depressed medical patients is twice that of nondepressed patients with similar levels of medical morbidity (Simon et al., 1995).

Dementing Disorders

Depressive symptoms of various intensity occur in approximately 50% of demented patients. The point prevalence of major depression or clinically significant depressive symptomatology is approximately 17% in patients with Alzheimer's disease (Wragg & Jeste, 1989). There is some evidence that family history of mood disorder predisposes patients with Alzheimer's disease to develop depression. Subcortical dementias (e.g., vascular dementia, Parkinson's disease, and Huntington's disease) are more likely to be complicated by depression than cortical dementias (e.g., Alzheimer's disease) (Sobin & Sacheim, 1997).

Depression is often a prodrome to dementing disorders. Individuals with late-life depression and dementia that subsides after remission of depression (pseudodementia) frequently develop dementia within a few years after the onset of depression (Alexopoulos, Meyers, et al., 1993; Kral & Emery, 1989; Reding et al., 1985). History of depression is associated with increased incidence of Alzheimer's disease (Jorm, van Duijn, et al., 1991; Kokmen et al., 1991; Speck et al., 1995). Depressive symptoms were associated with poorer cognitive function at baseline and with cognitive decline during follow-up (Bassuk et al., 1998; Devanand et al., 1996; Yaffe et al., 1999).

Depressive symptoms are common in elderly individuals who later develop dementia. Among elderly individuals with subclinical cognitive dysfunction, those who developed dementia 3 years later had more depressive symptoms (Ritchie et al., 1999). As subjects were progressing to dementia, they exhibited fewer affective symptoms and more agitation and psychomotor slowing. These changes paralleled reduction of cerebral blood flow in the left temporal region.

Depression earlier in life may be a risk factor for the later development of dementing disorders. Lifetime history of depression may increase the risk of Alzheimer's disease regardless of presence or absence of family history of dementing disorders (van Duijn et al., 1994). In elderly twins, depression was one risk factor for development of dementia regardless of the presence or absence of an apolipoprotein E4 (*APOE4*) allele (Steffens et al., 1997). Depressive symptoms and diagnoses were associated with cognitive decline and high risk for Alzheimer's disease (Geerlings et al., 2000). Depressive symptoms occurring more than 10 years from the onset of dementia were found to be a risk factor for Alzheimer's disease (Speck et al., 1995). In a meta-analytic study, history of depression was associated with onset of Alzheimer's disease after the age of 70 years only when depressive symptoms had appeared within 10 years before the onset of dementia (Jorm, van Duijn, et al., 1991). However, depression with onset more than 10 years before the diagnosis of dementia was associated with onset of Alzheimer's disease at any age, suggesting that previous depression can sometimes represent a risk factor in some patients and a prodromal expression of dementing illness in others.

Depression may contribute to development of dementia in patients with Alzheimer's disease. Lifetime duration of depression correlated with hippocampal volume reduction, although some disagreement exists (Davidson et al., 2002; Sheline et al., 1999). Excessive secretion of glucocorticoids and other stress-related hormones have been implicated. These hormones may reduce neurotrophic factors, inhibit neurogenesis, and promote amyloid neurotoxicity, thus accelerating the pathological cascade of Alzheimer's disease. Biological changes of depression may promote dementia; degenerative changes in brain stem aminergic nuclei that occur during Alzheimer's disease may lead to depression (Zubenko et al., 1990).

Finally, once depression develops as part of the brain changes of Alzheimer's disease, it may further accelerate the progression of Alzheimer's neuropathological changes. Several antidepressants elevate brain-derived neurotrophic factor (BDNF) in the rat hippocampus, an action perhaps mediated by the $5-HT_{2A}$ and the β-adrenoreceptor subtypes. Through this action, antidepressants may prevent stress-induced inhibition of neurogenesis and increase dendritic branching (Duman et al., 1997). It unclear, however, whether antidepressants delay the onset and slow the progress of Alzheimer's disease in depressed patients.

Disability

Disability consists of problems with self-care, household activities, getting around, understanding and communicating, getting along with others, and participating in society. Disability compromises quality of life and has various negative outcomes, such as high rate of hospital admissions (Harris et al., 1989), nursing home placement (Freedman et al., 1994), mortality (Gurialnik et al., 1991), and even morbidity for specific medical conditions (Pahor et al., 1994). Disability has a reciprocal relationship with psychiatric and medical disorders, and it constitutes a distinct functional dimension of health status.

Depression is the second leading cause of disability in the United States (Murray & Lopez, 1997). Depression may lead to disability in medically healthy elderly individuals directly (Bruce et al., 1994) and by contributing to and increasing the impact of medical burden. Moreover, disability resulting from medical or neurological illnesses has been found to be a risk factor for depressive disorders in late life. Therefore, depression and disability interact in a variety of ways with potentially detrimental consequences.

The course of disability parallels the course of depression. In community-residing individuals, residual depressive symptoms covary with disability over time (Ormel et al., 1993; von Korff et al., 1992). Reduction in the levels of depression was shown to result in approximately 50% reduction in days burdened by disability 1 year later (von Korff et al., 1992). In patients with chronic obstructive pulmonary disease, nortriptyline was superior to placebo in improving both depression and day-to-day function, although it did not influence the physiological measures of pulmonary insufficiency (Borson et al., 1992).

In elderly populations, disability often has been classified as impairment in self-maintenance functions (ability to eat, dress, groom, bathe, use the toilet, and ambulate) and impairment in IADLs, including ability to go to places out of walking distance, shop for groceries, prepare meals, do housework, launder clothes, use the telephone, take medications, and manage money. Clinical findings (i.e., severity of depression, cognitive impairment, medical burden) ascertained during a comprehensive clinical examination of depressed elderly patients appear to predict approximately 40% of the variance in IADLs (Alexopoulos, Vrontou, et al., 1996).

Self-maintenance is predicted by different demographic and clinical factors than IADLs in depressed elderly patients. Among older depressed adults, impairment in self-maintenance competence, for instance, was associated with increasing age, more severe chronic medical illness, psychomotor retardation, and lower subjective social support; depressed mood had a lower impact (Alexopoulos, Vrontou, et al., 1996; Steffens et al., 1999).

Unlike self-maintenance skills, IADLs are significantly influenced by depressive symptoms and signs (Alexopoulos, Vrontou, et al., 1996; Steffens et al., 1999). Specific depressive symptoms can uniquely contribute to IADL impairment. In depressed elderly psychiatric patients, IADL impairment was associated with high severity of depression and more specifically with anxiety, depressive ideation, apathy, psychomotor retardation, and weight loss, but less pathological guilt (Alexopoulos, Vrontou, et al., 1996; Steffens et al., 1999). Similar findings have been reported for community-residing elderly individuals, for whom IADL impairment was associated with dysphoria, sleep disturbance, appetite disturbance, feelings of guilt, death wishes and suicidal thoughts, loss of interest, concentration difficulties, psychomotor change, and loss of energy (Forsell et al., 1994).

Executive dysfunction (initiation-perseveration) seems to have a stronger relationship to IADL impairment than other cognitive impairments in depressed elderly patients (Alexopoulos, Vrontou, et al., 1996; Kiosses et al., 2000, 2001). A similar association between executive dysfunction and disability was reported in nondepressed patients with Alzheimer's disease of mild to moderate severity (Chen et al., 1998). Because both geriatric depression and executive dysfunction often occur in patients with frontostriatal impairment, these observations raise the question whether disability is an early indicator of impairment of the frontal and prefrontal areas.

Suicide

Suicide is more frequent in elderly individuals than any other population. In 1989, the suicide rate in the United States was 12.2/100,000 population (McIntosh et al., 1994; National Center for Health Statistics, 1992). Americans older than 65 years of age had a suicide rate of 20.1/100,000, almost twice that of the general population.

Suicide rates consistently increase in males and reach their highest level in the oldest age group. In contrast, female suicide rates increase slightly with age, peak in middle adulthood, and decline in late life. In 1989, the suicide rate for men older than 65 years was 40.7/100,000, and the suicide rate for women of similar age was 5.9/100,000. White men older than 65 years had the highest suicide rate (43.5/100,000), followed by non-white men (15.7/100,000), white women (6.3/100,000), and non-white women (2.8/100,000) (McIntosh et al., 1994; National Center for Health Statistics, 1992).

Although suicide is more frequent in elderly patients than in younger patients, the rate of suicide for elderly individuals steadily decreased from the 1930s to 1980. However, the suicide rate began to rise again in the 1980s (Allen & Blazer, 1991).

Demographic differences between persons who contemplate or attempt suicide and those who commit suicide suggest that these populations are dissimilar. About 60% of suicide victims are men, but 75% of those who attempt suicide are women. Suicide victims as a rule use guns or hang themselves, whereas 70% of suicide attempters take a drug overdose, and 22% cut or slash themselves.

Depression increases the risk for suicide in all age groups (Conwell, 1994). High severity of depression appears to be a predictor of suicidal behavior (Simon & von Korff, 1998). The suicide rate in individuals treated for depression within a health plan was 59 per 100,000 person-years of follow-up. Suicide risk per 100,000 person-years declined from 224 among patients who required psychiatric hospitalization for depression, to 64 among those who received outpatient psychiatric care, to 43 among those treated with anti-depressants in primary care, to 0 among those treated without antidepressants in primary care (Simon & von Korff, 1998).

Depression is the most common psychiatric diagnosis in elderly suicide victims, unlike younger adults, for whom substance abuse alone or with comor-bid mood disorders is the most frequent diagnosis (Conwell & Brent, 1995; Dennis & Lindesay, 1995; Henriksson et al., 1995). Major depression was identified in 80% of suicide victims older than 74 years of age, and its fre-quency ranged from 3.1% to 29.4% in younger victims (Conwell et al., 1996). These findings indicate that depression is the psychiatric disorder most likely to increase suicide risk in the elderly.

Despite the high frequency of suicide in late life, suicidal attempts and suicidal ideation decrease with aging (Moscicki, 1989; Wallace & Pfohl, 1995). Older adults commit more carefully planned and lethal self-destructive acts and give fewer indications of suicidal intent (Carney et al., 1994; Conwell et al., 1998). Therefore, although suicide attempts are more rare in old than young age, their lethality is increased.

Suicidal ideation is a risk factor for suicide in both young and elderly pa-tients. In younger psychiatric outpatients, suicidal ideation appears to predict completed suicide with 53% sensitivity, 83% specificity, and 4.2% predictive value (Beck et al., 1999). The sensitivity (80%) and predictive value (5.6%) of suicidal ideation is even higher in geriatric psychiatric outpatients.

The clinical profile of depressed elderly suicide victims suggests that, with treatment, their prognosis would be favorable. Most elderly suicide victims have a mild to moderately severe depression, no previous depressive episodes, and no comorbid substance abuse or personality disorders (Conwell, 1994; Conwell et al., 1996). These characteristics predict good response to treatment.

One third of elderly persons report loneliness as the principal reason for considering suicide. Approximately 10% of elderly individuals with suicidal ideation report financial problems, poor medical health, or depression as rea-sons for suicidal thoughts. Suicide victims are demographically different from individuals who attempt suicide. Psychological autopsy studies suggest that most elderly persons who commit suicide have had a psychiatric disorder, most com-monly depression. However, often psychiatric disorders of suicide victims do not receive medical or psychiatric attention.

More elderly suicide victims are widowed, and fewer are single, separated, or divorced than younger adults. Violent methods of suicide are more common in the elderly, but alcohol use and psychiatric histories appear to be less fre-quent. Most elderly persons who commit suicide communicate their suicidal thoughts to family or friends prior to the act of suicide.

The majority of elderly suicide victims see their physicians within a few months of their death and over a third within the week of their suicide (Diek-stra & van Egmond, 1989; Frierson, 1991). Therefore, reliable assessment of suicide risk is critical because protective measures may avert suicide.

Several clinical characteristics can be used to assess the risk for suicidal ideation in depressed elderly patients (Alexopoulos, Bruce, Hull, et al., 1999). During episodes of depression, suicidal ideation was associated with severity of depression, poor social support, and history of serious suicide attempts. Patients with severe depression and IADL impairment were more likely to have history of suicide attempts. Poor social support and history of serious suicide attempts were associated with suicidal ideation even in the context of mild depression.

Some clinical characteristics have been shown to predict the course of suicidal ideation (Alexopoulos, Bruce, Hull, et al., 1999). At the initial evaluation, suicidal ideation and history of serious suicide attempts were strong predictors of the evolution of suicidal ideation over time. During follow-up examinations, severity of depression, medical burden, disability, and social support predicted the longitudinal course of suicidal ideation. However, severity of concurrent depression was the main determinant of fluctuations in suicidal ideation over time. The relationship of geriatric depression to suicidal ideation suggests that identification and appropriate treatment of depression can improve suicidal ideation and ultimately lower the risk of suicide.

Older patients with major medical illnesses or a recent loss should be evaluated for depressive symptomatology and suicidal ideation and plans. Thoughts and fantasies about the meaning of suicide and life after death may reveal information that the patient is unable to share directly. There should be no reluctance to question patients about suicide because such questions do not increase the likelihood of suicidal behavior.

Bipolar Disorder

Mania or hypomania constitutes 5% to 10% of the diagnoses of elderly patients (Young & Klerman, 1992). However, limited information is available concerning the prevalence of bipolar disorders in the elderly community. Most patients with manic syndromes have bipolar mood disorder. Some cases of mania may be etiologically related to medical diseases and drugs (Krauthammer & Klerman, 1978). Manic symptoms and signs may be part of schizoaffective disorder, a condition related to bipolar disorder. Schizoaffective disorder is infrequently diagnosed in geriatric patients.

Klerman (1987) subcategorized bipolar disorder based on course and family history. Type I consists of patients who are hospitalized at least once for a manic episode and have a history of major depressive episodes. Type II includes patients with mild manic (hypomania) and depressive episodes. Type III patients have cyclothymic mood fluctuations without major depression or mania. Type IV patients have manic states resulting from medical illness or drugs; mania emerging during antidepressant treatment is not considered organic mood disorder. Type V patients have histories of major depression only with a family history of bipolar disorder.

Mania that first occurs in late life is a heterogeneous condition (Young & Klerman, 1992). A substantial subgroup of patients with late-onset mania consists of patients with unipolar major depression who changed polarity in late life. Some of these patients have had a family history of bipolar disorder and were classified as type V before they changed polarity. Bipolar disorders associated with medical illnesses or drugs (type IV) may be particularly prevalent among late-onset cases. The incidence of late-onset mania is unknown.

Studies of first hospital admissions suggest that the risk for mania declines with aging (Shulman & Post, 1980). However, there is some evidence that first admissions for mania increase after 60 years of age, especially in men (Eagles & Whalley, 1985). Patients with late-onset bipolar disorder have a lower rate of affective disorders among relatives compared with patients with early-onset mania (Rice & Reich, 1987). It has been suggested that mania associated with medical disorders or drug treatment as a rule has onset after 40 years of age (Krauthammer & Klerman, 1978). Mania with onset during senescence is associated with coarse brain disease. Cerebrovascular disease, especially right-sided lesions, has been implicated in late-onset mania (Starkstein et al., 1988).

The course and outcome of manic states in geriatric patients are unclear. As manic states in this age group probably represent various disorders with multiple biological determinants, no single characterization of mania can be considered prototypic (Young & Klerman, 1992). Disorientation, delirium, and reversible cognitive dysfunction have been described in patients with mania. It is unclear whether reversible cognitive dysfunction in mania leads to persistent cognitive dysfunction and dementia at follow-up as it does in depression. Older age appears to be associated with chronic mania, and there is a suggestion of an association between later age at onset and longer episode, as well as shorter intervals between episodes. However, further studies are needed to establish these relationships. There is no clear difference in relapse rate between patients with early-onset and those with late-onset geriatric mania, but prospective studies are needed (Young & Klerman, 1992). The mortality rate for elderly patients with bipolar disorder seems to be greater than the community base rate for this age group (Dhingra & Rabins, 1991) and appears to exceed that of geriatric patients with depression (Shulman et al., 1992). It remains to be determined whether patients with late-onset mania are at greater risk for the development of dementia than elderly patients with early onset.

BIOLOGICAL DYSFUNCTION

Studies using diverse methodology suggest that frontostriatal and limbic dysfunction contribute to the pathogenesis of at least some late-life depressive syndromes (Alexopoulos, 2002). The frontal lobe is connected to the basal ganglia through five contiguous, nonoverlapping parallel zones (cortico-striato-pallido-cortical pathways). Three cortico-striato-pallido-cortical pathways may be relevant to depression because damage to these pathways leads to behavioral abnormalities that resemble in part the depressive syndrome. Damage of the orbitofrontal circuit may lead to disinhibition, irritability, and diminished sensitivity to social cues. Damage of the anterior cingulate may result in apathy and reduced initiative. Damage of the dorsolateral circuit may result in difficulties in set shifting, learning, and word list generation.

Clinical studies have demonstrated that patients with disorders of subcortical structures often develop depression (Sobin & Sacheim, 1997). Moreover, the executive abnormalities of depressed elderly patients are similar to those of patients with basal ganglia disorders (Masserman & Cummings, 1997).

Structural neuroimaging studies of depressed elderly patients have revealed abnormalities consistent with frontostriatal impairment. Volume reduction in the subgenual anterior cingulate has been reported in familial major depression (Drevets et al., 1997). Bilateral white matter hyperintensities (WMHs) are prevalent in geriatric depression (Krishnan et al., 1997; Kumar et al., 2000) and mainly occur in subcortical structures and their frontal projections (Boone et al., 1992; Lesser et al., 1996). Lesions localized in the basal ganglia and their frontal projections (Chemerinski & Robinson, 2000) are associated with high incidence of depression.

Neuropathological studies identified abnormalities in frontal structures. Reduction in glia of the subgenual prelimbic anterior cingulate gyrus has been demonstrated in unipolar depressed patients (Lai et al., 2000; Rajkowska et al., 1999). Abnormalities in neurons of the dorsolateral prefrontal cortex have also been documented in unipolar disorder (Ongur et al., 1998; Rajkowska et al., 1999).

Functional neuroimaging studies suggest that depression is associated with abnormal metabolism (mostly increased) in limbic regions, including the amygdala, the pregenual and subgenual anterior cingulate, and the posterior orbital cortex, as well as the posterior cingulate and the medial cerebellum (Drevets, 2000). In contrast, the lateral and dorsolateral prefrontal cortex, the dorsal anterior cingulate (located posterior to the pregenual cingulate), and the caudate have reduced blood flow during depression (Drevets et al., 1992). Bilateral activation of the dorsal anterior cingulate and the hippocampus has been reported in severely depressed, nondemented elderly patients performing a word activation task (de Asis et al., 2001). Similarly, younger patients with mood disorders, when challenged with the Stroop response interference task, demonstrated blunted activation of the left anterior cingulate and minimal activation of the right anterior cingulate gyrus compared to normal controls (Rogers et al., 1998). Instead, patients with mood disorders showed increased activity in the left dorsolateral prefrontal and visual cortex. Taken together, these findings underscore the importance of subcortical neural systems in mediating development of depression.

Clinical and electrophysiological indices of frontostriatal dysfunction appear to influence the course of geriatric depression. Executive impairment, the neuropsychological expression of striatofrontal dysfunction, was reported to predict poor or delayed antidepressant response of geriatric major depression, and memory impairment did not influence the response to antidepressants (Kalayam & Alexopoulos, 1999). Poor or slow antidepressant response was associated with psychomotor retardation, a behavioral disturbance that may result from frontostriatal dysfunction. In addition to chronicity, executive dysfunction has been associated with relapse and recurrence of geriatric major depression and with residual depressive symptomatology (Alexopoulos et al., 2000). In these samples, memory impairment, disability, medical burden, social support, or number of previous episodes were not shown to influence the course of geriatric depression in this study. Therefore, the relationship of executive dysfunction to chronicity, relapse, and recurrence of geriatric depression appears to be specific to this disturbance. A preliminary study showed that microstructural abnormalities (revealed by diffusion tensor imaging) in white matter lateral to the anterior cingulate were correlated with executive dysfunction as well as poor or slow response to citalopram (Alexopoulos, Borson, et al., 2002). However, replication of these findings is needed.

The relationship between frontostriatal dysfunction and poor outcomes of depression is supported by structural and functional neuroimaging studies. White matter hyperintensities were found to predict chronicity of geriatric depression (Hickie et al., 1995). In the elderly, white matter abnormalities were associated with executive dysfunction (Boone et al., 1992), perhaps related to disruption of striatofrontal pathways. Functional neuroimaging studies have shown that remission of depression is associated with metabolic increases in dorsal cortical regions (dorsal anterior cingulate, posterior cingulate, dorsolateral, and inferior parietal) (Drevets, 2000). In contrast, decreases in ventral limbic and paralimbic structures (subgenual cingulate, ventral mid- and posterior insula, hippocampus, and hypothalamus) occur during remission (Mayberg, 2001).

Persistence of elevated amygdala metabolism during remission of depression was associated with high risk for relapse of depression (Drevets, 1999). Hypometabolism of the rostral anterior cingulate is associated with treatment-resistant depression in younger adults, and cingulate hypermetabolism is a predictor of favorable response (Mayberg, 2001). It has been proposed that disruption in the reciprocal relationship between dorsal cortical and ventral limbic regions contributes to depressive symptoms (Mayberg, 2001).

Microstructural abnormalities in white matter lateral to the anterior cingulate (medial frontal lobe) were found to predict poor or slow antidepressant response to citalopram. This effect was specific to this site because microstructural white matter abnormalities in other frontal areas or in a temporal area were not related to antidepressant response. White matter disruption in this area may lead to a "disconnection syndrome" that interferes with the reciprocal regulation between ventral limbic and dorsal neocortical structures and inhibits response to antidepressant treatment.

The causes of brain abnormalities in geriatric depression are multifactorial. It has been proposed that hypercortisolemia that occurs during depressive episodes leads to atrophy of the hippocampus (Sheline et al., 1996, 1999). APOE has been associated with late-life depression (Riley et al., 2000) and with hippocampal volume loss (Steffens et al., 2000). Among nondemented elderly individuals, the rate of volumetric loss was significantly greater among those with an *APOE4* allele compared to individuals without *APOE4* alleles (Moffat et al., 2000).

Depression is common in individuals with vascular diseases or vascular risk factors. Moreover, late-life depression is a frequent complication of stroke. Lacunar infarcts in the basal ganglia have the highest comorbidity with depression. Left hemisphere lesions, especially those close to the frontal pole, have been associated with poststroke depression, although this association was questioned by a meta-analysis (Carson et al., 2000). Subcortical atrophy appears to be a predisposing factor. These observations suggest that both degenerative and vascular processes contribute to the brain abnormalities identified in late-life depression.

DIAGNOSIS

Depression is underrecognized in elderly populations (*Mental Health*, 1999). Factors contributing to underrecognition of geriatric depression include underreporting of symptoms, uncertainty in defining clinically significant depression, and attributing symptoms to medical illness, disability, and dementing disorders (Alexopoulos, Borson, et al., 2002). The most important symptoms in diagnosing depression in an older patient include sad, downcast mood; frequent tearfulness; and recurrent thoughts of death and suicide (Alexopoulos, Kiosses, Klimstra, et al., 2002). Other symptoms include diminished interest in pleasurable activities; feelings of hopelessness, helplessness, or worthlessness or guilt; avoidance of social interactions or going out; psychomotor agitation or retardation; difficulty making decisions; and difficulty in planning daily activities.

Underreporting of Symptoms

The diagnosis of late-life depression is often complicated by underreporting of depressive symptoms (Gallo & Rabins, 1999). The current cohort of elderly patients is most likely to report physical symptoms such as lack of sleep, energy, appetite, and weight loss rather than sadness, feelings of guilt, suicidal ideation, hopelessness, and worthlessness. Depressed elderly patients often have anhedonia rather than sadness. Because these symptoms may originate from medical disorders, depression may be overlooked.

Depressive Syndromes Not Meeting Diagnostic Criteria

The majority of depressed elderly patients treated in primary care do not meet diagnostic criteria for depressive disorders. Katon and Schulberg (1992) estimated that 6% to 8% of primary care patients met criteria for major depression, and Oxman and coworkers (1990) observed that major depression occurs in 9% of elderly primary care patients. A larger subgroup had clinically significant depressive symptomatology. In medical populations, 25% of minor depressions evolve into major depression within a 2-year period (Katon & Schulberg, 1992). Minor depression has often been the diagnosis of elderly suicide victims (Conwell, 1994). These observations underscore the need for close follow-up and for use of antidepressants, psychotherapy, or both if depressive symptoms persist or worsen.

Medical Illness and Disability

Medical burden and disability accompanying late-life depression may overshadow the diagnosis of depression. In some cases, medical conditions predispose to or trigger depression (e.g., depression that first occurs after the onset of hypothyroidism or stroke). In other cases, the connection between the medical condition and the depression is less clear. Finally, medical conditions may mask the presence of depression. Older patients are likely to take a large number of medications, some of which (e.g., steroids, reserpine, methyldopa, antiparkinsonian medications, and β-blockers) can cause or exacerbate depressive symptoms. Patients with the depression–executive dysfunction syndrome have pronounced disability, loss of interest in activities, psychomotor retardation, and suspiciousness, but rather mild middle insomnia and diurnal mood variation (Alexopoulos, Kiosses, Klimstra, et al., 2002), a presentation that may obscure the identification of the depressive syndrome. In some patients with medical disorders or pronounced disability, the diagnosis of depression can only be made after successful antidepressant treatment. Even when an underlying medical condition is contributing to the depression, treatment of that condition alone is often not sufficient to resolve the depression. As a rule, both depression and the potentially contributing medical condition should be treated for optimal results.

Dementing Disorders

The similarity of depressive manifestations to symptoms and signs of dementing disorders often poses diagnostic problems (Alexopoulos, 1995). Patients with early-stage Alzheimer's disease show loss of interest, decreased energy, difficulty in concentration, agitation, or retardation. Apathy, a characteristic of frontal lobe syndrome, may be misidentified as retarded depression. Sad, downcast mood and psychic rather than vegetative features have been useful in distinguishing depressed-demented patients from patients with dementia alone.

It remains unclear whether depression is associated with the degree of cognitive impairment in demented patients. Demented patients may be unable to identify and express dysphoric feelings. For this reason, examination should rely on caregiver reports as well as examination of the patient. Identification of depression in demented patients is important because they may respond to drug therapy or electroconvulsive therapy (ECT).

Even when caregivers of demented patients are interviewed, the diagnosis of depression cannot be safely made. Reports of the rate of major depression in Alzheimer's patients have been highly discrepant, ranging from 0% to 87%, with most studies showing a range of 17% to 31% (Alexopoulos & Abrams, 1991). Patients with Alzheimer's disease report fewer depressive symptoms than collateral sources. This discrepancy is most influenced by lack of insight and medical burden in Alzheimer's patients and caregiver burden in collateral informants (Burke et al., 1998). Discrepancies in reporting symptoms of depression contribute to reduced or incorrect identification of depression in demented patients.

Scales that use only signs of depression have been developed (Katona & Aldridge, 1985), but they rate only part of the depressive syndrome. Scales that use information from patients and informants (Alexopoulos et al., 1988) offer a more comprehensive picture, but they are not free of bias inherent in patient and informant reports. In elderly community residents, structured instruments identified lower percentages of dementia (16.1%–28%) than clinicians who used *ICD-10* (*International Classification of Diseases, 10th Revision*) or *DSM-III-R* (APA, 1990) criteria and documented difficulties inherent in the current assessment methodology (Fichter et al., 1995). In a demented patient with an incomplete, yet persistent, depression syndrome, it is best to offer a trial of an antidepressant (for 6–8 weeks) rather than assume that the depressive symptoms are part of the dementia syndrome.

RECOGNITION AND TREATMENT
IN PRIMARY CARE SETTINGS

Unlike younger adults, most elderly patients receive treatment for depression in primary care settings (Schulberg et al., 1993) and resist referral to mental health professionals (Brody et al., 1997). Nonetheless, depression is underdiagnosed in medical settings (Alexopoulos, 2001b). General internists identified depression in approximately 6% of elderly patients (Luber et al., 2001). This percentage is two to three times lower that that expected from systematic studies (Alexopoulos, 1996a).

Multiple factors contribute to the underrecognition of geriatric depression in the primary care setting. These include the primary care physician's lack of confidence in diagnosing depression (Unutzer, Katon, Russo, et al., 1999; Unutzer, Katon, Sullivan, et al., 1999) and the tendency for depressed older persons to focus on somatic complaints (Gallo et al., 1999). Cultural stereotypes among physicians may lead to depression diagnoses less often in elderly African American patients (Cooper-Patrick et al., 1999). Depression is likely to receive less attention by primary care physicians when the patient has several medical problems (Nutting et al., 2000). Finally, limited training in interviewing techniques may make physicians less likely to offer the diagnosis of depression, especially in patients who are expected not to accept the diagnosis of depression and the recommended treatment.

The clinical profile of depressed patients seen in medical settings suggests that they can respond promptly to antidepressant treatment. Depressed patients in ambulatory medical settings have less-severe depression, briefer episodes, and more somatic symptoms than depressed patients seen in mental health settings (Borson et al., 1992; Koenig et al., 1992; Wells et al., 1992). A study found less psychiatric comorbidity, fewer patients with delusions, and a smaller number of past psychiatric hospitalizations in medical patients compared to mental health patients. Depressed medical patients were less likely to have chronic depression (23% vs. 34%) than mental health patients (Cooper et al., 1994).

Despite the fact that depressed elderly patients are likely to respond favorably to antidepressant treatment, depression remains undertreated in primary care settings. Approximately 11% of depressed high utilizers of primary care services received adequate antidepressant treatment, 34% received inadequate treatment, and 55% received no treatment (Katon & Schulberg, 1992). In a study of all patients seen over 1 year by a large university group primary care practice, approximately 41% of depressed patients received any antidepressant treatment regardless of age and medical comorbidity (Luber et al., 2000, 2001). Primary care physicians who were informed of depression diagnoses failed to provide any treatment to 27% of depressed patients (Schulberg et al., 1997). When physicians did prescribe antidepressants, the prescriptions were of insufficient dosage and duration.

Several models have been developed to improve the treatment of depression in the primary care setting. An example of such models is that developed by the PROSPECT (Prevention of Suicide in Primary Care Elderly: Collaborative Trial) study, which includes the placement of a depression care manager (health specialist) in primary care practices (Bruce & Pearson, 1999). The depression care manager assists the physician by providing timely and targeted patient-specific clinical strategies and encourages patient adherence to treatment through education and support.

The treatment algorithm used in PROSPECT was based on the Agency for Health Care Policy and Research (AHCPR) Practice Guidelines for the Treatment of Depression in Primary Care and was modified for treatment of the elderly at the primary care office. Guidelines used psychopharmacological (citalopram), psychosocial (interpersonal psychotherapy), and other interventions based on individual needs. Psychiatric consultation is offered only in complex cases. The guidelines provide for acute, continuation, and maintenance treatment over a 2-year period.

Preliminary analyses suggest large effects in reducing levels of depressive symptoms and suicidal ideation in practices implementing the PROSPECT intervention as compared practices offering usual care. Of note also are racial differences in remission rates: two thirds of elderly white patients treated in the intervention practices achieved remission of depression versus less than half of elderly African American patients. Differences in remission between African American and white elderly are complex and may include factors such as trust, stigma, failures in communication, adherence, and attrition from treatment.

TREATMENT

The main goals of treatment for geriatric depression include (1) remission of depression and (2) reduction in the risk of relapse and recurrence. Because depression often contributes to disability (Alexopoulos, Vrontou, et al., 1996) and excess medical morbidity, clinicians should expect an improvement in both these areas. Appropriate behavioral rehabilitation techniques should be combined with antidepressant treatment to enable elderly patients to regain function as the depressive syndrome subsides.

Drugs, medical illnesses, and dementing disorders may lead to depression. Steroids, reserpine, methyldopa, antiparkinsonian drugs, and β-blockers can cause depression. Viral infections; endocrinopathies such as thyroid, parathyroid, pituitary, and adrenal diseases; and malignancies such as lymphoma and pancreatic cancer often are complicated by depression. Although it is essential to diagnose and treat the underlying disease, depression may not remit until an antidepressant agent is used. For example, depression in an elderly patient with hypothyroidism rarely responds to thyroid supplementation alone. Similarly, an antidepressant trial often is ineffective before hypothyroidism is corrected. However, thyroid supplementation and an antidepressant drug offer the highest probability of antidepressant response. An overview of treatments for late-life mood disorders is described below. Each of these therapeutic approaches is reviewed thoroughly in chapters specifically devoted to them.

Pharmacotherapy

Antidepressants, regardless of class, lead to response (defined as at least 50% improvement of depressive symptoms) in approximately 60% of elderly patients, with a placebo response rate of 30% to 40% (Schneider, 1996). Even among responders, a significant number of elderly patients continue to have significant residual symptomatology.

Older patients can benefit from the same psychopharmacological agents as younger patients. However, the clinician must be aware that aging and medical conditions associated with aging have an impact on pharmacokinetics and increase the sensitivity to side effects even at low plasma concentrations of antidepressants (Schneider, 1996).

Four families of antidepressants are available for the treatment of geriatric depression. These are SSRIs, tricyclic antidepressants (TCAs), monoamine oxidase inhibitors (MAOIs), and atypical antidepressants. It is crucial that antidepressant drugs are given at adequate plasma levels or dosages for a sufficient length of time.

An adequate antidepressant trial in the elderly is longer than that for younger adults (Georgotas & McCue, 1989), although this view has been challenged. A complete response often occurs after 6 to 12 weeks of treatment. However, if there are no signs of improvement by the fourth week of treatment, most clinicians consider the antidepressant trial a failure.

SELECTIVE SEROTONIN REUPTAKE INHIBITORS Several studies have shown that SSRIs are more effective than placebo in depressed elderly outpatients (Schneider, 1996). The dosages of SSRIs should be increased gradually. The starting daily dosages may be fluoxetine 10 mg, paroxetine 10 to 20 mg, sertraline 25 to 50 mg, escitalopram 5 to 10 mg, and citalopram 10 to 20 mg. For most patients, daily dosages of fluoxetine 20 mg, paroxetine 20 to 30 mg, sertraline 75 to 100 mg, and citalopram 20 to 30 mg are sufficient, although higher dosages are required by some. The SSRI fluvoxamine may be effective in the treatment of geriatric depression, although research data are few.

The main advantage of SSRIs is their safety. With the exception of allergy, they have few, if any, dangerous side effects. Even when these drugs are not tolerated, the side effects consist of subjective discomfort rather than risk to the patient. Nausea, restlessness, insomnia, headache, diarrhea, and sexual dysfunction are the most frequent side effects in the elderly. Inappropriate secretion of antidiuretic hormone may lead to hyponatremia, confusion, and falls in the elderly, but these are rare.

SSRIs interact with drugs frequently used in the depressed elderly (De Vane, 1994). Fluoxetine, paroxetine, and to a lesser extent sertraline inhibit the cytochrome P450 2D6 liver cytochrome isoenzyme. This pathway is essential for the hydroxylation of nortriptyline and desipramine and the metabolism of antipsychotics and type 1_A antiarrhythmic drugs (encainide, flecanide), β-blockers, and verapamil, which have plasma levels that may be raised in SSRI-treated patients. Therefore, reduction of dosages and monitoring of plasma levels of tricyclic antidepressants and antipsychotic and antiarrhythmic drugs are required in patients treated with fluoxetine, paroxetine, and perhaps sertraline. Norfluoxetine, the metabolite of fluoxetine, inhibits the P450 3A4 isoenzyme. The 3A4 is responsible for the metabolism of alprazolam, triazolam, carbamazepine, quinidine, erythromycin, terfenazine, and astemizol and may lead to an increase in the plasma level of these agents.

For these reasons, when fluoxetine is prescribed, reduction and monitoring of dosages of drugs metabolized by the 2D6 and the 3A4 isoenzymes is required. Fluvoxamine inhibits the P450 3A4 and the 1A2 cytochrome isoenzyme, but does not significantly inhibit the 2D6 isoenzyme. Drugs metabolized by the 3A4 and the 1A2 should be cautiously prescribed in fluvoxamine-treated patients. Fluvoxamine may produce a threefold decrease in theophylline clearance by inhibiting the 1A2 isoenzyme responsible for its metabolism. Escitalopram and citalopram have a minimal effect on P450 2D6 and almost no effect on other liver isoenzymes.

TRICYCLIC ANTIDEPRESSANTS   The most commonly used tricyclic antidepressants are nortriptyline and desipramine because they have lower potential for sedation and weaker anticholinergic action than other tricyclics. Nortriptyline is the best-studied tricyclic in elderly patients; more than 300 subjects have been studied in 22 clinical trials, and patients older than 80 years of age have been included (Salzman et al., 1994). Nortriptyline rarely produces orthostatic hypotension and may be favored over other tricyclics for this reason.

Antidepressant response to tricyclics depends on their plasma levels and the duration of acute treatment (Alexopoulos & Salzman, 1998). Elderly patients require plasma levels similar to those of younger adults to respond to treatment with tricyclic antidepressants; dosages are 60 to 150 ng/mL for nortriptyline and above 115 ng/mL for desipramine. However, such plasma levels may be achieved with lower dosages in the elderly (nortriptyline 1–1.2 mg/kg and desipramine 1.5–2 mg/kg).

Tricyclics are contraindicated in patients with cardiac conduction defects. Nortriptyline and desipramine have properties similar to those of type 1_A antiarrhythmic drugs (quinidinelike drugs). When administered to patients with right or left bundle branch block, tricyclics may cause second-degree block in approximately 10% of cases (Roose et al., 1987). For this reason, an electrocardiogram (ECG) should always precede the use of tricyclics.

The type 1_A properties of tricyclics necessitate cautious use of these drugs in patients with ischemic heart disease. A multicenter study (Cardiac Arrhythmia Suppression Trial II [CAST-II]) demonstrated that type 1_A antiarrhythmics increase cardiac mortality in patients postmyocardial infarction (Cardiac Arrhythmia Suppression Trial Investigators, 1992). Although tricyclic antidepressants were not used in this study, the type 1_A antiarrhythmic properties of tricyclic antidepressants suggest cautious use in depressed patients with ischemic heart disease.

Tricyclic antidepressants have anticholinergic properties. For this reason, these drugs should be avoided in patients with prostatic hypertrophy or narrow-angle glaucoma. High intellectual functions, orthostatic blood pressure, the ECG, and the ability to urinate should be monitored frequently in depressed elderly patients receiving nortriptyline or desipramine. There is little justification for using the cyclic agents amitriptyline, imipramine, doxepin, maprotilene, and amoxapine as antidepressants in the elderly because they have stronger sedating and anticholinergic properties than secondary amines.

MONOAMINE OXIDASE INHIBITORS   The MAOI phenelzine may be effective in the treatment of major depression of patients in their mid- or late 60s (Schneider, 1996). However, there is limited research experience on MAOIs in old-old depressed patients. When MAOIs are used in the elderly, low dosages should be prescribed (e.g., phenelzine 30–45 mg daily or tranylcypromine 20–30 mg daily). Orthostatic hypotension is the most frequent side effect of MAO inhibitors. This side effect is of concern in the elderly because it may lead to falls and fractures, especially of the hip or the humerus. Other side effects include weight gain, lack of energy, insomnia, and daytime somnolence in phenelzine-treated patients and nervousness, insomnia, and excessive perspiration in tranylcypromine-treated patients. Peripheral neuropathy occurs in a small percentage of patients on MAO inhibitors and often responds to pyridoxine. Sympathomimetic amines, monoamine precursors, tricyclic antidepressants, SSRIs, venlafaxine, concomitant administration of two MAO inhibitors, and tyramine-rich food may cause a hypertensive crisis and should be avoided in patients on MAO inhibitors.

Drug interactions and diet restrictions often prevent the use of MAOIs in the elderly. Moclobemide, a reversible inhibitor of type A MAOs, has a mild interaction with tyramine-rich food because of its short elimination half-life and its reversible inhibition of MAO. For this reason, moclobemide is regarded as safer than the classical MAO inhibitors. Moclobemide appears to have neuroprotective properties through its antioxidant action. Studies are under way to examine the efficacy of moclobemide in patients with cerebrovascular and degenerative brain disorders. However, moclobemide is not available in the United States.

OTHER ANTIDEPRESSANTS Studies of younger adults suggest that bupropion is of comparable efficacy to tricyclics and SSRIs (Sweet et al., 1995), but limited research experience exists in depressed geriatric patients. Bupropion does not appear to influence cognitive function and heart rate heart rhythm. It has been found to be safe in a sample of patients with a variety of heart disorders (Roose et al., 1991).

Bupropion has few drug interactions, but it should not be prescribed in patients receiving MAO inhibitors. Bupropion may exacerbate preexisting hypertension. For this reason, blood pressure monitoring is required. Seizures have been reported in 0.4% of patients treated with bupropion. The risk of seizures can be minimized by use of a slow-release preparation, slow introduction of bupropion (100 mg daily), use of twice-a-day dosages, and restriction of the total daily dosage to 450 mg. Most elderly patients require 150 mg of bupropion two times daily, but higher dosages (e.g., 400 mg daily) may be used.

Venlafaxine, a reuptake inhibitor of serotonin and norepinephrine, was found effective in the treatment of younger adults with major depression resistant to drugs or ECT (Nierenberg et al., 1994; Schweitzer et al., 2001). A significant advantage of venlafaxine is its few drug-drug interactions; no clinically significant interactions have been reported except a life-threatening serotonin syndrome following coadministration with MAOIs. Frequent side effects include nausea, insomnia, sweating, and mild increases in blood pressure that require monitoring. Elderly patients appear to require dosages comparable to those of younger adults. Daily dosages of 75 to 200 mg are adequate for the majority of elderly patients. Nausea, a rather frequent side effect of venlafaxine, can be minimized by a slow increase of the daily dosage. Blood pressure should be monitored, especially in patients receiving dosages above 225 mg daily because venlafaxine can increase blood pressure. Extended-release preparations of venlafaxine should be favored because they can be administered once a day and lead to better compliance.

Mirtazapine, a sedating antidepressant, antagonizes the α_2-presynaptic inhibitory receptor as well as the 5-HT$_2$ and the 5-HT$_3$ serotonin receptors. However, it has no effect on the 5-HT$_{1A}$ or 5-HT$_{1B}$ receptors. Mirtazapine is an antagonist of histaminergic receptors and has a mild antagonist effect on the α_1-adrenergic and muscarinic receptors. These effects account for the sedative, hypotensive, and anticholinergic side effects of mirtazapine.

The elimination half-life of mirtazapine is 20 to 40 hours, and it is longer in women. Compared to younger adults, elderly patients have a 40% longer mirtazapine elimination half-life. Mirtazapine is metabolized in the liver by the cytochrome P450 2D6 and the 3A4 isoenzyme. Mirtazapine and its metabolites undergo phase II metabolism, during which they are glucuronized. Mirtazapine is not an inhibitor of the P450 cytochrome and does not influence the plasma levels of drugs metabolized by this system.

The side effects of mirtazapine include somnolence, dizziness, increased appetite, and weight gain. Agranulocytosis has been reported in approximately 1% of patients. Mild cholesterol and triglyceride increases have been observed in 15% and 6% of patients, respectively. The starting dosage of mirtazapine is 7.5 to 15 mg and should be administered at bedtime to reduce daytime sedation. Daily dosages up to 30 to 45 mg are sufficient for the treatment of geriatric depression.

Nefazodone, an antidepressant that has not been systematically studied in geriatric depression, promotes sleep and has anxiolytic effects. Nefazodone is well tolerated and safe in overdose, does not influence the sleep architecture, and does not cause sexual dysfunction. However, sedation and need for two daily doses may be a problem for some elderly patients. A total daily dosage of 150 to 300 mg is usually sufficient, but higher dosages (up to 500 mg) may be required. Cognitive function examination should be done in patients treated with nefazodone because this drug may lead to dose-related cognitive side effects (Van Laar et al., 1995). As of this writing, nefazodone has been taken off the market because of concerns about hepatotoxicity. Nefazodone inhibits the P450 3A4 isoenzyme of the liver. The 3A4 isoenzyme is responsible for the metabolism of alprazolam and triazolam. These drugs should be cautiously prescribed and preferably avoided in patients receiving nefazodone.

Dextroamphetamine and methylphenidate are relatively ineffective in elderly patients with primary major depression. However, psychostimulants appear to improve apathy and anergy in medical patients or cognitively impaired patients. Dextroamphetamine or methylphenidate at dosages of 5 to 10 mg in the morning and at noon is sufficient. In the elderly, psychostimulants have rapid onset of action, minimal side effects, limited potential for tolerance, and low risk for addiction (Satel & Nelson, 1989).

Electroconvulsive Therapy

ECT is equally effective as an acute treatment of severe depression and mania. ECT should be favored in patients with severe mood syndromes who may be unable to tolerate the long wait imposed by the gradual introduction of anti-depressants or mood stabilizers and the slow onset of drug action. ECT can also be prescribed for patients with cardiac conduction deficits, prostatic hypertrophy, or glaucoma, which increase the risk of treatment with tricyclics. The average number of ECT treatments required for the treatment of major depression is nine. Administration of three ECT treatments weekly appears to produce a more rapid recovery than ECT given once a week. Less-frequent ECT is associated with less cognitive impairment, but no differences were found 1 month after ECT comple-tion between the groups who had ECT three times or twice weekly.

ECT is a safe treatment, with a mortality rate of 0.01%. The majority of deaths (67%) related to ECT are because of cardiac complications, which oc-cur immediately after ECT or within a few hours after treatment (Alexopoulos et al., 1984, 1989). With adequate medical evaluation, monitoring during and after ECT, and appropriate intervention, most cardiovascular events related to ECT have a benign outcome. Geriatric patients sometimes develop prolonged confusion after ECT and may be prone to falls.

Dementing disorders are not a contraindication to ECT. Demented pa-tients are more prone to delirium and prolonged memory impairment than nondemented patients. However, administration of ECT once or twice a week may reduce the occurrence of these complications. There is no evidence that ECT accelerates the course of dementing disorders.

ECT is contraindicated in patients with recent myocardial infarction be-cause they have an increased risk of arrhythmias. ECT should not be adminis-tered in patients with intracranial tumors because it may lead to delirium, brain herniation, or death. ECT appears to be reasonably safe 1 month after a cere-brovascular accident.

Psychotherapy

Interpersonal therapy (IPT), cognitive-behavioral therapy (CBT), and perhaps psychodynamic psychotherapies have been found as effective as antidepressant drugs in the acute treatment of depressed elderly outpatients (Niederehe, 1994). IPT is a brief, focused psychotherapy. It addresses four factors that often are part of the interpersonal context of depressed patients: grief, role transitions, role disputes, and interpersonal deficits. Beyond its efficacy in the acute treat-ment of depression, use of antidepressant medication combined with monthly IPT sessions was superior to either treatment alone in preventing recurrence and prolonging recovery in elderly patients with recurrent unipolar depression (Reynolds et al., 1999). The superiority of combined treatment was especially evident in subjects aged 70 years and older.

CBT is based on the theory that cognitive and behavioral symptoms initiate and maintain the depressive syndrome. CBT uses a variety of approaches based on learning theory that seek to reduce pathological ideas and behaviors associated with depression. CBT alone (16–20 sessions), desipramine alone, and CBT combined with desipramine were all effective in the treatment of geriatric depression of mild to moderate severity (Thompson et al., 2001). CBT combined with desipramine was more effective than desipramine alone. Despite their efficacy and the lack of side effects, psychotherapies remain underutilized in geriatric depression.

Family interventions are useful in the treatment of geriatric mood disorders. Caregivers of elderly patients, especially caregivers of demented patients, often develop depression themselves that can be effectively addressed by psychotherapeutic or family interventions. Because most elderly depressed patients depend on family members for emotional support and for their day-to-day functioning, treatment approaches that include selected family members may be particularly effective.

Treatment Efficacy, Medical Burden, and Cognitive Impairment

There is evidence that medical burden does not significantly interfere with antidepressant response. In a large multicenter study, fluoxetine was well tolerated (11.6% discontinuation rate), but its efficacy was somewhat lower than that reported in younger adults (31.6% remission, 43.9% response) (Tollefson et al., 1995). History of medical illness (number of chronic medical conditions), but not current medical burden, was associated with greater response to fluoxetine and lower placebo response (Small et al., 1996). It has been shown that antidepressant treatment can improve mood, physical symptoms, and function in depressed patients with emphysema (Borson et al., 1992). Similarly, a variety of psychotherapies have been found effective both in the acute treatment of depressed elderly patients and in prevention of relapse and recurrence (Niederehe, 1994). Therefore, both antidepressants and psychotherapy have the potential to reduce depressive symptoms and disability.

Although limited information from systematic studies exists, most clinicians believe that depressed-demented patients respond favorably to antidepressant drugs (Alexopoulos, 1996b). Depressed-demented patients require dosages of antidepressants comparable to those of nondemented elderly depressed patients. Treatment of depression in demented patients has important implications. Effective treatment can reduce the suffering of depressed-demented patients and improve the quality of life of their families. Improvement of depression can reduce "excess disability" in demented patients and allow them to remain in the community. Finally, reduction of depressive symptoms can ameliorate the cognitive dysfunction contributed by depression and permit clinicians to determine the stage of dementia and advise patients and families about future treatment needs.

Continuation and Maintenance Somatic Treatments

Depression is a recurrent disorder. Once recovery is achieved, continuation treatment should be administered for at least 6 months with the same dosages of the antidepressant used during acute treatment. Failure to provide continuation treatment results in relapse in 30% to 35% of cases (reemergence of the index episode).

After 6 months of remission, patients remain at risk for a new episode of depression. Data from younger adults indicate that a history of three or more episodes is the strongest predictor of recurrence (Alexopoulos & Chester, 1992). Other predictors are high severity of the initial episode, persisting anxiety, and late age of illness (Alexopoulos, Meyers, et al., 1996). Patients at high risk for recurrence should have maintenance treatment for at least 1 to 2 years.

It is estimated that 70% of patients fail to take 25% to 50% of the dosages of their medications. Older patients and their families may not understand the importance of taking medications as prescribed. Concurrent medical illnesses can interfere with antidepressant response or attainment of adequate dosages. Alcoholism and other substance abuse may undercut pharmacotherapy. Difficulties accessing health care may hinder the ability of elderly, especially functionally impaired elderly, to obtain adequate treatment.

Treatment of Geriatric Mania

Lithium is an effective treatment for elderly manic patients who are able to tolerate it. However, lithium may be less effective and even less well tolerated in mania complicated by neurological and medical disorders than in uncomplicated mania. Elderly patients tend to show high lithium plasma levels at relatively low dosages because of an age-associated reduction in renal clearance.

About one half to two thirds of the dosage required for young adults is usually sufficient for elderly individuals. The half-life of lithium is about 24 hours in the seventh decade of life. Therefore, steady-state pharmacokinetics are anticipated 5 or more days after the stabilization of the daily dosage. Elderly persons have a high increase of pharmacodynamic sensitivity to lithium and tend to have a fine tremor and even myoclonus at plasma levels considered therapeutic for young adults. It has been suggested that lithium plasma levels of 0.3 to 0.6 mEq/L are clinically effective in elderly individuals. However, controlled studies are lacking. The onset of action of lithium is slow and may require several days or weeks.

Many elderly patients develop side effects when treated with lithium. Lithium may induce or worsen cognitive impairment, and this side effect is more prominent in dementia patients (Fann, 2002). In elderly patients with mania, delirium can develop at lithium levels at or even below the therapeutic lithium plasma level range. Patients with Parkinson's disease and patients receiving neuroleptics are prone to lithium-induced delirium (Patten et al., 2001). Delirium and cerebellar dysfunction may last for weeks after lithium discontinuation (Nambudiri et al., 1991). Sinoatrial block can be caused by lithium (Lai et al., 2000). Cardiac drugs, including digitalis and β-blockers, increase the risk for sinoatrial block. Salt depletion caused by vomiting or diarrhea, thiazide diuretics, nonsteroidal anti-inflammatory drugs, and angiotensin-converting enzyme inhibitors may raise lithium plasma levels and lead to toxicity.

Anticonvulsant drugs appear to have antimanic action in younger adults (Bowden, 2003). Anecdotal evidence suggests that sodium valproate (Gnam & Flint, 1993; Yassa & Cvejic, 1994) and carbamazepine (Kellner & Neher, 1991) are effective in elderly manic patients. A retrospective study of hospitalized manic elderly patients suggests that subjects receiving valproate (plasma levels 65–90 ng/mL) had a response rate similar (75% vs. 82%) to those treated with lithium (plasma levels above 0.79 mEq/L) (Chen et al., 1999). History of poor response to lithium does not preclude response to anticonvulsants (Bowden, 2003). Some evidence exists that valproate is more effective than lithium in rapidly cycling patients with dysphoric mania (Bowden, 2003). Patients with aggressive behavior resulting from dementing disorders maybe responsive to sodium valproate (Sival et al., 2002). Complete blood count and liver function tests should be obtained before treatment with carbamazepine and valproate. Carbamazepine may cause sedation, confusion, and ataxia in a dose-dependent fashion. Carbamazepine-treated patients should have frequent complete blood counts because carbamazepine can cause leukopenia (white blood cells counts below 4,000/mm^3) in approximately 2% of cases (Tohen et al., 1995). Approximately one half of the patients who develop carbamazepine-induced leukopenia have a drop in white count within the first 16 days of treatment. Valproate causes leukopenia in 0.4% of patients, a percentage comparable to that of tricyclic antidepressants.

Lithium and mood stabilizers have a delayed onset of action. For this reason, lorazepam or low dosages of atypical antipsychotics may be used in the early treatment of acutely agitated elderly manic patients. Haloperidol may be used in patients who are unable to take oral medications.

ECT is highly effective as an acute treatment of mania. Approximately 80% of ECT-treated patients with mania achieve remission or marked clinical improvement (Ciapparelli et al., 2001; Volpe & Tavares, 2003). ECT is effective even in patients with mania who are resistant to drug therapy. Clinical improvement after ECT is a primary therapeutic effect rather than a result of an ECT-induced organic brain syndrome. Patients with mania require a comparable number of ECT treatments to depressed patients. Patients with mania often have a lower seizure threshold than depressed patients. Because it is well tolerated by most geriatric patients, ECT is the treatment of choice for elderly manic patients who are unable to tolerate drug therapy or have a severe behavioral disturbance that requires control. It should be remembered that a sustained period of excited mania may be life threatening for a frail older person.

Treatment of Bereavement

The treatment of a bereaved elderly person depends on the severity of symptomatology. If major depression develops during the bereavement period, antidepressant treatment should be administered. Best outcomes for major depression associated with bereavement are achieved when psychotherapy is combined with a psychosocial intervention such as interpersonal therapy (Reynolds et al., 1999).

Bereaved persons with depressive symptomatology that does not meet criteria for major depression may benefit by brief focused psychotherapy. Interpersonal therapy lends itself well to this purpose because it addresses issues related to loss, depression, and change of roles.

Most elderly bereaved individuals do not develop depressive syndromes or clinically significant depressive symptoms. Therefore, prophylactic treatment is not recommended for the whole elderly bereaved population. However, psychoeducation self-help groups, counseling, group therapy, and individual dynamic psychotherapy may be helpful, and they should be considered for individuals with an intense reaction to loss or history of depression (Gallagher-Thompson, 1995).

RECOMMENDATIONS OF THE EXPERT CONSENSUS STUDY

Clinical research as well as meta-analytic studies provide reliable data for characterizing the clinical presentation of psychiatric syndromes and for testing the efficacy and safety of specific treatments. However, the clinical complexity of late-life depression and the number of possible combinations and sequences of available treatments make it difficult to provide clear recommendations based entirely on clinical trial data.

A method has been developed for describing expert opinion in a quantitative, reliable manner to fill some of the gaps in evidence-based guidelines. This method has been applied in late-life depression (Alexopoulos et al., 2001). Based on the literature, a 64-question survey (857 options) was prepared using a modified version of the RAND 9-point scale for rating appropriateness of medical decisions. The survey was sent to 50 national experts on geriatric depression (recipients of federal research grants in the past 5 years and authors of important publications), all of whom completed it. Consensus on each option was defined as a nonrandom distribution of scores by chi-square "goodness-of-fit" test. What follows are selected conclusions from the Expert Consensus Guideline.

1. Late-life depression occurs in the context of medical and neurological illnesses, disability, and psychosocial adversity. A comprehensive evaluation should include all these areas. Alcohol and substance abuse, medications that can cause mood disorders (e.g., prednisone), and dementing disorders were viewed as the most important comorbid conditions to assess in a depressed elderly patient. The goals of treatment should extend beyond reduction of depressive symptoms and suicidal ideation. Prevention of relapse and recurrence, improvement of cognitive and functional status, and development of skills needed for coping with handicaps and psychosocial stressors are important goals of treatment for late-life depression.

2. The symptom overlap of depression with medical and neurological disorders and the tendency of elderly patients to underreport somatic symptoms may obscure the diagnosis of late-life depression. Sad, downcast mood; poor spirits; frequently feeling like crying; and recurrent thoughts of death or suicide are the most important symptoms in making the diagnosis of geriatric depression. Rating scales, including the Hamilton Depression Rating Scale, the Cornell Scale for Depression in Dementia, the Geriatric Depression Scale, and the Mini-Mental State Examination can be useful in the assessment of depression.

3. Primary care physicians treat most depressed elderly patients. However, patients with psychotic depression, bipolar depression, and depression with suicidal ideation should be referred for specialized psychiatric care.

4. Elderly white men are at the highest risk for suicide. The risk markedly increases after the age of 80 years. High severity of depression, psychotic depression, alcoholism, recent loss or bereavement, abuse of sedatives, and recent development of disability are the most important risk factors in depressed elderly patients.

5. In nonpsychotic geriatric depression, a combination of antidepressants and psychotherapy is the preferred treatment for both severe and mild cases. Drug treatment alone or psychotherapy alone is an alternative in mild geriatric depression. Drug treatment or ECT are the alternatives in severe geriatric depression. ECT should be considered in patients who failed adequate antidepressant trials or who have severe depression with high suicide risk.

6. For pharmacological treatment of geriatric nonpsychotic depression, SSRIs followed by venlafaxine XR is the treatment of choice, followed by bupropion SR and mirtazapine. Among the SSRIs, the experts favored citalopram, followed closely by sertraline, followed by paroxetine; escitalopram was not available at the time of this study. Tricyclic antidepressants (nortriptyline or desipramine) are a reasonable alternative treatment in severe geriatric depression. Amitriptyline, imipramine, doxepin, amoxapine, maprotilene, trazodone, tranylcypromine,

and isocarboxazide should not generally be used for the treatment of depression in elderly patients. The minimal length of antidepressant trial should be 3 to 4 weeks, and the maximum length should be 6 to 7 weeks before switching to another antidepressant or an augmentation agent is used.

7. Cognitive-behavioral therapy, supportive psychotherapy, problem-solving therapy, and interpersonal therapy are the preferred psychotherapeutic approaches for older depressed patients. There is less support among the experts for psychodynamic psychotherapy.

8. Psychoeducational interventions were recommended as an adjunct treatment to help patients and their families improve treatment adherence.

9. In psychotic geriatric depression, combinations of antidepressants (SSRIs or venlafaxine XR) and atypical neuroleptics (except clozapine) were recommended by the experts, although research studies are lacking. ECT is another option. ECT should be considered either as a first choice or if the combination drug treatment fails.

10. There is no consensus on how to treat minor geriatric depression. Watchful waiting for at least 2 weeks or a trial of psychotherapy is favored. In minor depression persisting longer than 2 to 3 months, SSRI plus psychotherapy is the treatment of choice, although drug treatment alone or psychotherapy alone are reasonable alternatives. SSRI plus psychotherapy is the treatment of choice in geriatric dysthymia, but SSRI alone, venlafaxine XR alone, bupropion SR alone, and psychotherapy alone are acceptable alternatives.

11. For geriatric depression associated with a stressor, psychotherapy alone or combined with an antidepressant is recommended.

12. Residual insomnia in depressed elderly patients should be treated with trazodone and, if it fails, with zolpidem, zaleplon, mirtazapine, or lorazepam. Residual anxiety should be treated with an increase of the dosage of the antidepressant to maximum levels rather than prescription of an anxiolytic benzodiazepine.

13. If a patient has had little or no response to an antidepressant given at adequate dosages and for an adequate length of time, switching to a different antidepressant is appropriate. If a patient has had little or no response to an initial SSRI, the patient may be switched to venlafaxine XR or bupropion SR. If a patient has had little or no response to venlafaxine, the patient may be switched to an SSRI. If the patient has had little or no response to another antidepressant (e.g., a TCA, bupropion, nefazodone), switching to an SSRI or venlafaxine XR is appropriate. Other alternatives are a different SSRI, bupropion SR, nortriptyline, or mirtazapine. Although studies in geriatric subjects are lacking, research in younger patients suggests that switching from one SSRI to another is an effective strategy.

14. If the patient has had at least a partial response to the initial anti-

depressant, a second antidepressant or another augmenting agent of the first antidepressant should be added. If the initial antidepressant was an SSRI, bupropion, lithium, or nortriptyline may be added. If the initial antidepressant was a TCA, lithium or an SSRI may be added. If the patient was started on bupropion, an SSRI or lithium may be added.

15. For continuation and maintenance treatment, the dosages should be used that were effective during acute treatment. In patients with a single severe episode, antidepressant drug treatment should continue for 1 year, and longer treatment should be offered to patients with two episodes. Patients with three lifetime episodes should receive treatment for longer than 3 years. In a patient with psychotic depression who achieves remission following treatment with an antidepressant and an antipsychotic, the antipsychotic drug should be continued for 6 months. However, some experts recommend shorter or longer treatment. For a depressed patient who failed antidepressants but responded to ECT, antidepressants (other than the one to which the patient previously failed to respond) should be used for continuation/maintenance treatment. Continuation/maintenance ECT is another option. A study suggests that the combination of an antidepressant and a mood stabilizer (nortriptyline and lithium) is superior to monotherapy with nortriptyline in post-ECT continuation/maintenance treatment (Sackeim et al., 2001). Because many older patients cannot tolerate lithium, an anticonvulsant (divalproex or valproate) should be considered.

16. In an older patient with major depression and mild-to-moderate dementia, the treatment of choice is combination of an antidepressant with psychosocial intervention. Antidepressant medication alone is another option. Among the antidepressants, the experts considered citalopram, sertraline, and venlafaxine first-line choices. Among psychosocial interventions, caregiver-focused treatment and supportive psychotherapy should be favored.

17. If an older patient has major depressive disorder and a medical condition (e.g., hypothyroidism, vitamin B_{12} deficiency) likely to contribute to the depression, both an antidepressant and treatment for the comorbid condition should be offered. However, medical conditions likely to respond promptly to treatment (e.g., amphetamine withdrawal) should be treated first, and antidepressants should be used only if depression persists.

18. Depression can worsen the outcome of medical conditions requiring the patient's active participation in treatment (e.g., a depressed patient with chronic obstructive pulmonary disease who stops his or her exercise program, resulting in muscle deconditioning and increased disability). Such patients should be screened for depression; if they are

depressed, they should be treated with antidepressants and behavioral treatments aimed to increase their adherence to treatment.

19. Elderly patients often develop depression while receiving drugs that may increase depression. If the depression occurs in a patient receiving methyldopa, cimetidine, clonidine, hydralazine, propranolol, or reserpine, a switch to another medication is recommended. If the depression occurs in a patient treated with digitalis, estrogens, tamoxifen, vinblastine, or vincristin, this medication should be continued, and depression should be treated with antidepressants. There is no agreement on the best strategy for depression that occurs in patients treated with benzodiazepines, corticosteroids, progesterone, propoxyphene, or psychostimulants. Although it is desirable to discontinue benzodiazepines, many patients resist this recommendation.

20. Only a few combinations of antidepressants with other medications are contraindicated. A MAOI should not be combined with codeine, tramadol, or a tricyclic in older patients. Two tricyclics should not be concomitantly prescribed. Close monitoring of side effects is recommended when combining most SSRIs with tramadol, a tricyclic, codeine, or warfarin; bupropion SR with caffeine or a TCA; mirtazapine with tramadol, a TCA, or warfarin; trazodone with atenolol, captopril, codeine, tramadol, or a TCA; nefazodone with nifedipine, tramadol, or a TCA; and venlafaxine XR with atenolol, caffeine, tramadol, a TCA, or warfarin.

AKNOWLEDGMENT

This work was supported by National Institute of Mental Health grants RO1 MH42819, RO1 MH51842, RO1 MH59362, P30 MH68638, T32 MH19132; the Sanchez Foundation; and the Dr. I Foundation.

REFERENCES

Alexopoulos GS. Clinical and biological findings in late-onset depression. In: Tasman A, Goldfinger SM, Kaufmann CA, eds. *American Psychiatric Press Review of Psychiatry*. Vol. 9. Washington, DC: American Psychiatric Press; 1990:249–262.

Alexopoulos GS. Biological correlates of late-life depression. In: Schneider LS, Reynolds CF, Lebowitz BP, Friedhoff AJ, eds. *Diagnosis and Treatment of Depression in Late-Life: Results of the NIH Consensus Development Conference*. Washington, DC: National Institutes of Health; 1994:99–116.

Alexopoulos GS. Methodology of treatment studies in geriatric depression. *Am J Geriatr Psychiatry*. 1995;3:280–289.

Alexopoulos GS. Geriatric depression in primary care. *Int J Geriatr Psychiatry*. 1996a; 11:397–400.

Alexopoulos GS. The treatment of depressed-demented patients. *J Clin Psychiatry*. 1996b;57(Suppl.):14–20.

Alexopoulos GS. The depression–executive dysfunction syndrome of late life: a target for D3 receptor agonists. *Am J Geriatr Psychiatry.* 2001a;9:1–8.

Alexopoulos GS, PROSPECT group. Interventions for depressed elderly primary care patients. *J Geriatr Psychiatry.* 2001b;16:553–559.

Alexopoulos GS. Frontostriatal and limbic dysfunction in late-life depression. *Am J Geriatr Psychiatry.* 2002;10:687–695.

Alexopoulos GS, Abrams RC. Depression in Alzheimer's disease. *Psychiatr Clin North Am.* 1991;14:327–340.

Alexopoulos GS, Abrams RC, Young RC, Shamoian CA. Cornell Scale for Depression in Dementia. *Biol Psychiatry.* 1988;23:271–284.

Alexopoulos GS, Borson S, Cuthbert BN, et al. Assessment of late-life depression. *Biol Psychiatry.* 2002;52:164–174.

Alexopoulos GS, Bruce ML, Hull J, Kakuma T. Clinical determinants of suicidal ideation and behavior in geriatric depression. *Arch Gen Psychiatry.* 1999;56:1048–1053.

Alexopoulos GS, Bruce ML, Silbersweig D, Kalayam B, Stern E. Vascular depression: a new view of late-onset depression. *Dialog Clin Neurosci.* 1999;1:69–80.

Alexopoulos GS, Buckwalter K, Olin J, Martinez R, Wainscott C, Krishnan KR. Comorbidity of late-life depression: an opportunity for research in mechanisms and treatment. *Biol Psychiatry.* 2002;52:543–558.

Alexopoulos GS, Chester JG. Outcomes of geriatric depression. *Clin Geriatr Med.* 1992; 8:363–376.

Alexopoulos GS, Katz IR, Reynolds CF III, Carpenter D, Docherty JP. The expert consensus guideline series: pharmacotherapy of depressive disorders in older patients. *Postgrad Med.* October 2001:1–86.

Alexopoulos GS, Kiosses DN, Choi SJ, Murphy CF, Lim KO. Frontal white matter microstructure and treatment response of late-life depression: a preliminary study. *Am J Psychiatry.* 2002;159:1929–1932.

Alexopoulos GS, Kiosses D, Klimstra S, Kalayam B, Bruce ML. Clinical presentation of "depression–executive dysfunction syndrome" of late life. *Am J Geriatr Psychiatry.* 2002;10:98–102.

Alexopoulos GS, Meyers BS, Young RC, Campbell S, Sibersweig D, Charlson M. The "vascular depression" hypothesis. *Arch Gen Psychiatry.* 1997b;54:915–922.

Alexopoulos GS, Meyers BS, Young RC, Hull J, Sirey JA, Kakuma T. Executive dysfunction and risk for relapse and recurrence of geriatric depression. *Arch Gen Psychiatry.* 2000;57:285–290.

Alexopoulos GS, Meyers BS, Young RC, et al. Recovery in geriatric depression. *Arch Gen Psychiatry.* 1996;53:305–312.

Alexopoulos GS, Meyers BS, Young RC, Kakuma T, Silbersweig D, Charlson M. Clinically defined vascular depression. *Am J Psychiatry.* 1997a;154:562–565.

Alexopoulos GS, Meyers BS, Young RC, Mattis S, Kakuma T. The course of geriatric depression with "reversible dementia": a controlled study. *Am J Psychiatry.* 1993; 150:1693–1699.

Alexopoulos GS, Raue P, Arean P. Problem-solving therapy versus supportive therapy in geriatric major depression with executive dysfunction. *Am J Geriatr Psychiatry.* 2003;11:46–52.

Alexopoulos GS, Salzman C. Treatment of depression. In: Salzman C, ed. *Clinical Geriatric Psychopharmacology.* 3rd ed. Baltimore, MD: Williams and Wilkins; 1998: 184–244.

Alexopoulos GS, Shamoian CA, Lucas J, Weiser N, Berger H. Medical problems during ECT in geriatric patients and younger controls. *J Am Geriatr Soc.* 1984;32:651–654.

Alexopoulos GS, Vrontou C, Kakuma T, et al. Disability in geriatric depression. *Am J Psychiatry.* 1996;153:877–885.

Alexopoulos GS, Young RC, Abrams RC. ECT in the high-risk geriatric patient. *Conv Therapy.* 1989;26:551–554.

Alexopoulos G, Young R, Meyers B. Geriatric depression: age of onset and dementia. *Biol Psychiatry.* 1993;34:141–145.

Allen A, Blazer DG. Mood disorders. In: Sadavoy J, Lazarus LW, Jarvik LF, eds. *Comprehensive Review of Geriatric Psychiatry.* Washington, DC: American Psychiatric Press; 1991:337–351.

American Psychiatric Association. *Diagnostic and Statistical Manual of Mental Disorders.* 3rd ed., rev. Washington, DC: American Psychiatric Association; 1990.

American Psychiatric Association. *Diagnostic and Statistical Manual of Mental Disorders.* 4th ed. Washington, DC: American Psychiatric Association; 1994.

Armer J. Elderly relocation to a congregate setting: factors influencing adjustment. *Issues Ment Health Nurs.* 1993;14:157–172.

Bassuk SS, Berkman LF, Wypij D. Depressive symptomatology and incident cognitive decline in an elderly community sample. *Arch Gen Psychiatry.* 1998;55:1073–1081.

Baumgarten M, Battista R, Infante-Rivard C, Hanley J, Becker R, Gauthier S: The psychological and physical health of family members caring for an elderly person with dementia. *J Clin Epidemiol.* 1992;45:61–70.

Beck AT, Brown G, Steer RA, Dahlsgaard KK, Grisham J. Suicide ideation at its worst point: a predictor of eventual suicide in psychiatric outpatients. *Suicide Life Threat Behav.* 1999;29:1–9.

Boone KB, Miller BL, Lesser IM, et al. Neuropsychological correlates of white matter lesions in healthy elderly subjects. *Arch Neurol.* 1992;49:549–554.

Borson S, McDonald GJ, Gayle T, Deffenbach M, Lakshminarayan S, Van Tuinen C. Improvement in mood, physical symptoms, and function with nortriptyline for depression in patients with chronic obstructive pulmonary disease. *Psychosomatics.* 1992;33:190–201.

Bowden CL. Alproate. *Bipolar Disord.* 2003;5:189–202.

Brody DS, Khaliq AA, Thompson TL. Patients' perspectives on the management of emotional distress in primary care setting. *J Gen Intern Med.* 1997;12:403–406.

Bruce ML, Pearson JL. Designing an intervention to prevent suicide: PROSPECT (Prevention of Suicide in Primary Care Elderly: Collaborative Trial). *Dialog Neurosci.* 1999;1:100–112.

Bruce ML, Seeman TE, Merrill SS, Blazer DG; The impact of depressive symptomatology on physical disability: MacArthur studies of successful aging. *Am J Public Health.* 1994;84:1796–1799.

Burke WJ, Roccaforte WH, Wengel SP, McArthur-Miller D, Folks DG, Potter JF. Disagreement in the reporting of depressive symptoms between patients with dementia of the Alzheimer's type and their collateral source. *Am J Geriatr Psychiatry.* 1998; 6:308–319.

Burrows AB, Satlin A, Salzman C, Nobel K, Lipsitz L. Depression in a long-term care facility: clinical features and discordance between nursing assessment and patient interviews. *J Am Geriatr Soc.* 1995;43:1118–1122.

Butters MA, Becker JT, Nebes RD, et al. Changes in cognitive functioning following treatment of late-life depression. *Am J Psychiatry.* 2000;157:1949–1954.

Cardiac Arrhythmia Suppression Trial (CAST) Investigators. Effect of the antiarrhythmic agent moricizine on survival after myocardial infarction. *N Engl J Med.* 1992; 327:227–233.

Carney SS, Rich CL, Burke PA, Fowler RC. Suicide over 60: the San Diego Study. *J Am Geriatr Soc.* 1994;42:174–180.

Carson AJ, MacHale S, Allen K, et al. Depression after stroke and lesion location: a systematic review. *Lancet.* 2000;356:122–130.

Chemerinski E, Robinson RG. The neuropsychiatry of stroke. *Psychosomatics.* 2000; 41:5–14.

Chen ST, Altshuler LL, Melnyk KA, Erhart SM, Miller E, Minz J. Efficacy of lithium vs. valproate in the treatment of mania in the elderly: a retrospective study. *J Clin Psychiatry.* 1999;60:181–186.

Chen ST, Sultzer DL, Hinkin CH, Mahler ME, Cummings JL. Executive dysfunction in Alzheimer's disease: association with neuropsychiatric symptoms and functional impairment. *J Neuropsychiatr Clin Neurosci.* 1998;10:426–432.

Ciapparelli A, Dell'Osso L, Tundo A, et al. Electroconvulsive therapy in medication nonresponsive patients with mixed mania and bipolar depression. *J Clin Psychiatry.* 2001;62:552–555.

Clyburn LD, Stones MJ, Hajistravropoulos T, Tuokko H. Predicting caregiver burden and depression in Alzheimer's disease. *J Gerontol B Psychol Sci Soc Sci.* 2000;55: S2–S13.

Collins CE, Stommel M, Wang S, Given CW. Caregiving transitions: changes in depression among family caregivers of relatives with dementia. *Nurs Res.* 1994;43:220–225.

Conwell Y. Suicide in the elderly. In: Schneider LS, Reynolds CF, Lebowitz BD, Friedhoff AJ, eds. *Diagnosis and Treatment of Depression in Late Life: Results of the NIH Consensus Development Conference.* Washington, DC: American Psychiatric Press; 1994:397–418.

Conwell Y, Brent D. Suicide and aging I: patterns of psychiatric diagnoses. *Int Psychogeriatr.* 1995;7:149–164.

Conwell Y, Duberstein PR, Herrmann JH, Caine ED. Relationship of age and axis I diagnoses in victims of completed suicide: a psychological autopsy study. *Am J Psychiatry.* 1996;153:1001–1008.

Conwell Y, Duberstein PR, Herrmann J, Forbes N, Caine ED. Age differences in behaviors leading to completed suicide. *Am J Geriatr Psychiatry.* 1998;6:122–126.

Cooper PL, Crum RM, Ford DE. Characteristics of patients with major depression who received care in general medical and specialty mental health settings. *Med Care.* 1994;32:15–24.

Cooper-Patrick L, Gallo JJ, Gonzales JJ, et al. Race, gender, and partnership in the patient-physician relationship. *JAMA.* 1999;282:583–589.

Covinsky KE, Kahana E, Chin MH, Palmer RM, Fortinsky RH, Landefeld CS. Depressive symptoms and 3-year mortality in older hospitalized medical patients. *Ann Int Med.* 1999;130:563–569.

Covinsky KE, Palmer RM, Kresevic DM, et al. Improving functional outcomes in older patients: lessons from an acute care for elders unit. *J Qual Improv.* 1998;24:63–76.

Davidson RJ, Pizzagalli D, Nitschke JB, Putnam K. Depression: perspectives from affective neuroscience. *Annu Rev Psychol.* 2002;53:545–574.

de Asis JM, Stern E, Alexopoulos GS, et al. A hippocampal and anterior cingulate activation deficits in patients with geriatric depression. *Am J Psychiatry.* 2001;158:1321–1323.

Dennis MS, Lindesay J. Suicide in the elderly: the United Kingdom perspective. *Int Psychogeriatr.* 1995;7:263–274.

Devanand DP, Sano M, Tang MX, et al. Depressed mood and the incidence of Alzheimer's disease in the elderly living in the community. *Arch Gen Psychiatry.* 1996; 53:175–182.

DeVane CL. Pharmacokinetics of the newer antidepressants: clinical relevance. *Am J Med.* 1994;97(6A):13S–23S.

Diekstra RFW, van Egmond M. Suicide and attempted suicide in general practice, 1979–1985. *Acta Psychiatr Scand.* 1989;79:268–275.

Dinghra U, Rabins PV. Mania in the elderly: a five- to seven-year follow-up. *J Am Geriatr Soc.* 1991;39:581.

Drevets WC. Prefrontal cortical-amygdalar metabolism in major depression. *Ann N Y Acad Sci.* 1999;877:614–637.

Drevets WC. Neuroimaging studies of mood disorders. *Biol Psychiatry.* 2000;48:813–819.

Drevets WC, Price JL, Simpson JR, et al. Subgenual prefrontal cortex abnormalities in mood disorders. *Nature.* 1997;386:824–827.

Drevets WC, Videen TO, Price JL, Preskorn SH, Carmichael ST, Raichle ME. A functional anatomical study of unipolar depression. *J Neurosci.* 1992;12:3628–3641.

Duman RS, Heninger GR, Nestler EJ. A molecular and cellular theory of depression. *Arch Gen Psychiatry.* 1997;54:597–606.

Eagles JM, Whalley LJ. Ageing and affective disorders: the age at first onset of affective disorders in Scotland, 1966-1978. *Br J Psychiatry.* 1985;147:180.

Fann JR. Neurological effects of psychopharmacological agents. *Semin Clin Neuropsychiatry.* 2002;7:196–205.

Farran CJ, Miller BH, Kaufman JE, Davis L. Race, finding meaning, and caregiver distress. *J Aging Health.* 1997;9:316–333.

Fichter MM, Meller I, Schroppel H, Steinkirchner R. Dementia and cognitive decline in the oldest old in the community. Prevalence and comorbidity. *Br J Psychiatry.* 1995;166:621–629.

Forsell Y, Jorm AF, Winblad B. Association of age, sex, cognitive dysfunction and disability with major depressive symptoms in an elderly sample. *Am J Psychiatry.* 1994;151:1600–1604.

Freedman V, Berkman LF, Rapp S, Ostfeld A. Family networks: predictors of nursing home entry. *Am J Public Health.* 1994;84:843–845.

Frierson RL. Suicide attempts by the old and the very old. *Arch Intern Med.* 1991;151:141–144.

Gallagher-Thompson D. Clinical intervention strategies for distressed caregivers: rationale and development of psychoeducational approaches. In: Light E, Niederehe G,

Lebowitz BD, eds. *Stress Effects in Alzheimer's Disease Caregivers*. New York, NY: Springer; 1995:260–277.

Gallant MP, Connell CM. Predictors of decreased self-care among spouse caregivers of older adults with dementing illness. *J Aging Health*. 1997;9:373–395.

Gallo JJ, Rabins PV. Depression without sadness: alternative presentations of depression in late life. *Am Fam Physician*. 1999;60:820–826.

Gallo JJ, Rabins PV, Anthony JCL. Sadness in older persons: 13-year follow-up of a community sample in Baltimore, Maryland. *Psychol Med*. 1999;29:341–350.

Geerlings MI, Schoevers RA, Beekman AT, et al. Depression and risk of cognitive decline and Alzheimer's disease. Results of two community-based studies in the Netherlands. *Br J Psychiatry*. 2000;176:568–575.

Georgotas A, McCue RE. The additional benefit of extending an antidepressant trial past seven weeks in the depressed elderly. *Int J Geriatr Psychiatry*. 1989;4:191–195.

Gnam W, Flint AJ. New onset rapid cycling bipolar disorder in an 87 year old woman. *Can J Psychiatry*. 1993;38(5):324–326.

Gurialnik JM, LaCroix AZ, Branch LG, Kasl SV, Wallace RB. Morbidity and disability in older persons in the years prior to death. *Am J Public Health*. 1991;82:443–447.

Harris T, Kovar MG, Suzman R, Leinman JC, Feldmann JJ. Longitudinal study of physical ability in the oldest-old. *Am J Public Health*. 1989;79:698–702.

Hays JC, Landerman LR, George LK, et al. Social correlates of the dimensions of depression in the elderly. *J Gerontol B Psychol Sci Soc Sci*. 1998;53:P31–P39.

Henriksson MM, Marttunen MJ, Isometsä ET, et al. Mental disorders in elderly suicide. *Int Psychogeriatr*. 1995;7:275–286.

Hickie I, Scott E, Mitchell P, Wilhelm K, Austin MP, Bennett B. Subcortical hyperintensities on magnetic resonance imaging: clinical correlates and prognostic significance in patients with severe depression. *Biol Psychiatry*. 1995;37:151–160.

Jorm AF, Henderson AJ, Kaye DW, Jacomb PA. Mortality in relation to dementia, depression and social interaction in an elderly community sample. *Int J Geriatr Psychiatry*. 1991;6:5–11.

Jorm AF, van Duijn CM, Chandra V, et al. Psychiatric history and related exposures as risk factors for Alzheimer's disease: a collaborative re-analysis of case-control studies. *Int J Epidemiol*. 1991;20(Suppl 2):S43–S47.

Kalayam B, Alexopoulos GS. Prefrontal dysfunction and treatment response in geriatric depression. *Arch Gen Psychiatry*. 1999;56:713–718.

Katon W, Schulberg H. Epidemiology of depression in primary care. *Gen Hosp Psychiatry*. 1992;14:237–242.

Katona CLE, Aldridge CR. The dexamethasone suppression test and depressive signs in dementia. *J Affect Disord*. 1985;8:83–89.

Katz IR, Parmelee PA, Streim JE. Depression in older patients in residential care: significance of dysphoria and dimensional assessment. *Am J Geriatr Psychiatry*. 1995;3:161–169.

Kellner MB, Neher F. A first episode of mania after age 80. *Can J Psychiatry*. 1991;36:607–608.

Kindermann SS, Kalayam B, Brown GG, Burdick KE, Alexopoulos GS. Executive fucntions and P300 latency in elderly depressed patients and control subjects. *Am J Geriatr Psychiatry*. 2000;8:57–65.

Kiosses DN, Alexopoulos GS, Murphy C. Symptoms of striatofrontal dysfunction contribute to disability in geriatric depression. *Int J Geriatr Psychiatry.* 2000;15:992–999.

Kiosses DN, Klimstra S, Muphy C, Alexopoulos GS. Executive dysfunction and disability in elderly patients with major depression. *Am J Geriatr Psychiatry.* 2001;9:269–274.

Klerman GL. The classification of bipolar disorder. *Psychiatric Ann.* 1987;17(1):13–17.

Koenig HG, Meador K, Cohen HG, Blazer D. Depression in elderly men hospitalized with medical illness. *Arch Intern Med.* 1988;148:1929–1936.

Koenig HG, Veeraindar G, Shelp F, Kudler H, Cohen HJ, Blazer DG. Major depression in hospitalized medically ill older men: documentation, management, and outcome. *Int J Geriatr Psychiatry.* 1992;7:25–34.

Kokmen E, Beard CM, Chandra V, Offord KP, Schoenberg BS, Ballard DJ. Clinical risk factors for Alzheimer's disease: a population-based case-control study. *Neurology.* 1991;41:1393–1397.

Kral VA, Emery OB. Long-term follow-up of depressive pseudodementia of the aged. *Can J Psychiatry.* 1989;34:445–446.

Kramer M, German PS, Anthony JC, et al. Patterns of mental disorders among the elderly residents of eastern Baltimore. *J Am Geriatr Soc.* 1985;33:236–245.

Krauthammer C, Klerman GL. Secondary mania: manic syndromes associated with antecedent physical illness or drugs. *Arch Gen Psychiatry.* 1978;35:1333.

Krishnan KRR, Hays JC, Blazer DG. MRI-defined vascular depression. *Am J Psychiatry.* 1997;154:497–500.

Kumar A, Bilker W, Jin Z, et al. Atrophy and high intensity lesions: complementary neurobiological mechanisms in late-life depression. *Neuropsychopharmacology.* 2000;22:264–274.

Lacro JP, Jeste DV. Physical comorbidity and polypharmacy in older psychiatric patients. *Biol Psychiatry.* 1994;36:146–152.

Lai CL, Chen WJ, Huang CH, et al. Sinus node dysfunction in a patient with lithium intoxication. *J Formos Med Assoc.* 2000;99:66–68.

Lai T-J, Payne ME, Byrum CE, Steffens DC, Krishnan KRR. Reduction of orbital frontal cortex volume in geriatric depression. *Biol Psychiatry.* 2000;48:971–975.

Lesser I, Boone KB, Mehringer CM, Wohl MA, Miller BL, Berman NG. Cognition and white matter hyperintensities in older depressed adults. *Am J Psychiatry.* 1996;153:1280–1287.

Lockwood KA, Alexopoulos GS, Kakuma T, van Gorp WG. Subtypes of cognitive impairment in depressed older adults. *Am J Geriatr Psychiatry.* 2000;8:201–208.

Luber MP, Hollenberg JP, Williams-Russo P, et al. Diagnosis, treatment, comorbidity, and resource utilization in patients in a general medical practice. *Int J Psychiatry Med.* 2000;30:1–13.

Luber MP, Meyers BS, Williams-Russo PG, et al. Depression and service utilization in elderly primary care patients. *Am J Geriatr Psychiatry.* 2001;9:169–176.

Lutgendorf SK, Garand L, Buckwalter KC, Tripp-Reimer T, Hong SY, Lubaroff DM. Life stress, mood disturbance, and elevated interleukin-6 in healthy older women. *J Gerontol A Biol Sci Med Sci.* 1999;54:M434–M439.

Magaziner J, Simonsick EM, Kashner TM, et al. Predictors of functional recovery one year following hospital discharge for hip fracture: a perspective study. *J Gerontol.* 1990;45:101–107.

Masserman DL, Cummings JL. Frontal-subcortical circuits: the anatomical basis of executive, social, and motivated behaviors. *J Psychopharmacol.* 1997;11:107–114.

Mayberg HS. Depression and frontal-subcortical circuits. Focus on prefrontal-limbic interactions. In: Lichter DC, Cummings JL, eds. *Frontal-Subcortical Circuits in Psychiatric and Neurological Disorders.* New York, NY: Guilford Press; 2001:177–206.

McIntosh JL, Santos JF, Hubbard RW, Overholser, JC. *Elder Suicide: Research, Theory, and Treatment.* Washington, DC: American Psychological Association; 1994.

Meeks S, Murrell SA, Mehl RC. Longitudinal relationships between depressive symptoms and health in normal older and middle-aged adults. *Psychol Aging.* 2000;15:100–109.

Mental Health: A Report of the Surgeon General. Washington, DC: US Department of Health and Human Services; 1999.

Meyers BS. Late-life delusional depression: acute and long-term treatment. *Int Psychogeriatr.* 1995;7(Suppl):113–124.

Moffat SD, Szekely CA, Zonderman AB, Kabani NJ, Resnick SM. Longitudinal change in hippocampal volume as a function of apolipoprotein E genotype. *Neurology.* 2000;55:134–136.

Moscicki EK. Epidemiologic surveys as tools for studying behavior: a review. *Suicide Life Threat Behav.* 1989;19:131–146.

Mossey JM, Mutran E, Knott K, Craik R. Determinants of recovery 12 months after hip fracture: the importance of psychosocial factors. *Am J Public Health.* 1989;79:279–286.

Murphy E, Smith R, Lindesay J, Slattery J. Increased mortality rates in late-life depression. *Br J Psychiatry* 1988;152:347–353.

Murray CGL, Lopez AD. Alternative projections of mortality and disability by cause 1990–2020: global burden of disease study. *Lancet.* 1997;349:1498–1504.

Nambudiri DE, Meyers BS, Young RC. Delayed recovery from lithium neurotoxicity. *J Geriatr Psychiatry Neurol.* 1991;4:40–43.

National Center for Health Statistics. *Vital Statistics of the United States, 1988, Vol. 2: Mortality, Part A.* Washington, DC: US Public Health Service; 1991.

National Center for Health Statistics. Advance report of final mortality statistics, 1989. *NCHS Monthly Vital Stat Rep.* 1992;40(8, Suppl 2).

Nebes RD, Butters MA, Mulsant BH, et al. Decreased working memory and processing speed mediate cognitive impairment in geriatric depression. *Psychol Med.* 2000;30:679–691.

Niederehe GT. Psychosocial therapies with depressed older adults. In: Schneider LS, Reynolds CF, Lebowitz BD, Friedhoff AJ, eds. *Diagnosis and Treatment of Depression in Late Life.* Washington, DC: American Psychiatric Press; 1994:293–315.

Nierenberg AA, Feighner JP, Rudolph R, Cole JO, Sullivan J. Venlafaxine for treatment-resistant unipolar depression. *J Clin Psychopharmacol.* 1994;14:419–423.

NIH Consensus Conference. Diagnosis and treatment of depression in late life. *JAMA.* 1992;268:1018–1024.

Nutting PA, Rost K, Smith J, Werner JJ, Elliot C. Competing demands from physical problems: effect on initiating and completing depression care over six months. *Arch Fam Med.* 2000;9:1059–1064.

Olin JT, Schneider LS, Katz IR, et al. National Institute of Mental Health—provisional diagnostic criteria for depression of Alzheimer disease. *Am J Geriatr Psychiatry.* 2002;10:125–128.

Ongur D, Drevets WC, Price JL. Glial reduction in the prefrontal cortex in mood disorders. *Proc Natl Acad Sci U S A.* 1998;95:13290–13295.

Ormel J, Von Koroff M, Van Den Brink W, Katon W, Brilman E, Oldehinkel T. Depression, anxiety and social disability show synchrony of change in primary care patients. *Am J Public Health.* 1993;83:385–390.

Oxman TE, Barrett JE, Barrett J, Gerber P. Symptomatology of late-life minor depression among primary care patients. *Psychosomatics.* 1990;31:174–180.

Pahor M, Guralnik JM, Salive ME, Chrischilles EA, Manto A, Wallace RB. Disability and severe gastrointestinal hemorrhage: a prospective study of community-dwelling older persons. *J Am Geriatr Soc.* 1994;42:816–825.

Parmelee PA, Katz IR, Lawton MP. Depression among institutionalized aged: assessment and prevalence estimation. *J Gerontol.* 1989;44:M22–M29.

Parmelee PA, Katz IR, Lawton MP. Depression and mortality among institutionalized aged. *J Gerontol.* 1992;47:3–10.

Patten SB, Williams JV, Petcu R, et al. Delirium in psychiatric inpatients: a case-control study. *Can J Psychiatry.* 2001;46:162–166.

Rajkowska G, Miguel-Hidalgo LL, Wei J. Morphometric evidence for neuronal and glial prefrontal cell pathology in major depression. *Biol Psychiatry.* 1999;45:1085–1098.

Reding M, Haycox J, Blass J. Depression in patients referred to a dementia clinic: a three-year prospective study. *Arch Neurol.* 1985;42:894–896.

Reynolds CF, Frank E, Perel JM, et al. Nortriptyline and interpersonal psychotherapy as maintenance therapies for recurrent major depression: a randomized controlled trial in patients older than 59 years. *JAMA.* 1999;281:39–45.

Rice JP, Reich T. The familiar transmission of bipolar illness. *Arch Gen Psychiatry.* 1987;44:441–447.

Riley KP, Snowdon DA, Saunders AM, Roses AD, Mortimer JA, Nanayakkara N. Cognitive function and apolipoprotein E in very old adults: findings from the Nun Study. *J Gerontol B Psychol Sci Soc Sci.* 2000;55:S69–S75.

Ritchie K, Gilman C, Ledesert B, Touchon J, Kotzski PO. Depressive illness, depressive symptomatology, and regional cerebral blood flow in elderly people with subclinical cognitive impairment. *Age Ageing.* 1999;28:385–391.

Rogers MA, Bradshaw JL, Pantelis C, Phillips JG. Frontostriatal deficits in unipolar major depression. *Brain Res Bull.* 1998;47:297–310.

Roose SP, Dallack GW, Glassman AH, Woodring S, Walsh T, Giardina EGV. Cardiovascular effects of bupropion in depressed patients with heart disease. *Am J Psychiatry.* 1991;148:512–516.

Roose SP, Glassman AH, Giardina EGV, et al. Tricyclic antidepressants in depressed patients with cardiac conduction disease. *Arch Gen Psychiatry.* 1987;44:273–275.

Rovner BW. Depression and increased risk of mortality in the nursing home patient. *Am J Med.* 1993;94:19–22.

Sackeim HA, Haskett RF, Mulsant BH, et al. Continuation pharmacotherapy in the prevention of relapse following electroconvulsive therapy. *JAMA.* 2001;285:1299–1307.

Salzman C, Schneider LS, Alexopoulos GS. Pharmacological treatment of depression in late life. In: Bloom FE, Kupfer DJ, eds. *Psychopharmacology: Fourth Generation of Progress.* New York, NY: Raven Press; 1994:1471–1477.

Samuels SC, Katz IR, Parmelee PA, Boyce AA, Di Filippo. Use of the Hamilton and Montgomery-Asberg Depression Scales in institutionalized elderly patients. *Am J Geriatr Psychiatry*. 1996;4:237–246.

Satel SL, Nelson JC. Stimulants in the treatment of depression: a critical overview. *J Clin Psychiatry*. 1989;50:241–249.

Schneider LS. Pharmacologic considerations in the treatment of late life depression. *Am J Geriatr Psychiatry*. 1996;4(Suppl 1):S51–S65.

Schneider LS, Reynolds CF, Lebowitz BD, Friedhoff AJ, eds. *Diagnosis and Treatment of Depression in Late Life: Results of the NIH Consensus Development Conference.* Washington, DC: American Psychiatric Press; 1994.

Schulberg H, Couleman J, Block M, et al. Clinical trials of primary care treatments for major depression: issues in design, recruitment, and treatment. *Int J Psychiatry Med*. 1993;23:29–42.

Schulberg HC, Block MR, Madonia MJ, et al. The "usual care" of major depression in primary care practice. *Arch Fam Med*. 1997;6:334–339.

Schulz R, Williamson G. A 2-year longitudinal study of depression among Alzheimer's caregivers. *Psychol Aging*. 1991;6:569–578.

Schweitzer I, Burrows G, Tuckwell V, et al. Sustained response to open-label venlafaxine in drug-resistant major depression. *J Clin Psychopharmacol*. 2001;21:185–189.

Shamash K, O'Connell K, Lowy MM, Katona CLE. Psychiatric morbidity and outcome in elderly patients undergoing emergency hip surgery: a one year follow-up study. *Int J Geriatr Psychiatry*. 1992;7:505–509.

Sheline YI, Sanghavi M, Mintun MA, Gado MH. Depression duration but not age predicts hippocampal volume loss in medically healthy women with recurrent major depression. *J Neurosci*. 1999;19:5034–5043.

Sheline YI, Wang PW, Gado MH, Csernansky JG, Vannier MW. Hippocampal atrophy in recurrent major depression. *Proc Natl Acad Sci U S A*. 1996;93:3908–3913.

Shulman K, Post F. Bipolar affective disorder in old age. *Br J Psychiatry*. 1980;136:26.

Shulman KI, Tohen, Satlin A, et al. Mania compared with unipolar depression in old age. *Am J Psychiatry*. 1992;142:341–345.

Simon GE, von Korff M. Suicide mortality among patients treated for depression in an insured population. *Am J Epidemiol*. 1998;147:155–160.

Simon GE, von Korff M, Barlow W. Health care costs of primary care patients with recognized depression. *Arch Gen Psychiatry*. 1995;52:850–856.

Sival RC, Haffmans PM, Jansen PA, et al. Sodium valproate in the treatment of aggressive behavior in patients with dementia: a randomized placebo controlled clinical trial. *Int J Geriatr Psychiatry*. 2002;17:579–585.

Small GW, Birkett M, Meyers BS, Koran LM, Bystritsky A, Nemeroff CB. Impact of physical illness on quality of life and antidepressant response in geriatric major depression. Fluoxetine Collaborative Study Group. *J Am Geriatr Soc*. 1996;44:1220–1225.

Sobin C, Sacheim HA. Psychomotor symptoms of depression. *Am J Psychiatry*. 1997;154:4–17.

Speck CE, Kukull WA, Brenner DE, et al. History of depression as a risk factor for Alzheimer's disease. *Epidemiology*. 1995;6:366–369.

Starkstein SE, Boston JD, Robinson RG. Mechanisms of mania after brain surgery: twelve case reports and review of the literature. *J Nerv Ment Dis*. 1988;176:87–100.

Steffens DC, Byrum CE, McQuaid DR, et al. Hippocampal volume in geriatric depression. *Biol Psychiatry.* 2000;48:301–309.

Steffens DC, Hays JC, Krishnan KRR. Disability in geriatric depression. *Am J Geriatr Psychiatry.* 1999;7:34–40.

Steffens DC, Plassman BL, Helms MJ, Welsh-Bohmer KA, Saunders AM, Breitner JC. A twin study of late-onset depression and apolipoprotein E epsilon 4 as risk factors for Alzheimer's disease. *Biol Psychiatry.* 1997;41:851–856.

Sweet RA, Pollock BG, Kirshner M, Wright B, Altieri LP, De Vane CL. Pharmacokinetics of single- and multiple dose bupropion in elderly patients with major depression. *J Clin Psychopharmacol.* 1995;35:876–884.

Thompson LW, Coon DW, Gallagher-Thompson D, Sommer BR, Koin D. Comparison of desipramine and cognitive/behavioral therapy in the treatment of elderly outpatients with mild-to-moderate depression. *Am J Geriatr Psychiatry.* 2001;9:225–240.

Tohen M, Castillo J, Baldessarini RJ, Zarate V, Kando JC. Blood dyscrasias with carbamazepine and valproate: a pharmacoepidemiological study of 2,228 patients at risk. *Am J Psychiatry.* 1995;152:413–418.

Tollefson GD, Bosomworth JC, Heiligenstein JH, Potvin JH, Holman S. A double-blind, placebo-controlled clinical trial of fluoxetine in geriatric patients with major depression. The Fluoxetine Collaborative Study Group. *Int Psychogeriatr.* 1995;7:89–104.

Unutzer J, Katon W, Russo J, et al. Patterns of care for depressed older adults in a large-staff model HMO. *Am J Geriatr Psychiatry.* 1999;7:235–243.

Unutzer J, Katon W, Sullivan M, Miranda J. Treating depressed older adults in primary care: narrowing the gap between efficacy and effectiveness. *Milbank Q.* 1999;77:225–256, 174.

van Duijn CM, Clayton DG, Chandra V, et al. Interaction between genetic and environmental risk factors for Alzheimer's disease: a reanalysis of case-control studies. *Genet Epidemiol.* 1994;11:539–551.

Van Laar MW, Van Willigenburg APP, Volkerts ER. Acute and subchronic effects of nefazodone and imipramine on highway driving, cognitive function, and daytime sleepiness in healthy adult and elderly subjects. *J Clin Psychopharmacol.* 1995;15:30–40.

Volpe FM, Tavares A. Impact of ECT on duration of hospitalization for mania. *J ECT.* 2003;19:17–21.

von Korff M, Omel J, Katon W, Lin EHB. Disability and depression among high utilizers of health care: a longitudinal analysis. *Arch Gen Psychiatry.* 1992;49:91–100.

Wallace J, Pfohl B. Age-related differences in the symptomatic expression of major depression. *J Nerv Ment Dis.* 1995;183:99–102.

Wells KB, Burman MA. Caring for depression in America: lessons learned from early findings of the Medical Outcomes Study. *Psychiatr Med.* 1991;9:503–519.

Wells KB, Burman MA, Rogers W, Hays R, Camp P. The course of depression in adult outpatients. Results from the medical outcomes study. *Arch Gen Psychiatry.* 1992;49:788–794.

Wells KB, Stewart A, Hays RD, et al. The functioning and well-being of depressed patients: results from the medical outcomes study. *JAMA.* 1989;262:914–919.

West CG, Reed DM, Gildengorin GL. Can money buy happiness? Depressive symptoms in an affluent older population. *J Am Geriatr Soc.* 1998;46:49–57.

Wiener P, Alexopoulos GS, Kakuma T, Meyers BS, Rosendhal E, Chester J. The limits of history taking in geriatric depression. *Am J Geriatr Psychiatry*. 1997;5:116–125.

Wilson KC, Chen R, Taylor S, McCracken CF, Copeland JR. Socio-economic deprivation and the prevalence and prediction of depression in older community residents. The MRC-ALPHA Study. *Br J Psychiatry*. 1999;175:549–553.

Wragg RE, Jeste DV. Overview of depression and psychosis in Alzheimer's disease. *Am J Psychiatry*. 1989;146:577–589.

Yaffe K, Blackwell T, Gore R, Sands L, Reus V, Browner WS. Depressive symptoms and cognitive decline in nondemented elderly women: a prospective study. *Arch Gen Psychiatry*. 1999;56:425–430.

Yassa R, Cvejic J. Valproate in the treatment of post-traumatic bipolar disorder in a geriatric patient. *J Geriatr Psychiatry Neurol*. 1994;7:55–57.

Young RC, Klerman GL. Mania in late life: focus on age at onset. *Am J Psychiatry*. 1992;149:867–876.

Zisook S, Schuchter SR, Sledge R. Diagnostic and treatment considerations in depression associated with late-life bereavement. In: Schneider LS, Reynolds CF, Lebowitz BD, Friedhoff AJ, eds. *Diagnosis and Treatment of Depression in Late Life. Results of the NIH Consensus Development Conference*. Washington, DC: American Psychiatric Press; 1994:419-435.

Zubenko GS, Moosy J, Kopp U. Neurochemical correlates of major depression in primary dementia. *Arch Neurol*. 1990;47:209–214.

22

Psychoses

Dilip V. Jeste, MD
Laura B. Dunn, MD
Laurie A. Lindamer, PhD

Psychoses are among the most serious psychiatric disorders in any age group, including the elderly. These disorders are characterized by delusions, hallucinations, thought disorder, bizarre behavior, or other evidence of loss of touch with reality. Most types of psychosis that occur in younger persons can be seen in older patients. There are, however, some important epidemiological and clinical differences between early-onset and late-onset psychoses. In older patients, secondary psychoses (due to underlying medical or neurological conditions) are more common than primary psychotic disorders. The most common type of chronic secondary psychosis in this population is psychosis related to dementia. This chapter deals with psychosis of Alzheimer's disease (AD) and other dementias and the prototypical primary psychotic disorders, such as schizophrenia and delusional disorder; secondary psychotic illnesses due to other general medical conditions and mood disorders with psychotic features are described elsewhere. We will then discuss the prototypical primary psychotic disorders such as schizophrenia and delusional disorder.

PSYCHOSIS OF ALZHEIMER'S DISEASE AND OTHER DEMENTIAS

Alzheimer's disease is the most common type of dementia in the elderly. A sizable proportion of patients with AD manifest psychotic symptoms and disruptive behaviors, frequently resulting in substantial distress to family members and caregivers. In a retrospective review of over 1,700 consecutive admissions to a psychogeriatric unit, Webster and Grossberg (1998) found that 10% of cases exhibited late-life onset of psychotic symptoms; of these cases, 40% were caused by AD or vascular dementia.

Psychosis of AD is believed to be a distinct syndrome that differs markedly from schizophrenia in older patients (Jeste & Finkel, 2000). A number of neuropsychological and neurobiological differences between patients with AD with and without psychosis have been reported. A greater prevalence of extrapyramidal symptoms (EPS) and a more rapid rate of cognitive decline have been reported in patients with AD with psychosis compared to patients with AD without psychosis (Stern et al., 1994); greater impairment on neuropsychological tests of frontal lobe functioning has also been reported in patients with AD with psychosis compared to those without (Jeste et al., 1992). Other kinds of dysfunction in the frontal temporal cortex (e.g., greater cholinergic loss) have also been associated with delusions in dementia (Sultzer, 1996).

The presence of psychosis in patients with AD has been shown to have important clinical correlates: psychosis in patients with AD is associated with an increased risk of aggressive behavior, wandering, agitation, disruptive behavior, family problems, and lack of self-care in comparison with patients with AD without psychosis (Rockwell, Jackson, et al., 1994). This may help explain the high rate of institutionalization among patients with AD with delusions (Steele et al., 1990; Stern et al., 1997).

When delusions are present, the *Diagnostic and Statistical Manual of Mental Disorders, Fourth Edition (DSM-IV)* recommends, but does not provide criteria for, coding them as a predominant feature of dementia (American Psychiatric Association [APA], 1994a). The text revision to the *DSM-IV (DSM-IV-TR)* now provides for coding of psychotic features in AD using the additional diagnosis of psychotic disorder due to Alzheimer's disease, with delusions (or hallucinations) (APA, 2000).

Moreover, diagnostic criteria for psychosis of AD and related dementias have recently been proposed to further epidemiological and treatment studies of these phenomena (Jeste & Finkel, 2000). The criteria require (1) a primary diagnosis of AD, (2) the presence of hallucinations (visual or auditory) or delusions (not present prior to the diagnosis of AD), (3) a duration of psychotic symptoms at least intermittently for 1 month or longer, and (4) symptoms "severe enough to cause some disruption in functioning" (Jeste & Finkel, 2000, p. 32). Exclusion criteria include ever having met criteria for schizophrenia or a related psychotic disorder (including mood disorder with psychotic features), occurrence of psychotic symptoms during the course of a delirium, or the presence of other causes of psychotic symptoms, such as a general medical condition or medication-induced psychosis. Specifiable associated features are "with agitation," "with negative symptoms" (e.g., apathy, avolition, or motor slowing), or "with depression" (when prominent depressive symptoms are present). It is hoped that these criteria will spur and enable research to further the understanding of the epidemiology, clinical course, and treatment potential for these disabling symptoms.

Dementias other than AD are also associated with psychosis. Dementia with Lewy bodies (DLB), considered to be the second most common cause of dementia, is frequently associated with prominent visual hallucinations and, often, secondary delusions (Schneider, 1999). Patients with DLB may have a higher prevalence of hallucinations and delusions compared to patients with AD (Rockwell et al., 2000). Vascular dementia also may be associated with hallucinations or delusions.

Psychotic symptoms (delusions and hallucinations) were found in approximately one third of a sample of patients with Parkinson's disease (PD) (Naimark et al., 1996). These psychoses have been usefully classified into six syndromes: (1) hallucinations with preserved insight, (2) medication-induced psychotic disorders (with clear consciousness), (3) delirium, (4) schizophrenia-like psychotic disorders (with clear consciousness and in the absence of medication treatment), (5) schizophrenia with subsequent development of PD, and (6) other psychotic disorders (Peyser et al., 1998). In the second syndrome, medication-induced psychotic disorders, dopaminergic agents can place patients at risk for development of psychotic symptoms. In these cases, hallucinations and delusions may occur with partial or total lack of insight. Patients frequently show no other evidence of a thought disorder or a delirium.

Prevalence

In 329 patients with clinically diagnosed probable AD, Paulsen and colleagues (2000) found a cumulative incidence of new-onset psychotic symptoms of 20% at 1 year, 36% at 2 years, 50% at 3 years, and 51% at 4 years. Estimates of the prevalence of psychotic symptoms in patients with AD range from approximately 30% to 50% (Jeste & Finkel, 2000). In a review of psychiatric features occurring in patients with AD, Wragg and Jeste (1989) noted that about 30% of patients (range 10%–73%) exhibited delusions, often of a persecutory nature. Hallucinations were reported to occur in about 21%–49% of the patients, with a tendency toward a higher incidence in hospitalized and nursing home populations.

Diagnosis and Symptomatology

Psychotic symptoms in the demented patient may present as disordered perception and thought content. Delusions are usually concrete, simple, paranoid, and nonbizarre and may be stimulated by environmental stress. The more common types of delusions refer to specific persons stealing things or spying on the patient or someone impersonating the spouse or a significant other (Burns et al., 1990). Complex, elaborate, or systematized delusions that characterize schizophrenia or delusional disorder are rarely seen in patients with AD. Because of cognitive impairment, the patient may be unable to verbalize thoughts or perceptions properly. In such cases, the occurrence of delusions or hallucinations can only be inferred from the patient's behavior (e.g., responses to a visual or auditory hallucination). Visual hallucinations are somewhat more frequent than auditory hallucinations. Patients with PD with psychosis appear to be more likely to experience hallucinations than delusions (Naimark et al., 1996).

Pathogenesis/Etiology

As discussed above, psychotic symptoms in AD have been reported to be associated with specific neuropsychiatric features, including an increased incidence of extrapyramidal signs and cognitive decline, frontotemporal dysfunction, and visual and auditory deficits. Psychotic symptoms appear to be more common in the middle stages of AD. Other investigators have reported that patients with AD and psychosis had increased densities of senile plaques, neurofibrillary tangles, and paired helical filament (PHF)–tau protein in specific cortical areas compared to patients with AD without psychosis (Mukaetova-Ladinska et al., 1995; Zubenko et al., 1991).

Differential Diagnosis

In patients with dementia, it is not uncommon for psychotic symptoms to develop due to intervening medical illnesses or the use of any of numerous medications. Prior to initiating a treatment plan, these potential causes or exacerbating factors should be investigated by psychiatric and medical history, physical examination, review of medications, and laboratory testing as indicated. Collateral information from family or caregivers is often crucial in a careful evaluation. The onset of AD or other dementing illness prior to the development of psychotic symptoms should help differentiate these patients from elderly patients with schizophrenia or delusional disorder who have subsequently developed some cognitive impairment.

Treatment

Until the introduction of the atypical antipsychotic medications, the primary pharmacological treatment for psychosis of AD and other dementias involved the use of conventional neuroleptics. Although past studies of the treatment of psychosis in dementia were hampered by methodological limitations, including high dropout rates secondary to drug side effects and short study duration, conventional neuroleptics were shown to be at least moderately effective in the management of psychotic or agitated patients with dementia.

Several important considerations now limit the use of conventional neuroleptics in the elderly. These agents carry a significant risk of undesirable side effects, particularly EPS and tardive dyskinesia. The risk of EPS is higher in elderly patients compared to younger patients on administration of a given amount of neuroleptic (Jeste et al., 1999). Furthermore, the incidence of persistent tardive dyskinesia has been shown to be much higher in patients who begin treatment with conventional neuroleptics in later life (Jeste, Caligiuri et al., 1995). Other side effects that are of particular concern in elderly patients include anticholinergic and cardiovascular effects. The clinician should advise the patient and family of the possibility of adverse effects, including sedation, anticholinergic effects, parkinsonian reactions, postural hypotension, neuroleptic malignant syndrome, and tardive dyskinesia, and evaluate the patient frequently to detect these side effects. Periodic assessment (at least once every several months) for the emergence of involuntary movements is also recommended.

Although data are still somewhat limited, the atypical antipsychotics, including risperidone, olanzapine, quetiapine, ziprasidone, and clozapine, have emerged in recent years as promising agents for the pharmacological treatment of psychosis and severe agitation in patients with dementia. While the atypical agents are generally well tolerated by older individuals, recommended dose ranges are considerably lower than for younger patients; dose titration should also be carried out more gradually in older patients. In addition, starting and maintenance doses should be even lower for elderly patients with psychosis complicating AD or other dementias than for older patients with schizophrenia (Jeste et al., 1999).

Several large, placebo-controlled trials of the treatment of AD accompanied by psychosis or severe agitation reported that risperidone and olanzapine were associated with significant improvements and were well tolerated at appropriately low doses (Katz et al., 1999; Street, Clark, et al., 2000). Katz and associates compared 0.5, 1, and 2 mg of risperidone per day with placebo in nursing home patients. While the 1-mg and 2-mg doses were each more effective than placebo in the treatment of psychosis and aggressive behavior, the 2-mg dose was associated with greater risk of EPS. De Deyn and associates (1999) compared the efficacy and tolerability of haloperidol, risperidone, and placebo and found greater reduction in aggressive behaviors in patients receiving risperidone compared to those on haloperidol or placebo. Street and colleagues compared placebo to 5, 10, and 15 mg per day of olanzapine for the treatment of AD-related psychosis and behavioral disturbances in nursing home patients; 5 mg per day was the most effective dose in this population.

Side effects of atypical antipsychotic medications that occur with clinically significant frequency include sedation (particularly with clozapine, olanzapine, and quetiapine), orthostatic hypotension, and, at higher dose ranges, EPS (especially with risperidone). The risk of developing tardive dyskinesia is likely to be much lower for patients taking atypical antipsychotics than for patients taking typical antipsychotic medications (Jeste, 2000).

For example, in a large, open-label, multisite trial of risperidone in the treatment of dementia (AD, vascular, or mixed), Jeste and colleagues found a 1-year cumulative incidence of persistent emergent tardive dyskinesia of 2.6%, a rate much lower than has been reported in elderly patients taking conventional neuroleptics (Jeste et al., 2000). In this study, the average optimal daily dose of risperidone was 0.75 to 1.5 mg per day. Long-term side effects that are of concern include weight gain and the risk of developing hyperglycemia and new-onset diabetes (Allison et al., 1999; Wirshing et al., 1998).

Although effective, particularly for PD-related psychosis, the use of clozapine in older individuals is considered problematic because of the risk of leukopenia and agranulocytosis and the substantial risk of orthostasis, sedation, and anticholinergic effects. In addition, the necessity of weekly blood draws may make compliance difficult for some elderly patients.

In patients with psychosis associated with dementia with Lewy bodies, caution is warranted when prescribing antipsychotic medications. These patients are particularly sensitive to antipsychotic medications: a severe neuroleptic sensitivity syndrome can develop in which patients can experience severe parkinsonism, autonomic instability, falls, and even death (a 3-fold increase in mortality has been reported) (Campbell et al., 2001; McKeith et al., 2000). Dosages of antipsychotics, even the atypical ones, thus generally should be even lower than those used in patients with AD. Anticholinergic medications also are more likely to cause side effects in these patients and so should be avoided as much as possible (Stoppe et al., 1999). Some studies, most of them small, indicate potential benefits of cholinesterase inhibitors for improvement of psychotic symptoms in patients with DLB; some investigators would recommend these as first-line agents given the hazards associated with antipsychotic use (Campbell et al., 2001; McKeith et al., 2000).

Patients with parkinsonian dementia also are more vulnerable to EPS. For Parkinson-related psychosis, clozapine has demonstrated efficacy at reducing psychotic symptoms without worsening motor function; there is also evidence that clozapine may improve resting and postural tremor in some patients (Bonuccelli et al., 1997; Masand, 2000). It is important that very low initial doses (e.g., 6.25 mg per day) and target doses (e.g., 50 mg per day) and very slow titration schedules be used to avoid adverse effects on motor symptoms.

Initial studies (with small numbers of enrolled patients) on the potential of olanzapine to treat PD-related psychosis have been inconsistent, with some investigators finding symptomatic improvement, but worsened parkinsonism (Graham et al., 1998), and still others reporting that low doses of olanzapine were associated with a decrease in psychotic symptoms and no worsening of parkinsonian symptoms (Wolters et al., 1996). Early studies of quetiapine for the treatment of PD-related psychosis suggest that this agent improves psychotic symptoms and does not worsen motor functioning (Yeung et al., 2000). As newer atypical antipsychotics continue to be introduced, further investigation of their effectiveness and tolerability for these conditions is warranted.

A number of other, non-antipsychotic pharmacological options have been used with varying success in patients with dementia and psychosis, although these options have generally been recommended for the treatment of agitation rather than for delusions or hallucinations per se. It is important to document the specific problematic behaviors and monitor these carefully during any trial with one of these pharmacotherapeutic agents. These agents include antidepressants such as citalopram, trazodone, and sertraline; mood stabilizers such as valproic acid and carbamazepine; and anxiolytics such as benzodiazepines and buspirone (Tariot, 1996). Most studies of the use of these medications in patients with dementia have been small and uncontrolled, however. Further research is needed to clarify the potential roles of these treatments in the management of dementia with psychosis or agitation.

Recently, several investigators have focused on the potential effectiveness of cholinergic agents for the treatment of psychosis and behavioral disturbances in patients with AD. Cummings and colleagues (2000) assessed the potential role of the cholinesterase inhibitor donepezil in a large cross-sectional study of community-dwelling patients with AD. In 84 patients who had taken donepezil for 6 months, caregiver-reported behavioral disturbances were significantly less severe compared to those of 248 patients not taking donepezil. In particular, caregivers reported that patients taking donepezil displayed the following behaviors significantly less often than patients not taking donepezil: threatening to hurt others, talking loudly and rapidly, and destroying property. The newest approved cholinesterase inhibitors, rivastigmine and galantamine, also have shown promise in initial placebo-controlled studies for the treatment of psychosis and behavioral disturbances in patients with AD (Kindermann et al., 2002; Olin & Schneider, 2001; Tariot et al., 2000).

Donepezil has also been studied for potential utility in the treatment of cognitive deficits and psychopathology in patients with DLB. In a small study, Samuel and colleagues (2000) found that, compared to patients with AD, those with DLB demonstrated significantly greater cognitive improvement over a 6-month period. Patients with DLB also showed significantly greater declines in paranoid and delusional ideation and affective disturbance compared to the patients with AD. Similar results were obtained by McKeith and colleagues (2000) in a placebo-controlled study of the effects of rivastigmine on 120 patients with DLB; those receiving active treatment had significantly fewer delusions and hallucinations and less apathy and anxiety while on medication compared to those taking placebo.

Nonpharmacological interventions also can be beneficial. Evaluating the patient's environment for potentially modifiable factors that may be exacerbating symptoms is an important first step. Supportive psychotherapy may be beneficial for patients in the earlier stages of dementia, and behavioral management can be valuable in various stages of the illness. Families can benefit considerably from support, education, and assistance with appropriate ways of coping with the afflicted family member.

Course and Prognosis

Although there have been few systematic studies of the course of psychosis of AD, some naturalistic data exist. In a large, prospective study of the course of psychopathology in patients with early-stage AD followed for up to 5 years, Devanand and colleagues (1997) reported on the likelihood of the development and persistence of behavioral disturbance and psychotic symptoms. These investigators found that behavioral disturbances, particularly agitation, had the greatest likelihood of developing and persisting. Hallucinations and paranoid delusions showed a moderate degree of persistence and were more likely than depressive symptoms to continue over time.

After the early stages of dementia, however, symptom patterns may change. As the severity of the dementia increases, psychotic symptoms tend to decrease (Cummings et al., 1987). This apparent remission may represent a "pseudo-remission," rather than a real one, because patients in the later stages of AD may lack the cognitive and verbal abilities to express their delusions or hallucinations.

The prognosis for psychosis and behavioral disturbances associated with AD and other dementias can be improved through the use of appropriate interventions such as those described above. Medications should not be prescribed indefinitely, however, especially given the possibility of improvement in psychotic symptoms as dementia progresses.

LATE-ONSET SCHIZOPHRENIA

Historical Background

A century ago, Kraepelin (1919/1971) used the term *dementia praecox* to refer to a disorder we now know as schizophrenia. Dementia praecox suggested an onset in youth and a deterioration of function in the "emotional and volitional spheres of mental life"(p. 3). Kraepelin later came to doubt the appropriateness of his terminology because the "dementia" of dementia praecox was not always accompanied by permanent deterioration; remissions seemed to occur in some cases. In addition, not all of the patients first presented symptoms in youth. There was a subset of patients with onset of symptoms well into the fifth, sixth, or seventh decades of life. Kraepelin applied the diagnosis of paraphrenia to those patients with a (usually, but not always) relatively late onset of delusions and hallucinations, characterized by a predominance of paranoid symptoms. Although Kraepelin stressed the disintegration of personality in dementia praecox as opposed to paraphrenia, he described some patients with paraphrenia who had a predominantly downhill course, while a subset of patients with dementia praecox did not suffer a marked deterioration in social and personal functioning. Indeed, follow-up studies of Kraepelin's patients with paraphrenia by other investigators indicated that some of the patients diagnosed as having paraphrenia had features similar to those of dementia praecox (Mayer, 1921).

The initial classification systems, *DSM-I* and *DSM-II* (APA, 1952, 1968), did not include age at onset of schizophrenia as a criterion. It was not until the *DSM-III* (APA, 1980) that it was first stipulated that the onset of symptoms for schizophrenia must be before age 45 years. *DSM-III-R* (APA, 1987), on the other hand, allowed an onset of schizophrenic symptoms after age 45 years and used the terminology late-onset schizophrenia for diagnosing these individuals. None of the *DSM* systems included paraphrenia as a diagnostic entity. Most recently, *DSM-IV* (APA, 1994b) eliminated altogether any age cutoff for the diagnosis of schizophrenia.

Recent studies suggest that schizophrenia with onset in middle age is similar in a number of important ways to early-onset schizophrenia, yet represents a distinct subtype of the disorder (Jeste et al., 1997; Palmer et al., 2001; Pearlson et al., 1993). In particular, patients with late-onset schizophrenia (onset after age 40 or 45 years) are similar to those with early-onset schizophrenia in terms of clinical features (Howard et al., 1993), family history, neuropsychological characteristics, and brain imaging findings; at the same time, there are interesting gender and other differences.

Some researchers (Andreasen, 1999) believe that psychotic symptoms that emerge for the first time after 40 years of age represent not schizophrenia, but rather a late-onset psychosis arising from heterogeneous causes. As evidence of this assertion, it is stated that, in contrast to the typical constellation of clinical features seen in early-onset schizophrenia, patients with the onset of psychotic symptoms after age 40 years usually lack predominant negative symptoms (particularly affective blunting) or thought disorder. In addition, because patients with the onset of psychosis in very late life (i.e., the seventh and eighth decades) often have structural brain diseases (e.g., strokes or tumors), the psychotic symptoms may represent a neurodegenerative disease mechanism.

A neurodegenerative model would be used to explain a disorder in which an individual begins to exhibit symptoms in adulthood, after previously established normal neurobiological development, and there are progressive neurodegenerative changes. A neurodevelopmental model, on the other hand, would posit that the disorder results from abnormal brain development—that is, it is rooted in brain insults (e.g., malnutrition, infection) or lesions occurring during the pre- or perinatal period of neurobiological development or even, as some have proposed, may result from abnormal synaptic pruning during adolescence (i.e., later in development).

Murray, Castle, and colleagues (Castle & Murray, 1993; Murray et al., 1992) suggest that a neurodegenerative model would explain late-onset schizophrenia. However, studies by Jeste and colleagues (Jeste et al., 1997) and others, supported in a recent international consensus statement (Howard et al., 2000) favor the notion that schizophrenia with onset in middle age (onset after 40 years of age) is likely to be neurodevelopmental in origin, while schizophrenia-like psychosis with a very late onset (onset after 60 years of age) represents a heterogeneous group of neurodegenerative conditions.

This consensus panel concluded that these diagnoses have both face validity and clinical utility (Howard et al., 2000). The agreed-upon terminology, however, is meant to clarify these patients' diagnoses and to spur research efforts rather than to serve as a definitive statement about the etiology, pathophysiology, course, or outcome of these entities. It should also be noted that the consensus panel did not achieve unanimity in deciding on specific age cutoffs (e.g., 40 or 60 years). Clearly, further research is needed to delineate better the spectrum of disorders that can present with psychotic symptoms in middle age and later.

Epidemiology

Although the literature on late-onset schizophrenia dates to 1913, several important problems exist with its interpretation. No general agreement on the definition of late onset has existed, with some studies choosing 40 years of age and others evaluating patients with onset after 45, 60, or 65 years of age. Other problems include a lack of consistency in diagnostic criteria for schizophrenia and the frequent difficulty of defining the age of onset of schizophrenia.

A review by Harris and Jeste (1988) that analyzed data from the psychiatric literature estimated that 13% of all hospitalized schizophrenic patients were reported to have onset of the illness in their 40s, 7% experienced onset in their 50s, and 3% first presented after 60 years of age. Based on the epidemiologic catchment area data, Keith and colleagues (1991) estimated a 0.6% 1-year prevalence rate of schizophrenia in individuals between 45 and 64 years of age. Rates of schizophrenia in people older than 65 years range from 0.1% to 0.5% (Howard et al., 2000). Some investigators have suggested that the prevalence of late-onset schizophrenia may be higher as most of the studies have used treated samples of patients; many patients with paranoid symptoms, however, may not seek treatment (Castle, 1999).

Most studies of late-onset schizophrenia show a 2 to 10 times higher proportion of women compared to men (Bland, 1977; Bleuler, 1943; Castle & Murray, 1993; Kay & Roth, 1961). The observed differences between men and women in age of onset, clinical course, and outcome have led some researchers to propose that there may be distinct subtypes of schizophrenia in men and women.

Lewine (1981) discussed this possibility, as well as the alternative possibility of a timing model of schizophrenia. According to the subtype model, men are differentially susceptible to a typical subtype of the illness, involving an early onset, while women are more susceptible to the atypical subtype, more frequently characterized by a later onset (Lewine, 1981). According to the alternative, timing model, men and women have either an earlier (in men) or delayed (in women) onset of schizophrenia because of biological or psychosocial gender differences. Several factors, such as neuroendocrine changes, greater longevity of women, psychosocial stressors, and differences in care-seeking and role expectations, have been suggested as possible explanations for the higher prevalence of late-onset schizophrenia in women. Psychosocial factors such as care-seeking and role expectations have not been shown, however, to be important determinants of gender differences.

Diagnosis

The patient should meet all the *DSM-IV* (APA, 1994b) criteria for schizophrenia, with the additional requirement that onset of symptoms, including the prodrome, must occur at or after age 40 years (Howard et al., 2000). It is important to note that there is no universally agreed-on age cutoff for diagnosing late-onset schizophrenia. While *DSM-III-R* (APA, 1987) used 45 years as the age criterion, a recent international consensus panel chose 40 years of age. It is important to make certain that there were no prodromal symptoms of schizophrenia (e.g., marked social isolation, blunted or inappropriate affect, marked impairment in personal hygiene, etc.) occurring before the specified age to exclude earlier-onset schizophrenia. Documentation of a decrease in functioning markedly below the highest level achieved may be difficult in older patients, who may be retired, widowed, or socially less active.

Symptomatology

Delusions and hallucinations are the most prominent psychotic symptoms in patients with late-onset schizophrenia. While patients with late-onset schizophrenia have symptoms similar to those of patients with an early onset, some differences have been noted. Compared to patients with early-onset schizophrenia, those with late-onset schizophrenia are more likely to have paranoid schizophrenia. Formal thought disorder and inappropriate, flattened, or blunted affect are present, but tend to be less prominent than in younger patients with schizophrenia (Howard et al., 2000; Jeste et al., 1988).

Etiology and Pathophysiology

The etiology and pathophysiology of late-onset schizophrenia are not well understood. The following aspects have been explored in some detail: genetics, premorbid personality, neuropsychology, brain imaging, and sensory deficits.

GENETICS Studies that have examined the prevalence of schizophrenia in families of patients with late-onset schizophrenia have had methodological problems (Harris & Jeste, 1988). For example, not all family members have been followed into old age to ensure that every case of late-onset schizophrenia in other family members is detected. Physical illness and geographic relocation of relatives also make it difficult to conduct such studies. Some studies suggest that the prevalence of schizophrenia is approximately 7% in siblings and 3% in parents of all probands with late-onset schizophrenia (Bleuler, 1943; Herbert & Jacobson, 1967; Kay & Roth, 1961; Larson & Nyman, 1970; Rokhlina, 1975). Other studies have found a higher prevalence of family history of schizophrenia, with approximately 10% to 15% of patients with middle-age onset having a first-degree relative with schizophrenia (Jeste, Harris, et al., 1995; Jeste et al., 1997). In patients with schizophrenia-like psychosis with a very late onset (after 60 years of age), available data do not support a genetic association with schizophrenia in first-degree relatives (Howard et al., 1997).

PREMORBID PERSONALITY   Some studies (Herbert & Jacobson, 1967; Kay & Roth, 1961) noted that a sizable proportion of patients with late-onset schizophrenia had abnormal premorbid personality traits of a paranoid or schizoid nature. Many patients were never married and were considered by neighbors to be eccentric. Nevertheless, when compared to patients with earlier-onset schizophrenia, those whose onset was in middle age are more likely to have been married, held a job, and have children (Jeste, Harris, et al., 1995).

NEUROPSYCHOLOGY   Heaton and colleagues (1994) compared neuropsychological performance of patients with late-onset schizophrenia with that of two groups of patients with early-onset schizophrenia (currently younger than 45 years and older than 45 years), patients with AD, and normal older comparison subjects. The three schizophrenia groups performed more poorly than the normal comparison subjects on each of the neuropsychological ability areas except for memory; no schizophrenia group showed memory (delayed recall) impairment. In contrast, the AD group was worse than the normal comparison group on memory as well as on all the other ability areas. Furthermore, the AD group demonstrated greater learning and memory impairments than the schizophrenia groups; the three schizophrenia groups did not differ from one another. Another study compared, using the Mini-Mental State Examination (MMSE) and Mattis's Dementia Rating Scale (DRS), the rates of change over 1 year of patients with late-onset schizophrenia and patients with AD (Palmer et al., 2000). While patients with AD lost a mean of 3.5 points on the MMSE and 13.6 points on the DRS, those with late-onset schizophrenia gained a mean of 0.5 points on the MMSE and 0.22 points on the DRS. These data suggest that cognitive deficits in most patients with late-onset schizophrenia are nonprogressive.

Other studies have found certain differences between patients with early-onset and those with late-onset schizophrenia. For instance, semantic memory organization was found to be significantly impaired in patients with early onset, but almost normal in patients with late onset (Paulsen et al., 1996). Other research has reported that patients with late-onset schizophrenia demonstrate less severe impairments in learning, psychomotor tasks, and abstraction compared to patients with early-onset schizophrenia, while the overall pattern of cognitive impairments in the two groups is similar (Jeste et al., 1997).

BRAIN IMAGING   Although the available data are relatively limited, findings tend to support the notion that patients with both early-onset and late-onset schizophrenia show similar nonspecific structural brain abnormalities (Jeste et al., 1997; Pearlson, 1999). Several groups of investigators have reported that patients with late-onset schizophrenia have increased ventricle-to-brain ratios by magnetic resonance imaging (MRI) or computerized tomographic (CT) scan (Krull et al., 1991; Naguib & Levy, 1987; Rabins, 1989) as well as third-ventricle enlargement (Pearlson et al., 1993). Other investigators have found similarities between patients with early-onset and late-onset schizophrenia in reduced superior temporal gyrus size (Pearlson et al., 1997). On the other hand, Barta and colleagues (1997) compared patients with late-onset schizophrenia to age-matched patients with Alzheimer's disease and found that the patients with schizophrenia showed a greater reduction of volume in both superior temporal gyri compared to those patients with AD. Together, these findings suggest that changes in the superior temporal lobes in patients with late-onset schizophrenia are similar to those seen in patients with early-onset schizophrenia.

Electroencephalographic (EEG) evidence indicates that patients with late-onset schizophrenia do not have an underlying dementing illness: in a study comparing patients with late-onset schizophrenia with age-matched healthy controls, the patients with late onset had similar electroencephalograms, except for having more generalized slowing. This slowing was thought to be accounted for, at least in part, by the effects of antipsychotic medications (Sachdev et al., 1999).

Several reports have also documented large areas of subcortical white matter hyperintensities (in the periventricular regions as well as elsewhere) in patients with late-onset schizophrenia and related psychoses compared to age-matched normal comparison subjects (Breitner et al., 1990; Coffey et al., 1990; Lesser et al., 1991, 1992; Miller et al., 1991; Miller & Lesser, 1988) and to patients with early-onset schizophrenia (Tonkonogy & Geller, 1999). In addition, some reports have noted an increased number of vascular lesions in patients with a variety of late-life psychoses (Breitner et al., 1990; Flint et al., 1991). Other investigators, however, have not found differences in white matter hyperintensities between patients with late onset and those with early onset or normal comparison subjects (Symonds et al., 1997). Thus, the consistency of such findings and their possible etiopathological significance for late-onset cases is yet to be determined.

In the few studies of functional brain imaging conducted in patients with late-onset schizophrenia, single-photon emission computed tomography (SPECT) findings have revealed lower global cortical uptake (particularly in the left posterior frontal region and bilateral inferior temporal regions) in late-life schizo-phrenic patients than in normal comparison subjects (Dupont et al., 1994; Lesser et al., 1993). The uptake did not correlate with age of onset, duration of illness, current daily neuroleptic dose, severity of psychopathology, or global cognitive impairment. In a study of positron emission tomography (PET) in late-onset schizophrenia, Pearlson and colleagues (1993) reported elevated B_{max} (receptor density) values for dopamine D_2 receptors in 13 patients who were antipsychotic naive with late-onset schizophrenia compared to age and gender norms; this indicated that the higher D_2 values in the patients were not second-ary to antipsychotic effects. Thus, important questions remain regarding the possible pathogenetic significance of the brain abnormalities associated with late-onset schizophrenia.

SENSORY DEFICITS   Several studies have reported an association between sensory impairment and late-onset schizophrenia. One review found that over 85% (23/27) of published studies suggested a positive association between sensory (visual or hearing) impairment and a somewhat heterogeneous group of late-life psychoses with paranoid symptoms (Prager & Jeste, 1993). Methodological limitations in much of the available literature, however, require caution when making generalizations regarding the relative contribution of sensory deficits to late-onset schizophrenia.

Prager and Jeste (1993) found that, although middle-aged and elderly patients with early-onset schizophrenia, late-onset schizophrenia, or mood dis-orders had greater impairments on measures of corrected visual acuity and in self-reported hearing deficits compared to normal comparison subjects, impair-ment levels on uncorrected visual acuity or on pure-tone audiometry were simi-lar to those of the normal comparison group. These findings suggest that the observed relationship between sensory deficits and late-life psychosis may be due, at least in part, to inadequate correction of sensory deficits (e.g., not get-ting the appropriate eyeglasses) in older psychiatric patients. Although a causal relationship between sensory impairment and late-life psychosis remains to be elucidated, interventions designed to increase correction of sensory impairment in the elderly could be potentially effective in decreasing the morbidity of late-life psychotic disorders.

Differential Diagnosis

Whenever an aged patient presents with psychotic symptoms, pathology related to medical illnesses or medications must first be ruled out. This is especially important because a number of medical illnesses (for example, electrolyte im-balances, thyroid disorders, Parkinson's disease, hyperglycemia, urinary tract infections, and delirium) can present with psychotic symptoms (Webster & Grossberg, 1998). Many medications also can place elderly patients at risk for the development of psychotic symptoms, mediated primarily through delirium.

Commonly found causes include alcohol and benzodiazepines. A careful neuro-logical examination accompanied by complete blood chemistry, including tests of thyroid function and vitamin deficiencies (e.g., B_{12} and folic acid), CT or MRI of the brain, as well as serological tests for syphilis, are usually part of the assessment. Other appropriate laboratory tests may be needed in individual patients (see Chapter 11).

Another important differential diagnosis is early-onset schizophrenia. It is prudent to obtain a detailed history of the disorder from the patient as well the patient's family or friends because some patients may have had prodromal or even overt psychotic symptoms for some time prior to the first hospitalization. The prodrome differs from premorbid personality traits in that it requires clear deterioration from a previous level of functioning. Also, some patients with an apparently late-onset psychosis may have had a more benign psychotic illness that never required hospitalization until age 40 or 45 years.

Mood disorders with psychotic features may present for the first time in middle or old age and can be confused with late-onset schizophrenia. The pre-dominance of affective symptoms and periodicity of the illness should lead the clinician to consider a mood disorder.

Delusional disorder may mimic late-onset schizophrenia, but the latter diagnosis is more likely in the presence of bizarre delusions or prominent audi-tory hallucinations, Schneiderian first-rank symptoms, deteriorated function-ing, and flattening of affect (see the section on late-life delusional disorder for further discussion).

Treatment

The general principles outlined in the section on treatment of dementia-related psychoses apply. Available studies have suggested that a majority of patients with late-onset schizophrenia improve symptomatically with appropriate phar-macotherapy (Jeste et al., 1996). The newer, atypical antipsychotic medications such as risperidone, olanzapine, and quetiapine have become the treatment of choice for schizophrenia and other psychoses in both older and younger patients due to their efficacy and a reduced risk of both EPS and tardive dyskinesia.

In studies of mainly younger patients with schizophrenia, the atypical agents have been shown to be effective for the treatment of positive and nega-tive symptoms (Howard et al., 2000; McClure & Jeste, 1999). While data on the use of these medications in older patients have recently begun to be col-lected, treatment studies of older patients with schizophrenia have primarily enrolled patients with early-onset schizophrenia. Nevertheless, the findings should be generalizable to patients with late-onset schizophrenia, with the ca-veat that patients with late onset generally require even lower doses of antipsy-chotic medications than age-comparable patients with early onset.

In reviewing available literature on the use of risperidone in elderly patients with schizophrenia and related disorders, Madhusoodanan and associates (2000) concluded that available data support the use of this agent as a first-line pharmacological treatment for schizophrenia and related disorders in older patients. Olanzapine has also demonstrated overall efficacy and tolerability at an average daily dose of 12.4 mg in geriatric patients with schizophrenia (Street, Tollefson et al., 2000).

For patients with late-onset schizophrenia, the starting dose should generally be one quarter to one half of the usual adult starting dose; for patients over age 60 or those with schizoprenia-like psychosis of very late onset, even lower doses may be effective (Howard et al., 2000; Jeste, 2000). Since the introduction of the atypical antipsychotics, a frequent dilemma facing clinicians involves whether and how best to switch patients from a conventional to an atypical agent. Because of the high risk of relapse when antipsychotic drugs are withdrawn, it is recommended that the dose of the conventional neuroleptic be slowly titrated down while the atypical is slowly titrated up (Jeste et al., 1999). The lowest effective maintenance dose should be used once the patient is clinically stable.

Nonpharmacological treatment for schizophrenia is also indicated in the majority of cases. A large body of research, conducted primarily in younger patients with schizophrenia, has shown that psychosocial therapies for schizophrenia play a vital role in the treatment and rehabilitation of patients with schizophrenia, although further studies are warranted to clarify the most useful elements (or active ingredients) of these treatments, to improve matching of patients to treatments, to evaluate the best combinations of these treatments with one another and with pharmacological treatments, and to determine how best to consolidate treatment gains. In social skills training (SST), patients learn skills to improve social competence and problem solving. Interventions based on the SST model have demonstrated efficacy using a variety of outcome measures, including independent living skills and relapse rates; it appears that the benefits of SST may require "booster" sessions to be maintained (Lauriello et al., 1999).

Cognitive-behavioral therapy (CBT) for schizophrenia teaches patients to cope more adaptively with their symptoms, beliefs, and feelings. Patient and therapist work together to discuss symptoms, reduce emotional distress, and find alternative ways of viewing events or beliefs (e.g., a delusional belief would be reframed as one possible way of interpreting events). In a review of empirical studies of CBT for schizophrenia, the authors concluded that CBT showed some benefits for helping patients better cope with their symptoms, particularly delusions (Dickerson, 2000). Patients with more clearly focused symptoms and accompanying distress appeared to benefit the most. Again, it remains unclear how lasting and robust the gains made with CBT are, and the predictors of response to CBT need further clarification. Degree of insight into one's illness, for example, appears to be associated with response to CBT, but it is unclear whether severity of psychopathology is associated with treatment response.

Recent work has evaluated the benefits of a novel, integrated cognitive-behavioral, social skills training (CBSST) intervention in groups of older patients with primarily early-onset schizophrenia (McQuaid et al., 2000). As the name suggests, CBSST combines the SST elements of problem solving and role playing with the CBT techniques of thought identification and challenging. Results of a small, randomized controlled pilot study comparing CBSST plus pharmacotherapy to CBSST alone demonstrated the intervention's feasibility in an older population of patients with schizophrenia and suggested that augmentation of pharmacotherapy with CBSST may lead to further symptom reduction (Granholm et al., 2001).

Family interventions for schizophrenia have been studied extensively, mainly in younger patients. Numerous studies have shown the benefits of family interventions (lasting from 6 weeks to 9 months) for relapse prevention. Successful interventions utilizing various approaches have several underlying principles in common, including psychoeducation about schizophrenia, improving family assistance with medication adherence, and family stress reduction through communication skills and outreach to extended social support networks (Lauriello et al., 1999). Fruitful avenues for future research would include clarifying the active ingredients for efficacy of family interventions and exploring potential combinations of family interventions with other psychosocial interventions and pharmacotherapies.

Course and Prognosis

Studies of the course of late-onset schizophrenia have generally found it to be chronic. The risk of suicide in the first 10 years of the illness is elevated to a level approximately equivalent to that found in patients with early-onset schizophrenia. Spontaneous remissions appear to be uncommon, and discontinuation of antipsychotic medications (frequently due to nonadherence) tends to exacerbate psychosis. With good adherence and supportive psychosocial therapies, the outlook can be better.

SCHIZOAFFECTIVE DISORDER

For schizoaffective disorder, patients must have an uninterrupted period of illness in which they have symptoms that meet Criterion A for schizophrenia as well as a major depressive episode, a manic episode, or a mixed episode. During this period, there must also have been delusions or hallucinations for at least 2 weeks in the absence of prominent mood symptoms. Recent research suggests that schizoaffective disorder may be a subcategory of schizophrenia (rather than affective disorders) as the two disorders share a number of epidemiological, clinical, and neuropsychological features (Evans et al., 1999).

AGING OF PATIENTS WITH EARLIER-ONSET SCHIZOPHRENIA

Many patients with early-onset schizophrenia survive into old age, yet comparatively little is known about the long-term course and outcome of schizophrenia. A long-held, yet overly narrow, notion of the long-term course of schizophrenia views the illness as resulting in progressive decline and dementia. In Kraeplin's (1919/1971) initial conceptualization of dementia praecox, the onset of illness in adolescence or early adulthood was followed thereafter by progressive functional decline. Davidson and colleagues (1995) provided data consistent with this view, noting that more than 60% of the institutionalized patients with schizophrenia they studied showed signs of dementia. Institutionalized patients, however, are not representative of the majority of patients with schizophrenia (Cohen, 1990); therefore, these findings cannot be taken as a definitive view of long-term outcome in older patients with schizophrenia.

In fact, much of the literature is suggestive of improvement over time in many patients with schizophrenia. Whereas approximately 20% of patients appear to experience the functional decline described by Kraepelin (1919/1971), another 20% to 30% are found to show substantial improvement and even remission (Belitsky & McGlashan, 1993; Bleuler, 1978; Ciompi, 1980; Harding et al., 1987; McGlashan, 1988). Thus, in available long-term studies, heterogeneity of outcome is a constant finding. Available data suggest that, in the majority of patients, initial deterioration usually occurs shortly after the onset of the disorder and is often limited to the first 5 or 10 years after illness, while aging is accompanied by stability or even improvement in symptoms (Belitsky & McGlashan, 1993). One well-known example of recovery involved the case of John Nash. Dr. Nash, a mathematician who won a Nobel Prize, developed schizophrenia in his late 20s, suffered from a severe form of the illness for many years, then experienced a remission later in life, allowing him to return to a productive academic career (Nasar, 1998).

Recent studies of neuropsychological deficits in chronic schizophrenia suggest that cognitive dysfunction typically remains stable following the initial deterioration (Eyler Zorrilla et al., 2000; Heaton et al., 2001). In a large longitudinal study, Heaton and colleagues followed outpatients with schizophrenia for an average of 3 years (range 6 months to 10 years) with annual neuropsychological evaluations and compared these patients with normal subjects. Although the patients with schizophrenia had more baseline neuropsychological impairment, there was no evidence of cognitive deterioration over time, which was in contrast to variability in clinical symptoms observed over time. Eyler-Zorrilla and colleagues compared cognitive functioning of community-dwelling patients aged 40 to 85 years with early-onset schizophrenia with that of normal comparison subjects. In this cross-sectional study, while measures of cognitive functioning were lower in the schizophrenia group, there were no differences between the patients and the normal comparison groups in age-related variation of scores. The results of these studies suggest that, in the noninstitutionalized majority of patients with schizophrenia, neuropsychological deficits remain stable over time.

In contrast, in a study of over 300 inpatients with schizophrenia older than 65 years who were followed over 30 months, Harvey and colleagues (1999) found that a subset (approximately 30%) experienced a decline in their overall cognitive and functional status. More severe positive symptoms at baseline, older age, and lower educational level were risk factors for greater impairment over time.

The differences in findings between outpatients and inpatients with chronic schizophrenia have not been explained satisfactorily by duration of institutionalization or the presence of other dementing disorders. It thus appears that, while the majority of patients with schizophrenia do not experience an overall decline in cognitive functioning as they age, there may be a small minority (who are more likely to be institutionalized) who do show a progressive decline.

The notion of *schizophrenic burnout*, a proposed pattern of age-related change in patients with schizophrenia in which positive symptoms remit while negative symptoms increase, also is challenged by long-term data. In a study of nearly 400 chronically institutionalized patients aged 25 to 85 years with schizophrenia, Davidson and colleagues (1995) found that, while positive symptoms abated somewhat with age, they were still present, raising doubt about the concept of complete burnout, at least in institutionalized patients. Only patients older than 85 years showed a reduction of positive symptoms that was at the 30th percentile of the normative scores for patients with schizophrenia. Moreover, in this study, negative symptoms were more severe in older patients compared to younger patients. Other investigators have found that a minority of patients experience improvement in both positive and negative symptoms, while a majority continues to have both kinds of symptoms (Jeste et al., 1997).

Many attempts have been made to uncover associations between specific factors and outcome in schizophrenia. A number of patient-related factors (e.g., better prognosis in women, those ever married, those with good premorbid adjustment, and those with normal neurological evaluations) and illness-related factors (e.g., better prognosis with acute-onset, short-duration illness with affective symptoms and fewer negative symptoms) have been associated with outcome in the literature, but most of these findings are of uncertain predictive value for individual patients. An ongoing area of investigation involves the question of whether early intervention during a first psychotic episode is associated with a better long-term outcome (Wyatt, 1991).

Research is needed to examine the impact of changes in social structure and other age-related changes on the course and outcome of schizophrenia. While most older patients with schizophrenia remain disabled to some degree, research also indicates that many patients experience improvements in certain realms of social functioning with increasing age. For example, improved coping strategies, more active participation in recovery, and greater support from patients' families can contribute to more adaptive social functioning (Cohen et al., 2000). One of the strongest predictors of adaptive functioning is social support, while negative symptoms, cognitive impairment, and abnormal movements are associated with poorer community functioning. Biological factors, such as hormonal changes in the climacterium, also may be important, although the role of such factors have only recently begun to be elucidated.

LATE-LIFE DELUSIONAL DISORDER

Persecutory delusions in the elderly patient usually occur in the context of another, underlying neuropsychiatric disorder (e.g., schizophrenia, mood disorder, or dementia). Occasionally, however, a primary delusional disorder is implicated. Conceptualization and study of this disorder have been hampered by inconsistencies in nomenclature and diagnostic criteria.

Kraepelin (1919, 1919/1971) defined *paranoia* as an often incurable disorder characterized by the development of a chronic, well-systematized, delusional state of nonbizarre quality with little or no impairment of orientation, memory, or intellect and an absence of hallucinations, thought disorder, disturbed volition, or personality deterioration. Kraepelin's paraphrenia, on the other hand, included both paranoid delusions and systematized hallucinations and typically had its onset in later life.

Prevalence

The *DSM-IV* (APA, 1987) estimated the population prevalence of delusional disorder at 0.03%, with a lifetime risk of 0.05% to 0.1%. In a retrospective, postmortem case review of 1,849 patients who had died while in state hospitals or nursing homes over a 20-year period, Heston (1987) found that, while only about 2% of patients satisfied *DSM-III* (APA, 1980) criteria for paranoid disorder, another 13% had paranoid ideation.

Delusional disorder can occur in young adults, but usually presents first in mid to late adulthood. The average age of onset is somewhat earlier for men (40–49 years) than for women (60–69 years).

Diagnosis and Symptomatology

The patient should meet the *DSM-IV* (APA, 1994a) criteria for delusional disorder. The occurrence of nonbizarre delusions (defined by *DSM-IV* as delusions involving situations that may occur in real life, e.g., being followed, having a disease, being deceived by one's spouse or lover) is fundamental to this illness. The symptoms must have been present for at least 1 month. Tactile or olfactory hallucinations, if present, must be related to the delusional theme, and affective symptoms, if any, must be brief. The predominant theme or themes of the delusion may be erotomanic, grandiose, jealous, persecutory, somatic, or of unspecified or mixed types. As distinct from patients with schizophrenia, patients with delusional disorder do not have prominent auditory hallucinations and do not display personality deterioration.

Pathogenesis and Etiology

Several factors have been postulated to contribute to the development of delusional disorder, although the available evidence in favor of each needs verification.

GENETICS   Some investigators have found an increased incidence of schizophrenia in families of patients with paranoid or delusional disorder (Kendler & Davis, 1981).

PREMORBID PERSONALITY   Persons with certain premorbid personality disorders, such as schizotypal or paranoid, may be more likely to develop delusional disorder.

NEUROPSYCHOLOGICAL AND BRAIN IMAGING FINDINGS   Using MRI, Rockwell, Krull, and colleagues (1994) compared three groups of patients (those with late-onset psychosis with somatic delusions, those with late-onset psychosis without somatic delusions, and normal comparison subjects) and found no significant differences in degree of atrophy or presence of white matter hyperintensities. Patients with somatic delusions had lower scores on a full-scale IQ test, however. One study compared middle-aged and older patients with delusional disorder to those with schizophrenia. In this study, the patients with delusional disorder had nonsignificantly lower levels of neuropsychological impairment but overall more severe psychopathology compared to the patients with schizophrenia (Evans et al., 1996).

SENSORY DEFICITS   Some studies have demonstrated an association between hearing loss and paranoia in the elderly (Cooper & Curry, 1976), while other systematic studies have failed to confirm this relationship (Moore, 1981).

SOCIOECONOMIC STATUS   There is some evidence that immigration or low socioeconomic status can predispose to delusional disorder (APA, 1994a; Gurian et al., 1992).

Differential Diagnosis

To make the diagnosis of delusional disorder, organic causes must first be investigated and excluded. Delusional syndromes associated with early dementia can resemble delusional disorder (APA, 1994a). The absence of severe cognitive impairment in delusional disorder should help to rule out dementia. The differentiation from late-onset schizophrenia was discussed above.

Delusions can accompany mood disorders. Therefore, for a diagnosis of delusional disorder to be made, it must be established that the delusions preceded the onset of mood disorder.

In cases with unclear diagnosis, psychotic disorder, not otherwise specified (NOS), may be considered (discussed below).

Treatment

Antipsychotic drugs are often efficacious, especially in agitated delusional patients, but they must be administered cautiously in the elderly patient. Patients with delusional disorder are sometimes refractory to antipsychotic pharmacotherapy. One common problem in the treatment of these patients is nonadherence, particularly because the symptoms are frequently more distressing to others than to the patient. Raskind and colleagues (1979) suggested that parenteral depot neuroleptics might be preferable to oral daily medication because of problems with adherence. From the viewpoint of therapeutic efficacy, however, there is little evidence that any one type of antipsychotic agent is superior to others.

Supportive psychotherapy is an important modality of treatment. Difficulty in establishing rapport with these patients is common (Evans et al., 1996). Thus, for some delusional patients, especially those who are paranoid, a somewhat distant, medical-type approach may be more acceptable and less threatening. Antidepressant drugs, electroconvulsive therapy, and psychotherapeutic approaches have all been tried with limited success.

Course and Prognosis

The data on prognosis are limited, making it difficult to draw conclusions. The course may be chronic, especially in those with persecutory delusions, whereas others may have remissions and relapses. The diagnostic consistency of the disorder over a long period has been questioned. Kraepelin (1919, 1919/1971) noticed that diagnostic inconsistency was extremely high, with 80% of the patients later meeting his criteria for dementia praecox or paraphrenia. In other studies, diagnostic consistency ranged from 3% to 56% (Koehler & Hornstein, 1986; Winokur, 1977). The wide range is probably due, at least in part, to differences in the length of follow-up.

PSYCHOTIC DISORDERS NOT ELSEWHERE CLASSIFIED

The *DSM-IV* (APA, 1994b) describes several other psychotic disorders that are less well defined. There is a relative paucity of literature on the characterization of these disorders in the elderly. The conditions in this category include the following: brief psychotic disorder, schizophreniform disorder, shared psychotic disorder, and psychotic disorder NOS.

Brief Psychotic Disorder

Brief psychotic disorder is characterized by sudden onset of psychotic symptoms of less than 1 month duration, which may or may not have been precipitated by a marked stressor, with eventual return to the premorbid level of functioning.

Schizophreniform Disorder

Schizophreniform disorder is similar to schizophrenia except that the duration of symptoms (including the prodromal and residual phases) is at least 1 month, but less than 6 months.

Shared Psychotic Disorder

The shared psychotic disorder diagnosis is used when a close relationship with a person (or persons) with an already present delusion results in the new development of a similar delusion in the second person. One review of published case reports found that the disorder was equally prevalent in younger and older patients and in men and women; that comorbid dementia, depression, mental retardation, and hallucinations were common; and that social isolation appeared to be a risk factor (Silveira & Seeman, 1995). McNiel and colleagues (1972) described shared psychotic disorder (also called folie à deux) in two elderly persons with shared persecutory delusions. The authors noted that the disorder in their patients was similar to that in younger persons, except for an unusually strong interdependence in the elderly couple.

Psychotic Disorder, Not Otherwise Specified

The *DSM-IV* (APA, 1994a) describes psychotic disorder NOS as a disorder with clearly psychotic symptoms about which insufficient information is available to make a specific diagnosis or with symptoms that do not meet the criteria for any other specific psychotic disorder. In essence, this is a residual category to be used in those situations in which either the patient's history and symptoms do not fit into any other category or not enough information is available to make a diagnosis. This diagnosis is often applied in cases in which psychotic symptoms are present, but it is unclear whether the symptoms are due to a medical condition, substances, or a primary psychotic disorder.

In a case series study of 16 patients with late-onset psychotic symptoms after age 45 years who met criteria for psychotic disorder NOS, Lesser and colleagues (1992) reported that 7 patients had pure hallucinatory symptoms (6 with auditory, 1 with visual symptoms) without delusions, and these hallucinations were unable to be attributed adequately to a medical or neurological condition or medications. Another 6 patients had both hallucinations and delusions, but there was insufficient evidence from the history of a decline in functioning for the patients to be classified as having schizophrenia. Finally, 3 patients had delusions without hallucinations. The delusions were bizarre and complex, ruling out the possibility of delusional disorder; again, these 3 patients also did not demonstrate markedly impaired functioning below their previously achieved highest level, although this criterion was more difficult to establish because many of the patients were retired or living alone. On MRI examination, two thirds of the patients had abnormal findings; these findings were nonspecific and could not be used to differentiate these patients from those with other late-onset psychotic disorders.

Some investigators have reported an association between the presence of visual disorders (such as age-related macular degeneration) and visual hallucinations (Holroyd et al., 1994). Visual hallucinations in patients with macular degeneration were not associated with progressive cognitive impairment in a follow-up study; in this same study, 60% of patients experienced improvement of their visual hallucinations over time, and 2 patients reported cessation of their hallucinations after laser eye surgery (Holroyd & Rabins, 1996).

The prevalence of visual hallucinosis in patients with eye pathology ranges from 18% to 57%, and many of these patients do not have insight. Therefore, such physical disorders must be carefully ruled out as factors causing and maintaining the disturbance before considering the diagnosis of psychosis NOS (Beck & Harris, 1994).

CONCLUSION

Psychotic symptoms can develop in the elderly as a result of a variety of conditions. With increasing research in this area, the terminology and classification have improved, although much remains to be learned about the etiopathology of these disorders. It is of utmost importance to exclude neurological, endocrine, and other medical conditions in evaluating an older patient with new onset of psychosis in the absence of a past history of a psychotic disorder. The psychosis of AD is a specific syndrome with important public health implications, such as caregiver distress, higher rates of institutionalization, and an increased risk of agitation, wandering, and other disruptive behaviors. As such, the syndrome requires careful evaluation and management. Schizophrenia with onset in middle age appears to be a distinct form of schizophrenia, while schizophrenia-like psychosis with very late onset tends to be a heterogeneous group of neurodegenerative conditions.

ACKNOWLEDGMENTS

This work was supported, in part, by the National Institute of Mental Health (5R37-MH43693, MH45131, P30MH49671) and by the Department of Veterans Affairs.

REFERENCES

Allison DB, Mentore JL, Heo M, et al. Antipsychotic-induced weight gain: a comprehensive research synthesis. *Am J Psychiatry*. 1999;156:1686–1696.

American Psychiatric Association. *Diagnostic and Statistical Manual of Mental Disorders*. 1st ed. Washington, DC: American Psychiatric Press; 1952.

American Psychiatric Association. *Diagnostic and Statistical Manual of Mental Disorders*. 2nd ed. Washington, DC: American Psychiatric Press; 1968.

American Psychiatric Association. *Diagnostic and Statistical Manual of Mental Disorders*. 3rd ed. Washington, DC: American Psychiatric Press; 1980.

American Psychiatric Association. *Diagnostic and Statistical Manual of Mental Disorders*, 3rd ed., rev. Washington, DC: American Psychiatric Press; 1987.

American Psychiatric Association. *Diagnostic and Statistical Manual of Mental Disorders*. 4th ed. Washington, DC: American Psychiatric Association; 1994b.

American Psychiatric Association. *Diagnostic and Statistical Manual of Mental Disorders*. 4th ed., text revision. Washington, DC: American Psychiatric Association; 2000.

American Psychiatric Association. *Diagnostic Criteria From* DSM-IV. Washington, DC: American Psychiatric Association; 1994a.

Andreasen NC. I don't believe in late onset schizophrenia. In: Howard R, Rabins PV, Castle DJ, eds. *Late-Onset Schizophrenia*. Philadelphia, PA: Wrightson Biomedical Publishing; 1999:111–123.

Barta PE, Powers RE, Aylward WH, et al. Quantitative MRI volume changes in late-onset schizophrenia and Alzheimer's disease compared to normal controls. *Psychiatry Res*. 1997;68:65–75.

Beck J, Harris MJ. Visual hallucinosis in non-psychotic elderly. *Int J Geriatr Psychiatry*. 1994;9:531–536.

Belitsky R, McGlashan TH. The manifestations of schizophrenia in late life: a dearth of data. *Schizophr Bull*. 1993;19:683–685.

Bland RC. Demographic aspects of functional psychoses in Canada. *Acta Psychiatr Scand*. 1977;55:369–380.

Bleuler M. Late schizophrenic clinical pictures. *Fortschr Neurol Psychiatr*. 1943;15:259–290.

Bleuler M. *The Schizophrenic Disorders: Long-term Patient and Family Studies*. Clemens SM, trans. New Haven, CT: Yale University Press; 1978.

Bonuccelli U, Ceravolo R, Salvetti S, et al. Clozapine in Parkinson's disease tremor. Effects of acute and chronic administration. *Neurology*. 1997;49:1587–1590.

Breitner J, Husain M, Figiel G, et al. Cerebral white matter disease in late-onset psychosis. *Biol Psychiatry*. 1990;28:266–274.

Burns A, Jacoby R, Levy R. Psychiatric phenomena in Alzheimer's disease. I: Disorders of thought content. *Br J Psychiatry*. 1990;157:72–76.

Campbell S, Stephens S, Ballard C. Dementia with Lewy bodies: clinical features and treatment. *Drugs Aging*. 2001;18:397–407.

Castle DJ. Epidemiology of late onset schizophrenia. In: Howard R, Rabins PV, Castle DJ, eds. *Late Onset Schizophrenia*. Philadelphia, PA: Wrightson Biomedical Publishing; 1999:139–146.

Castle DJ, Murray RM. The epidemiology of late-onset schizophrenia. *Schizophr Bull*. 1993;19:691–700.

Ciompi L. Catamnestic long-term study on the course of life and aging of schizophrenics. *Schizophr Bull*. 1980;6:606–618.

Coffey CE, Figiel GS, Djang WT, et al. Subcortical hyperintensity on magnetic resonance imaging: a comparison of normal and depressed elderly subjects. *Am J Psychiatry*. 1990;47:187–189.

Cohen CI. Outcome of schizophrenia into later life: an overview. *Gerontologist*. 1990; 30:790–797.

Cohen CI, Cohen GD, Blank K, et al. Schizophrenia and older adults: an overview: directions for research and policy. *Am J Geriatr Psychiatry.* 2000;8:19–28.

Cooper AF, Curry AR. The pathology of deafness in the paranoid and affective psychoses of later life. *J Psychosom Res.* 1976;20:97–105.

Cummings JL, Donohue JA, Brooks RL. The relationship between donepezil and behavioral disturbances in patients with Alzheimer's disease. *Am J Geriatr Psychiatry.* 2000;8:134–140.

Cummings JL, Miller B, Hill MA, et al. Neuropsychiatric aspects of multi-infarct dementia and dementia of the Alzheimer type. *Arch Neurol.* 1987;44:389–393.

Davidson M, Harvey PD, Powchik P, et al. Severity of symptoms in chronically institutionalized geriatric schizophrenic patients. *Am J Psychiatry.* 1995;152:197–207.

De Deyn P, Rabheru K, Rasmussen A, et al. A randomized trial of risperidone, placebo, and haloperidol for behavioral symptoms of dementia. *Neurology.* 1999;53:946–955.

Devanand DP, Jacobs DM, Tang MX, et al. The course of psychopathologic features in mild to moderate Alzheimer disease. *Arch Gen Psychiatry.* 1997;54:257–263.

Dickerson FB. Cognitive behavioral psychotherapy for schizophrenia: a review of recent empirical studies. *Schizophr Res.* 2000;43:71–90.

Dupont RM, Lehr P, Lamoureaux G, et al. Preliminary report: cerebral blood flow abnormalities in older schizophrenic patients. *Psychiatry Res.* 1994;55:121–130.

Evans JD, Heaton RK, Paulsen JS, et al. Schizoaffective disorder: a form of schizophrenia or affective disorder? *J Clin Psychiatry.* 1999;60:874–882.

Evans JD, Paulsen JS, Harris MJ, et al. A clinical and neuropsychological comparison of delusional disorder and schizophrenia. *J Neuropsychiatry Clin Neurosci.* 1996;8:281–286.

Eyler Zorrilla LT, Heaton RK, McAdams LA, et al. Cross-sectional study of older outpatients with schizophrenia and healthy comparison subjects: no differences in age-related cognitive decline. *Am J Psychiatry.* 2000;157:1324–1326.

Flint AJ, Rifat SI, Eastwood MR. Late-onset paranoia: distinct from paraphrenia? *Int J Geriatr Psychiatry.* 1991;6:103–109.

Graham JM, Sussman JD, Ford DS, et al. Olanzapine in the treatment of hallucinosis in idiopathic Parkinson's disease: a cautionary note. *J Neurol Neurosurg Psychiatry.* 1998;65:774–777.

Granholm E, McQuaid JR, McClure FS, et al. A randomized controlled pilot study of cognitive behavioral social skills training for older patients with schizophrenia. *Schizophr Res.* 2001;53:167–169.

Gurian BS, Wexler D, Baker EH. Late-life paranoia: possible association with early trauma and infertility. *Int J Geriatr Psychiatry.* 1992;7:277–284.

Harding CM, Brooks GW, Ashikaga T, et al. The Vermont longitudinal study: II. Long-term outcome of subjects who once met the criteria for *DSM-III* schizophrenia. *Am J Psychiatry.* 1987;144:727–735.

Harris MJ, Jeste DV. Late-onset schizophrenia: an overview. *Schizophr Bull.* 1988;14:39–55.

Harvey PD, Silverman JM, Mohs RC, et al. Cognitive decline in late-life schizophrenia: a longitudinal study of geriatric chronically hospitalized patients. *Biol Psychiatry.* 1999;45:32–40.

Heaton R, Paulsen J, McAdams LA, et al. Neuropsychological deficits in schizophrenia: relationship to age, chronicity and dementia. *Arch Gen Psychiatry.* 1994;51:469–476.

Heaton RK, Gladsjo JA, Palmer BW, et al. Stability and course of neuropsychological deficits in schizophrenia. *Arch Gen Psychiatry*. 2001;58:24–32.

Herbert ME, Jacobson S. Late paraphrenia. *Br J Psychiatry*. 1967;113:461–469.

Heston LL. The paranoid syndrome after mid life. In: Miller NE, Cohen GD, eds. *Schizophrenia and Aging*. New York, NY: Guilford Press; 1987:249–257.

Holroyd S, Rabins PV. A 3-year follow-up study of visual hallucinations in patients with macular degeneration. *J Nerv Ment Dis*. 1996;184:188–189.

Holroyd S, Rabins PV, Finkelstein D, et al. Visual hallucinations in patients from an opthalmology clinic and medical clinic population. *J Nerv Ment Dis*. 1994;182: 273–276.

Howard R, Castle D, Wessely S, et al. A comparative study of 470 cases of early and late-onset schizophrenia. *Br J Psychiatry*. 1993;163:352–357.

Howard R, Graham C, Sham P, et al. A controlled family study of late-onset non-affective psychosis (late paraphrenia). *Br J Psychiatry*. 1997;170:511–514.

Howard R, Rabins PV, Seeman MV, et al. Late-onset schizophrenia and very-late-onset schizophrenia-like psychosis: an international consensus. *Am J Psychiatry*. 2000; 157:172–178.

Jeste DV. Tardive dyskinesia in older patients. *J Clin Psychiatry*. 2000;61:27–32.

Jeste DV, Caligiuri MP, Paulsen JS, et al. Risk of tardive dyskinesia in older patients: a prospective longitudinal study of 266 patients. *Arch Gen Psychiatry*. 1995;52: 756–765.

Jeste DV, Eastham JH, Lacro JP, et al. Management of late-life psychosis. *J Clin Psychiatry*. 1996;57(suppl 3):39–45.

Jeste DV, Finkel SI. Psychosis of Alzheimer's disease and related dementias: diagnostic criteria for a distinct syndrome. *Am J Geriatr Psychiatry*. 2000;8:29–34.

Jeste DV, Harris MJ, Krull A, et al. Clinical and neuropsychological characteristics of patients with late-onset schizophrenia. *Am J Psychiatry*. 1995;152:722–730.

Jeste DV, Harris MJ, Pearlson GD, et al. Late-onset schizophrenia: studying clinical validity. *Psychiatr Clin North Am*. 1988;11:1–14.

Jeste DV, Okamoto A, Napolitano J, et al. Low incidence of persistent tardive dyskinesia in elderly patients with dementia treated with risperidone. *Am J Psychiatry*. 2000; 157:1150–1155.

Jeste DV, Rockwell E, Harris MJ, et al. Conventional versus newer antipsychotics in elderly patients. *Am J Geriatr Psychiatry*. 1999;7:70–76.

Jeste DV, Symonds LL, Harris MJ, et al. Non-dementia non-praecox dementia praecox? Late-onset schizophrenia. *Am J Geriatr Psychiatry*. 1997;5:302–317.

Jeste DV, Wragg RE, Salmon DP, et al. Cognitive deficits of patients with Alzheimer's disease with and without delusions. *Am J Psychiatry*. 1992;149:184–189.

Katz IR, Jeste DV, Mintzer JE, et al. Comparison of risperidone and placebo for psychosis and behavioral disturbances associated with dementia: a randomized, double-blind trail. *J Clin Psychiatry*. 1999;60:107–115.

Kay DWK, Roth M. Environmental and hereditary factors in the schizophrenias of old age ("late paraphrenia") and their bearing on the general problem of causation in schizophrenia. *J Ment Sci*. 1961;107:649–686.

Keith SJ, Regier DA, Rae DS. Schizophrenic disorders. In: Robins LN, Regier DA, eds. *Psychiatric Disorders in America: The Epidemiologic Catchment Area Study*. New York, NY: Free Press; 1991:33–52.

Kendler S, Davis KL. The genetics and biochemistry of paranoid schizophrenia and other paranoid psychoses. *Schizophr Bull.* 1981;7:689–709.

Kindermann SS, Dolder CR, Bailey A, et al. Pharmacologic treatment of psychosis and agitation in elderly patients with dementia: four decades of experience. *Drugs Aging.* 2002;19:257–276.

Koehler K, Hornstein C. 100 years of *DSM-III* paranoia—how stable a diagnosis over time? *Eur Arch Psychiatry Neurol Sci.* 1986;235:255–258.

Kraepelin E. *Dementia Praecox and Paraphrenia.* Barclay RM, trans. Robertson GM, ed. Huntington, NY: Krieger; 1971. (Originally published 1919.)

Kraepelin E. On paranoid diseases [in German]. *Z Gesamte Neurol Psychiatrie.* 1919; 11:617–638.

Krull AJ, Press G, Dupont R, et al. Brain imaging in late-onset schizophrenia and related psychoses. *Int J Geriatr Psychiatry.* 1991;6:651–658.

Larson CA, Nyman GE. Age of onset in schizophrenia. *Hum Hered.* 1970;20:241–247.

Lauriello J, Bustillo J, Keith SJ. A critical review of research on psychosocial treatment of schizophrenia. *Biol Psychiatry.* 1999;46:1409–1417.

Lesser IM, Jeste DV, Boone KB, et al. Late-onset psychotic disorder, not otherwise specified: clinical and neuroimaging findings. *Biol Psychiatry.* 1992;31:419–423.

Lesser IM, Miller BL, Boone KB, et al. Brain injury and cognitive function in late-onset psychotic depression. *J Neuropsychiatry Clin Neurosci.* 1991;3:33–40.

Lesser IM, Miller BL, Swartz JR, et al. Brain imaging in late-life schizophrenia and related psychoses. *Schizophr Bull.* 1993;19:773–782.

Lewine R. Sex differences in schizophrenia: timing or subtype? *Psychol Bull.* 1981;90: 432–444.

Madhusoodanan S, Brenner R, Cohen CI. Risperidone for elderly patients with schizophrenia or schizoaffective disorder. *Psychiatr Ann.* 2000;30:175–180.

Masand PS. Atypical antipsychotics for elderly patients with neurodegenerative disorders and medical conditions. *Psychiatr Ann.* 2000;30:203–208.

Mayer W. On paraphrenic psychoses [in German]. *Z Gesamte Neurolog Psychiatrie.* 1921;71:187–206.

McClure FS, Jeste DV. Treatment of late onset schizophrenia and related disorders. In: Howard R, Rabins PV, Caste DJ, eds. *Late Onset Schizophrenia.* Philadelphia, PA: Wrightson Biomedical Publishing; 1999:217–232.

McGlashan TH. A selective review of recent North American long-term follow-up studies of schizophrenia. *Schizophr Bull.* 1988;14:515–542.

McKeith I, Del Ser T, Spano P, et al. Efficacy of rivastigmine in dementia with Lewy bodies: a randomised, double-blind, placebo-controlled international study. *Lancet.* 2000;356:2031–2036.

McNiel JN, Verwoerdt A, Peak D. Folie a deux in the aged: review and case report of role reversal. *J Am Geriatr Soc.* 1972;20:316–323.

McQuaid JR, Granholm E, McClure FS, et al. Development of an integrated cognitive-behavioral and social skills training intervention for older patients with schizophrenia. *J Psychother Res Pract.* 2000;9:149–156.

Miller BL, Lesser IM. Late-life psychosis and modern neuroimaging. *Psychiatr Clin North Am.* 1988;11:33–46.

Miller BL, Lesser IM, Boone KB, et al. Brain lesions and cognitive function in late-life psychosis. *Br J Psychiatry.* 1991;158:76–82.

Moore NC. Is paranoid illness associated with sensory defects in the elderly? *J Psychosom Res.* 1981;25:69–74.

Mukaetova-Ladinska EB, Harrington CR, Xuereb J, et al. Treating Alzheimer's and other dementias. In: Bergener M, Finkel SI, eds. *Treating Alzheimer's and Other Dementias.* New York, NY: Springer; 1995:57–80.

Murray RM, O'Callaghan E, Castle DJ, et al. A neurodevelopmental approach to the classification of schizophrenia. *Schizophr Bull.* 1992;18:319–332.

Naguib M, Levy R. Late paraphrenia: neuropsychological impairment and structural brain abnormalities on computed tomography. *Int J Geriatr Psychiatry.* 1987;2: 83–90.

Naimark D, Jackson E, Rockwell E, et al. Psychotic symptoms in Parkinson's disease patients with dementia. *J Am Geriatr Soc.* 1996;44:296–299.

Nasar S. *A Beautiful Mind.* New York, NY: Simon & Schuster; 1998.

Olin J, Schneider L. Galantamine for Alzheimer's disease. *Cochrane Database Syst Rev.* 2001;4:CD001747.

Palmer BW, Bondi MW, Gladsjo JA, et al. Stability of performance on cognitive measures among patients with late-onset schizophrenia versus probable Alzheimer disease [abstract]. *Am J Geriatr Psychiatry.* 2000:8:46–47.

Palmer BW, McClure F, Jeste DV. Schizophrenia in late-life: findings challenge traditional concepts. *Harvard Rev Psychiatry.* 2001;9:51–58.

Paulsen JS, Heaton RK, Sadek JR, et al. The nature of learning and memory impairments in schizophrenia. *J Int Neuropsychol Soc.* 1996;1:88–99.

Paulsen JS, Salmon DP, Thal LJ, et al. Incidence of and risk factors for hallucinations and delusions in patients with probable AD. *Neurology.* 2000;54:1965–1971.

Pearlson GD. Brain imaging in late onset schizophrenia. In: Rabins HR, Castle DJ, eds. *Late Onset Schizophrenia.* Philadelphia, PA: Wrightson Biomedical Publishing; 1999:191–204.

Pearlson GD, Barta PE, Powers RE, et al. Ziskind-Somerfeld Research Award 1996. Medial and superior temporal gyral volumes and cerebral asymmetry in schizophrenia versus bipolar disorder. *Biol Psychiatry.* 1997;41:1–14.

Pearlson GD, Tune LE, Wong DF, et al. Quantitative D_2 dopamine receptor PET and structural MRI changes in late onset schizophrenia. *Schizophr Bull.* 1993;19:783–795.

Peyser CE, Naimark D, Langston JW, et al. Psychotic syndromes in Parkinson's disease. *Semin Clin Neuropsychiatry.* 1998;3:41–50.

Prager S, Jeste DV. Sensory impairment in late-life schizophrenia. *Schizophr Bull.* 1993; 19:755–772.

Rabins P. Coexisting depression and dementia. *J Geriatr Psychiatry.* 1989;22:17–24.

Raskind M, Alvarez C, Herlin S. Fluphenazine enthanthate in the outpatient treatment of late paraphrenia. *J Am Geriatr Soc.* 1979;27:459–463.

Rockwell E, Choure J, Galasko D, et al. Psychopathology at initial diagnosis in dementia with Lewy bodies versus Alzheimer disease: comparison of matched groups with autopsy-confirmed diagnoses. *Int J Geriatr Psychiatry.* 2000;15:819–823.

Rockwell E, Jackson E, Vilke G, et al. A study of delusions in a large cohort of Alzheimer's disease patients. *Am J Geriatr Psychiatry.* 1994;2:157–164.

Rockwell E, Krull AJ, Dimsdale J, et al. Late-onset psychosis with somatic delusions. *Psychosomatics.* 1994;35:66–72.

Rokhlina ML. A comparative clinico-genetic study of attack-like schizophrenia with late and early manifestations with regard to age [in Russian]. *Zh Nevropatol Psikhiatr.* 1975;75:417–424.

Sachdev P, Brodaty H, Roubina S, et al. An electroencephalographic investigation of late-onset schizophrenia. *Int Psychogeriatr.* 1999;11:421–429.

Samuel W, Caligiuri M, Galasko D, et al. Better cognitive and psychopathologic response to donepezil in patients prospectively diagnosed as dementia with Lewy bodies: a preliminary study. *Int J Geriatr Psychiatry.* 2000;15:794–802.

Schneider LS. Pharmacologic management of psychosis in dementia. *J Clin Psychiatry.* 1999;60:54–60.

Silveira JM, Seeman MV. Shared psychotic disorder: a critical review of the literature. *Can J Psychiatry.* 1995;40:389–395.

Steele C, Rovner B, Chase GA, et al. Psychiatric symptoms and nursing home placement of patients with Alzheimer's disease. *Am J Psychiatry.* 1990;147:1049–1051.

Stern Y, Albert M, Brandt J, et al. Utility of extrapyramidal signs and psychosis as predictors of cognitive and functional decline, nursing home admission, and death in Alzheimer's disease: prospective analyses from the predictors study. *Neurology.* 1994;44:2300–2307.

Stern Y, Tang M, Albert MS, et al. Predicting time to nursing home care and death in individuals with Alzheimer's disease. *JAMA.* 1997;277:806–812.

Stoppe G, Brandt CA, Staedt JH. Behavioural problems associated with dementia: the role of newer antipsychotics. *Drugs Aging.* 1999;14:41–54.

Street JS, Clark WS, Gannon KS, et al. Olanzapine treatment of psychotic and behavioral symptoms in patients with Alzheimer disease in nursing care facilities: a double-blind randomized, placebo-controlled trial. The HGEU Study Group. *Arch Gen Psychiatry.* 2000;57:968–976.

Street JS, Tollefson GD, Tohen M, et al. Olanzapine for psychotic conditions in the elderly. *Psychiatr Ann.* 2000;30:191–196.

Sultzer DL. Neuroimaging and the origin of psychiatric symptoms in dementia. *Int Psychogeriatr.* 1996;8(suppl 3):239–243.

Symonds LL, Olichney JM, Jernigan TL, et al. Lack of clinically significant structural abnormalities in MRIs of older patients with schizophrenia and related psychoses. *J Neuropsychiatry Clin Neurosci.* 1997;9:251–258.

Tariot P. Treatment strategies for agitation and psychosis in dementia. *J Clin Psychiatry.* 1996;57:21–56.

Tariot PN, Solomon PR, Morris MD, et al. A 5-month, randomized, placebo-controlled trial of galantamine in AD. *Neurology.* 2000;54:2269–2276.

Tonkonogy JM, Geller JL. Late-onset paranoid psychosis as a distinct clinicopathologic entity: magnetic resonance imaging data in elderly patients with paranoid psychosis of late onset and schizophrenia of early onset. *Neuropsychiatry.* 1999;12:230–235.

Webster J, Grossberg GT. Late-life onset of psychotic symptoms. *Am J Geriatr Psychiatry.* 1998;6:196–202.

Winokur G. Delusional disorder (paranoia). *Compr Psychiatry.* 1977;18:511–521.

Wirshing DA, Spellberg BJ, Erhart SM, et al. Novel antipsychotics and new onset diabetes. *Biol Psychiatry.* 1998;44:778–783.

Wolters EC, Jansen ENH, Tuynman-Qua HG, et al. Olanzapine in the treatment of dopaminomimetic psychosis in patients with Parkinson's disease. *Neurology.* 1996; 47:1085–1087.

Wragg R, Jeste DV. Overview of depression and psychosis in Alzheimer's disease. *Am J Psychiatry.* 1989;146:577–587.

Wyatt RJ. Neuroleptics and the natural course of schizophrenia. *Schizophr Bull.* 1991; 17:325–351.

Yeung PP, Tariot PN, Schneider LS, et al. Quetiapine for elderly patients with psychotic disorders. *Psychiatr Ann.* 2000;30:197–201.

Zubenko GS, Moossy J, Martinez AJ, et al. Neuropathologic and neurochemical correlates of psychosis in primary dementia. *Arch Neurol.* 1991;48:619–624.

23

Anxiety Disorders

Alastair J. Flint, MB, FRCP (C), FRANZCP

Anxiety disorders fall into the following categories: phobic disorders, panic disorder, generalized anxiety disorder, obsessive-compulsive disorder (OCD), and posttraumatic stress disorder (PTSD). Anxiety disorders are less prevalent in the elderly than in younger adults (Flint, 1994; Jorm, 2000). Nevertheless, they are relatively common in later life. Between 5% and 10% of older people living in the community meet *Diagnostic and Statistical Manual* (DSM) criteria for a current anxiety disorder (Beekman et al., 1998; Regier et al., 1988; Uhlenhuth et al., 1983). Rates of subsyndromal anxiety (that is, symptoms of anxiety that do not meet full criteria for a disorder, yet still have the potential to cause distress and disability) are even higher. For example, Copeland and coworkers (1987b) found that 22% of people aged 65 years or older living in Liverpool, England, had primary subsyndromal symptoms of obsessive, phobic, or generalized anxiety.

Throughout the adult life span, anxiety disorders are more common in women than men (Flint, 1994). As a group, anxiety disorders have a peak age of onset in adolescence and early adulthood (Antony & Swinson, 1996). With the exception of agoraphobia, it is unusual for a primary anxiety disorder to begin in late life (Flint, 1994). Anxiety that starts for the first time in late life (late-onset anxiety) is frequently associated with another condition, such as depression, dementia, physical illness, or medication toxicity or withdrawal.

PRIMARY ANXIETY DISORDERS

Phobic Disorders

Phobias are persistent and irrational fears of situations, objects, or activities that result in a compelling desire to avoid the phobic stimulus. Phobic disorders are subdivided into specific phobias, agoraphobia, and social phobia. A specific phobia is a fear of a circumscribed stimulus such as animals, heights, or blood. In agoraphobia, the phobic stimulus is a situation in which there might be difficulty or embarrassment in escaping. Agoraphobic situations in the elderly are similar to those for younger individuals and include being out of the home alone, being in an enclosed space, being in a crowd, or traveling (Lindesay, 1991). Social phobia is a fear of situations in which the individual fears humiliation or embarrassment when under the scrutiny of others; examples of these situations are public speaking, eating in public, or attending social gatherings.

Depending on the study, phobias are either the most common or second most common anxiety disorder among elderly people living in the community (Flint, 1994). Agoraphobia is more prevalent than specific phobia or social phobia (Lindesay, 1991; Manela et al., 1996; Uhlenhuth et al., 1983). However, it is possible that epidemiological surveys underestimate the prevalence of social phobia in the elderly in that people with this condition may be less willing to be interviewed. Most older people with a specific phobia have had the disorder since childhood or early adolescence (Lindesay, 1991; Livingston et al., 1997); in general, the phobia causes little, if any, social impairment (Lindesay, 1991). On the other hand, agoraphobia in late life frequently has its onset after the age of 60 years (Lindesay, 1991; Livingston et al., 1997), and it is often associated with moderate to severe social impairment (Lindesay, 1991).

It is argued that agoraphobia in younger adults is usually a conditioned response to panic attacks (Klein, 1980). Older people with agoraphobia, however, rarely report a current or past history of panic attacks (Burvill et al., 1995; Lindesay, 1991; Manela et al., 1996). Lindesay (1991) and others (Livingston et al., 1997) have found that most people with late-onset agoraphobia attribute the start of their disorder to an abrupt onset of physical illness or some other traumatic event, such as a fall or being mugged. This finding is supported by the observation of Burvill and coworkers (Burvill et al., 1995) that agoraphobia was significantly more common in female survivors of stroke than in normal comparison subjects, and in the majority of cases, the agoraphobia began after the stroke. Lindesay (1991) also found an association between phobic disorders and early parental loss due to separation or death, suggesting that these early life experiences may confer a vulnerability to the development of agoraphobia in old age.

Generalized Anxiety Disorder

Generalized anxiety disorder is characterized by excessive uncontrollable worries accompanied by symptoms of motor tension (shakiness, muscle tension, restlessness, fatigue) and hypervigilance (feeling keyed up, difficulty concentrating, initial insomnia, irritability, and heightened startled response). According to *DSM-IV* (American Psychiatric Association [APA], 1994) criteria, the symptoms are chronic, occurring most days for 6 months or more. Symptoms of autonomic hyperarousal (for example, palpitations, dry mouth, dizziness, hot flashes, gastrointestinal distress) also can be a feature of generalized anxiety disorder in older people (Blazer et al., 1991).

Some epidemiological studies have found that generalized anxiety disorder is the most prevalent anxiety disorder in later life, whereas others have found that it is less common than phobic disorders (Flint, 1994). Throughout the life span, generalized anxiety disorder has a high frequency of comorbidity with depression and with other anxiety disorders (Blazer et al., 1991). Consistent with this finding, generalized anxiety disorder seldom starts as a "pure" disorder in late life. The Epidemiologic Catchment Area study found that when people with major depression and panic disorder were excluded, only 3% of cases of generalized anxiety disorder started after the age of 64 years (Blazer et al., 1991). Other studies have found that, when generalized anxiety disorder starts for the first time in late life, it is usually associated with a depressive illness (Lindesay et al., 1989; Manela et al., 1996; Parmelee et al., 1993). Thus, an important clinical point is that symptoms of generalized anxiety disorder in an older person should always prompt a careful search for an associated depressive disorder.

Panic Disorder

Panic disorder is characterized by recurrent panic attacks. A panic attack is a discrete period of intense fear or discomfort during which a number of somatic and cognitive symptoms of anxiety develop abruptly and reach a peak within 10 minutes. Epidemiological surveys consistently report a low (less than 0.5%) period prevalence of panic disorder among older people living in the community (Flint, 1994). These studies also suggest that panic disorder rarely starts for the first time in later life (Flint, 1994). When panic attacks do occur in the elderly, the symptoms are qualitatively similar to those described by younger people (Sheikh et al., 1991). However, the elderly may have fewer and less severe symptoms and may be less avoidant (Sheikh et al., 1991). Among clinical populations, late-onset panic attacks are frequently comorbid with a depressive illness or medical condition, particularly cardiovascular, gastrointestinal, or chronic pulmonary diseases (Hassan & Pollard, 1994).

Obsessive-Compulsive Disorder

The essential feature of obsessive-compulsive disorder is recurrent obsessions or compulsions. Obsessions are ideas, thoughts, or impulses that are experienced as senseless and intrusive and persist despite attempts to suppress them. The person recognizes that the obsessions are a product of his or her mind and not imposed from without. Compulsions are repetitive, purposeful behaviors that are performed in response to an obsession or in a stereotyped fashion, with the goal of reducing the distress or preventing some other dreaded event or situation. However, either the activity is not connected in a realistic way with what it is designed to prevent or it is clearly excessive.

Similar to panic disorder, OCD has a low prevalence in late life (Flint, 1994). Most community-based epidemiological studies have found period prevalence rates of between 0% and 0.8% among older people (Flint, 1994). Only about 5% of people attending specialty OCD clinics are aged 60 years or older (Jenike, 1991; Kohn et al., 1997). OCD seldom begins in late life; most elderly people with this disorder have had symptoms for decades (Jenike, 1991; Kohn et al., 1997). Preliminary data suggest that the clinical presentation of OCD does not significantly differ between younger and older people (Kohn et al., 1997). Common obsessions in older patients are contamination fears, pathological doubt, and fear of harming others (Kohn et al., 1997). Common compulsions are checking, counting, and washing rituals (Kohn et al., 1997).

Ruminative thoughts are common in late-life depression (Lyness et al., 1997) and, at times, can take the form of obsessions. From the point of view of treatment, it is important to differentiate between obsessions and delusions in depressed patients. The recommended treatment for delusional depression is electroconvulsive therapy or a combination of antidepressant and antipsychotic medications (APA, 1993). On the other hand, depression with associated obsessions may well respond to antidepressant monotherapy.

Posttraumatic Stress Disorder

Posttraumatic stress disorder develops in people who have been exposed to markedly distressing trauma that is outside the range of normal human experience. The trauma is then reexperienced in a variety of ways, including distressing recollections, dreams, or flashbacks. Other symptoms of PTSD include persistent avoidance of stimuli associated with the trauma, numbing of general responsiveness (for example, feeling detached from others, restricted range of affect, diminished interest in activities), and symptoms of hyperarousal. The symptoms usually begin soon after the trauma, but can be delayed for a number of months or years. The *DSM-IV* (APA, 1994) also includes the category *acute stress disorder*, which is symptomatically similar to PTSD but lasts for a shorter period of time (from a minimum of 2 days to a maximum of 4 weeks) and occurs within 4 weeks of the traumatic event.

The period prevalence and incidence of PTSD in the general elderly population is not known. Several studies have examined PTSD in Holocaust survivors and veterans who were prisoners of war during World War II. In these groups, symptoms of PTSD are often chronic, persisting into late life in 20%–50% of cases (Kluznik et al., 1986; Kuch & Cox, 1992; Rosen et al., 1989; Speed et al., 1989). The intensity and chronicity of symptoms is positively correlated with the severity of the trauma (Kluznik et al., 1986; Kuch & Cox, 1992; Rosen et al., 1989; Speed et al., 1989). Some investigators have found an association between the presence of stressful life events in old age, such as reminders of the war experience, bereavement, or a significant change in physical health, and worsening or reemergence of symptoms of PTSD (Kaup et al., 1993; Macleod, 1994).

Late-onset PTSD has been reported in older people who have been victims of, or witnessed, natural disasters such as earthquakes or other types of disasters such as aircraft accidents (Goenjian et al., 1994; Livingston et al., 1994). In most of these late-onset cases, the symptoms improve with time. However, a significant minority of individuals continues to report symptoms at least 2 years after the disaster (Livingston et al., 1994).

ANXIETY ASSOCIATED WITH OTHER CONDITIONS

Depression

Throughout the life span, anxiety and depression frequently coexist. Major depression is present in up to 70% of older people with generalized anxiety disorder (Copeland, Davidson, et al., 1987; Manela et al., 1996; Parmelee et al., 1993) and a significant minority of older people with other anxiety disorders (Beekman et al., 2000; Lindesay, 1991; Livingston et al., 1994; Manela et al., 1996). Longitudinal data suggest that when generalized anxiety and depression coexist in the elderly, the anxiety is usually secondary to the depression (Aström, 1996; Castillo et al., 1995; Parmelee et al., 1993). Anxiety that is symptomatic of depression will usually resolve with appropriate treatment of the depression (Flint & Rifat, 1997b). Occasionally, however, symptoms of anxiety persist despite resolution of other depressive symptoms. In such cases, there may be an increased risk of relapse or recurrence of the depression (Flint & Rifat, 1997b). It is also important to recognize that when depression is complicated by a high level of anxiety, it may take longer to respond to treatment than depression with a low level of anxiety (Flint & Rifat, 1997a).

Dementia

Among people living in the community, dementia is not associated with an increased prevalence of anxiety disorders (Forsell & Winblad, 1997; Skoog, 1993). Anxious mood and subsyndromal symptoms of generalized anxiety, however, are often present in clinical samples of people with dementia (Ballard et al., 1996; Orrell & Bebbington, 1996; Wands et al., 1990). Consistent with findings in the general elderly population, anxiety in dementia is frequently associated with depression (Forsell & Winblad, 1998; Orrell & Bebbington, 1996). For example, in a study of elderly people with memory problems, anxiety symptoms were present in 9% of those with a diagnosis of dementia, 36% of those with a diagnosis of major depression, and 43% of those with both dementia and depression (Eisdorfer et al., 1981).

Restlessness or hyperactivity (agitation) frequently complicates dementia. Agitation is not synonymous with anxiety, but in some people with dementia, it may be a behavioral manifestation of anxiety that cannot be communicated verbally. The clinician should suspect anxiety as a contributor to agitation in dementia if the patient has a history of anxiety or depression or is manifesting signs of depression (Cherminski et al., 1998; Forsell & Winblad, 1998).

The sudden onset of anxiety, fear, or agitation in a person with dementia, especially if it occurs in the evening or at night and is associated with an abrupt decline in cognitive function and visual hallucinations, should always make one suspect a superimposed delirium.

Physical Illness and Medications

Anxiety and physical illness are related in several ways. First, anxious mood may be an appropriate response to the onset or consequences of physical illness. Second, pathological anxiety may complicate a medical or neurological illness. For example, an elderly patient may develop agoraphobia following a myocardial infarction or stroke or suffer prominent symptoms of generalized anxiety in the context of physical ill health and depression. Third, medications used to treat physical disorders may, at times, contribute to anxiety-like symptoms. Anxiety-like symptoms may be a complication of therapeutic doses of dopamine agonists, steroids, and some antihypertensive drugs. They also may be a consequence of toxicity from sympathomimetics, β-adrenergic agonists (for example, salbutamol), theophylline, digoxin, or thyroxine.

Conversely, anxiety can contribute to medical morbidity and mortality. People with a high level of anxiety are at increased risk of hypertension (Bowen et al., 2000; Jonas et al., 1997), cardiac arrhythmias (Moser & Dracup, 1996), ischemic heart disease (Bowen et al., 2000; Haines et al., 1987; Kawachi et al., 1994), and death from cardiovascular causes (Haines et al., 1987; Kawachi et al., 1994). In addition, anxiety has been associated with an increased risk of gastrointestinal and respiratory disorders (Bowen et al., 2000) and death from neoplasms and chronic obstructive airway disease (Harris & Barraclough, 1998). Symptoms of anxiety also may contribute to excess disability and impaired recovery in patients with cardiac or cerebrovascular disease (Aström, 1996; Sullivan et al., 1997). Finally, benzodiazepines, frequently taken by older people with anxiety, can contribute to falls, hip fractures, and cognitive impairment (APA, 1990).

TREATMENT

Cognitive and Behavioral Therapies

Cognitive and behavioral therapies have well-established efficacy in the treatment of anxiety disorders in younger adults (Antony & Swinson, 1996). Specifically, cognitive therapy has been found to be consistently more effective than no therapy or placebo for panic disorder with or without agoraphobia, social phobia, PTSD, and generalized anxiety disorder (Antony & Swinson, 1996). Its efficacy in the treatment of obsessions is less clear (James & Blackburn, 1995). Exposure therapy is the psychological treatment of choice for phobic avoidance and the rituals of obsessive-compulsive disorder (Antony & Swinson, 1996).

There has been little evaluation of cognitive-behavioral therapies in older patients with anxiety. Case reports have described the use of exposure therapy for successful treatment of older people suffering from OCD or phobic avoidance (Calamari et al., 1994; Leng, 1985; King & Barrowclough, 1991). Preliminary uncontrolled data suggest that some older patients with panic disorder can benefit from cognitive therapy, even when symptoms have been present for a number of years (Swales et al., 1996). As mentioned, most elderly people with agoraphobia do not have a history of panic attacks. There is no evidence that pharmacotherapy is an effective treatment for agoraphobia that is not associated with panic. Exposure therapy, therefore, is the treatment of choice for most people with late-onset agoraphobia. In these individuals, it is important to ensure that exposure therapy is accompanied by the withdrawal of unnecessary domiciliary support services because the ongoing presence of those services can reinforce the phobic behavior and likely undermine the behavioral intervention (Lindesay & Banerjee, 1994).

Cognitive-behavioral treatments obviously need to be tailored to a person's physical and cognitive capacity. These treatments may not be feasible for elderly people with severe physical limitations or moderate to severe intellectual impairment.

Pharmacological Treatments

ANTIDEPRESSANTS In recent years, there has been growing awareness that antidepressant medications have a broad spectrum of efficacy in the treatment of anxiety disorders (Antony & Swinson, 1996). Controlled studies in mixed-age patients have found that selected antidepressants are beneficial in the treatment of panic disorder with or without agoraphobia, generalized anxiety disorder,

OCD, PTSD, and social phobia (Antony & Swinson, 1996) (Table 23-1). There have been no controlled trials of antidepressant pharmacotherapy for older people with a primary anxiety disorder. However, case reports and uncontrolled trials suggest that older people with these disorders can benefit from antidepressants (Calamari et al., 1994; Hassan & Pollard, 1994; Wylie et al., 2000). A retrospective analysis of data pooled from 5 randomized controlled trials found that venlafaxine had similar efficacy in younger and older patients in the treatment of generalized anxiety disorder (Katz et al., 2002). Chronicity of symptoms should not deter attempts at treatment. Skoog and Skoog (1999) reported that clomipramine resulted in symptomatic improvement in 10 of 17 (59%) patients with chronic OCD, 6 of whom recovered. This was despite the

TABLE 23-1.   Medications found effective in controlled studies treating anxiety disorders in patients of various ages

Disorder	Medication
Panic disorder with or without agora-phobia	TCA: clomipramine, desipramine, imipramine
	SSRI: citalopram, fluoxetine, fluvoxamine, paroxetine, sertraline
	MAOI: brofaromine, phenelzine
	Benzo: alprazolam, clonazepam, diazepam, lorazepam
Generalized anxiety disorder	TCA: imipramine
	SSRI: paroxetine
	Other antidepressants: trazodone, venlafaxine
	Benzo: various
	Azapirone: buspirone
Obsessive-compulsive disorder	TCA: clomipramine
	SSRI: fluoxetine, fluvoxamine, paroxetine, sertraline
Posttraumatic stress disorder	TCA: amitriptyline, imipramine
	SSRI: fluoxetine, paroxetine, sertraline
	MAOI: phenelzine
Social phobia	SSRI: fluvoxamine, paroxetine, sertraline
	MAOI: brofaromine, phenelzine
	Benzo: alprazolam, clonazepam

Source: From Flint (2000), with permission from Medworks Media.

Data from reviews by Antony and Swinson (1996) and the American Psychiatric Association (1998) and from trials by Rocca et al. (1997), Davidson et al. (1999), Brady et al. (2000), Marshall et al. (2001), Stein et al. (1998, 1999).

None of these studies were specific to the elderly. TCA, tricyclic antidepressant; SSRI, selective serotonin reuptake inhibitor; MAOI, monoamine oxidase inhibitor; Benzo, benzodiazepine.

fact that the clomipramine was initiated several decades after the onset of the disorder.

The selective serotonin reuptake inhibitors (SSRIs) are preferable first-line antidepressants for anxiety disorders in the elderly. If started at too high a dose, SSRIs may initially exacerbate symptoms of anxiety; therefore, a lower starting dose (for example, 5–10 mg per day of paroxetine or 25 mg per day of sertraline) is often indicated in elderly anxious individuals. Once it has been established that the patient is tolerating the starting dose, the dose should then be gradually increased to the usual therapeutic range.

BENZODIAZEPINES   Benzodiazepines are an effective treatment for panic disorder, generalized anxiety disorder, social phobia, and adjustment disorder with anxious mood (acute situational anxiety) (Antony & Swinson, 1996). As previously noted, most elderly people with symptoms of generalized anxiety also have a depressive illness, and in this situation, the primary pharmacological treatment should be antidepressant medication. Some patients with anxious depression may, however, also require short-term treatment with a benzodiazepine until the antidepressant becomes effective.

All benzodiazepines have the capacity to cause cognitive impairment, psychomotor impairment, instability of gait, and falls and hip fractures (APA, 1990). In situations for which benzodiazepines are indicated, lorazepam and oxazepam are preferred for the elderly because these medications have relatively short elimination half-lives (10–15 hours) and no active metabolites, and they do not undergo oxidative metabolism in the liver (thus, their clearance is not affected by age) (APA, 1990). As a result, these drugs do not have the potential for cumulative toxicity in the elderly, which is a risk associated with longer acting compounds such as diazepam or clonazepam.

Most elderly patients who are prescribed a benzodiazepine do not require the drug on an ongoing basis. However, there are instances when long-term benzodiazepine treatment may be necessary. In particular, some patients with chronic primary generalized anxiety disorder who have been maintained on a benzodiazepine for years experience a significant worsening of anxiety when an attempt is made to withdraw the medication. In such cases, if the benzodiazepine is not causing significant side effects, it is usually least disruptive to patients to leave them on the medication and monitor them on a regular basis. If side effects do become an issue as the person grows older, dose reduction rather than complete discontinuation of the drug may be the best compromise.

BUSPIRONE   Although buspirone can be an effective treatment for generalized anxiety disorder (Table 23-1), it has a limited role in the management of anxiety in later life. First, buspirone is not a substitute for antidepressant medication in the treatment of generalized anxiety secondary to depression. Second, buspirone has a delayed onset of action of 2 weeks or more, so it is not suitable for the acute treatment of anxiety (Steinberg, 1994). Buspirone does not cause sedation, psychomotor impairment, cognitive impairment, or depressed respiration (Steinberg, 1994). Thus, it may be preferred to a benzodiazepine in the ongoing management of generalized anxiety in nondepressed patients who have chronic obstructive airway disease, sleep apnea, or a neurological disorder. However, selected antidepressant medications (Table 23-1) also may be effective for these patients.

Sometimes, a physician chooses to switch a patient from long-term benzodiazepine therapy to buspirone. Because buspirone has a delayed onset of action and it does not suppress benzodiazepine withdrawal symptoms (Schweizer & Rickels, 1986), a patient should not be abruptly switched from a benzodiazepine to buspirone. Instead, the patient should take a therapeutic dose of buspirone for 2–4 weeks before the benzodiazepine is gradually tapered. Despite this approach, however, some patients may be less satisfied with the anxiolytic effect of buspirone compared with that of a benzodiazepine (DeMartinis et al., 2000).

REFERENCES

American Psychiatric Association. *Benzodiazepine Dependence, Toxicity and Abuse.* Washington, DC: American Psychiatric Association; 1990.

American Psychiatric Association. *Diagnostic and Statistical Manual of Mental Disorders.* 4th ed. Washington, DC: American Psychiatric Association; 1994.

American Psychiatric Association. Practice guideline for major depressive disorder in adults. *Am J Psychiatry.* 1993;150(4 suppl), 1–26.

American Psychiatric Association. Practice guidelines for the treatment of patients with panic disorder. *Am J Psychiatry.* 1998;155:1–34.

Antony MM, Swinson RP. *Anxiety Disorders and Their Treatment: A Critical Review of the Evidence-Based Literature.* Ottawa, Canada: Health Canada; 1996.

Aström M. Generalized anxiety disorder in stroke patients. A 3-year longitudinal study. *Stroke.* 1996;27:270–275.

Ballard C, Boyle A, Bowler C, Lindesay J. Anxiety disorders in dementia sufferers. *Int J Geriatr Psychiatry.* 1996;11:987–990.

Beekman ATF, Bremmer MA, Deeg DJH, et al. Anxiety disorders in later life: a report from the longitudinal aging study Amsterdam. *Int J Geriatr Psychiatry.* 1998;13: 717–726.

Beekman ATF, de Beurs E, van Balkom AJLM, Deeg DJH., van Dyck R, van Tilburg W. Anxiety and depression in later life: co-occurrence and communality of risk factors. *Am J Psychiatry.* 2000;157:89–95.

Blazer D, George LK, Hughes D. Generalised anxiety disorder. In: Robins LN, Regier DA, eds. *Psychiatric Disorders in America: The Epidemiological Catchment Area Study.* New York, NY: Free Press; 1991:180–203.

Bowen RC, Senthilselvan A, Barale A. Physical illness as an outcome of chronic anxiety disorders. *Can J Psychiatry.* 2000;45:459–464.

Brady K, Pearlstein T, Asnis GM, et al. Efficacy and safety of sertraline treatment of posttraumatic stress disorder: a randomized controlled trial. *JAMA.* 2000;283: 1837–1844.

Burvill PW, Johnson GA, Jamrozik KD, Anderson CS, Stewart-Wynne EG, Chakera TM. Anxiety disorders after stroke: results from the Perth Community Stroke Study. *Br J Psychiatry*. 1995;166:328–332.

Calamari JE, Faber SD, Hitsman BL, Poppe CJ. Treatment of obsessive compulsive disorder in the elderly: a review and case example. *J Behav Ther Exp Psychiatry*. 1994; 25:95–104.

Castillo CS, Schultz SK, Robinson RG. Clinical correlates of early-onset and late-onset poststroke generalized anxiety. *Am J Psychiatry*. 1995;152:1174–1179.

Cherminski E, Petracca G, Manes F, Leiguarda R, Starkstein SE. Prevalence and correlates of anxiety in Alzheimer's disease. *Depress Anxiety*. 1998;7:166–170.

Copeland JRM, Davidson IA, Dewey ME. The prevalence and outcome of anxious depression in elderly people aged 65 and over living in the community. In: Racagni G, Smeraldi E, eds. *Anxious Depression: Assessment and Treatment*. New York, NY: Raven Press; 1987:43–47.

Copeland JRM, Dewey ME, Wood N, Searle R, Davidson IA, McWilliam C. Range of mental illness among the elderly in the community: prevalence in Liverpool using the GMS-AGECAT package. *Br J Psychiatry*. 1987;150:815–823.

Davidson JRT, DuPont RL, Hedges D, Haskins JT. Efficacy, safety, and tolerability of venlafaxine extended release and buspirone in outpatients with generalized anxiety disorder. *J Clin Psychiatry*. 1999;60:528–535.

DeMartinis N, Rynn M, Rickels K, Mandos L. Prior benzodiazepine use and buspirone response in the treatment of generalized anxiety disorder. *J Clin Psychiatry*. 2000; 61:91–94.

Eisdorfer C, Cohen D, Keckich W. Depression and anxiety in the cognitively impaired aged. In: Klein DF, Rabkin J, eds. *Anxiety: New Research and Changing Concepts*. New York, NY: Raven Press; 1981:425–430.

Flint AJ. Anxiety and its disorders in later life. *Prim Psychiatry*. 2000;7(9):56–61.

Flint AJ. Epidemiology and comorbidity of anxiety disorders in the elderly. *Am J Psychiatry*. 1994;151:640–649.

Flint AJ, Rifat SL. Effect of demographic and clinical variables on time to antidepressant response in geriatric depression. *Depress Anxiety*. 1997a;5:103–107.

Flint AJ, Rifat SL. Two-year outcome of elderly patients with anxious depression. *Psychiatr Res*. 1997b;66:23–31.

Forsell Y, Winblad B. Anxiety disorders in non-demented and demented elderly patients: prevalence and correlates. *J Neurol Neurosurg Psychiatry*. 1997;62:294–295.

Forsell Y, Winblad B. Feelings of anxiety and associated variables in a very elderly population. *Int J Geriatr Psychiatry*. 1998:13;454–458.

Goenjian AK, Najarian LM, Pynoos RS, et al. Posttraumatic stress disorder in elderly and younger adults after the 1988 earthquake in Armenia. *Am J Psychiatry*. 1994; 151:895–901.

Haines AP, Imeson JD, Meade TW. Phobic anxiety and ischaemic heart disease. *Br Med J*. 1987;295:297–299.

Harris E, Barraclough B. Excess mortality of mental disorder. *Br J Psychiatry*. 1998; 173:11–53.

Hassan R, Pollard CA. Late-life-onset panic disorder: clinical and demographic characteristics of a patient sample. *J Geriatr Psychiatry Neurol*. 1994;7:86–90.

James IA, Blackburn I-M. Cognitive therapy with obsessive-compulsive disorder. *Br J Psychiatry*. 1995;166:444–450.

Jenike MA. Geriatric obsessive-compulsive disorder. *J Geriatr Psychiatry Neurol*. 1991; 4:34–39.

Jonas BS, Franks P, Ingram DD. Are symptoms of anxiety and depression risk factors for hypertension? *Arch Fam Med*. 1997;6:43–49.

Jorm AF. Does old age reduce the risk of anxiety and depression? A review of epidemiological studies across the adult life span. *Psychol Med*. 2000;30:11–22.

Katz IR, Reynolds CF, Alexopoulos GS, Hackett D. Venlaxafine ER as a treatment for generalized anxiety disorder in older adults: pooled analysis of five randomized placebo-controlled clinical trials. *J Am Geriatr Soc*. 2002;50:18–25.

Kaup BA, Ruskin PE, Nyman G. Significant life events and PTSD in elderly World War II veterans. *Am J Geriatr Psychiatry*. 1993;2:239–243.

Kawachi I, Sparrow D, Vokonas PS, Weiss ST. Symptoms of anxiety and risk of coronary heart disease. The normative aging study. *Circulation*. 1994;90:2225–2229.

King P, Barrowclough C. A clinical pilot study of cognitive-behavioural therapy for anxiety disorders in the elderly. *Behav Psychother*. 1991;19:337–345.

Klein DF. Anxiety reconceptualized. *Compr Psychiatry*. 1980;21:411–427.

Kluznik JC, Speed N, Van Valkenburg C, Magraw R. Forty-year follow-up of United States prisoners of war. *Am J Psychiatry*. 1986;143:1443–1446.

Kohn R, Westlake RJ, Rasmussen SA, Marsland RT, Norman WH. Clinical features of obsessive-compulsive disorder in elderly patients. *Am J Geriatr Psychiatry*. 1997;5: 211–215.

Kuch K, Cox BJ. Symptoms of PTSD in 124 survivors of the Holocaust. *Am J Psychiatry*. 1992;149:337–340.

Leng N. A brief review of cognitive-behavioural treatments in old age. *Age Ageing*. 1985;14:257–263.

Lindesay J. Phobic disorders in the elderly. *Br J Psychiatry*. 1991;159:531–541.

Lindesay J, Banerjee S. Generalized anxiety and phobic disorders. In: Chiu E, Ames D, eds. *Functional Psychiatric Disorders of the Elderly*. Cambridge, UK: Cambridge University Press; 1994:78–92.

Lindesay J, Briggs K, Murphy E. The Guy's/Age Concern Survey: prevalence rates of cognitive impairment, depression and anxiety in an urban elderly community. *Br J Psychiatry*. 1989;155:317–329.

Livingston G, Watkin V, Milne B, Manela MV, Katona C. The natural history of depression and the anxiety disorders in older people: the Islington community study. *J Affect Disord*. 1997;46:255–262.

Livingston HM, Livingston MG, Fell S. The Lockerbie disaster: a 3-year follow-up of elderly victims. *Int J Geriatr Psychiatry*. 1994;9:989–994.

Lyness JM, Conwell Y, King DA, Cox C, Caine ED. Ruminative thinking in older inpatients with major depression. *J Affect Disord*. 1997;46:273–277.

Macleod AD. The reactivation of post-traumatic stress disorder in later life. *Aust N Z J Psychiatry*. 1994;28:625–634.

Manela M, Katona C, Livingston G. How common are the anxiety disorders in old age? *Int J Geriatr Psychiatry*. 1996;11:65–70.

Marshall RD, Beebe KL, Oldham M, Zaninelli R. Efficacy and safety of paroxetine treatment for chronic PTSD: a fixed-dose, placebo-controlled study. *Am J Psychiatry*. 2001;158:1982–1988.

Moser DK, Dracup K. Is anxiety early after myocardial infarction associated with subsequent ischemic and arrhythmic events? *Psychosom Med*. 1996;58:395–401.

Orrell M, Bebbington P. Psychosocial stress and anxiety in senile dementia. *J Affect Disord.* 1996;39:165–173.

Parmelee PA, Katz IR, Lawton MP. Anxiety and its association with depression among institutionalized elderly. *Am J Geriatr Psychiatry.* 1993;1:46–58.

Regier DA, Boyd JH, Burke JD Jr, et al. One-month prevalence of mental disorders in the United States: based on five epidemiologic catchment area sites. *Arch Gen Psychiatry.* 1988;45:977–986.

Rocca P, Fonzo V, Scotta M, Zanalda E, Ravizza L. Paroxetine efficacy in the treatment of generalized anxiety disorder. *Acta Psychiatr Scand.* 1997;95:444–450.

Rosen J, Fields RB, Hand AM, Falsettie G, Van Kammen DP. Concurrent posttraumatic stress disorder in psychogeriatric patients. *J Geriatr Psychiatry Neurol.* 1989;2: 65–69.

Schweizer E, Rickels K. Failure of buspirone to manage benzodiazepine withdrawal. *Am J Psychiatry.* 1986;1483:1590–1592.

Sheikh JI, King RJ, Taylor CB. Comparative phenomenology of early-onset versus late-onset panic attacks: a pilot study. *Am J Psychiatry.* 1991;148:1231–1233.

Skoog G, Skoog I. A 40-year follow-up of patients with obsessive-compulsive disorder. *Arch Gen Psychiatry.* 1999;56:121–127.

Skoog I. The prevalence of psychotic, depressive and anxiety syndromes in demented and non-demented 85-year-olds. *Int J Geriatr Psychiatry.* 1993;8:247–253.

Speed N, Engdahl B, Schwartz J, Eberly R. Posttraumatic stress disorder as a consequence of the POW experience. *J Nerv Ment Dis.* 1989;177:147–153.

Stein MB, Fyer AJ, Davidson JRT, Pollack MH, Wiita B. Fluvoxamine treatment of social phobia (social anxiety disorder): a double-blind, placebo-controlled study. *Am J Psychiatry.* 1999;156:756–760.

Stein MB, Liebowitz MR, Lydiard RB, Pitts CD, Bushnell W, Gergel I. Paroxetine treatment of generalized social phobia (social anxiety disorder): a randomized controlled trial. *JAMA.* 1998;280:708–713.

Steinberg JR. Anxiety in elderly patients. A comparison of azapirones and benzodiazepines. *Drugs Aging.* 1994;5:335–345.

Sullivan MD, LaCroix AZ, Baum C, Grothaus LC, Katon WJ. Functional status in coronary artery disease: a 1-year prospective study of the role of anxiety and depression. *Am J Med.* 1997;103:348–356.

Swales PJ, Solvin JF, Sheikh JI. Cognitive-behavioural therapy in older panic disorder patients. *Am J Geriatr Psychiatry.* 1996;4:46–60.

Uhlenhuth EH, Balter MB, Mellinger GD, Cisin IH, Clinthorne J. Symptom checklist syndromes in the general population: correlations with psychotherapeutic drug use. *Arch Gen Psychiatry.* 1983;40:1167–1173.

Wands K, Merskey H, Hachinski VC, Fisman M, Fox H, Boniferro M. A questionnaire investigation of anxiety and depression in early dementia. *J Am Geriatr Soc.* 1990; 38:535–538.

Wylie ME, Miller MD, Shear MK, et al. Fluvoxamine pharmacotherapy of anxiety disorders in later life: preliminary open-trial data. *J Geriatr Psychiatry Neurol.* 2000;13: 43–48.

24

Personality Disorders

Robert C. Abrams, MD
Joel Sadavoy, MD, FRCPC

INTRODUCTION

Personality disorders in the elderly are poorly understood, but have increasingly been appreciated for their potential to cause emotional suffering and disability in patients and frustration among those who attempt to care for them. While most clinicians encounter florid borderline or antisocial psychopathology only rarely, data show that the overall prevalence of personality disorders in old age remains substantial; what is changed is the distribution of individual disorders and clusters. In addition, personality dysfunction that does not fully meet criteria for a diagnosis of a personality disorder may take on greater importance in the later decades of life. Geriatric personality disorders are also important as comorbid conditions that contribute to or influence the presentation and course of affective disorders or as precursors of late-onset psychoses.

This chapter begins with a discussion of relationships between aging and the personality traits proposed by psychological investigators and then moves to a review of the clinical literature that considers personality disorders and traits in terms of standard diagnostic categories. The clinical sections include discussion of how comorbid psychiatric, medical, and neurological disorders that occur in later life may affect the phenomenology of the subthreshold and diagnosable personality disorders. The last sections of the chapter cover assessment issues and management, with an emphasis on how personality dysfunction can adversely affect an older person's ability to adapt to specific settings and can mar relationships with family members, physicians, and other important caregivers.

The reader should consider that two principal methods have been used to study relationships between personality and aging. The first, a cross-sectional approach, is most common. This methodology assesses different cohorts of individuals (e.g., young, middle-aged, and older adults) for the prevalence and severity of personality disorders and traits. Although cross-sectional comparisons are relatively easy to conduct, they can only suggest, but not prove, effects of aging. For example, patients who are currently in their 80s represent a different birth cohort than individuals in their 20s and have experienced different child-rearing practices and had different life experiences (ranging from the Great Depression and World War II to an increase in divorce rates and single-parent households). The effect of aging in cross-sectional comparisons is thus by implication.

In contrast, the second method, prospective longitudinal studies of groups of people, can demonstrate how these individuals change in basic personality attributes or in traits associated with personality disorders. Using clinical samples, longitudinal studies can clarify relationships between aging and factors associated with diagnosable personality disorders. These studies are more difficult to conduct and are therefore less frequent. The chapter's review includes both types of study.

DEFINITIONS

We conceptualize personality as a set of characteristic ways an individual responds to both internal stimuli, such as affects, and external stimuli, such as stress, relationships, or tasks. An individual's personality characteristics result from both constitutional factors and life experiences, particularly those that occurred in childhood, and represent a pattern of responses. Particular response patterns, not necessarily pathological except in extremes, are known as *personality traits*. Relationships between specified personality traits and aging have been studied through systematic investigations of nonclinical as well as clinical populations.

In contrast to personality traits, *personality disorders* are constellations of specific traits, pathological by definition or in their extent, that are associated with dysfunctional relationships and behavior. Clinical investigators have begun to address how aging affects the prevalence, symptom presentation, comorbid relationships, and severity of personality disorders. The perspective of these studies differs from that of the psychological studies carried out in "normal" populations to determine how aging affects personality.

CHANGES IN PERSONALITY ASSOCIATED WITH AGING

Underlying the study of personality disorders in the elderly are the fundamental, and not completely answered, questions of whether and how personality changes over time. A scientific answer to the question of whether personality changes depends partly on methodology, and here it is of particular relevance whether cross-sectional or longitudinal studies are cited. Large-scale population studies and other cross-sectional investigations have tended to support the notion of interiority (Neugarten, 1979) and related conceptions (Bee, 1986) that characterize normal aging as a progression toward a quiet, inner-directed attitude.

For example, the classical cross-sectional Minnesota Multiphasic Personality Inventory (MMPI) literature, involving large age-stratified populations of medical patients, showed that older medical patients scored higher on scales that measured introversion, concern with health, immaturity, and depression than younger patients and scored lower on scales that measured impulsivity, sociopathy, and hostility than younger patients (Swenson et al., 1973). These findings are consistent with the declines in criminality and sociopathy with aging found by Woodruff and others in the 1970s (Woodruff et al., 1971) and with more recent reports of age-related moderation of impulsivity (Stevenson et al., 2003) and increases in affective control (LaBouvie-Vief et al., 1989).

Eysenck and Eysenck (1985) found that, in age-stratified samples, three fundamental traits used to define personality (psychoticism, extraversion, and neuroticism) all declined with age from a peak at the teenage years. Men started with higher levels of extraversion and lower levels of neuroticism than women, but the decline in extraversion among men was steeper, so that a crossover occurred; older men then had less extraversion, that is, they were less outgoing, than older women, the opposite of the picture in young adulthood. The notion that aging is associated with increasing androgyny has also found support by others (Helson & Wink, 1992).

In contrast to cross-sectional comparisons, longitudinal studies using MMPI data (Gynther, 1979) and more recent studies of normative aging using a comprehensive five-factor model of personality (McCrae & Costa, 1990, 1997) have demonstrated a general stability of personality traits in later life. These findings suggest that it is mainly in illness—e.g., depression, dementia, or chronic medical conditions—that significant personality change is to be found in the elderly. The data emphasizing longitudinal stability of key personality dimensions are congruent with original psychoanalytic theories, which held that, after childhood, major psychological structures were mutable only with extensive therapeutic intervention, if then (Freud, 1923/1962).

However, other investigators using prospective or longitudinal methodology have emphasized psychological maturation over the life span rather than stability. Vaillant (1977) studied vignettes of behavior collected at different ages to investigate the maturation of psychological defenses; he concluded that the findings basically supported the Eriksonian conceptualization of maturation as a sequence of responses to the developmental challenges occurring at different phases of life (Erikson, 1963). In a prospective study of 173 college men from ages 18 to 65 years, Vaillant and colleagues also showed that, while dysfunctional personality traits may persist over many decades, their detrimental effects on adjustment and personal happiness become less obvious with time (Vaillant & Milofsky, 1980).

Of course, other factors may influence the maturation of the personality and provide additional exceptions to the rule of stability, some of them positive and others negative. For example, psychotherapy aims to advance the process of personal growth, while catastrophic life events and disadvantages associated with gender, social class, certain social roles, and alcoholism can all inhibit the maturation of the personality (Costa & McCrae, 1992b; Helson & Stewart, 1994).

In considering the potential for personality change or stability, the age-related evolution of personality disorders should be distinguished from normal personality development. Based on a cross-sectional regression analysis of the relationships of different personality disorder traits with age, Tyrer (1988) proposed a distinction between "mature" and "immature" disorders. Based on Tyrer's analyses, the mature disorders include the obsessive-compulsive, schizotypal, schizoid, and paranoid categories; these personality disorders are presumed to be chronic conditions that show more stability and less variation over time than others. The immature disorders according to Tyrer include the borderline, antisocial, narcissistic, histrionic, and passive-aggressive categories; these personality disorders are more evident in younger individuals, may have earlier onset than mature personality disorders, and may become less obvious with time. However, Tyrer's cross-sectional analyses did not specifically address how personality disorders classified according to levels of maturity are affected by aging.

Other authors, such as Vaillant and Perry (1990), found longitudinal observations to generally support the idea that the immature or flamboyant personality disorders, particularly the histrionic, show gradual improvement over time, whereas conditions like avoidant and dependent disorders are more chronic. Similarly, McGlashan (1986) and Stone (1993) each observed, based on follow-up data, that the most florid borderline symptomatology in young adults tends to be attenuated by about 30 years of age. However, McGlashan also warned that the disturbance in interpersonal relationships seen in young patients with borderline disorder, even after a period of relative quiescence, may persist as a potential nidus for serious difficulties in the later decades of life.

PREVALENCE OF PERSONALITY DISORDERS
IN OLDER PERSONS

For several reasons, it has been difficult to get an accurate picture of the prevalence of personality disorders in the geriatric population. Historically, there has been some ambivalence about the appropriateness of the personality disorder designation in elderly patients. For example, the framers of the *Diagnostic and Statistical Manual of Mental Disorders, Third Edition* (*DSM-III*) expressed the view that personality disorders could not be found in substantial numbers among the elderly. The introduction to Axis II in *DSM-III* noted that personality disorders are present for most of adult life, but become "attenuated" by middle age (American Psychiatric Association [APA], 1980); at the same time, *DSM-III* required symptoms to be present currently to make the diagnosis, thereby signaling that they intended these diagnoses to be assigned infrequently. Only in the organic personality syndrome of *DSM-III* and the revised third edition, *DSM-III-R* (APA, 1987) were there no restrictions on age or duration of symptoms in the criteria for personality disorder. However, organic personality syndrome and its successor, personality change due to a general medical syndrome, in the fourth edition (*DSM-IV*; APA, 1994) and text revision to the fourth edition (*DSM-IV-TR*; APA, 2000), have been classified apart from the traditional personality disorders, mainly because a known organic etiology is required.

Additional categories in the *DSM* nosology, such as personality traits or coping style affecting medical condition, phase of life problem, or other or unspecified personality disorders may capture one or more elements of dysfunctional personality change with aging, but do not by themselves constitute a nosology for personality disorders in geriatric patients. The introduction in *DSM-IV* and *DSM-IV-TR* of personality disorder Criterion D, which requires that dysfunctional personality traits be stable, of long duration, and specifically traceable to adolescence or early adulthood, has provided greater clarity. However, future research may show that the requirement for early onset is excessively limiting with respect to the elderly population and contributes to underdiagnosis in this age group.

Another difficulty in assessing the prevalence of personality disorder in the elderly is that some criteria for the individual disorders may have limited relevance or be difficult to apply to the experiences of elderly patients. Axis II criteria have been criticized for allowing insufficient consideration of changes in the types of interpersonal relationships that older persons have and in the domains in which they function (Fogel & Westlake, 1990). Thus, personality disorders in older adults will not be expressed in the context of separating from parents, developing intimate relationships, or functioning in the workplace, but in the setting of widowhood, contraction of one's social network, and retirement. Also, clinicians might underestimate recklessness or impulsivity in older patients because the usual avenues for such behavior are not readily available in the lives of the elderly. Conversely, clinicians might overestimate the pathological aspects of realistically dependent behavior in disabled older patients.

In addition, studies of personality disorder diagnoses in elderly patients have been difficult to compare. Comparability has been limited because the studies used different designs, populations, and methods (e.g., structured interview, chart review, etc.). Thus, it is not surprising that the literature on personality disorders in late life is relatively inconclusive. Individual studies have suggested a lower prevalence of personality disorders in old, versus young, adults, especially in Cluster B (Casey, 1988; Kroessler, 1990; Kunik et al., 1994) and no differences between elderly males and elderly females (Ames & Molinari, 1994).

However, a meta-analysis based on 30 studies published from 1980 to 1997 that examined personality disorders in older adults produced only minimal differences based on age. The overall prevalence rate for a diagnosis of personality disorder was 20% for the patients in the studies over 50 years of age, versus 22% for those younger than 50 years (Abrams & Horowitz, 1999). This type of analysis does not rule out the possibility of a true age effect, but it does support the impression that personality disorders are to be found in older adults in numbers greater than formerly thought. Aging may not, after all, necessarily imply a linear reduction in prevalence or severity of personality disorders. In support of this notion, an epidemiological study of personality disorders conducted by Reich and coworkers (1988) found Cluster B symptoms to be prevalent in a reverse J-shaped curve; core traits declined to 60 years of age, then took a smaller but distinct upturn. The meta-analytic data cited above also tended to support gender differences in the distribution of individual personality disorders; that is, the female predominance in young adult populations of histrionic, borderline, and dependent personality disorders was retained in the geriatric age group, as was the male predominance in narcissistic, antisocial, paranoid, schizoid, and schizotypal personality disorders.

Within geriatric populations, rates of personality disorder appear to be highest in patients with depressive disorders, about 33% in those with major depressive disorder and 31% in elderly patients with dysthymic disorder (Devanand et al., 2000). In at least some studies of elderly depressives or dysthymics, avoidant and dependent personality disorders have been the most frequent, a finding that seems intuitive given the higher rates of personality disorder in depressed populations and the close relationships between depressive and anxious-fearful phenomena (Abrams et al., 1994; Devanand et al., 2000). However, Abrams and Horowitz (1999) found paranoid personality disorder to be the most prevalent across all studies; this seems consistent with Tyrer's (1988) maturation hypothesis, in which suicidality and impulsiveness, key characteristics of the immature or Cluster B disorders, would diminish over time, leaving Cluster A disorders more numerically prevalent in old age.

An important gap in knowledge concerns information on the prevalence of personality traits that do not meet full diagnostic criteria for a personality disorder and how these traits change with age. Such traits may be remnants of previously existing personality disorder diagnoses that have "burned out" over time, or they may have persisted over many years at a subthreshold level. Whatever their origin, the dysfunctional traits that do not meet diagnostic criteria for a personality disorder because of insufficient severity or duration may well represent the most numerous and the most clinically important personality "disorders" in the elderly population. Personality disorders not otherwise specified (NOS) (i.e., those conditions that meet the general criteria for personality disorder diagnosis, but not for any of the specific entities) may also prove important in the elderly.

To summarize, knowledge of the epidemiology of personality disorders in the elderly is based on a relatively narrow database from which it is premature to draw definite conclusions. However, the data suggest the following hypotheses:

1. The overall prevalence of personality disorders in clinical populations may be only slightly lower in elderly than in younger adults.
2. Rates of personality disorder diagnoses are highest in patients with Axis I depressive disorders.
3. Personality disorders from Clusters C and A may be the most numerically important in older adults.
4. Elderly patients with personality disorders, like younger ones, have a high frequency of Axis I–Axis II comorbidity, with especially close associations between Cluster C personality disorders and major depression or dysthymic disorder.
5. The distributions of individual disorders according to gender seen in young adults (i.e., more numerous borderline, histrionic, and dependent personality disorders among females and more narcissistic, antisocial, paranoid, schizoid, and schizotypal personality disorders among males) may persist into old age, although it is not clear that personality disorders overall are more prevalent in either gender.
6. Personality dysfunction that does not meet full diagnostic criteria for personality disorder and personality disorder NOS may be particularly important entities in elderly populations.

RELATIONSHIPS BETWEEN PERSONALITY DISORDERS AND COMORBIDITIES THAT OCCUR IN LATER LIFE

Comorbid personality conditions are a complicating feature of the presentation and management of primary conditions. While depression is the most common comorbid condition, other Axis I disorders, including anxiety disorders, posttraumatic states, and somatization disorders, also frequently interact with personality disorder (Sadavoy, 1999).

Late-Life Personality Disorders and Depression

As suggested in the section above, personality disorders in the elderly are concentrated in depressed populations. For example, while the overall rate of personality disorder in the elderly was estimated to be about 20% based on published studies, the prevalence of personality disorder comorbidity among elderly patients with depressive disorders was 33% (Abrams & Horowitz, 1999).

What is the significance of personality disorder–major depressive disorder comorbidity in the elderly? In younger adults with major depressive disorder, comorbid personality disorders have been associated with earlier onset of depression, multiple depressive episodes, and longer duration of episodes (Black et al., 1988), as well as with more frequent suicide attempts compared to other depressives. The presence of comorbid personality disorder in younger adults also appears to negatively influence the short-term outcome of pharmacotherapy of major depressive disorder (Pfohl et al., 1984), particularly in patients with Cluster C personality disorders (Frank et al., 1987).

In elderly patients with depression, personality disorders have been associated with chronicity of affective symptoms (Devanand et al., 1994), completed suicide (Loebel, 1990), and poor short-term outcome in psychotherapy (Thompson et al., 1988), although the relationship of personality disorder with length of depressive episodes remains uncertain. As in younger adults, when personality disorder and major depressive disorder coexist, the first major depressive episode tends to occur earlier in life (Abrams et al., 1994). Some geriatric samples show a predominance of avoidant and dependent (Cluster C) personality disorders (e.g., Abrams et al., 1987), although, as noted earlier, paranoid personality disorder was the most prevalent in a meta-analytic review of recent studies (Abrams & Horowitz, 1999).

In elderly patients with dysthymia, personality disorders have been found to occur in about the same rate as in elderly patients with major depressive disorder (31.2%) (Devanand et al., 2000). In geriatric dysthymia, personality disorders were associated with an earlier age at onset and greater symptomatic severity of depression, greater frequency of other Axis I disorders, and lower socioeconomic status (Devanand et al., 2000). The findings in both major depressive disorder and dysthymia of a lower frequency of personality disorder comorbidity with increasing age of depression onset support the notion that these late-life depressive disorders are fundamentally different entities from those found in younger populations.

Despite the organization of DSM nosology into separate axes since 1980, personality and depressive disorders have long been viewed as related and, when depression is nonmelancholic, difficult to distinguish. DSM-IV-TR (APA, 2000) describes how acute mood or anxiety disorders may produce cross-sectional symptoms that "mimic" personality traits and impede the diagnostic process by distorting the individual's view of his or her long-term functioning. At their core, personality disorders involve long-term difficulties in self-concept, regulation of affect and impulses, and the quality of interpersonal relationships, all of which could be affected by mood or in turn produce effects on mood. Thus, the relationships among depressive episodes, personality characteristics, and functioning are necessarily complex.

Personality disorders and depression may be orthogonal or etiologically independent even if concurrent (Hirschfeld & Klerman, 1979), but multiple interactions are possible. Clinicians have long noted that, in both young and older adult patients, personality dysfunction seems to be exacerbated by depressive disorder; that is, depression makes the already difficult personality even harder to manage and tolerate. Also, it has been suggested that the experience of episodes of depression can "scar" the personality, leading to diminished self-esteem and increased dependency (Hirschfeld & Klerman, 1979). Given the cumulative impact of repeated depressive episodes, older persons would be most vulnerable to this effect.

Another model proposes a synergistic or interactive relationship between personality and depression, one in which their combined effects lead to prolonged impairments in functioning and adaptation (Abrams et al., 2001). In elderly patients, the presence of residual depressive symptoms after treatment of a major depressive episode might continue to exacerbate personality disorder symptoms, resulting in prolongation of depression-related disability (poorer global functioning 1 year after remission from the acute episode) (Abrams et al., 2001). Thus, elderly patients with both depressive and personality disorders represent a sizable population having particular vulnerability for protracted depression-related disability.

Personality Disorders and Cognitive Decline

There remains some doubt whether the passivity, withdrawal, loss of interest, lability, and immaturity of emotional responses observed in patients with Alzheimer's disease should be viewed as personality phenomena rather than behavioral manifestations of central nervous system dysfunction. The changes in coping that accompany dementia may also be seen as part of the underlying neurological disorder. However, Cummings et al. (1990) argued that changes in the manner of emotional expression, ways of relating to others, enthusiasm, and maturity all reflect alterations in long-standing behavioral style and thus can legitimately be viewed as personality phenomena.

In senile dementia of the Alzheimer type (SDAT), a recognizable sequence of personality changes has begun to emerge. However, these personality changes do not seem to have a simple linear relationship to the severity of cognitive impairment. What has been found is an early disengagement and increase in passivity, including loss of interest in hobbies and overall loss of spontaneity (Petry et al., 1989). Based on the five-factor model of personality (McCrae & Costa, 1990), there is an early increase in neuroticism, with reductions in extraversion and conscientiousness; these trends continue as the disease progresses, along with smaller decreases in openness and agreeableness (Welleford et al., 1995). Early SDAT may also be associated with more anxiety and dysphoria than more advanced stages, when patients' awareness of the illness seems to recede (Chatterjie et al., 1992). In vascular dementia, patients at a comparable phase of illness may show greater maturity and control than individuals with SDAT, but over time, both show deterioration of functioning and loss of integrity of the personality (Cummings et al., 1990).

ASSESSMENT OF PERSONALITY DISORDERS
IN OLDER PERSONS

The diagnosis of personality disorder in elderly patients requires considerable effort. First, the clinician should be sensitive to the need to translate some of the diagnostic criteria—particularly for the borderline and antisocial personality disorders—into the experiences and surroundings of the elderly. Older persons exist in different life circumstances than young adults. For example, older adults may have more stable relationships and lack the stresses associated with beginning a career. These differences in circumstances may obscure dysfunctional personality traits such as those that are most likely be to be expressed in new interpersonal relationships and those that unmask an unstable sense of self. Also, because symptoms are required to be present more or less continuously from late adolescence through adulthood, the clinician must ask elderly patients or informants to provide history over a lengthy time frame; in practice, it is difficult and unusual to obtain information of this nature.

Assessment in the Context of Depression

Contamination of personality disorder assessment by the effects of mood state, usually depression, poses another problem. Congruent with their mood state, depressed patients may exaggerate negative aspects of their behavior, or certain features of their depressed mood state may be difficult to distinguish from dysfunctional personality traits. Depressed elderly patients may not only distort their histories as younger patients do, but often lack the motivation and energy to engage in a retrospective evaluation of their long-term personality functioning, which naturally covers a longer time than with younger adults. For these reasons, assignment of Axis II disorders has been thought to be best deferred until resolution of the acute depressive episode.

This state-trait confound has been widely recognized as a methodological problem in research using younger subjects (for example, Reich et al., 1987), but not definitively investigated in the elderly. Consequently, in studies of elderly depressed patients for whom personality features also need to be examined, measures of dimensional personality traits, such as the five factors elaborated by McCrae and Costa (1990, 1997), have increasingly been used in lieu of categorical personality disorder diagnoses. These five factors—neuroticism, extraversion, openness, agreeableness, and conscientiousness—are operationalized in the NEO Personality Inventory–Revised (NEO-PI-R) instrument (Costa & McCrae, 1992a) and may be both more reliable and less influenced by affective state than traditionally diagnosed personality disorders. The NEO-PI-R has also lent itself to novel uses in studies relevant to geriatric depression, for example, as a structured interview allowing relatives of suicide completers to provide postmortem personality profiles of the victim (Duberstein et al., 1994).

Another approach that could be considered for both investigative and clinical work is the use of structured instruments for the assessment of *DSM* personality disorders, some of which, like the Personality Disorder Examination (Loranger et al., 1987), are relatively resistant to state effects and can yield both categorical diagnoses and dimensional scores for each personality disorder. Informants, if available, may provide some degree of corroborative validation for any assessment method.

Assessment in Persons With Cognitive Impairment

Personality dysfunction in elderly patients with cognitive impairment has generally not been assessed using categorical personality disorder criteria. However, a growing literature suggests that caregivers or close relatives can provide reliable and valid information with the NEO-PI-R about the patient's premorbid functioning (Chatterjie et al., 1992; Siegler et al., 1994; Strauss et al., 1993). These studies have used a technique in which informants are interviewed twice—first to report on the subject's personality functioning before the onset of dementia and again to describe the individual's present personality functioning. Findings suggest that the onset of dementia is associated with increases in neuroticism and decreases in extraversion, openness, and conscientiousness. However, confirmatory longitudinal studies are lacking.

Research into relationships between premorbid personality characteristics and changes in dementia can lead to better understanding of which of these factors are clinical predictors of the behavioral disturbances, such as agitation, that often occur in association with cognitive deterioration. It is also hoped that this kind of research will delineate clear targets for the development of pharmacological and environmental interventions.

CLINICAL IMPACT OF PERSONALITY
DYSFUNCTION IN OLD AGE

There are many settings and situations in which personality disorders or subsyndromal personality dysfunction in the elderly may be evident. One of the most typical is in general medical practice, in which personality dysfunction can create troubling disturbances in the doctor-patient relationship. Patients may induce frustration in their physicians by refusing or thwarting much-needed medical interventions, while at the same time complaining of illness or even exaggerating physical symptoms. They may have little motivation to improve. They may refuse to acknowledge the need for social interventions such as home care, assisted living, or nursing home care, sometimes creating a crisis by insisting on conditions that threaten their safety. They may also become unreasonably litigious, disrupting the doctor-patient relationship entirely. Individuals with personality disorders or personality dysfunction are likely to be well represented among the patients described by hospital and nursing home staffs as "difficult," "demanding," "hateful," or other pejoratives.

Elderly individuals may be chronically angry or dissatisfied, rejecting or rejection sensitive, or merely misanthropic, unable to reach out to others or to allow themselves to be consoled. These characteristics are expressed in many aspects of their personal lives, including in relationships with family members and with the caregivers who become more essential as people age. Disturbances in personality-disordered patients' interactions with other people are also likely to undermine their relationships with physicians and impact negatively on their attitudes toward treatment and adherence to medical recommendations. Because the goal of having home health aides is to help elders compensate for diminished functional independence, disturbance in those relationships is especially costly to the individual. The overall cost of personality dysfunction to the patients, to their families, and to society has never been reckoned.

In short, individuals with personality disorders age badly. Rather, they become unable or unwilling to acknowledge the limitations imposed by the passing of time, unable or unwilling to accept help, and unable or unwilling to make reasonable decisions about their health care, finances, and day-to-day maintenance.

CLINICAL PROFILES

Below, we offer some overall clinical profiles, organized according to cluster, of the presentation of personality disorder symptomatology in older adults.

The elderly patient with Cluster A disorders or subthreshold symptomatology (paranoid, schizoid, schizotypal) is typically an elderly person who has been a loner or reclusive and in some instances iconoclastic or rebellious. What most defines these individuals is the lifelong avoidance of emotionally taxing one-on-one relationships, a feature that often seals their general isolation from the rest of society. Such people can function fairly well throughout much of adult life by going their own way and steering clear of demanding or intimate relationships. Their difficulties often do not become apparent until they need to live communally, such as in a nursing home or other institutional setting, in which they cannot avoid intensive human contact and must comply with rules. The need for assistance in bathing or dressing is often poorly tolerated because of the intimacy that is implied.

Cluster A personality disorders are sometimes referred to or included within the category of schizophrenia-spectrum disorders; they are often found to have been premorbid conditions among patients with late-onset schizophrenia or delusional disorder (Harris & Jeste, 1988). As discussed in previous sections of this chapter, Cluster A symptomatology is thought to start relatively late and persist throughout adult life. Accordingly, these conditions have been described as mature personality disorders, partly to distinguish them from the Cluster B or immature disorders, which start early, but may diminish in intensity over time (Tyrer, 1988).

Cluster B is represented by the borderline, narcissistic, antisocial, and histrionic disorders. Again, these have traditionally been viewed as disorders of immaturity (i.e., with early onset and progressive diminution in intensity of symptoms). Indeed, the image of the typical seductive, manipulative, or chronically self-injurious borderline young woman is rarely matched to the clinical presentation of older adults; occasional case reports in the literature of patients who do meet this profile, if anything, serve to reinforce their rarity. In addition, the decline in criminality with age in both populations and individuals has long been established (Woodruff et al., 1971). However, various symptoms in this cluster do persist and have considerable clinical and human importance. For example, the person with significant narcissistic features is faced with particular difficulties as he or she ages (Sadavoy, 1992).

To varying degrees, individuals with high degrees of narcissistic trait have difficulty accepting a loss of physical beauty and desirability, especially if it has been a major source of their self-esteem or they cannot relinquish a position of control at work. Thus, they do not focus on giving to the next generation, passing along whatever wealth or wisdom they have accumulated. Generally, they cannot sublimate their reluctance to withdraw from active professional life by promoting a worthy cause that might live on after them; instead, they remain intent on holding on to beauty, power, or wealth. Such individuals cannot genuinely feel pride and enthusiasm for the accomplishments of their younger protégés or even their own children, but instead feel envy. This may translate into such behaviors as allowing children to fight over an anticipated inheritance, playing one against the other with the carrot of money or possessions, or making last-ditch efforts to stay in control by refusing medical or nursing services that are truly needed. Narcissism and envy tend to cause an older person to experience their adult children's growing independence with resentment or feelings of abandonment. Narcissistic traits may even prevent a person from preparing or accepting his or her eventual death, perhaps placing the individual at risk for significant depression when that reality can no longer be avoided. In some or all of these ways, pathological narcissism and envy may deprive the individual of the pleasures that can be experienced in maturity.

Remnants of borderline and narcissistic personality disorder features may be found in older patients' manipulative use of physical illness and disability. For example, they may seek help, then reject it, or in other ways create conflicts among family members or institutional staff members over their care. A form of narcissism is sometimes seen in which pride is taken at experiencing the very worst suffering, based on a fear of loneliness and abandonment and predicated on the notion that the need for assistance is the only claim that can legitimately be made on others.

Cluster C anxiety phenomena may be represented by a generalized fearfulness and pessimism. In the context of coping with fears of illness and dependency, individuals with Cluster C traits would be expected to demonstrate heightened controlling or passive-aggressive behaviors or exaggerated dependency and needs for reassurance. Sometimes, such individuals in old age may mask their underlying fearfulness with a pervasive veneer of dissatisfaction, through which nothing they can experience in the present is good or sufficient, especially compared to what they knew in the past. Of course, these manifestations also contain narcissistic elements.

MANAGEMENT AND TREATMENT

This overview of management and treatment borrows the useful structure of published guidelines (APA, 2001) on treatment of borderline personalities to consider the issues of old age. Treatment of personality disorders in old age is both similar to and different from therapies for younger patients, but age-specific issues require substantial modification or refocusing of these principles to address more age-specific factors of diagnosis and treatment. Treatment of personality disorder in old age gets short shrift in both the general psychogeriatric literature and the personality disorder literature. Indeed, there is little acknowledgment of this problem anywhere in the mainstream writings on treatment on the subject and few if any studies to guide clinical practice.

General Assessment Considerations

All therapy of personality disorder begins with full assessment. As with all geriatric therapies, this may have to be repeated from time to time as the patient's condition evolves. In elders, treatment is complicated by comorbid factors that are virtually always present. Hence, assessment includes:

1. Careful examination of physical problems. A full physical examination is usually best performed by a family doctor or other physician. Important for many reasons, this examination also helps the therapist determine what the realistic physical issues may be. When the therapist is anxious along with the patient, for example, about the potential that serious physical problems have emerged, poor decisions are made. The best defense against these common issues in treatment of the patient with personality disorder is a comprehensive assessment. Because these patients often use physical complaints as the language of communication with the therapist, an alternative to the ability to describe psychological pain, it is a ready source of manipulation. By knowing what the reality is, the therapist is able to redirect the patient's somatized complaints accurately to the source of the patient's conflict and symptomatic behavior. This reduces the potential for defensive manipulation.
2. Suicidal potential. When older patients with personality disorder become desperate, they often invoke desperate solutions, including threats of suicide or strong wishes for death. Careful inquiry at the outset helps identify this issue and brings it into the treatment situation. Patients who have been chronically self-destructive or suicidal as a feature of

their personality disorders require an exploration of what increases their suicidal impulses, how they have coped with them, and what factors have prevented them from completing suicide previously. Access to a variety of lethal means of suicide, including both prescribed and over-the-counter medications, underscores the importance of identifying the risk for suicide and aggressively managing these individuals. Lethality of prescribed medications readily available to the patient and other available means of suicide need to be assessed and corrective measures taken as necessary.

3. Assessment of concurrent medications and factors that affect the use and metabolism of medication. Medication review also involves knowing where the patient obtains his or her medications, including sometimes making direct contact with other prescribers or pharmacies to confirm the information.

4. Assessment of complaints of sleep problems and nocturnal anxiety. These are common problems around which manipulation occurs. They present greater challenges in therapy of elders because they are often reality based and cannot simply be interpreted away. Management poses special problems because the medications used to manage these problems are subject to abuse. Moreover, the side effects are problematic in elders, with the induction of cognitive slippage, gait instability associated with falls, and sometimes paradoxical increase in anxiety because of feelings of loss of control induced by anxiolytic drugs.

5. Assessment of alcohol or other substance abuse. Substance abuse is especially problematic in old age because the elderly patient becomes increasingly less able to tolerate doses and patterns of use of younger years. The age-related, stress-induced motivation to drink or self-medicate, however, often increases in these patients, leading to a vicious circle. Substance abuse is often hidden by the patient and requires collateral information when available.

6. Assessment of cognitive impairment. Impairment reduces control over impulses, may contribute to increased perception of loss of control over self and environment, and may produce clinging agitated behavior or overreliance on medical intervention.

7. Assessment of social and environmental factors. These are more complex in elders. Examination of family relationships and conducting a social review as well as a family interview when necessary reduce the chance of the therapist buying into the patient's long-standing distortions and beliefs about family interactions. The nursing home or other custodial environment is a breeding ground for personality disorder–based psychopathology because of the frequent indifference of such places to the individual needs of patients and the tendency to reject the difficult behaviors of patients with personality disorder. The most common effect of the custodial environment, especially in the first weeks or

months after admission, is to increase stress on the narcissistically vulnerable patient or those prone to rejection sensitivity and abandonment fears. Residence in extended-care facilities provides a fertile ground for rekindling conflict with authority figures and emotions associated with personality-based fears of others, mistrust of intimacy, and loss of personal control.

Perceptions of abandonment by caregivers and family are common among patients with personality disorder and may lead them to perceive a lower level of support than is actually there. IADL/ADL capacities and home environment should also be examined because the PD patient may become quite dysfunctional at home as a result of anxiety or depressive reactions. This latter assessment may require a home visit by the therapist or other team member.

Management and Treatment Considerations

COORDINATION OF CARE   Elders generally have a number of professional caregivers in their lives. A hallmark of the behavior of many elderly patients with more severe forms of personality disorder is manipulation of the system, examples of which include "multiple doctoring" and "splitting" of health care aides, family caregivers, physicians, pharmacists, and other personnel by encouraging conflicts among them or otherwise engendering confusion. Coordination of care is essential, but very difficult even in a closed system like a nursing home, in which staff communication among team members is often fragmentary. The successful therapist will need to spend more time than desired on coordinating the system of care and ensuring that there is adequate communication among the caregiving group. This is one indication for family conferences. In the nursing home environment, communication meetings are important to discuss diagnosis, team tensions generated by the patient, treatment plans, and consistency of the interventions among all members of the team.

USE OF GROUP THERAPY SETTINGS   Elders sometimes do well in group settings, such as a day hospital, that serve both a specific therapeutic function and important social support functions. They also provide brief, but important, periods of respite for other caregivers. Generally, however, these group formats are more effective if composed only of elders rather than mixing elderly patients with personality disorders into a general adult group setting.

EMPLOYMENT OF INDIVIDUAL PSYCHOTHERAPIES   Some form of individual therapy is usually necessary in treating elders with personality disorder. Crisis intervention alone is sometimes sufficient, but occasionally more intensive therapy is necessary when the patient can no longer cope with the array of life-transforming events encountered. Overwhelming life change is not amenable to short-term crisis intervention and may require longer term therapy that incorporates individual and other psychosocial interventions.

INVOLVEMENT OF THE FAMILY   Family involvement in therapy is often important, but complicated by long-standing conflicts in which adult children continue to be locked into unresolved patterns of interaction that stem from years past and have little relationship to the current problems of old age with which the parent is struggling. Managing the family thus typically involves helping children begin to place the parent into a more age-appropriate context. From the patient's viewpoint, therapy helps them to develop a more appropriate set of expectations. For example, the therapist is effective if he or she can act as an interpersonal coach, reviewing scenarios of interaction between parents and children (or other close caregivers) and working out a more effective request/response pattern.

RESPONSE TO CRISES AND SAFETY MANAGEMENT   Personality disorder–based crises in old age tend to be less dramatic than in younger years and more focused on health-related issues or family/caregiver conflicts. Elders who are reliant on caregivers may strain their relationships to the breaking point and cause caregivers to abandon them when they need them the most. Some elders are at true risk of suicide if pushed to desperation by a system that will not or cannot respond to their needs (e.g., because of inattentive children or professional staff that fails to diagnose new psychopathology such as the emergence of a depressive disorder or a medication side effect such as akathisia). This last issue becomes most relevant in long-term care settings or in family interactive situations when the patient's agitation, suicidal desperation, or somatic complaints are labeled as part of the familiar lifelong personality-derived manipulations that the patient may have exhibited for years. Inherent in this rejection are often the hostility and underlying rage of caregivers toward a difficult or therapeutically unresponsive patient. Patients with a pattern of help-rejecting, yet complaining, behavior are at particular risk for not receiving adequate treatment for a real medical syndrome.

Dealing with Special Issues: Splitting and Limit Setting

Splitting is a great danger with elders because of the various avenues for manipulation of others that exist. Splitting is a construct derived from psychoanalytic theory that offers a useful model for understanding certain behaviors found in personality disorder.

Splitting refers to the patient's tendency to behave toward others as though they are either all good or all bad, that is, as either idealized or having no value. This oversimplified good-versus-bad perception of significant others is complicated by the fact that patients with borderline personality disorders frequently, and often without much provocation, shift individuals from one of these categories into the other. In a confined environment, such as an assisted-living facility, elders with a propensity for splitting are likely to perceive staff as either helpful or harmful and to play one staff member against others (e.g., befriending the idealized staff member while speaking against devalued others). Disputes within the caregiver group can arise as different caregivers or family members assume strongly felt, but opposing, views of the patient's care. Awareness of this process, the reasons behind it, and a resident's propensity to behave this way can enable staff to respond more objectively toward residents and avoid becoming involved in conflicts that result from a resident's distorted perceptions.

Setting limits and boundaries with elders is sometimes more complicated than with younger patients. For example it can be hard for therapists and other caregivers to determine when it is appropriate to respond to patient demands or requests of staff (e.g., for increased personal attention or medication) or complaints about other residents in a long-term care facility and what is the result of patients' personality-based behavior.

Boundaries must be established around the form and frequency of patient communication, such as limits on impulsive, desperate, or importuning phone calls. An added issue in treating personality disorder in elders is attending to boundaries for their families. Families often adopt the patient's infectious anxiety, for example, by calling the doctor inappropriately. The therapist therefore needs to take family members' distress, and sometimes psychopathology, into account during the treatment. This involves allowing the family time to discuss issues, placing therapeutic limits on them, remaining alert to and heading off issues that may induce litigiousness, or intervening at the systemic level if families begin to become too disruptive (e.g., trying to bypass the system, overusing emergency facilities, or making complaints to nursing home or hospital management).

REFERENCES

Abrams RC. The aging personality [editorial]. *Int J Geriatr Psychiatry*. 1991;6:1–3.

Abrams RC, Alexopoulos GS, Spielman LA, Klausner E, Kakuma T. Personality disorder symptoms predict declines in global functioning and quality of life in elderly depressed patients. *Am J Geriatr Psychiatry*. 2001;45:111–119.

Abrams RC, Alexopoulos GS, Young RC. Geriatric depression and *DSM-III-R* personality disorder criteria. *J Am Geriatr Soc*. 1987;35:383–386.

Abrams RC, Horowitz SV. Personality disorders after age 50: a meta-analytic review of the literature. In: Rosowsky E, Abrams RC, Zweig RA, eds. *Personality Disorders in Older Adults: Emerging Issues in Diagnosis and Treatment*. Mahwah, NJ: Lawrence Erlbaum; 1999.

Abrams RC, Rosendahl E, Card C, Alexopoulos GS. Personality disorder correlates of late and early onset depression. *J Am Geriatr Soc*. 1994;42:727–731.

American Psychiatric Association. *Diagnostic and Statistical Manual of Mental Disorders*. 3rd ed. Washington, DC: American Psychiatric Association; 1980.

American Psychiatric Association. *Diagnostic and Statistical Manual of Mental Disorders*. 3rd ed., rev. Washington, DC: American Psychiatric Association; 1987.

American Psychiatric Association. *Diagnostic and Statistical Manual of Mental Disorders*. 4th ed. Washington, DC: American Psychiatric Association; 1994.

American Psychiatric Association. *Diagnostic and Statistical Manual of Mental Disorders*. 4th ed., text rev. Washington, DC: American Psychiatric Association; 2000.

American Psychiatric Association. Practice guidelines for the treatment of patients with borderline personality disorder. *Am J Psychiatry*. 2001;158(suppl):4–52.

Ames A, Molinari V. Prevalence of personality disorders in community-living elderly. *J Geriatr Psychiatry Neurol*. 1994;7:189–194.

Bee HL. Changes in personality, motivations and values over the adult years. In: Bee HL, ed. *The Journey of Adulthood*. New York, NY: Macmillan; 1986.

Black DW, Bell S, Hulbert J, Nasrallah A. The importance of Axis II in patients with major depression: a controlled study. *J Affect Disord*. 1988;14:115–122.

Casey P. The epidemiology of personality disorder. In: Tyrer P, ed. *Personality Disorders: Diagnosis, Management and Course*. London, England: Wright; 1988:74–81.

Chatterjie A, Strauss ME, Smyth KA, Whitehouse PJ. Personality changes in Alzheimer's disease. *Arch Neurol*. 1992;49:486–491.

Costa PT, McCrae RR. *Revised NEO Personality Inventory and NEO Five Factor Inventory: Professional Manual*. Odessa, FL: Psychological Assessment Resources; 1992a.

Costa PT, McCrae RR. Trait psychology comes of age. In: Sonderegger T, ed. *Nebraska Symposium on Motivation 1991*. Lincoln, NE: University of Nebraska Press; 1992b:169–204.

Cummings JL, Petry S, Dian L, Shapira J, Hill MA. Organic personality disorder in dementia syndromes: an inventory approach. *J Neuropsychiatry Clin Neurosci*. 1990;2:261–267.

Devanand DP, Nobler MS, Singer T, et al. Is dysthymia a different disorder in the elderly? *Am J Psychiatry*. 1994;151:1592–1599.

Devanand DP, Turret N, Moody BJ, et al. Personality disorders in elderly patients with dysthymic disorder. *Am J Geriatr Psychiatry*. 2000;8:188–195.

Duberstein PR, Conwell Y, Caine ED. Age differences in the personality characteristics of suicide completers: preliminary findings from a psychological autopsy study. *Psychiatry*. 1994;57:213–224.

Erikson EH. *Childhood and Society*. 2nd ed. New York, NY: Norton; 1963.

Eysenck HJ, Eysenck MW. *Personality and Individual Differences*. New York, NY: Plenum; 1985.

Fogel BS, Westlake R. Personality disorder diagnoses and age in inpatients with major depression. *J Clin Psychiatry*. 1990;51:232–235.

Frank E, Kupfer DJ, Jacob M, Jarret D. Personality features and response to acute treatment in recurrent depression. *J Pers Disord*. 1987;1:14–26.

Freud S. *The Ego and the Id*. Riviere J, trans. New York, NY: Norton; 1962. (Original work published 1923.)

Gynther MD. Aging and personality. In: Butcher JN, ed. *New Developments in the Use of the MMPI*. Minneapolis: University of Minnesota Press; 1979.

Harris MJ, Jeste DV. Late-onset schizophrenia: an overview. *Schizophr Bull*. 1988;14: 39.

Helson R, Stewart A. Personality change in adulthood. In: Heatherton TF, Weinberger JL, eds. *Can Personality Change?* Washington, DC: American Psychological Association; 1994:201–225.

Helson R, Wink P. Personality change in women from the early forties to the early fifties. *Psychol Aging.* 1992;7:46–55.

Hirschfeld RMA, Klerman GL. Personality attributes and affective disorders. *Am J Psychiatry.* 1979;136:67–70.

Kroessler D. Personality disorders in the elderly. *Hospital Community Psychiatry.* 1990; 41:1325–1329.

Kunik ME, Mulsant BH, Rifai AH, et al. Diagnostic rate of comorbid personality disorders in elderly psychiatric inpatients. *Am J Psychiatry.* 1994;151:603–605.

LaBouvie-Vief G, DeVoe M, Bulka D. Speaking about feelings: conceptions of emotion across the life span. *Psychol Aging.* 1989;4:425–437.

Loebel JP. Competed suicide in the elderly. In: Greenbelt MD, ed. *Abstracts, Third Annual Meeting and Symposium, American Association for Geriatric Psychiatry.* San Diego, CA: American Association for Geriatric Psychiatry; 1990:2.

Loranger AW, Susman VL, Oldham JM, Russakoff LM. The personality disorder examination: a preliminary report. *J Pers Disord.* 1987;1:1–13.

McCrae RR, Costa PT. *Personality in Adulthood.* New York, NY: Guilford; 1990.

McCrae RR, Costa PT. Personality trait structure as a human universal. *Am Psychol.* 1997;52:509–516.

McGlashan TH. The Chestnut Lodge follow-up study. III. Long-term outcome of borderline personalities. *Arch Gen Psychiatry.* 1986;43:20–30.

Neugarten B. Time, age, and the life cycle. *Am J Psychiatry.* 1979;136:887–894.

Petry S, Cummings JL, Hill MA, Shapira J. Personality alterations in dementia of the Alzheimer type: a three-year follow-up study. *J Geriatr Psychiatry Neurol.* 1989;2: 203–207.

Pfohl B, Stangl D, Zimmerman M. The implications of *DSM-III* personality disorders for patients with major depression. *J Affect Disord.* 1984;7:309–318.

Reich J, Nduaguba M, Yates W. Age and sex distribution of *DSM-III* personality cluster traits in a community population. *Compr Psychiatry.* 1988;29:298–303.

Reich J, Noyes R, Hirschfeld RMA, Coryell W, O'Gorman T. State and personality in depressed and panic patients. *Am J Psychiatry.* 1987;144:184–187.

Sadavoy, J. Borderline personality disorders in the elderly. In: Silver D, Rosenbluth M, eds. *The Handbook of Borderline Disorders.* Madison, CT: International Universities Press; 1992.

Sadavoy, J. The effect of personality disorder on Axis I disorders in the elderly. In: Duffy M, ed. *Handbook of Counselling and Psychotherapy With Older Adults.* New York, NY: Wiley and Sons; 1999:397–413.

Sadavoy, J. The symptom expression of personality disorder in old age. *Clin Gerontol.* 1996;16(3):19–36.

Siegler IC, Dawson DV, Welsh KA. Caregiver ratings of personality change in Alzheimer's disease patients: a replication. *Psychol Aging.* 1994;9:464–466.

Strauss ME, Pasupathi M, Chatterjee A. Concordance between observers in descriptions of personality change in Alzheimer's disease. *Psychol Aging.* 1993;8:475–480.

Swenson WM, Pearson JS, Osoborne D. *An MMPI Source Book: Basic Item, Scale and Pattern Data on 50,000 Medical Patients.* Minneapolis: University of Minnesota Press; 1973.

Stevenson J, Meares R, Comerford A. Diminished impulsivity in older patients with borderline personality disorder. *Am J Psychiatry*. 2003;160:165–166.

Stone MH. Long-term outcome in personality disorders [abstract]. *Br J Psychiatry*. 1993;162:229–313.

Thompson LW, Gallagher D, Czirr R. Personality disorder and outcome in the treatment of late-life depression. *J Geriatr Psychiatry*. 1988;21:133–146.

Tyrer P. *Personality Disorders: Diagnosis, Management and Course*. London, England: Wright; 1988.

Vaillant GE. *Adaptation to Life*. Boston, MA: Little, Brown; 1977.

Vaillant GE, Milofsky E. Natural history of male psychological health: IX. Empirical evidence for Erikson's model of the life cycle. *Am J Psychiatry*. 1980;137:1348–1359.

Vaillant GE, Perry JC. Personality disorders. In: Kaplan HI, Sadock BJ, eds. *Comprehensive Textbook of Psychiatry*. Vol. 2. 5th ed. Baltimore, MD: Williams and Wilkins; 1990:1352–1387.

Welleford EA, Harkins SW, Taylor JR. Personality change in dementia of the Alzheimer's type: relations to caregiver personality and burden. *Exp Aging Res*. 1995;21:295–314.

Woodruff RA, Guze SE, Clayton PJ. The medical and psychiatric implications of antisocial personality (sociopathy). *Dis Nerv Syst*. 1971;32:712–714.

25

Substance Abuse

Roland M. Atkinson, MD

INTRODUCTION

Over the past 20 years, studies have indicated that substance abuse—particularly alcohol and tobacco abuse—is a significant source of psychiatric and physical morbidity in aging individuals. The elderly are a highly heterogeneous population with substantial variability in physical and functional status. As such, the presentations, consequences, and complications of substance abuse among aging persons are wide ranging. In this chapter, I review the literature on the use and abuse by elderly persons of alcohol, prescription psychoactive drugs (especially benzodiazepines), nonprescription drugs, tobacco products, and illicit drugs.

In Table 25-1, several terms are defined as they are used in this chapter. Current criteria for diagnosing substance dependence and abuse are listed in Table 25-2. Close reading of these criteria reveals that not all are applicable to many elderly individuals. There is no reason why criteria for substance abuse should not also include recurrent use that causes or aggravates adverse medical reactions; in fact, there are common medical manifestations of substance abuse in later life (Moore et al., 1999). Risk factors for substance abuse in the elderly population are listed in Table 25-3. For further information and a general overview of the field of substance abuse, refer to standard texts (Lowinson et al., 1997; Schuckit, 2000).

TABLE 25-1.   Definitions of terms used in the substance abuse field

Psychoactive: Any chemical (alcohol, therapeutic agent, industral compound, or illicit drug) with important effects on the central nervous system.

Substance: A psychoactive that typically is associated with a substance use disorder. The term includes alcohol; opioids; sedative-hynotics; antianxiety agents of the barbiturate and benzodiazepine types; psycomotor stimulants, especially amphetamines and cocaine; tobacco products; and certain over-the-counter psychoactives. The terms *chemical* and *drug* in this context are synonymous with substance (e.g., chemical dependence, drug abuse).

Standard drink: A standard drink of beverage alcohol is equivalent to a 12-ounce domestic beer (alcohol content about 4%), a 5-ounce glass of table wine (about 12% alcohol), or a mixed drink containing 1 to 1.5 ounces hard liquor (about 40% alcohol).

Use: Appropriate medical or social consumption of a psychoactive in a manner that minimizes the potential for dependence or abuse.

Heavy use: Use of a substance in greater quantity than the usual norms, but without obvious negative social, behavioral, or health consequences. Heavy alcohol or tobacco users may be dependent on the substance. *At-risk or risky* drinkers refers to heavy consumers of alcohol, usually in later life, at rates of $\geq$5–21 drinks/week for men, $\geq$10–14 for women, or binges in which $\geq$4–5 drinks are consumed on a single drinking occasion. *Safe drinking levels* for elderly persons are recommended by the US National Institute on Alcohol Abuse and Alcoholism not to exceed 7 drinks/week or 2 drinks on a single drinking occasion.

Misuse: Use of a prescribed drug in a manner other than directed. The term can mean overuse, underuse, improper dose sequencing, lending or borrowing another's medication, with or without harmful consequences.

Problem use: Use of a substance in a manner that induces negative social, behavioral, or health consequences. A problem user may or may not meet criteria for substance dependence or abuse, although many do. Alcohol problems or drug problems are categories often used by epidemiologists in community prevalence surveys.

Abuse: A less-pervasive form of substance use disorder than substance dependence, with problems perhaps restricted to a particular area of difficulty (see Table 25-2).

Dependence: Dependence on a substance is defined by explicit diagnostic criteria, such as those listed in *DSM-IV* (see Table 25-2). Serious and persistent involvement in the heavy use of the substance is the rule. These approaches set aside the older distinction between *physical dependence* and *psychological dependence*, which are now viewed as differing manifestations of similar disorders. The terms *alcoholism* and *addiction* are usually used as synonyms for dependence on alcohol and other drugs, respectively.

Substance use disorder: A clinical condition in which substance abuse or substance dependence can be diagnosed. An *alcohol use disorder* (AUD) refers collectively to alcohol dependence and alcohol abuse.

Substance abuse, chemical dependence, and *addictions*: These terms are often used to refer to the entire professional/scientific field.

TABLE 25-2. *DSM-IV* **criteria for substance dependence and abuse**

Substance Dependence*
A maladaptive pattern of substance use, leading to clinically significant impairment or distress, as manifested by three [or more] of the following, occurring at any time in the same 12-month period:
1. Tolerance, as defined by either of the following:
    a. need for markedly increased amounts of the substance to achieve intoxication or desired effect; or
    b. markedly diminished effect with continued use of the same amount of the substance
2. Withdrawal, as manifested by either of the following:
    a. characteristic withdrawal syndrome for the substance; or
    b. the same [or a closely related] substance is taken to relieve or avoid withdrawal symptoms
3. The substance is often taken in larger amounts or over a longer period than was intended
4. There is a persistent desire or unsuccessful efforts to cut down or control substance use
5. A great deal of time is spent in activities necessary to obtain the substance [e.g., visiting multiple doctors or driving long distances], use the substance [e.g., chain smoking], or recover from its effects
6. Important social, occupational, or recreational activities are given up or reduced because of substance use
7. Substance use is continued despite knowledge of having a persistent or recurrent physical or psychological problem that is likely to have been caused or exacerbated by the substance [e.g., current cocaine use despite recognition of cocaine-induced depression, or continued drinking despite a peptic ulcer made worse by alcohol consumption]

Substance Abuse†
A. A maladaptive pattern of substance use leading to clinically significant impairment or distress, as manifested by one [or more] of the following, occurring within a 12-month period:
    1. Recurrent substance use resulting in a failure to fulfill major role obligations at work, school, or home [e.g., repeated absences or poor work performance related to substance use; substance-related absences, suspensions, or expulsions from school; neglect of children or household]
    2. Recurrent substance use in situations in which it is physically hazardous [e.g., driving an automobile or operating a machine when impaired by substance use]
    3. Recurrent substance-related legal problems [e.g., arrest for substance-related disorderly conduct]
    4. Continued substance use despite having persistent or recurrent social or interpersonal problems caused or exacerbated by the effects of the substance [e.g., arguments with spouse about consequences of intoxication, physical fights]
B. The symptoms have never met the criteria for Substance Dependence for this class of substance

*From American Psychiatric Association (1994, p. 181).
†From American Psychiatric Association (1994, pp. 182–183).

TABLE 25-3.   Risk factors for substance abuse in the elderly

Predisposing factors
  Family history (alcohol)
  Previous substance abuse
  Previous pattern of substance consumption (individual and cohort effects)
  Personality traits (sedative-hypnotics, anxiolytics)
Factors that may increase substance exposure and consumption level
  Gender (men: alcohol, illicit drugs; women: sedative-hypnotics, anxiolytics)
  Chronic illness associated with pain (opioid analgesics), insomnia (hypnotics), or
    anxiety (anxiolytics)
  Long-term prescribing (sedative-hypnotics, anxiolytics)
  Caregiver overuse of as-needed medication (institutionalized elderly)
  Life stress, loss, social isolation
  Negative affects (depression, grief, demoralization, anger) (alcohol)
  Family collusion and drinking partners (alcohol)
  Discretionary time, money (alcohol)
Factors that may increase the effects and abuse potential of substances
  Age-associated drug sensitivity (pharmacokinetic, pharmacodynamic factors)
  Chronic medical illnesses
  Other medications (alcohol-drug, drug-drug interactions)

ALCOHOL USE DISORDERS;
PROBLEM AND RISKY DRINKING

Epidemiology

PREVALENCE   Alcohol use and alcohol problems decline with age, but still constitute a significant public health problem. Community surveys show that alcohol use in the US is most prevalent in the age group 25 to 45 years and declines stepwise in older age cohorts to 12-month prevalence levels, among persons aged 55 years and older, of 46% who reported any alcohol use (Ruchlin, 1997) and 30% who reported consuming at least 12 drinks in the past 12 months (Grant, 1997). Rates of any recent alcohol use continue to decline after age 55 years to 25% of persons age 85 and older (Ruchlin, 1997). Rates for *risky* (heavy, nonproblem) drinking and problem drinking, which may or may not meet *DSM-IV* (*Diagnostic and Statistical Manual of Mental Disorders, Fourth Edition*, American Psychiatric Association [APA], 1990) criteria for an alcohol use disorder, by older adults vary widely depending on the population sampled and definitions of use (Atkinson, 1990). In one survey of primary care office practice rolls, the prevalence of risky drinking in patients aged 65 years and older was 15% for men and 12% for women (Adams et al., 1996).

Because older adults with alcohol problems also have high rates of comorbid medical disorders, they are represented much more commonly in clinical settings than in community surveys. Reports of elderly clinical cohorts show rates of current problem drinking that can vary from 4% to 23%, depending on the setting where studied (reviewed in Atkinson, 2000). Community prevalence rates for alcohol dependence are lower: In household surveys, only about 2% to 3% of elderly men and less than 1% of women in the United States currently suffer from these disorders (Grant, 1997; Helzer et al., 1991). The spectrum of current and potential alcohol-related problems far exceeds the clinical population who are alcohol dependent—those traditionally termed *alcoholic* patients.

Older men are twice as likely to use alcohol currently as older women and two to six times more likely than women to be problem drinkers. These patterns hold true across diverse ethnic and racial groups (reviewed in Atkinson, 2000). Once alcohol dependence develops, it is more likely to persist in older men than in women. Several factors contribute to the apparent decline in drinking and drinking problems with age, including premature deaths of early-onset alcoholics, moderation or cessation of drinking with age by surviving alcoholics and social drinkers, reticence to report drinking accurately by older patients, both underrecognition and underreporting of cases by clinicians, and cohort and period effects (Atkinson et al., 1992). This said, for many elderly individuals, drinking patterns established in early adult or middle life persist into old age or may even increase in tempo (Liberto et al., 1992; Schutte et al., 1998).

LATE-ONSET ALCOHOL PROBLEMS Retrospective studies of community-dwelling elderly have noted subsets who report increasing alcohol consumption in later life, either for the first time or in a fluctuating pattern established earlier. Household surveys and clinical reports demonstrated that onset of initial drinking problems at age 50 years or older is not uncommon, although there are "intermittent" cases—in which persons with early-onset alcoholism achieved prolonged abstinence in middle life but relapsed later—that can be mistaken for late onset (Atkinson, 1994). Studies showed that, on average, at least one third of older patients with alcohol use disorders (AUDs) have onset after middle life, although in treatment samples, the proportion of patients with onset after age 60 years can vary from 30% to over 60%, depending on the setting and demographic factors.

The notion that late-onset alcohol dependence usually occurs secondary to a mood or cognitive disorder has not been upheld by systematic studies (Atkinson, 1994), although many persons with late-onset alcohol problems were risky or reactive drinkers in the past (Schutte et al., 1998). Late-onset alcohol problems are typically milder and more circumscribed than those beginning in earlier life. Compared with early-onset cases, late-onset problem drinkers also tend to have less alcoholism among relatives, less psychopathology, and higher socioeconomic status; more women report late onset than men (Atkinson, 1994; Liberto & Oslin, 1995).

Although there is clinical evidence to support the view that late-onset drinking problems sometimes begin in reaction to life stress, it is not true that this group exhibits more reactive drinking than lifelong alcoholics, who are notorious for their tendency to drink more in response to any significant life event. Compared with alcoholism of long duration, late-onset problems tend to resolve more often without formal treatment (Moos et al., 1991), but there is little evidence to suggest that they respond more favorably to alcoholism treatment than patients with early onset (Blow, Walton, Chermack, et al., 2000; Atkinson, 1994).

RISK FACTORS   A family history of alcoholism, personal history of previous heavy or reactive consumption, or prior episode of an AUD increases the risk of a new episode of problem drinking (see Table 25-3). Frailty, dysfunction, and need for multiple prescription medications all increase the vulnerability of elderly patients to adverse alcohol effects, as do certain symptoms, such as insomnia, pain, and depression, for which some elders take alcohol as self-medication. At the same time, in community surveys, alcohol consumption tends to be greater in older adults who are physically fit and mobile, economically well off, and married (reviewed in Atkinson et al., 1992).

Response to a given alcohol load increases with age. Pharmacokinetics play a role. In the fasted state, a nonalcoholic man in his 60s may have a peak blood alcohol level 20% to 25% higher than a man in his 30s after a standard alcohol load; for women, this difference is even greater (Lucey et al., 1999). These changes are largely attributable to reduced volume of distribution for alcohol because of decline in lean body mass and body water with age and to reduced alcohol dehydrogenase activity in the gut wall, allowing absorption of a larger portion of ingested alcohol. Even when controlling for blood alcohol level, performance is more impaired with age after a standard alcohol load, indicating an increasing neuropharmacodynamic effect of alcohol with age. This has been demonstrated on measures of subjective intoxication experience, memory, performance on divided attention tasks, and measures of coordination—body sway and hand dexterity—after single alcohol doses (reviewed in Atkinson, 2000).

Diagnosis and Symptomatology

CLINICAL PRESENTATIONS   In an elderly individual, an alcohol-related problem may not be suspected because the presenting picture often does not correspond with stereotypes based on younger patients. Severe primary alcohol dependence certainly is seen in older adults, but antisocial behavior and lower socioeconomic status are less common, and clinical manifestations may be variable.

Circumscribed or "focal" alcohol problems most typically present as biomedical symptoms or problems. Alcohol excess can cause, aggravate, or complicate the management of problems as diverse as hypertension, diabetes mellitus, osteoporosis, gastritis, macrocytic anemia, hypercholesterolemia, parkinsonism, and gout (for more information, see Gambert & Katsoyannis, 1995; Smith, 1995). A number of cancers (mouth, esophagus, pharynx, larynx, liver, colorectal) are caused or aggravated by alcohol dependence. Breast cancer in one large survey was 1.3 times more common in women who currently drink than in nondrinkers (Thun et al., 1997). Alcohol-drug interactions can confound medical prescribing: Acute alcohol intake reduces the action of many drugs; conversely, chronic high alcohol consumption may increase drug metabolism by inducing hepatic microsomal drug-metabolizing enzyme activity. Alcohol can potentiate the sedating effects of prescribed benzodiazepines and opioids, and some drugs (e.g., chlorpromazine and histamine H_2 blockers) reduce alcohol dehydrogenase activity in the gut wall, permitting greater alcohol absorption and increasing susceptibility to intoxication when drinking (for more information, see Adams, 1995; Fraser, 1997; Korrapati & Vestal, 1995). Other commonly encountered circumscribed problems in older patients include repeated arrest for driving an automobile while under the influence of alcohol and recurrent family conflict caused by alcoholism.

Older patients with *uncomplicated mild alcohol dependence*, including many daily risky drinkers, may have no specific complaints or findings (Blow, Walton, Barry, et al., 2000). Tolerance may accompany this pattern. Because of risk of later medical or psychiatric sequelae of sustained heavy drinking, intervention is justified.

Medically complex dependence is often the presentation of aging alcoholics who are admitted to the emergency department or acute medical inpatient unit. The symptoms, although obvious, may be nonspecific and thus easily attributed to a cause other than alcohol abuse; indeed, alcohol may be just one of several factors contributing to the clinical picture. Presenting features may include delirium, dementia, lack of self-care, dehydration, malnutrition, gastrointestinal complaints, bladder and/or bowel incontinence, muscle weakness or frank myopathy, gait disorder, recurring falls, burns, head trauma, or accidental hypothermia. Hypoglycemia, congestive heart failure, and aspiration pneumonia can also be caused or aggravated by alcohol dependence.

Psychiatrically complex dependence is seen in those patients who have an alcohol use disorder associated with another psychiatric disorder (dual diagnoses). Mood disorders, mainly depression and cognitive and anxiety disorders are the most common psychiatric comorbidities in this age group (Atkinson et al., 2001; Atkinson & Misra, 2002b). Accurate differential diagnosis often requires repeated assessment over time.

COMPLICATIONS AND ASSOCIATED FEATURES   Alcohol intoxication may occur at lower dose levels in older persons because of increased biological sensitivity. While there is no evidence that alcohol withdrawal disorders (the tremulous syndrome, hallucinosis, seizures, and delirium tremens) occur at different rates in the elderly, alcohol withdrawal can be more severe and more difficult to treat with age and may be associated with greater mortality (Brower et al., 1994;

Liskow et al., 1989). Other central nervous system complications include reversible cognitive impairment; Wernicke-Korsakoff syndrome; dementia associated with alcoholism; and deterioration of another form of dementia, such as Alzheimer's (King, 1986), among others (for more information, see Atkinson, 2000). Alcohol-associated insomnia resembles the age-associated pattern of sleep disorganization; both show frequent awakenings, especially from deep, slow-wave sleep, and reduced rapid eye movement (REM) sleep (Dustman, 1984).

Medical complications have already been described. Psychosocial complications are diverse. Alcohol problems are found in 7% to 30% of older suicides (Blazer, 1982; Conwell et al., 1990; Martin & Streissguth, 1982). The association of alcoholism with suicide may be stronger in men in late middle age than in elderly men or women of any age (Conwell et al., 1990). A 50-year longitudinal study of men demonstrated that the strong association between poor social support and premature mortality is significantly mediated by alcohol abuse, among several other variables (Vaillant et al., 1998). Case material has demonstrated problems of alcohol-related divorce and homelessness, and that alcohol intoxication may be a factor in geriatric pedophilia and other sexual misconduct and in violent events (e.g., abuse or attacks by and on elderly individuals).

Among substance-related comorbidities, active tobacco dependence—principally cigarette smoking—is highly prevalent in elderly alcoholics (about 50%–70%); active dependence on prescribed sedatives, anxiolytics, and opioid analgesics varies (from 2% to 14%), depending on the cohort studied (studies reviewed in Atkinson, 2000). Recent illicit drug abuse is uncommon in most clinical settings, but can be highly prevalent—as high as 25% of cases—in some culturally diverse urban patient groups (Schonfeld et al., 2000).

COURSE Based on retrospective reports, the span from onset of the first alcohol problem to recognition of current problems can be as long as 50 years. Over this course, drinking may have been steady, progressive, or variable; in some cases, sober periods of 10 years or longer occur between problem drinking episodes. In one prospective 4-year repeated telephone survey of over 1,600 community-dwelling late-middle-aged drinkers and nondrinkers, 37% reported one or more current alcohol problems initially (Moos et al., 1991). Resolution of current problems within the next year occurred in 29% of the problem drinkers. Early-onset problem drinkers remitted less often than recent-onset problem drinkers (24% vs. 41%). Gains made at 1 year were sustained at the 4th year resurvey in 70% of the remitted problem group (Schutte et al., 1994). Among nonproblem drinkers at baseline, 8% developed one or more alcohol-related problems in the next year.

There is evidence that social drinkers tend to modify their consumption downward with age, while problem drinkers are more likely to choose to abstain. The prevalence of problem drinking after 85 years of age is very low. Mortality rates are very high when active drinking continues in the face of frank dementia or active alcohol-related liver disease.

Approaches to Diagnosis

INTERVIEWS   Diagnosis of AUDs and problem drinking requires openness to the possibility of the problem; skillful interviewing, sometimes aided by screening tests and home visits; physical and neurological examination; and appropriate laboratory tests. Information elicited from interviews provides the foundation for accurate diagnosis. The task of acquiring information is by no means easy and may be especially daunting in elderly individuals. Sensitive inquiry about drinking practices is sometimes necessary to elicit this information and should be a routine part of the geriatric psychiatric workup. Denial of alcohol problems and defensiveness when asked about drinking are common in alcoholic patients. Reasons include alcohol-related amnesia for intoxication episodes, shame about reliance on alcohol, pessimism about recovery, and the desire to continue drinking. Comorbid depression or cognitive disorder can also influence veracity. For these reasons, careful rapport building through repeated contacts; thorough inquiry with relatives, caregivers, and others in the social network; reviews of medical records; and home visitation are especially useful assessment methods.

SCREENING INSTRUMENTS   The CAGE test and the geriatric version of the Michigan Alcoholism Screening Test (MAST-G) (Table 25-4) have both shown promise as preliminary screens for alcohol problems in older clinical populations (Blow et al., 1992; Buchsbaum et al., 1992; Joseph et al., 1995), although not all studies find these measures sufficiently sensitive in elderly patients (Luttrell et al., 1997). Among risky drinkers, only about 40% were CAGE+ in one study (Adams et al., 1996). A positive result on either measure does not make the diagnosis of an AUD, but these tests can help identify patients who need more detailed assessment.

PHYSICAL AND LABORATORY FINDINGS   Physical stigmata of alcoholic liver disease, peripheral polyneuropathy, and cerebellar ataxia are among physical findings that may help confirm a diagnosis, but these are often absent. Laboratory data may be helpful, especially in mild dependence or in differential diagnosis of complex cases. Findings from one large group of older alcoholic patients are compared with findings for younger patients in Table 25-5. Macrocytic red blood cells, with or without anemia, and liver transferase enzyme elevations are the most typical findings. Toxicological examination of blood or breath samples for alcohol may help establish a diagnosis of severe alcohol intoxication in the moribund patient. In the ambulatory patient, a high blood alcohol level (>150 mg/100 mL) in the presence of a relatively normal mental

TABLE 25-4. Screening measures for alcohol problems

CAGE screening measure*
1. Have you ever felt you ought to Cut down on your drinking?
2. Have people Annoyed you by criticizing your drinking?
3. Have you ever felt bad or Guilty about your drinking?
4. Have you ever had a drink first thing in the morning to steady your nerves or get rid of a hangover ("Eye-opener")?
(Positive answers to two or more questions suggest an alcohol problem at some time, although the problem may not be currently active.)

Short Michigan Alcoholism Screening Test—Geriatric Version (SMAST-G)†
In the past year:
1. When talking with others, do you underestimate how much you actually drink?
2. After a few drinks, have you sometimes not eaten or been able to skip a meal because you didn't feel hungry?
3. Does having a few drinks help decrease your shakiness or tremors?
4. Does alcohol sometimes make it hard for you to remember parts of the day or night?
In the past year:
5. Do you usually take a drink to relax or calm your nerves?
6. Do you drink to take your mind off your problems?
7. Have you ever increased your drinking after experiencing a loss in your life?
8. Has a doctor or nurse ever said they were worried or concerned about your drinking?
9. Have your ever made rules to manage your drinking?
10. When you feel lonely, does having a drink help?
(Three or more positive responses indicative of a recent or current alcohol use problem.)

*Modified from Ewing (1984).
†From Blow (1991).

and neurological examination is strong evidence for tolerance and physical dependence.

DIFFERENTIAL DIAGNOSIS Two problems, depression and cognitive impairment, deserve special emphasis because they commonly occur in aging patients, but also can be sequelae of sustained heavy drinking in persons otherwise not mentally ill.

DEPRESSION As in younger patients, depressive symptoms are present in a majority of older alcoholic patients entering treatment after recent heavy drinking (Atkinson, 1999). More often than not, such depressive symptoms appear to be alcohol induced, even in cases meeting criteria for major depression; scores on depression measures usually fall to normal levels without specific antidepressant treatment after 2 to 4 weeks sobriety (Brown et al., 1995). But, there is also a strong comorbid association between true (nonalcohol-induced)

TABLE 25-5. Frequency of laboratory abnormalities in elderly and younger inpatients with alcoholism

Blood tests*	Results†			
	Patients ≥65 years‡		Younger patients‡	
	Number	%	Number	%
MCH increased	213	71	123	57§
AST increased	214	56	123	42‖
GGT increased	123	55	101	48
MCV increased	213	44	124	17§
Glucose increased	206	32	124	36
Uric acid increased	201	21	123	<1§
Albumin decreased	186	17	115	3§
Alkaline phosphatase increased	213	11	123	15
Triglycerides increased	191	16	122	19
Phosphorous increased	198	9	124	11

Source: Adapted from Hurt et al. (1988).

*MCH, mean corpuscular hemoglobin; AST, aspartate aminotransferase; GGT, γ-glutamyltransferase; MCV, mean corpuscular volume.

†Number = number of patients tested in each age group; % = percentage of patients tested in the age group who had an abnormal value.

‡Older patients: N = 216, mean age 69.6 years, age range 65 to 83 years. Younger patients: N = 125, mean age 44.3 years, age range 19 to 64 years.

§$P < .01$ using Wilcoxon two-sample rank sum test to compare age groups for proportion having an abnormal value.

‖$P < .05$; for others, $P > .3$.

major depression and alcohol dependence across the lifespan, including older adults (Grant & Harford, 1995). Studies of older patients in treatment for alcohol use disorders showed that comorbid depressive disorders are diagnosed in 12% to 25% of cases (Atkinson et al., 2001; Finlayson et al., 1988). While there is no convincing evidence that depression causes alcoholism in persons not predisposed to an AUD (Dawson & Grant, 1998; Grant et al., 1996), once a pattern of excessive alcohol use has been established, negative emotional states associated with depression (e.g., sadness, boredom, anger, tension) may trigger repeated drinking episodes (Dupree & Schonfeld, 1998). While such alcohol use may afford brief respite from emotional distress (self-medication), over time it can further aggravate a comorbid depressive condition. Factors that may help differentiate between alcohol-induced and true comorbid depression are listed in Table 25-6.

Recently drinking patients judged to suffer from true comorbid depression should, of course, be treated promptly and vigorously with antidepressants, as should any patient suffering severely from depressive symptoms or judged seri-

TABLE 25-6.   Alcohol-induced depression versus comorbid depression*

Feature	Alcohol-induced depression	Comorbid (persistent) depression
May meet criteria for major depression	+	+
Prior episodes occurred while drinking	+	+
Begins to improve after just a few days' sobriety	+	−
May take 2–3 weeks to resolve if untreated	+	−
Tends to persist more than 3 weeks if untreated	−	+
First episode may have pre-dated alcohol problems	−	+
Prior episodes occurred during abstinent periods	−	+
Family history of depression/suicide more likely	−	+
Current major life problems/stressors more likely	−	+

Source: Based on Atkinson (1999); Brown et al. (1995).
*The two conditions may co-occur.

ously suicidal. Effective treatment of coexisting depression often results in reduced alcohol consumption, as demonstrated in studies of mixed-age alcoholic patients (Litten & Allen, 1998) and heavy-drinking elderly depressed patients (Oslin et al., 2000). However, in cases of mild to moderate depression in recently drinking alcoholic patients—cases in which it is unclear whether depressive symptoms are simply alcohol-induced—antidepressant medication should be withheld for up to 2 to 3 weeks if possible so that remission is not falsely attributed to medication, and an unjustified diagnosis of (nonalcohol-induced) depressive disorder can be avoided.

COGNITIVE IMPAIRMENT AND DEMENTIA In early sobriety, recovering alcoholic patients often show defects in memory, visual-spatial skills, abstraction, and problem solving that increase with age in frequency, severity, and duration. Such deficits may not fulfill criteria for dementia, yet may only resolve over a protracted course of months to years (Brandt et al., 1983; Grant et al., 1984). In mild cases, residual deficits after a few weeks of sobriety can be sufficiently subtle that a coarse screen for dementia such as the Mini-Mental State Examination (MMSE) will not indicate them.

Frank dementia is also commonly associated with alcohol excess (Table 25-7). In the Liverpool (United Kingdom) community epidemiological survey of the elderly, men with a history of very heavy drinking were 4.6 times more likely to have current dementia than other men (Saunders et al., 1991). Among elderly alcoholic patients in treatment, 13% to 25% have coexisting dementia (Atkinson et al., 2001; Finlayson et al., 1988). In dementia registries, more than 20% of patients may have a history of alcoholism or heavy drinking (studies summarized in Oslin et al., 1998).

Neuropsychological and neuroimaging studies point to widespread dam-

TABLE 25-7. *DSM-IV* **diagnostic criteria for alcohol-induced persisting dementia**

A. The development of multiple deficits manifested by both:
  (1) memory impairment (impaired ability to learn new information or to recall pre-
       viously learned information); and
  (2) one or more of the following cognitive disturbances:
       (a) aphasia [language disturbance];
       (b) apraxia [impaired ability to carry out motor activities despite intact motor
           function];
       (c) agnosia [failure to recognize or identify objects despite intact sensory func-
           tion]; and/or
       (d) disturbance in executive functioning [i.e., planning, organization, sequenc-
           ing, abstracting].
B. The cognitive deficits in criteria A1 and A2 each cause significant impairment in social or occupational functioning and represent a significant decline from a previous
   level of functioning.
C. The deficits do not occur exclusively during the course of a delirium and persist beyond the usual duration of alcohol intoxication or withdrawal.
D. There is evidence from the history, physical examination, or laboratory findings
   that the deficits are etiologically related to the persisting effects of alcohol use.

Source: From American Psychiatric Association (1994, p. 154).

age to the central nervous system (CNS) in chronic alcoholic patients (reviewed in Atkinson, 2000). Age, rather than duration of alcoholism, tends to be the most critical factor in the extent of CNS damage. Cortical atrophy reflects loss of both gray and white matter, occurs in older alcoholic individuals beginning about the fifth decade, and is over and above the changes associated with normal aging (Jernigan et al., 1991; Pfefferbaum et al., 1992, 1997). Morphological changes are especially evident in frontal areas, and many of the deficits in cognitive performance suggest the prominence of frontal lobe dysfunction in chronic alcoholic patients (Kril et al., 1997; Pfefferbaum et al., 1997). Compromised metabolism in frontal and prefrontal areas in older chronic alcoholic patients (hypofrontality) is also suggested by positron emission tomographic studies and studies of regional cerebral blood flow and event-related potentials (reviewed by Atkinson, 2000).

Differential diagnosis between dementia associated with alcoholism and Alzheimer's dementia (AD) can be difficult; some findings potentially useful in differentiating these conditions are offered in Table 25-8. Alcohol might also be a risk factor, like hypertension, that increases vulnerability to various forms of dementia. Apart from the neurotoxic effects of alcohol and associated vitamin deficiency states, alcoholics are known to be at high risk for repeated head trauma and infectious diseases that could predispose to dementia. Heavy drinking also aggravates cardiovascular diseases and thus could contribute indirectly to a vascular presentation of dementia (Fisman et al., 1996).

TABLE 25-8. Features that may distinguish between alcohol-related and Alzheimer's dementias*

Feature	Alcohol-induced persisting dementia	Alzheimer's dementia
Meets criteria for dementia	+	+
Cortical atrophy on MRI	+	+
Long history of heavy drinking	+	−
Ataxia may be present	+	−
Peripheral polyneuropathy may be present	+	−
Cerebellar atrophy may be present on MRI	+	−
Abstinence halts cognitive decline	+	−
Cortical atrophy can be reversed	+	−
Anomia/dysnomia prominent	−	+
Cognitive decline continues despite abstinence	−	+
CSF tau protein may be elevated	−	+

Source: Based on Morikawa et al. (1999); Oslin et al. (1998); Smith and Atkinson (1995).

MRI, magnetic resonance imaging of the brain; CSF, cerebrospinal fluid.

*Symbols "+" and "−" mean that the finding is more (+) or less (−) likely to be associated with this form of dementia.

Treatment, Prognosis, and Outcome

BRIEF INTERVENTION FOR RISKY DRINKERS Brief intervention is based on the finding that a clinician's simple advice to cut down on alcohol consumption can modify patients' drinking behavior (Edwards, 1988). It is further based on the public health model of harm reduction and can be effective in reducing alcohol consumption to safe levels without the need for total abstinence or formal alcoholism treatment. This approach is indicated in heavy drinkers who do not yet have significant alcohol-related problems and probably in many mild cases of dependence and circumscribed mild problem drinking.

After confirming a pattern of risky drinking, the clinician explains to the patient that the drinking level exceeds safe norms, solicits the patient's willingness to establish a lower consumption goal, has the patient make a contract to pursue this goal and to keep a drinking diary, and then follows up in a few months to review whether the new drinking limit has been achieved. Typically, a primary care physician conducts this intervention, although any clinician can do so.

In one randomized controlled trial in which 146 risky drinking elderly outpatients in 24 primary care practice sites were assigned either to receive brief intervention or a control intervention (in which generalized health promotion advice was given), drinking was reduced by 36% in patients receiving advice to cut down compared to no change in controls (Fleming et al., 1999).

Another multisite trial found comparable results; it used home visitation by a psychologist or social worker to deliver a similar intervention (Blow, 1999).

GENERAL ISSUES IN THE TREATMENT OF ALCOHOL USE DISORDERS   Once the diagnosis of an AUD is established, it is important to present the information thoroughly and objectively to the patient and spouse or other close relative or caregiver as a basis for urging an appropriate course of action. It is helpful to reassure the patient and family that older persons with drinking problems actually have fared as well as or better than younger persons in a variety of treatment settings (Atkinson, 1995).

The treatment has three aims: (1) reduce or cease alcohol use; (2) treat medical and psychiatric comorbidities; and (3) engender psychological changes to reduce the risk of relapse. The person with more pervasive alcohol problems should receive outpatient psychosocial alcoholism treatment (Atkinson et al., 1998; Dupree et al., 1984; Schonfeld et al., 2000). Ambulatory, gradual detoxification is often achieved without resorting to medications or hospital admission. Medications to reduce craving, such as naltrexone, may be helpful.

In the most serious cases, including those involving patients who have not been helped by outpatient treatment, such patients should be referred to an inpatient chemical dependency treatment unit, ideally one that specializes in treating older adults (Blow, Walton, Chermack, et al., 2000; Kashner et al., 1992). If severe medical or psychiatric complications are present or major withdrawal is anticipated or already occurring, initial treatment should take place in an acute inpatient medical or psychiatric unit, followed by transfer to a chemical dependency unit after stabilization.

Intractable heavy drinking in the presence of dementia or other coexisting major mental disorder may force placement of the patient in long-term residential care, where, unfortunately, alcoholic patients are not always welcomed. In a few locales, alcohol-free foster homes and other residential facilities have been established; these are staffed by personnel trained to care for recovering alcoholic patients in an accepting manner. Comprehensive guides to treatment of older alcohol- and drug-abusing patients are available (Center for Substance Abuse Treatment, 1998; Gurnack et al., 2002).

PSYCHOSOCIAL TREATMENTS   Motivational counseling (Center for Substance Abuse Treatment, 1999; Fleming, 2002; Miller & Rollnick, 1991) has generally displaced more confrontive crisis-precipitation techniques as the preferred approach to the older alcoholic patient who initially resists advice to enter treatment. Age-specific group treatment is indicated whenever it is possible to aggregate several older patients in the same program. Such arrangements can foster peer bonding, shared reminiscence, longer retention in treatment, and improved drinking outcomes (Atkinson et al., 1998; Center for Substance Abuse Treatment, 1998; Kashner et al., 1992; Kofoed et al., 1987).

When group treatment is not possible, individual case management is the

PSYCHIATRIC DISORDERS OF THE ELDERLY

best approach, ideally using nursing or other clinical personnel trained in gerontology and addictions (Atkinson & Misra, 2002a; Kaempf et al., 1999). Case management is also required for many patients in elder-specific, group-based treatment programs. Family engagement in the program may enhance treatment retention and efficacy (Atkinson et al., 1993, 1998). Cognitive-behavioral psychotherapeutic and educational methods, using very specific, manual-assisted techniques, have also proven useful with older adult alcoholics (Dupree et al., 1984; Dupree & Schonfeld, 1998; Schonfeld et al., 2000). Participation in Alcoholics Anonymous is often beneficial, especially at meetings organized exclusively for this age group (Atkinson & Misra, 2002a).

PHARMACOLOGICAL TREATMENTS   Use of the deterrent drug disulfiram can be hazardous in older patients because of the risk of a cardiovascular crisis precipitated by acetaldehyde toxicity if the patient drinks while taking disulfiram. Naltrexone appears to be safe in geriatric cases and has shown some promise for reducing the extent of drinking lapses (Oslin et al., 1997a, 1997b). Reports are lacking on the safety and efficacy of acamprosate in elderly persons, but it could prove equal to naltrexone in reducing craving and severe drinking lapses in this population (Paille et al., 1995; Sass et al., 1996). While antidepressant drugs appear to reduce drinking in alcoholic elders who have current comorbid depression (see discussion above), there is little evidence that these agents deter drinking in nondepressed patients (Litten & Allen, 1998).

TREATMENT ADHERENCE AND OUTCOME   As a group, older alcoholic patients seem to respond to alcoholism treatment as well as or better than younger alcoholic patients (Atkinson, 1995). Older patients are more likely to continue in longer term outpatient treatment than younger patients (Atkinson et al., 1993), especially when grouped with age peers (Kofoed et al., 1987). Court-supervised older drinking drivers and married elders whose spouses participate in treatment are more likely to continue in treatment than their age peers who lack such third-party involvement (Atkinson et al., 1993, 1998). In a study comparing 1-year drinking outcomes of older alcoholics randomly assigned either to an age-specific inpatient alcoholism treatment unit (ATU) or to an age-heterogeneous ATU in the same facility, patients treated in the age-specific program were more likely to be abstinent a year later (Kashner et al., 1992). In Project MATCH, a large multisite outpatient alcoholism treatment study, patients aged 60 years and older (7% of the sample) fared well (Atkinson & Misra, 2002a; Project MATCH Research Group, 1997). Their 12-month posttreatment drinking outcomes were highly favorable—as successful as younger patients' outcomes—and equally successful for each of the three treatment conditions compared in the study: a cognitive-behavioral condition; motivational counseling; and a 12-step counseling model adapted from Alcoholics Anonymous (each modality was randomly assigned and individually administered in weekly sessions for 3 months).

Alcohol and Health Maintenance

MODERATE DRINKING AND MAINTAINING GOOD HEALTH   The use of small amounts of beverage alcohol has been advocated as a safe social adjuvant in elder residential care facilities, but more comprehensive management of the facility milieu may better ensure optimal socialization (Atkinson & Kofoed, 1984). Alcohol has also long been touted as an appetite stimulant. In healthy elderly persons, caloric intake and blood levels of some micronutrients may increase with alcohol intake, although other micronutrient levels decrease (Jacques et al., 1989). Use of alcohol to aid sleep is problematic because regular alcohol late in the evening is apt to disorganize sleep (Dustman, 1984).

If moderate drinking is advised, several cautions apply. The list of potentially hazardous interactions of alcohol with chronic medical disorders and medications is lengthy (see "Pharmacological Treatments" above). Clinicians who advise outpatients to use alcohol should recall that, in the residential studies, quantity was carefully regulated and use within a social context was ensured (Atkinson & Kofoed, 1984). The National Institute on Alcohol Abuse and Alcoholism (1995) advises that healthy elderly persons should limit themselves to no more than seven standard drinks per week and no more than two drinks per drinking occasion.

MODERATE ALCOHOL USE AND THE PREVENTION OF CORONARY HEART DISEASE   An intriguing aspect of the alcohol and health maintenance debate is the well-validated association of regular, but moderate, alcohol use (one to two drinks per day) with lower morbidity and mortality from coronary heart disease (CHD), especially in men, when compared to heavy alcohol users and abstainers. Why should teetotalers have higher rates of severe CHD than moderate drinkers?

One possible explanation is that the heterogeneous abstainer group might include subgroups at high risk for CHD (e.g., former alcoholics and others in poor health). Indeed, this tends to be the case. A history of alcohol dependence also nullifies health-protective effects of current light or moderate alcohol use (Dawson, 2000). In one large study, older persons who had experienced adverse health events or who demonstrated fewer adaptive coping skills were more commonly represented among abstainers than among moderate drinkers (Mertens et al., 1996). Unfortunately, a number of studies have not controlled for such variables, including the two studies to date that focused exclusively on elderly samples and that reported a "protective" effect of alcohol against CHD (Colditz et al., 1985; Scherr et al., 1992).

More recent mixed-age studies have provided such controls and still demonstrated a protective effect of alcohol in CHD. Studies suggest a number of biological mechanisms that might help explain the protective effects of alcohol in CHD, including alcohol-induced increase in an antiatherogenic fraction of circulating high-density lipoprotein cholesterol (Davidson, 1989; Srivastava et al., 1994); anticoagulant effects (Davidson 1989); antioxidant effects (Artaud-

Wild et al., 1993; Soleas et al., 1997); decreases in circulating fasting insulin and fasting insulin resistance index values (Lazarus et al., 1997); and increased activation of epsilon protein kinase C in cardiac muscle (Chen et al., 1999; Miyamae et al., 1998).

MODERATE DRINKING PROTECTION AGAINST OTHER LATE-LIFE HEALTH PROBLEMS   A smaller, more general, apparent protective effect of moderate drinking on mortality from all causes has been demonstrated in several studies (e.g., Colditz et al., 1985; Mertens et al., 1996; Thun et al., 1997). Much of this overall effect is attributable to reduced mortality from cardiovascular diseases. Aggregated all-cause mortality rates obscure the fact that several important causes either have no association with alcohol consumption (e.g., deaths from colorectal cancer, hemorrhagic stroke, pneumonia, and respiratory diseases) or a linear relationship in which any level of consumption is more likely to be associated with mortality than not drinking at all (e.g., deaths from alcoholism, accidents, and liver cirrhosis) (Thun et al., 1997).

Several reports suggest that moderate alcohol intake may have a beneficial effect on cognitive status (Cerhan et al., 1998; Christian et al., 1995; Dufouil et al., 1997; Galanis et al., 2000; Letenneur et al., 1993; Orgogozo et al., 1997) and even a possible protective effect against development of age-related retinal macular degeneration (Obisesan et al., 1998). These phenomena require further study.

BENZODIAZEPINE DEPENDENCE

Epidemiology and Long-Term Benzodiazepine Use

BENZODIAZEPINE USE BY COMMUNITY-DWELLING ELDERLY PERSONS   The benzodiazepine class of sedative-hypnotics has achieved dominance over the past 30 years because of the relative safety and efficacy of these agents in the treatment of insomnia and anxiety. The number of benzodiazepine prescriptions peaked in the mid-1970s and has since been in decline worldwide, but contrary to this general trend, use of these drugs in the elderly has not changed appreciably, even though the individual agents change.

In 1991, persons aged 65 years and older represented 13% of the US population, but received 27% of all benzodiazepine prescriptions and 38% of prescriptions for benzodiazepine hypnotic agents (Woods & Winger, 1995). Surveys of community-dwelling elderly suggest that 5% to 15% have on hand currently prescribed benzodiazepines. The mere occurrence of an acute hospital care episode, for any cause, increases the likelihood that an elderly patient will receive a new outpatient benzodiazepine prescription (Grad et al., 1999).

Young adult abusers of benzodiazepines consume these drugs outside medical supervision, use them for euphoriant effects, escalate the dose over time, and continue use despite adverse consequences, but such behaviors are very uncommon in older people, and misuse tends toward underuse. Most older persons use these agents as directed. Unfortunately, long-term daily use of benzodiazepines at conventionally prescribed doses can produce physical dependence with characteristic "discontinuance symptoms" when the drug is stopped, and chronic toxicity from long-term exposure to these agents at therapeutic doses is also more likely in old age.

LONG-TERM BENZODIAZEPINE USE AND THE DEVELOPMENT OF DEPENDENCE It is now well established that regular, daily therapeutic doses of any benzodiazepine, if prolonged beyond 4 to 12 months and depending on the pharmacokinetics of the particular drug, can result in the development of physical dependence without dose escalation (APA, 1990; Higgitt, 1988). There is little tolerance to the anxiolytic and antipanic effects of diazepam, alprazolam, or other drugs in this class. Tolerance to their hypnotic effects, on the other hand, is well documented, so that addiction to increasingly high doses is also possible, especially in persons who take a benzodiazepine over a protracted period for chronic insomnia.

Clinical surveys have long indicated that the elderly are more likely to receive benzodiazepines for prolonged periods than younger persons. Indeed, within the general population, the most likely long-term benzodiazepine user is an elderly woman (Ancill & Carlyle, 1993). Prescription surveys show continuing evidence of this pattern (e.g., Isacson et al., 1992; Simon et al., 1996; Thomson & Smith, 1995). Although receipt of a prescription does not ensure that the patient uses the drug daily, these studies demonstrate that many elderly patients are placed at risk for developing benzodiazepine dependence by the manner in which these drugs are prescribed (Egan et al., 2000).

The prevalence of drug dependence disorders of all types in persons aged 65 years and older reported in community surveys is very slow, but such data almost certainly do not reflect low-dose benzodiazepine dependence, which is typically unrecognized by the patient and poorly measured by the dependence criteria. True withdrawal signs and symptoms have been reported to occur in 20% to 50% of chronic benzodiazepine users after discontinuation (Roy-Byrne & Hommer, 1988; Schweizer et al., 1990).

INSTITUTIONAL BENZODIAZEPINE USE Concern has been widely expressed that, in nursing homes and residential care facilities, older patients may be particularly likely to be dosed with excessive sedatives to control behavior. Needless dosing with benzodiazepines and neuroleptics for agitation has been demonstrated (Cohen-Mansfield et al., 1999). The practice of open-ended dispensing of nightly benzodiazepines for sleep also is certainly to be discouraged. Most cases of benzodiazepine-induced or benzodiazepine-aggravated cognitive impairment and ataxia are seen in this circumstance.

Efforts to rationalize and curb use of these agents in nursing homes have produced mixed results. Reduced use of benzodiazepines has been demonstrated in some settings (e.g., Avorn et al., 1992; Gilbert et al., 1993; Schmidt et al., 1998). Elsewhere, perhaps because of improved recognition of anxiety disorders or reduction in use of neuroleptics brought about by the enforcement of federal regulations for use of psychoactive medications in nursing homes contained in the Congressional Omnibus Budget Reconciliation Act of 1987 (OBRA 87), benzodiazepine use has in fact increased in the past few years, to levels approaching 30% to 40% of residents regularly receiving these agents in some nursing homes (Borson & Doane, 1997; Lasser & Sunderland, 1998).

RISK FACTORS FOR BENZODIAZEPINE DEPENDENCE Pharmacological factors increasing the likelihood of dependence, besides duration of treatment, include higher drug dose level, shorter pharmacokinetic elimination half-life, and higher milligram potency of the agent (APA, 1990). Patient factors include prior or concurrent alcoholism or sedative drug dependence, chronic insomnia (rather than anxiety) as the target symptom for which the drug is prescribed, and coexisting chronic pain or personality disorder.

Diagnosis and Symptomatology

DIAGNOSING DEPENDENCE AND WITHDRAWAL Benzodiazepine dependence and withdrawal may be overlooked initially in hospitalized elderly patients who do not or cannot disclose their daily use of these agents, and the deteriorating course that ensues may be misdiagnosed as myocardial infarction, hypertensive crisis, or infection (Whitcup & Miller, 1987). Delirium may be a more common presentation of withdrawal in older patients and be misattributed to other causes. In one study of 45 medical inpatients aged 60 years and older who developed a delirium while in the hospital, benzodiazepine use was implicated in 29% of the cases (Foy et al., 1995). Withdrawal delirium occurred in 13% (7 of 52) of elderly long-term benzodiazepine users withdrawing abruptly from a mean dose of 7.75 mg/day of diazepam in another study (Foy et al., 1986).

When initiating benzodiazepine treatment or stepping up the dose, there is a transitional period before a new plasma steady-state drug level is achieved, during which toxic effects may occur transiently, consisting of one or more of the following symptoms: sedation, ataxia, and increased reaction time. Age-related pharmacokinetic and pharmacodynamic changes render elderly individuals especially susceptible to these effects, and the duration until steady state is more protracted with age as well. Once steady state is achieved at a maintenance dose level that is continued long term, varying degrees of chronic toxicity may build up, especially in elderly users, but in many cases, low doses for long periods will cause few, if any, obvious physical or behavioral sequelae as long as the drug is taken regularly.

Among outpatients, many cases of dependence on benzodiazepines are evident only when noting a long-standing prescription. Low-dose dependence is not proven, however, merely by the pharmacy record. One patient may not take the agent regularly, while another may also be surreptitiously consuming supplies garnered from multiple sources. Benzodiazepine toxicity and possible dependence should always be considered when patients have poorly explained sedation, ataxia, depression, or cognitive impairment. When there is strong suspicion of surreptitious benzodiazepine use, a search for undisclosed prescription bottles should be conducted, with the aid of relatives and home visitation, and a urine examination for benzodiazepines should be obtained.

COMPLICATIONS: CHRONIC BENZODIAZEPINE TOXICITY Chronic toxicity has subtle manifestations at low doses and becomes more obvious when dose escalation follows the development of tolerance. In an older person, even at therapeutic dose levels, toxicity may be manifested by persistent ataxia, leading to falls; depressed mood, which can be mistaken for an affective disorder; oversedation; memory impairment and other cognitive dysfunction; and possibly frank dementia (reviewed in APA, 1990; Atkinson, 2000; Woods & Winger, 1995).

Memory impairment typically is the consequence of drug disruption of memory consolidation (transfer of newly learned information from short-term to long-term memory) (Barbee, 1993). While the effect size may be small because of baseline deficits in recall in elderly patients, the additional impairment produced by benzodiazepines can compromise memory more severely than the same dose given to younger persons (Woods & Winger, 1995). Benzodiazepines can also induce anterograde amnesia. Functional decline was associated with benzodiazepine use in two large US studies (Ried et al., 1998; Sarkisian et al., 2000).

MECHANISMS UNDERLYING AGE-ASSOCIATED CHANGES IN RESPONSE TO BENZODIAZEPINES As a person ages, alterations occur in the volume of distribution, elimination half-life, and clearance of metabolized benzodiazepines, producing higher steady-state plasma drug concentrations than those produced by giving the same drug load to a younger individual (Greenblatt et al., 1991a, 1991b; Ozdemir et al., 1996). However, even controlling for plasma drug concentration, the elderly develop more sedation, psychomotor impairment, and memory problems (Bertz et al., 1997; Greenblatt et al., 1991a, 1991b), suggesting an increased neuropharmacodynamic effect with age, as well as more marginal baseline brain function (Woods & Winger, 1995). Basic mechanisms accounting for age-associated increased sensitivity to benzodiazepines have not been determined, but may involve postreceptor mechanisms in GABAergic neurons and second-messenger systems (Ozdemir et al., 1996).

COMPLICATIONS ASSOCIATED WITH COMORBID DISORDERS AND MEDICATION INTERACTIONS Benzodiazepines may contribute to respiratory insufficiency in patients with pulmonary disorders, increased falls and incoordination in patients with cerebellar disease or compromised vascular supply to the posterior fossa, or deteriorating status in demented or depressed patients. These agents potentiate the effects of alcohol and opioids. Cimetidine and propanolol interfere with the metabolism of benzodiazepines and can raise their blood levels, but the clinical importance of these effects appears to be small.

BENZODIAZEPINE DISCONTINUANCE SYMPTOMS   Following abrupt termination of benzodiazepines after long-term use, clinically significant discontinuance symptoms occur in as many as 90% of patients who have been taking low daily doses; these symptoms are summarized in Table 25-9. Often, symptoms can be quite distressing and sometimes very serious. Symptoms occurring after cessation of long-term benzodiazepines often represent a mixture of rebound, reoccurrence, and true withdrawal symptoms (APA, 1990).

Rebound symptoms are identical to those for which the drug was originally prescribed, but they reoccur rapidly, are more severe or intense than in the past, and resolve in a few days. *Reoccurrence symptoms* are also identical to the original symptoms, but they appear gradually, never exceed their original intensity, and persist. They represent a return to the chronic symptom pattern suppressed by drug therapy. Some symptoms, like restlessness or irritability, are common and can represent any of the three types of discontinuance phenomena, depending on the history, intensity, and time course. Other symptoms, like psychosis, seizures, or delirium, are uncommon and almost always represent true *withdrawal phenomena*, defined as new or novel symptoms for that patient, with early or late onset, but typically lasting only 2 to 4 weeks. There is evidence that older adults experience discontinuance symptoms with similar or less intensity, compared to younger adults, when the drug dose is tapered gradually and thus may tolerate such withdrawal reasonably well (Cantopher et al., 1990; Schweizer et al., 1989).

TABLE 25-9.   Benzodiazepine discontinuance symptoms (specific symptoms by frequency)

Frequent	Common	Uncommon*
Anxiety	Flulike symptoms (nausea, coryza, lethargy,	Delirium
Insomnia	diaphoresis)	Seizures
Restlessness	Sensitivity to sound, touch, or light	Persistent tinnitus
Agitation	Aches and pains	Depsersonalization
Irritability	Blurred vision	Derealization
Muscle tension	Depression	Paranoid delusions
	Nightmares	Hallucinations
	Hyperreflexia	Psychosis
	Ataxia	
	Autonomic hyperactivity	

Source: Adapted from American Psychiatric Association (1990).

*Typically when present these represent true withdrawal symptoms.

Treatment, Prognosis and Outcome

DRUG DISCONTINUATION IN THE DEPENDENT PATIENT   Gradual discontinuation of the drug is indicated, at least in those dependent patients who suffer from chronic toxicity or other complications or who have developed tolerance with dose escalation above the therapeutic range (APA, 1990; Higgitt et al., 1985). The goal is to proceed slowly enough in decremental reductions to avoid major withdrawal and minimize other discontinuance symptoms. Some patients, especially those who have developed lengthy, high-dose habits, may require many months of tapering to avert serious discontinuance symptoms. As the dose reaches lower levels, the size and frequency of decrements may have to be reduced even further, especially for high-potency drugs with a short half-life like alprazolam.

In the end, the reduction schedule must be tailored to meet individual needs, although a period of 1 to 4 months is often sufficient. It is no small feat to persuade some elderly persons to give up benzodiazepines, and various intervention strategies may be needed. In some cases, reduction to very low drug doses rather than complete discontinuation may have to be the solution. In cases of high-dose dependence or mixed prescription drug and alcohol dependence, specialized inpatient treatment may be required (Center for Substance Abuse Treatment, 1998; Finlayson & Hofmann, 2002).

ADJUNCTIVE MEASURES IN MANAGING DRUG DISCONTINUATION   Several drug substitutes, including propanolol, clonidine, carbamazepine, buspirone, and barbiturates, have been studied, but none clearly merits widespread use (APA, 1990; Roy-Byrne & Ballenger, 1993). Psychological therapies (Gilbert et al., 1993; Golombok & Higgitt, 1993) and self-help groups (Tattersall, 1993) can be useful adjuncts for drug-dependent persons withdrawing from benzodiazepines.

OUTCOME OF MEDICALLY SUPERVISED BENZODIAZEPINE WITHDRAWAL   Despite evidence that old age is not associated with more severe withdrawal, studies of mixed-age patient groups show that older persons have a poorer outcome following therapeutic attempts to discontinue benzodiazepines after long-standing use (studies reviewed in Atkinson, 2000). Older age was associated with both difficulty completing withdrawal protocols and increased likelihood of relapse to benzodiazepine use despite completion of a cessation program. The mean age of subjects in these follow-up studies was 40 to 50 years, and numbers of elderly persons were small. Risk factors for relapse in such studies of mixed-aged patients, besides older age, include casual efforts to discontinue (as opposed to participation in a formal protocol), personality pathology, dependence on agents with short half-lives, higher drug doses, higher caffeine intake, and continued psychiatric symptomatology (see Atkinson, 2000).

For long-term benzodiazepine users who do succeed in discontinuing use of these agents, several studies indicate the possibility of at least some improvement in cognitive functioning (Golombok et al., 1988; Salzman et al., 1992; Tonne et al., 1995) and improvement, or at least no deterioration, in symptoms of anxiety, depression, and insomnia (Rickels et al., 1990; Salzman et al., 1992; Schweizer et al., 1990). A study of 76 patients (mean age 62 years) successfully withdrawn from chronic benzodiazepine use found that medical and mental health visits fell from 25.4 per year before detoxification to 4.4 per year afterward (Burke et al., 1995). But other studies suggested that the majority of patients who successfully withdraw from benzodiazepines may continue to experience significant anxiety, depression, and insomnia and thus remain at risk for return to use of these agents (Atkinson, 2000).

MANAGING LONG-TERM BENZODIAZEPINE USE   Ideally, daily-dose regimens of benzodiazepines should be used over short periods of time (i.e., no more than several weeks) for acute episodes of anxiety or insomnia. However, some patients might benefit from longer term treatment. Deciding when to prescribe long-term treatment can be quite difficult, requiring consideration of the extent of the patient's relief from morbid anxiety symptoms balanced against the hazards of chronic toxicity and physical dependence (Ancill & Carlyle, 1993).

Long-term, low-dose therapy may be justified, especially for patients whose anxiety responds better to a benzodiazepine than to alternative therapies and who are reliable, have no history of alcoholism or drug addiction, and who can be well supervised medically (APA, 1990). In these circumstances, however, the physician should anticipate the likelihood of inducing physical dependence and seek the informed consent of patient and family in deciding how to proceed. Moreover, as in the case of the epileptic or diabetic patient, steps should be taken to protect the patient from inadvertent abrupt drug withdrawal (e.g., by clearly documenting the status of the patient as a long-term benzodiazepine user in the medical record, by educating patient and family never to stop the drug abruptly and to inform all new health care providers of this long-standing medication).

TOBACCO AND OTHER DRUG USE DISORDERS

Tobacco (Nicotine) Dependence

EPIDEMIOLOGY AND SIGNIFICANCE   Although older adults are less likely to smoke than younger adults, tobacco dependence is the most common of all substance use disorders in the elderly; is entirely obvious, thus taking no special effort to establish the diagnosis; and arguably accounts for far more medical disability and mortality in the elderly than abuse of all other substances combined. Because of its low behavioral toxicity, however, tobacco dependence has held little interest for psychiatrists. Compulsive tobacco use is rooted, nonetheless, in an abnormal behavior pattern that merits the attention of mental health professionals. There has been debate about whether smoking might exert a protective effect against the development of dementia. US community survey data for 1994 showed that, among persons aged 65 years and older, 13% of men and 11% of women were regular daily cigarette smokers (National Center for Health Statistics, 1996).

DIAGNOSIS OF TOBACCO DEPENDENCE; SYMPTOMS OF NICOTINE WITHDRAWAL Nicotine dependence is characterized by pursuit of pleasurable effects from nicotine use, a compulsive pattern of use despite knowledge of health hazards, withdrawal symptoms, tolerance, and craving and relapse with abstinence. The usual criteria for substance dependence (Table 25-2) are not very satisfactory because low behavioral toxicity and easy access to cheap tobacco products make several of these criteria irrelevant.

When moderate-to-heavy daily use of tobacco is discontinued, smokers experience a variety of unpleasant mood and physical symptoms that begin within hours of abstinence. Psychological symptoms include irritability, anxiety, depression, and craving. Physiological symptoms include low energy, concentration difficulties, headache, increased appetite, and nonspecific somatic complaints. There is little investigation into age-related changes in the prevalence or severity of these withdrawal symptoms.

NEUROPHARMACOLOGY OF NICOTINE DEPENDENCE Nicotine has numerous effects on the CNS, which are mediated via widely distributed nicotinic receptors on cholinergic neurons innervating various structures (reviewed in Atkinson, 2000). These effects include increases in cerebral glucose uptake, epinephrine, norepinephrine, arginine, vasopressin, adrenocorticotropic hormone, cortisol, growth hormone, and prolactin; increase in dopamine biovailability; and release of endogenous opioids (reviewed in Brautbar, 1995). Of greatest importance from the standpoint of tobacco dependence are the well-established effects of nicotine on midbrain dopamine systems (reviewed in Jarvik & Schneider, 1992; Nisell et al., 1995).

ADVERSE HEALTH CONSEQUENCES OF SMOKING If the pleasures of smoking are immediate, the complications are long delayed. Indeed, 75% of the years of potential life lost because of premature smoking-attributable deaths in the United States are estimated to occur in the period from age 65 years on (US Public Health Service, 1988). Smoking doubles the risk of death from combined causes in persons aged 35 to 70 years (Thun et al., 1997). Major health problems associated with tobacco dependence are well known and include various cancers; heart, peripheral, and cerebrovascular disease; chronic obstructive lung disease; peptic ulcer; osteoporosis; burns; reduced body weight; impaired sense of taste and smell; loss of mobility; and poorer physical functioning (studies reviewed in Atkinson, 2000). Smoking also interferes with the metabolism of many drugs (Dawson & Vestal, 1984).

POSITIVE HEALTH CONSEQUENCES OF SMOKING CESSATION   After stopping tobacco use, elderly persons experience greater longevity, reduced morbidity and mortality from myocardial infarction, reduced risk of death from smoking-related cancers and chronic obstructive lung disease, and improvement in pulmonary function and hip bone mineral density compared to their contemporaries who continue smoking. The reduced risk of death becomes evident within 1 to 2 years after quitting and approaches that of never-smokers after 15 to 20 years of abstinence (LaCroix & Omenn, 1992).

ATTITUDES TOWARD SMOKING AMONG OLDER ADULTS   It is not certain whether older smokers are more or less successful than younger persons in quitting, but it is clear that most successful quitters achieve this goal spontaneously without participating in a specialized treatment program. Successful quitters often cite health concerns, death of loved ones who smoked, or a physician's advice as motivating factors. Of those continuing to smoke, many say they want to quit, and up to half have tried recently.

Nevertheless, currently smoking elders may be less likely than younger smokers to believe in the health hazards of smoking and more likely to view smoking as a positive habit to enhance coping, reduce stress, or control weight (Orleans, Jepson, et al., 1994; Schoenbaum, 1997). Older smokers report the same reasons as younger smokers for return to smoking after quitting: irritability, weight gain, fear of weight gain, friction with family members, and inability to concentrate.

SMOKING CESSATION APPROACHES   Among smoking cessation methods, some, like rapid smoking aversion therapy or medicinal nicotine substitutes (polacrilex gum, transdermal patches), may be contraindicated in older patients with coronary heart disease, cardiac arrhythmias, hypertension, or diabetes mellitus. Brief intervention in primary care medical settings and self-help guides, when appropriately tailored to elderly individuals, can produce 6-month to 1-year quit rates as high as 20% compared to spontaneous quit rates of 5% to 10% (Morgan et al., 1996; Rimer & Orleans, 1994). Transdermal nicotine patch therapy yielded a 6-month quit rate of 29% in one naturalistic study of elderly smokers (Orleans, Resch, et al., 1994).

Bupropion favorably affected smoking cessation in several careful studies of mixed-age nondepressed smokers (Hurt et al., 1997; Jorenby et al., 1999), doubling the 12-month quit rate compared to placebo controls. Bupropion appears to be equal in effects to nicotine replacement methods (Hughes et al., 1999). Unfortunately, the use of this drug specifically in aging smokers has not received attention.

Quit rates by any method are influenced favorably by more frequent contact with supervising personnel, although elderly patients prefer minimal-contact approaches, which for economic reasons should be tried first in most cases.

SMOKING PROTECTION AGAINST DEMENTIA   Since the early 1980s, more than 30 studies have examined whether smoking is associated with lower rates for AD and dementia in general, but most are not reliable because they tended to be relatively small, retrospective, cross-sectional case-control surveys of prevalent cases (Doll et al., 2000). In one review, 4 of 17 such studies demonstrated a protective effect of regular smoking against AD (Lee, 1994). Confounding variables, such as differential mortality (Ott et al., 1998; Wang et al., 1999) and smoking-related nondementing illnesses that increase the proportion of smokers among control cases (Doll et al., 2000), have often made results of such studies difficult to interpret.

Prospective, population-based studies of incident cases were consistent in demonstrating that current regular smoking either has little or no association with AD or overall dementia rates (Broe et al., 1998; Doll et al., 2000; Wang et al., 1999) or is associated with greater, not lesser, risk of AD and other dementias (Merchant et al., 2000; Ott et al., 1998). These findings are consistent with other studies that failed to show any protective effect of smoking on cognitive performance in nondemented middle-aged and older adults (Cerhan et al., 1998; Edelstein et al., 1998; Leibovici et al., 1999).

Still, new reports, based on prevalent case series, of a protective effect of smoking in AD continue to appear (Hillier & Salib, 1997; Tyas et al., 2000). Two additional findings may stimulate continuing interest in this theme. There is evidence that nicotine inhibits amyloid formation (Salomon et al., 1996), and that senile plaque formation is less prominent in the brains of patients with AD who were smokers than in brains of nonsmoking AD case controls (Ulrich et al., 1997). There is also evidence from the prospective studies cited above that risk of AD is lower in smokers who possess the apolipoprotein ε4 (APOE ε4) allele than in those who lack this allele (Merchant et al., 2000; Ott et al., 1998; Van Duijn et al., 1995).

OTHER DRUG USE DISORDERS

Prescription Opioid Analgesic Dependence

Greater sensitivity with age to the analgesic effects of opioids is suggested by some clinical reports (Honari et al., 1997; Woodhouse & Mather, 1998). Dependence on prescribed opioids is less common than benzodiazepine dependence, tends to be long standing (beginning typically before old age), and is often associated with chronic pain disorders and high levels of psychopathology (Finlayson & Davis, 1994). Whether opioid dependence liability changes with age is uncertain (Ozdemir et al., 1996). Treatment is tailored to individual patient needs (Finlayson & Hofmann, 2002).

Over-the-Counter Drugs

Use of psychoactive over-the-counter (OTC) drugs by the elderly is common, especially use of analgesics (Chrischiles et al., 1990, 1992; Stoehr et al., 1997) and hypnotics (Johnson, 1997; Sproule et al., 1999). Herbal medicines are also increasingly popular in the aging population, especially for enhancement of mood (e.g., hypericum [St. John's wort]), sleep (e.g., valerian), and cognition (e.g., gingko biloba) (Ernst, 1999; Riedel & Jorissen, 1998). There is a potential for medical and behavioral problems from habitual overuse of the many available nostrums containing antihistamines, anticholinergics, caffeine, aspirin, or the newer nonsteroidal antiinflammatory agents (Kofoed, 1985). Anticholinergics may impair cognition (Miller et al., 1988; Peters, 1989; Rovner et al., 1988) or cause delirium (Gustafson et al., 1988; Tune & Bylsma, 1991). Chronic salicylate toxicity increases with age and may produce a dementialike syndrome associated with tinnitus and irritability (Bailey & Jones, 1989; Grigor et al., 1987). No data exist about the true extent of OTC drug dependence and complications among older adults.

Illicit Drug Use Disorders

Abuse of illicit drugs by the elderly is very uncommon by most reports. Combined results of three national representative household surveys, conducted during 1991–1993 ($N = 87,915$), showed 1-year prevalence rates for persons aged 50 years and older of 0.6% for marijuana (tetrahydrocannabinol, THC) use (0.8% in men, 0.5% in women) and 0.1% for cocaine use (0.2% in men, 0.1% in women) (Kandel et al., 1997). Sporadic use of these substances by older persons has been reported (Abrams & Alexopoulos, 1988), especially by patients who are alcohol dependent (Miller et al., 1991).

A study of 565 geriatric psychiatry inpatients at one Veterans Affairs medical center found that 1% were diagnosed with illicit drug use disorders (Edgell et al., 2000). Another Veterans Affairs study of 110 culturally diverse patients (nearly half were ethnic/racial minorities) treated in an urban elder-specific substance abuse program found illicit drug abuse as the sole addictive disorder in 9% of cases and illicit drug abuse together with abuse of alcohol or prescription psychoactive drugs in an additional 29% (Schonfeld et al., 2000). Older persons tend to acquire these drugs from their adult children or from younger sexual partners (Atkinson et al., 1998). Use of illegal drugs may impair social functioning and expose the user to legal and health risks. Clinical disorders vary by drug class (opioids, stimulants, sedative-hypnotics of the barbiturate type, marijuana, and hallucinogens).

OPIOID ADDICTION   Opioid addiction is the most thoroughly described form of illicit drug abuse in older persons (studies reviewed in Atkinson et al., 1992). Typical addicts are men who have survived their addiction for many years, led socially isolated lives, and been secretive about drug use. They tend to avoid law enforcement agents and often continue to support their drug habits through legal employment into their 60s. They tend to practice scrupulous hygiene with needles and syringes and may substitute "cleaner" drugs like hydromorphone for heroin when available. They enter methadone maintenance as they become too old to "hustle," and the methadone clinic may become their main social network. Some older addicts tolerate methadone poorly. Few, however, accept or do well in drug-free treatment.

MARIJUANA (TETRAHYDROCANNABINOL)   Both recreational and medical users of marijuana are represented among the older population (Sussman, 1997). There is evidence for the potential therapeutic value of THC in illnesses requiring pain relief, control of nausea and vomiting, and appetite stimulation, although effect size is typically not large; purified products and safe, reliable dose delivery systems are not yet available; and more efficacious drugs are indicated before marijuana is tried (Institute of Medicine, 1999).

In contrast to the anxiety reduction and euphoria often demonstrated by younger and more experienced users, elderly persons, especially those not previously exposed, are more likely to report increased anxiety or unpleasant, dysphoric mood, which is more prominent after taking purified THC than after smoking marijuana (Institute of Medicine, 1999). In Oregon—one of nine states at this writing that permit medical usage of marijuana—among the first 1,247 registrants, 35 (2.8%) were aged 65 and older, compared to a proportion of 16.8% for this age group among the state's general population (Oregon Medical Marijuana Program, personal communication, November 2000). Thus, the elderly are underrepresented in this patient-initiated program despite their likelihood of suffering from several of the conditions for which the Oregon law permits marijuana use (e.g., cancer, cancer chemotherapy side effects, glaucoma, cachexia, severe pain, and severe nausea from any cause, among others). Overall, marijuana use by the elderly appears to be low and in general not problematic.

REFERENCES

Abrams RC, Alexopoulos GS. Substance abuse in the elderly: over-the-counter and illegal drugs. *Hosp Community Psychiatry*. 1988;39:822–823, 829.

Adams WL. Interactions between alcohol and other drugs. *Int J Addictions*. 1995;30: 1903–1923.

Adams WL, Barry KL, Fleming MF. Screening for problem drinking in older primary care patients. *J Am Med Assoc*. 1996;276:1964–1967.

American Psychiatric Association. *Benzodiazepine Dependence, Toxicity, and Abuse*. Washington, DC: American Psychiatric Press; 1990.

American Psychiatric Association. *Diagnostic and Statistical Manual of Mental Disorders.* 4th ed. Washington, DC: American Psychiatric Press, 1994.

Ancill RJ, Carlyle WW. Benzodiazepine use and dependency in the elderly: striking a balance. In: Hallstrom C, ed. *Benzodiazepine Dependence.* Oxford, UK: Oxford University Press; 1993:238–251.

Artaud-Wild SM, Sonnor SL, Sexton G, Connor WE. Differences in coronary mortality can be explained by differences in cholesterol and saturated fat intake in 40 countries but not in France and Finland. *Circulation.* 1993;88:2771–2779.

Atkinson RM. Aging and alcohol use disorders: diagnostic issues in the elderly. *Int Psychogeriatr.* 1990;2:55–72.

Atkinson RM. Late onset problem drinking in older adults. *Int J Geriatr Psychiatry.* 1994;9:321–326.

Atkinson RM. Treatment programs for aging alcoholics. In: Beresford TP, Gomberg ESL, eds. *Alcohol and Aging.* New York, NY: Oxford University Press, 1995:186–210.

Atkinson RM. Depression, alcoholism and ageing: a brief review. *Int J Geriatr Psychiatry.* 1999;14:905–910.

Atkinson RM. Substance abuse. In: Coffey CE, Cummings JL, eds. *Textbook of Geriatric Neuropsychiatry.* 2nd ed. Washington, DC: American Psychiatric Press; 2000: 367–400.

Atkinson RM, Ganzini L, Bernstein MJ. Alcohol and substance-use disorders in the elderly. In: Birren JE, Sloane RB, Cohen GD, eds. *Handbook of Mental Health and Aging.* 2nd ed. New York, NY: Academic Press; 1992:515–555.

Atkinson RM, Kofoed LL. Alcohol and drug abuse. In: Cassell CK, Walsh JR, eds. *Geriatric Medicine. Vol 2. Fundamentals of Geriatric Care.* New York, NY: Springer-Verlag; 1984:219–235.

Atkinson RM, Misra S. Further strategies in the treatment of aging alcoholics. In: Gurnack AM, Atkinson RM, Osgood NJ, eds. *Treating Alcohol and Drug Abuse in the Elderly.* New York, NY: Springer-Verlag; 2002a:131–151.

Atkinson RM, Misra S. Mental disorders and symptoms in older alcoholics. In: Gurnack AM, Atkinson RM, Osgood NJ, eds. *Treating Alcohol and Drug Abuse in the Elderly.* New York, NY: Springer-Verlag; 2002b:50–71.

Atkinson RM, Ryan SC, Turner JA. Variation among aging alcoholics in treatment. *Am J Geriat Psychiatry.* 2001;9:275–282.

Atkinson RM, Tolson RL, Turner JA. Factors affecting outpatient treatment compliance of older male problem drinkers. *J Stud Alcohol.* 1993;54:102–106.

Atkinson RM, Turner JA, Tolson RL. Treatment of older adult problem drinkers: lessons learned from "The Class of '45." *J Ment Health Aging.* 1998;4:197–214.

Avorn J, Soumerai SB, Everitt DE, et al. A randomized trial of a program to reduce the use of psychoactive drugs in nursing homes. *N Engl J Med.* 1992;327:168–173.

Bailey RB, Jones SR. Chronic salicylate intoxication: a common cause of morbidity in the elderly. *J Am Geriatr Soc.* 1989;37:556–561.

Barbee JG. Memory, benzodiazepines, and anxiety: integration of theoretical and clinical perspectives. *J Clin Psychiatry.* 1993;54(10 suppl):86–97.

Bertz RJ, Kroboth PD, Kroboth FJ, et al. Alprazolam in young and elderly men: sensitivity and tolerance to psychomotor, sedative and memory effects. *J Pharmacol Exp Ther.* 1997;281:1317–1329.

Blazer DG. *Depression in Late Life.* St. Louis, MO: Mosby, 1982.

Blow FC. *Michigan Alcoholism Screening Test—Geriatric Version (MAST-G)*. Ann Arbor: University of Michigan Alcohol Research Center; 1991.

Blow FG. The effectiveness of an elder-specific brief alcohol intervention for older hazardous drinkers. *Gerontologist*. 1999;39(Special issue 1):S569–S570.

Blow FC, Brower KJ, Schulenberg JE, Demo-Dananberg LM, Young JP, Beresford TP. The Michigan Alcoholism Screening Test—Geriatric Version (MAST-G): a new elderly-specific screening instrument. *Alcoholism (New York)*. 1992;16:372.

Blow FC, Walton MA, Barry KL, Coyne JC, Mudd SA, Copeland LA. The relationship between alcohol problems and health functioning of older adults in primary care settings. *J Am Geriatr Soc*. 2000;48:769–774.

Blow FC, Walton MA, Chermack ST, Mudd SA, Brower KJ. Older adult treatment outcome following elder-specific inpatient alcoholism treatment. *J Subst Abuse Treat*. 2000;19:67–75.

Borson S, Doane K. The impact of OBRA-87 on psychotropic drug prescribing in skilled nursing facilities. *Psychiatr Serv*. 1997;48:1289–1296.

Brandt J, Butters N, Ryan C, Bayog R. Cognitive loss and recovery in long-term alcohol abusers. *Arch Gen Psychiatry*. 1983;40:435–442.

Brautbar N. Direct effects of nicotine on the brain: evidence for chemical addiction [editorial]. *Arch Environ Health*. 1995;50:263–266.

Broe GA, Creasey H, Jorn AF, et al. Health habits and risk of cognitive impairment and dementia in old age: a prospective study on the effects of exercise. *Aust N Z J Public Health*. 1998;22:621–623.

Brower KJ, Mudd S, Blow FC, Young JP, Hill EM. Severity and treatment of alcohol withdrawal in elderly versus younger patients. *Alcoholism (New York)*. 1994;18:196–201.

Brown SA, Inaba RK, Gillin JC, Schuckit MA, Steward MA, Irwin MR. Alcoholism and affective disorder: clinical course of depressive symptoms. *Am J Psychiatry*. 1995;152:45–52.

Buchsbaum DG, Buchanan RG, Welsh J, Centor RM, Schnoll SH. Screening for drinking disorders in the elderly using the CAGE questionnaire. *J Am Geriatr Soc*. 1992;40:662–665.

Burke KC, Meek WJ, Krych R, et al. Medical services used by patients before and after detoxification from benzodiazepine dependence. *Psychiat Serv*. 1995;46:157–160.

Cantopher T, Olivieri S, Cleave N, Edwards JG. Chronic benzodiazepine dependence: a comparative study of abrupt withdrawal under propanolol cover versus gradual withdrawal. *Br J Psychiatry*. 1990;156:406–411.

Center for Substance Abuse Treatment. *Substance Abuse Among Older Adults: Treatment Improvement Protocol 26*. Rockville, MD: US Dept of Health and Human Services, Public Health Service, Substance Abuse and Mental Health Services Administration; 1998. DHHS Publication 98-3179.

Center for Substance Abuse Treatment. *Brief Interventions and Brief Therapies for Substance Abuse: Treatment Improvement Protocol 34*. Rockville, MD: US Dept. of Health and Human Services, Public Health Service, Substance Abuse and Mental Health Services Administration; 1999. DHHS Publication 99-3353.

Cerhan JR, Folsom AR, Mortimer JA, et al. Correlates of cognitive function in middle-aged adults. Atherosclerosis Risk in Communities (ARIC) Study Investigators. *Gerontology*. 1998;44:95–105.

Chen CH, Gray MO, Mochly-Rosen D. Cardioprotection from ischemia by a brief exposure to physiological levels of ethanol: role of epsilon protein kinase C. *Proc Natl Acad Sci U S A.* 1999;96:12784–12789.

Chrischilles EA, Foley DJ, Wallace RB, et al. Use of medications by persons 65 and over: data from the established populations for epidemiologic studies of the elderly. *J Gerontol Med Sci.* 1992;47:M137–M144.

Chrischilles EA, Lemke JH, Wallace RB, Drube GA. Prevalence and characteristics of multiple analgesic drug use in an elderly study group. *J Am Geriatr Soc.* 1990;38: 979–984.

Christian JC, Reed T, Carmelli D, Page WF, Norton JA Jr, Breitner JC. Self-reported alcohol intake and cognition in aging twins. *J Stud Alcohol.* 1995;56:414–416.

Cohen-Mansfield J, Lipson S, Werner P, Billig N, Taylor L, Woosley R. Withdrawal of haloperidol, thioridazine, and lorazepam in the nursing home: a controlled, double-blind study. *Arch Intern Med.* 1999;159:1733–1740.

Colditz GA, Branch LG, Lipnick RJ, et al. Moderate alcohol and decreased cardiovascular mortality in an elderly cohort. *Am Heart J.* 1985;109:886–889.

Conwell Y, Rotenberg M, Caine ED. Completed suicide at age 50 and over. *J Am Geriatr Soc.* 1990;38:640–644.

Davidson DM. Cardiovascular effects of alcohol. *West J Med.* 1989;151:430–439.

Dawson DA. Alcohol consumption, alcohol dependence, and all-cause mortality. *Alcoholism (New York).* 2000;24:72–81.

Dawson DA, Grant BF. Family history of alcoholism and gender: their combined effects on *DSM-IV* alcohol dependence and major depression. *J Stud Alcohol.* 1998;59: 97–106.

Dawson GW, Vestal RE. Smoking, age, and drug metabolism. In: Bosse R, Rose CL, eds. *Smoking and Aging.* Lexington, MA: Lexington Books; 1984:131–156.

Doll R, Peto R, Boreham J, Sutherland I. Smoking and dementia in male British doctors: a prospective study. *BMJ.* 2000;320:1097–1102.

Dufouil C, Ducimetiere P, Alperovitch A. Sex differences in the association between alcohol consumption and cognitive performance. *Am J Epidemiol.* 1997;146:405–412.

Dupree LW, Broskowski H, Schonfeld L. The Gerontology Alcohol Project: a behavioral treatment program for elderly alcohol abusers. *Gerontologist.* 1984;24:510–516.

Dupree LW, Schonfeld L. Cognitive-behavioral and self-management treatment of older problem drinkers. *J Ment Health Aging.* 1998;4:215–232.

Dustman RE. Alcoholism and aging: electrophysiological parallels. In: Hartford JT, Samorajski T, eds. *Alcoholism in the Elderly. Social and Biomedical Issues.* New York, NY: Raven; 1984:201–225.

Edelstein SL, Kritz-Silverstein D, Barrett-Connor E. Prospective association of smoking and alcohol use with cognitive function in an elderly cohort. *J Womens Health.* 1998;7:1271–1281.

Edgell RC, Kunik ME, Molinari VA, Hale D, Orengo CA. Nonalcohol-related use disorders in geropsychiatric patients. *J Geriat Psychiatry Neurol.* 2000;13:33–37.

Edwards G. Which treatments work for drinking problems? *BMJ.* 1988;296:4–5.

Egan M, Moride Y, Wolfson C, Monette J. Long-term continuous use of benzodiazepines by older adults in Quebec: prevalence, incidence and risk factors. *J Am Geriatr Soc.* 2000;48:811–816.

Ernst E. Herbal medications for common ailments in the elderly. *Drugs Aging*. 1999;15: 423–428.

Ewing JA. Detecting alcoholism: the CAGE questionnaire. *JAMA*. 1984;252:1905–1907.

Finlayson RE, Davis LJ Jr. Prescription drug dependence in the elderly population: demographic and clinical features of 100 inpatients. *Mayo Clin Proc*. 1994;69:1137–1145.

Finlayson RE, Hofmann V. Prescription drug misuse: treatment strategies. In: Gurnack AM, Atkinson RM, Osgood NJ, eds. *Treating Alcohol and Drug Abuse in the Elderly*. New York, NY: Springer-Verlag; 2002:155–174.

Finlayson RE, Hurt RD, Davis LJ Jr, Morse RM. Alcoholism in elderly persons: a study of the psychiatric and psychosocial features of 216 inpatients. *Mayo Clin Proc*. 1988;63:761–768.

Fisman M, Ramsay D, Weiser M. Dementia in the elderly alcoholic—a retrospective clinico-pathological study. *Int J Geriatr Psychiatry*. 1996;11:209–218.

Fleming MF. Identification and treatment of alcohol use disorders in older adults. In: Gurnack AM, Atkinson RM, Osgood NJ, eds. *Treating Alcohol and Drug Abuse in the Elderly*. New York, NY: Springer-Verlag; 2002:85–108.

Fleming MF, Barry KL, Adams WL, Stauffacher EA. Brief physician advice for alcohol problems in older adults: a randomized community-based trial. *Am J Fam Pract*. 1999;48:378–384.

Foy A, Drinkwater V, March S, Mearrick P. Confusion after admission to hospital in elderly patients using benzodiazepines. *BMJ (Clin Res Ed)*. 1986;293:1072.

Foy A, O'Connell D, Henry D, Kelly J, Cocking S, Halliday J. Benzodiazepine use as a cause of cognitive impairment in elderly hospital inpatients. *J Gerontol*. 1995;50A: M99–106.

Fraser AG. Pharmacokinetic interactions between alcohol and other drugs. *Clin Pharmacokinetics*. 1997;33:79–90.

Galanis DJ, Joseph C, Masaki KH, Petrovich H, Ross GW, White L. A longitudinal study of drinking and cognitive performance in elderly Japanese American men: the Honolulu-Asia Aging Study. *Am J Public Health*. 2000;90:1254–1259.

Gambert SR, Katsoyannis KK. Alcohol-related medical disorders of older heavy drinkers. In: Beresford TP, Gomberg ESL, eds. *Alcohol and Aging*. New York, NY: Oxford University Press; 1995:70–81.

Gilbert A, Innes JM, Owen N, Sansom L. Trial of an intervention to reduce chronic benzodiazepine use among residents of aged-care accommodation. *Aust N Z J Med*. 1993;23:343–347.

Golombok S, Higgitt A. Psychological treatments for benzodiazepine dependence. In: Hallstrom C, ed. *Benzodiazepine Dependence*. Oxford, UK: Oxford University Press; 1993:296–309.

Golombok S, Moodley PJ, Lader M. Cognitive impairment in long-term benzodiazepine users. *Psychol Med*. 1988;18:365–374.

Grad R, Tamblyn R, Holbrook AM, Hurley J, Feightner J, Gayton D. Risk of a new benzodiazepine prescription in relation to recent hospitalization. *J Am Geriatr Soc*. 1999;47:184–188.

Grant BF. Prevalence and correlates of alcohol use and *DSM-IV* alcohol dependence in the United States: results of the National Longitudinal Alcohol Epidemiologic Survey. *J Stud Alcohol*. 1997;58:464–473.

Grant BF, Harford TC. Comorbidity between *DSM-IV* alcohol use disorders and major depression: results of a national survey. *Drug Alcohol Depend.* 1995;39:197–206.

Grant BF, Hasin DS, Dawson DA. The relationship between *DSM-IV* alcohol use disorders and *DSM-IV* major depression: examination of the primary-secondary distinction in a general population sample. *J Affect Disord.* 1996;38:113–128.

Grant I, Adams KM, Reed R. Aging, abstinence, and medical risk factors in the prediction of neuropsychologic deficit among long-term alcoholics. *Arch Gen Psychiatry.* 1984;41:710–718.

Greenblatt DJ, Harmatz JS, Shader RI. Clinical pharmacokinetics of anxiolytics and hypnotics in the elderly: therapeutic considerations (Part I). *Clin Pharmacokinet.* 1991a;21:165–177.

Greenblatt DJ, Harmatz JS, Shader RI. Clinical pharmacokinetics of anxiolytics and hypnotics in the elderly: therapeutic considerations (Part II). *Clin Pharmacokinet.* 1991b;21:262–273.

Grigor RR, Spitz PW, Furst DE. Salicylate toxicity in elderly patients with rheumatoid arthritis. *J Rheumatol.* 1987;14:60–66.

Gurnack AM, Atkinson RM, Osgood NJ, eds. *Treating Alcohol and Drug Abuse in the Elderly.* New York, NY: Springer-Verlag; 2002.

Gustafson Y, Berggren D, Brannstrom B, et al. Acute confusional states in elderly patients treated for femoral neck fracture. *J Am Geriatr Soc.* 1988;36:525–530.

Helzer JE, Burnam A, McEvoy LT. Alcohol abuse and dependence. In: Robins LN, Regier DA, eds. *Psychiatric Disorders in America. The Epidemiologic Catchment Area Study.* New York, NY: Free Press; 1991:81–115.

Higgitt A. Indications for benzodiazepine prescriptions in the elderly [editorial]. *Int J Geriatr Psychiatry.* 1988;3:239–243.

Higgitt AC, Lader MH, Fonagy P. Clinical management of benzodiazepine dependence. *BMJ.* 1985;291:688–690.

Hillier V, Saib E. A case-control study of smoking and Alzheimer's disease. *Int J Geriatr Psychiatry.* 1997;12:295–300.

Honari S, Patterson DR, Gibbons J, et al. Comparison of pain control medication in three age groups of elderly patients. *J Burn Care Rehab.* 1997;18:500–504.

Hughes JR, Goldstein MG, Hurt RD, Shiffman S. Recent advances in the pharmacotherapy of smoking. *JAMA.* 1999;281:72–76.

Hurt RD, Finlayson RE, Morse RM, Davis LJ. Alcoholism in elderly persons: medical aspects and prognosis of 216 inpatients. *Mayo Clin Proc.* 1988;63:753–760.

Hurt RD, Sachs DPL, Glover ED, et al. A comparison of sustained-release bupropion and placebo for smoking cessation. *N Engl J Med.* 1997;337:1195–1202.

Institute of Medicine. *Marijuana and Medicine: Assessing the Science Base.* Washington, DC: National Academy Press; 1999.

Isacson D, Carsjo K, Bergman U, et al. Long-term use of benzodiazepines in a Swedish community: an 8-year follow-up. *J Clin Epidemiol.* 1992;45:429–436.

Jacques PF, Sulsky S, Hartz SC, Russell RM. Moderate alcohol intake and nutritional status in nonalcoholic elderly subjects. *Am J Clin Nutr.* 1989;50:875–883.

Jarvik ME, Schneider NG. Nicotine. In: Lowinson JH, Ruiz P, Millman RB, Langrod JG, eds. *Substance Abuse: A Comprehensive Textbook.* 2nd ed. Baltimore, MD: Williams and Wilkins; 1992:334–356.

Jernigan TL, Butters N, DiTraglia G, et al. Reduced cerebral grey matter observed in alcoholics using magnetic resonance imaging. *Alcoholism (New York)*. 1991;15: 418–427.

Johnson JE. Insomnia, alcohol, and over-the-counter drug use in old-old urban women. *J Community Health Nurs*. 1997;14:181–188.

Jorenby DE, Leischow SJ, Nides MA, et al. A controlled trial of sustained-release bupropion, a nicotine patch, or both for smoking cessation. *N Engl J Med*. 1999;340: 685–691.

Joseph C, Ganzini L, Atkinson R. Screening for alcohol use disorders in the nursing home. *J Am Geriatr Soc*. 1995;43:368–373.

Kaempf G, O'Donnell C, Oslin DW. The BRENDA model: a psychosocial addiction model to identify and treat alcohol disorders in elders. *Geriatr Nurs*. 1999;20:302–304.

Kandel D, Chen K, Warner LA, Kessler RC, Grant B. Prevalence and demographic correlates of symptoms of last year dependence on alcohol, nicotine, marijuana and cocaine in the US population. *Drug Alcohol Depend*. 1997;44:11–29.

Kashner TM, Rodell DE, Ogden SR, Guggenheim FG, Karson CN. Outcomes and costs of two VA inpatient treatment programs for older alcoholic patients. *Hosp Community Psychiatry*. 1992;43:985–989.

King MB. Alcohol abuse and dementia. *Int J Geriatr Psychiatry*. 1986;1:31–36.

Kofoed LL. OTC drug overuse in the elderly: what to watch for. *Geriatrics*. 1985;55: 55–60.

Kofoed LL, Tolson RL, Atkinson RM, Toth RL, Turner JA. Treatment compliance of older alcoholics: an elder-specific approach is superior to "mainstreaming" [published correction appears in *J Stud Alcohol*. 1987;48:183]. *J Stud Alcohol*. 1987; 48:47–51.

Korrapati MR, Vestal RE. Alcohol and medications in the elderly: complex interactions. In: Beresford TP, Gomberg ESL, eds. *Alcohol and Aging*. New York, NY: Oxford University Press; 1995:42–55.

Kril JJ, Halliday GM, Svoboda MD, Cartwright H. The cerebral cortex is damaged in chronic alcoholics. *Neuroscience*. 1997;79:983–998.

LaCroix AZ, Omenn GS. Older adults and smoking. *Clin Geriatr Med*. 1992;8:69–87.

Lasser RA, Sunderland T. Newer psychotropic medication use in nursing home residents. *J Am Geriatr Soc*. 1998;46:202–207.

Lazarus R, Sparrow D, Weiss ST. Alcohol intake and insulin levels. The Normative Aging Study. *Am J Epidemiol*. 1997;145:909–916.

Lee PN. Smoking and Alzheimer's disease: a review of the epidemiological evidence. *Neuroepidemiology*. 1994;13:131–144.

Leibovici D, Ritchie K, Ledesert B, Touchon J. The effects of wine and tobacco consumption on cognitive performance in the elderly: a longitudinal study of relative risk. *Int J Epidemiol*. 1999;28:77–81.

Letenneur L, Dartigues JF, Orgogozo JM. Wine consumption in the elderly. *Ann Intern Med*. 1993;118:317–318.

Liberto JG, Oslin DW. Early versus late onset of alcoholism in the elderly. *Int J Addict*. 1995;30:1799–1818.

Liberto JG, Oslin DW, Ruskin PE. Alcoholism in older persons: a review of the literature. *Hosp Community Psychiatry*. 1992;43:975–984.

Liskow BI, Rinck C, Campbell J, DeSouza C. Alcohol withdrawal in the elderly. *J Stud Alcohol*. 1989;50:414–421.

Litten RZ, Allen JP. Pharmacologic treatment of alcoholics with collateral depression: issues and future directions. *Psychopharm Bull.* 1998;34:107–110.

Lowinson JH, Ruiz P, Millman RB, Langrod JG, eds. *Substance Abuse: A Comprehensive Textbook.* 3rd ed. Baltimore, MD: Williams and Wilkins; 1997.

Lucey MR, Hill EM, Young JP, Demo-Dananberg L, Beresford TP. The influence of age and sex on blood ethanol levels in healthy humans. *J Stud Alcohol.* 1999;60:103–110.

Luttrell S, Watkin V, Livingston G, et al. Screening for alcohol misuse in older people. *Int J Geriatr Psychiatry.* 1997;12:1151–1154.

Martin JC, Streissguth AP. Alcoholism and the elderly: an overview. In: Eisdorfer C, Fann WE, eds. *Treatment of Psychopathology in the Aging.* New York, NY: Springer; 1982:242–280.

Merchant C, Tang MX, Albert S. Manly J, Stern Y, Mayeux R. The influence of smoking on the risk of Alzheimer's disease. *Neurology.* 2000;54:777–778.

Mertens JR, Moos RH, Brennan PL. Alcohol consumption, life context, and coping predict mortality among late-middle-aged drinkers and former drinkers. *Alcoholism (New York).* 1996;20:313–319.

Miller NS, Belkin BM, Gold MS. Alcohol and drug dependence among the elderly: Epidemiology, diagnosis, and treatment. *Compr Psychiatry.* 1991;32:153–165.

Miller PS, Richardson JS, Jyu CA, et al. Association of low serum anticholinergic levels and cognitive impairment in elderly presurgical patients. *Am J Psychiatry.* 1988; 145:342–345.

Miller WR, Rollnick S. *Motivational Interviewing: Preparing People to Change Addictive Behavior.* New York, NY: Guilford; 1991.

Miyamae M, Rodriguez MM, Camacho SA, Diamond I, Mochly-Rosen D, Figueredo VM. Activation of epsilon protein kinase C correlates with a cardioprotective effect of regular ethanol consumption. *Proc Natl Acad Sci U S A.* 1998;95:8262–8267.

Moore AA, Morton SC, Beck JC, et al. A new paradigm for alcohol use in older persons. *Med Care.* 1999;37:165–179.

Moos RH, Brennan PL, Moos BS. Short-term processes of remission and nonremission among late-life problem drinkers. *Alcoholism (New York).* 1991;15:948–955.

Morgan GD, Noll EL, Orleans CT, Rimer BK, Amfoh K, Bonney G. Reaching midlife and older smokers: tailored interventions for routine medical care. *Prev Med.* 1996; 25:346–354.

Morikawa Y-I, Arai H, Matsuschita S, et al. Cerebrospinal fluid tau protein levels in demented and nondemented alcoholics. *Alcoholism (New York).* 1999;23:575–577.

National Center for Health Statistics. Cigarette smoking among adults—United States, 1994. *MMWR Morb Mortal Wkly Rep.* 1996;45:588–590.

National Institute on Alcohol Abuse and Alcoholism. *The Physician's Guide to Helping Patients With Alcohol Problems.* Washington, DC: US Dept of Health and Human Services, Public Health Service, National Institutes of Health, National Institute on Alcohol Abuse and Alcoholism; 1995. NIH Publication 95-3769.

Nisell M, Nomikos GG, Svensson TH. Nicotine dependence, midbrain dopamine systems and psychiatric disorders. *Pharmacol Toxicol.* 1995;76:157–162.

Obisesan TO, Hirsch R, Kosoko O, Carlson L, Parrott M. Moderate wine consumption is associated with decreased odds of developing age-related macular degeneration in NHANES-1. *J Am Geriatr Soc.* 1998;46:1–7.

Orgogozo JM, Dartigues JF, Lafont S, et al. Wine consumption and dementia in the elderly: a prospective community study in the Bordeaux area. *Revue Neurol (Paris)*. 1997;153:185–192.

Orleans CT, Jepson C, Resch N, Rimer BK. Quitting motives and barriers among older smokers. *Cancer*. 1994;74:2055–2061.

Orleans CT, Resch N, Noll E, Keintz MK, Rimer BK, Brown TV, Snedden TM. Use of transdermal nicotine in a state-level prescription plan for the elderly. *JAMA*. 1994; 271:601–607.

Oslin D, Atkinson RM, Smith DM, Hendrie H. Alcohol related dementia: proposed clinical criteria. *Int J Geriatr Psychiatry*. 1998;13:203–212.

Oslin DW, Katz IR, Edell WS, Ten Have TR. Effects of alcohol consumption on the treatment of depression among elderly patients. *Am J Geriatr Psychiatry*. 2000;8: 215–220.

Oslin D. Liberto JG, O'Brien J, Krois S. The tolerability of naltrexone in treating older, alcohol dependent patients. *Am J Addict*. 1997a;6:266–270.

Oslin D, Liberto JG, O'Brien J, Krois S, Norbeck J. Naltrexone as an adjunctive treatment for older patients with alcohol dependence. *Am J Geriatr Psychiatry*. 1997b; 5:324–332.

Ott A, Slooter AJC, Hofman A, et al. Smoking and risk of dementia and Alzheimer's disease in a population-based cohort study: the Rotterdam Study. *Lancet*. 1998; 351:1840–1843.

Ozdemir V, Fourie J, Busto U, Naranjo CA. Pharmacokinetic changes in the elderly: do they contribute to drug abuse and dependence? *Clin Pharmacokinet*. 1996;31: 372–385.

Paille FM, Guelfi JD, Perkins AC, Royer RJ, Steru L, Parot P. Double-blind randomized multicentre trial of acamprosate in maintaining abstinence from alcohol. *Alcohol Alcohol*. 1995;30:239–247.

Peters NL. Snipping the thread of life: antimuscarinic side effects of medications in the elderly. *Arch Intern Med*. 1989;149:2414–2420.

Pfefferbaum A, Lim KO, Zipursky RB, et al. Brain gray and white matter volume loss accelerates with aging in chronic alcoholics: a quantitative MRI study. *Alcoholism (New York)*. 1992;16:1078–1089.

Pfefferbaum A, Sullivan EV, Mathalon DH, Lim KO. Frontal lobe volume loss observed with magnetic resonance imaging in older chronic alcoholics. *Alcoholism (New York)*. 1997;21:521–529.

Project MATCH Research Group. Matching alcoholism treatments to client heterogeneity: Project MATCH posttreatment drinking outcomes. *J Stud Alcohol*. 1997;58: 7–29.

Rickels K, Schweizer E, Case WG, Greenblatt DJ. Long-term therapeutic use of benzodiazepines, I: effects of abrupt discontinuation. *Arch Gen Psychiatry*. 1990;47:899–907.

Ried LD, Johnson RE, Gettman DA. Benzodiazepine exposure and functional status in older people. *J Am Geriatr Soc*. 1998;46:71–76.

Riedel WJ, Jorissen BL. Nutrients, age and cognitive function. *Curr Opin Clin Nutr Metab Care*. 1998;1:579–585.

Rimer BK, Orleans CT. Tailoring smoking cessation for older adults. *Cancer*. 1994;74: 2051–2054.

Rovner BW, David A, Lucas-Blaustein MJ, et al. Self-care capacity and anticholinergic drug levels in nursing home patients. *Am J Psychiatry*. 1988;145:107–109.

Roy-Byrne PP, Ballenger JC. Pharmacological treatments for benzodiazepine dependence. In: Hallstrom C, ed. *Benzodiazepine Dependence.* Oxford, UK: Oxford University Press; 1993:310–322.

Roy-Byrne PP, Hommer D. Benzodiazepine withdrawal: overview and implications for treatment of anxiety. *Am J Med.* 1988;84:1041–1052.

Ruchlin HS. Prevalence and correlates of alcohol use among older adults. *Prev Med.* 1997;26:651–657.

Salomon A, Jao S-C, Marcinowski K, et al. Nicotine inhibits amyloid formation by the beta peptide. *Biochemistry.* 1996;35:13568–13578.

Salzman C, Fisher J, Nobel K, Glassman R, Wolfson A, Kelley M. Cognitive improvement following benzodiazepine discontinuation in elderly nursing home residents. *Int J Geriatr Psychiatry.* 1992;7:89–93.

Sarkisian CA, Liu H, Gutierrez PR, Seeley DG, Cummings SR, Mangione CM. Modifiable risk factors predict functional decline among older women: a prospectively validated clinical prediction tool. The Study of Osteoporotic Fractures Research Group. *J Am Geriatr Soc.* 2000;48:170–178.

Sass H, Soyka M, Mann K, Zieglgansberger W. Relapse prevention by acamprosate: results from a placebo-controlled study on alcohol dependence. *Arch Gen Psychiatry.* 1996;53:673–680.

Saunders PA, Copeland JRM, Dewey ME, et al. Heavy drinking as a risk factor for depression and dementia in elderly men. *Br J Psychiatry.* 1991;159:213–216.

Scherr PA, LaCroix AZ, Wallace RB, et al. Light to moderate alcohol consumption and mortality in the elderly. *J Am Geriatr Soc.* 1992;40:651–657.

Schmidt I, Claesson CB, Westerholm B, Nilsson LG, Svarstad BL. The impact of regular multidisciplinary team interventions on psychotropic prescribing in Swedish nursing homes. *J Am Geriatr Soc.* 1998;46:77–82.

Schoenbaum M. Do smokers understand the mortality effects of smoking? Evidence from the Health and Retirement Survey. *Am J Public Health.* 1997;87:755–759.

Schonfeld L, Dupree LW, Dickson-Fuhrmann E, et al. Cognitive-behavioral treatment of older veterans with substance abuse problems. *J Geriatr Psychiatry Neurol.* 2000;13:124–129.

Schuckit MA. *Drug and Alcohol Abuse.* 5th ed. New York, NY: Kluwer Academic/Plenum; 2000.

Schutte KK, Brennan PL, Moos RH. Remission of late-life drinking problems: a 4-year follow-up. *Alcoholism (New York).* 1994;18:835–844.

Schutte KK, Brennan PL, Moos RH. Predicting the development of late-life late-onset drinking problems: a 7-year prospective study. *Alcoholism (New York).* 1998;22:1349–1358.

Schweizer E, Case WG, Rickels K. Benzodiazepine dependence and withdrawal in elderly patients. *Am J Psychiatry.* 1989;146:529–531.

Schweizer E, Rickels K, Case WG, Greenblatt DB. Long-term therapeutic use of benzodiazepines. II: effects of gradual taper. *Arch Gen Psychiatry.* 1990;47:908–915.

Simon GE, VanKorff M, Barlow W, Pabiniak C, Wagner E. Predictors of chronic benzodiazepine use in a health maintenance organization sample. *J Clin Epidemiol.* 1996;49:1067–1073.

Smith DM, Atkinson RM. Alcoholism and dementia. *Int J Addictions.* 1995;30:1843–1869.

Smith JW. Medical manifestations of alcoholism in the elderly. *Int J Addictions.* 1995; 30:1749–1798.

Soleas GJ, Diamandis EP, Goldberg DM. Resveratrol: a molecule whose time has come? And gone? *Clin Biochem.* 1997;30:91–113.

Sproule BA, Busto UE, Buckle C, Herrmann N, Bowles S. The use of non-prescription sleep products in the elderly. *Int J Geriatr Psychiatry.* 1999;14:851–857.

Srivastava LM, Vasisht S, Agarwal DP, Goedde HW. Relation between alcohol intake, lipoproteins and coronary artery disease: the interest continues. *Alcohol Alcohol.* 1994;29:11–24.

Stoehr GP, Ganguli M, Seaberg EC, Echement DA, Belle S. Over-the-counter medication use in an older rural community: the moVIES Project. *J Am Geriatr Soc.* 1997;45: 158–165.

Sussman S. Marijuana use in the elderly. *Clin Geriatr.* 1997;5(3):109–112, 117–119.

Tattersall M. Self-help groups and benzodiazepine dependence. In: Hallstrom C, ed. *Benzodiazepine Dependence.* Oxford, UK: Oxford University Press; 1993:323–336.

Thomson M, Smith WA. Prescribing benzodiazepines for noninstitutionalized elderly. *Can Fam Physician.* 1995;41:792–798.

Thun MJ, Peto R, Lopez AD, et al. Alcohol consumption and mortality among middle-aged and elderly US adults. *N Engl J Med.* 1997;337:1705–1714.

Tonne U, Hiltunen AJ, Vikander B, et al. Neuropsychological changes during steady-state drug use, withdrawal and abstinence in primary benzodiazepine-dependent patients. *Acta Psychiatr Scand.* 1995;91:299–304.

Tunc LE, Bylsma FW. Benzodiazepine-induced and anticholinergic-induced delirium in the elderly. *Int Psychogeriatr.* 1991;3:397–408.

Tyas SL, Koval JJ, Pederson LL. Does an interaction between smoking and drinking influence the risk of Alzheimer's disease? Results from three Canadian data sets. *Stat Med.* 2000;19:1685–1696.

Ulrich J, Johannson-Locher G, Seiler WO, Stahelin HB. Does smoking protect from Alzheimer's disease? Alzheimer-type changes in 301 unselected brains from patients with known smoking history. *Acta Neuropathol (Berl).* 1997;94:450–454.

US Public Health Service: state-specific estimates of smoking-attributable mortality and years of potential life lost—United States, 1985. *MMWR Morb Mortal Wkly Rep.* 1988;37:689–693.

Vaillant GE, Meyer SE, Mukamal K, Soldz S. Are social supports in late midlife a cause or a result of successful physical ageing? *Psychol Med.* 1998;28:1159–1168.

Van Duijn CM, Havekes LM, Van Broeckhoven C, et al. Apolipoprotein E genotype and association between smoking and early onset Alzheimer's disease. *BMJ.* 1995; 310:627–631.

Wang HX, Fratiglioni L, Frisoni GB, Viitanen M, Winblad B. Smoking and the occurrence of Alzheimer's disease: cross-sectional and longitudinal data in a population-based study. *Am J Epidemiol.* 1999;149:640–644.

Whitcup SM, Miller F. Unrecognized drug dependence in psychiatrically hospitalized elderly patients. *J Am Geriatr Soc.* 1987;35:297–301.

Woodhouse A, Mather LE. The influence of age upon opioid analgesic use in the patient-controlled analgesia (PCA) environment. *Anaesthesia.* 1998;52:949–955.

Woods JH, Winger G. Current benzodiazepine issues. *Psychopharmacology.* 1995;118: 107–115.

26

Sleep Disorders in Geriatric Psychiatry

Joseph Kwentus, MD

Complaints of either disturbed nighttime sleep or excessive daytime sleepiness are common in geriatric patients. These complaints may be caused by primary sleep disorders such as sleep apnea and insomnia, or sleep complaints may suggest the presence of other psychiatric or medical disorders. Depression, mania, and substance abuse and other psychiatric disorders disrupt the sleep of older people as they do in their younger counterparts. Moreover, dementia, delirium, and the sleep problems that accompany these conditions are decidedly prevalent in elderly individuals. Coronary disorders, renal failure, pulmonary failure, hepatic failure, and pain adversely affect sleep independent of associated delirium. Further complexity is added because older people residing in institutional settings are subject to environmentally induced sleep problems not under their own control. In addition, sleep disturbance can be induced by the myriad medications that elderly people take.

Sleep patterns and circadian rhythms of normal elderly are different from those of younger people. These normal age-related changes in sleep patterns cause apprehension in some elderly people. As a result, some older people turn to sedative medications to help them sleep. These medications have predictable short-term results on the sleep disorders of elderly people, but may cause daytime problems and may be difficult to withdraw. In addition, the long-term effects of these interventions have not been studied. This discussion focuses on the interaction between sleep physiology of normal aging and the ailments to which elderly people are subject.

NORMAL SLEEP CHANGES WITH AGE

Polysomnography allows viewing of three distinct physiological states that occur throughout 24 hours. These states are wake, NREM (non–rapid eye movement or slow-wave), and REM (rapid eye movement) sleep. Predictable changes in these physiological patterns begin at birth and continue throughout life. The electroencephalogram (EEG) helps define these physiological stages.

NREM sleep is the restorative phase of sleep. At the initiation of sleep, the EEG becomes slower. The background rhythm changes from about 10 Hz to 6 Hz. At the same time, the electrooculogram demonstrates slow rolling movements, and muscle tone becomes quieter. Gradually, two sleep-specific waveforms emerge: sleep spindles and K complexes. Sleep spindles are bursts of activity at frequencies of 12 to 14 Hz on EEG. The K complexes are high-amplitude triphasic waves. Sleep spindles and K complexes are the hallmark of Stage 2 sleep. During Stage 3 and 4 sleep, the prominence of sleep spindles and K complexes diminishes, and the EEG becomes dominated by delta waves consisting of high-amplitude activity that occurs at about 2 to 4 Hz. As the EEG slows, the depth of sleep increases, and the person is less arousable. Metabolic activity diminishes, and autonomic discharges decrease. With advancing age, the deeper stages of NREM sleep tend to occur earlier in the night, sleep consolidation declines, and time of awakening and the rhythms of body temperature, plasma melatonin, insulin, and cortisol shift to an earlier clock hour (Dijk & Duffy, 1999).

Normal aging decreases the amount of NREM sleep and changes its characteristics. In particular, there is less delta sleep (Dijk & Duffy, 1995; Prinz et al., 1982). At the same time, the lighter stages of sleep may increase somewhat. Despite this increase in the lighter stages of sleep, there are generally fewer spindles and K complexes. Spindles and K complexes also change in configuration and are generally less well defined (Jankel & Niedermeyer, 1985). These changes in slow-wave sleep are more prominent in older women than in older men (Gigli et al., 1996).

REM sleep represents another distinct physiological state. During REM sleep, the EEG speeds up. Rapid eye movements appear. Muscle tone reaches its lowest level, causing virtual paralysis. Any remaining muscle activity occurs as bursts during eye movements. REM sleep is a highly active sleep associated with dramatic physiological changes. Oxygen requirements and autonomic activity increase. Body temperature falls toward the ambient room temperature. The metabolic controls of respiration are dramatically altered, and the upper airway becomes much more relaxed. These changes combine to make the individual more vulnerable to sleep apnea during REM sleep.

The function of REM sleep remains unknown, but one of the most fascinating aspects of REM is the fact that dreams are experienced. Dreams are usually accompanied by autonomic discharges. REM sleep reaches its peak early in life and gradually diminishes. In spite of this, REM sleep remains well intact into the 90s in normal individuals.

During a 24-hour cycle, a person advances through cycles of wake, NREM, and REM sleep. In normal aging, the relationship among these physiological cycles changes dramatically. The waking state is characterized by a tendency to more frequent naps. It takes older people a longer time to fall asleep. At the same time, there are more frequent awakenings during sleep cycles. In addition, the overall amount of time spent asleep is decreased even though the amount of time spent in bed may remain the same or even increase. Sleep efficiency is therefore decreased, and the depth of sleep is reduced. REM sleep tends to occur earlier in the night (Reynolds et al., 1985). These changes that are seen in the laboratory are reflected in the subjective reports of elderly persons, who say that they take longer to fall asleep despite earlier bedtimes. Normal elderly also report earlier morning awakenings and more arousals during the night.

Older adults often report that they need less sleep than they formerly needed. Although older people sleep less than younger people, they have decreased sleep efficiency and tend to spend just as much time in bed as younger people. This decreased need for sleep should not be confused with the symptoms of primary sleep disorders. Even in older people, persistent daytime sleepiness usually indicates the presence of a sleep disorder. As in any area of geriatric medicine, it is important to distinguish pathology from normal development. In fact, the changes in sleep that occur normally in aging make the older person more vulnerable to sleep disorders.

Older people may have several coexisting sleep disorders that increase the challenge for the physician. The physician who is sensitive to these issues and knowledgeable about sleep can address the causes of sleep problems, thereby improving the nighttime sleep and daytime functioning of the older adult. Sleep is an important health consideration in older people. Habitual sleep patterns may affect morbidity and mortality independently from vascular disease (Qureshi et al., 1997). Sleep apnea affects the outcome of pulmonary disease, and nocturnal esophageal reflux can lead to cancer. On the other hand, preserved sleep architecture and the absence of sleep disorder predict more successful aging and less-severe physical and cognitive decline (Spiegel et al., 1999).

SLEEP DISTURBANCES IN ELDERLY PERSONS

Epidemiology

Problems with sleep increase with age. From 30% to 60% of older people have some kind of sleep complaint (Almeida et al., 1999; Miles & Dement, 1980). These problems range from sleep apnea to bad sleep habits. Snoring and sleep apnea are associated with structural abnormalities of the airway, obesity, and male sex. Insomnia is associated with low family income, retirement, disability, depression, living alone, and female sex. In addition, sleep disturbance is a major and debilitating symptom of bereavement (Prigerson et al., 1995). However, the most significant association with insomnia is depression. One of the best predictors of future depression in older people who are not currently depressed is current sleep disturbance.

Some older people develop poor sleep habits, and up to one half of elderly persons intermittently use some kind of sleeping medicine. Elderly people are prone to develop sleep phase disorder and may sleep during the day and stay awake at night. Some of the change in sleep patterns is because of alteration in the circadian rhythm. However, many factors are involved, including the fact that many older people no longer have structured activities during retirement. Older people may live in settings that are not conducive to uninterrupted sleep. Poor sleep is highly correlated with poor health status, and poor health is more common in the elderly. Finally, many elderly people are caregivers for spouses and other relatives. These caregiving roles may require them to be up all night.

Diagnosis

Most sleep complaints can be classified as insomnia, hypersomnolence, parasomnias (disorders of arousal, partial arousal, and sleep stage transition), and disturbance of the sleep-wake cycle. Presenting symptoms are the first clue to cause and can be classified as primarily insomnia or hypersomnolence. In younger people, insomnia is usually secondary to psychiatric or neurological illness, and hypersomnolence is associated with sleep apnea or narcolepsy. In older patients, the picture is far more complex, and multifactorial etiology is common. As in any other area of medicine, diagnosis is based on a thorough history, a complete physical exam, a review of medical and psychiatric symptoms, and laboratory testing. The principal laboratory tests are the all-night polysomnogram and the multiple sleep latency test. These tests are expensive. History and a physical are usually adequate to diagnose the cause of insomnia alone. Hypersomnolence is more difficult to quantitate without polysomnography.

Methods other than polysomnography to measure sleep have been developed and are used more extensively in studies of sleep in older people. For example, the wrist actigraph is a device that estimates sleep versus wakefulness on the basis of wrist activity. The wrist actigraph may be used to determine the efficacy of a particular treatment when compared to baseline in elderly persons with insomnia. The actigraph is not adequate as a diagnostic tool. It overestimates sleep in psychiatric cases and underestimates it in others.

Another nonintrusive measure of sleep developed for home sleep monitoring is a pressure-sensitive pad that reports signals from respiration and movement. There are a variety of other devices aimed at diagnosing and monitoring breathing disorders at home or in nursing home settings. These devices may serve a purpose when polysomnography is not available.

Insomnia

Insomnia is an important issue for elderly people. Older adults are more likely than younger adults to live in situations in which behavioral conditioning can lead to insomnia. In addition, older adults already suffer from inefficient sleep and frequent awakenings. These problems are somewhat more prevalent in women, who generally report their complaints accurately and have abnormalities that can be documented on sleep monitoring. Sleep problems tend to get worse after menopause and are ameliorated somewhat by estrogen replacement (Polo-Kantola et al., 1999). Because many women are discontinuing hormone therapy in response to concerns about safety, there may be an increase in sleep complaints. In spite of this, the sleep complaints of older people, particularly the complaints of older women, are often dismissed. This may even be truer in managed-care settings (Hatoum et al., 1998).

Insomniacs tend to suffer from hyperarousal and anxiety during the day. Because psychophysiological insomnia is a behavioral response to certain conditions, it is best treated behaviorally. Both insomniacs and their significant others are more willing to accept psychological intervention than pharmacological intervention if they are given the option. The most important intervention is educating the insomniac about the principles of sleep hygiene (see Table 26-1).

The initial approach is to adhere to a regular schedule of going to bed and arising. If the patient takes daytime naps, it is important to clarify the reason. Although napping is more common in older people, it is helpful to explain to the patient that daytime naps will decrease nighttime sleep. Cognitive behavior therapy, relaxation therapy, and sleep restriction also have a definite role in the treatment of the older insomniac. Regular aerobic exercise may enhance the quality and depth of sleep in late life.

As there are often multiple contributing factors, insomnia should be considered a symptom and not a diagnosis. Depression, poor health, and lack of physical activity are associated with insomnia in elderly people (Morgan & Clarke, 1997b). Sleep apnea, periodic limb movements, gastroesophageal reflux, pulmonary disease, coronary disease, and a host of other medical problems produce insomnia in elders. Psychiatric disorders contribute significantly to insomnia in the elderly. Anxiety and affective disorders are important, but dementia also contributes to the problem. Finally, the patient's drugs should be evaluated to determine if insomnia is an adverse effect of a pharmacological intervention for a medical problem. Even with appropriate evaluation and treatment, insomnia is more persistent and enduring in older people. Older insomniacs are more likely to have significant physical or mental problems than younger insomniacs (Morgan & Clarke, 1997b).

In spite of this, nonpharmacological treatments of insomnia are effective in the elderly. Treatment methods such as stimulus control and sleep restriction, which target maladaptive sleep habits, are especially beneficial for older insomniacs, whereas relaxation-based interventions aimed at decreasing arousal

TABLE 26-1.   Sleep hygiene rules

Do not go to bed and try to sleep until you are sleepy.

Perform bedtime rituals (brushing teeth, washing up, etc.) at the same time every night.

Get up at the same time every morning.

Do not nap.

Exercise daily early in the day.

Do not use your bedroom during the day. Reserve it for sleep and sex.

Do not review the day's worries at bedtime; do that when you wake up.

Avoid heavy meals at bedtime. If you are really hungry, have a light snack.

Stop smoking if you can. Initially, your sleep will be worse, but later it will improve.

Have caffeine in the morning only and in limited amounts.

Do not drink alcohol 4 hours prior to bed.

Try to take medicines that cause activities such as urination (diuretics) early enough to avoid nighttime arousal.

Ask your doctor if any medicines you are taking might keep you up and then ask if there are substitutes. Take medicines only as directed.

If you wake up at night because of pain, ask your doctor for a longer acting pain medicine.

Make sure that supports such as eye glasses, walker, or hearing aid are at the bedside.

Empty your bladder before bed.

Control the nighttime environment. Temperature should be comfortable. Eliminate noise. Replace uncomfortable mattress. Make sure there is only enough light to enable you to walk safely to the bathroom.

Do not watch the clock.

If it helps, use soothing noise such as a fan or other appliance or a "white noise" machine.

If unable to fall asleep within 30 minutes, get out of bed and perform soothing activity, such as listening to soft music or reading.

Have adequate exposure to bright light during the day.

Do not exercise before bedtime.

If you are a caregiver, do not place unrealistic demands on yourself regarding your caregiving attentiveness.

---

produce more limited effects. Cognitive and educational interventions are instrumental in altering age-related dysfunctional beliefs and attitudes about sleep. Daytime exercise or other vigorous activity is helpful for some, while taking a siesta seems to impair nighttime sleep and increase mortality. Only a few older adults will resume "normal" sleep patterns after treatment, but most report greater satisfaction with their sleep patterns, use fewer medications, and display less psychological distress (Morin et al., 1999).

Elderly people are prone to changes in sleep phase. Delayed sleep phase syndrome involves undesirably late bedtimes and equally late wake-up times (Dijk & Duffy, 1999). The chief complaint is usually early night insomnia. The opposite problem is advanced sleep phase syndrome. Unnecessary early bed-times partially account for the high prevalence of early morning awakening in healthy older people.

The circadian temperature rhythm exerts powerful effects on the regulation of sleep. Insomnia in the geriatric population is associated with diminished amplitude in the body temperature rhythm. Although elderly people tend to go to sleep earlier than younger people, the chief complaint is usually early night insomnia.

One treatment involves a paradigm of phase advancing by having the patient retire a couple of hours later each day. Chronotherapy has generally been abandoned because of lack of efficacy. Treatment with melatonin or vitamin B_{12} and timed exposure to bright light have been suggested as treatments for circadian sleep disturbances in nondemented as well as demented older persons Although these interventions sometimes succeed, sleep phase syndromes have a worse treatment outcome than other sleep disorders (Regestein & Monk, 1995).

Dementia and Depression

Depression and dementia cause the most difficulty in managing sleep disturbances that require medical attention. In these conditions, both sleep initiation and sleep maintenance are affected. Depression causes difficulty going asleep, sleep fragmentation, decreased sleep efficiency, and early morning awakening. Sleep architecture, including the timing and intensity of the REM cycle and the timing and depth of slow-wave sleep, are affected. Early morning awakening is the sleep symptom most consistently related to depressed mood and is least related to dementia (Reynolds et al., 1988). People who are earlier in their depressive episodes have their sleep impaired more than those later in their episode (Dew et al., 1996).

The depressed older person spends many hours in bed awake and half-asleep. This inactivity can lead to dehydration, disuse atrophy, decubitus, and a variety of other medical problems. The earlier the treatment, the better.

Antidepressants are the treatment of choice for sleep disturbances associated with depression. The selective serotonin reuptake inhibitors (SSRIs) are the most commonly prescribed antidepressants for older people. However, SSRIs sometimes increase sleep complaints. If sleep disorder is a major feature of the depression, then consideration should be given to a more sedating agent rather than a more activating agent. If a tricyclic is chosen, the prescriber must consider the effects on the heart and the risk of falls.

Ironically, a night of sleep deprivation potentiates antidepressant effect. Even after treatment for depression, symptoms of sleep disorder may persist. Behavioral treatments are preferred in these circumstances, but the addition of a sedative may be necessary. Older people who have been treated for depression often continue to have EEG evidence of sleep disturbance. These changes are most frequently reflected in NREM sleep and include continued difficulty with sleep maintenance.

Sleep disorders associated with dementia depend on the etiology of the dementia. Alzheimer's disease is associated with sleep fragmentation and decreased sleep spindles and K complexes. An important contrast between a depressed person and a person with Alzheimer's disease is in the production of REM sleep. Depressed people often experience excessive REM in the early portion of the sleep cycle. Time between sleep onset and first REM is often decreased in depression. In Alzheimer's disease, on the other hand, there is often a decrease in the total amount of REM sleep. The difference in the REM in these two conditions is probably related to neurotransmitter changes, particularly of acetylcholine.

Depression and dementia, particularly dementia of the Alzheimer's type, demonstrate decreased amounts of Stage 3 and Stage 4 sleep. This is the restorative phase of sleep; therefore, both depressed and mildly demented people are likely to complain of fatigue. When demented and nondemented elderly persons are compared, demented patients are found to have more sleep disruption and arousals, lower sleep efficiency, a higher percentage of Stage 1 sleep, and decreases in Stage 3 and 4 sleep. These findings worsen as the dementia progresses. Later in the course of the dementia, patients also have increased daytime sleepiness (Pat-Horenczyk et al., 1998). The result is complete fragmentation of sleep/wakefulness during the night and day (Pat-Horenczyk et al., 1998).

Sleep disorder in vascular dementia and Lewy body dementias are less well studied. Because vascular dementia can be associated with pathology in the brain stem reticular formation, a variety of sleep effects can be seen. Sleep apnea may occur in patients with cerebrovascular disease because of damage to respiratory control mechanisms. Lewy body dementia, Parkinson's disease, and cerebrovascular disorders have been associated with REM sleep behavior disorder (Olson et al., 2000). REM sleep behavior disorder is one of the more dramatic parasomnias. In this disorder, the sufferers act out their dreams because the mechanism for muscle activity suppression is not functioning properly. These people can become quite violent during the episode. People with diffuse Lewy body dementia often suffer from hallucinations. These often occur at sleep onset or at the time of awakening.

Prion infection usually causes a rapidly fatal dementia (Creutzfeldt-Jakob disease); however, the thalamic form of this disease causes a sleep disorder referred to as fatal insomnia. There is also a familial variety, fatal familial insomnia. The illness ends in dementia and death.

Sleep Apnea and Snoring

Sleep apnea is a well-established sleep disorder with high morbidity. Several studies have suggested that sleep apnea is extremely frequent in the elderly, with its prevalence estimated at 18% (Partinen, 1995). The prevalence of obstructive sleep apnea increases with age in both sexes, with an odds ratio of 2.2 for each 10-year increase.

There is a causal association between sleep apnea in the elderly and cardiovascular disease (Peker et al., 2000). Elderly sleep apnea patients have more sleep disturbances, are more depressed, and have more cognitive deficits compared to normal old persons. These cognitive effects appear to be related to the degree of hypoxemia. A high level of sleep-disordered breathing is a risk factor for mortality during REM sleep phase in these patients. In addition, untreated sleep apnea causes loss of daytime cognitive abilities. Sleepiness may lead to mistakes in judgment, motor vehicle accidents, falls, and other misfortunes and deleteriously affect social and marital life (Ohayon et al., 1997).

The evaluation of sleep apnea in older people is complicated by the fact that there is a high level of nonsymptomatic respiratory dysregulation in older people (Phillips et al., 1996). Central apneas occur frequently in subjects with neurological disorders, such as infarction, tumor, and encephalopathy, or in those with chronic heart failure or chronic obstructive pulmonary disease (COPD). Central apnea is so common in nursing homes that the condition is ignored; staff sit by and patiently wait for the patient to start breathing again. There is no evidence that evaluation and treatment would help these people. However, treatment with nocturnal oxygen is warranted in symptomatic cases when there is associated nocturnal desaturation (Franklin et al., 1997). However, obstructive pulmonary disease is extremely common in older people with obstructive apnea (Rossi et al., 1996). Therefore, the risk of respiratory depression associated with hypercapnia must also be considered in any potential intervention.

On the other hand, snoring and obstructive apnea deserve attention. As obstructive sleep apnea worsens, it contributes significantly to the morbidity and mortality of several common medical conditions, including hypertension (Bixler et al., 2000); cardiac disease (Peker et al., 2000); and cerebral vascular disease (Parra et al., 2000). Sinus arrest and atrioventricular block have been demonstrated in as many as 30% of patients with sleep apnea (Becker et al., 1995). Sleep apnea worsens hypoventilation at night in several respiratory conditions, leading to increased hypoxemia (Becker et al., 1999). Repeated apneic events cause cerebral damage over time (Kamba et al., 1997) and contribute to cognitive deterioration (Dealberto et al., 1996).

Overweight individuals may be helped by weight loss, but this is usually impossible to accomplish in geriatric populations. Alcohol or other sedatives (e.g., benzodiazepines and antihistamines) should be avoided before going to bed. An appropriate specialist should treat allergy and nasopharyngeal pathology. Several intranasal sprays (e.g., intranasal corticosteroid or cromolyn sprays) are available if allergic rhinitis is contributing to snoring.

More severe cases require more aggressive management, ranging from the application of dental devices (Hans et al., 1997) and nasal strips to surgery. The most common surgery is uvulopalatopharyngeoplasty, which may be conducted by a variety of different techniques (Aboussouan et al., 1995). A more conservative therapy is positive airway pressure delivered by a variety of different machines designed to splint the airway during sleep to keep it open (Redline et al., 1998). Oxygen may be used in selected cases, either with or without positive-pressure devices. Modafinil reduces daytime sleepiness in patients with obstructive sleep apnea who continue to complain of fatigue. Unfortunately, predicting which patients will respond to which treatment remains difficult.

Narcolepsy

Narcolepsy usually starts during adolescence; however, there is great variability in the clinical presentation of narcolepsy, and genetic forms of the disorder may present with mild disease severity and not be recognized until later in life. It has been discovered that genetic varieties of narcolepsy resuilt from the absence of neuroexcitation in the hypocretin system (Chakravorty & Rye, 2003). Narcolepsy persists throughout the life cycle and continues to require treatment. Secondary forms of narcolepsy may be caused by a variety of neurological insults, including head trauma and stroke. Older individuals are prone to these types of neurological insults.

Symptoms of narcolepsy include excessive somnolence, hypnagogic hallucinations, cataplexy, and sleep paralysis. Diagnosis of narcolepsy is based on the clinical presentation of appropriate symptoms and confirmation of sleeponset REM during the multiple sleep latency test. Polysomnography is used to rule out other sleep disorders.

Treatment for narcolepsy usually includes stimulant medication, usually amphetamines. Treatment with modafinil produced significant improvement in the multiple sleep latency test and the maintenance of wakefulness test.

Movement Disorders

Periodic limb movements of sleep (PLMS) is a condition of debilitating, repetitive, stereotypic leg movements that occur in NREM sleep. The leg movements occur every 20 to 40 seconds and can last much of the night. Each movement may be associated with an arousal. The occurrence of PLMS seems to increase with age and is associated with peripheral neuropathy. PLMS usually causes difficulty initiating and maintaining sleep. PLMS is extremely common in elderly patients (Coleman et al., 1981).

Restless legs syndrome is a condition involving an uncontrollable urge to move the legs at night. The patient can usually report this symptom. There may be a family history of the condition; in some cases, an underlying medical disorder (e.g., renal, neurological, or cardiovascular disease) seems associated.

No medication has been uniformly effective in treating PLMS. Suggested medications include nighttime doses of trazodone (50 to 150 mg) for sedation. This treatment is usually combined with a dose of controlled-release L-dopa/carbidopa. Dosing is started low and titrated upward gradually. Morning leg restlessness can develop, which suggests that the treatment has worn off or the presence of drug withdrawal. Nausea is the most common side effect. Psychiatric side effects and dyskinesia are rare. A 70% long-term response rate is typical, but tolerance and daytime withdrawal effects are common.

Other treatments for PMLS include benzodiazepines and low doses of narcotic analgesics given at an appropriate time prior to bedtime. Drug choice is based on minimizing side effects. Patients with restless legs syndrome or PMLS benefit from avoiding caffeine, tricyclic antidepressants, antipsychotic medications, and antihistamines. Restless legs syndrome may be relieved in a small number of patients by high dosages of vitamin E (800–1,200 IU per day).

Medical Problems

Medical conditions are extremely important contributors to the sleep problems of older individuals. Difficulty maintaining sleep is often related to a variety of organic conditions. Gastroesophageal reflux is a common medical condition that causes older people to wake up in the middle of the night with coughing and sometimes with an acid taste in the mouth. Aspiration pneumonia is common and can be serious. Gastroesophageal reflux can be treated in some cases by elevating the head of the bed or changing sleep position (Khoury et al., 1999). The right lateral decubitus is associated with most severe reflux. The prescription of famotidine (Mann et al., 1995), ranitidine, or a proton pump inhibitor may reduce the effects of the reflux. Patients with gastroesphageal reflux often have coexisting obstructive sleep apnea that should be treated (Ing et al., 2000).

Patients with strokes and degenerative neurological conditions often have a variety of sleep disturbances, commonly sleep apnea. Again, this can produce frequent nighttime awakenings. Sleep apnea may also increase the risk of future strokes through a variety of mechanisms. Pain from arthritis, cancer, disc disease, and a number of other conditions is common in older people. It is important that analgesia is sufficient to allow for adequate sleep. Congestive heart failure can produce paroxysmal nocturnal awakening and orthopnea.

Chronic obstructive pulmonary disease also produces symptoms incompatible with sleep. In these patients, sleep efficiency waxes and wanes depending on the severity of the underlying condition. Cerebrovascular disease can cause both obstructive and central sleep apnea (Good et al., 1996). Patients who are on renal dialysis have problems with periodic leg movements, sleep apnea, and insomnia (Benz et al., 1999). In patients with end-stage renal disease, these sleep problems may be associated with increased mortality (Benz et al., 2000). Nighttime urination is often associated with poor quality of sleep, thirst at night, and increased fatigue in the daytime (Donahue & Lowenthal, 1997). In men, prostate problems can cause difficulty with nocturia (see Table 26-2).

Certain medications and other agents such as diuretics or stimulating agents (e.g., caffeine, sympathomimetics, bronchodilators) taken near bedtime can exacerbate symptoms. Certain medications can induce nightmares and impair sleep, such as some antidepressants, antiparkinson agents, and anti-

TABLE 26-2. Common medical problems and sleep

Disorder	Sleep effect	Implications	Treatment
Renal failure	Sleep anpnea; hypersomnia; periodic limb movement; insomnia	Poor overall prognosis. Screen for apnea	Treat sleep disorder; adequate hemodialysis; correct anemia
Functional bowel disorder	Nonrestorative sleep	Lowered visceral perception	Low-dose tricyclics
Gastroesophageal reflux	Frequent arousals with inability to maintain sleep	Common cause of recurrent pneumonia	Proton pump inhibitor; elevate bed; reduce evening meal; lose weight
Coronary artery disease	Cheyne-Stokes respirations and nocturnal dyspnea in chronic heart failure and atrial fibrillation	Nocturnal dyspnea; Cheyne-Stokes causes daytime sleepiness and implies poor prognosis	Increase daytime activity; avoid sedatives; treat sleep apnea; nocturnal O_2 for some
Chronic pulmonary disease	Insomnia caused by cough; increase in central and obstructive apnea	Increased oxygen desaturation from decreased drive	Avoid sedatives and alcohol; continuous positive airway pressure (CPAP) or O_2 may help
Head trauma	Posttraumatic insomnia or hypersomnia; posttraumatic narcolepsy	May limit rehabilitation	Assess symptoms and treat
Degenerative neurological disease	Sleep apnea; Parkinson's disease and Lewy body dementia associated with rapid eye movement (REM) sleep behavior disorder; periodic movements in degenerative diseases	Multiple sleep problems based on location of lesion or lesions; associated psychiatric illnesses common (i.e., depression in Parkinson's disease)	Rational approach based on understanding of sleep effects of the neurological illness; diagnose and treat psychiatric illness
Hepatic disease (cirrhosis)	Periodic limb movement syndrome; circadian rhythm abnormalties; myoclonic jerks	Difficulty initiating and maintaining sleep	Treat hepatic encephalopathy; be aware of drug metabolism
Urinary tract disorders	Nocturia	Difficulty maintaining sleep	Treat urinary tract infections, benign prostatic hypertrophy, etc.
Cancer	Insomnia related to treatment or bereavement	Multifactorial; sleep history neglected in cancer patients	Assess psychological, behavioral, and health impact, then treat

(continued)

TABLE 26-2. *Continued*

Disorder	Sleep effect	Implications	Treatment
Chronic pain	Difficulty initiating and maintaining sleep; patients with rheumatic disease (especially with widespread pain) have greater sleep disturbance	May cause secondary psychophysiological insomnia; attitude toward pain contributes to sleep; improving sleep tends to decrease pain	Treatment should consider medication that will provide adequate analgesia at night; primary sleep disorder should be treated; cognitive therapy
Delirium	Sleep disorder is part of diagnosis	Differential diagnosis is key to appropriate treatment	Treat underlying cause; symptomatic treatment

hypertensives. Sedation should be given at bedtime rather than during the day, if possible.

Multifactorial Sleep Problems

Elderly people often have more than one cause for difficulty in initiating and maintaining sleep. The reasons may include psychological and physical reasons. Therefore, a person who has dementia may also suffer from behavioral conditioning effects that result in a psychophysiological insomnia. Similarly, this person may also be depressed and have PLMS. Because elderly people are prone to a multiplicity of factors that contribute to insomnia, a careful analysis of sleep, sleep conditions, and medical issues must be undertaken. With the proper diagnosis, the appropriate therapy can be developed that addresses major issues involved in the person's difficulty sleeping.

Elderly people may complicate sleep through attempts at treatment. Some older people try to treat their insomnia with alcohol. In fact, some older physicians even recommend that their patients have a nightcap before retiring. Alcohol can actually cause rebound insomnia in the middle of the night.

Sundowning

Disturbances of the sleep-wake cycle that result in daytime sleep and nighttime wakefulness are common with dementia. The baseline slowing of EEG activity often seen with dementia can make interpretation of sleep versus wakefulness and discrimination between stages of NREM sleep difficult. One of the most difficult sleep disturbances in demented people is a psychiatric phenomenon known as sundowning (McGaffigan & Bliwise, 1997). Sundowners increase restless and verbal behavior as evening approaches.

In nursing homes, sundowners tend to be more demented than nonsundowners (Evans, 1987). Among physiological factors, odor of urine, being awakened frequently on the evening shift, and fewer medical diagnoses are significantly associated with sundowning. Significant psychosocial factors are current room residence less than 1 month, more recent admission to the facility, and higher evening levels of confusion. Sundowning can occur in people with mild dementia who appear relatively normal in the day, but who become confused in the late afternoon or evening. More severely demented people appear relatively calm during the day, but become agitated, restless, or aggressive during the night. Problems with sleeping and sundowning are often a stage in the dementing illness.

Although it most commonly occurs in institutionalized demented patients, sundowning can occur in persons not otherwise manifesting frank dementia and in homes. Sundowning has a more profound impact than confusion or agitation during the day. If these nocturnal behaviors persist, they can have a profound effect on the caregiver and may result in placement in a nursing facility (Gallagher-Thompson et al., 1992).

Sundowning is probably a nonspecific reaction to an assortment of causes. There is no single underlying mechanism. It has been suggested that sometimes a lack of clues from light and dark cycles may precipitate sundowning. Alzheimer's disease causes disturbances of circadian rhythms, and sundowning in the patients with this disease may be related to a phase delay of body temperature. Other factors that have been implicated include sensory deprivation, lack of structure, and reaction to novel environments.

There is also a possibility that, in some cases, sundowning reflects disruptive behaviors that occur with identical frequency throughout the day, but with differential impact on nursing staff or caregiver at night. Decreased daytime activity and increased nighttime motor activity may reflect the fact that sleep-wake rhythms are flatter in older adults than in caregivers. Decreased daytime activity may result from deficient physical stimulation or frailty. Depression, sleep-schedule disturbances, restless legs, or other sleep disorders can explain increased nighttime activity in some.

The sudden onset of sundowning may also indicate the presence of some occult medical problem, such as a urinary tract infection, pulmonary infection, a disturbance in blood chemistry, or the introduction of a new medication. Sundowning may result from the sedation given to quiet patients, especially on evening shifts, in many health care facilities. In institutional care, managing those who disturb others at night can be the bane of the staff and may result in increased sedation with the increased risk of falls and sometimes significant worsening of dementia from either residual sedation or other drug side effects (see Table 26-3).

Sleep of Elderly Persons in Institutional Settings

Insomnia may be a more important factor that leads to nursing home placement than cognitive disturbance. A large percentage of caregivers report that

TABLE 26-3.   Checklist to reduce sundowning

Provide orientation cues
Give adequate daytime stimulation
Medical evaluation to rule out treatable causes of delirium
Maintain adequate levels of light
Establish bedtime routine and ritual
Allow the same staff member to care for the same residents every day
Investigate any environmental factors that might keep the individual awake
Use exercise to expend energy to help the body feel more fatigued at bedtime
Have resident avoid drinking any stimulant like coffee or avoid smoking cigarettes
    close to bedtime
Give diuretics and laxatives early in the day to prevent elimination at night
Provide care (baths, meals, activities) at the same time every day
Be sure residents have glasses and hearing aids in place and functioning
Familiar objects at bedside or on the bed may help assure the resident of personal
    safety
Monitor amount of sensory stimulation in the environment
Consider exposure to bright light in the late afternoon
"As needed" medication should be avoided
If medication is required for disturbing behavior, establish a regular dose
Caregiver may need to use respite help

nocturnal difficulties played an important role in their decision to institutional-ize an elderly relative (Pollak et al., 1997). The caregiver may be awakened numerous times with the elderly person's complaints of incontinence, pain, and sleeplessness. Fatigue contributes significantly to agitation on the part of the patient and irritability on the part of the caregiver.

When the primary reason for placement is sleep disturbance, a thorough sleep assessment is indicated. Treatable disorders are best dealt with in advance. Older people have a high prevalence of sleep apnea, periodic limb movements, and gastroesophageal reflux. Occasionally, treatment of a sleep disorder can effectively delay placement.

Not only are nursing home residents likely to have a sleep disorder before placement, but also sleep disturbance becomes more common as patients become more impaired in the institution. People in nursing homes regularly use sedatives for sleep (Monane et al., 1996). Nonetheless, they have abnormal sleep-wake patterns and increased amounts of time spent in bed.

Unfortunately, the nursing home environment may be partially responsible for some of these problems. Nighttime arousals of residents are often associated with noise and light disturbances (Schnell et al., 1999). The major source of these disturbances is often the nursing staff. More than one half of nursing home residents may wake up as often as two to three times per hour during the night. Nursing practices related to incontinence are particularly disruptive. On average, nursing home residents only get 40 minutes of sleep for every hour spent in bed.

In some nursing homes, residents remain asleep much of the day. There may be little exposure to natural light in these facilities. As a result, there is a tendency to develop phase shift problems. Improving sleep hygiene in the nursing home setting requires successful implementation of a multifaceted environmental intervention that provides sufficient stimulus and light during the day and the elimination of nocturnal interruption.

Most nursing homes spend considerable time and effort in assessing risk of falls. Many falls occur at night because patients tend to get up in the middle of the night and wander. If an effort is made to survey the nursing home environment for unwanted nocturnal stimuli and hindrances to sleep, there may be attendant cost savings in terms of reduced risk of falls. Nursing homes should be able to provide adequate education and supervision for staff to reduce their impact on the sleep of residents. In addition, environmental rounds should be made to ensure a quiet and comfortable sleeping area. Nursing home residents are subject to behavioral conditioning. Staff should not put residents to bed early in the night when they are not sleepy. In addition, there should be some consideration for a nighttime ritual for those who are able to benefit from such an intervention.

Even in the best of environments, sleep disruption for nursing home residents will remain endemic because the cause is usually multifactorial. Solutions require effort and thought. Solutions must take into account the health problems of the elderly resident to ensure that sleep problems are not secondary to treatable conditions such as urinary tract infection, untreated congestive heart failure, or even pain (Gentili et al., 1997). Affective disorder should always be treated.

Up to 40% of institutionalized elderly are on some sort of hypnotic. Psychopharmacological assistance for sleep may help some residents, but care should be taken to ensure that the therapy is justified in terms of the patient's condition rather than the staff's complaint (Monane et al., 1996). Ongoing pharmacy audits can substantially reduce overprescribing (Griffith & Robinson, 1996). If a specific sleep therapy will likely impair daytime performance, an alternative should be considered. In demented patients, therapy for sleep should take into account the type of the dementia. Therefore, anticholinergics should be avoided in patients with Alzheimer's disease, neuroleptics in patients with Lewy body dementia, and benzodiazepines in patients with multiinfarct dementia and problems with coordination. Sedatives dampen circadian rhythms and may add to problems with sleep-wake cycles.

Patients, physicians, and nurses view sleep problems in different ways. A format that focuses on sleep disturbances during treatment planning meetings can help bridge these gaps. The staff can then think through the multiple factors that contribute to sleep disturbance. These factors include the environment, current medicines, the patient's medical treatments, incontinence care, psychosocial stresses, and behavioral reinforcements. The treatment team can also consider prior sleep history and the presence of primary sleep disorders.

Mood disorders can be reevaluated and treated. Simple interventions for psychophysiological insomnia may include relaxation groups or even backrubs. Some of the sleep problems of patients with Alzheimer's disease may not respond consistently to behavioral and pharmacological therapy. These patients may function better on specialized units. Placement of problem patients on specialized units prevents disruption of the general nursing home population.

PHARMACOLOGY OF SLEEP DISORDERS

Transient, situational insomnia may respond to sedatives. Treatment of elderly people with sedatives is fraught with danger. In fact, the use of medication to promote sleep is associated with higher mortality. Older patients with chronic sleep complaints should not be started on a sedative hypnotic agent without a careful clinical assessment to identify the cause of the sleep disturbance. Sedative hypnotics cause falls both at night and during the day. Daytime symptoms of sedative hypnotic use in elderly patients include cognitive problems, performance problems, and irritability. Tolerance often develops to longer acting sedative hypnotics. In the patient with chronic insomnia, it is imperative for the clinician to exclude primary sleep disorders and review medications and other medical conditions that may be contributory.

If the initial history and physical examination do not suggest a serious underlying cause for the sleep problem, a trial of improved sleep hygiene is the best initial approach. Commonly recommended measures are listed in Table 26-1.

Sedative/hypnotic drugs for the treatment of chronic insomnia are generally considered ineffective by most experts, but helpful by many patients. Elderly people in these situations may use over-the-counter sleeping pills. Some commonly used over-the-counter preparations, such as *Valeriana officinalis*, have not been shown effective for insomnia. Other preparations contain anticholinergic drugs and are more dangerous than some prescribed medications.

Late-life insomnia shows a level of chronicity incompatible with hypnotic drug therapy as currently recommended. Because elderly people may be on sleeping pills for an extended period, choice of appropriate therapy is crucial (Morgan & Clarke, 1997a). Older women are more likely to have chronic insomnia and therefore more likely to become dependent on sedatives. Poor health is associated with insomnia, and habitual use of hypnotics and the use of sedatives are associated with higher mortality (Seppala et al., 1997).

In spite of this, these drugs are often used carelessly. Physicians tend to give out large quantities of sedative hypnotics in a single prescription. In addition, there is usually little attempt to monitor the use of these compounds. At times, prescriptions are continued even if the patient complains they are not working. The nature of the sleep disorder that prompted the prescription is often not well documented. Cognitive side effects of the medicine are rarely examined.

Chloral hydrate is relatively safe for older people and is available as a capsule, syrup, or suppository. Although it is the sedative preferred by many psychiatrists, it is difficult to determine its particular advantage over other agents also helpful in promoting sleep in older people. Although choral hydrate can induce hepatic microsomal enzymes, it usually does not prolong the prothrombin time in patients who are on coumadin. However, it may increase the level of some anticonvulsants. Demented patients may show daytime confusion with chloral hydrate, but this is true of almost any sedative. Daytime effects in most elderly people are minimal, but there can be rebound insomnia if the drug is withdrawn after prolonged use. It should be used with caution in depressed people because an overdose can be fatal. The overdose potential of choral hydrate is often overlooked.

Benzodiazepines remain the most commonly suggested agents for sleep. Apparent clinical differences among benzodiazepine hypnotics in their effect on sleep latency are based on pharmacokinetic properties of absorption and distribution. The residual unwanted daytime effects depend on the drug's elimination and clearance. These should be used as briefly as possible, not to exceed 2 to 3 weeks of therapy or, if used longer, for only 2 or 3 nights per week. Care must be taken with these agents to avoid dependence because continued use results in increasing tolerance and increasing doses. Long-acting agents (e.g., flurazepam) should not be used in older patients because of associated daytime sedation, lethargy, ataxia, falls, and cognitive and psychomotor impairment. The short-acting agent triazolam may be useful for patients who have difficulty falling asleep, but is not effective in maintaining sleep. Triazolam causes nocturnal amnesia and confusion, and it is not used very often.

People who take the intermediate-acting agents (e.g., temazepam, estazolam, and lorazepam) have less daytime drowsiness than those who take flurazepam. Benzodiazepines suppress both REM sleep and delta sleep. These agents should be given 30 minutes before bedtime so that the effect occurs when the patient attempts to sleep. Because the differences between these drugs are not very great, the physician is best served by becoming familiar with one intermediate-acting agent. Lorazepam is particularly useful because it is commonly used for generalized anxiety and also for agitation in elderly people. Lorazepam improves sleep in patients with insomnia associated with moderately severe anxiety or depression. If lorazepam is used for nighttime sedation, it obviates the need for multiple benzodiazepine preparations. It is particularly useful in hospitalized patients because an intramuscular form is available. One of the major advantages of lorazepam on an outpatient basis is that it is available in a generic, less-expensive preparation.

Benzodiazepine treatment of insomnia is associated with a significant increase in sleep duration, but this is countered by a number of adverse effects that may be significant in older people (Holbrook et al., 2000). These include objective memory deficits, performance impairment, and problems with balance. Benzodiazepines are the most commonly implicated medications in institutional falls with injury. A withdrawal syndrome occurs after discontinuation of long-term therapeutic use of benzodiazepines (Hajak et al., 1998). However, many older individuals on chronic benzodiazepine therapy can be withdrawn without deleterious effects on their sleep (Petrovic et al., 1999). Some elderly benzodiazepine users would like to discontinue benzodiazpines. Patients need information and advice on how to discontinue these drugs (Barter & Cormack, 1996).

Zolpidem is a short-acting hypnotic of a new chemical class (imidazopyridines) that has demonstrated efficacy in elderly insomniacs. Elderly people who take zolpidem report improved sleep latency, total sleep time, and sleep quality. Adverse effects on memory or performance appear to be minimal, and there is no evidence of daytime sleepiness. Most studies demonstrated that rebound insomnia on drug discontinuation is not a significant factor. On polysomnography evaluation, zolpidem shows a shift of slow-wave sleep to an earlier period of the night, with a more physiological sleep structure.

There have been case reports of psychosis following the use of zolpidem. Zolpidem does not have prominent anxiolytic properties. Lorazepam may be preferred in patients with prominent anxiety symptoms. In some older patients, zolpidem may cause agitation, leading to a cycle of pharmacological interventions.

Zaleplon is a pyrazolopyrimidine with properties similar to zolpidem. Zolpidem and zaleplon are particularly well tolerated in patients with medical problems such as COPD or end-stage renal disease. Long-term administration of zolpidem and zaleplon appear to be well tolerated. Zaleplon has a very short half-life. Zaleplon shortens sleep latency, but is not very useful for sleep maintenance and early awakening. Zaleplon does not consistently increase total sleep time. Like benzodiazepines, zaleplon and zolpidem are recommended for short-term (2–3 weeks) use only and, if used longer, for only 2 or 3 nights per week.

Because benzodiazepines have significant morbidity in older people, particularly those with dementia, there has been a tendency to use fewer of these drugs (Lopez et al., 1999). The use of sedating antidepressants has become more popular. Antidepressants with anticholinergic side effects should be avoided because of risk of memory loss. Risk of falls should also be considered. Antidepressants have demonstrated efficacy in older persons with major depression and sleep difficulties, with or without bereavement. Some antidepressants are effective sleeping agents in nondepressed insomniacs.

Trazodone is not anticholinergic, has moderate orthostatic effects, and is not associated with tolerance or morning hangover. Trazodone has been used as a hypnotic in depressed patients receiving other antidepressant medications. Nefazodone has many of the advantages of trazodone. In addition, it has greater anxiolytic properties and produces less orthostasis.

Sedating antihistamines are common ingredients in over-the-counter sleeping products. Most of these drugs have potent anticholinergic effects, and tolerance develops after several weeks. Although these drugs are popular with geriatric patients, their use should be discouraged by responsible clinicians.

TABLE 26-4. Pharmacology of initiating and maintaining sleep in elderly persons

Drug	Class	Dosing	Half-life	Drug interactions	Advantages	Disadvantages
Chloral hydrate	Mechanism of action through metabolite trichloroethanol	250 mg to start, may be increased to 1,000 mg	8 hours (active metabolite)	May increase anticonvulsant levels; flushing and tachycardia with intravenous furosemide	Effectively administered by capsule, syrup, suppository); usually well tolerated without morning hangover or next-day effects	Hypnotic effect lost after 2 weeks of continuous use; contraindicated in marked hepatic cardiac or renal impairment; rebound insomnia; potentially fatal in overdose
Depakote	Anticonvulsant; mood stabilizer	500–1,500 at bedtime	6–10 hours	Alters serum concentrations of protein-bound drugs; enzyme induction increases blood levels of other anticonvulsants	Most useful in elderly patients with manic symptoms or agitation with manic quality; available as Depakote Sprinkles, which can be given with food	Nausea and vomiting occur at start of treatment; thrombocytopenia; may increase serum ammonia; sleep-promoting properties best reserved for patients with mania or agitation
Lorazepam	Intermediate-acting benzodiazepine	0.25 mg to start; may be increased to 2 mg	12 hours	Potentiates sedative effect of other drugs	Effective in initiating and maintaining sleep; intramuscular form available; metabolism predictable in older people	Associated with falls, memory loss, irritability, and performance problems; some rebound insomnia

Melatonin	Pineal hormone	2–10 mg		Rapid	Wake time after sleep onset significantly shorter; tendency for shorter sleep latency	
Nefazodone	Sedating antidepressant	50–200 mg	2–4 hours	Potentiates triazolam; serotonin syndrome with MAOIs	Antianxiety effect; less gastrointestinal upset and hypotension than with trazodone	Mild orthostasis or over sedation
Risperidone	Atypical neuroleptic	0.25–3 mg	3–20 hours; longer in elderly	Hypotension with some antihypertensives	Useful when psychosis is the cause of insomnia in institutional settings	May cause over sedation; sometimes causes akathisia
Trazodone	Sedating antidepressant (heterocyclic)	25–150 mg	Biphasic half-life; first peak at 3 hours; second peak at 5–9 hours	Increased levels of phenytoin and digoxin; serotonin syndrome with MAOIs	Effective for insomnia with or without depression; sometimes used with an SSRI for depression with insomnia	Orthostasis; dosing after food minimizes sedation and hypotension; sedation may be profound immediately after dosing and lead to falls if the patient is not in bed; risk of priapism
Zaleplon	Pyrazolopyrimidine	5–20 mg	1 hour	Potentiates sedative effect of other drugs	Rapid onset of action; no hangover; tolerance/rebound insomnia uncommon	More effective in initiating sleep than increasing sleep duration
Zolpidem	Imidazopyridine	5 mg to 10 mg	2.5 hours in healthy elderly	Potentiates sedative effect of other drugs	Rapid onset; no hangover; tolerance/rebound insomnia uncommon	Psychosis has been reported; confusion rare; mild anxiolytic

MAOI, monoamine oxidase inhibitors; SSRI, selective serotonin reuptake inhibitor.

Anticholinergic agents interfere with new learning, access to semantic memory, vigilance, and continuous performance. Barbiturates are not indicated for insomnia.

Melatonin has been used to treat sleep problems in elderly people (Avery et al., 1998). Although impairment of melatonin production is not always associated with sleep problems, melatonin sometimes improves sleep quality and efficiency in the elderly (Brusco et al., 1999). Melatonin may effectively facilitate discontinuation of benzodiazepine therapy and maintain good sleep quality. Melatonin appears helpful for sleep in some depressed patients, but may not be as effective with sleep disorders associated with dementia.

Sometimes, a sleep problem is a manifestation of an overall problem with agitation. In these instances, medications that have a sedating effect can be given primarily at night. These medications include sodium valproate, certain SSRIs, and some antipsychotics. Risperidone has a particularly sedating effect in elderly agitated people. It has the advantage of promoting delta sleep and may be particularly useful in insomnia associated with dementia and psychosis. Dosing should begin at a very low dose in elderly people. Increases should be slow. Fortunately, there is a liquid form of the drug that allows low doses in small incremental increases. At low doses, risperidone has a favorable clinical profile in older people (Falsetti, 2000).

Depakote has hypnotic action that is independent of its mood-stabilizing properties. This may be increased by the concomitant use of sedatives. Patients who have manic-like symptoms will probably do better with depakote than with a sedative hypnotic alone (see Table 26-4).

CONCLUSION

The sleep history is essential for recognizing clinically important sleep disorders. An appropriate history leads to an effective evaluation and treatment plan. Taking care of sleep problems of the elderly improves their quality of life and appreciably benefits general health.

REFERENCES

Aboussouan LS, Golish JA, Wood BG, Mehta AC, Wood DE, Dinner DS. Dynamic pharyngoscopy in predicting outcome of uvulopalatopharyngoplasty for moderate and severe obstructive sleep apnea. *Chest.* 1995;107:946–951.

Almeida OP, Tamai S, Garrido R. Sleep complaints among the elderly: results from a survey in a psychogeriatric outpatient clinic in Brazil. *Int Psychogeriatr.* 1999;11: 47–56.

Avery D, Lenz M, Landis C. Guidelines for prescribing melatonin. *Ann Med.* 1998;30: 122–130.

Barter G, Cormack M. The long-term use of benzodiazepines: patients' views, accounts and experiences. *Fam Pract.* 1996;13:491–497.

Becker H, Brandenburg U, Peter JH, Von Wichert P. Reversal of sinus arrest and atrioventricular conduction block in patients with sleep apnea during nasal continuous positive airway pressure. *Am J Respir Crit Care Med.* 1995;151:215–218.

Becker HF, Piper AJ, Flynn WE, McNamara SG, Grunstein RR, Peter JH, Sullivan CE. Breathing during sleep in patients with nocturnal desaturation. *Am J Respir Crit Care Med.* 1999;159:112–118.

Benz RL, Pressman MR, Hovick ET, Peterson DD. A preliminary study of the effects of correction of anemia with recombinant human erythropoietin therapy on sleep, sleep disorders, and daytime sleepiness in hemodialysis patients (the SLEEPO study). *Am J Kidney Dis.* 1999;34:1089–1095.

Benz RL, Pressman MR, Hovick ET, Peterson DD. Potential novel predictors of mortality in end-stage renal disease patients with sleep disorders [see comments]. *Am J Kidney Dis.* 2000;35:1052–1060.

Bixler EO, Vgontzas AN, Lin HM, et al. Association of hypertension and sleep-disordered breathing. *Arch Intern Med.* 2000;160:2289–2295.

Brusco LI, Fainstein I, Marquez M, Cardinali DP. Effect of melatonin in selected populations of sleep-disturbed patients. *Biol Signals Recept.* 1999;8:126–131.

Chakravorty S, Rye D. Narcolepsy in the older adult: epidemiology, diagnosis and management. *Drugs Aging.* 2003;20(5):361–376.

Coleman RM, Miles LE, Guilleminault CC, Zarcone VP Jr, van den Hoed J, Dement WC. Sleep-wake disorders in the elderly: polysomnographic analysis. *J Am Geriatr Soc.* 1981;29:289–296.

Dealberto MJ, Pajot N, Courbon D, Alperovitch A. Breathing disorders during sleep and cognitive performance in an older community sample: the EVA Study [see comments]. *J Am Geriatr Soc.* 1996;44:1287–1294.

Dew MA, Reynolds CF III, Buysse DJ, et al. Electroencephalographic sleep profiles during depression: effects of episode duration and other clinical and psychosocial factors in older adults. *Arch Gen Psychiatry.* 1996;53:148–156.

Dijk DJ, Duffy JF. Sleep and sleep disorders in older adults. *J Clin Neurophysiol.* 1995; 12:139–146.

Dijk DJ, Duffy JF. Circadian regulation of human sleep and age-related changes in its timing, consolidation and EEG characteristics. *Ann Med.* 1999;31:130–140.

Donahue JL, Lowenthal DT. Nocturnal polyuria in the elderly person. *Am J Med Sci.* 1997;314:232–238.

Evans LK. Sundown syndrome in institutionalized elderly. *J Am Geriatr Soc.* 1987;35: 101–108.

Falsetti AE. Risperidone for control of agitation in dementia patients. *Am J Health Syst Pharm.* 2000;57:862–870.

Franklin KA, Eriksson P, Sahlin C, Lundgren R. Reversal of central sleep apnea with oxygen. *Chest.* 1997;111:163–169.

Gallagher-Thompson D, Brooks JO III, Bliwise D, Leader J, Yesavage JA. The relations among caregiver stress, "sundowning" symptoms, and cognitive decline in Alzheimer's disease. *J Am Geriatr Soc.* 1992;40:807–810.

Gentili A, Weiner DK, Kuchibhatil M, Edinger JD. Factors that disturb sleep in nursing home residents. *Aging (Milano).* 1997;9:207–213.

Gigli GL, Placidi F, Diomedi M, Maschio M, Silvestri G, Scalise A, Marciani MG. Sleep in healthy elderly subjects: a 24-hour ambulatory polysomnographic study. *Int J Neurosci.* 1996;85:263–271.

Good DC, Henkle JQ, Gelber D, Welsh J, Verhulst S. Sleep-disordered breathing and poor functional outcome after stroke. *Stroke.* 1996;27:252–259.

Griffith DN, Robinson M. Prescribing practice and policy for hypnotics: a model of pharmacy audit. *Age Ageing.* 1996;25:490–492.

Hajak G, Clarenbach P, Fischer W, et al. Rebound insomnia after hypnotic withdrawal in insomniac outpatients. *Eur Arch Psychiatry Clin Neurosci.* 1998;248:148–156.

Hans MG, Nelson S, Luks VG, Lorkovich P, Baek SJ. Comparison of two dental devices for treatment of obstructive sleep apnea syndrome (OSAS). *Am J Orthod Dentofacial Orthop.* 1997;111:562–570.

Hatoum HT, Kania CM, Kong SX, Wong JM, Mendelson WB. Prevalence of insomnia: a survey of the enrollees at five managed care organizations. *Am J Manag Care.* 1998;4:79–86.

Holbrook AM, Crowther R, Lotter A, Cheng C, King D. Meta-analysis of benzodiazepine use in the treatment of insomnia. *CMAJ.* 2000;162:225–233.

Ing AJ, Ngu MC, Breslin AB. Obstructive sleep apnea and gastroesophageal reflux. *Am J Med.* 2000;108(Suppl 4a):120S–125S.

Jankel WR, Niedermeyer E. Sleep spindles. *J Clin Neurophysiol.* 1985;2:1–35.

Kamba M, Suto Y, Ohta Y, Inoue Y, Matsuda E. Cerebral metabolism in sleep apnea: evaluation by magnetic resonance spectroscopy. *Am J Respir Crit Care Med.* 1997; 156:296–298.

Khoury RM, Camacho-Lobato L, Katz PO, Mohiuddin MA, Castell DO. Influence of spontaneous sleep positions on nighttime recumbent reflux in patients with gastroesophageal reflux disease. *Am J Gastroenterol.* 1999;94:2069–2073.

Lopez OL, Wisniewski SR, Becker JT, Boller F, DeKosky ST. Psychiatric medication and abnormal behavior as predictors of progression in probable Alzheimer disease. *Arch Neurol.* 1999;56:1266–1272.

Mann SG, Murakami A, McCarroll K, et al. Low dose famotidine in the prevention of sleep disturbance caused by heartburn after an evening meal. *Aliment Pharmacol Ther.* 1995;9:395–340.

McGaffigan S, Bliwise DL. The treatment of sundowning: a selective review of pharmacological and nonpharmacological studies. *Drugs Aging.* 1997;10:10–17.

Miles LE, Dement WC. Sleep and aging. *Sleep.* 1980;3:119–220.

Monane M, Glynn RJ, Avorn J. The impact of sedative-hypnotic use on sleep symptoms in elderly nursing home residents. *Clin Pharmacol Ther.* 1996;59:83–92.

Morgan K, Clarke D. Longitudinal trends in late-life insomnia: implications for prescribing. *Age Ageing.* 1997a;26:179–184.

Morgan K, Clarke D. Risk factors for late-life insomnia in a representative general practice sample. *Br J Gen Pract.* 1997b;47:166–169.

Morin CM, Mimeault V, Gagne A. Nonpharmacological treatment of late-life insomnia. *J Psychosom Res.* 1999;46(2):103–116.

Ohayon MM, Caulet M, Philip P, Guilleminault C, Priest RG. How sleep and mental disorders are related to complaints of daytime sleepiness. *Arch Intern Med.* 1997; 157:2645–2652.

Olson EJ, Boeve BF, Silber MH. Rapid eye movement sleep behaviour disorder: demographic, clinical and laboratory findings in 93 cases. *Brain.* 2000;123(Pt 2):331–339.

Parra O, Arboix A, Bechich S, et al. Time course of sleep-related breathing disorders in first-ever stroke or transient ischemic attack. *Am J Respir Crit Care Med.* 2000; 161(2 Pt 1):375–380.

Partinen M. Epidemiology of obstructive sleep apnea syndrome. *Curr Opin Pulm Med.* 1995;1:482–487.

Pat-Horenczyk R, Klauber MR, Shochat T, Ancoli-Israel S. Hourly profiles of sleep and wakefulness in severely versus mild-moderately demented nursing home patients. *Aging (Milano).* 1998;10:308–315.

Peker Y, Hedner J, Kraiczi H, Loth S. Respiratory disturbance index: an independent predictor of mortality in coronary artery disease. *Am J Respir Crit Care Med.* 2000; 162:81–86.

Petrovic M, Pevernagie D, Van Den Noortgate N, Mariman A, Michielsen W, Afschrift M. A programme for short-term withdrawal from benzodiazepines in geriatric hospital inpatients: success rate and effect on subjective sleep quality. *Int J Geriatr Psychiatry.* 1999;14:754–760.

Phillips BA, Berry DT, Lipke-Molby TC. Sleep-disordered breathing in healthy, aged persons: fifth and final year follow-up. *Chest.* 1996;110:654–658.

Pollak CP, Stokes PE, Wagner DR. Nocturnal interactions between community elders and caregivers, as measured by cross-correlation of their motor activity. *J Geriatr Psychiatry Neurol.* 1997;10:168–173.

Polo-Kantola P, Erkkola R, Irjala K, Pullinen S, Virtanen I, Polo O. Effect of short-term transdermal estrogen replacement therapy on sleep: a randomized, double-blind crossover trial in postmenopausal women. *Fertil Steril.* 1999;71:873–880.

Prigerson HG, Frank E, Kasl SV, et al. Complicated grief and bereavement-related depression as distinct disorders: preliminary empirical validation in elderly bereaved spouses. *Am J Psychiatry.* 1995;152:22–30.

Prinz P, Peskind ER, Vitaliano PP. Changes in the sleep and waking EEGs of non demented and demented elderly subjects. *J Am Geriatr Soc.* 1982;30:86–93.

Qureshi AI, Giles WH, Croft JB, Bliwise DL. Habitual sleep patterns and risk for stroke and coronary heart disease: a 10-year follow-up from NHANES I. *Neurology.* 1997;48:904–911.

Redline S, Adams N, Strauss ME, Roebuck T, Winters M, Rosenberg C. Improvement of mild sleep-disordered breathing with CPAP compared with conservative therapy. *Am J Respir Crit Care Med.* 1998;157:858–865.

Regestein QR, Monk TH. Delayed sleep phase syndrome: a review of its clinical aspects [see comments]. *Am J Psychiatry.* 1995;152:602–608.

Reynolds CF, Kupfer DJ, Tasksa LS. EEG sleep in healthy elderly, depressed, and demented subjects. *Biol Psychiatry.* 1988;20:431–442.

Reynolds CF III, Kupfer DJ, Taska LS, Hoch CC, Sewitch DE, Spiker DG. Sleep of healthy seniors: a revisit. *Sleep.* 1985;8:20–29.

Rossi A, Ganassini A, Tantucci C, Grassi V. Aging and the respiratory system. *Aging (Milano).* 1996;8:143–161.

Schnelle JF, Alessi CA, Al-Samarrai NR, Fricker RD Jr, Ouslander JG. The nursing home at night: effects of an intervention on noise, light, and sleep. *J Am Geriatr Soc.* 1999;47:430–438.

Seppala M, Hyyppa MT, Impivaara O, Knuts LR, Sourander L. Subjective quality of sleep and use of hypnotics in an elderly urban population. *Aging (Milano).* 1997; 9:327–334.

Spiegel R, Herzog A, Koberle S. Polygraphic sleep criteria as predictors of successful aging: an exploratory longitudinal study. *Biol Psychiatry.* 1999;45:435–442.

27

Sexuality and Aging

Marc E. Agronin, MD

Sexuality in late life is often viewed with humor by younger individuals. This stems, no doubt, from underlying feelings of discomfort and sometimes even denial of its presence in older individuals, especially in long-term care settings. Why is this? One reason may be that the idea of sexuality clashes with stereotypes of mom and dad or grandma and grandpa. The denial of sexuality in parents and grandparents is then generalized to all older individuals. Our culture reflects this denial and discomfort in popular media, in which sexuality is typically portrayed in television, magazines, and movies by young and attractive individuals. These defensive and distorted ways of thinking about sexuality in late life—denial, generalization, and humor—represent a form of ageism or the belief that elderly individuals are not as capable of being sexual by virtue of their age. Sexual dysfunction is thus seen as a normal and untreatable part of aging.

The extent of these attitudes can be alarming. In a letter to a popular advice columnist several years ago, an older woman calling herself "worn out in California" wrote to complain that her husband "is in his 80s and refuses to give up on sex." She went on to complain that despite some mild erectile dysfunction, he continued to request sex with her weekly. The columnist's response was short and harsh: "Tell that inconsiderate, horny old coot *no* unless *you* feel like it" (Landers, 1996). The fact that such an insensitive and misinformed comment about late-life sexuality could appear in the media, written by a wise and beloved columnist, illustrates just how far ageist stereotypes have penetrated our culture.

Despite these stereotypes, several factors have begun changing societal views of sexuality in late life. Both the sexual and the feminist revolutions of the 1960s and 1970s changed attitudes toward sexuality in general, laying the groundwork for perspectives on late-life sexuality that were more open minded. Since then, one of the most influential factors in further broadening perspectives toward late-life sexuality has been the growth of hormone replacement therapy (HRT) for postmenopausal women. As a result of HRT, many women are able to maintain more vital and enjoyable sexual function well beyond menopause. This may change, however, depending on the impact of new data reassessing the benefits of HRT and highlighting the potentially increased risk of breast and ovarian cancer (Lacey et al., 2002; Writing Group for the Women's Health Initiative Investigators, 2002).

For men, the advent of numerous treatments for erectile dysfunction (ED), a relatively common sexual dysfunction in late life, has also ensured the persistence of sexual function in later years. In particular, the discovery of oral erectogenic agents such as Viagra (sildenafil) has revolutionized the treatment of ED. The very name of this medication conjures up images of vigor and vitality with the power of Niagara Falls and serves as a distinct contrast to the connotations of powerlessness and shame surrounding the term impotence. The availability of Viagra and the high-profile ad campaign featuring former Senator Robert Dole has made the topics of both ED and sexuality in late life more common and comfortable items of everyday conversation. In turn, the destigmatization of ED has no doubt brought many older couples into treatment who otherwise might have suffered in silence and shame.

Attitudes toward sexuality in late life will continue to change. A century ago, the expected life span of an adult in the United States was 40 years; now, men and women routinely live into their 80s. Futurists predict that, while the absolute life span will not go much past 100 years, the span of active and healthy living is expected to increase (Dychtwald & Flower, 1989). Thus, what it means to be an 80-year-old in the year 2000 will likely be vastly different in the 2020s. At the same time, the percentage of individuals older than 65 years will nearly double—from 12% to 20%—by 2010. This increase is represented largely by baby boomers, those individuals who brought about both the sexual and feminist revolutions. These demographic changes will have a tremendous impact on both sexual behaviors and sexual attitudes in late life, however late life will be defined in the future.

SEXUAL BEHAVIORS IN LATE LIFE

A perspective on sexuality in late life must reflect more than demographic necessity and be based on empirical research. In fact, there have been numerous studies of sexual behaviors in late life that quite convincingly counter the many ageist stereotypes that late-life sexuality either does not exist or is inevitably burdened with sexual dissatisfaction or dysfunction. Several general themes have emerged from such research and are covered in this chapter:

- Sexual activity continues into late life, although the frequency of sexual activity declines.
- Normal aging slows sexual response, but not the capacity to enjoy sex.
- Sexual dysfunction is not a normal part of aging, but is a common result of pathological aging.
- Sexual dysfunction, no matter what the cause, can be treated across the life span.

The state of sexuality in late life was perhaps best summarized by Kligman (1991), who wrote, "With reasonable personal health and an available partner, most elderly persons continue sexual relations into their eighth and ninth decade" (p. 18). His words are reflected in the findings of several major studies over the last 20 years, which have all shown quite convincingly that a majority of individuals older than 60 years are sexually active, albeit with modest declines determined in part by gender and the availability of partners. Such studies have indicated that older men are more sexually active than older women, and individuals with steady partners are more active than single individuals. In general, the major predictors of sexual interest and activity in late life include the previous level of sexual activity; the availability, health, and sexual interest of a partner; and an individual's overall physical health (Comfort & Dial, 1991; Kligman, 1991).

One of the most recent studies of late-life sexuality was conducted by the AARP (formerly the American Association of Retired Persons) and its *Modern Maturity* (*MM*) magazine (Jacoby, 1999); the study consisted of a mail survey by which researchers gathered responses from 1,384 men and women aged 45 years and older. The survey found that three quarters of both men and women older than the age of 45 years remained sexually active. Comparing cohorts, the AARP/*MM* findings indicated that 84% of men and 78% of women aged 45 to 59 years had steady sexual partners, compared to 58% of men and 21% of women older than 75 years. In terms of frequency, 50% of individuals aged 45 to 59 years reported having sex at least once a week, compared to 30% of men and 24% of women aged 60 to 74 years who reported the same weekly frequency. Of the respondents, the majority of men without partners said they masturbated, while over 77% of women did not.

The AARP/*MM* study also examined attitudes toward specific aspects of sexuality. Underscoring the importance of sexuality in later life, 60% of men and 35% of women said that sexual activity was important to their overall quality of life. Two thirds of all respondents were extremely or somewhat satisfied with sex. Attitudes toward partners were generally favorable, with a majority of both sexes describing their partners with terms that included "best friend," "kind and gentle," and "physically attractive." There were several generational differences in attitudes toward sex. Individuals older than 60 years were less likely than younger respondents to approve of oral sex, masturbation, and sex between unmarried partners.

Results from the AARP/MM study were consistent with several earlier studies. The *Starr-Weiner Report on Sex and Sexuality in the Mature Years* (Starr and Weiner, 1981) found that 80% of men and women aged 60 to 91 years were sexually active, defined as having sex at least once a month. Marsiglio and Donnelly (1991) studied over 800 married men and women aged 60 years and older and found that over 50% had sex at least monthly, with a mean frequency of 4.26 times per month between the ages of 60 and 75 years. This frequency decreased to a mean of 2.75 times per month for those 76 years and older. These figures can be compared to rates of sexual frequency among younger individuals (N = 3,432, aged 19–59 years) from an influential University of Chicago Study (Michael et al., 1994) in which men had sex an average of 6.5 times per month and women 6.2 times per month.

In a mail survey of 1,292 individuals aged 60 to 90 years, the National Council on the Aging (1998) found that 80% of respondents with sexual partners had sex at least once a month. By gender, 61% of men remained sexually active compared to 37% of women. Of the women, 85% sought partners who were financially secure, while 79% of men sought partners who were interested in sex. In addition, men were twice as likely as women to want more sex than they were already having. Satisfaction with sex remained quite high in late life, with 61% of respondents with partners indicating that sex was as physically satisfying as in their 40s. A sizable number of respondents attributed lower satisfaction to the fact that they or a partner had less physical desire, a medical condition that interfered with sex, or medications that reduced desire.

THE SEXUAL RESPONSE CYCLE AND AGING

To understand the impact of the aging process on sexual function, it is important first to review a general model of sexual function. In the 1960s, sex researchers Masters and Johnson (1966) pioneered the modern field of sexology by studying in detail several hundred heterosexual couples during sexual activity. They developed a four-stage model known as the *sexual response cycle* to illustrate the physiological changes that take place in the body during sexual activity. These four stages include (1) excitement or arousal, (2) plateau, (3) orgasm, and (4) resolution. Kaplan (1974) and Snarch (1991) have added to this model a fifth stage, labeled desire, to account for a fundamental psychological and physiological component of sexuality that underlies sexual response. In general, sexual response is not a linear process, but rather a waxing-and-waning pattern of sexual arousal that may culminate in orgasm, depending on a host of factors. All of these factors can be influenced by age-related changes in sexual function.

The first stage of desire corresponds in its most basic definition to physical and psychological urges (including thoughts and fantasies) to seek out and respond to sexual interaction. This drive is centered in the limbic system of the brain, particularly in the hypothalamus, and is stimulated in both sexes by testosterone. Desire is intimately linked to the physiological process of sexual excitement or arousal as it is difficult for one to exist without the other.

For both sexes, sexual arousal can be triggered by thoughts and fantasies or direct physical stimulation. Autonomic nervous stimulation leads to predictable physiological responses in both sexes, including increased muscle tone, increases in heart and respiratory rates, and increased blood flow (termed *vasocongestion*) to the genitals. In men, this results in penile erection, while in women it results in vaginal lubrication and swelling of breast and genital tissues, especially the clitoris. The relatively brief plateau stage is characterized by a sense of impending orgasm, followed by orgasm and then a refractory period of relaxation called *resolution*. In both sexes, orgasm is characterized by sensations of euphoria associated with rhythmic contractions of genital muscles. In men, orgasm is brief and accompanied by ejaculation, while in women orgasm tends to last longer and may involve multiple successive occurrences.

Normal aging brings several changes to the sexual response cycle in both sexes, summarized in Table 27-1. In women, the most significant changes occur during menopause, a period of 2 to 10 years that usually ends in the early 50s. The decline and eventual cessation of ovarian estrogen production during menopause leads to important changes in sexual function, including atrophy of urogenital tissue (which increases risks for urinary tract infections) and decreased vaginal size. During sexual response, there are decreases in vaginal lubrication, vasocongestion, and erotic sensitivity of nipple, clitoral, and vulvar tissue. As a result, sexual desire may decline, and sexual arousal may require more time. Sexual intercourse may be more uncomfortable due to vaginal and clitoral tissue being less lubricated and more sensitive, and orgasms may be felt as less intense. Up to 85% of women during menopause also experience symptoms such as hot flashes, head and neck aches, mood changes, and excess fatigue.

The use of hormone replacement therapy will, to a large degree in most women, reverse these age-associated changes in sexual function. Estrogen can be taken orally or in the form of a slow-release skin patch. It is often prescribed together with progesterone to replicate previous hormone levels. Estrogen cream can also be applied directly to genital tissues to relieve irritation and enhance lubrication. Declines in testosterone production during menopause also affect sexuality, leading to loss of libido (Sherwin et al., 1985), thinning of pubic hair, and decreased production of bodily oils that moisturize skin and hair. In addition, testosterone receptors in erogenous zones such as the nipples, vulva, and clitoris are less sensitized to sexual stimulation (Rako, 1996).

Some researchers have questioned whether there is a male menopause or *andropause*. Research indicates, however, that there is no significant decrease

TABLE 27-1. Normal age-related changes in sexual function

Men
  Modest decline in testosterone production with unpredictable effect on sexual func-
    tion
  Minimal change in sperm count, but less functional sperm and decreased rate of
    conception
  No predictable changes in sexual desire (libido)
  Sexual arousal requires more tactile stimulation; psychological arousal may be inad-
    equate
  Erections take longer to achieve and are more difficult to sustain
  Decreased penile rigidity due to decreases in blood flow and smooth muscle relax-
    ation
  Ejaculation requires more stimulation and involves a diminished sensation of ur-
    gency during the plateau stage
  Ejaculation is less forceful with decreased ejaculate volume
  Refractory period (when the penis is unable to respond to stimulation) increases by
    hours to days
Women
  Predictable decline and eventual cessation of estrogen production during meno-
    pause
  Sexual desire (libido) may decline due to a decrease in testosterone levels
  Reduced blood supply to pelvic region
  Vaginal size shortens and narrows; vaginal mucosa is thinner and less lubricated
  Vaginal lubrication and swelling during arousal is slower and decreased
  Sexual arousal may take longer and require increased stimulation
  Strength and amount of vaginal contractions during orgasm decrease

Sources: Goodwin and Agronin (1997); Metz and Miner (1985); Spector et al. (1996).

in testosterone levels with age (Metz & Miner, 1995), and slow declines in testicular function result in only a mild decrease in fertility. Any decreases in testosterone that do occur may not have any predictable negative effects on sexual desire or function. As a result, the normal sexual changes in aging men are gradual and tend to be more modest compared to those of women (Metz & Miner, 1995). As men age, desire may involve less anticipatory physical arousal, and sexual arousal and orgasm may take longer to achieve. Erections require more physical stimulation and in general tend to be less frequent, less durable, and less reliable, with decreased volume of ejaculate during orgasm. However, there are no clear decreases in physical pleasure. In older men, the resolution or refractory stage is much longer, lasting hours to days instead of minutes to hours as in younger men.

In both sexes, the impact of physiological changes in sexual function will be mediated by a number of psychosocial factors. The more knowledge that an individual has about what constitutes normal age-associated changes in their sexual function, the easier it may be to accept these changes. For example, a man who does not understand the normal changes in erectile function may misinterpret them and believe that he is suffering from a sexual problem. Similarly, a woman may misinterpret the experience of vaginal dryness to mean that she does not want to have sex. Such overreactions to normal changes can lead an individual to engage in less frequent or more limited sexual activity. Research has shown that a lack of information about changes in sexual function in later life can lead to excess fear and pain (Boyer & Boyer, 1982).

Many older individuals also buy into ageist stereotypes about sexuality, seeing their behaviors as inappropriate or potentially harmful, despite having relatively normal sexual desire and capacity. Other individuals may lose self-confidence and feel less sexy, especially as they struggle to cope with age-associated changes in physical appearance, strength, and endurance. Such attitudinal barriers may be more damaging to sexuality than actual physiological changes (Starr & Weiner, 1981).

The quality of an individual's relationship with a partner will also be influential. As discussed below, couples often have to adapt sexual technique and refocus more time on foreplay to preserve previous levels of sexual function and enjoyment. A couple that is not able to work together may thus experience difficulty with sex and perhaps even sexual dysfunction. On the other hand, aging can also open many new possibilities for sexuality in later life. Couples may have more time to spend with each other once children have left home or after retirement. For postmenopausal women, sex without the possibility of pregnancy can reduce a degree of anxiety previously associated with sex.

SEXUAL DYSFUNCTION IN LATE LIFE

Despite the fact that a majority of older individuals continue to engage in sexual activity, the prevalence of sexual dysfunction does increase with age (Spector et al., 1996). The classification of sexual disorders according to the *Diagnostic and Statistical Manual of Mental Disorders, Fourth Edition Text Revision* (*DSM-IVTR*; American Psychiatric Association, 2000) is listed in Table 27-2. Erectile dysfunction is the most common form of sexual dysfunction in older men, affecting over 50% of men aged 40 to 70 years and nearly 70% of men aged 70 years (Althof & Seftel, 1995; Feldman et al., 1994). In older women, the most common forms of sexual dysfunction include hypoactive sexual desire, inhibited orgasm, and dyspareunia (Bachmann & Leiblum, 1991; Renshaw, 1996). Unfortunately, physicians often fail to inquire about sexual function in older patients, perhaps due to their own stereotypes or discomfort. As a result, many older individuals suffer with treatable forms of sexual dysfunction and are either too ashamed to inquire or ignorant or pessimistic about the prospects for treatment. Luckily, attitudes are changing. It is critical for clinicians to understand how vital a role they can play in providing support, education, and treatment to such individuals.

Although medical and psychiatric problems and medication effects usually

TABLE 27-2.   *DSM-IVTR* classification of sexual dysfunction

Sexual desire disorders
   Hypoactive sexual desire disorder: persistent or recurrent deficiency of sexual fanta-
     sies and desire for sex
   Sexual aversion disorder: extreme aversion to and avoidance of genital sexual con-
     tact
Sexual arousal disorders
   Female sexual arousal disorder: persistent or recurrent difficulty to attain or main-
     tain vaginal swelling and lubrication during sexual activity
   Male erectile disorder (impotence): persistent or recurrent inability to attain or main-
     tain an erection adequate for sexual activity
Orgasmic disorders
   Female/male orgasmic disorder: persistent or recurrent delay in or absence of or-
     gasm in response to sexual stimulation
   Premature ejaculation: persistent or recurrent, uncontrollable, rapid ejaculation
     that occurs just prior to or shortly after penetration.
Sexual pain disorders
   Dyspareunia: recurrent or persistent genital pain associated with sexual intercourse
   Vaginismus: recurrent or persistent involuntary spasm of vaginal muscles that limits
     or prohibits vaginal penetration

Source: American Psychiatric Association (2000).

serve as the main causes of sexual dysfunction in late life, numerous psychological factors must be considered. They include performance anxiety, the presence of another sexual disorder in one or both partners, fears of self-injury or
death due to medical conditions (e.g., history of myocardial infarction, shortness of breath), sensitivity to loss of personal appearance or control of hygiene
(e.g., due to incontinence or the presence of a colostomy), relationship problems, and life stress. The first occurrence of psychogenic sexual dysfunction
often follows a major stress such as the loss of a loved one, a divorce, a financial or occupational strain, or a major health scare. Such major stresses may
break sexual patterns and lead to uncertainty of how to resume sexual activity.
As noted, the availability of partners is an acute issue for women, who outnum-
ber men by over 2 to 1 by the age of 85.

   Medical and psychiatric disorders that serve as the most common causes
of sexual dysfunction in geriatric patients are listed in Table 27-3. In both
sexes, major risk factors for sexual dysfunction include diabetes mellitus,
peripheral vascular disease, cancer, chronic obstructive pulmonary disease, depression, stroke, dementia, Parkinson's disease, and substance abuse. These
and other medical disorders exert both primary and secondary effects on sexual
function. For example, primary effects would include impaired sexual arousal
due to diabetic neuropathy or impaired genital vasocongestion due to peripheral vascular disease. Secondary effects such as fatigue, pain, and physical

TABLE 27-3. **Common medical and psychiatric conditions associated with sexual dysfunction in late life**

Anxiety disorders (generalized anxiety disorder, obsessive-compulsive disorder, panic disorder)
Arthritis and other degenerative joint diseases
Atherosclerosis (peripheral vascular disease, cerebrovascular accident [CVA])
Cardiac disease (coronary artery disease, congestive heart failure, myocardial infarct)
Cancer (especially urologic and genital cancers and their treatments)
Chronic organ failure (renal, hepatic)
Chronic obstructive pulmonary disease (COPD)
Dementia (Alzheimer's disease, vascular dementia, etc.)
Diabetes mellitus
Major depressive disorder and other mood disorders
Multiple sclerosis
Parkinson's disease
Prostate disease/prostate surgery
Schizophrenia and other chronic psychotic disorders
Substance abuse

disability due to medical illness can make individuals feel less sexy and less confident in their sexual ability, which in turn can lead to hypoactive desire.

Medications also serve as fundamental causes of sexual dysfunction and can affect both sexes at any point in the sexual response cycle (Crenshaw & Goldberg, 1996; Goodwin & Agronin, 1997). The most common problematic medications include antihypertensives such as β-blockers and diuretics, anti-androgens, and many psychotropic medications (Gitlin, 1994). Some of the most common medications associated with sexual dysfunction in late life are listed in Table 27-4.

Sexual dysfunction in late life is often comorbid with other psychiatric disorders. Symptoms may range from transient dysfunction present only during episodes of illness to full-blown sexual disorders independent of the primary psychiatric disorder. Major depression often involves loss of libido as a cardinal symptom, but may also be associated with inhibited arousal and erectile dysfunction. Symptomatic anxiety and anxiety and panic disorder are frequently associated with sexual dysfunction, in particular with sexual phobias and aversion (Kaplan, 1987). Unfortunately, many of the antidepressants used to treat both mood and anxiety disorders can cause or exacerbate sexual dysfunction (see Table 27-4). Anywhere from 10% to 40% of men on selective serotonin reuptake inhibitors (SSRIs) and tricyclic antidepressants (TCAs) may experience some degree of decrease in desire, erectile dysfunction, or delayed or inhibited orgasm (Segraves, 1998). The same holds for benzodiazepines, which have been associated with decreased sexual desire and erectile dysfunction, in particular when combined with lithium.

Schizophrenia and other psychotic disorders often involve sexual prob-

TABLE 27-4.   Medications associated with sexual dysfunction in late life

Adrenal corticosteroids
α-Adrenergic blockers (e.g., prazosin, phentolamine)
Antiandrogens (leuprolide, ketoconazole)
Antidepressants (monoamine oxidase inhibitors [MAOIs], tricyclic antidepressants
    [TCAs], selective serotonin reuptake inhibitors [SSRIs], venlafaxine)
Antihistamines
Antihypertensives (thiazide diuretics, β-blockers, angiotensin-converting enzyme [ACE]
    inhibitors, clonidine, spironolactone, calcium channel blockers, reserpine)
Antipsychotics (conventional and atypical agents)
Benzodiazepines
Cancer chemotherapeutic agents
Cardiac medications (digoxin, amiodarone)
Disopyramide
H_2 blockers
L-Dopa
Mood stabilizers (e.g., lithium, valproic acid, carbamazepine)

Sources: Goodwin and Agronin (1997); Kligman (1991).

lems. Individuals with negative symptoms, including social withdrawal or discomfort in the presence of others, apathy, and blunted emotional affect, may have relatively little interest in sexual relationships. Those with positive symptoms such as delusions, hallucinations, and bizarre thought patterns may have difficulty relating to others and interacting in sexually comfortable or appropriate ways. During periods of symptom remission, however, sexual relationships can be more appropriate. All of the antipsychotic medications can cause sexual dysfunction, usually in proportion to the dose being used (Crenshaw & Goldberg, 1996; Gitlin, 1994). As with antidepressant and anxiolytic medications, antipsychotics can decrease libido, interfere with sexual arousal, and inhibit or block erections, ejaculation, and orgasm.

Erectile Dysfunction

As a model of sexual dysfunction in late life, consider the most common ailment—erectile dysfunction. Erectile dysfunction, a disorder of sexual arousal, is characterized by the inability to achieve or sustain an erection that is adequate for sexual function. Historically, ED was seen as a psychological problem; currently, it is believed that up to 80% of erectile dysfunction is primarily caused by a physical problem with erectile physiology (Althof & Seftel, 1995; Feldman et al., 1994). There are, however, important psychological components involved in both cause and effects of ED. For many men, erections are equated with masculinity, potency, and vitality. As a result, ED in late life is often experienced by men as an alarming harbinger of physical and sexual decline. Performance anxiety, stress, depression, and relationship problems can trigger or exacerbate ED. In turn, ED is associated with feelings of anger, anxiety, powerlessness, shame, and humiliation in front of one's partner. Recurrent erectile dysfunction can ultimately lead to depression.

It is necessary to understand penile erectile anatomy and physiology to understand how things can go wrong. The penis contains three cylindrical bodies: two corpora cavernosa lie atop the corpus spongiosum, which contains the urethra. These bodies contain spongy erectile tissue, composed of vascular spaces or sinusoids surrounded by smooth muscle. Erections occur when autonomic nervous innervation leads to relaxation of cavernosal smooth muscle, thus allowing blood flow into the vascular spaces.

This muscle relaxation is mediated by the release of the neurotransmitter nitric oxide, with subsequent activation of cyclic guanosine monophosphate (GMP). As the vascular spaces in the spongy erectile tissue expand, the penile veins that drain them are compressed against the surrounding collagenous sheath or tunica albuginea, thus preventing outflow. The erection subsides when smooth muscles surrounding the vascular spaces contract, mediated by the breakdown of cyclic GMP back to GMP via the phosphodiesterase enzyme (PDE) type 5.

Erectile dysfunction results from one of three physiological problems: (1) failure of initiation due to psychological or neurological inhibition of nervous stimulation, (2) failure to attain penile arterial filling, or (3) failure to maintain penile veno-occlusion. The last two causes are frequently associated with peripheral vascular disease, which in turn is associated with hypertension, hyperlipidemia, and tobacco use.

Sexual Function and Dysfunction in Dementia

Sexuality continues to play an important role in the lives of many individuals suffering from dementia, often by providing a nonverbal means of communication and intimacy. Depending on the degree of dementia, however, the ability to initiate sexual activity and sustain performance may become impaired. Agitation, disinhibition, and psychosis associated with dementia may give rise to sexually aggressive or inappropriate behaviors. There are also ethical issues that complicate sexuality associated with dementia, such as when one partner is not fully competent to consent to sex, especially with another demented individual (Haddad & Benbow, 1993), or when the nonaffected partner seeks to fulfill sexual needs outside the relationship. It is important to understand these issues when assessing and treating patients with dementia and their caregivers. Unfortunately, health care professionals often fail to inquire about such issues despite how commonly they affect couples (Duffy, 1995).

Dementia will affect sexuality in several ways. On the one hand, sexual desire may remain strong, and even increase, especially if previous inhibitions are reduced by cognitive impairment. As the dementia progresses, a cognitively intact partner may develop considerable concern as to whether the affected individual is truly consenting to sexual activity (Hanks, 1992). They may also feel frustrated with a partner who does not always recognize them or who requests sex repeatedly because he or she cannot remember when they last had sex (Davies et al., 1992; Redinbaugh et al., 1997). As a result, the cognitively intact partner's sexual desire may decline because the partner's dementia and associated changes in behavior and personality are viewed as a sexual turnoff. Partners may be further confused by conflicting feelings of love and fidelity for their demented spouse and guilt over their desires for extramarital intimacy.

It is not surprising, then, that there is an overall decrease in sexual activity in affected couples. In one study, only 27% of couples with a partner suffering from Alzheimer's disease were sexually active, compared to 82% of couples with partners without dementia (Wright, 1991). This decrease may also be attributed in part to sexual dysfunction associated with the dementing process. For example, cognitive impairment may reduce attentional capacity during sex, as well as the ability to sequence and initiate components of lovemaking (Duffy, 1995; Redinbaugh et al., 1997). This impairment may explain why men with Alzheimer's disease suffer from high rates of erectile dysfunction—over 50% in one sample (Zeiss et al., 1990)—due in part to their inability to maintain a cognitive focus on physical and mental stimulation during sex. Such reasoning may also explain why inhibited orgasm (or anorgasmia) is common in women with dementia (Wright, 1991). In general, there have been few studies that looked at sexual dysfunction in dementia, so the rates of specific sexual disorders within different types of dementia are not known.

Although the percentage of individuals suffering from dementia who demonstrate sexually aggressive or inappropriate behaviors is relatively small, these individuals tend to generate a disproportionate amount of anxiety among caregivers and clinical attention from long-term care staff. The problematic behaviors associated with dementia include inappropriate sexual comments or demands, hypersexual behaviors (e.g., repeated requests for sexual gratification, compulsive masturbation), disinhibition (e.g., exposing oneself, disrobing, or masturbating in public areas), and sexually aggressive behaviors such as attempts to grope, fondle, or force sex on another person.

These behaviors have been seen in 2% to 7% of various samples of individuals with Alzheimer's disease (Burns et al., 1990; Kumar et al., 1988; Rabins et al., 1982), although these rates may be higher in institutionalized populations (Mayers, 1994). For example, one study found that 25% of residents on a dementia unit engaged in sexually inappropriate behaviors (Hashmi et al., 2000). Because frontal and temporal regions of the brain are involved in behavioral control and inhibition, individuals with dementia affecting these areas of the brain may be particularly vulnerable to demonstrating such inappropriate behaviors (Haddad & Benbow, 1993; Lishman, 1987; Raji et al., 2000). Other factors associated with inappropriate or hyperactive sexual behaviors include mania, psychosis, alcohol or drug abuse, stroke, head trauma (Hashmi et al., 2000), and the use of L-dopa (Bowers et al., 1971).

When assessing an individual who has allegedly demonstrated problematic behaviors, it is critical to identify the context of the behaviors. For example, public disrobing or touching of genitals in public may not be due to sexual urges, but instead may reflect underlying confusion, delirium, motor restlessness, or stereotypy associated with dementia. However, caregivers or long-term care staff sometimes misinterpret innocuous behaviors as reflecting sexual disinhibition (Redinbaugh et al., 1997). A good example would be the demented and aphasic individual in a wheelchair who reaches or grabs for attention, inadvertently hitting someone in the waist or chest area. The individual is simply reaching out for help from the height of the wheelchair, but the staff who is touched in the groin or breast area may wrongly view this as sexual aggression. It is also important to recognize that even individuals with severe dementia have legitimate needs for physical stimulation and intimacy (Spector et al., 1996) and may be reacting out of frustration and confusion because they lack the ability to communicate their needs verbally.

How can these challenging issues of sexuality in dementia be addressed? Anyone working with or caring for individuals with dementia must understand that they have a right to engage in sexual relationships if they still have the capacity to understand the nature of the relationship and provide reasonable consent. If the cognitively intact partner is concerned about the competency of his or her spouse to engage in sexual activity, a psychiatric or psychological consultation may shed light on the affected individual's understanding of the relationship. Lichtenberg and Strzepek (1990) have proposed several questions to be addressed in any interview that seeks to determine an individual's competency to consent to a sexual relationship:

1. Does the individual know who is initiating sexual contact? Can she or he describe his or her preferred degree of intimacy?
2. Is the sexual activity consistent with previous beliefs and values? Can the individual say "No" to unwanted activity?
3. Does the individual have an understanding that a sexual relationship with someone other than his or her spouse may be temporary? Can the individual describe how he or she would react if it were to end?

Responses to these questions will help determine the demented individual's awareness of the relationship, ability to avoid coercion and exploitation, and awareness of the possible risks.

One main purpose of psychological or psychiatric intervention is to provide education about sexuality to caregivers in the community as well as to staff in long-term care settings. This will help to optimize appropriate interpretation of and response to apparent inappropriate sexual behaviors. In addition, educational programs for long-term care staff may foster more open-minded attitudes (White & Catania, 1982). Behavioral approaches for inappropriate sexual comments may include setting verbal limits and redirecting the individual to a different topic. Staff and caregivers must be careful to avoid reinforcing inappropriate comments, such as by laughing at off-color jokes or teasing patients in a seductive manner in response to sexual comments.

For inappropriate or aggressive sexual advances, staff may need to remove the individual physically from the situation or restrict the person from contact with vulnerable individuals. Sometimes, restrictive clothing (e.g., pants without zippers, suspenders to keep pants up) can cut down on public displays of genitals, although caution must be given not to inadvertently restrain the individual. Because sexual advances may reflect unmet sexual needs, existing partners can be asked to consider providing more physical and perhaps sexual intimacy in hopes that this will remove the drive toward inappropriate behaviors.

When behavioral approaches are insufficient, psychiatric consultation is needed to provide better control through pharmacotherapy. The choice of medication will depend on the nature and severity of the behaviors and on the presence of underlying psychopathology. In general, however, much sexual aggression can be viewed like any other form of agitation associated with dementia and treated accordingly. As such, a variety of psychotropic agents, in particular atypical antipsychotics, have been shown to be efficacious for treating agitation (Tariot, 1999) and sexual problems associated with dementia.

Medications may also be used to target specific underlying psychopathology. For example, overactive libido can sometimes be reduced by many of the antidepressants with sexual side effects, such as the SSRIs or the tricyclic antidepressants (Raji et al., 2000; Segraves, 1998), or by β-blockers. If the inappropriate sexual behaviors are felt to reflect hypersexuality due to mania, the use of an antipsychotic or a mood stabilizer is indicated.

Another pharmacological strategy to decrease libido and sexual aggression has been the use of hormone therapy. Estrogen has been shown to reduce aggression in demented men (Kyomen et al., 1999), which would be applicable with sexually aggressive behaviors. Two steroid hormones with both progesterone and antiandrogen activity include medroxyprogesterone (MPA; sold as Provera and Depo-Provera) and cyproterone acetate (CA). MPA works by blocking synthesis of testosterone in the testes. Both agents have been shown to reduce sexually aggressive behaviors in demented individuals (Brown, 1998; Cooper, 1987; Nadal & Allgulander, 1992), although CA is only available in several European countries. Side effects from both CA and MPA may include weight gain, glucose intolerance, and liver dysfunction.

SEXUALITY IN LONG-TERM CARE

The role of sexuality for residents in long-term care is not only stigmatized by the fact that they are elderly, but even more so by the fact they are no longer living independently and often suffer from multiple medical and psychiatric problems, including cognitive impairment. As a result, both residents and staff tend to view sexuality in a negative manner. Residents often feel sexually unattractive and are pessimistic about whether sex would even be possible or enjoyable (Kaas, 1978; Wasow & Loeb, 1979). Not surprisingly, the rate of sexual activity is low in most nursing facilities (Mulligan & Palguta, 1991). For many residents, however, the desire for sexual relationships still exists. In a 1982 study of 250 nursing home residents, White (1982) found that 91% were not sexually active in the last month, but 17% wanted to be sexually active but lacked privacy or a partner. Other common barriers to sexuality among long-term care residents include loss of interest, chronic illness, sexual dysfunction, and negative attitudes of staff (Richardson & Lazur, 1995; Wasow & Loeb, 1979).

When a couple involves one or more partners who are living in a long-term care facility, it is important for staff to be aware of residents' rights to sexual expression and to accommodate a couple's privacy when appropriate. There are several ways in which mental health consultants can help remove barriers to sexuality in long-term care settings. First, it is important to educate staff about sexuality in late life to dispel stereotypes, provide an understanding of residents' rights to sexual expression, and provide a conceptualization of sexuality as helping residents to meet needs for intimacy and physical contact (Spector et al., 1996). By federal law, residents have the right to associate with and communicate privately with individuals of their own choosing (Federal Regulations, 1990). Residents should also be educated about sexuality in later life, and their sexual rights. One way to facilitate these education goals for residents and staff in long-term care settings is to develop and promote a policy on sexuality. One such policy, developed by the Hebrew Home for the Aged in Riverdale, New York, is outlined in Table 27-5.

To carry out such a policy, long-term care clinical staff should ensure that a sex history is incorporated into intake and routine nursing, medical, and mental health evaluations. These evaluations can also serve to assess residents' concerns and capacity with respect to sexual function and relationships. Long-

TABLE 27-5.   Resident sexual rights and staff and organizational responsibilities, Hebrew Home for the Aged at Riverdale, New York (1997)

1. Residents have rights to seek out and engage in sexual expression among other residents or visitors.
2. Residents have the right to obtain materials with sexually explicit content.
3. Residents may have access to private space and professional counseling in support of sexual expression.
4. Staff members have the responsibility to uphold and facilitate residents' sexual expression. This would restrict intervention in sexual activity without specific indications.
5. The organization has the responsibility to ensure privacy, provide staff education, and maintain oversight of rights.

Source: Reingold (1997).

term care facilities must ensure adequate privacy for couples who wish to be intimate and help facilitate conjugal or home visits. To this end, facilities should, when feasible, provide private rooms for married couples or other partners to share. Adequate privacy can be increased by the use of "Do Not Disturb" signs, locks on doors, and reminders to staff and residents to knock before entering another resident's room (Spector et al., 1996). Finally, facilities can provide beauty services such as hairdressers and manicurists (Richardson & Lazur, 1995).

ASSESSMENT OF SEXUAL DYSFUNCTION IN LATE LIFE

The assessment of sexual dysfunction in late life depends to a large degree on a comfortable and productive doctor-patient relationship in which an individual and his or her partner feel secure enough to disclose adequate history and the physician has both the knowledge and the openness to ask the right questions and pursue sufficient tests. Spouse or partner involvement and cooperation are critical and can make or break a successful outcome. The evaluation of sexual dysfunction in late life first involves identifying the specific problem and then obtaining a comprehensive medical, psychiatric, and sex history to identify potential causes as well as potential pitfalls during treatment (Cheadle, 1991).

A comprehensive sex history will examine an individual's prior sexual experiences, current sexual functioning, sexual relationships, and attitudes toward sexuality and toward any current partner. With older couples, interviewers must be able to identify relevant age-appropriate issues (Sbrocco et al., 1995). It is important to balance the need to gather sexual history with the responsibility to be sensitive to the fact that this may be some of the most personal information that a patient will ever divulge.

The medical workup for sexual dysfunction involves a physical exam, laboratory testing, and sometimes specialized diagnostic testing. The physical exam focuses on genital and urologic anatomy and function and tries to assess underlying vascular and neurological function. Lab testing will examine routine blood chemistry (e.g., blood count, electrolytes, glucose, lipid profile), testosterone and prolactin levels, thyroid function, and (in men) prostate-specific antigen (PSA). The most common specialized diagnostic tests for erectile dysfunction include nocturnal penile tumescence and rigidity (NPTR; a test to determine whether natural erections occur during sleep) and penile ultrasound (a test to assess blood flow in the penis).

TREATMENT OF SEXUAL DYSFUNCTION IN LATE LIFE

The preservation and enhancement of sexual activity in geriatric patients requires an understanding and sensitivity to the fact that many of these individuals want and intend to continue with sex despite changes in physical and sexual function. Once an evaluation is complete, it is important to provide both partners with education about normal and dysfunctional sexuality. This information helps to reassure the affected individual that he or she is not alone with the problem, that it has specific causes, and that it can be treated.

In addition, clinicians can help patients gain an expanded perspective of sexuality as a form of physical and psychological intimacy and not solely as sexual intercourse. The process of providing such information to patients and discussing suggestions will build trust between patient and clinician, and this relationship will lay the basis for the patient to feel comfortable with seeking follow-up and with being open about emotional reactions to the problem. Many treatments fail at this point, not because the treatment will not work, but because the patient and clinician—whether urologist, nurse, psychiatrist, or sex therapist—never establish a solid working relationship. Treatment can also fail when one partner refuses to cooperate with treatment or when problems within the entire relationship become insurmountable.

Couples with one or both partners suffering from chronic medical illness or disability will face unique challenges. They often need to shift focus from intercourse to foreplay and to adapt sexual practices to account for physical limitations such as fatigue, loss of muscle strength, and pain. Physicians should work to maximize both rehabilitative and palliative treatments, such as the use of analgesics for pain, inhalers for shortness of breath, and physical therapy for joint immobility or muscle weakness.

Organizations such as the American Cancer Society, the United Ostomy Organization, and the National Jewish Center for Immunology and Respiratory Medicine have published excellent brochures on maintaining sexual function despite specific medical illness. In addition, appropriate treatment of depression, anxiety, or psychosis can often lead to significant improvement in sexual function, assuming that the medications used to treat these disorders do not themselves cause problems. Several ways in which an older couple can enhance sexual function and cope with disability are outlined in Table 27-6.

When medication side effects impair sexual function, physicians can consider several options (Goodwin & Agronin, 1997; Margolese & Assalian, 1996). The first step would be to continue the medication and wait for tolerance of the side effect to develop because many side effects diminish or go away after several weeks. If there is no change, a dose reduction can be tried. An attempt to simplify the overall regimen might also be helpful because combinations of medications can cause more sexual side effects than each medication alone. For certain medications, such as antidepressants, with short half-lives, a "drug holiday" in which the medication is temporarily stopped for a day or two (such as on weekends) can result in transient improvement in sexual function (Rothschild, 1995). However, there is the risk of recurrent psychiatric symptoms during this holiday.

Ultimately, a clinician may have to consider stopping the medication and substituting an alternative agent that has less potential for sexual side effects.

TABLE 27-6.   Ten ways to enhance sexual function in late life

1. Cultivate a positive attitude toward sexuality in later life.
2. Maintain optimal health and fitness. Avoid use of tobacco and excess alcohol.
3. Maintain open and honest communication with your partner about how your sexual responsiveness has changed over time.
4. Focus on foreplay as much as on intercourse. Be open-minded about adapting sexual practices to your needs.
5. Maximize treatment of medical problems or disability that is interfering with sexual function. Consult a physician with any concerns about excess exertion during sex. For concerns about adequate stamina, use appropriate exercise to build up strength and self-confidence.
6. Maximize treatment of symptoms that impact sex prior to sex. For pain, consider taking a warm shower or bath, having a relaxing massage, or taking analgesics prior to sex. For shortness of breath, adapt sexual activity to minimize exertion and use prescribed inhalers ahead of time. Choose times of day for sex when pain is at a minimum.
7. Hormone replacement therapy can relieve vaginal dryness and improve vasocongestion for peri- or postmenopausal women. Tender genital or breast tissue may require more gentle stimulation, sometimes with the use of an external lubricant.
8. Identify problematic medications and investigate alternative agents or strategies.
9. Avoid unrealistic expectations that sex must be the same as when you were younger.
10. Explore sexual positions to decrease exertion or to account for equipment such as oxygen tanks or ostomy bags. Suggested positions for intercourse include lying side by side, sitting face to face, or the male kneeling behind with the female resting her knees on the ground and her arms on a bed.

Sources: Butler and Lewis (1986); Goodwin and Agronin (1997).

For example, the antidepressants bupropion (Walker et al., 1993), mirtazapine (Gelenberg et al., 2000), and nefazodone (Feiger et al., 1996) have not been associated with the degree of sexual dysfunction seen with tricyclics and SSRIs. For antipsychotics, more potent agents (e.g., risperidone, haloperidol) with less anticholinergic side effects may cause less dysfunction.

When sexual dysfunction is due to antidepressant medications, clinicians can also consider the use of antidotes to reverse sexual side effects (Gitlin, 1994; Segraves, 1998). Several antidotes include yohimbine, amantadine, cyproheptadine (use with caution because this medication can also reverse the antidepressant effect of SSRIs), bethanecol, methylphenidate, buspirone, bromocriptine (for antipsychotic-induced sexual dysfunction), and the antidepressants bupropion, nefazodone, mirtazapine, and trazodone. More recently, Viagra (sildenafil) has also been shown to reverse antidepressant-induced erectile dysfunction (Nurnberg et al., 1999). Depending on the antidote, it can be taken anywhere from 30 to 60 minutes prior to anticipated sex (on an "as needed" basis) and in increasing doses until success is achieved. If as-needed use of an antidote does not work, a regularly scheduled daily dose should be considered.

If none of these strategies work, clinicians have to consider the trade-off between the benefits of the medication and the resultant sexual side effect. For some individuals, going off the medication poses too great a risk for recurrent psychiatric symptoms, and there may not be adequate alternatives. This is a frustrating situation, and affected individuals have to choose between discontinuing a needed medication and coping with persistent sexual dysfunction.

Hypoactive sexual desire is a significant sexual problem for women across the life span and involves multiple psychological and physical factors. For some older women, loss of libido results from a poor self-image brought about by age-associated losses of physical strength and beauty and changes in sexual function that result from the cessation of estrogen production during menopause. An older woman's ability to see herself as a sexual being can be further eroded by exposure to negative societal attitudes and images of sexuality in late life. Unfortunately, many women internalize these distorted, ageist beliefs. Treatment of low desire must begin by providing sex education and counseling to counter those psychological barriers. Estrogen replacement may help improve sexual arousal and comfort, which in turn may lead to increased desire.

The critical physiologic cause of low desire in women, however, appears to be the reduction in levels of free testosterone associated with menopause. Testosterone replacement in women with hypoactive sexual desire has been beneficial (Basson, 1999; Rako, 1996), although side effects can include weight gain, virilization (e.g., growth of facial and chest hair, lowering of the voice), suppression of clotting factors, and even liver damage. Using lower doses of testosterone to avoid supraphysiological levels and avoiding alkylated testosterone can sometimes avoid these side effects (Basson, 1999).

Sildenafil has also been studied in women with sexual dysfunction (hypoactive desire, orgasmic disorder, or dyspareunia) associated with female sexual arousal disorder, and although it was well tolerated, it did not lead to improvement (Basson et al., 2000).

Treatment Modalities for Erectile Dysfunction

Treatment of ED in geriatric patients involves all of the same approaches as with younger men and has certainly been revolutionized with the advent of oral erectogenic agents. However, there are several major reversible causes of erectile dysfunction that, if present, must be addressed before other treatments are considered. Hypogonadism with testosterone deficiency is a cause of erectile dysfunction in around 5% of cases. Testosterone replacement is usually given topically through use of a patch. It should be avoided in men with a history of prostate or bladder cancer or bladder outlet obstruction. Some men suffer from erectile dysfunction as a result of vascular damage and may benefit from microsurgical revascularization. Peyronie's disease, characterized by curvature of the penis during erection due to scarring, can also be treated, with resultant improvement in erectile function.

Penile intracavernosal self-injection was the first pharmacological treatment for erectile dysfunction. Injectable agents work by increasing smooth muscle relaxation and arterial dilatation in the penis. Two of the available agents (Caverject, Edex) are preparations of alprostadil, which is a synthetic form of prostaglandin E_1. Injection of these agents directly into the base of the penis 10 to 20 minutes before sex leads to erections in 70% to 80% of men (Althof & Seftel, 1995). Injection therapy with alprostadil has been associated with local pain, scar tissue formation with chronic use, and (rarely) prolonged erections or priapism. Other injectable agents have included VIP (vasoactive intestinal polypeptide), phentolamine, and papaverine hydrochloride, sometimes in combination. Alprostadil may also be given in the form of a urethral suppository called MUSE (*medicated urethral stimulation of erection*), which takes away the need to use a needle but can also be associated with some penile discomfort and is rarely associated with hypotension (Padma-Nathan et al., 1997).

Sildenafil (Viagra) was the first oral erectogenic agent available for men with ED, followed by tadalafil (Cialis), and more recently vardenafil (Levitra). All three agents improve erectile function in men with both organic and psychogenic ED by serving as selective inhibitors of phosphodiesterase type 5 (PDE 5), the key enzyme found in penile erectile tissue. Each agent can be taken 30 to 60 minutes prior to anticipated sexual activity. Erections do not occur spontaneously on the medications, but require adequate physical stimulation. Their obvious advantages are ease of use and high rate of success in up to 70% to 80% of affected men (Boolel et al., 1996; Porst, Padma-Nathan, et al., 2003; Porst, Young, et al., 2003). Potential side effects for these agents include headache, skin flushing, dizziness, gastrointestinal discomfort, blurred vision, and the potential for blood pressure increases when combined with nitrates (e.g, sublingual nitroglycerin, isosorbide, etc.). In addition, the PDE 5 inhibitors should be used with caution in men with abnormal penile shape, a history of orthostatic hypotension, severe renal or hepatic disease, concomitant use of certain antiviral and antifungal medications, and diseases that increase the risk of priapism such as sickle cell anemia, multiple myeloma, and leukemia.

Another type of oral erectogenic medication is sublingual apomorphine (Uprima), currently available outside of the United States. It serves as a centrally active dopamine agonist and affects the area of the brain that causes erections (Seagraves, 2000). Apomorphine is rapidly absorbed and can help men achieve an erection in response to stimulation within 20 to 30 minutes. Potential side effects include nausea and the potential for hypotension and even syncope in a small percentage of users. Despite the efficacy of all oral erectogenic agents, it is important for older men to realize that these medications are not substitutes for poor sexual or marital relationships, and can pose risks for men with brittle cardiovascular disease and/or deconditioned bodies now seeking sexual exertion (Mobley & Baum, 1999).

Two other important treatments for ED are vacuum constriction devices and penile implants (Sison et al., 1997). Vacuum constriction devices restore erectile function by utilizing a plastic vacuum tube and pump placed over the penis to create a vacuum that causes blood flow into the penis. Once an erection is achieved, a ring is placed around the base of the penis to maintain rigidity, and the tube is removed. Although quite effective, the use of vacuum constriction devices requires some dexterity and can cause numbing, bruising, and delayed ejaculation (Dutta & Eid, 1999). Penile implants are an effective, but less frequently used, treatment for erectile dysfunction. There are a number of devices on the market, some which are semirigid and others that consist of inflatable tubes with implantable pumps (Evans, 1998). Aside from the risks of surgery and infection, the main complication for these devices is mechanical failure, with an incidence that ranges from 5% to 20% (Lewis, 1995). Because surgical placement leads to destruction of erectile tissue, a prosthetic device will always be needed to achieve an erection. They can, however, be surgically repaired or reimplanted.

Sex Therapy in Late Life

For some older couples, sexual dysfunction has clear psychological roots, often in the context of a dysfunctional relationship. Sex therapy is always best when done *conjointly*, meaning that both partners are involved because both are considered an integral part of the problem and solution. Although historically sex therapy has utilized a psychodynamic model to uncover underlying unconscious conflicts responsible for erectile dysfunction, current treatment models view that as less successful and instead rely on cognitive-behavioral techniques (Kaplan, 1974, 1983; Rosen & Leiblum, 1988). Brief supportive and educational counseling is first step in treatment and can help dispel distorted and uninformed attitudes toward sexuality in general and a sexual problem in particular. Sometimes, an individual or couple needs some minor problem solving on how to reorient their sexual practices to resolve a problem. In other cases, more intensive couples therapy is needed to resolve long-standing relationship issues before work on a sexual problem can even begin.

Sex therapy itself involves both cognitive and behavioral techniques, with an overall goal to build an association between relaxed and sensual physical intimacy and sexual relations. The same principles can be applied across the life span, with several refinements in late life. Using cognitive therapy techniques, the therapist tries to understand how the individual's thought process during sexual activity is leading to dysfunction and then attempts to refocus distorted cognitive attitudes toward sexual activity into more practical ones.

For example, many men with ED find it difficult to remove themselves from the role of a spectator during sex, watching themselves with their partner and constantly taking note of the status of their erection. This spectator role, as first described by Masters and Johnson (1970), only produces anxiety and distracts a man from concentrating on pleasurable sensations, thus reinforcing his erectile dysfunction. To counter this, a man is taught to shift his mental focus from his erection to other pleasurable aspects of the encounter (Kaplan, 1974).

Erectile dysfunction may also be perpetuated by a cognitive distortion such as *catastrophizing*, in which a man thinks that if he does not achieve an erection during sex he will be rejected not only by his partner, but also by all women. Another common cognitive distortion is *all-or-nothing thinking*, in which a man thinks that he must achieve an erection immediately during sex or the whole thing is pointless. The problem with such cognitive distortions is that, while they are unrealistic, the force of belief often leads them to become self-fulfilling prophecies. The therapist helps the patient gain insight into the negative impact of such thoughts and then to practice replacing them with more realistic and hopeful ones, sometimes even with positive assertions or affirmations of success (Goodwin & Agronin, 1997).

Behavioral techniques used during sex therapy begin with exercises called *sensate focus*, in which a couple learns physical relaxation techniques and then applies these to nonpressured sensual touching. Sensate focus helps to reduce performance anxiety and restore the natural flow of the sexual response cycle. Once a couple is able to feel relaxed and physically intimate without sexual stimulation, they gradually progress to genital stimulation and then intercourse. Several adjustments in these exercises may be required for the older couple. For example, older patients with physical problems that involve some degree of disability may express concerns about being able to exert themselves adequately during sexual activity. The therapist might recommend one of several positions that minimize exertion, such as with partners side by side or with one partner kneeling on pillows and braced on a low bed. Other suggestions outlined in Table 27-6 might also apply. Such simple suggestions may remove some of the most anxiogenic barriers for an older couple, especially the common, but unfounded, belief that they lack the stamina or dexterity for sexual activity.

During the process of behavioral sex therapy, the therapist continues to work with the couple on their relationship and tries to identify and confront resistance that inevitably arises during treatment. Such resistance to these seemingly innocuous exercises often serves to identify key problems in the relationship that are either causing the sexual dysfunction or impeding its treatment. Regardless of age, many couples find that sexual interest, pleasure, and improved function reemerges during sex therapy, thus allowing them to again enjoy such a fundamental component of their relationship.

REFERENCES

Althof SE, Seftel AD. The evaluation and management of erectile dysfunction. *Psychiatr Clin North Am.* 1995;18(1):171–192.

American Psychiatric Association. *Diagnostic and Statistical Manual of Mental Disorders.* 4th ed. *Text Revision.* Washington, DC: American Psychiatric Association; 2000.

Bachmann GA, Leiblum SR. Sexuality in sexagenarian women. *Maturitas.* 1991;13:43–50.

Basson R. Androgen replacement for women. *Can Fam Physician.* 1999;45:2100–2107.

Basson R, McInnes R, Smith MD, et al. Efficacy and safety of sildenafil in estrogenized women with sexual dysfunction associated with female sexual arousal disorder. *Obstet Gynecol.* 2000;95(4, suppl 1):S54.

Boolell M, Gepi-Attee S, Gingell JC, Allen MJ. Sildenafil, a novel effective oral therapy for male erectile dysfunction. *Br J Urol.* 1996;78:257–261.

Bowers MB, Woert MV, Davis L. Sexual behavior during L-dopa treatment for parkinsonism. *Am J Psychiatry.* 1971;127:1691–1693.

Boyer G, Boyer J. Sexuality and aging. *Nursing Clin North Am.* 1982;17:421–427.

Brown FW. Case report: sexual aggression in dementia. *Ann Long-Term Care.* 1998;6:248–249.

Burns A, Jacoby R, Levy R. Psychiatric phenomena in Alzheimer's disease: IV. Disorders of behavior. *Br J Psychiatry.* 1990;157:86–94.

Butler RN, Lewis MI. *Love and Sex After 40: A Guide for Men and Women for Their Mid and Later Years.* New York, NY: Harper & Row; 1986.

Cheadle MJ. The screening sexual history: getting to the problem. *Clin Geriatr Med.* 1991;7:9–13.

Comfort A, Dial LK. Sexuality and aging: an overview. *Clin Geriatr Med.* 1991;7:1–7.

Cooper AJ. Medroxyprogesterone acetate (MPA) treatment of sexual acting out in men suffering from dementia. *J Clin Psychiatry.* 1987;48:368–370.

Crenshaw TL, Goldberg JP. *Sexual Pharmacology: Drugs That Affect Sexual Function.* New York, NY: Norton; 1996.

Davies HD, Zeiss A, Tinklenberg JR. 'Til death do us part: intimacy and sexuality in the marriages of Alzheimer's patients. *J Psychosoc Nurs.* 1992;30:5–10.

Duffy LM. Sexual behavior and marital intimacy in Alzheimer's couples: a family theory perspective. *Sexuality Disabil.* 1995;13:239–254.

Dutta TC, Eid JF. Vacuum constriction devices for erectile dysfunction: a long-term, prospective study of patients with mild, moderate, and severe dysfunction. *Urology.* 1999;54:891–893.

Dychtwald K, Flower J. *Agewave: The Challenges and Opportunities of an Aging America.* Los Angeles, CA: Jeremy P. Tarcher; 1989.

Evans C. The use of penile prostheses in the treatment of impotence. *Br J Urol.* 1998;81:591–598.

Federal Regulations, Code 42: The Patient's Bill of Rights. Chapter 4, Section 483, 1990.

Feiger A, Kiev A, Shrivastava RK, Wisselink PG, Wilcox CS. Nefazodone versus sertraline in outpatients with major depression: focus on efficacy, tolerability, and effects on sexual function and satisfaction. *J Clin Psychiatry.* 1996;57(suppl 2):53–62.

Feldman HA, Goldstein I, Hatzichristou DG, Krane RJ, McKinlay JB. Impotence and its medical and psychosocial correlates: results of the Massachusetts Male Aging Study. *J Urol.* 1994;151:54–61.

Gelenberg AJ, Laukes C, McGahuey C, et al. Mirtazepine substitution in SSRI-induced sexual dysfunction. *J Clin Psychiatry.* 2000;61:356–360.

Gitlin MJ. Psychotropic medications and their effects on sexual function: diagnosis, biology, and treatment approaches. *J Clin Psychiatry.* 1994;55:406–413.

Goodwin AJ, Agronin ME. *A Women's Guide to Overcoming Sexual Fear and Pain.* Oakland, Calif: New Harbinger Press; 1997.

Haddad P, Benbow S. Sexual problems associated with dementia: Part 2. Aetiology, assessment and treatment. *Int J Geriatr Psychiatry.* 1993;8:631–637.

Hanks N. The effects of Alzheimer's disease on the sexual attitudes and behaviors of married caregivers and their spouses. *Sexuality Disabil.* 1992;10:137–151.

Hashmi FH, Krady AI, Qayum F, Grossberg GT. Sexually disinhibited behavior in the cognitively impaired elderly. *Clin Geriatr.* 2000;8(11):61–68.

Jacoby S. Great sex. What's age got to do with it? *Modern Maturity* [serial online]. September/October 1999. Available at: www.aarp.org/press/1998/nr100198.html. Accessed November 1, 2000.

Kaas MJ. Sexual expression of the elderly in nursing homes. *Gerontologist.* 1978;18: 372–378.

Kaplan HS. *The Evaluation of Sexual Disorders: Psychological and Medical Aspects.* New York, NY: Brunner/Mazel; 1983.

Kaplan HS. *The New Sex Therapy.* New York, NY: Brunner/Mazel; 1974.

Kaplan HS. *Sexual Aversion, Sexual Phobias, and Panic Disorder.* New York, NY: Brunner/Mazel; 1987.

Kligman EW. Office evaluation of sexual function and complaints. *Clin Geriatr Med.* 1991;7:15–39.

Kumar A, Koss E, Metzler D, et al. Behavioral symptomatology in dementia of the Alzheimer type. *Alzheimer's Dis Assoc Disord.* 1988;2:363–365.

Kyomen HH, Satlin A, Hennen J, Wei JY. Estrogen therapy and aggressive behavior in elderly patients with moderate-to-severe dementia. *Am J Geriatr Psychiatry.* 1999; 7:339–348.

Lacey JV Jr, Mink PJ, Lubin JH, et al. Menopausal hormone replacement therapy and risk of ovarian cancer. *JAMA.* 2002;288:334–341.

Landers, A. *Ann Landers.* Newspaper advice column. September, 1996.

Lewis RW. Long-term results of penile prosthetic implants. *Urol Clin North Am.* 1995; 22:847–856.

Lichtenberg PA, Strzepek DM. Assessments of institutionalized dementia patient's competencies to participate in intimate relationships. *Gerontologist.* 1990;30:117–120.

Lishman WA. Cardinal psychological features of cerebral disorder. In: Lishman WE, ed. *Organic Psychiatry: The Psychological Consequences of Cerebral Disorder.* 2nd ed. Oxford, UK: Blackwell; 1987:3–20.

Margolese HC, Assalian P. Sexual side effects of antidepressants: a review. *J Sex Marital Ther.* 1996;22:209–224.

Marsiglio W, Donnelly D. Sexual relations in later life: a national study of married persons. *J Gerontol.* 1991;46:S338–S344.

Masters WH. Sex and aging: expectations and reality. *Hosp Pract.* 1986;15:175–198.

Masters WH, Johnson VE. *Human Sexual Inadequacy.* Boston, MA: Little, Brown; 1970.

Masters WH, Johnson VE. *Human Sexual Response.* Boston, MA: Little, Brown; 1966.

Mayers KS. Sexuality and the patient with dementia. *Sexuality Disabil.* 1994;12:213–219.

Metz ME, Miner MH. Male "menopause," aging, and sexual function: a review. *Sexuality Disabil.* 1995;13:287–307.

Michael RT, Gagnon JH, Laumann EO, Kolata G. *Sex in America: A Definitive Survey.* Boston, MA: Little, Brown; 1994.

Mobley DF, Baum N. Sildenafil in elderly men: advice and caveats. *Clin Geriatr.* 1999; 7(12):34–41.

Mulligan T, Palguta RF Jr. Sexual interest, activity, and satisfaction among male nursing home residents. *Arch Sex Behav.* 1991;20:199–204.

Nadal M, Allgulander S. Normalization of sexual behavior in a female with dementia after treatment with cyproterone. *Int J Geriatr Psychiatry.* 1992;8:265–267.

National Council on the Aging. *Healthy Sexuality and Vital Aging. Executive Summary.* Washington DC: National Council on the Aging; 1998.

Nurnberg HG, Lauriello J, Hensley PL, et al. Sildenafil for iatrogenic serotonergic antidepressant medication-induced sexual dysfunction in 4 patients. *J Clin Psychiatry.* 1999;60:33–35.

Porst H, Padma-Nathan H, Giuliano F, Anglin G, Varanese L, Rosen R. Efficacy of tadalafil for the treatment of erectile dysfunction at 24 and 36 hours after dosing: a randomized controlled trial. *Urology.* 2003;62(1):121–125.

Porst H, Young JM, Schmidt AC, Buvat J. International Vardenafil Study Group. Efficacy and tolerability of vardenafil for treatment of erectile dysfunction in patient subgroups. *Urology.* 2003;62(3):519–523.

Padma-Nathan H, Hellstrom WJG, Kaiser FE, et al. Treatment of men with erectile dysfunction with transurethral alprostadil. *N Engl J Med.* 1997;336:1–7.

Rabins PV, Mace NL, Lucas MJ. The impact of dementia on the family. *JAMA.* 1982; 248:333–335.

Raji M, Liu D, Wallace D. Case report: sexual aggressiveness in a patient with dementia: sustained clinical response to citalopram. *Ann Long-Term Care.* 2000;8:81–83.

Rako, S. *The Hormone of Desire: The Truth About Sexuality, Menopause, and Testosterone.* New York, NY: Harmony Books; 1996.

Redinbaugh EM, Zeiss AM, Davies HD, Tinklenberg JR. Sexual behavior in men with dementing illnesses. *Clin Geriatr.* 1997;5(13):45–50.

Reingold DA. Rights of nursing home residents to sexual expression. *Clin Geriatr.* 1997; 5(4):52–63.

Renshaw D. Sexuality and aging. In: Sadavoy J, Lazarus LW, Jarvik LF, Grossberg GT, eds. *Comprehensive Review of Geriatric Psychiatry.* 2nd ed. Washington, DC: American Psychiatric Press; 1996:713–729.

Richardson JP, Lazur A. Sexuality in the nursing home patient. *Am Fam Physician.* 1995;51:121–124.

Rosen RC, Leiblum SR. *Principles and Practice of Sex Therapy: Update for the 1990s.* New York, NY: Guilford Press; 1988.

Rothschild AJ. Selective serotonin reuptake inhibitor-induced sexual dysfunction: efficacy of a drug holiday. *Am J Psychiatry.* 1995;152:1514–1516.

Sbrocco T, Weisberg BA, Barlow DH. Sexual dysfunction in the older adult: assessment of psychosocial factors. *Sexuality Disabil.* 1995;13:201–218.

Schover LR, Jensen SB. *Sexuality and Chronic Illness.* New York, NY: Guilford Press; 1988.

Segraves RT. Antidepressant-induced sexual dysfunction. *J Clin Psychiatry.* 1998; 59(suppl 4):48–54.

Segraves RT. New treatment for erectile dysfunction. *Curr Psychiatry Rep.* 2000;2:206–210.

Sherwin BB, Gelfand MM, Brender W. Androgen enhances sexual motivation in females: a prospective crossover study of sex steroid administration in the surgical menopause. *Psychosom Med.* 1985;47:339–351.

Sison AS, Godschalk MF, Mulligan T. Erectile dysfunction in the elderly: treatment recommendations from the recent American Urological Association Guidelines. *Clin Geriatr.* 1997;5(7):73–76.

Snarch D. *Constructing the Sexual Crucible: An Integration of Sexual and Marital Therapy.* New York, NY: Norton; 1991.

Spector IP, Rosen RC, Leiblum SR. Sexuality. In: Reichman WE, Katz PR, eds. *Psychiatric Care in the Nursing Home.* New York, NY: Oxford University Press; 1996: 133–150.

Starr BD, Weiner MB. *The Starr-Weiner Report on Sex and Sexuality in the Mature Years.* New York, NY: McGraw-Hill; 1981.

Tariot PN. Treatment of agitation in dementia. *J Clin Psychiatry.* 1999;60(suppl 8): 11–20.

Walker PW, Cole JO, Gardner EA, et al. Improvement in fluoxetine-associated sexual dysfunction in patients switched to bupropion. *J Clin Psychiatry.* 1993;54:459–465.

Wasow M, Loeb MB. Sexuality in nursing homes. *J Am Geriatr Soc.* 1979;27:73–79.

White CB. Sexual interests, attitudes, knowledge, and sexual history in relation to sexual behavior in the institutionalized aged. *Arch Sex Behav.* 1982;11:11–21.

White CB, Catania JA. Psychoeducational intervention for sexuality with the aged, family members of the aged, and people who work with the aged. *Int J Aging Hum Dev.* 1982;15:121–138.

Wright LK. The impact of Alzheimer's disease on the marital relationship. *Gerontologist.* 1991;31:224–237.

Writing Group for the Women's Health Initiative Investigators. Risks and benefits of estrogen plus progestin in healthy postmenopausal women. Principal results from the Women's Health Initiative randomized controlled trial. *JAMA.* 2002;288:321–333.

Zeiss AM, Davies HD, Wood M, Tinklenberg JR. The incidence and correlates of erectile problems in patients with Alzheimer's disease. *Arch Sex Behav.* 1990;19:325–332.

SECTION IV

Treatment

28

The Practice of Evidence-Based Geriatric Psychiatry

Stephen J. Bartels, MD, MS
Aricca R. Dums, BA
Thomas E. Oxman, MD
Sarah I. Pratt, PhD

The field of geriatric psychiatry has come of age. The recent surgeon general's report on mental health (US Department of Health and Human Services, 1999) and the report of the Administration on Aging (2001), *Older Adults and Mental Health,* underscore the dramatic development in knowledge over the past decade on the causes and treatments of geriatric mental health disorders. Despite these advances, older adults with mental disorders are at increased risk to receive treatments that are inappropriate or inadequate (Bartels, 2002). Bridging the gap between research and clinical services has been highlighted in reports from the Institute of Medicine (2001) and the National Institute of Mental Health (1999) as one of the most important priorities in contemporary health care.

Over the last several decades, the field of medicine has developed systematic methods to support the implementation of proven or "evidence-based" treatments into routine clinical care. However, the field of psychiatry, especially geriatric psychiatry, lags behind medicine in teaching and using evidence-based strategies.

In this chapter, we highlight the current state of evidence-based practices for older adults with mental health problems. We discuss the emergence and rationale for evidence-based practices; the hierarchical characteristics, quality, and methodology associated with the identification of evidence-based practices; established and emerging interventions for common geriatric mental disorders; barriers to implementation in health care settings in which older adults commonly seek treatment; approaches to overcoming these barriers based on practice change research; and a strategy that the individual clinician can employ to practice evidence-based medicine.

THE DIFFERENCE BETWEEN EVIDENCE-BASED
MEDICINE AND TRADITIONAL PARADIGMS

The primary difference between evidence-based medicine and traditional medical paradigms rests on the methods for evaluating treatment interventions and applying this information to clinical care and decision-making processes. Traditional medicine emphasizes clinical experience and local opinion on preferred practices. Under this approach, the practitioner draws on knowledge gained from prior cases, colleagues, and a nonsystematic appraisal of the value of new treatments. Available clinical practice guidelines are based on the clinical wisdom and opinion of experts without reference to a systematic evaluation of the quality of the research data (Friedland et al., 1998). In contrast, evidence-based medicine utilizes a different set of principles to aid decision-making processes. A hierarchy of evidence is used to guide clinical decision making and to classify the level of evidence that supports an intervention. Evidence-based medicine draws heavily on the use of external evidence to support, but not replace, internal clinical skills, judgment, and experience (Friedland et al., 1998; Guyatt & Rennie, 2002; Sackett et al., 1996).

DEFINING EVIDENCE-BASED PRACTICES

Over the past two decades, the field of medicine has led the charge to identify and disseminate evidence-based practices. These efforts were spurred by the insight of Cochrane (1972) and the ensuing development of the Cochrane Collaboration. Cochrane (Cochrane Collaboration, 2002) asserted that limited health care resources should be applied to the provision of interventions that had been proven effective through properly designed evaluation trials, with emphasis on randomized controlled trials (RCTs).

The development of an evidence-based practice begins with the collection and critical evaluation of the best evidence to address a given clinical question. Assessing the potential worth of an intervention is a complex process, especially in the context of many studies with conflicting results, potential bias associated with conflicts of interest, or different methodologies, samples, and outcome measures.

Several strategies exist to address this challenge. Reviewing the strength of evidence for a clinical practice requires evaluation of the quality (including minimization of bias), quantity (including magnitude of effect, sample size, power), and consistency (similar findings reported using similar and different experimental designs) of studies. These elements help to characterize the level of confidence that can be assigned to a body of knowledge (West et al., 2002).

TABLE 28-1. Hierarchical classification of evidence for effectiveness of research studies

1. A meta-analysis or systematic review of well-designed randomized controlled trials
2. A single, properly designed randomized controlled trial
3. Studies without randomization (i.e., single group pre-post, cohort, time series, or matched case-control studies)
4. Other quasi-experimental studies from more than one center or research group
5. Expert reports and authorities' recommendations based on descriptive studies or clinical evidence

In developing fields, such as geriatric psychiatry, the empirical research base is limited, but principles of evidence-based decision making can still be applied. The best *available* evidence is used to direct decision-making processes. Hence, the range of potential sources of evidence may be considered, from randomized clinical trials (if available) to single case reports. Systematic approaches to evaluate the treatment literature use hierarchical models that rate the quality of evidence that supports a specific treatment. For example, a widely used approach to ranking medical treatment research studies (Gray, 1997) is shown in Table 28-1.

Evaluating the evidence base for psychosocial treatments, such as psychotherapy, presents special challenges. In contrast to pharmacological trials in which the intervention and control conditions are clearly identified and measured (a specific dose of a medication compared to a placebo or comparison medication), uniform delivery of psychosocial interventions is less certain. Furthermore, identifying a valid "placebo" or comparison condition is also more complicated for psychosocial treatments. Finally, there is less agreement on common outcome measures to be used in assessing treatment effectiveness, thereby making comparisons between different studies more difficult.

Criteria developed by the American Psychological Association (Chambless & Hollon, 1998; Chambless & Ollendick, 2001) to evaluate the effectiveness of psychosocial interventions (see Table 28-2) require that studies report

TABLE 28-2. American Psychological Association criteria to rank effectiveness

Highest support:
1. Efficacy from at least two well-designed, prospective, randomized controlled studies by different investigators with clearly described interventions
2. A large series (>9) of single case design experiments

Probable effectiveness:
1. Two studies showing that treatment was superior to a waiting-list control group
2. A small series (>3) of single case design experiments
3. One or more studies that meet criteria for the highest level of evidence, but have not yet been replicated by different investigators

on measures used to standardize treatments and outcomes. For example, to be included in an analysis of an evidence base, studies must meet certain criteria for quality, including use of fidelity measures, replication of trials following a manualized protocol, valid outcome measures, and use of appropriate data analytic techniques (Chambless & Hollon, 1998).

Evidence-based medicine is designed to optimize care for individual patients by linking research and practice with clinical education and decision-making processes (Gambrill, 1999). Efforts to apply a systematic approach to evaluating geriatric mental health interventions can help provide older adults with effective interventions that facilitate recovery and improve functional outcomes.

THE NEED FOR A GERIATRIC EVIDENCE
BASE IN PSYCHIATRY

Although older adults often have similar outcomes compared to younger adults when given the same treatment, attention toward mental health interventions tailored for older adults is based on the premise that aging is associated with a variety of changes in physiological, cognitive, and social functioning that may affect response to treatment. The importance of evidence-based practices for older adults is supported both by differential response to psychotherapeutic interventions according to level of cognitive impairment and by age-associated differences in pharmacological response and sensitivity to medication side effects (Banerjee & Dickinson, 1997).

For example, due to declining cholinergic nervous system activity associated with aging, use of the most highly anticholinergic tricyclic antidepressants (e.g., amitriptyline) is generally contraindicated in older persons (Oxman, 1996). Similarly, the use of long-acting benzodiazepines in older persons has been associated with a variety of adverse outcomes, including increased incidence of falls, hip fractures, and cognitive impairment (Burke et al., 1998).

An additional and important feature of geriatric psychopharmacology is the increased risk of drug-drug interactions and the common presence of medical comorbidity in older persons. On average, older adults use up to 6 prescribed medications and 3.4 nonprescribed medications on a regular basis (Larsen & Hoot Martin, 1999). The risk of an adverse reaction increases with each additional drug (Beers & Ouslander, 1989). This is further complicated by widespread use of over-the-counter drugs, which may have additive effects or interact with prescribed drugs.

Among the mentally ill, older adults are at greater risk than younger adults for medical comorbidity and, in turn, drug-drug interactions (Beyth & Shorr, 1999). Furthermore, older adults with mental disorders are more likely to receive inappropriate or inadequate medication prescriptions compared to younger adults with mental disorders (Bartels et al., 1997) and compared to other older adults without mental disorders (Druss et al., 2001; Giron et al.,

2001). In general, older adults with mental disorders are at increased risk for poorer quality care (Bartels, 2002), underscoring the need to promote the use of evidence-based practices by clinicians.

A final (although perhaps counterintuitive) rationale for critically evaluating the evidence base is illustrated by instances in which the data have not supported conventional wisdom recommending against the use of specific agents in older persons due to assumed greater problems with side effects, treatment adherence, or tolerability. For instance, sensitivity to lithium may be more problematic in older persons because of declining renal function and increased blood levels on doses commonly used for younger adults. Although some reports indicate greater difficulty managing older patients on lithium, others report similar effects in younger and older persons (Bendz et al., 1994; Fahy & Lawlor, 2001; Hussain et al., 1997). According to clinical lore, antihypertensive β-blockers, commonly used in older persons, are contraindicated due to their alleged propensity to induce depression. However, reviews of the evidence do not support this contention (Gerstman et al., 1996; Kohn, 2001; Perez-Stable et al., 2000; Ried et al., 1998). Finally, the potentially more severe adverse side effects associated with tricyclic antidepressants (TCAs; e.g., anticholinergic, cardiovascular effects) in comparison to those of selective serotonin reuptake inhibitors (SSRIs) have been cited in claims that SSRIs are better tolerated than TCAs in older persons. Despite appropriate cautions regarding potentially serious adverse events associated with TCAs, meta-analyses failed to find significant differences between SSRIs and TCAs with respect to efficacy or discontinuation due to side effects (Anderson, 2000; Gerson et al., 1999; McCusker et al., 1998; Mittmann et al., 1997; Mulrow et al., 1999; Wilson et al., 2001).

Regrettably, until recently, clinicians have been left to extrapolate the evidence base on efficacy and tolerability of medications from studies with limited relevance to general clinical practice with older persons. Conventional drug trials typically excluded people over 65 years of age. Furthermore, when pharmaceutical industry studies do include older adults, they commonly select individuals who are the healthiest and least physically disabled to minimize required reports of adverse events and withdrawal from pharmaceutical trials (Banerjee & Dickinson, 1997). Models of medication effectiveness research designed to remedy some of these limitations include recent multisite studies sponsored by the National Institute of Mental Health, including the Clinical Antipsychotic Trials in Intervention Effectiveness (CATIE) study for Alzheimer's disease (Schneider et al., 2001) and the Sequenced Treatment Alternatives to Relieve Depression (STAR*D) (Lavori et al., 2001). These studies have few exclusionary criteria and include older individuals with medical comorbidity, multiple medications, and treatment by individuals in nonacademic (routine) clinical practice settings. These studies, and others currently under way, will provide the next generation of effectiveness studies to define the evidence base for pharmacological treatment of older adults with mental disorders.

EVIDENCE-BASED MEDICINE APPLIED TO GERIATRIC
PSYCHIATRY: AN OVERVIEW OF META-ANALYSES
AND EVIDENCE-BASED REVIEWS

The following section provides an overview of the best-established interventions for the most common psychiatric problems among older adults (including dementia, depression, substance abuse, anxiety, and schizophrenia). In reviewing the treatment literature, we examined the highest level of evidence, consisting of meta-analytic studies that utilized accepted statistical procedures to determine empirical support and systematic evidence-based review articles that use standardized criteria to evaluate the evidence base (Guyatt, Haynes, et al., 2000). This overview is not intended to be an exhaustive summary of the empirical evidence base, but rather provides a foundation for discussing the implementation of evidence-based geriatric mental health practices. In conducting this review, we searched MEDLINE, PsychInfo, and Cochrane Library databases for English language review articles published through the year 2001. Based on this approach, we identified 25 meta-analytic studies and 8 evidence-based reviews (Bartels, Dums, et al., 2002; Bartels, Haley, et al., 2002).

Treatments for the cognitive and behavioral symptoms of dementia and for major depression were among the most highly examined and empirically supported interventions in geriatric mental health. Less attention has been paid to systematic reviews of the treatment of other geriatric mental health problems, such as alcohol abuse, anxiety, and psychotic disorders.

The Evidence Base for Treatment of Dementia

Our search of published systematic reviews identified a substantial series of meta-analyses (Birks, Grimley, et al., 2000; Birks, Melzer, et al., 2000; Birks & Flicker, 2003; Fioravanti & Flicker, 2001; Fioravanti & Yanagi, 2000; Higgins & Flicker, 2000; Oken et al., 1998; Olin & Schneider, 2001; Qizilbash et al., 1998; Spector et al., 2001) and evidence-based reviews (American Psychiatric Association, 1997; Brodaty et al., 2001; Doody et al., 2001; Emre & Hanaoasi, 2000; Gatz et al., 1998; Kasl-Godley & Gatz, 2000; National Institute for Clinical Excellence, 2001) on treatment of the cognitive symptoms in dementia. Overall, there is consensus among these literature reviews that cholinesterase inhibitors have a significant (although modest) effect in diminishing the rate of cognitive decline among individuals with mild to moderate Alzheimer's dementia when compared to placebo over a period of 6 to 12 months (Brodaty et al., 2001; Doody et al., 2001; National Institute for Clinical Excellence, 2001). Evidence-based reviews and meta-analysis of other agents, such as antioxidants (Tabet et al., 2000), anti-inflammatories, estrogen replacement (Hogervorst et al., 2002), and gingko biloba (Birks et al., 2002), did not support treatment effectiveness or were inconclusive and warrant further studies (Doody et al., 2001). Psychosocial interventions such as cognitive retraining programs can temporarily slow decline in functional skills for a limited subset of individuals, but do not result in sustained effects (Gatz et al., 1998; Spector et al., 2001).

Treatment effectiveness of pharmacological and psychosocial interventions for behavioral and psychotic symptoms of dementia was assessed in several meta-analyses (Kirchner et al., 2001; Lanctot et al., 1998; Lonergan et al., 2001; Olin et al., 2001; Schneider et al., 1990) and evidence-based reviews (American Psychiatric Association, 1997; Doody et al., 2001; Gatz et al., 1998; Kasl-Godley & Gatz, 2000). In general, these systematic reviews of pharmacological interventions found that conventional antipsychotic agents are effective in reducing agitation and psychosis among individuals with dementia, although effect sizes are relatively small (Doody et al., 2001; Lanctot et al., 1998; Schneider et al., 1990). A series of individual RCTs examined the effectiveness of novel antipsychotics as well as the use of anticonvulsants and antidepressants for reducing agitation, depression, and other behavioral symptoms of dementia (De Deyn et al., 1999; Katz et al., 1999; Pollock et al., 2002; Porsteinsson et al., 2001; Street et al., 2000; Sultzer, 2000). However, with the exception of one meta-analysis of antidepressant agents that yielded inconclusive results (Bains et al., 2002), there are no meta-analytic or evidence-based reviews that evaluated the effectiveness of these types of agents.

Systematic reviews found that nonpharmacological interventions can be effective in reducing behavioral symptoms of dementia (Doody et al., 2001; Gatz et al., 1998; Kasl-Godley & Gatz, 2000). Behavioral interventions, environmental modifications, and stimulus control procedures have been shown to improve problem behaviors, such as urinary incontinence, self-care skills, and wandering (Doody et al., 2001; Gatz et al., 1998). However, treatment gains are difficult to maintain in the absence of continuous teaching and consistent reinforcement of target behaviors (Allen-Burge et al., 1996). Finally, psycho-education and counseling for caregivers can decrease caregiver burden and depression and can delay nursing home admission (Doody et al., 2001; Mittelman et al., 1996; Sorensen et al., 2002).

The Evidence Base for Treatment of Geriatric Major Depression

Meta-analytic (Anderson, 2000; Gerson et al., 1999; McCusker et al., 1998; Mittmann et al., 1997; Mulrow et al., 1999; Wilson et al., 2001) and evidence-based (Thorpe et al., 2001) reviews support the effectiveness of pharmacological treatment for geriatric major depression. Over half of older adults treated with antidepressants experience at least a 50% reduction in depressive symptoms (Wilson et al., 2001). At the same time, it should be noted that a recent meta-analysis of antidepressant studies (including all age groups) determined that the effect of antidepressants may be only 20% better than placebo treatment combined with physician and research assistant visits (Kirsch et al., 2002).

Among studies that compared different types of antidepressants in the treatment of geriatric depression, comparable efficacy and tolerability has been reported among TCAs, SSRIs, and non-SSRI norepinephrine reuptake inhibitors (NSSRIs) (Wilson et al., 2001). However, clinically significant differences in side effect profiles between TCAs and SSRIs exist (Gerson et al., 1999).

In addition, 7 meta-analytic studies (Cuijpers, 1998; Engels & Verney, 1997; Gerson et al., 1999; Koder et al., 1996; McCusker et al., 1998; Pinquart & Soerensen, 2001; Scogin & McElreath, 1994) and three evidence-based reviews (Gatz et al., 1998; Laidlaw, 2001; Thorpe et al., 2001) reported on the effectiveness of psychotherapy. Effective psychosocial interventions for geriatric depression include cognitive therapy, behavioral therapy, cognitive-behavioral therapy (CBT), and interpersonal therapy (Cuijpers, 1998; Engels & Verney, 1997; Gatz et al., 1998; Koder et al., 1996; McCusker et al., 1998; Pinquart & Soerensen, 2001; Scogin & McElreath, 1994).

A meta-analysis found similar effectiveness of pharmacological and psychological treatments among depressed patients over age 55 years (Gerson et al., 1999). Furthermore, findings from several RCTs suggest that the combined use of pharmacological and psychosocial interventions may be more effective in preventing the recurrence of major depression than either intervention alone (Lenze et al., 2002; Reynolds et al., 1999).

The Evidence Base for Treatment of Other Geriatric Mental Disorders

Alcohol abuse and anxiety are common problems among older adults. Psychotic disorders, although less common, often have particularly debilitating outcomes. To date, with the exception of one evidence-based review of the effectiveness of psychotherapy that included studies of alcohol use disorders and anxiety (Gatz et al., 1998), meta-analytic studies and evidence-based reviews are lacking.

The evidence-based review suggested that CBT, age-specific group treatment, and supportive and nonconfrontational treatment approaches are effective in the treatment of geriatric alcohol abuse (Gatz et al., 1998). Findings from RCTs suggest that brief, motivationally oriented cognitive-behavioral interventions that include education on the impact of alcohol on older persons appear to be particularly effective (Blow & Barry, 2000; Fleming et al., 1999).

In contrast, pharmacological interventions for geriatric alcohol abuse have less support (Center for Substance Abuse Treatment, 1998; Fingerhood, 2000). For instance, naltrexone can help prevent recidivism when used as a component of alcohol rehabilitation; however, additional research with larger group sizes is needed (Oslin et al., 1997).

Treating older anxiety-disordered adults with either pharmacological or psychosocial treatments has not been extensively researched. Although abundant research exists to support the effectiveness of psychosocial and pharmacological agents among younger adults, the literature provides a limited perspective on the effectiveness of treatments for geriatric anxiety disorders (Krasucki et al., 1999; Sheikh & Cassidy, 2000; Stanley & Beck, 2000). Benzodiazepines are a commonly prescribed treatment; however, few RCTs have been conducted with this population (Stanley & Beck, 2000). CBT is the only psychosocial intervention with empirical support in treating geriatric anxiety (Gatz et al., 1998; Stanley & Novy, 2000). Although several promising psychotherapeutic interventions exist (e.g., supportive group psychotherapy and individual behavior therapy), these interventions have been inadequately studied among older adults with anxiety disorders (Gatz et al., 1998).

Finally, meta-analytic studies or evidence-based reviews that evaluated the treatment of geriatric schizophrenia are lacking. Several RCTs of atypical and conventional antipsychotics among older adults with schizophrenia suggested treatment effectiveness (Howanitz et al., 1999; Verma et al., 2001); however, these studies have not yet been reviewed in aggregate. Although systematic reviews suggested that atypical and conventional agents have similar efficacy among younger patients (Geddes et al., 2000; Leucht et al., 1999), older persons are more susceptible to adverse side effects of conventional antipsychotics (Maixner et al., 1999). In contrast, atypical agents produce fewer motor side effects (e.g., tardive dyskinesia) in older persons (Jeste et al., 2000). However, they are not free from more serious cardiac side effects, including prolonged QTc interval, leading to potential lethal torsades de pointes (Glassman & Bigger, 2001). The only psychosocial interventions designed for older adults with schizophrenia that have been described to date in the research literature were controlled pilot studies that suggested potential benefits of a combination of CBT and skills training (Granholm et al., 2002) and a combination of health management and skills training (Bartels et al., in press).

The Evidence Base for Geriatric Mental Health Services

The literature is limited with respect to the effectiveness of different models of service delivery. A single evidence-based review was identified that found support for the effectiveness of community-based, multidisciplinary geriatric mental health treatment teams (Draper, 2000). In addition, a recent RCT suggested that multidisciplinary psychogeriatric teams may be more cost-effective than usual care due to reduced utilization of inpatient care (Kominski et al., 2001). Hospital-based geriatric psychiatry consultation-liaison services appear to be effective, although further research is necessary to evaluate such programs comprehensively. In contrast, this evidence-based review found no RCTs that assessed the effectiveness of geropsychiatric inpatient units or day hospital programs (Draper, 2000). Finally, a review of the effectiveness of geriatric consul-

tation services to nursing homes (Bartels, Moak, et al., 2002) found one RCT
that indicated a lack of clinically different outcomes between geriatric psychiatry consultation services and usual care.

Summary of the Evidence Base and Limitations

Table 28-3 illustrates selected geriatric mental health interventions supported
by different degrees of evidence, including meta-analyses, evidence-based re-

TABLE 28-3. Selected evidence-based geriatric mental health interventions

Dementia
  Cognitive symptoms
  • Cholinesterase inhibitors.*,†
  • Cognitive retraining/reality orientation.*,†
  Behavioral symptoms
  • Environmental and behavioral modification.*,†
  • Antipsychotics.*,†
  • SSRI antidepressants, anticonvulsants, cholinesterase inhibitors may reduce de-
    pression, agitation, and behavioral problems.‡,§
Geriatric depression
  • Antidepressants (SSRIs, NSSRIs, TCAs).*,†
  • Psychotherapy (cognitive therapy, behavior therapy, cognitive-behavioral
    therapy).*,†
  • Problem-solving therapy, interpersonal therapy, brief psychodynamic therapy, and
    reminiscence therapy may reduce symptoms.*,†
Geriatric alcohol abuse
  • Age-specific, nonconfrontational, brief motivational, and cognitive-behavioral ther-
    apies may be effective.†,‡,§
Geriatric anxiety
  • Limited empirical evidence.
  • Conventional antianxiety agents (e.g., benzodiazepines).§
  • Cognitive-behavioral therapy.†,‡
Geriatric schizophrenia
  • Limited empirical evidence.
  • Efficacy of antipsychotics supported by individual studies and general reviews.‡,§
  • Skills training, community support, and family psychoeducation are recom-
    mended.§
Geriatric mental health services
  • Community-based, multidisciplinary, geriatric mental health teams.†

Source: From Bartels, Dums, et al. (2002). NSSRI, non-SSRI norepinephrine reuptake inhibitors; SSRI,
selective serotonin reuptake inhibitor; TCA, tricyclic antidepressant.
*Meta-analysis.
†Evidence-based review.
‡Individual randomized controlled trial.
§Expert consensus statement or clinical guideline.

views, individual RCTs, and expert consensus panels or clinical guidelines. A growing number of meta-analytic studies and evidence-based reviews demonstrated empirical support for the effectiveness of pharmacological and psychosocial interventions for geriatric mental disorders.

Pharmacological treatment of Alzheimer's disease indicated modest effectiveness of cholinesterase inhibitors in temporarily decreasing cognitive decline and enhancing cognitive function for 6 to 12 months and suggested that antipsychotic agents are modestly effective in the treatment of co-occurring psychosis and agitation. The use of antidepressants was supported in the treatment of geriatric depression.

CBT has established efficacy in the treatment of geriatric depression, alcohol abuse, and anxiety. Environmental modifications and behavioral interventions represent effective psychosocial interventions for behavioral problems in dementia. Caregiver psychoeducation and support can delay nursing home admission of older persons with dementia. Finally, community-based, multidisciplinary geriatric mental health treatment teams are effective in improving clinical outcomes (Bartels, Dums, et al., 2002).

It is important to recognize that the identification of evidence-based practices is, in some respects, a starting point for improving the quality of care. Evidence-based practice literature should be continuously updated to reflect recent research findings. Furthermore, meta-analytic procedures that evaluate interventions must be weighted for methodological rigor and clinical significance. Aggregate analyses are prone to excluding informative studies and may cluster studies without sufficient attention to important differences. These reviews can be affected by small sample sizes, lack of interchangeable instruments and extractable data, and duration of studies (Schneider et al., 1990). Most important, clinical trials do not always generalize to clinical practice due to methodological constraints (Sackett et al., 1996). Although there is controversy surrounding the role and reliability of meta-analyses in clinical decision making, a rigorous meta-analysis of multiple studies has the advantage of using quantitative methods to provide a single best estimate of the effect of an intervention (Friedland et al., 1998; Guyatt & Rennie, 2002).

CHALLENGES TO IMPLEMENTING GERIATRIC MENTAL HEALTH EVIDENCE-BASED PRACTICES

While the evidence base supporting geriatric mental health interventions is growing, there is substantial unmet need for mental health services. Specifically, nearly half of older adults with a recognized mental disorder do not utilize mental health services (George et al., 1988). Although this problem is not unique to older adults, this group is particularly vulnerable to age-related economic and physical barriers to care, gaps in services, and inadequate financing of mental health treatments and services (Administration on Aging, 2001; Fields, 2000; Pace, 1989). A lack of providers with geriatric expertise or spe-

TABLE 28-4. Primary settings and providers within the geriatric mental health services system

• Primary care	• Aging network services
• Long-term care	• Home care
• Specialty mental health care	• Family caregiver
• Hospitals	• Criminal justice system

cialization represents a significant challenge to providing effective mental health services. Although community-based service providers are increasing their capacity to respond to the mental health concerns of older adults, they often continue to lack adequate reimbursement and the staff necessary to provide appropriate prevention and treatment services (Administration on Aging, 2001).

One of the greatest challenges to improving treatment of mental disorders in older persons lies in the fragmentation of the mental health service delivery system (see Table 28-4). Significant differences between providers in these settings complicate the implementation of evidence-based treatments (Burns & Taube, 1990; Gatz & Smyer, 1992). For example, over half of older persons who receive mental health care are treated by primary care physicians (Burns & Taube, 1990; George et al., 1988), yet they often have inadequate time to address psychiatric problems and the full range of competing patient needs (Klinkman, 1997). The implications of these barriers are particularly problematic for older primary care patients with psychiatric disorders, who are at increased risk to receive inappropriate pharmacological treatment and are less likely to be treated with psychotherapeutic interventions compared to younger patients (Bartels et al., 1997).

RESEARCH ON EFFECTIVE APPROACHES TO CHANGING CLINICAL PRACTICE

There is a well-recognized disparity between research that defines the most effective and advanced treatments and actual clinical practice in usual care for both pharmacological and psychosocial interventions. Effective training of clinicians in evidence-based practices is an essential component of mainstreaming these practices into usual care and enhancing the mental health services that older adults receive. Several innovative practice change technologies hold promise for improving the implementation of evidence-based interventions.

Traditional educational programs designed to have an impact on the mental health practices of primary care providers have failed to change physician behavior and improve the outcome of late-life mental illness (Callahan, 2001). For example, simply providing practice guidelines to clinicians without additional measures is ineffective (Grimshaw & Russell, 1993; Oxman, 1998). However, educational interventions that incorporate multiple techniques to actively involve the learner appear to be effective (Oxman, 1998). Academic detailing, consisting of brief, one-on-one physician dialogues and individualized feedback on treatment practices have resulted in short-term improvement in rates of diagnosing depression (Pond et al., 1994) and decreases in inappropriately prescribed medications (Soumerai, 1998; Thomson O'Brien et al., 2000).

System change interventions that modify the process of care within primary care offices have also resulted in significant improvements in quality of care and patient outcomes (Callahan, 2001). Effective interventions include the use of standardized symptom severity measures for treatment response, treatment flow sheets to monitor patient progress (Brody et al., 2000), and registries for scheduling routine follow-up visits (Lin et al., 1995). Care management models in which psychiatric specialists provide supervision to nurse care managers and limited consultation to the prescribing physician also improve the quality of mental health treatment (Oxman & Dietrich, 2002; Rost et al., 2001; Simon et al., 2000). Finally, providing collaborative and integrated geriatric mental health and primary care services in the same setting can improve the implementation and outcomes of evidence-based mental health assessment and treatment (Katon et al., 1995; Katzelnick et al., 2000). Several multicenter randomized trials are currently testing the effectiveness of such models of collaborative care for older primary care patients (Bartels, Coakley, et al., 2002; Coyne et al., 2001; Unützer et al., 2001).

Little is known about improving adherence to empirically based geriatric mental health practices by community mental health providers. Most community-based mental health clinicians lack training in assessment and treatment of mental disorders of aging. A recent study found that less than half of older adults receiving community-based mental health services were routinely assessed for common symptoms and functional problems. However, use of an assessment and treatment planning instrument resulted in broad-based clinician adherence to standardized geriatric assessment practices (Bartels, Miles, et al., 2002).

In summary, an evolving practice research literature identifies several approaches to improving both the knowledge of mental health providers and the clinical care of mentally ill older adults. Successful techniques emphasize educational programs that actively involve the learner and systems change interventions such as integrated care management, assessment and treatment tool kits, automated reminders, and decision support technologies.

PRACTICING AS AN EVIDENCE-BASED CLINICIAN

Despite a growing body of research documenting empirically supported treatments, a substantial gap remains between the knowledge base and services provided in routine clinical settings. Practicing clinicians are only too familiar with the challenge of remaining current in a rapidly changing and expanding field of knowledge. Conventional approaches include subscribing to a number of selected journals and scanning tables of contents and abstracts to identify articles that are relevant to clinical questions that arise in practice. This nonsystematic process is augmented by periodic attendance at selected continuing medical education sessions.

Despite these efforts, the average clinician is unlikely to be exposed to current studies or reviews that directly guide them in implementing evidence-based practices. In turn, the clinician is often left feeling overwhelmed by the demands of too little time and a limited capacity to review and retain a wealth of new and changing information.

In response to this dilemma, recent reforms in medical education have called for clinicians to be trained as competent and facile users of medical knowledge (Carraccio et al., 2002), including computer-based information. For example, Guyatt and Rennie (2002) provided an excellent step-by-step manual with detailed instruction on using and appraising the evidence base, including conducting Web-based searches, reviewing resources that synthesize research, and locating and evaluating individual research studies.

Mental health providers can utilize several information sources to improve understanding of evidence-based practices and implementation of evidence-based protocols (see Table 28-5). The greatest benefit from evidence-based practices is gained when these materials are reliable and readily translatable to clinical practice and when the knowledge base is regularly updated (Lawrie et al., 2001).

Some clinicians turn to treatment practice guidelines, decision trees, or algorithms as the foremost resource for providing quality care (Addis & Krasnow, 2000). Although clinical practice guidelines are readily available for a variety of geriatric mental heath disorders, their use is complicated by several factors. Guidelines typically rely on consensus among a panel of experts, who

---

TABLE 28-5. Information sources for understanding and implementing evidence-based practices

Clinical guidelines
  Example: American Psychiatric Association guidelines.
  Advantage: Rely on consensus among a panel of experts, who weigh the evidence.
  Disadvantage: Clinical guidelines may vary in quality; may be poorly constructed; may under- or overestimate effects or side effects.

Prefiltered databases of systematic reviews
  Example: Cochrane Collaboration, *Evidence-based Mental Health*, Best Evidence.
  Advantage: Authors search, summarize, and evaluate published evidence.
  Disadvantage: A subscription is often required for access; geriatric mental health reviews are limited.

Unfiltered databases of published medical literature
  Example: MEDLINE.
  Advantage: Comprehensive and readily accessible database of medical literature.
  Disadvantage: Care is needed in conducting the search and evaluating the literature.

weigh the evidence supporting different treatment options and recommend specific approaches. However, guidelines and unsystematic reviews, including those from specialty societies, may be poorly constructed and may underestimate or overestimate treatment effects or side effects (Grilli et al., 2000; Shaneyfelt et al., 1999).

Valid guidelines should be based on the presence of a supporting systematic review of evidence linking treatment options to outcomes, discussion of relevant patient groups and preferences or values associated with treatment recommendations, and an indication of the strength of the authors' recommendations (Guyatt & Rennie, 2002). Unfortunately, many conventional unstructured reviews do not apply these criteria. Thus, other approaches are potentially more appropriate.

A practical approach to evaluating the evidence is to consult electronic prefiltered databases, such as the Cochrane Collaboration, *Evidence-Based Mental Health*, or Best Evidence. The authors of these systematic reviews have searched, summarized, and evaluated the published evidence. The Cochrane Collaboration is an international organization that prepares, maintains, and provides quarterly updates of systematic reviews of health care interventions by evaluating RCTs and some high-quality observational studies. *Evidence-Based Mental Health* is a journal consisting of systematic reviews exclusively in the area of mental health. This journal summarizes original articles and reviews that have been published elsewhere, evaluates them using standard criteria, and includes commentary by clinical experts. Finally, Best Evidence provides a restricted review of 170 medical journals that focus on common diseases. Since 1995, this has included selected psychiatric journals and topics in mental health. Similar to the Cochrane products, articles included within Best Evidence meet basic standards of methodological quality (Guyatt & Rennie, 2002).

Despite the potential benefit of these prefiltered databases, these resources have limited applicability in developing fields such as geriatric psychiatry, and access to these products is limited to individuals who either are affiliated with major medical hospitals or educational institutions or are fiscally capable of individually subscribing to or purchasing the product. In general, prefiltered systematic reviews of the mental health literature have only recently been developed. Synopses of the literature from geriatric psychiatry are quite limited, with the most developed systematic reviews available for Alzheimer's disease and depression. However, these resources are likely to increase in capacity and practical value over the coming years.

Unfiltered databases, such as MEDLINE, assist in finding information when prefiltered resources do not provide satisfactory results. MEDLINE is a relatively comprehensive (containing over 11 million citations) and readily accessible database of medical literature. However, the comprehensiveness of MEDLINE necessitates both care in selecting the search strategy (i.e., how to combine, expand, or limit searches) and a thorough understanding of how the database is structured. In addition, MEDLINE places the burden on the searcher to separate the wheat from the chaff to identify studies of similar quality. The provider must precisely specify what information is required to resolve a defined patient problem, conduct an efficient search of the literature, select the best of the relevant studies, apply rules of evidence to determine the study validity, and extract the clinical message and apply it to the problem. Several tips for improving the quality of MEDLINE searches are available in recent publications (Friedland et al., 1998; Gray, 1997; Greenhalgh, 1997; Guyatt & Rennie, 2002; Sackett et al., 1996).

Few data are available that provide an indication of the time needed to train clinicians to become evidence-based practitioners or of available outcome measures that judge the degree to which a clinician practices evidence-based medicine. However, preliminary findings suggest that it is feasible to train early-career physicians to develop skills to access prefiltered resources by incorporating such skills into the overall residency training program (Guyatt, Meade, et al., 2000). In addition, surveys of physicians in general practice suggest that developing the skills to use evidence-based reviews is feasible and requires minimal additional education or training.

For instance, a study of British general practitioners found that most currently use evidence-based summaries (72%) and evidence-based practice guidelines or protocols (84%), yet only 5% believe that learning the skills required to identify and appraise individual original studies is the most effective way to move toward practicing evidence-based medicine (McColl et al., 1998). Efforts to encourage the use of evidence-based medicine may be best focused on improving availability and access to evidence-based summaries and guidelines for geriatric mental health practices. Finally, although it appears that the field of medicine is widely embracing use of evidence-based summaries, the field of psychiatry lags well behind in adopting this systematic approach to practice.

IMPLEMENTATION KITS: A FACILITATED APPROACH TO HELPING CLINICIANS AND SYSTEMS TO DELIVER EVIDENCE-BASED SERVICES

As described above, one approach to becoming an evidence-based clinician is to become skilled in locating and using computer-based systematic reviews of the research literature, augmented by targeted electronic searches. However, for many clinicians, the demands of practice are likely to limit the regular use of this approach. An alternative strategy consists of using prepackaged implementation resource kits. These integrated manuals and resource materials provide clinicians with detailed descriptions of how to deliver a specific evidence-based practice.

Evidence-based implementation resource kits have been piloted in younger populations with severe mental illness, but are yet to be developed for geriatric populations. However, there are several potential advantages to this approach (Drake et al., 2001; Torrey et al., 2001). First, implementation kits are only developed for practices with proven efficacy. Second, practice improvement materials designed for the clinician meet the needs of providers with varying degrees of assessment and treatment expertise. Third, the kits clearly identify evidence-based practices and include clinical decision support systems and guidelines that promote the use of evidence-based practices in the health care setting. Finally, these materials are supplemented by separate implementation resources for other major stakeholder groups, including public mental health authorities, administrators of provider organizations, consumers, and family members (Torrey et al., 2001).

In the future, routine implementation of evidence-based mental health treatments is likely to be facilitated by the widespread use of electronic medical record systems linked to databases with information on effective treatment protocols. Models that are currently in use in medical practices hold promise for improved implementation of mental health evidence-based practices, including automated decision support mechanisms and treatment algorithms that are integrated into computer-based treatment plans and electronic medical records.

LIMITATIONS OF EVIDENCE-BASED PRACTICE METHODOLOGY

Several caveats are in order with respect to evidence-based practice (see Table 28-6). First, evidence alone is inadequate to guide treatment selections. Decisions need to incorporate patient values or preferences. For example, an extensive psychiatric hospitalization accompanied by an intensive course of electroconvulsive therapy may be helpful in addressing treatment-resistant depression in a person with a significant medical illness accompanied by major depression. However, the acceptability of such a treatment is likely to be viewed differently by an 85-year-old man receiving hospice care for terminal cancer who wishes to spend his last months at home compared to a 30-year-old father of young children with a diagnosis of adult-onset diabetes. Second, there is a shortage of

---

TABLE 28-6.   Limitations of the evidence-based practice methodology

1. Evidence alone is inadequate to guide clinical decisions.
2. There is a shortage of consistent scientific evidence of effectiveness.
3. Unique characteristics of the patient challenge generalizability of aggregate evidence.
4. Limited financial resources exist to apply scientifically based advances to broad populations.
5. Evidence-based reviews and meta-analyses are limited to conventional experimental studies of a single intervention.
6. Regardless of the level of evidence, treatment should be guided by consumer preferences, values, and clinical presentation.
7. Conflicts of interest have the potential to bias reporting of research on the effectiveness of interventions.

---

consistent scientific evidence of the effectiveness of interventions for many geriatric mental health problems. It is not uncommon for clinicians to encounter situations for which there is no direct evidence to guide treatment decisions. Third, the unique biological characteristics of the specific patient will always challenge the generalizability and application of aggregate evidence. Fourth, limited financial resources for health care inevitably limit the application of scientifically based advances to broad populations.

A final and important limitation of evidence-based reviews and meta-analyses is that they are limited to data that are largely based on conventional experimental designs that compare single interventions. In this respect, they are unlikely to inform more complex clinical decisions, such as determining the best next agent in a series of failed trials or the use of complex combination therapies. Furthermore, these studies are unlikely to cover the full range of diagnostic subtypes and are also unlikely to consider common comorbid disorders as variables in decision making. Overall, the sheer number of possible sequences and combinations of available treatments for the large number of different clinical conditions makes it impossible to provide clinical recommendations based entirely on data from RCTs (Djulbegovic & Hadley, 1998; Shekelle et al., 1998).

One approach to address gaps left by available evidence-based guidelines uses standardized surveys and quantitative methods to derive expert consensus (Brook et al., 1986). Guidelines on the pharmacotherapy of depression in older patients by Alexopoulos and colleagues (Alexopoulos et al., 2001) provide an example of this method applied to geriatric psychiatry. Using a 9-point rating of the appropriateness of the treatment choice, the authors were able to inquire about a variety of clinical questions, including recommended assessment procedures, acute and maintenance treatment strategies, dosing and duration of treatment, strategies for treatment-resistant conditions, combination therapy, and drug selection in the context of medical comorbidity. As such, this approach represents an alternative guide for clinical decision making when empirically derived data are unavailable or not feasible. However, as always, caution is indicated when using guidelines that are not directly supported by data-based studies and that are derived from expert opinion.

In summary, it is important to stress that the evidence base for treatment consists of a hierarchy of different types of studies and quality of data. There is a misperception that only RCTs or systematic reviews comprise the evidence base for effective treatments. Although RCTs are preferred in evaluating the effectiveness of treatment interventions, evidence-based medicine supports the use of evidence from the best *available* studies corresponding to the clinical situation, complemented by an understanding of the limits of the existing data. In some instances, well-designed, nonrandomized observational outcome studies or small individual trials may constitute the evidence base. In other situations, the clinician is left to rely cautiously on well-designed surveys of experts and consensus guidelines. Regardless of the level of certainty regarding the evidence, final treatment decisions should be informed by knowledge of the patient's unique clinical presentation, values, and preferences (Guyatt & Rennie, 2002).

CONFLICTS OF INTEREST, ETHICAL CONSIDERATIONS, AND POTENTIAL COMPROMISE IN THE OBJECTIVITY OF RESEARCH FINDINGS

As clinicians, researchers, and the general public seek to interpret the results of clinical efficacy studies, they rely on investigators to employ impartiality and integrity in conducting and reporting scientific research. However, the potential for biased actions and reporting of data is a legitimate concern. Industry provides 70% of the financial resources for clinical drug trials conducted in the United States (Bodenheimer, 2000). Interactions with pharmaceutical representatives have been associated with (1) requests for additions to formularies (some of which have little to no advantage over existing formulary drugs); (2) increased awareness, preference, and prescribing of new drugs (combined with decreased prescribing of generic drugs); (3) higher prescribing costs; (4) attitudes that support interactions with pharmaceutical representatives; (5) favorable publications and research findings; and (6) underpublication of unfavorable findings (Choudhry et al., 2002; Wazana, 2000).

Current policies for reporting conflicts of interest vary widely across institutions (Lo et al., 2000). Furthermore, less than half of the leading 48 medical or scientific journals (as measured by the number and rate of citations) reported disclosure of financial interests in published research reports (McCrary et al., 2000). Among 100 authors of clinical guidelines published between 1991 and 1999 for common medical diseases, 87% had a relationship with at least 1 pharmaceutical manufacturer (Choudhry et al., 2002). Despite significant financial interests held by these individuals, only 7% felt that their relationship with the pharmaceutical industry influenced their treatment recommendations (yet, 19% believed that their coauthors were influenced by such a relationship) (Choudhry et al., 2002). Of the 44 published guidelines for which the authors were surveyed, the authors of only 1 reported a financial conflict of interest with the pharmaceutical industry, authors for 1 reported no conflicts of interest, and the remaining 42 did not indicate the existence of potential conflicts of interest (Choudhry et al., 2002). As such, readers cannot assume that conflicts of interest are uniformly disclosed (McCrary et al., 2000).

In summary, conflicts of interest have the potential to bias reporting of research on effectiveness of interventions. Clinicians should take care in reviewing published reports to identify and weigh potential conflicts of interest of the investigators. To counteract biased reporting, it is recommended that clinicians search prefiltered databases, such as the Cochrane database, of systematic reviews that examine the methods, measures, and outcomes of studies and provide an objective, independent analysis of published findings by reviewers who lack conflicts of interest.

CONCLUSION

Several future directions for the field of geriatric psychiatry are suggested by the preceding overview of the rationale, development, and implementation of evidence-based practices in geriatric mental health. First, the gap between empirically supported treatments and their current availability for older persons with mental disorders must be addressed to ensure that older adults have access to the most effective interventions. The failure of conventional educational approaches necessitates the development and use of novel approaches to improving care.

Second, improving the quality of routine clinical practice includes using methods that assist the clinician in making use of current data from an evolving medical literature. For some clinicians, using approaches from evidence-based medicine will include developing the skills to access prefiltered systematic reviews of the research literature, complemented (when necessary) by efficient and focused electronic searches of primary sources. However, for others, the promise of evidence-based medicine is most likely to be realized when evidence-based practices are clearly identified, summarized, and integrated into systems that are used to plan, evaluate, and document care.

The field of geriatric psychiatry has rapidly developed over the past decade and now consists of a spectrum of treatments and services supported by a growing body of empirical research. Enhancing outcomes for the growing number of older persons affected by mental disorders will necessitate that "bridging science and service" (National Institute of Mental Health, 1999) becomes a priority for researchers and clinicians alike.

REFERENCES

Addis ME, Krasnow AD. A national survey of practicing psychologists' attitudes toward psychotherapy treatment manuals. *J Consult Clin Psychol.* 2000;68(2):331–339.

Administration on Aging. *Older Adults and Mental Health: Issues and Opportunities.* Rockville, MD: Dept of Health and Human Services; 2001.

Alexopoulos GS, Katz IR, Reynolds CF, Carpenter D, Docherty JP. The expert consensus guideline series: pharmacotherapy of depressive disorders in older patients. *Postgrad Med Spec Rep.* October 2001:1–86.

Allen-Burge R, Stevens AB, Burgio LD. Effective behavioral interventions for decreasing dementia-related challenging behavior in nursing homes. *Int J Geriatr Psychiatry.* 1996;14:213–228.

American Psychiatric Association. Practice guideline for the treatment of patients with Alzheimer's disease and other dementias of late life. *Am J Psychiatry.* 1997; 154(suppl 5):1–39.

Anderson IM. Selective serotonin reuptake inhibitors versus tricyclic antidepressants: a meta-analysis of efficacy and tolerability. *J Affect Disord.* 2000;58:19–36.

Bains J, Birks JS, Dening TR. The efficacy of antidepressants in the treatment of depression in dementia (Cochrane Review). In: *The Cochrane Library.* Oxford: Update Software;2002, Issue 4.

Banerjee S, Dickinson E. Evidence based health care in old age psychiatry. *Int J Psychiatry Med.* 1997;27:283–292.

Bartels SJ. Quality, costs, and effectiveness of services for older adults with mental disorders: a selective overview of recent advances in geriatric mental health services research. *Curr Opin Psychiatry.* 2002;15:411–416.

Bartels SJ, Coakley E, Oxman TE, et al. Suicidal and death ideation in older primary care patients with depression, anxiety and at-risk alcohol use. *Am J Geriatr Psychiatry.* 2002;10:417–427.

Bartels SJ, Dums AR, Oxman TE, et al. Evidence-based practices in geriatric mental health care. *Psychiatr Serv.* 2002;53:1419–1431.

Bartels SJ, Forester BP, Meuser KT, et al. Enhanced skills training and health care management for older persons with severe mental illness. *Community Ment Health J.* In press.

Bartels SJ, Haley WJ, Dums AR. Implementing evidence-based practices in geriatric mental health. *Generations.* 2002;26:90–98.

Bartels SJ, Horn S, Sharkey P, Levine K. Treatment of depression in older primary care patients in health maintenance organizations. *Int J Psychiatry Med.* 1997;27:215–231.

Bartels SJ, Miles KM, Dums AR. Improving the quality of care for older adults with mental disorders. The outcomes-based treatment planning system of the NH-Dartmouth Psychiatric Research Center. *Home Care Res Initiative.* Spring 2002:1–6.

Bartels SJ, Moak GS, Dums AR. Models of mental health services in nursing homes. *Psychiatr Serv.* 2002;53:1390–1396.

Beers MH, Ouslander JG. Risk factors in geriatric drug prescribing. *Drugs.* 1989;37:105–112.

Bendz H, Aurell M, Balldin J, Mathe AA, Sjodin I. Kidney damage in long-term lithium patients: a cross-sectional study of patients with 15 years or more on lithium. *Nephrol Dial Transplant.* 1994;9:1250–1254.

Beyth RJ, Shorr RI. Epidemiology of adverse drug reactions in the elderly by drug class. *Drugs Aging.* 1999;14:231–239.

Birks J, Flicker L. Selegiline for Alzheimer's disease (Cochrane Review). In: *The Cochrane Library.*Oxford: Update Software; 2003, Issue 1.

Birks J, Grimley EJ, Iakovidou V, Tsolaki M. Rivastigmine for Alzheimer's disease (Cochrane Review). In: *The Cochrane Library.* Oxford: Update Software; 2000, Issue 4.

Birks J, Grimley EJ, Van Dongen M. Ginkgo biloba for cognitive impairment and dementia (Cochrane Review). In: *The Cochrane Library.* Oxford: Update Software; 2002, Issue 4.

Birks JS, Melzer D, Beppu H. Donepezil for mild and moderate Alzheimer's disease (Cochrane Review). In: *The Cochrane Library.* Oxford: Update Software; 2000: Issue 4.

Blow FC, Barry KL. Older patients with at-risk and problem drinking patterns: new developments in brief interventions. *J Geriatr Psychiatry Neurol.* 2000;13:115–123.

Bodenheimer T. Uneasy alliance—clinical investigators and the pharmaceutical industry. *N Engl J Med.* 2000;342:1539–1544.

Brodaty H, Ames D, Boundy KL, et al. Pharmacological treatment of cognitive deficits in Alzheimer's disease. *Med J Aust*. 2001;175:324–329.

Brody D, Dietrich AJ, deGruy F. The Depression in Primary Care Tool Kit. *Int J Psychiatry Med*. 2000;30:99–110.

Brook RH, Chassin MR, Fink A, Solomon DH, Kosecoff J, Park RE. A method for the detailed assessment of the appropriateness of medical technologies. *Int J Technol Assess Health Care*. 1986;2:53–63.

Burke WJ, Folks DG, McNeilly DP. Effective use of anxiolytics in older adults. *Clin Geriatr Med*. 1998;14:47–65.

Burns BJ, Taube CA. Mental health services in general medical care and nursing homes. In: Fogel B, Furino A, Gottlieb G, eds. *Mental Health Policy for Older Americans: Protecting Minds at Risk*. Washington, DC: American Psychiatric Press; 1990: 63–84.

Callahan CM. Quality improvement research on late life depression in primary care. *Med Care*. 2001;39:772–784.

Carraccio C, Wolfsthal SD, Englander R, Ferentz K, Martin C. Shifting paradigms: from Flexner to competencies. *Acad Med*. 2002;77:361–367.

Center for Substance Abuse Treatment. *Treatment Improvement Protocol (TIP) #26. Substance Abuse Among Older Adults*. Rockville, MD: US Dept of Health and Human Services. Public Health Service, Substance Abuse and Mental Health Services Administration, Center for Substance Abuse Treatment; 1998.

Chambless DL, Hollon SD. Defining empirically supported therapies. *J Consult Clin Psychol*. 1998;66:7–18.

Chambless DL, Ollendick TH. Empirically supported psychological interventions: controversies and evidence. *Annu Rev Psychol*. 2001;52:685–716.

Choudhry NK, Stelfox HT, Detsky AS. Relationships between authors of clinical practice guidelines and the pharmaceutical industry. *JAMA*. 2002;287:612–617.

Cochrane AL. *Effectiveness and Efficiency. Random Reflections on Health Services*. London, England: Nuffield Provincial Hospitals Trust; 1972. (Reprinted in 1989 in association with the *BMJ*; reprinted in 1999 for Nuffield Trust by the Royal Society of Medicine Press, London.)

Cochrane Collaboration. Why the "Cochrane" Collaboration? June 21, 2002. Available at: http://www.cochrane.org/cochrane/archieco.htm. Accessed August 1, 2002.

Coyne JC, Brown G, Datto C, Bruce ML, Schulberg HC, Katz I. The benefits of a broader perspective in case-finding for disease management of depression: early lessons from the PROSPECT Study. *Int J Geriatr Psychiatry*. 2001;16:570–576.

Cuijpers P. Psychological outreach programmes for the depressed elderly: a meta-analysis of effects and dropouts. *Int J Geriatr Psychiatry*. 1998;13:41–48.

De Deyn P, Rabheru K, Rasmussen A, et al. A randomized trial of risperidone, placebo, and haloperidol for behavioral symptoms of dementia. *Neurology*. 1999;53:946–955.

Djulbegovic B, Hadley TR. Evaluating the quality of clinical guidelines: linking decisions to medical evidence. *Oncology*. 1998;12:310–314.

Doody RS, Stevens JC, Beck C, et al. Practice parameter: management of dementia (an evidence-based review): report of the Quality Standards Subcommittee of the American Academy of Neurology. *Neurology*. 2001;56:1154–1166.

Drake RE, Goldman HH, Leff HS, et al. Implementing evidence-based practices in routine mental health service settings. *Psychiatr Serv*. 2001;52:179–182.

Draper B. The effectiveness of old age psychiatry services. *Int J Geriatr Psychiatry*. 2000; 15:687–703.

Druss BG, Bradford WD, Rosenheck RA, Radford MJ, Krumholz HM. Quality of medical care and excess mortality in older patients with mental disorders. *Arch Gen Psychiatry*. 2001;58:565–572.

Emre M, Hanaoasi HA. Evidence-based pharmacological treatment of dementia. *Eur J Neurol*. 2000;7:247–253.

Engels GI, Verney M. Efficacy of nonmedical treatments of depression in elders: a quantitative analysis. *J Clin Geropsychol*. 1997;3:17–35.

Fahy S, Lawlor BA. Lithium use in octogenarians. *Int J Geriatr Psychiatry*. 2001;16: 1000–1003.

Fields SD. Clinical practice guidelines: finding and appraising useful, relevant recommendations for geriatric care. *Geriatrics*. 2000;55:59–63.

Fingerhood M. Substance abuse in older people. *J Am Geriatr Soc*. 2000;48:985–995.

Fioravanti M, Flicker L. Efficacy of nicergoline in dementia and other age associated forms of cognitive impairment (Cochrane Review). In: *The Cochrane Library*. Oxford: Update Software; 2001, Issue 4.

Fioravanti M, Yanagi M. Cytidinediphosphocholine (CDP choline) for cognitive and behavioral disturbances associated with chronic cerebral disorders in the elderly (Cochrane Review). *Cochrane Library*. Oxford: Update Software; 2000, Issue 4.

Fleming MF, Manwell LB, Barry KL, Adams W, Stauffacher EA. Brief physician advice for alcohol problems in older adults: a randomized community-based trial. *J Fam Pract*. 1999;48:378–384.

Friedland DJ, Go AS, Davoren JB, et al. *Evidence-Based Medicine: A Framework for Clinical Practice*. Stamford, CT: Appleton & Lange; 1998.

Gambrill E. Evidence-based clinical behavior analysis, evidence-based medicine and the Cochrane collaboration. *J Behav Ther Exp Psychiatry*. 1999;30:1–14.

Gatz M, Fiske A, Fox LS, et al. Empirically validated psychological treatments for older adults. *J Ment Health Aging*. 1998;4:9–46.

Gatz M, Smyer MA. The mental health system and older adults in the 1990s. *Am Psychol*. 1992;47:741–751.

Geddes J, Freemantle N, Harrison P, Bebbington P. Atypical antipsychotics in the treatment of schizophrenia: systematic overview and meta-regression analysis. *BMJ*. 2000;321:1371–1376.

George LK, Blazer DG, Winfield-Laird I, Leaf PJ, Fischbach RL. Psychiatric disorders and mental health service use in later life. In: Brody JA, Maddox GL, eds. *Epidemiology and Aging*. New York, NY: Springer; 1988:189–221.

Gerson S, Belin TR, Kaufman A, Mintz J, Jarvik L. Pharmacological and psychological treatments for depressed older patients: a meta-analysis and overview of recent findings. *Harv Rev Psychiatry*. 1999;7:1–28.

Gerstman BB, Jolson HM, Bauer M, Cho P, Livingston JM, Platt R. The incidence of depression in new users of β-blockers and selected antihypertensives. *J Clin Epidemiol*. 1996;49:809–815.

Giron MS, Wang HX, Bernsten C, Thorslund M, Winblad B, Fastbom J. The appropriateness of drug use in an older nondemented and demented population. *J Am Geriatr Soc*. 2001;49:277–283.

Glassman AH, Bigger JTJ. Antipsychotic drugs: prolonged QTc interval, torsade de pointes, and sudden death. *Am J Psychiatry*. 2001;158:1774–1782.

Granholm E, McQuaid JR, McClure FS, Pedrelli P, Jeste DV. A randomized controlled pilot study of cognitive behavioral social skills training for older patients with schizophrenia. *Schizophr Res.* 2002;53:167–169.

Gray JAM. *Evidence-Based Healthcare: How to Make Health Policy and Management Decisions.* New York, NY: Churchill Livingston; 1997.

Greenhalgh T. How to read a paper: the MEDLINE database. *BMJ.* 1997;315:180–183.

Grilli R, Margrini N, Penna A, Mura G, Liberati A. Practice guidelines developed by specialty societies: the need for a critical appraisal. *Lancet.* 2000;355:103–106.

Grimshaw JM, Russell IT. Effect of clinical guidelines on medical practice: a systematic review of rigorous evaluations. *Lancet.* 1993;342:1317–1322.

Guyatt G, Rennie D. *Users' Guides to the Medical Literature: A Manual for Evidence-Based Clinical Practice/The Evidence-Based Medicine Working Group.* Chicago, IL: AMA Press; 2002.

Guyatt GH, Haynes RB, Jaeschke RZ, et al. for the Evidence-Based Medicine Working Group. Users' guides to the medical literature: XXV. Evidence-based medicine: principles for applying the users' guides to patient care. *JAMA.* 2000;284:1290–1296.

Guyatt GH, Meade MO, Jaeschke RZ, Cook DJ, Haynes RB. Practitioners of evidence based care. *BMJ.* 2000;320:954–955.

Higgins JPT, Flicker L. Lecithin for dementia and cognitive impairment (Cochrane Review). In: *The Cochrane Library.* Oxford: Update Software; 2000, Issue 4.

Hogervorst E, Yaffe K, Richards M, Huppert F. Hormone replacement therapy to maintain cognitive function in women with dementia. (Cochrane Review). In: *The Cochrane Library.* Oxford: Update Software; 2002, Issue 3.

Howanitz E, Pardo M, Smelson DA, et al. The efficacy and safety of clozapine versus chlorpromazine in geriatric schizophrenia. *J Clin Psychiatry.* 1999;60:41–44.

Hussain KM, Kostandy G, Kurz L, Pachter BR. Hemodynamic, electrocardiographic, metabolic, and hematologic abnormalities resulting from lithium intoxication. A case report. *Angiology.* 1997;48:351–354.

Institute of Medicine. *Crossing the Quality Chasm: A New Health System for the 21st Century.* Washington, DC: Institute of Medicine; March 2001.

Jeste DV, Okamoto A, Napolitano J, Kane JM, Martinez RA. Low incidence of persistent tardive dyskinesia in elderly patients with dementia treated with risperidone. *Am J Psychiatry.* 2000;157:1150–1155.

Kasl-Godley J, Gatz M. Psychosocial interventions for individuals with dementia: an integration of theory, therapy, and a clinical understanding of dementia. *Clin Psychol Rev.* 2000;20:755–782.

Katon W, Von Korff M, Lin E, et al. Collaborative management to achieve treatment guidelines. Impact on depression in primary care. *JAMA.* 1995;273:1026–1031.

Katz IR, Jeste DV, Mintzer JE, Clyde C, Napolitano J, Brecher M. Comparison of risperidone and placebo for psychosis and behavioral disturbances associated with dementia: a randomized, double-blind trial. Risperidone Study Group. *J Clin Psychiatry.* 1999;60:107–115.

Katzelnick DJ, Simon GE, Pearson SD, et al. Randomized trial of a depression management program in high utilizers of medical care. *Arch Fam Med.* 2000;9:345–351.

Kirchner V, Kelley CA, Harvey RJ. Thioridazine for dementia (Cochrane Review). In: *The Cochrane Library.* Oxford: Update Software; 2001, Issue 3.

Kirsch A, Moore TJ, Scoboria A, Nicholls SS. The emperor's new drugs: an analysis of antidepressant medication data submitted to the US Food and Drug Administration. *Prev Treat.* 2002;5; July 15. Available at http://journals/apa.org/prevention/volume5/pre0050023a.html. Accessed August 1, 2002.

Klinkman M. Competing demands in psychosocial care: a model for the identification and treatment of depressive disorders in primary care. *Gen Hosp Psychiatry.* 1997; 19:98–111.

Koder DA, Brodaty H, Anstey KJ. Cognitive therapy for depression in the elderly. *Int J Geriatr Psychiatry.* 1996;11:97–107.

Kohn R. β-Blockers an important cause of depression: a medical myth without evidence. *Med Health R I.* 2001;84:92–95.

Kominski G, Andersen R, Bastani R, et al. UPBEAT: the impact of a psychogeriatric intervention in VA medical centers. Unified Psychogeriatric Biopsychosocial Evaluation and Treatment. *Med Care.* 2001;39:500–512.

Krasucki C, Howard R, Mann A. Anxiety and its treatment in the elderly. *Int Psychogeriatr.* 1999;11:25–45.

Laidlaw K. An empirical review of cognitive therapy for late life depression: does research evidence suggest adaptations are necessary for cognitive therapy with older adults. *Clin Psychol Psychother.* 2001;8:1–14.

Lanctot KL, Best TS, Mittmann N, et al. Efficacy and safety of neuroleptics in behavioral disorders associated with dementia. *J Clin Psychiatry.* 1998;59:550–561.

Larsen PD, Hoot Martin JL. Polypharmacy and the elderly. *AORN J.* 1999;69:619–628.

Lavori PW, Rush AJ, Wisniewski SR, et al. Strengthening clinical effectiveness trials: equipoise-stratified randomization. *Biol Psychiatry.* 2001;50:792–801.

Lawrie SM, Scott AIF, Sharpe MC. Implementing evidence-based psychiatry: whose responsibility? *Br J Psychiatry. Special Issue.* 2001;178:195–196.

Lenze EJ, Dew MA, Mazumdar S, et al. Combined pharmacotherapy and psychotherapy as maintenance treatment for late-life depression: effects on social adjustment. *Am J Psychiatry.* 2002;159:466–468.

Leucht S, Pitschel-Walz G, Abraham D, Kissling W. Efficacy and extrapyramidal side-effects of the new antipsychotics olanzapine, quetiapine, risperidone, and sertindole compared to conventional antipsychotics and placebo. A meta-analysis of randomized controlled trials. *Schizophr Res.* 1999;35:51–68.

Lin EH, Von Korff M, Katon W, et al. The role of the primary care physician in patients' adherence to antidepressant therapy. *Med Care.* 1995;33:67–74.

Lo B, Wolf LE, Berkeley A. Conflict-of-interest policies for investigators in clinical trials. *N Engl J Med.* 2000;343:1616–1620.

Lonergan E, Luxenberg J, Colford J. Haloperidol for agitation in dementia (Cochrane Review). In: *The Cochrane Library.* Oxford: Update Software; 2002, Issue 2.

Maixner SM, Mellow AM, Tandon R. The efficacy, safety, and tolerability of antipsychotics in the elderly. *J Clin Psychiatry.* 1999;60(suppl 8):29–41.

McColl A, Smith H, White P, Field J. General practitioner's perceptions of the route to evidence based medicine: a questionnaire survey. *BMJ.* 1998;316:361–365.

McCrary SV, Anderson CB, Jakovljevic J, et al. A national survey of policies on disclosure of conflicts of interest in biomedical research. *N Engl J Med.* 2000;343:1621–1626.

McCusker J, Cole M, Keller E, Bellavance F, Berard A. Effectiveness of treatments of depression in older ambulatory patients. *Arch Int Med.* 1998;158:705–712.

Mittelman MS, Ferris SH, Shulman E, Steinberg G, Levin B. A family intervention to delay nursing home placement of patients with Alzheimer disease: a randomized controlled study. *JAMA.* 1996;276:1725–1731.

Mittmann N, Herrmann N, Einarson TR, et al. The efficacy, safety and tolerability of antidepressants in late life depression: a meta-analysis. *J Affect Disord.* 1997;46: 191–217.

Mulrow CD, Williams JW, Trivedi M, et al. *Treatment of Depression—Newer Pharmacotherapies; Evidence Report/Technology Assessment Number 7.* Rockville, MD: Agency for Health Care Policy and Research; 1999. AHCPR Publication 99-E014.

National Institute for Clinical Excellence. *Technology Appraisal Guidance No. 19: Guidance on the Use of Donepezil, Rivastigmine and Galantamine for the Treatment of Alzheimer's Disease.* London, England: National Institute for Clinical Excellence; 2001.

National Institute of Mental Health. *Bridging Science and Service.* Rockville, MD: National Institute of Mental Health; 1999.

Oken BS, Storzbach DM, Kaye JA. The efficacy of Ginkgo biloba on cognitive function in Alzheimer disease. *Arch Neurol.* 1998;55:1409–1415.

Olin J, Schneider L. Galantamine for Alzheimer's disease (Cochrane Review). In: *The Cochrane Library.* Oxford: Update Software; 2002: Issue 3.

Olin J, Schneider L, Novit A, Luczak S. Hydergine for dementia (Cochrane Review). In: *The Cochrane Library.* Oxford: Update Software; 2001, Issue 2.

Oslin D, Liberto JG, O'Brien J, Krois S, Norbeck J. Naltrexone as an adjunctive treatment for older patients with alcohol dependence. *Am J Geriatr Psychiatry.* 1997;5: 324–332.

Oxman TE. Antidepressants and cognitive impairment in the elderly. *J Clin Psychiatry.* 1996;57(suppl 5):38–44.

Oxman TE. Effective educational techniques for primary care providers: application to the management of psychiatric disorders. *Int J Psychiatry Med.* 1998;28:3–9.

Oxman TE, Dietrich AJ. The key role of primary care physicians in mental health care for elders. *Generations.* 2002;11:59–65.

Pace WD. Geriatric assessment in the office setting. *Geriatrics.* 1989;44(6):29–35.

Perez-Stable EJ, Halliday R, Gardiner PS, et al. The effects of propranolol on cognitive function and quality of life: a randomized trial among patients with diastolic hypertension. *Am J Med.* 2000;108:359–365.

Pinquart M, Soerensen S. How effective are psychotherapeutic and other psychosocial interventions with older adults? A meta-analysis. *J Ment Health Aging.* 2001;7: 207–243.

Pollock BG, Mulsant BH, Rosen J, et al. Comparison of citalopram, perphenazine, and placebo for the acute treatment of psychosis and behavioral disturbances in hospitalized, demented patients. *Am J Psychiatry.* 2002;159:460–465.

Pond C, Mant A, Kehoe L, Hewitt H, Brodaty H. General practitioner diagnosis of depression and dementia in the elderly: can academic detailing make a difference? *Fam Pract.* 1994;11:141–147.

Porsteinsson AP, Tariot PN, Erb R, et al. Placebo-controlled study of divalproex sodium for agitation in dementia. *Am J Geriatr Psychiatry.* 2001;9:58–66.

Qizilbash N, Whitehead A, Higgins J, Wilcock G, Schneider L, Farlow M for the Dementia Trialists' Collaboration. Cholinesterase inhibition for Alzheimer disease: a meta-analysis of the tacrine trials. *JAMA.* 1998;280:1777–1782.

Reynolds CF, Frank E, Perel JM, et al. Nortriptyline and interpersonal psychotherapy as maintenance therapies for recurrent major depression: a randomized controlled trial in patients older than 59 years. *JAMA*. 1999;281:39–45.

Ried LD, McFarland BH, Johnson RE, Brody KK. β-Blockers and depression: the more the murkier? *Ann Pharmacother*. 1998;32:699–708.

Rost K, Nutting P, Smith J, Werner J, Duan N. Improving depression outcomes in community primary care practice: a randomized trial of the QUEST intervention. *J Gen Intern Med*. 2001;16:143–149.

Sackett DL, Rosenberg WM, Gray JA, Haynes RB, Richardson WS. Evidence based medicine: what it is and what it isn't. *BMJ*. 1996;312:71–72.

Schneider LS, Pollock VE, Lyness SA. A meta-analysis of controlled trials of neuroleptic treatment in dementia. *J Am Geriatr Soc*. 1990;38:553–563.

Schneider LS, Tariot PN, Lyketsos CG, et al. NIMH-Clinical Antipsychotic Trials in Intervention Effectiveness (CATIE): Alzheimer's disease trial methodology. *Am J Geriatr Psychiatry*. 2001;9:346–360.

Scogin F, McElreath L. Efficacy of psychosocial treatments for geriatric depression: a quantitative review. *J Consult Clin Psychol*. 1994;62:69–74.

Shaneyfelt TM, Mayo-Smith MF, Rothwangl J. Are guidelines following guidelines? The methodological quality of clinical practice guidelines in the peer-reviewed medical literature. *JAMA*. 1999;281:1900–1905.

Sheikh JI, Cassidy EL. Treatment of anxiety disorders in the elderly: issues and strategies. *J Anxiety Disord*. 2000;14:173–190.

Shekelle PG, Kahan JP, Bernstain SJ, Leape LL, Kamberg CJ, Park RE. The reproducibility of a method to identify the overuse and underuse of medical procedures. *N Engl J Med*. 1998;338:1888–1895.

Simon GE, VonKorff M, Rutter C, Wagner E. Randomised trial of monitoring, feedback, and management of care by telephone to improve treatment of depression in primary care. *BMJ*. 2000;320:550–554.

Sorensen S, Pinquart M, Duberstein P. How effective are interventions with caregivers? An updated meta-analysis. *Gerontologist*. 2002;423:356–372.

Soumerai SB. Principles and uses of academic detailing to improve the management of psychiatric disorders. *Int J Psychiatry Med*. 1998;28:81–96.

Spector A, Orrell M, Davies S, Woods B. Reality orientation for dementia (Cochrane Review). In: *The Cochrane Library*. Oxford: Update Software; 2000: Issue 4.

Stanley MA, Beck JG. Anxiety disorders. *Clin Psychol Rev*. 2000;20:731–754.

Stanley MA, Novy DM. Cognitive-behavior therapy for generalized anxiety in late life: an evaluative overview. *J Anxiety Disord*. 2000;14:191–207.

Street JS, Clark WS, Gannon KS, et al. Olanzapine treatment of psychotic and behavioral symptoms in patients with Alzheimer disease in nursing care facilities: a double-blind, randomized, placebo-controlled study. *Arch Gen Psychiatry*. 2000;57:968–976.

Sultzer DL. Selective serotonin reuptake inhibitors and trazodone for treatment of depression, psychosis, and behavioral symptoms in patients with dementia. *Int Psychogeriatr*. 2000;12(suppl 1):245–251.

Tabet N, Birks J, Grimley Evans J, Orrel M, Spector A. Vitamin E for Alzheimer's disease (Cochrane Review). In: *The Cochrane Library*. Oxford: Update Software; 2000, Issue 4.

Thomson O'Brien MA, Oxman AD, Davis DA, et al. Educational outreach visits: effects on professional practice and health care outcomes (Cochrane Review). In: *The Cochrane Library*. Oxford: Update Software; 2000, Issue 2.

Thorpe L, Whitney DK, Kutcher SP, Kennedy SH. Clinical guidelines for the treatment of depressive disorders 6. Special populations. *Can J Psychiatry*. 2001;46:63S–76S.

Torrey WC, Drake RE, Dixon L, et al. Implementing evidence-based practices for persons with severe mental illnesses. *Psychiatr Serv*. 2001;52:45–50.

Unützer J, Katon W, Williams JWJ, et al. Improving primary care for depression in late life: the design of a multicenter randomized trial. *Med Care*. 2001;39:785–799.

US Department of Health and Human Services. *Mental Health: A Report of the Surgeon General*. Rockville, MD: US Dept of Health and Human Services, Substance Abuse and Mental Health Services Administration, Center for Mental Health Services, National Institutes of Health, National Institute of Mental Health; 1999.

Verma S, Orengo CA, Kunik ME, Hale D, Molinari VA. Tolerability and effectiveness of atypical antipsychotics in male geriatric inpatients. *Int J Geriatr Psychiatry*. 2001;16:223–227.

Wazana A. Physicians and the pharmaceutical industry: is a gift ever just a gift? *JAMA*. 2000;283:373–380.

West S, King V, Carey TS, et al. *Systems to Rate the Strength of Scientific Evidence. Evidence Report/Technology Assessment No. 47*. Rockville, MD: Agency for Healthcare Research and Quality; April 2002. AHRQ Publication 02-E016.

Wilson K, Mottram P, Sivanranthan A, Nightingale A. Antidepressant versus placebo for depressed elderly (Cochrane Review). In: *The Cochrane Library*. Oxford: Update Software; 2001, Issue 2.

29

Electroconvulsive Therapy

Charles H. Kellner, MD
C. Edward Coffey, MD
Robert M. Greenberg, MD

M ajor depression is one of the most common and serious illnesses in the elderly. In addition to death from suicide, depressive illness is associated with substantial mortality from medical illness (Avery & Winokur, 1976). Electroconvulsive therapy (ECT) remains the "gold standard" treatment for serious depression and, as such, requires careful consideration as a therapeutic modality. Such consideration is particularly relevant because there is evidence that ECT is safe and particularly effective in elderly patients (Consensus Conference, 1985; Sackeim, 1998) and because of the sensitivity to the side effects of antidepressant medication experienced by the geriatric population. With the burgeoning of psychopharmacological treatments for depression, many may have believed that ECT was well on its way to extinction; however, we are no longer sanguine about the efficacy of antidepressant medications for all patients. Even with the most sophisticated psychopharmacological treatment combinations, a substantial proportion of patients remain severely ill. For these patients, it is fortunate that ECT remains a viable treatment option.

The case for ECT is strengthened by its record of safety. ECT compares

This chapter is an updated version of a chapter by C. Edward Coffey, MD, and Charles Kellner, MD, "Electroconvulsive Therapy," which appeared in *Textbook of Geriatric Neuropsychiatry*, 2nd ed., American Psychiatric Press (http://www.appi.org), Washington, DC, 2000, pp. 829–860. Used with permission of the publisher.

favorably with other medical procedures for its low morbidity and mortality. With advances in ECT technique, the safety profile of the treatment continues to be refined (Abrams, 1997a, 1997b), and ECT has enjoyed a resurgence as a mainstream treatment. Furthermore, it has a predictably rapid onset of effect (Segman et al., 1995) and can be performed in both inpatient and outpatient settings (Fink et al., 1996).

ECT is most commonly used for the treatment of severe depression. We discuss its use for this indication and evaluate ECT as a treatment for mania, psychosis, and mood disorders because of general medical and neurological conditions, such as poststroke depression and Parkinson's disease. As the mind-body dualism separating the fields of psychiatry and neurology dissolves, investigators and clinicians will have further opportunities to explore the potent effects of ECT on functions of the brain as well as of the mind.

ELECTROCONVULSIVE THERAPY IN GERIATRIC PRACTICE

Considerable evidence suggests that a large proportion of patients receiving ECT are elderly. Kramer (1985) reviewed patterns of ECT use in California between 1977 and 1983 and found that the probability of receiving ECT increased with age of the patient. Patients 65 years and older were given ECT at a rate of 3.86/10,000 population, compared with 0.85/10,000 in those 25 to 44 years old. In an analysis of the data on ECT use in California between 1984 and 1994, Kramer (1999) found similar patterns.

Lambourn and Barrington (1986) surveyed the use of ECT from 1972 to 1983 in a British population of 3 million and found that ECT use was more common in patients (especially female patients) 60 years or older. In a study of 5,729 psychiatric admissions over 3 years, Malla (1988) found that patients who received ECT in general hospitals were significantly older than patients who did not receive ECT.

Babigian and Guttmacher (1984) reviewed a massive data set from the Monroe County (New York) Psychiatric Case Register over three 5-year periods. They found that, among patients hospitalized for the first time, those who received ECT were older than those who did not. Thompson and co-workers (1994) analyzed data from the National Institute of Mental Health Sample Survey program for 1980 and 1986, which included representative samples of psychiatric inpatients in the United States. These researchers found that approximately one third of ECT recipients were 65 years or older, a figure far out of proportion to the representation of that age group in the sample (8.2%).

Several aspects of the natural history, clinical features, and sequelae of major depressive illness help explain the frequent use of ECT in elderly patients. Although age per se does not constitute a particular indication for ECT, a combination of clinical features, alterations in medical sensitivity and responsiveness, and natural history of depression in the elderly may help explain the frequent use of ECT in this population.

Depression in the elderly may be a more severe illness (Post, 1992) with higher rates of psychotic features, particularly in late-onset depression (Meyers & Greenberg, 1986), and higher suicide rates than any other populations (Centers for Disease Control and Prevention [CDC], 1988). The elderly may be more sensitive to medication side effects and may be less tolerant of the combination of antidepressants and antipsychotics typically required to treat psychotic depression. This combination of illness severity and relative medication intolerance may lead to early ECT referral. At least in terms of the morbidity and mortality associated with traditional tricyclic antidepressants, ECT may present less medical risk.

ECT may also be preferred when rapid, definite response is critical, such as in the case of elderly patients whose medical status is compromised by complications of depression, including dehydration and malnutrition. There is some evidence that later life depression may be more resistant to medications, particularly late-onset major depression (Alexopoulos et al., 1996). In contrast, most studies that looked at age as a variable have found greater age to be a positive predictor of ECT response (Black et al., 1993; Coryell & Zimmerman, 1984; O'Connor et al., 2001; Tew et al., 1999).

Without effective treatment, major depression in the elderly may become a severe, frequently relapsing, or chronic disorder with high associated morbidity and mortality. A number of studies have found that the use of ECT is one of the most important variables associated with a positive outcome in later life depression (Bosworth et al., 2002; Philbert et al., 1995; Rubin et al., 1991; Zubenko et al., 1994).

MEDICAL PHYSIOLOGY OF ELECTROCONVULSIVE THERAPY IN ELDERLY PATIENTS

The data on the physiology of ECT have been compiled largely from mixed-age samples, and to our knowledge, few data focus specifically on the physiology of ECT in elderly patients. Clearly, the myriad physiological changes that accompany an ECT seizure take on particular importance in elderly individuals, for whom medical illnesses involving multiple organ systems are common. Of greatest importance are the physiological effects of ECT on the brain and the cardiovascular system. As described separately in this chapter, modifications in ECT technique may be required for patients with brain or cardiovascular disease.

Cerebral Physiology

With ECT, an electrical stimulus is used to depolarize cerebral neurons and thereby produce a generalized cerebral seizure. The mechanism by which

ECT seizures are propagated is not well understood. Bilateral ECT appears to lead to seizure generalization through direct stimulation of the diencephalon, whereas seizures induced with unilateral stimulation may begin focally in the stimulated cortex and then generalize via corticothalamic pathways (Staton, 1981).

During the initial phase of the induced seizure, electroencephalographic activity is variable, consisting of patterns of low-voltage fast activity and polyspike rhythms. These patterns correlate with tonic or irregular clonic motor movements. With seizure progression, electroencephalographic activity evolves into a pattern of hypersynchronous polyspikes and waves that characterize the clonic motor phase. These regular patterns begin to slow and eventually disintegrate as the seizure ends, sometimes terminating abruptly in a flat electroencephalogram (EEG) (Weiner & Krystal, 1993).

The ictal EEG has been the focus of much research aimed at identifying markers of therapeutic response (discussed in a separate section). These studies indicated that age has a major impact on a number of ictal EEG measures and is associated with shorter seizure duration, shorter duration of the slow-wave phase, weaker overall strength and patterning, and lower early ictal, midictal, and postictal amplitudes (Krystal et al., 1995, 1998; Nobler et al., 1993).

The ECT-induced seizure is also associated with a variety of transient and benign changes in cerebral physiology, including increases in cerebral blood flow, cerebral blood volume (resulting in a transient increase in intracranial pressure), and cerebral metabolism of oxygen and glucose (Bolwig et al., 1977; Brodersen et al., 1973; Prohovnik et al., 1986). The brief increase in intracranial pressure is rarely of clinical consequence, but it is the reason for extreme caution when ECT is used in patients with space-occupying mass lesions. Postictally, cerebral flow and metabolism are decreased globally and regionally for at least several hours, and then they return to normal values (Nobler et al., 1994; Rosenberg et al., 1988; Scott et al., 1994; Volkow et al., 1988). Conflicting data exist regarding the interictal effects of ECT, with both reduced (Nobler et al., 1994) and increased (Bonne et al., 1996) cerebral blood flow reported approximately 1 week after a course of ECT. The effects of age on these changes have not been described.

Large, albeit transient, increases in blood–brain barrier permeability and cerebral blood flow also occur during the seizure (Bolwig et al., 1977; Devanand, Dwork, et al., 1994; Ingvar et al., 1983) and may account for the short-lived increase in T_1 relaxation times demonstrated by brain magnetic resonance (MR) imaging after ECT (Mander et al., 1987; Scott et al., 1990). The effects of age and associated brain changes on these blood–brain barrier alterations have not been described in humans, but in animals, age is associated with increased blood–brain permeability changes after 10 electroconvulsive seizures (Oztas et al., 1990).

Cardiovascular Physiology

ECT results in a marked activation of the autonomic nervous system, and the relative balance of parasympathetic and sympathetic nervous system activity determines the observed cardiovascular effects (Applegate, 1997). Vagal (parasympathetic) tone is increased during and immediately after administration of the electrical stimulus, and this may be manifested by bradycardia or even a brief period of asystole. With development of the seizure, activation of the sympathetic nervous system occurs, resulting in a marked increase in heart rate, blood pressure, and cardiac workload. Peripheral stigmata of sympathetic activation may also be observed and include piloerection and gooseflesh.

The tachycardia and hypertension continue through the ictus and generally end along with the seizure. Shortly after the seizure, there may be a second period of increased vagal tone that may be manifested by bradycardia and various dysrhythmias, including ectopic beats. As the patient awakens from anesthesia, there may be an additional period of increased heart rate and blood pressure as a result of arousal and further sympathetic outflow (Welch & Drop, 1989).

The cardiovascular responses during ECT combine to produce an increase in myocardial oxygen demand and a decrease in coronary artery diastolic filling time. Transient electrocardiographic changes in the ST and T waves are seen in some patients during the procedure, but it is unclear whether these findings are related to myocardial ischemia (Gould et al., 1983; McCall, 1997; Wesner, 1986; Zvara et al., 1997). A direct effect of central nervous system stimulation on cardiac repolarization has been proposed as an alternative mechanism (Welch & Drop, 1989). No corresponding increase in levels of cardiac enzymes has been found to accompany these electrocardiographic changes (Braasch & Demaso, 1980). In a study of patients receiving ECT, Messina and colleagues (1992) obtained echocardiograms during and after ECT treatments and found transient regional wall motion abnormalities more often in patients with ST-T changes on electrocardiograms (ECGs), suggesting a period of demand myocardial ischemia. The clinical importance of these findings remains to be evaluated.

The effects of age on the cardiovascular response to ECT have been examined in only a few modern studies. Shettar and coworkers (1989) randomly assigned 19 patients (mean age $\pm$ SD was 51 ± 21 years; range 19–84 years) to ECT with pretreatment with glycopyrrolate or with placebo, the alternate pretreatment drug used for the subsequent ECT treatment (i.e., each patient served as his or her own control). For both types of pretreatment, there was no correlation between age and length of poststimulus asystole. In two controlled studies of mixed-age samples that included elderly patients (Prudic et al., 1987; Webb et al., 1990), no relationship was found between age and ECT-induced changes in heart rate, blood pressure, or rate-pressure product. In a study of relatively younger patients (mean age 43 years, range 20–64 years), Huang and associates (1989) noted a significant inverse correlation between age and increases in blood pressure and rate-pressure product.

Although these results suggest that age per se is not associated with the extent of the cardiovascular response to ECT, these findings must be interpreted cautiously. Some of the subjects in these studies (especially those who were older) were also receiving antihypertensive drug therapy that may have attenuated their cardiovascular response to the treatments (as discussed in the section on cardiovascular side effects). Other clinical observations suggest that at least some elderly patients with cardiovascular disease may be at risk for marked increases in pulse and blood pressure during ECT (Applegate, 1997; Bodley & Fenwick, 1966; Gerring & Shields, 1982; Zielinski et al., 1993).

DIAGNOSTIC INDICATIONS AND EFFICACY

Major Depression

The most common indication for ECT in the elderly population remains depression, both unipolar and bipolar. In elderly patients with depression, ECT is typically used as a second-line treatment, after patients have failed to respond to a trial of medication or have exhibited intolerance of the side effects of medication. ECT should be considered a first-line intervention, however, in certain situations: severe suicidality, severe delusional depression, inanition and malnutrition, history of previous response to ECT, or patient preference (American Psychiatric Association [APA], 2000).

Several clinical studies involving mixed-age samples and various diagnoses have found increasing age to be associated with a favorable outcome from ECT (Black et al., 1993; Carney et al., 1965; Coryell & Zimmerman, 1984; Folstein et al., 1973; Gold & Chiarella, 1944; Kahn et al., 1959; Mendels, 1965; O'Connor et al., 2001; Roberts, 1959; Strömgren, 1973). Investigators in other studies involving older patients have reported a diminished response to unilateral, but not bilateral, ECT (Heshe et al., 1978; Pettinati et al., 1986; Strömgren, 1973) or a requirement for longer courses of treatment (Ottosson, 1960; Rich et al., 1984b). These studies did not, however, take into account the issue of stimulus dosing, which we now know is critical for effective unilateral ECT and an important variable in the rate of response with both unilateral and bilateral ECT (see section on stimulus dosing).

The effects of ECT in elderly patients with depression have been directly examined in a small number of studies, but results are somewhat difficult to compare because of differences in patient samples (e.g., size and diagnosis), ECT technique (e.g., stimulus waveform, dosage, and electrode placement), and assessment methodology (Table 29-1). Nevertheless, reported response rates range from 63% to 98%, clearly demonstrating that increasing age per se does not have a negative impact on the effectiveness of ECT for depressive illness. In fact, there is evidence to suggest that ECT is even more effective in the elderly than in younger age groups (O'Connor et al., 2001). Indeed, other data (although uncontrolled) indicated that ECT is associated with reduced chronicity, decreased morbidity, and decreased mortality (Avery & Winokur, 1976; Babigian & Guttmacher, 1984; Wesner & Winokur, 1989).

There are no controlled, prospective, randomized studies comparing the efficacy and side effects of ECT versus drug therapy for treatment of depression in elderly patients. In a retrospective chart review of 112 consecutive geriatric hospital admissions, Meyers and Mei-Tal (1985–1986) compared outcome in depressed patients who had received ECT with outcome in those who had received tricyclic antidepressants (nonrandom assignment) and found that ECT was associated with a better response rate (81% vs. 62%) and a lower morbidity rate (0% vs. 27%).

Because major depression in elderly patients appears to respond well to ECT, there may be little need to correlate specific clinical features with ECT response. However, in the case of data derived largely from mixed-age samples, a particularly good response to ECT has been associated with the presence of psychosis, catatonia, pseudodementia, pathological guilt, anhedonia, agitation, and neurovegetative signs (Greenberg & Fink, 1992; Hickie et al., 1996; Salzman, 1982; Zorumski et al., 1988).

In a prospective study involving 29 elderly patients (Fraser & Glass 1980), guilt, anhedonia, and agitation were identified as positive prognostic signs. In multiple studies, response to ECT has been particularly good in patients with delusional depression compared with a nonpsychotic group (Hickie et al., 1996; Mulsant et al., 1991; Pande et al., 1990; Petrides et al., 2001; Wilkinson et al., 1993), although other studies have found no difference (O'Leary et al., 1995; Rich et al., 1984a, 1986; Sobin, Prudic, et al., 1995; Solan et al., 1988).

The use of ECT in agitated or psychotic elderly patients may spare them exposure to neuroleptic agents. This consideration is important, given the high risk of tardive dyskinesia and drug-induced parkinsonism in elderly patients (Jenike, 1985), although this risk is likely diminished since the introduction of atypical antipsychotics.

Several authors have also attempted to identify predictors of nonresponse to ECT. In a retrospective study, Magni and coworkers (1988) compared elderly patients who responded to ECT and those who did not respond and found that physical illness during the index episode, fewer negative life events preceding the onset of the index episode, and prior depressive episodes of long duration were predictive of nonresponse to ECT. Other investigators have found that longer duration of the index episode predicts poorer outcome (Fraser & Glass, 1980; Karlinsky & Shulman, 1984).

Previous courses of ECT and increased age at the time of first treatment with ECT have been linked with a slower response rate to ECT, with no effect

TABLE 29-1. Studies of electroconvulsive therapy (ECT) as a treatment for geriatric depression

Study	Subjects	Methods	Findings
Fraser and Glass, 1980	29 patients (8 men, 21 women); age 64–86 years; depressive illness by Feighner criteria*	Prospective; ECT two times/ week; chopped sine wave; randomized assignment to bilateral ($n = 16$) or right unilateral ($n = 13$) electrode placement; blinded outcome rating	Both groups had significant reductions in HRSD score 3 weeks after last treatment, at which point 28 patients (97%) showed "satisfactory" clinical outcome; no group differences in therapeutic response; average time to reorientation after fifth ECT treatment was 32.8 minutes for bilateral ECT and 9.5 minutes for right unilateral ECT; WMS scores improved during ECT, and 3 weeks after ECT all scores were normal; no group differences
Gaspar and Samarasinghe, 1982	33 patients (9 men, 24 women); age 66–88 years (mean ± SD, 73.9 ± 5.7 years); depression in 28 (85%) of 33 patients; diagnostic criteria unspecified	Prospective; ECT two times/week for 3–4 weeks, then one time/ week; mean number of ECT treatments 8.7 (range 2–29); bilateral; outcome rated as good, intermediate poor	Good outcome in 26 patients (79%), intermediate outcome in 3 (9%), poor outcome in 4 (12%)
Karlinsky and Shulman, 1984	33 inpatients (11 men, 22 women); age 62–85 years (mean ± SD, 73.2 ± 5.0 years); DSM-III major depression, single episode, in 12 patients (36.4%); major depression, recurrent, in 18 (54.5%); bipolar disorder in 3 (9.1%)	Retrospective; ECT two or three times/week; sine wave; unilateral ($n = 23$, 69.7%), bilateral ($n = 3$, 9.1%), or both ($n = 7$, 21.2%); nonblinded outcome rating by author consensus from clinical progress notes; follow-up at 3 and 6 months	Immediate "good" response in 14 patients (42.4%), "moderate" response in 12 (36.4%), "poor" response in 7 (21.2%); during 6-month follow-up, 23 patients (69.7%) remained out of hospital, and 6 (18.2%) received more ECT; only one complication (pneumonia), and even this patient was able to complete ECT course

Burke et al., 1985	30 patients (7 men, 23 women); age 60–82 years (mean 72 years); *DSM-III* major depression in 24 patients, bipolar disorder in 5	Retrospective; average number of ECT treatments 9 (range 1–25); brief pulse; bilateral in 70%; outcome rating (4-point scale) determined by review of medical records	92% of patients with major depression improved, and 69% showed complete symptom resolution
Burke et al., 1987	136 patients (39 men, 97 women); mean age of total sample 48 years; 96 subjects <60 years (mean ± SD, 39 ± 12.19 years), 40 subjects >60 years (mean ± SD, 69 ± 6.43 years); 81% of total sample had a major affective disorder; diagnoses of elderly subgroup unspecified	Sine wave; bilateral in 87%, unilateral in 73%; mean number (±SD) of ECT treatments 9 ± 3.6	70% of total sample had complete resolution of affective symptoms (61% <60 years, 75% >60 years); complication rates increased with age (35% in older group, 18% in younger group)
Kramer, 1987	50 inpatients (9 men, 41 women); age 61–88 years (mean 74.1 years); *DSM-III* major depression in 49 patients, schizophrenia in 1	Retrospective; ECT three times/week; brief pulse; bilateral all patients; nonblinded assessment by author's chart review	46 patients (92%) "much improved" after ECT; no serious medical complications
Godber et al., 1987	163 patients (43 men, 120 women); mean age 86 years; all >65 years; primary depression by Feighner criteria* in 153 patients (94%), psychotic symptoms in 80 (49%)	ECT two times/week for most patients, three times/week for those slow to respond; sine wave; right unilateral in 155 patients (95%); mean number of ECT treatments 11.2	83 patients (51%) "fully recovered," 37 (23%) "much improved," 34 (21%) poor response

(continued)

853

TABLE 29-1. *Continued*

Study	Subjects	Methods	Findings
Magni et al., 1988	30 patients (14 men, 16 women); mean age 73.9 years; *DSM-III* major depression	Retrospective; ECT two or three times/week initially, then once weekly; bilateral in all patients; minimum of 7 ECT treatments (range 7–12); independent clinical rating by two psychiatrists	19 patients (63%) responded to ECT
Coffey et al., 1988	44 inpatients (18 men and 26 women) with leukoencephalopathy; age 60–86 years (mean 73 years); *DSM-III* major depression in all patients	Retrospective; ECT three times/ week; brief-pulse, "moderately suprathreshold" stimulus; average number of ECT treatments 9 (range 6–14); nonblinded global ratings of clinical response	"Excellent" response in 54%, "good" response in 44%
Coffey et al., 1989	51 inpatients (15 men, 36 women); age 60–90 years (mean 71.3 years); *DSM-III* major or bipolar depression in 49 patients, organic affective disorder in 2	Prospective; ECT three times/ week; brief pulse; unilateral ($n = 38$), bilateral ($n = 3$), or both ($n = 10$); mean number of ECT treatments 9 (range 5–18); nonblinded observer and patient self-rating	42 patients (82%) met criteria for full therapeutic response; no association between ECT response and brain white matter abnormalities on magnetic resonance images

Study	Sample / Methods	Design	Results
Mulsant et al., 1991	42 inpatients (7 men, 35 women); age 60–89 years (mean ± SD, 73.5 ± 7.3 years); *DSM-III* major depression	Prospective; ECT three times/week; brief pulse; unilateral ($n = 29$, 69%), bilateral ($n = 3$, 7%), or unilateral and then bilateral ($n = 10$, 24%); mean number of ECT treatments 8.3 (range 4–13); HRSD, BPRS, and MMSE scores used for outcome rating, obtained by research nurses	28 patients (67%) had excellent response to ECT (50% decrease in HRSD score); 38 patients had decrease in BPRS score; no significant change in mean MMSE scores for group
Rubin et al., 1991	101 inpatients (19 men, 82 women); mean age (±SD) 76.0 ± 6.4 years; *DSM-III* unipolar depression	Retrospective; 46 patients (46%) received ECT (technique not described), some in combination with antidepressant drug therapy; 65 (64%) received antidepressant drug therapy only; nonrandomized; nonblinded retrospective outcome rating by unit director	Relative to patients treated with drug therapy, those who received ECT had significantly lower final BDI scores and higher frequency of ratings of "major improvement" (78% vs. 42% for non-ECT group)
Kellner et al., 1992	15 patients (11 men, 4 women); age 53–87 (mean 69.9 years); *DSM-III* major depression	Prospective; blinded rating of outcome measures, including cognitive assessment and antidepressant response; randomized assignment to ECT one time/week or three times/week for 3 weeks; brief pulse; bilateral	All patients improved; mean HRSD scores decreased from 27 to 12 in three times/week group and from 29 to 20 in one time/week group; no difference in cognitive effects between groups

(continued)

855

TABLE 29-1. *Continued*

Study	Subjects	Methods	Findings
Wilkinson et al., 1993	78 patients (23 men, 55 women); four age groups (18–39, 40–64, 65–74, and 75–88 years); 43 patients >65 years (mean 68.96 years in age 65–74 years group and and 79.50 years in age 75–88 years group); *DSM-III* major depression with melancholia or psychosis	Prospective; ECT two times/ week; right unilateral in 5 patients (6%), bilateral in remainder; mean number of ECT treatments 7.9; nonblinded cognitive and affective ratings; positive response to ECT defined as >50% reduction in Montgomery Asberg Depression Rating Scale	Positive response to ECT in 73% of patients >65 years and 54% of patients <65 years; age associated with response to ECT and with more improvement in cognition on MMSE with ECT
Casey and Davis, 1996	19 patients (8 men, 16 women); mean age 79.5 years; *DSM-III* major depression in 18 patients; bipolar disorder in 1	Retrospective; brief-pulse ECT (22 courses); nonrandomized electrode placement (bilateral, $n = 13$; unilateral, $n = 1$; both $n = 8$); nonblinded assessment of "complication," "confusion," and clinical response (4-point scale)	Clinical response (rating >3) achieved in 19 (86.3%) courses; response associated with younger age, lower ASA rating, and absence of neurological disorder; dental (1), cardiovascular (2), urinary retention (1), and confusion (1)
Tomac et al., 1997	34 patients >85 years old (79% female); mean age 81 years (range 85–96); *DSM-III* major depression (85%), bipolar disorder (9%), depressive disorder NOS (3%), delusional disorder (3%), and dementia NOS (59%)	Retrospective; brief-pulse ECT three times/week (mean 7 ECTs); nonrandomized electrode placement (unilateral, 65%; bilateral, 18%; and both, 17%); stimulus dosage at 150%–200% initial seizure threshold; nonblinded assessment of therapeutic response and treatment complications	Significant increase in GAF (mean 8.2 points, $n = 30$) and significant decrease in HRSD (mean 5.7 points, $n = 16$) and BPRS (mean 47.2 points, $n = 18$); significant increase in MMSE scores (mean 2.6 points, $n = 20$); treatment complications in 27 (79%), with most common confusion or delirium (32%), transient hypertension (67%), and arrhythmia (24%)

Study	Patients	Methods	Results
Gormley et al., 1998	67 patients >75 years old (73% female); mean age 79.4 years (range 75–91); ICD-10 recurrent depression (78%), bipolar disorder (15%), or depressive disorder (7%)	Retrospective; brief-pulse ECT twice weekly (mean 6.7 ECTs); nonrandomized electrode placement (bilateral, 95%; unilateral, 2%; both, 3%); nonblinded assessment of therapeutic response (4-pont scale), "complications," "confusion," and "memory impairment"	Marked improvement in 53% and moderate improvement in 32%; complications in 11% (prolonged confusion, 6.5%; hypomania, 4%; hypertension, 2%; headache, 2%)
Tew et al., 1999	268 women; 133 adult patients (<60 years); 63 young-old patients (age 60–74 years); 72 old-old patients (>75 years); DSM-III-R major depression	Prospective; brief-pulse ECT three times/week; nonrandomized electrode placement (bilateral, $n = 22$; unilateral, $n = 136$; both, $n = 87$); stimulus dosage at 2.5 times initial seizure threshold; nonblinded assessment of therapeutic response (HRSD score <10 at 3 days after last ECT) and of MMSE scores	Adult group had lower response rate (54%) than young-old group (73%), whereas old-old group had an intermediate rate of response (67%); no relation of response to burden of medical illness; only adult group showed significant decline in MMSE scores at 3 days post-ECT

on eventual positive outcome (Rich et al., 1984b; Salzman, 1982; Shapira & Lerer, 1999). Sackeim and others have demonstrated lower response rates and higher post-ECT relapse rates in patients who had pre-ECT relative medication resistance (Flint & Rifat, 1998; Prudic et al., 1990, 1996; Sackeim et al., 1990; Shapira et al., 1995).

These limited data should not discourage the clinician from initiating a trial of ECT in patients with any of the aforementioned predictors of non-response. The fact that patients who receive ECT come from a selected population that is less responsive to antidepressant medication and generally at greater risk for relapse underscores the value of this treatment for the most difficult to treat elderly patients.

Efforts at using biological markers to predict ECT response in elderly patients have met with equivocal success. A variety of probes have been investigated in mixed-age samples, including the dexamethasone suppression test (DST), the thyrotropin-releasing hormone (TRH) test, and other neuroendocrine tests (Decina et al., 1987; Kamil & Joffe, 1991; Kirkegaard et al., 1975; Krog-Meyer et al., 1984; Papakostas et al., 1981; Swartz, 1993), as well as polysomnographic studies (Coffey et al., 1988; Grunhaus et al., 1996). None of these laboratory studies appears to be strong "state-specific" markers for major depressive illness, and data are inconsistent (Devanand et al., 1991) on whether they can be used serially to follow the course of ECT, predict outcome, or predict early relapse.

Several reports have focused on the efficacy and safety of ECT in the old-old (variably defined as between 75 and 85 years of age and older) (Casey & Davis 1996; Cattan et al., 1990; Gormley et al., 1998; Manly et al., 2000). These reports extend the general conclusions that ECT remains a highly effective and well-tolerated procedure even in the most elderly population. There was a trend in some case series, although not others, toward a higher rate of post-ECT confusion or generally mild cardiovascular complications. Generalizability is limited by the retrospective design of the reports and wide variability in patient characteristics, treatment techniques, assessment methods, and definitions of "complications" vis-à-vis common, transient physiological effects of ECT. In summary, the preponderance of data and clinical experience suggest that the response rate of major depression to ECT is at least as high, if not higher, in older than in younger patients.

Although few studies have directly compared residual depressive symptoms following ECT and pharmacotherapy, it is likely that full remission is more common following ECT (Hamilton, 1982). Residual depressive symptoms have a serious impact on the quality of life and may result in chronicity of depression in the elderly and increase the likelihood of relapse (Prien & Kupfer, 1986). A number of studies have suggested that use of ECT is one of the most important variables in predicting a positive outcome of depression in the elderly, with reduced chronicity, decreased morbidity, and possibly decreased mortality (Avery & Winokur, 1976; Babigian & Guttmacher, 1984; Philbert et al., 1995; Wesner & Winokur, 1989; Zubenko et al., 1994).

Mania

Although extensive clinical experience indicates that ECT is effective for treating both the manic and depressed phases of bipolar illness in elderly patients, formal data for this population are lacking. A small number of controlled studies involving relatively young mixed-age samples have found ECT to be superior to drug therapy (Mukherjee, 1988; Mukherjee et al., 1994; Small et al., 1988, 1991). ECT appeared to be particularly effective in mixed bipolar states and agitated mania, conditions that may become more prevalent as the illness becomes more chronic and refractory (Calabrese et al., 1993). ECT may be particularly suitable for elderly patients who have this more severe form of bipolar disorder. Also, morbidity from ECT is likely to be less risky than the cardiovascular risks of a sustained period of mania in an older person.

Anticonvulsant medications are often effective in mixed bipolar disorder (Calabrese et al., 1993), although we are not aware of efficacy studies testing this use of anticonvulsants in elderly patients. ECT itself also has powerful anticonvulsant properties (Coffey et al., 1995b; Sackeim et al., 1983). Whether bilateral ECT is more effective than nondominant unilateral ECT in the treatment of mania remains controversial (Black et al., 1986; Milstein et al., 1987; Mukherjee et al., 1988, 1994; Small et al., 1991).

Schizophrenia and Other Psychotic Disorders

No controlled data exist on the use of ECT in elderly patients with schizophrenia. ECT has been used in relatively younger patients with this illness, and in these patients, the presence of affective or catatonic features, an acute onset of illness with relatively brief duration, or a history of response to ECT correlate with good outcome (APA, 2000). ECT is not very effective for treating the chronic, residual phase of the illness with predominant negative features (Weiner & Coffey, 1988). These "deficit" states become more common as the illness progresses (Kaplan & Sadock, 1988) and thus should be highly represented in elderly schizophrenic populations, although controlled data on this issue are lacking. To the best of our knowledge, there are no systematically collected data on the efficacy of ECT in patients with late-onset functional psychoses, such as late-onset schizophrenia.

Affective Disorder in Dementia

Of patients with dementia, 20% to 30% have marked concomitant depression, and 10% to 15% of patients with a diagnosis of dementia actually have reversible cognitive impairment associated with depression (Price & McAllister, 1989; Rummans et al., 1999). Depression may be difficult to diagnose in demented patients. Some patients with dementia may be too ill to generate depressive complaints. Affective disorder may manifest itself as agitated, screaming behavior with neurovegetative signs in such patients. Determining whether there is a personal or family history of affective disorder may be helpful in diagnosing depression in these patients (Fogel, 1988). Thorough treatment of depression in patients with dementia often does much to enhance quality of life and functional status (Benbow, 1988; Carlyle et al., 1991; Fogel, 1988; Grant & Mohan, 2001; Holmberg et al., 1996; Krystal & Coffey 1997; Nelson & Rosenberg, 1991; Price & McCallister, 1989; Weintraub & Lippmann, 2001; Zwil et al., 1992).

In a literature review of 56 patients with dementia and depression treated with ECT, Price and McAllister (1989) found a 73% rate of response of depression. ECT effectively treated depression in several subtypes of dementia, including senile dementia of the Alzheimer's type, multiinfarct dementia, and normal-pressure hydrocephalus, as well as the dementias of Parkinson's disease and Huntington's disease (Price & McAllister, 1989). Location of the electrodes was not specified in the majority of the cases reviewed. Nearly one third of patients with dementia also had an improvement in cognition after ECT. Delirium was a relatively infrequent complication of ECT in these patients (overall occurrence, 21%), clearing by the time of discharge in all but one patient.

To minimize cognitive side effects of ECT, physicians of patients with dementia may need to pay special attention to issues of concomitant medications, electrode placement, and frequency of treatments (discussed separately below). Prospective studies are needed to address the efficacy and side effects of ECT in depressed patients with dementia. Particular attention needs to be paid to issues of informed consent or proxy consent (see section on pretreatment evaluation) in this population.

Parkinson's Disease

Because of the limited treatment options for patients with Parkinson's disease, particularly when medication fails or cannot be tolerated, ECT has been assessed as a treatment option (Table 29-2). Case reports suggest that ECT may be an effective treatment for both the motor manifestations of Parkinson's disease and the commonly associated depression (for a review, see Kellner & Bernstein, 1993). Interestingly, some patients experience improvement in motor symptoms, but not improvement in mood, or vice versa (Kellner & Bernstein, 1993; Young et al., 1985).

A group of Swedish investigators (Andersen et al., 1987) performed the most methodologically rigorous trial of ECT in Parkinson's disease. In this double-blind, controlled, crossover design comparison of real ECT and sham ECT, 9 (82%) of 11 nondepressed elderly patients with the on-off phenomenon experienced substantial improvement in parkinsonian symptoms with ECT, with the improvement lasting 2 to 6 weeks. Sham ECT was ineffective. Bilateral ECT was received by 9 patients (8 responded, 1 did not respond), and 2 patients received right unilateral ECT (1 responded, 1 did not respond). Five to six treatments were given during the active phase of the trial. The stimulus-dosing strategy was not fully detailed in the report.

In a prospective naturalistic study, Douyon and associates (1989) studied seven patients with both Parkinson's disease and major depression. Substantial improvement in motor function was noted after only two bilateral treatments. Following an average of seven bilateral ECT treatments, with "just-above-threshold" stimulus dosing, mean New York University Parkinson's Disease Rating Scale scores decreased from 65 to 32 (51% improvement). Patients remained well, without further ECT, for 4 weeks to 6 months. Although initial Hamilton Depression Scale scores were determined for all patients (all scores were above 20), follow-up scores were determined for only four. Depression scores decreased by a mean of 50% in these patients.

In the report of another prospective naturalistic study, Zervas and Fink (1991) described the ECT treatment of four nondepressed elderly patients with severe, refractory Parkinson's disease. Three of the four patients received bilateral ECT. Stimulus-dosing strategies were not specified. Improvement in parkinsonism rating scores of 20% to 40% was observed. Two patients were successfully treated with ongoing maintenance ECT, but once it was discontinued, both patients relapsed within 4 to 6 weeks. Finally, ECT has also been found to be effective for neuroleptic-induced parkinsonism (Hermesh et al., 1992).

Rasmussen and Abrams (1991) suggested that the primary indication for ECT in Parkinson's disease is refractoriness to, or intolerance of, antiparkinsonian medication in patients with severe disability from the disease. They recommended that ECT for Parkinson's disease be initiated with right unilateral placement at substantially suprathreshold electrical dosage, with a switch to bilateral ECT if no response is seen after three unilateral treatments. However, some patient's with Parkinson's disease may be at increased risk of developing delirium during ECT (Figiel et al., 1991; Nymeyer & Grossberg, 1997), a complication that could be worsened using bilateral electrode placement. For patients who have clearly benefited from ECT, Rasmussen and Abrams (1991) recommended maintenance ECT administered just frequently enough to maintain improvement. Aarsland and coworkers (1997) reported on two additional patients whose Parkinson's disease was successfully treated with maintenance ECT, and others have reported its utility for this purpose as well (Krystal & Coffey, 1997; Wengel et al., 1998).

Poststroke Depression

Approximately one third of patients develop marked depression in the 2 years after a stroke (Robinson & Price, 1982; Rummans et al., 1999). In a placebo-

TABLE 29-2. Electroconvulsive therapy (ECT) for the treatment of Parkinson's disease

Study	Number of subjects	Diagnosis	ECT course	Treatment response
Fromm, 1959	8	Parkinson's disease	5–6 bilateral ECT treatments	Improvement: 5 patients Mild improvement: 2 patients No improvement: 1 patient
Brown, 1973	7	Parkinson's disease and major depression	Average of 8 ECT treatments (electrode placement unknown)	No improvement in Parkinson's symptoms No improvement in depression
Lebensohn and Jenkins, 1975	2	Parkinson's disease and depression 1 patient Parkinson's disease and bipolar disorder, depressed: 1 patient	4–6 ECT treatments (electrode placement unknown)	Improvement in Parkinson's symptoms: 2 patients Improvement in depressive symptoms: 2 patients
Lipper and Bermanzohn, 1975	1	Parkinson's disease and psychotic depression	7 ECT treatments (electrode placement unknown)	Marked improvement in depression Improvement in Parkinson's symptoms
Dysken et al., 1976	1	Parkinson's disease and depression	12 bilateral ECT treatments	Improvement in Parkinson's symptoms Improvement in depressive symptoms
Asnis, 1977	1	Parkinson's disease and psychotic depression	6 bilateral ECT treatments	Improvement in Parkinson's symptoms Improvement in depressive symptoms

Reference	N	Diagnosis	Treatment	Outcome
Yudofsky, 1979	1	Parkinson's disease and psychotic depression	10 ECT treatments (electrode placement unknown)	Improvement in Parkinson's symptoms Improvement in depressive symptoms
Balldin et al., 1980	5	Parkinson's disease: 5 patients Parkinson's disease and depression: 3 patients	4–8 bilateral ECT treatments	Improvement in Parkinson's symptoms: 5 patients Improvement in depressive symptoms: 3 patients
Balldin et al., 1981	9	Parkinson's disease	3–8 bilateral ECT treatments	Marked improvement: 5 patients Slight improvement: 2 patients No improvement: 2 patients
Ward et al., 1980	5	Parkinson's disease	6 bilateral ECT treatments	No improvement: 5 patients
Holcomb et al., 1983	1	Parkinson's disease and depression	14 ECT treatments (electrode placement unknown)	Improvement in Parkinson's symptoms Improvement in depressed mood
Levy et al., 1983	1	Parkinson's disease and major depression	10 ECT treatments (electrode placement unknown)	Improvement in Parkinson's symptoms Resolution of depressive symptoms
Young et al., 1985	1	Parkinson's disease, major depression, and dementia	7 right unilateral ECT treatments	Improvement in Parkinson's symptoms No improvement in depressed mood or cognitive function

(continued)

TABLE 29-2. *Continued*

Study	Number of subjects	Diagnosis	ECT course	Treatment response
Jaeckle and Dilsaver, 1986	1	Parkinson's disease and bipolar disorder, depressed	9 bilateral ECT treatments	Improvement in Parkinson's symptoms Improvement in depressed mood
Andersen et al., 1987	11	Parkinson's disease	Sham control Bilateral: 9 patients Right unilateral: 2 patients	Improvement: 9 patients
Burke et al., 1988	3	Parkinson's disease and depression	5–8 right unilateral ECT treatments	Improvement in Parkinson's symptoms: 2 patients Improvement in depressed mood: 3 patients
Arte-Vaidya and Jampala, 1988	1	Parkinson's disease and mania	12 bilateral ECT treatments	Improvement in Parkinson's symptoms Resolution of manic symptoms
Roth et al., 1988	1	Parkinson's disease and bipolar disorder, manic	10 right unilateral ECT treatments	Improvement in Parkinson's symptoms Resolution of manic symptoms
Birkett, 1988	5	Parkinson's disease and major depression	Right unilateral ECT (number of treatments unknown)	Improvement in Parkinson's symptoms: 4 patients Improvement in depressive symptoms: 4 patients

Study	N	Diagnosis	Treatment	Outcome
Douyon et al., 1989	7	Parkinson's disease and major depression	Average of 7 bilateral ECT treatments	Improvement in depressed mood: 7 patients Improvement in Parkinson's symptoms: 7 patients
Lauterbach and Moore, 1990	1	Parkinson's disease and major depression	9 ECT treatments (electrode placement unknown)	Improvement in Parkinson's symptoms Improvement in depression
Zervas and Fink, 1991	4	Parkinson's disease	8–12 ECT treatments Bilateral: 3 patients Right unilateral: 1 patient	Improvement in Parkinson's symptoms: 4 patients
Friedman and Gordon, 1992	5	Parkinson's disease and major depression	7–12 ECT treatments Bilateral: 1 patient Right unilateral: 3 patients Electrode placement unknown: 1 patient	Improvement in depressed mood: 4 patients Improvement in Parkinson's symptoms: 3 patients
Holzer et al., 1992	1	Parkinson's disease and major depression	8 right unilateral ECT treatments	Improvement in Parkinson's symptoms Improvement in depressed mood
Oh et al., 1992	11	Parkinson's disease and major depression (10 patients) or mania (1 patient)	3–9 ECT treatments Bilateral: 1 patient Right unilateral: 9 patients Unilateral, then bilateral: 1 patient	Minor improvement in Parkinson's symptoms: 2 patients Improved psychiatric symptoms: 6 patients Post-ECT delirium: 7 patients

controlled trial, Lipsey and colleagues (1984) found a statistically significant improvement in poststroke depression treated with nortriptyline. In other uncontrolled studies, the response rate to psychostimulants in this population was 47% to 52% (Finklestein et al., 1987; Lingam et al., 1988). However, patients with stroke are often quite medically ill and debilitated and may be intolerant of pharmacotherapy. In the study by Lipsey and coworkers (1984), 35% of patients assigned to receive nortriptyline dropped out because of medication intolerance.

Clinical reports suggest that ECT may also be effective for treating poststroke depression. In a retrospective chart review of 14 patients with poststroke depression (mean age 66 years) treated with ECT at Massachusetts General Hospital in Boston, Murray and colleagues (1986) found that 86% had marked improvement in depression after ECT. Apparently, no patient exhibited any worsening of neurological deficit, and although formal measures of cognitive status were not reported, 5 of the 6 patients with "cognitive impairment" before ECT showed lessening of this deficit after ECT.

Currier and associates (1992) published retrospective data on 20 geriatric patients with poststroke depression treated with ECT at the same hospital, with predominantly nondominant unilateral electrode placement used. A "marked or moderate response" to ECT was observed in 95% of patients. No patient experienced any exacerbation of preexisting neurological deficits, but 3 patients exhibited "minor encephalopathic complications" (prolonged postictal confusion and amnesia), and 2 patients developed "severe interictal delirium requiring neuroleptics." Of note, 7 of their patients (35%) relapsed within a mean of 4 months of discontinuation of ECT despite ongoing maintenance drug therapy.

Elderly psychiatric patients with no clinical history of stroke often have subcortical white matter hyperintensities on magnetic resonance images; these are believed to be evidence of ischemic cerebrovascular disease. Coffey and coworkers (1989) found a high rate (82%) of response to ECT in depressed patients with these MRI findings; many of these patients had been refractory to antidepressant drug therapy. In addition, the majority of the patients tolerated the course of ECT without major systemic or cognitive side effects. This positive outcome with ECT is especially notable given other data that suggest subcortical ischemic disease may be associated with depressive illness resistant to treatment with antidepressant medications (Fujikawa et al., 1996).

In summary, ECT may be effective for poststroke depression, but controlled prospective data are needed to confirm this clinical impression and to identify patients potentially at risk for the adverse effects of the treatment.

ISSUES OF ELECTROCONVULSIVE THERAPY TECHNIQUE RELEVANT TO ELDERLY PATIENTS

Pretreatment Evaluation

When a patient is referred for ECT, a focused evaluation of indications and risk factors for the treatment should ensue (APA, 2000; Coffey, 1998). The patient's current mental status, neuropsychiatric history (including recent somatic therapies and history of treatment with ECT), and family psychiatric history should be reviewed. In the evaluation of medical risk factors for the treatment, the focus should be on the brain, the cardiovascular system, the musculoskeletal system, and the upper gastrointestinal tract. Any history of head trauma or surgery, seizures, focal or general neurological complaints, angina, congestive heart failure, bony fractures, osteoporosis, spinal disease or trauma, or esophageal reflux should be elicited. Any personal or family history of problems with anesthesia should be noted.

Handedness should be assessed because of its relevance to nondominant unilateral electrode placement (Kellner et al., 1997). Because the hand used for writing is a fallible indicator, patients should be asked which hand they use to throw a ball, cut with a knife, and so on (APA, 2000). A minority of left-handed patients and patients with mixed dominance may have language localized to the right hemisphere. For this reason, if substantial confusion is observed in a left-handed patient after the first right unilateral ECT treatment, consideration should be given to the use of left unilateral electrode placement at the next session. The time required for the patient to become fully oriented after the treatment can be measured for each type of electrode placement, and the series can then be continued using the placement associated with less confusion (Pratt et al., 1971).

A careful documentation of baseline affective and cognitive status is essential in elderly patients before initiation of ECT. The Hamilton or Montgomery Asberg Depression Rating scales and the Mini-Mental State Examination are often helpful standardized instruments that may be used at intervals throughout the ECT course.

A physical examination should be performed and serum electrolytes and an ECG obtained before ECT is initiated in elderly patients. Special care should be given to the neurological examination, including the fundoscopic examination to rule out papilledema. Further studies such as hemogram, other serum chemistries, spine x-rays, EEGs, brain computed tomographic (CT) scans or magnetic resonance images, and cardiac functional evaluations (Applegate, 1997; Coffey, 1998; Rayburn, 1997) should be ordered as clinically indicated. Elderly patients have an increased occurrence of clinically important incidental brain findings (e.g., aneurysm, subdural hematoma, undiagnosed primary metastatic brain tumor, and evidence of increased intracranial pressure), and brain imaging may have predictive value as a tool to detect increased risk for some ECT side effects (discussed in the section on amnesia) (Coffey, 1996).

In the presence of a mass lesion associated with increased intracranial pressure, the further increase in intracranial pressure associated with ECT could lead to brain herniation. Such events are rare (Kellner, 1996), and the type, size, and location of brain tumor correlate with the degree of risk. Smaller, slow-growing tumors that have no associated edema and do not obstruct cerebrospinal fluid flow present less risk. There are several case reports of successful ECT in the presence of meningiomas (Greenberg et al., 1988; Kellner et al., 1991b; Malek-Ahmadi & Sedler, 1989; McKinney et al., 1998).

For patients with serious cardiovascular disease, consultation with a cardiologist may be indicated. Once the decision to proceed with ECT has been made, the cardiologist should suggest how best to maximize the patient's cardiovascular function in preparation for, and during, ECT (Applegate, 1997; Dolinski & Zvara, 1997; McCall, 1997; Rayburn, 1997; Weiner et al., 2000).

The patient's medications should be carefully reviewed. Typically, all psychotropics are stopped before ECT, although neuroleptics may be used if necessary (Farah et al., 1995). Lithium taken around the time of ECT has been linked to an increased occurrence of delirium and prolonged seizures (Weiner et al., 1980). Most patients should not receive lithium for at least 1 day prior to ECT, with serum lithium levels kept as low as clinically feasible (Kellner, Nixon, et al., 1991). Discontinuation of lithium may be appropriate for some patients receiving an ECT series. However, complete discontinuation of lithium may not be advisable for other patients with severe and recurrent mood disorder, particularly when ECT is used as a continuation/maintenance treatment. Thus, lithium use concurrent with ECT must be made on a case-by-case basis.

Antidepressants are usually stopped to avoid cumulative cardiac and central nervous system side effects (Kellner, Nixon, et al., 1991), although this practice is under reconsideration (APA, 2000). Studies in the early 1960s found no added benefit with tricyclic antidepressant and ECT combination therapy (Seager & Bird, 1962).

However, in a retrospective chart review of 84 geriatric patients with depression, Nelson and Benjamin (1989) found improved outcome (i.e., the need for fewer treatments) with combination therapy with a tricyclic antidepressant and ECT. No increase in side effects occurred in the group receiving combination therapy. The study was severely limited by its retrospective design and by the fact that the ECT-only group presumably included more medically ill patients, in whom antidepressant therapy may have been stopped for fear of complication (Nelson & Benjamin, 1989).

Lauritzen and associates (1996) demonstrated the safety of ECT combined with paroxetine or imipramine, as well as the ability of both antidepressants to decrease relapse in the 6 months after index treatment (although paroxetine was more effective for relapse prevention than was imipramine). Interestingly, these authors also showed that concurrent imipramine treatment increased the response rate to acute ECT.

Benzodiazepines may impair the intensity of the therapeutic seizure, thereby potentially decreasing treatment response (Kellner, 1997b; Pettinati et al., 1986). The use of these agents in elderly patients may also theoretically increase their susceptibility to cognitive side effects from ECT. Benzodiazepine use should be minimized or stopped, whenever possible, before ECT. When necessary, the use of the lowest feasible doses of agents with relatively short half-lives and no active metabolites (e.g., lorazepam, oxazepam) has been recommended (APA, 2000; Greenberg & Pettinati, 1993).

In patients with epilepsy, the anticonvulsant effect of ECT itself may allow a temporary decrease in anticonvulsant dose. There are few reported data about the effects of carbamazepine and valproate on the efficacy of ECT. However, because anticonvulsant medications could interfere with the induction of adequate ECT seizures, anticonvulsants prescribed for psychiatric indications (i.e., not for epilepsy) should usually be tapered and discontinued before ECT (Fink & Sackeim, 1998; Kellner et al., 1997).

Several other specific pharmacological issues require attention. Theophylline levels should be monitored closely because high blood levels during ECT have been associated with status epilepticus (Abrams, 1997a; Devanand et al., 1998). Metrifonate and echothiophate are organophosphate medications that irreversibly inhibit cholinesterase and pseudocholinesterase and may cause prolonged apnea when combined with succinylcholine and should not be given (Zorumski et al., 1988). In theory, rivastigmine (Exelon), a pseudoirreversible inhibitor, and donepezil (Aricept), tacrine (Cognex), galantamine (Reminyl) (reversible cholinesterase inhibitors used in patients with Alzheimer's disease) could increase the duration of succinylcholine muscle relaxation. However, initial case report literature (Zink et al., 2002) and growing clinical experience suggest that acetylcholinesterase inhibitors may be continued safely during ECT. Otherwise, patients should take any required cardiac, antireflux, or other medications with a sip of water the morning of the ECT session.

A final and critically important component of the pre-ECT evaluation is the informed consent procedure. According to the 2000 American Psychiatric Association task force report on the practice of ECT, adequately informed consent should involve "1) the provision of adequate information, 2) a patient who is capable of understanding and acting intelligently upon such information, and 3) the opportunity to provide consent in the absence of coercion" (p. 97).

Compared with younger patients, those older than 65 years appear to be less aware that they can refuse ECT (Malcolm, 1989). With the increased prevalence of cognitive impairment in elderly patients, competency to consent becomes a major issue, and the education of both patient and family becomes essential. This is also a time in the patient's life cycle when children are becoming increasingly responsible for their parents, and the patient's children should be involved in the consent process whenever possible. Incompetent patients may require the judicial appointment of a legal guardian for consent. (For a pertinent sample of an informed consent document, see APA, 2000.)

There has been a shift to performing ECT on an outpatient basis. Many centers have found this to be a viable and efficient way to offer the treatment as long as certain precautions are taken (Fink et al., 1996). First, the patient's psychiatric illness must allow safe management outside the hospital. Clearly, acute suicidality or agitated psychosis will often require inpatient hospitalization. Second, the patient's medical status should be stable enough for safe outpatient management. In addition, strong social support is required; family members or others must transport the patient to and from the treatment facility, ensure the patient takes nothing by mouth (NPO) for at least 8 hours before a treatment session, and provide supervision between treatments (with particular attention paid to ensuring that the patient refrains from driving and making important financial or personal decisions while experiencing cognitive side effects) (Fink, 1994). For some patients, it is helpful to administer the first (or several initial) ECT treatment on an inpatient basis and then switch to outpatient treatments once it has been established that outpatient treatments can be administered safely and comfortably.

Electroconvulsive Therapy Technique

In the United States, ECT is commonly given as a series of single treatments on alternate mornings. Elderly individuals typically receive ECT initially in an inpatient setting. Patients have been previously evaluated for coexisting medical conditions and indications for treatment, and the consent process has been initiated. The treatment team consists of a psychiatrist, an anesthesiologist, and specially trained nursing personnel. ECT is typically given in either a special treatment suite or the recovery area of an operating room suite. Patients should have nothing to eat or drink for at least 8 hours before treatment.

Once baseline vital signs and an ECG have been obtained and pulse oximetry has been performed, the short-acting barbiturate methohexital is given intravenously at a dosage of approximately 1 mg/kg body weight, followed by the depolarizing neuromuscular blocker succinylcholine, which is given intravenously at a dosage of 0.75 to 1.5 mg/kg body weight. Adequacy of neuromuscular blockade is monitored using a peripheral nerve stimulator or by clinical assessment of relaxation, including loss of reflexes and tone.

Throughout the procedure, the patient is ventilated with 100% oxygen, and blood oxygen saturation is monitored using a pulse oximeter. Heart rate and blood pressure are also closely monitored. After a specially designed bite block is inserted into the patient's mouth, a predetermined electrical stimulus is delivered across electrodes placed on the patient's properly prepared scalp. Typically, a generalized seizure ensues, lasting from 20 to 90 seconds. The seizure is monitored by electroencephalography and by observation of the motor manifestations of the seizure, with a blood cuff inflated above systolic pressure on the right ankle to prevent access of the succinylcholine to the right foot.

Ventilatory support is continued until the patient emerges from the anesthesia, and further recovery is provided in an environment with as little stimulation as possible. The entire procedure takes about 20 minutes, and patients are often able to have breakfast within an hour of the time of treatment.

A typical course of ECT consists of 6 to 12 treatments, although occasionally patients may require fewer or more treatments to achieve full response. The treatment schedule is often modified in elderly patients to lessen cognitive side effects, with treatments given once or twice per week rather than three times per week (APA, 2000; Freeman, 1995; Lerer et al., 1995; Zervas et al.,

1993). ECT is stopped when maximal clinical improvement is thought to have been achieved or when further improvement is not noted between treatments. Special attention is then given to continuation/maintenance treatment with either medication or ECT (discussed in the section Continuation/Maintenance Electroconvulsive Therapy).

Anesthesia Considerations

Brief, light general anesthesia is used during ECT to render the patient unconscious during (and thus amnesic for) the procedure. Methohexital is the agent of choice because it has a rapid onset and a brief duration of action, and it induces minimal postanesthesia confusion. Methohexital also appears to have a decreased anticonvulsant effect than thiopental or propofol (Bergsholm & Swartz, 1996). Still, because methohexital is an anticonvulsant and because the seizure threshold is often increased in elderly patients (see the following section), the lowest effective anesthetic dose is desirable. Because methohexital dosing is based on a lean body mass, the required methohexital dosage in many elderly patients may be less than 1 mg/kg total body weight (Fragen & Avram, 1990).

Etomidate is a reasonable alternative to methohexital, especially in cases of severe cardiovascular disease, but it is more expensive and is associated with pain on infusion, longer cognitive recovery time, and short-term adrenocortical suppression. Propofol, another alternative anesthetic agent, is well tolerated, but has anticonvulsant properties and may be associated with shorter seizures (APA, 2000) (whether this characteristic impedes clinical antidepressant efficacy is unknown).

The preferred neuromuscular blocking agent for ECT is succinylcholine, primarily because it has rapid onset and a brief duration of action. The use of succinylcholine may require special consideration in the elderly patient. Succinylcholine indirectly stimulates muscarinic cholinergic receptors in the sinus node, causing prolonged depolarization, followed by a depolarized state that is resistant to further stimulation. The initial depolarization causes fasciculations and may contribute to bradycardia, especially if serial doses are required. This effect may be pronounced in patients receiving β-blockers and those with evidence of preexisting conduction delay on ECGs, both frequently the case among elderly patients. Pretreatment with anticholinergics, such as atropine or glycopyrrolate, will block this bradycardiac effect (the use of anticholinergic premedication is discussed in greater detail in the section on cardiovascular side effects). Myalgia following ECT may be because of either fasciculation caused by succinylcholine or excessive motor movement during the seizure. Fasciculation may be blocked in subsequent ECT treatments by administering a small pretreatment dose (e.g., 3 mg) of d-tubocuranine.

Intragastric pressure also increases with the use of succinylcholine and is related to abdominal skeletal muscle fasciculation; however, the risk of gastric reflux and aspiration is reduced by a concomitant increase in esophageal pressure above the lower esophageal sphincter (Miller & Savarese, 1990). Certain groups of elderly patients (e.g., those with hiatal hernia, gastroparesis, or morbid obesity) are at risk for substantial gastroesophageal reflux during the procedure, with subsequent risk for aspiration pneumonitis (Zibrak et al., 1988). Smokers are particularly prone to morbidity from aspiration (Lichtor, 1990). In these patients, additional strategies beyond requiring NPO status before a session may be considered to decrease gastric volume and acidity during ECT. Premedication with histamine, subtype 2 (H_2), receptor antagonists or sodium citrate decreases gastric acidity, and metoclopramide increases lower esophageal sphincter tone and promotes gastric emptying (Lichtor, 1990).

Stimulus Dosing

Seizure threshold (the amount of electricity required to elicit a seizure) increases with age (Coffey et al., 1995a; Sackeim et al., 1991). This effect is believed to be the result of a decrease in the excitability of the brain, but may also be partially because of increases in skull thickness (electrical resistance) with aging. Older patients thus require higher ECT stimulus intensities (doses) than do younger patients, but the optimal stimulus dosage for ECT has yet to be determined. Data from mixed-age samples suggest that barely suprathreshold stimulus intensities may be ineffective (especially for unilateral, nondominant ECT), whereas excessive stimulus dosing has been linked to more cerebral toxicity (Sackeim et al., 1993; Weiner et al., 1986).

Speed of response in ECT was shown to be related to stimulus dose intensity relative to seizure threshold with both unilateral and bilateral electrode placements (Sackeim et al., 1993). Data from Sackeim and coworkers (2000) and McCall and associates (2000) suggest that, with right unilateral electrode placement, stimulus doses should be much higher (e.g., up to 6 times seizure threshold) than with bilateral ECT to maximize antidepressant efficacy.

Given these data, patients treated with unilateral ECT generally should receive moderately to markedly suprathreshold stimulation, defined as 2.5 times to 6 or more times their seizure threshold (APA, 2000). This method of stimulus dosing requires a determination of the patient's seizure threshold, which may be done routinely at the first ECT session by increasing stimulus intensity in fixed increments over successive stimulations until a seizure results (Coffey et al., 1995a; Kellner et al., 1997; Sackeim et al., 1987). Alternatively, formulas that estimate seizure threshold based on variables such as age, sex, and electrode placement or the use of high fixed-dose unilateral stimuli are clinically acceptable options for stimulus dosing (Abrams & Swartz, 1989; McCall et al., 1995, 2000; APA, 2000). For bilateral ECT, moderately suprathreshold stimulus dosing at 1.5 to 2.5 times seizure threshold is recommended because the efficacy of this modality appears to be less sensitive to dosing effects than that of unilateral ECT and because higher stimulus doses may cause more cognitive impairment (APA, 2000).

A renewed interest in alternative electrode placement (e.g., bifrontal) (Bailine et al., 2000) may lead to development of techniques that optimize antidepressant efficacy with more acceptable cognitive profiles. There has been much interest in using ictal EEG characteristics as a predictor of treatment "adequacy" or subsequent dosing adjustments (Abrams, 2001; Krystal & Weiner, 1993). However, such strategies are still in the experimental stages.

Seizure threshold increases during ECT (the well-known anticonvulsant effect), at times necessitating increases in stimulus dose during the course of therapy (Coffey et al., 1990, 1995b; Kellner et al., 1997; Sackeim, 1991; Sackeim et al., 1991). This effect does not appear to be more pronounced in elderly patients, but because this population has a higher initial seizure threshold, some older patients may eventually require stimulus intensities during their course of treatment that exceed the maximal settings of the ECT device (Krystal et al., 2000). Although previously recommended as an agent to increase seizure duration (and possibly decrease seizure threshold), the use of caffeine has fallen into disfavor as its utility and safety have come into question (Enns et al., 1996). Higher-powered ECT devices (available in some European countries) are also helpful. The effects of cerebral disease and age-related changes in brain structure on ECT seizure threshold have not been described, but are currently under study.

Electrode Placement

The choice of unilateral or bilateral ECT in the elderly patient is often a complex one. Studies in mixed-age samples suggest that right unilateral ECT has fewer cognitive side effects (Weiner et al., 1986). However, a study involving mixed samples found bilateral ECT administered at 1.5 times the seizure threshold was equal to right unilateral ECT at 8 times threshold in mood and memory effects over a 1-month follow-up (McCall et al., 2002). Most research has also found unilateral and bilateral ECT to be equally effective (APA, 2000); however, in those studies in which differences have been noted, bilateral ECT has consistently been found to be more effective (for a review, see Abrams, 1997a).

Few studies have addressed the issue of electrode placement specifically in elderly patients. In a meta-analysis of the literature, Pettinati and colleagues (1986) found a trend for improved efficacy in elderly patients receiving bilateral treatment. In the only reported randomized study, 29 elderly patients with depression were assigned either to unilateral or bilateral ECT two times a week (Fraser & Glass, 1980). Stimulus-dosing strategies were unclear. No group differences were observed in terms of therapeutic response or memory performance after ECT, but those subjects randomly given bilateral electrode placement required more time to become reoriented after the fifth ECT treatment (Table 29-1). Whether the effects of cerebral disease or age-related structural brain changes modify the therapeutic or adverse effects of unilateral versus bilateral ECT in elderly patients has not been studied.

Thus, limited data exist to guide the choice of ECT electrode placement in elderly patients with neuropsychiatric illness. A reasonable approach is to begin with right unilateral ECT in elderly patients, switching to bilateral ECT if minimal or no response is seen by the fifth or sixth treatment. However, if right unilateral ECT was not initiated at a high stimulus dose relative to seizure threshold, a high dosage increase might be considered prior to switching to bilateral electrode placement (Tew et al., 2002). Because bilateral ECT may be associated with a statistically greater likelihood of response, it may be considered the treatment of choice in patients in urgent need of care. If intolerable cognitive side effects develop with bilateral ECT, the treatment may be changed to unilateral ECT once the affective disorder has begun to respond. Finally, atypical electrode placements (e.g., left unilateral, right frontotemporal–left frontal, or bifrontal) may be clinically useful in some elderly patients (Bailine et al., 2000; Kellner 1997a, 2000; Letemendia et al., 1993; Manly & Swartz, 1994).

Seizure Monitoring

The seizure may be monitored indirectly by observation of the convulsive motor response of a "cuffed" extremity, but more direct monitoring with ictal electroencephalography is preferred. The ECT seizure is monitored to confirm that a seizure has occurred and to determine when it has ended (Kellner et al., 1997; Weiner & Krystal, 1993). The ictal EEG has been studied using sophisticated computer analysis to determine whether various indices, such as amplitude, regularity, or coherence, may be predictive of treatment efficacy (Krystal et al., 1995, 1996; Weiner & Krystal, 1993). These studies suggest that such measures hold promise for indicating seizure adequacy during treatment sessions.

Continuation/Maintenance Electroconvulsive Therapy

Major depression is increasingly recognized as a chronic, relapsing condition. Some studies have found 6-month relapse rates as high as 50% for patients initially responsive to antidepressant medications who are then given no form of continuation/maintenance therapy (Prien & Kupfer, 1986). Similarly high rates of relapse have been noted after response to ECT if no form of continuation/maintenance therapy is given (Imlah et al., 1965; Jarvie, 1954). Frank and coworkers (1990) found that recurrence rates after response to pharmacotherapy can be substantially reduced by maintenance of antidepressant medication at full dose.

ECT is one of the few treatments in modern medicine that is commonly stopped as soon as it has proven effective. Usual clinical practice involves administration of continuation/maintenance pharmacotherapy after successful ECT. Because these patients often failed to respond to medication therapy before ECT, it is not surprising that a 50% relapse rate at 1 year was found for patients receiving maintenance pharmacotherapy after response to ECT (Sackeim et al., 1990). In that study, there was a particular propensity to relapse within 4 months after successful ECT.

Results of a growing number of studies involving mixed-age samples indicate that continuation/maintenance ECT is safe and effective for the prevention of depressive relapse, and there are several promising retrospective studies involving elderly patients (for a review, see Monroe, 1991). Thienhaus and colleagues (1990) described the cases of six elderly patients with major mood disorder treated with maintenance ECT for a period of 1 to 6 years. While receiving maintenance ECT, patients spent significantly fewer days in the hospital per year on average compared with the interval prior to beginning maintenance ECT.

Dubin and associates (1992) reported the successful use of maintenance ECT for an average of 22 months in a group of eight patients older than 75 years. No major adverse events were associated with maintenance ECT in this case series.

Loo and coworkers (1991) described the use of maintenance ECT in seven elderly patients over an average of 3 years. Mean time in the hospital during this 3-year period decreased to 3 weeks, compared with 27 weeks for patients treated during the 3 years before the introduction of maintenance ECT. Patients had 1.4 recurrences of illness during the maintenance ECT period, compared with 4.7 recurrences for patients during the 3 years preceding maintenance ECT.

In one of the few prospective studies to date, Clarke and colleagues (1989) evaluated 27 patients (mean age 65 years, range 26–90 years) not taking psychotropic medications who were assigned to a continuation ECT protocol after initial response to ECT. Only 8% of patients who completed the continuation ECT protocol required rehospitalization, whereas 47% relapsed among those who did not complete the protocol (a statistically significant difference).

A multisite study comparing treatment with nortriptyline, nortriptyline-lithium, and placebo after successful ECT was carried out by Sackeim and colleagues (2001). Over the 24-week trial, the relapse rates were placebo 84%, nortriptyline 60%, and nortriptyline-lithium 39%. Their study indicates the absolute need for active treatment after successful ECT. Another multisite study, complementary to the Sackeim and associates (2001) study, in which a fixed schedule of continuation ECT is compared to nortriptyline-lithium over 24 weeks is nearing completion (Petrides et al., 2001). The data from this study will inform the field about the relative efficacy of continuation/maintenance ECT as a relapse prevention strategy.

Continuation/maintenance ECT typically involves single treatments given initially at weekly intervals, with the frequency gradually reduced to every 4 to 8 weeks as the patient's depressive symptoms allow. The increased interval between maintenance treatments results in fewer cognitive side effects than with an index course of ECT, leading to the suggestion that bilateral treatment may be the modality of choice for continuation/maintenance ECT (Kellner et al., 1991a). However, in the absence of data to guide the choice of electrode placement for continuation/maintenance ECT, it is equally appropriate to continue the same placement that led to recovery of the index episode.

Several factors determine whether the treatments can be given on an outpatient basis. Patients must reliably follow NPO orders for 6 to 8 hours before treatment (patients are permitted only a sip of water to take any required premedications). Patients must also have an adequate support system to ensure observation and care for several hours after treatment. If these criteria cannot be met or if the patient has complex medical or recovery needs, an overnight stay in the hospital may be required.

ADVERSE EFFECTS OF ELECTROCONVULSIVE THERAPY AND THEIR MANAGEMENT

The safety of ECT compares favorably with that of any treatment requiring general anesthesia. The mortality is variously reported as approximating 3 deaths per 100,000 treatments (the same as for general anesthesia for minor surgery) and may actually be decreasing with improved management of underlying medical illnesses (Abrams, 1997a). To put these data into perspective, Abrams (1997b) noted that ECT is 10 times safer than childbirth.

Koessler and Fogel (1993) compared the mortality during long-term follow-up of 65 depressed patients aged 80 years or older who had been treated with ECT or antidepressant medication. The 2-year survival rate was 54% in the group treated with ECT versus 90% in the group treated with medication. However, this group difference was probably related to more severe depression and physical illness in the patients who had received ECT. The course of ECT itself was remarkably well tolerated by these elderly patients, with a 20-month median interval between ECT and time of death. The authors called for further attention to medical comorbidity as a prognostic factor in future outcome studies of geriatric depression. Abrams (1997b) noted that the estimated mortality rate among community-dwelling elderly patients (approximately 0.26% every 3 weeks) was an order of magnitude higher than that observed after a 3-week course of eight ECT treatments in elderly patients (approximately 0.016%).

Cardiovascular Side Effects

A proportion of elderly patients referred for ECT have serious preexisting cardiovascular disease. Common cardiac conditions such as hypertension, angina, previous myocardial infarction, atrial and ventricular arrhythmia, aneurysm, and conduction system disease require evaluation and optimized treatment before ECT to minimize any adverse effects from the hemodynamic events that occur during ECT.

Uncontrolled retrospective studies comparing the cardiovascular complication rate of ECT in older and younger patients have found an increase in transient and treatable complications in elderly patients. In a nonblinded, retrospective chart review of 293 patients, Alexopoulos and associates (1984) found cardiovascular complications in 9% of the patients aged 65 years and older compared with 1% of the patients younger than 65 years. Cardiac ischemia, arrhythmia, hypertension, and congestive heart failure were the most common complications, although the vast majority of complications were not clearly temporally related to ECT and did not prevent the completion of treatment.

Burke and colleagues (1987) conducted a similar retrospective chart review of 136 subjects, 30% of whom were aged 60 years and older. Sine wave bilateral ECT was used in 85% of cases. These investigators found a cardiorespiratory complication rate of 15% in patients aged 60 years and older compared with 3% in those younger than 60 years. Complications were correlated with the number of cardiovascular medications the patient was receiving, with more medication presumably marking those with more cardiovascular illness. These complications did not affect treatment response.

In a chart review of 81 elderly patients, Cattan and coworkers (1990) found a 36% cardiovascular complication rate with ECT in patients older than age 80 years compared with 12% in younger geriatric patients. As would be expected, the older patients had notably more medical diagnoses and were receiving more cardiovascular medication than the younger patients.

Two controlled studies of ECT in a total of 66 high-risk patients with cardiovascular disease demonstrated the safety of ECT in elderly individuals. Zielinski and associates (1993) compared the rate of cardiac complications in a group of 40 depressed patients (mean age 68.9 years, range, 54–84 years) with serious preexisting cardiac disease (left ventricular impairment, conduction delay, and ventricular arrhythmias) with the rate of such complications in a group of 40 depressed patients (mean age 68.3 years, range 55–83 years) without cardiac disease. Not surprisingly, the group with preexisting cardiac disease had more complications. Most of the complications were transient (e.g., brief arrhythmias or increases in ectopy), however, and 38 of the 40 cardiac patients were able to complete their course of ECT. The group of depressed patients with cardiac disease had even more difficulty with adverse cardiac effects from prior trials of tricyclic antidepressants; 11 of the 21 patients had been forced to stop tricyclic treatment because of cardiovascular complications.

Rice and coworkers (1994) used a case-control design to compare two groups of patients older than 50 years of age who were receiving ECT. One group consisted of 26 patients at increased risk for cardiac complications, and 27 patients at standard risk made up the other group. Compared with the patients at standard risk for cardiac complications, patients in the high-risk group were older, had received more medical consultations before ECT, and experienced more minor medical complications from ECT. However, the two groups did not differ in terms of frequency of major medical complications, and no patients died or experienced permanent cardiac morbidity from ECT.

The data reviewed above suggest that ECT is a low-risk procedure, even in elderly patients (Applegate, 1997). Still, prospective studies, carefully controlled for severity of cardiovascular and other medical disease, are needed to evaluate the effects of age on cardiovascular complications of ECT.

Increasingly sophisticated medical management during ECT should decrease the cardiovascular risk of treatment in elderly patients (Applegate, 1997). The primary areas of concern are bradycardia, tachycardia, hypertension, and ventricular arrhythmia. Anticholinergic premedications (atropine and glycopyrrolate) may be used to prevent vagally induced bradycardia, but in elderly patients, their use may be more complicated by confusion, tachycardia, constipation, and urinary retention. The method of serial electrical stimulations to determine a patient's seizure threshold (described in the section on stimulus dosing) may involve administration of subconvulsive stimuli, with a vagal surge unaccompanied by the sympathetic outflow associated with a seizure. The use of this method, as well as the presence of conduction delay on the ECG, may indicate the need for premedication with an anticholinergic, particularly if the patient is also receiving a β-blocker medication. Outside of these clinical scenarios, some practitioners reserve the use of anticholinergic premedication for patients who develop unusually prolonged or severe bradyarrhythmias during ECT.

Hypertension and tachycardia during ECT in elderly patients may be attenuated by short-acting intravenous β-blockers such as labetalol, esmolol, or nitroglycerine preparations (Howie et al., 1990; Stoudemire et al., 1990). It should be kept in mind that β-blockers have anticonvulsant effects, and their use during ECT may limit the intensity of the ECT seizure and, in turn, its therapeutic potency. Although the hemodynamic responses to ECT are robust, they are well tolerated by most patients, including elderly individuals (Webb et al., 1990). In addition, indiscriminate use of antihypertensive medication may lead to clinically significant hypotension in elderly patients. Therefore, it is usually unnecessary to routinely blunt the cardiovascular response to ECT in elderly patients unless such changes are extreme or are clearly associated with evidence of cardiovascular compromise. Finally, in patients receiving adrenergic blockers, anticholinergic premedication should be considered to prevent a disproportionate decrease of sympathetic tone below parasympathetic tone, with resultant bradycardia (Abrams, 1997a).

Marked posttreatment ventricular ectopy (multifocal premature ventricular contractions [PVCs] or several consecutive PVCs) may be treated with lidocaine (1–1.5 mg/kg body weight). Because of its anticonvulsant properties, lidocaine should be given after termination of the seizure (Drop & Welch,

1989). Stoudemire and coworkers (1990) found that ventricular ectopy could also be reduced by pretreatment with labetalol.

Cerebral Side Effects

There is no evidence that ECT causes structural brain damage (Devanand, Dwork, et al., 1994; Weiner, 1984). Carefully controlled prospective brain imaging studies in humans revealed no changes in brain structure for up to 6 months after a course of ECT (Coffey, 1993; Coffey et al., 1991). Neuropathological studies in animals, including cell counts in regions thought to be at risk, revealed no evidence of brain damage when the seizures were induced under conditions that approximated standard clinical practice (i.e., when the seizures were temporally spaced, relatively brief, and modified by oxygenation and muscle relaxation). Furthermore, studies of the pathophysiology of seizure-induced structural brain damage in animals indicated that the conditions necessary for injury do not apply to the modern practice of ECT (Weiner, 1984).

The incidence of cerebrovascular complications with ECT is exceedingly rare. ECT has been given successfully to patients with cerebral aneurysms, with close management of blood pressure elevation (Krystal & Coffey, 1997). An intracerebral hemorrhage reported in a normotensive patient during ECT was probably related to cerebral amyloid angiopathy (Weisberg et al., 1991). We know of no other reported case of intracerebral hemorrhage with ECT or of any documented case of ischemic stroke during the treatment.

The amount of time that must elapse before ECT can be safely administrated after an acute cerebral infarction is unclear. Alexopoulos and associates (1984) reported the uneventful delivery of ECT 4 days after a cerebral infarct (whether it was hemorrhagic or ischemic was not specified), and others (Currier et al., 1992; Murray et al., 1986) reported successful ECT 1 to 2 months after ischemic stroke. These patients require time for cerebral vessels to heal before ECT, as well as careful management of blood pressure during the procedure. Titratable agents with short half-lives (e.g., esmolol or nitrates) are helpful in this situation. Care must be taken to avoid hypotension in all elderly patients with cerebrovascular disease.

Other intracranial processes are risk factors for ECT. As described in the section on pretreatment evaluation, intracranial mass lesions and increased intracranial pressure are among the most serious risk factors for ECT. In a retrospective literature review, Maltbie and colleagues (1980) examined 28 patients (mean age 47 years, range 20–80 years) with brain tumors who were treated with ECT. Only 34% of patients improved, and 74% showed neurological deterioration, with 29% dying from neurological complications within a month of ECT. A form of recall bias flawed this study, with cases involving dramatic outcomes more likely to be reported.

As well, a previously undiagnosed brain tumor would more likely be diagnosed during a treatment course involving complications than during an uneventful ECT course. Abrams (1997a) and Kellner (1996) reviewed reports of several cases of safe delivery of ECT to patients with brain tumors, mostly meningiomas, and ascribed the lessened risk to the fact that the tumors were small, slow growing, and had no associated increased intracranial pressure.

There is no report of safely delivered ECT prospectively given to a patient with documented increased intracranial pressure (Abrams, 1997a). Subdural hematomas may require evacuation before ECT (Abrams, 1997a).

Side Effects in Other Organ Systems

Other organ systems that may be impaired in the elderly need to be evaluated before ECT, including the lungs, bones, eyes, and teeth (Weiner et al., 2000). Pulmonary status should be optimized before ECT. Patients with severe chronic obstructive pulmonary disease and carbon dioxide retention may require special ventilatory strategies during the treatment (Abrams, 1997a). Pneumonia secondary to aspiration of gastric contents may occur rarely during ECT (Alexopoulos et al., 1989; Karlinsky & Shulman, 1984).

Patients with osteoporosis, spinal disc disease, or spondylosis may require increased muscular relaxation during ECT. Such patients should receive succinylcholine doses of at least 1.0 to 1.5 mg/kg body weight, and they require careful attention to clinical evidence of adequate relaxation (e.g., loss of reflexes or tone and disappearance of fasciculation) before delivery of the stimulus. Kellner, Tollhurst, and Burns (1991) reported the safe treatment, using succinylcholine doses of 1.3 mg/kg weight, of a patient with osteoporosis and cervical spondylosis with multiple subluxations of the cervical spine.

Because ECT produces a transient increase in intraocular pressure, patients with chronic open-angle glaucoma should receive their eyedrops before ECT. As noted, treatment with echothiophate, an irreversible cholinesterase inhibitor, should be stopped several days before ECT. Patients with acute closed-angle glaucoma or retinal detachment should be stabilized before ECT and watched closely by an ophthalmologist during an ECT course.

When a patient's teeth are loose, decayed, or asymmetrical, the risk of dental injury during ECT may be increased. A major portion of malpractice litigation with ECT is related to dental issues (Slawson, 1985). A specially designed bite block must be inserted before delivery of the ECT stimulus. The tongue, cheeks, and lips must be kept clear of the clenching teeth. The bite block should be used even in edentulous patients. Occasionally, upper or lower dentures may be kept in place during the treatment to facilitate airway management. In patients with only a few remaining, and possibly loose, teeth, dental consultation or alternative bite block strategies (with the aim of shifting bite pressure to the molars) may be helpful (Welch, 1993).

Cognitive Side Effects

The cognitive side effects of ECT include acute postictal confusion, impaired retrograde and anterograde memory, and occasionally interictal delirium. The severity of these adverse effects is increased with bilateral electrode placement, sine waveform, higher stimulus dose relative to seizure threshold, and more frequent treatments. Conversely, cognitive side effects are reduced with right unilateral electrode placement, brief-pulse waveform, lower stimulus dose relative to seizure threshold, and longer intervals between treatments (APA, 2000). Although it has been suggested that elderly patients may be at greater risk for these cognitive side effects than are younger patients, controlled data on this issue are limited.

ACUTE POSTICTAL DISORIENTATION   In studies involving mixed-age samples of adults, increasing age has been associated with longer or more severe disorientation immediately after ECT (Burke et al., 1987; Calev et al., 1991; Daniel et al., 1987; Miller et al., 1986; Sackeim et al., 1987). Pre-ECT global cognitive status and the duration of postictal disorientation are reported to be strong predictors of the magnitude of retrograde amnesia up to 2 months after the course of ECT (Sobin, Sackheim, et al., 1995). Additional risk factors for post-ECT confusion in elderly patients may include presence of major medical illness or use of psychotropic medications during ECT.

In a study that focused on elderly patients, Fraser and Glass (1978) measured time to recovery of full orientation in nine elderly patients with depression who received ECT in which electrode placement alternated (i.e., unilateral placement in one treatment followed by bilateral placement in the next treatment, and so on). When comparing these reorientation times with those reported in the literature for younger patients, the investigators observed that recovery in elderly patients took five times longer for unilateral treatment and nine times longer for bilateral treatment. Recovery time after bilateral ECT increased cumulatively over the course of ECT and with closer spacing of treatments. No such relationship was found for unilateral ECT.

In a subsequent study of 29 elderly patients with depression randomly assigned to courses of either unilateral ($n = 13$) or bilateral ($n = 16$) sine wave ECT, Fraser and Glass (1980) found significantly longer reorientation times after the fifth ECT session among patients receiving bilateral treatments (32.8 minutes) than among those receiving unilateral treatments (9.5 minutes) (Table 29-1). In contrast to the group undergoing bilateral ECT, patients receiving unilateral ECT had a significant reduction in recovery time from the first to the last treatment.

In a study of subjective side effects during ECT, Devanand and colleagues (1995) found that older patients actually reported fewer severe cognitive symptoms (i.e., confusion/disorientation and amnesia) than did younger patients.

AGITATED DELIRIUM ON EMERGENCE FROM ANESTHESIA Approximately 10% of patients receiving ECT experience an acute agitated delirium on emergence from anesthesia; this is characterized by restlessness, disorientation, combativeness, and poor response to commands. Age does not appear to be a risk for this complication (Devanand et al., 1989). The complication is usually effectively treated with intravenous benzodiazepines (e.g., midazolam or diazepam) or other sedatives (e.g., droperidol or methohaxital).

INTERICTAL DELIRIUM In a small proportion of patients, ECT is associated with more prolonged disorientation and even frank interictal delirium. Most studies evaluating interictal delirium in elderly patients have used disorientation rather than the full *DSM-III-R* (APA, 1987) or *DSM-IV* (APA, 1994) criteria as a measure for delirium. In a retrospective study involving 136 patients receiving mainly bilateral sine wave ECT, Burke and associates (1987) found disorientation (confusion severe enough to alter the treatment plan) in 18% of patients older than 60, but in 13% of younger patients. This incidence increased to 25% for patients older than 75 years.

In a retrospective study in which mostly bilateral (waveform not specified) ECT was administered, Alexopoulos and coworkers (1984) found a somewhat greater incidence of confusion (disorientation to time, place, and person) in elderly patients (12.6%) than in younger patients (9.6%). Cattan and colleagues (1990) conducted a study involving primarily bilateral or combination bilateral-unilateral sine wave ECT and found a nonsignificant trend for more frequent severe disorientation (defined functionally by interference in ward activities) in elderly patients older than 80 years (59%, $n = 39$) compared with those patients 65 to 80 years old (45%, $n = 42$).

In the study of Alexopoulos and associates (1984), elderly patients with a history of underlying organic brain disease were found to have higher levels of severe post-ECT confusion than the young patients did, suggesting that baseline cerebral impairment may increase the risk of adverse cognitive effects of ECT.

In several studies, subcortical structural disease has been implicated in the development of interictal delirium with ECT. We have found subcortical gray and white matter lesions more extensive in elderly patients who developed a prolonged interictal delirium during a course of ECT (Figiel et al., 1990). The majority of these patients were able to continue ECT with no decline in expected treatment response. All patients were free of delirium 1 week after ECT (Coffey et al., 1989; Figiel et al., 1990).

The importance of subcortical disease in producing delirium after ECT was further suggested by Martin and coworkers. (1992), who found that patients with ischemic lesions of the caudate nucleus had a 92% incidence of delirium during ECT. Patients with a previous stroke in other brain regions had the same incidence of delirium as did a group of elderly depressed control (no stroke) subjects receiving ECT (Martin et al., 1992). In a prospective study of seven consecutive patients with Parkinson's disease, Figiel and associates (1991) found a 100% incidence of interictal delirium during a course of ECT. The delirium lasted 7 to 21 days, longer than is typical, but 86% of patients recovered from depression.

In summary, although the duration and severity of acute post-ECT disorientation may increase with age, the majority of elderly patients appear to recover their orientation within 60 to 120 minutes of the treatment. In the small percentage of elderly patients who develop more prolonged confusion or frank delirium, underlying cerebral impairment, especially dysfunction of the basal ganglia, may be contributory. Clearly, more research is needed in a larger number of elderly patients to characterize post-ECT confusion and to identify its risk factors, including the effects of preexisting cerebral impairment.

AMNESIA   A course of ECT is associated with transient disturbances in memory, including both retrograde and anterograde amnesia. Retrograde amnesia (forgetting of material known before the ECT) may extend back several months before ECT and is more pronounced with bilateral electrode placement, sine waveform, grossly suprathreshold stimulus intensity, and increased treatment frequency (Abrams, 1997a). These same factors also increase anterograde amnesia (forgetting of information acquired after the start of ECT). These side effects subside within weeks of completion of ECT, but some patients may have permanent loss of specific memories for some events that occurred before, during, or shortly after the treatment course. Although some patients report persistent memory difficulties, objective testing has demonstrated that ECT is not likely to produce persistent impairment in the ability to remember past information or acquire new information (APA, 2000). Rarely, persistent and severe retrograde amnesia may occur following ECT (Sackeim, 2000), but this remains controversial (Abrams, 2002).

Given the large body of data on the amnestic effects of ECT, it is surprising that there has been relatively little controlled research on age as a risk factor (Abrams, 1997a; Calev et al., 1993; Fink, 1979). Some (Fromholt et al., 1973; Heshe et al., 1978), but not all (d'Ellia & Raotma, 1977; Strömgren et al., 1976) early studies found that ECT-induced amnesia was worse in older patients.

Zervas and coworkers (1993) examined age effects on memory in a study comparing twice-weekly and three-times-a-week bilateral ECT administered using contemporary techniques (pulse waveform given at "moderately suprathreshold" stimulus intensity). The sample consisted of 42 inpatients with a mean age (±SD) of 53.5 ± 16.1 years; no patient was older than 65 years, however. Correlations were found between age and decrements in retrograde memory 1 to 3 days after the end of ECT, but not 1 month or 6 months posttreatment. Age was also correlated with decrements in verbal anterograde memory acutely and 1 month after ECT (but not 6 months after ECT) and with changes in figural anterograde memory acutely and 6 months after ECT.

McElhiney and colleagues (1995) examined autobiographical memory in a mixed-age sample (mean age [±SD] 54 ± 13.9 years) of 75 patients with depression; the patients were randomly assigned with regard to electrode placement and stimulus intensity. Age was a predictor of decreased recall of autobiographical memories after ECT. In a follow-up report on this sample, the pre-ECT modified Mini-Mental State Examination score was predictive of the extent of retrograde autobiographical amnesia both 1 week and 2 months after ECT (Sobin, Sackheim, et al., 1995). This study provided evidence in support of the conventional clinical wisdom that preexisting cognitive deficit is a risk factor for more severe ECT-induced amnesia.

Work is under way to determine whether age-related structural changes on brain images might also be predictive of cognitive impairment after ECT (Coffey, 1996). Lisanby and colleagues (2000) demonstrated that ECT tends to effect impersonal memory more than personal (autobiographical) memory.

Successful ECT may improve memory performance in elderly patients with the pseudodementia of depression (Reynolds et al., 1987; Stoudemire et al., 1995). In the study of Fraser and Glass (1980) described above (also see Table 29–1), all elderly patients showed impairment of memory function before ECT, but during treatment, memory improved and was normal in all patients by 3 weeks after completion of the ECT course. No group differences were found on the basis of electrode placement.

There has been relatively little research into the effects of age on subjective memory complaints after ECT (Prudic et al., 2000). As noted, Devanand and colleagues (1995) found that older patients actually reported fewer severe cognitive symptoms (i.e., confusion/disorientation and amnesia) than did younger patients.

In summary, controlled data appear to support the clinical wisdom that elderly patients are at greater risk for the amnestic side effects of ECT. More work is needed in a larger number of elderly patients (especially very old patients) to characterize the extent and severity of ECT-induced amnesia and to identify relevant risk factors, including the effects of preexisting cerebral impairment. Recommendations for decreasing ECT amnesia in elderly patients include using unilateral electrode placement and brief-pulse stimuli, avoiding maximally suprathreshold stimulus dosing with bilateral ECT, and decreasing the frequency of treatments (e.g., giving ECT on Monday and Friday instead of Monday, Wednesday, and Friday). A variety of pharmacological agents have shown antiamnestic activity in animal models of ECT, but clinical trials in humans have been limited by methodological issues (Prudic et al., 1998).

PSYCHOSOCIAL ISSUES

In addition to its myriad biological effects, ECT has important intrapsychic and interpersonal effects. A powerful treatment, during which the patient is put to sleep and has an electrical stimulus delivered to the head, may arouse predictable fears and fantasies in the patient. Issues of trust and autonomy over one's body while in a vulnerable position may predominate, especially in patients with a history of trauma. Patient education—particularly educational videotapes—may reduce these fears.

Patients who are vulnerable to idealized fantasies of a nurturing, all-caring, supportive other may overvalue the ECT procedure and practitioner. Conversely, these patients may excessively devalue the treatment when their distorted expectations are not realized. Such patients may be at increased risk for a bad psychological outcome from the treatment. The ECT practitioner should challenge overidealization of the treatment, and the informed consent process should be firmly grounded in factual information.

Patient attitude surveys indicate that those undergoing ECT typically find the experience no more upsetting than a trip to the dentist (Fox, 1993; Hughes et al., 1981; Malcolm, 1989). In the only study that has systematically examined the effects of age on patients' perception and knowledge of ECT, Malcolm (1989) found that patients older than 65 years had less knowledge of the procedure before treatment and were also less fearful of it. In addition, fewer elderly patients viewed the treatment as frightening after completing a course of ECT.

Medicolegal issues surrounding the use of ECT in elderly patients include the informed consent process (discussed in the pretreatment evaluation section), do not resuscitate (DNR) orders, and consideration of driving after ECT. A patient with DNR status may still experience improved quality of life with aggressive treatment of his or her affective disorder and may still be considered for ECT (Sullivan et al., 1992). In such cases, strategies for the management of major complications that could occur during ECT should be discussed with the patient and the family before treatment. Patients should not drive until such time after a ECT course when cognitive side effects have substantially resolved (Fink, 1994). This issue may be an especially sensitive one for elderly patients who consider driving a means of maintaining their mobility and functional independence.

Financial concerns are of increasing importance in today's cost-conscious health care marketplace. A growing body of literature suggests that ECT has economic advantages over other forms of treatment for severe mood disorders. The cost-effectiveness of ECT has been demonstrated for both inpatient treatment of the index episode as well as for maintenance therapy on an ambulatory basis (Markowitz et al., 1987; McDonald et al., 1998; Olfson et al., 1998; Steffens et al., 1995). Despite these advantages, there remains much variation in ECT reimbursement patterns, and it is not uncommon to encounter payers who will reimburse only for ECT when it is given on an inpatient basis. In addition, reimbursement rates are very low, thus discouraging the use of this safe and highly effective treatment.

TRANSCRANIAL MAGNETIC STIMULATION

Transcranial magnetic stimulation (TMS) is a relatively new technology that uses an electrically induced magnetic field to generate small electrical currents that can depolarize brain neurons. Repeated TMS (rTMS) can cause repeated neuronal firing that (depending on a variety of technical factors related to the TMS and possible host factors) can either augment or suppress neuronal network functioning. Many ECT research groups throughout the world are investigating rTMS as a possible antidepressant treatment. Most studies have open trials, relatively few elderly patients have been studied, and results indicate that there are minimal side effects, but only modest improvements in mood (for a concise review, see George, 1998). Although it is unclear what role rTMS will play in the management of elderly patients who are candidates for ECT, rTMS holds great promise as a tool for understanding the neurobiology of mood regulation (George et al., 1999).

CONCLUSION

Sixty years after its introduction, ECT remains a cornerstone of the treatment of severe affective disorder and selected other neuropsychiatric illnesses in elderly patients. Modifications in ECT technique have reduced the risk of severe side effects in this population. There is, however, a paucity of controlled studies comparing the efficacy and safety of ECT versus pharmacotherapy in elderly patients. ECT also appears to be an effective treatment in patients with preexisting brain disease and in some cases may even have a beneficial effect on the underlying neurological disorder. Further study is needed to determine the impact of age-related changes in brain structure or function and of preexisting cerebral disease on the beneficial effects of ECT in the elderly.

REFERENCES

Aarsland D, Larsen JP, Waage O, et al. Maintenance electroconvulsive therapy for Parkinson's disease. *Convuls Ther.* 1997;13:274–277.

Abrams R. *Electroconvulsive Therapy*. 3rd ed. New York, NY: Oxford University Press; 1997a.

Abrams R. The mortality rate with ECT. *Convuls Ther.* 1997b;13:125–127.

Abrams R. Quantitative EEG during seizures induced by ECT. *J ECT.* 2001;17(3):226–227.

Abrams R. Does brief-pulse ECT cause persistent or permanent memory impairment? *J ECT.* 2002;18(2):71–73.

Abrams R, Swartz CM. *ECT Instruction Manual for the Thymatron DG*. Chicago, IL: Somatics; 1989.

Alexopoulos GS, Meyers B, Young R, et al. Recovery in geriatric depression. *Arch Gen Psychiatry.* 1996;53:305–312.

Alexopoulos GS, Shamoian CJ, Lucas J, et al. Medical problems of geriatric psychiatric patients and younger controls during electroconvulsive therapy. *J Am Geriatr Soc.* 1984;32:651–654.

Alexopoulos GS, Young RG, Abrams RC. ECT in the high-risk geriatric patient. *Convuls Ther.* 1989;5:75–87.

American Psychiatric Association. *Diagnostic and Statistical Manual of Mental Disorders.* 3rd ed., rev. Washington, DC: American Psychiatric Association; 1987.

American Psychiatric Association. *Diagnostic and Statistical Manual of Mental Disorders.* 4th ed. Washington, DC: American Psychiatric Association; 1994.

American Psychiatric Association. *The Practice of Electroconvulsive Therapy: Recommendations for Treatment, Training and Privileging.* 2nd ed. Washington, DC: American Psychiatric Association; 2000.

Andersen K, Balldin J, Gottfries CG, et al. A double-blind evaluation of electroconvulsive therapy in Parkinson's disease with "on-off" phenomena. *Acta Neurol Scand.* 1987;76:191–199.

Applegate RJ. Diagnosis and management of ischemic heart disease in the patient scheduled to undergo electroconvulsive therapy. *Convuls Ther.* 1997;13:128–144.

Asnis G. Parkinson's disease, depression, and ECT: a review and case study. *Am J Psychiatry.* 1977;134:191–195.

Atre-Vaidya N, Jampala V. Electroconvulsive therapy in parkinsonism with affective disorder. *Br J Psychiatry.* 1988;152:55–58.

Avery E, Winokur G. Mortality in depressed patients treated with electroconvulsive therapy and antidepressants. *Arch Gen Psychiatry.* 1976;33:1029–1037.

Babigian HM, Guttmacher LB. Epidemiologic considerations in electroconvulsive therapy. *Arch Gen Psychiatry.* 1984;41:246–253.

Bailine SH, Rifkin A, Kayne E, et al. Comparison of bifrontal and bitemporal ECT for major depression. *Am J Psychiatry.* 2000;157:121–123.

Balldin J, Eden S, Granerus A-K, et al. Electroconvulsive therapy in Parkinson's syndrome with "on-off" phenomenon. *J Neural Transm.* 1980;47:11–21.

Balldin J, Granerus A-K, Lindstedt G, Modigh K, Walinder J. Predictors for improvement after electroconvulsive therapy in parkinsonian patients with on-off symptoms. *J Neural Transm.* 1981;52(3):199–211.

Benbow SM. ECT for depression in dementia. *Br J Psychiatry.* 1988;152:859.

Bergsholm P, Swartz CM. Anesthesia in electro convulsive therapy and alternatives to barbiturates. *Psychiatr Ann.* 1996;26:709–712.

Birkett DP. ECT in parkinsonism with affective disorder [letter]. *Br J Psychiatry.* 1988; 152:712–713.

Black DW, Winokur G, Nasrallah A. ECT in unipolar and bipolar disorders: a naturalistic evaluation of 460 patients. *Convuls Ther.* 1986;2:231–237.

Black DW, Winokur G, Nasrallah A. A multivariate analysis of the experience of 423 depressed inpatients treated with electroconvulsive therapy. *Convuls Ther.* 1993;9:112–120.

Bodley PO, Fenwick PBC. The effects of electro convulsive therapy on patients with essential hypertension. *Br J Psychiatry.* 1966;112:1241–1249.

Bolwig T, Hertz M, Paulson O, et al. The permeability of the blood-brain barrier during electrically induced seizures in man. *J Clin Invest.* 1977;7:87–93.

Bonne O, Krausz Y, Shapira B, et al. Increased cerebral blood flow in depressed patients responding to electroconvulsive therapy. *J Nucl Med.* 1996;37:1075–1080.

Bosworth HB, McQuoid DR, George LK, Steffens DC. Time-to-remission from geriatric depression: psychosocial and clinical factors. *Am J Geriatr Psychiatry.* 2002;10: 551–559.

Braasch ER, Demaso DR. Effect of electroconvulsive therapy on serum isoenzymes. *Am J Psychiatry.* 1980;137:625–626.

Brodersen P, Paulson OB, Bolwig TG, et al. Cerebral hyperemia in electrically induced epileptic seizures. *Arch Neurol.* 1973;28:334–338.

Brown G. Parkinsonism, depression and ECT [letter]. *Am J Psychiatry.* 1973;132: 1084.

Burke WJ, Peterson J, Rubin E. Electroconvulsive therapy in the treatment of combined depression and Parkinson's disease. *Psychosomatics.* 1988;29:341–346.

Burke WJ, Rubin EH, Zorumski CF, et al. The safety of ECT in geriatric psychiatry. *J Am Geriatr Soc.* 1987;35:516–521.

Burke WJ, Rutherford JL, Zorumski CF, et al. Electro convulsive therapy and the elderly. *Compr Psychiatry.* 1985;26:480–486.

Calabrese JR, Woyshville MJ, Kimmel SE, et al. Mixed states and bipolar rapid cycling and their treatment with divalproex sodium. *Psychiatr Ann.* 1993;23:70–78.

Calev A, Cohen R, Tubi N, et al. Disorientation and bilateral moderately suprathreshold titrated ECT. *Convuls Ther.* 1991;7:99–110.

Calev A, Pass HL, Shapira B, et al. ECT and memory. In: Coffey CE, ed. *The Clinical Science of Electroconvulsive Therapy.* Washington, DC: American Psychiatric Press; 1993:125–142.

Carlyle W, Killick L, Ancil R. An effective treatment in the screaming demented patient. *J Am Geriatr Soc.* 1991;39:637–639.

Carney MWP, Roth M, Garside RF. The diagnosis of depressive syndromes and the prediction of ECT response. *Br J Psychiatry.* 1965;111:659–674.

Casey DA, Davis MH. Electroconvulsive therapy in the very old. *Gen Hosp Psychiatry.* 1996;18:436–439.

Cattan RA, Barry PP, Mead G, et al. Electroconvulsive therapy in octogenarians. *J Am Geriatr Soc.* 1990;38:753–758.

Centers for Disease Control and Prevention. Recommendations for a community plan for the prevention and containment of suicide clusters. *MMWR Morb Mortal Wkly Rep.* 1988;37(Suppl 6):1–12.

Clarke TB, Coffey CE, Hoffman GW, et al. Continuation therapy for depression using outpatient electroconvulsive therapy. *Convuls Ther.* 1989;5:330–337.

Coffey CE. Structural brain imaging and electroconvulsive therapy. In: Coffey CE, ed. *The Clinical Science of Electroconvulsive Therapy.* Washington, DC: American Psychiatric Press; 1993:73–92.

Coffey CE. Brain morphology in primary mood disorders: implications for ECT. *Psychiatr Ann.* 1996;26:713–716.

Coffey CE. The pre ECT evaluation. *Psychiatr Ann.* 1998;28:506–508.

Coffey CE, Figiel GS, Djang WT, et al. Leukoencephalopathy in elderly depressed patients referred for ECT. *Biol Psychiatry.* 1988;24:143–161.

Coffey CE, Figiel GS, Djang WT, et al. White matter hyperintensity on magnetic resonance imaging: clinical and neuroanatomic correlates in the depressed elderly. *J Neuropsychiatry Clin Neurosci.* 1989;1:135–144.

Coffey CE, Figiel GS, Weiner RD, et al. Caffeine augmentation of ECT. *Am J Psychiatry.* 1990;147:579–585.

Coffey CE, Lucke J, Weiner RD, et al. Seizure threshold in electroconvulsive therapy. I. Initial seizure threshold. *Biol Psychiatry.* 1995a;37:713–720.

Coffey CE, Lucke J, Weiner RD, et al. Seizure threshold in electroconvulsive therapy. II. The anticonvulsant effect of ECT. *Biol Psychiatry.* 1995b;37:777–788.

Coffey CE, Weiner RD, Djang WT, et al. Brain anatomic effects of ECT: a prospective magnetic resonance imaging study. *Arch Gen Psychiatry.* 1991;48:1013–1021.

Consensus Conference. Electroconvulsive therapy. *JAMA.* 1985;254:2103–2108.

Coryell W, Zimmerman M. Outcome following ECT for primary unipolar depression: a test of newly proposed response predictors. *Am J Psychiatry.* 1984;141:862–867.

Currier MB, Murray GB, Welch CC. Electroconvulsive therapy for post-stroke depressed geriatric patients. *J Neuropsychiatry Clin Neurosci.* 1992;4:140–144.

Daniel WF, Crovitz HF, Weiner RD. Neuropsychological aspects of disorientation. *Cortex.* 1987;23:169–187.

Decina P, Sackeim HA, Kahn DA, et al. Effects of ECT on the TRH stimulation test. *Psychoneuroendocrinology.* 1987;12:29–34.

d'Ellia G, Raotma H. Memory impairment after convulsive therapy: influence of age and number of treatments. *Acta Psychiatr Nerenkr.* 1977;223:219–226.

Devanand DP, Briscoe KM, Sackeim HA. Clinical features and predictors of postictal excitement. *Convuls Ther.* 1989;5:140–146.

Devanand DP, Decina P, Sackeim HA, et al. Status epilepticus during ECT in a patient receiving theophylline. *J Clin Psychopharmacol.* 1988;8:153.

Devanand DP, Dwork AJ, Hutchinson MSE, Bolwig TG, Sackeim HA. Does ECT alter brain Structure? *Am J Psychiatry.* 1994;151:957–970.

Devanand DP, Fitzsimons L, Prudic J, et al. Subjective side effects during electroconvulsive therapy. *Convuls Ther.* 1995;11:232–240.

Devanand DP, Nobler MS, Singer T, et al. Is dysthymia a different disorder in the elderly? *Am J Psychiatry.* 1994;151:1592–1599.

Devanand DP, Sackeim HA, Lo ES, et al. Serial dexamethasone suppression tests and plasma dexamethasone levels. *Arch Gen Psychiatry.* 1991;48:525–533.

Dolinski SY, Zvara DA. Anesthetic considerations of cardiovascular risk during electroconvulsive therapy. *Convuls Ther.* 1997;13:157–164.

Douyon R, Serby M, Klutchko B, et al. ECT and Parkinson's disease revisited: a "naturalistic" study. *Am J Psychiatry.* 1989;146:1451–1455.

Drop LJ, Welch CA. Anesthesia for electroconvulsive therapy in patients with major cardiovascular risk factors. *Convuls Ther.* 1989;5:88–101.

Dubin WR, Jaffe R, Roemer R, et al. The efficacy and safety of maintenance ECT in geriatric patients. *J Am Geriatr Soc.* 1992;40:706–709.

Dysken M, Evans H, Chan C, et al. Improvement of depression and parkinsonism during ECT: a case study. *Neuropsychobiology.* 1976;2:81–86.

Enns M, Peeling J, Sutherland GR. Hippocampal neurons are damaged by caffeine-augmented electroshock seizures. *Biol Psychiatry.* 1996;40:642–647.

Farah A, Beale MD, Kellner CH. Risperidone and ECT combination therapy: a case series. *Convuls Ther.* 1995;11:280–282.

Feighner JP, Robins E, Guze SB, et al. Diagnostic criteria for use in psychiatric research. *Arch Gen Psychiatry.* 1972;26:57–63.

Figiel GS, Coffey CE, Djang WT, et al. Brain magnetic resonance imaging findings in ECT-induced delirium. *J Neuropsychiatry Clin Neurosci.* 1990;2:53–58.

Figiel GS, Hassen MA, Zorumski C, et al. ECT-induced delirium in depressed patients with Parkinson's disease. *J Neuropsychiatry Clin Neurosci.* 1991;3:405–411.

Fink M. *Convulsive Therapy: Theory and Practice.* New York, NY: Raven; 1979.

Fink M. Convalescence and ECT. *Convuls Ther.* 1994;10:301–303.

Fink M, Abrams R, Bailine S, et al. Ambulatory electroconvulsive therapy: report of a task force of the Association for Convulsive Therapy. Association for Convulsive Therapy. *Convuls Ther.* 1996;12:42–55.

Fink M, Sackeim HA. Theophylline and the risk of status epilepticus in ECT. *J ECT.* 1998;14:286–290.

Finklestein SD, Weintraub RJ, Karmooz N, et al. Antidepressant drug treatment for post-stroke depression: a retrospective study. *Arch Phys Med Rehabil.* 1987;68:772–778.

Flint AJ, Rifat SL. Two-year outcome of psychotic depression in late life. *Am J Psychiatry.* 1998;155:178–183.

Fogel BS. Electroconvulsive therapy in the elderly: a clinical research agenda. *Int J Geriatr Psychiatry.* 1988;3:181–190.

Folstein MF, Folstein S, McHugh PR. Clinical predictors of improvement after electroconvulsive therapy of patients with schizophrenic, neurotic reactions, and affective disorders. *Biol Psychiatry.* 1973;7:147–152.

Fox HA. Patients' fear of and objection to electroconvulsive therapy. *Hosp Community Psychiatry.* 1993;44:357–360.

Fragen RJ, Avram MJ. Barbiturates. In: Miller RD, ed. *Anesthesia.* Vol. 1. 3rd ed. New York, NY: Churchill Livingstone; 1990:225–242.

Frank E, Kupfer DJ, Perel JM, et al. Three year outcomes for maintenance therapies in recurrent depression. *Arch Gen Psychiatry.* 1990;47:1093–1099.

Fraser RM, Glass IB. Recovery from ECT in elderly patients. *Br J Psychiatry.* 1978;133:524–528.

Fraser RM, Glass IB. Unilateral and bilateral ECT in elderly patients: a comparative study. *Acta Psychiatr Scand.* 1980;62:13–31, 1980.

Freeman CP, ed. *The ECT Handbook: The Second Report of the Royal College of Psychiatrists' Special Committee on ECT.* London, England: Royal College of Psychiatrists; 1995.

Friedman J, Gordon N. Electroconvulsive therapy in Parkinson's disease: a report of five cases. *Convuls Ther.* 1992;8:204–210.

Fromholt P, Christensen AL, Strömgren LS. The effects of unilateral and bilateral electroconvulsive therapy on memory. *Acta Psychiatr Scand.* 1973;49:466–478.

Fromm GH. Observations on the effects of electroshock treatment in patients with parkinsonism. *Bull Tulane Univ.* 1959;18:71–73.

Fujikawa T, Yokota N, Muraoka M, et al. Response of patients with major depression and silent cerebral infarction to antidepressant drug therapy, with emphasis on central nervous system adverse reactions. *Stroke.* 1996;27:2040–2042.

Gaspar A, Samarasinghe LA. ECT in psychogeriatric practice—a study of risk factors, indications and outcome. *Compr Psychiatry.* 1982;23:170–175.

George MS. Why would you ever want to? Toward understanding the antidepressant effect of prefrontal rTMS. *Hum Psychopharmacol.* 1998;13:307–313.

George MS, Nahas Z, Kozel FA, Goldman J, Molloy M, Oliver N. Improvement of depression following transcranial magnetic stimulation. *Curr Psychiatry Rep.* 1999; 1:114–124.

Gerring JP, Shields HM. The identification and management of patients with high risk for cardiac arrhythmias during modified ECT. *J Clin Psychiatry.* 1982;43:140–143.

Godber C, Rosenvinge H, Wilkinson D, et al. Depression in old age: prognosis after ECT. *Int Geriatr Psychiatry.* 1987;2:19–24.

Gold L, Chiarella CJ. The prognostic value of clinical findings in cases treated with electric shock. *J Nerv Ment Dis.* 1944;100:577–583.

Gormley N, Cullen C, Walters L, et al. The safety and efficacy of electroconvulsive therapy in patients over age 75. *Int Geriatr Psychiatry.* 1998;13:871–874.

Gould L, Gopalaswamy C, Chandy F, et al. Electroconvulsive therapy-induced ECG changes simulating a myocardial infarction. *Arch Intern Med.* 1983;143:1786–1878.

Grant JE, Mohan SN. Treatment of agitation and aggression in four demented patients using ECT. *J ECT.* 2001;17:205–209.

Greenberg L, Fink M. The use of electroconvulsive therapy in geriatric patients. *Clin Geriatr Med.* 1992;8:349–354.

Greenberg LB, Mofson R, Fink M. Prospective electroconvulsive therapy in a delusional depressed patient with a frontal meningioma: a case report. *Br J Psychiatry.* 1988; 153:105–107.

Greenberg RM, Pettinati HM. Benzodiazepines and electroconvulsive therapy. *Convuls Ther.* 1993;9:262–273.

Grunhaus L, Shipley JE, Eiser A, et al. Polysomnographic studies in patients referred for ECT: pre-ECT studies. *Convuls Ther.* 1996;12:224–231.

Hamilton M. The effect of treatment on the melancholia (depressions). *Br J Psychiatry.* 1982;140:223–230.

Hermesh H, Aizenberg D, Friedberg G, et al. Electroconvulsive therapy for persistent neuroleptic-induced akathisia and parkinsonism: a case report. *Biol Psychiatry.* 1992;31:407–411.

Heshe J, Roder E, Theilgaard A. Unilateral and bilateral ECT: a psychiatric and psychological study of therapeutic effect and side effects. *Acta Psychiatr Scand Suppl.* 1978;275:1–180.

Hickie I, Mason C, Gordon P, et al. Prediction of ECT response: validation of a sign-based (CORE) system for defining melancholia. *Br J Psychiatry.* 1996;169:68–74.

Holcomb H, Sternberg D, Heninger G. Effects of electroconvulsive therapy on mood, parkinsonism and tardive dyskinesia in a depressed patient: ECT and dopamine systems. *Biol Psychiatry.* 1983;18:865–873.

Holmberg SK, Tariot PN, Challapalli R. Efficacy of ECT for agitation in dementia. *Am J Geriatr Psychiatry.* 1996;4:330–334.

Holzer JC, Giakas WJ, Mazure CM, et al. Dysarthria during ECT given for Parkinson's disease and depression. *Convuls Ther.* 1992;8:201–203.

Howie MB, Black HA, Zvar AD, et al. Esmolol reduces autonomic hypersensitivity and length of seizures induced by electroconvulsive therapy. *Anesth Analg.* 1990;71: 384–388.

Huang KC, Lucas LF, Tsueda K, et al. Age-related changes in cardiovascular function associated with electroconvulsive therapy. *Convuls Ther.* 1989;5:17–25.

Hughes J, Barraclough BM, Reeve W. Are patients shocked by ECT? *J R Soc Med.* 1981; 74:283–285.

Imlah NW, Ryan E, Harrington JA. The influence of antidepressant drugs on the response to electroconvulsive therapy and on subsequent relapse rates. *Neuropsychopharmacology.* 1965;4:438–442.

Ingvar M, Siesjö BK. Local blood flow and glucose consumption in the rat brain during sustained bicuculine-induced seizures. *Acta Neurol Scand.* 1983;68:129–144.

Jaeckle R, Dilsaver S. Covariation of depressive symptoms, parkinsonism, and post-dexamethasone plasma cortisol levels in a bipolar patient: simultaneous response to ECT and lithium carbonate. *Acta Psychiatr Scand.* 1986;74:68–72.

Jarvie H. Prognosis of depression treated by electric convulsive therapy. *BMJ.* 1954;1: 132–134.

Jenicke MA. *Handbook of Geriatric Psychopharmacology.* Littleton, MA: PSG Publishing; 1985.

Kahn RL, Pollack M, Fink M. Sociopsychologic aspects of psychiatric treatment in a voluntary mental hospital: duration of hospitalization, discharge ratings and diagnosis. *Arch Gen Psychiatry.* 1959;1:566–574.

Kamil R, Joffe RT. Neuroendocrine testing in electroconvulsive therapy. *Psychiatr Clin North Am.* 1991;14:961–970.

Kaplan HI, Sadock BJ, eds. *Synopsis of Psychiatry.* 5th ed. Baltimore, MD: Williams and Wilkins; 1988:253–269.

Karlinsky H, Shulman KI. The clinical use of electroconvulsive therapy in old age. *J Am Geriatr Soc.* 1984;32:183–186.

Kellner CH. The CT scan (or MRI) before ECT: a wonderful test has been overused [editorial]. *Convuls Ther.* 1996;12:79–80.

Kellner CH. Left unilateral ECT: still a viable option? *Convuls Ther.* 1997a;13:66–67.

Kellner CH. Seizure interference by medications: how big a problem [editorial]? *Convuls Ther.* 1997b;13:1–3.

Kellner CH. Towards the modal ECT treatment. *J ECT.* 2001;17:1–2.

Kellner CH, Bernstein HJ. ECT as a treatment for neurological illness. In: Coffey CE, ed. *The Clinical Science of Electroconvulsive Therapy.* Washington, DC: American Psychiatric Press; 1993:183–210.

Kellner CH, Burns CM, Bernstein HJ, et al. Electrode placement in maintenance electroconvulsive therapy. *Convuls Ther.* 1991a;7:61–62.

Kellner CH, Burns CM, Bernstein HJ, et al. Safe administration of ECT in a patient with a calcified frontal mass. *J Neuropsychiatry Clin Neurosci.* 1991b;3:353–354.

Kellner CH, Coffey CE, Beale MD, et al. *Handbook of ECT.* Washington, DC: American Psychiatric Press; 1997.

Kellner CH, Monroe RR, Pritchett J, et al. Weekly ECT in geriatric depression. *Convuls Ther.* 1992;8:246–252.

Kellner CH, Nixon DW, Bernstein HJ. ECT-drug interactions: a review. *Psychopharmacol Bull.* 1991;27:596–609.

Kellner CH, Tollhurst JE, Burns CM. ECT in the presence of severe cervical spine disease. *Convuls Ther.* 1991;7:52–55.

Kirkegaard C, Norlem N, Lauridsen UB, et al. Protirelin stimulation test and thyroid function during treatment of depression. *Arch Gen Psychiatry.* 1975;32:1116–1118.

Koessler D, Fogel B. Electroconvulsive therapy for major depression in the oldest old. *Am J Geriatr Psychiatry.* 1993;1:30–37.

Kramer BA. Use of ECT in California, 1977–1983. *Am J Psychiatry.* 1985;142:1190–1192.

Kramer BA. Electroconvulsive therapy use in geriatric depression. *J Nerv Ment Dis.* 1987;175:233–235.

Kramer BA. Use of ECT in California, revised: 1984–1994. *J ECT.* 1999;15:246–251.

Krog-Meyer I, Kirkegaard C, Kijne B, et al. Prediction of relapse with the TRH test and prophylactic amitriptyline in 39 patients with endogenous depression. *Am J Psychiatry.* 1984;141:946–948.

Krystal AD, Coffey CE. Neuropsychiatric considerations in the use of electroconvulsive therapy. *J Neuropsychiatry Clin Neurosci.* 1997;9:283–292.

Krystal AD, Coffey CE, Weiner RD, et al. Changes in seizure threshold over the course of electroconvulsive therapy affect therapeutic response and are detected by ictal EEG ratings. *J Neuropsychiatry Clin Neurosci.* 1998;10:178–186.

Krystal AD, Dean MD, Weiner RD, et al. ECT stimulus intensity: are present ECT devices too limited? *Am J Psychiatry.* 2000;157:963–967.

Krystal AD, Weiner RD. Low-frequency ictal EEG activity and ECT therapeutic impact. *Convuls Ther.* 1993;9:220–224.

Krystal AD, Weiner RD, Coffey CE. The ictal EEG as a marker of adequate stimulus intensity with unilateral ECT. *J Neuropsychiatry Clin Neurosci.* 1995;7:296–303.

Krystal AD, Weiner RD, Gassert D, et al. The relative ability of 3 ictal EEG frequency bands to differentiate ECT seizures on the basis of electrode placement, stimulus intensity, and therapeutic response. *Convuls Ther.* 1996;12:13–24.

Lambourn J, Barrington PC. Electroconvulsive therapy in a sample British population in 1982. *Convuls Ther.* 1986;2:169–177.

Lauritzen L, Odgaard K, Clemmesen L, et al. Relapse prevention by means of paroxetine in ECT-treated patients with major depression: a comparison with imipramine and placebo in medium term continuation therapy. *Acta Psychiatr Scand.* 1996;94:241–251.

Lauterbach E, Moore N. Parkinsonism-dystonia syndrome and ECT. *Am J Psychiatry.* 1990;147:1249–1250.

Lebensohn Z, Jenkins R. Improvement of parkinsonism in depressed patients treated with ECT. *Am J Psychiatry.* 1975;132:283–285.

Lerer B, Shapira B, Calev A, et al. Antidepressant and cognitive effects of twice- versus three-times-weekly ECT. *Am J Psychiatry.* 1995;152:564–570.

Letemendia FJ, Delva NJ, Rodenburg M, et al. Therapeutic advantage of bifrontal electrode placement in ECT. *Psychol Med.* 1993;23:349–360.

Levy L, Savit J, Hodes M. Parkinsonism: improvement by electroconvulsive therapy. *Arch Phys Med Rehabil.* 1983;64:432–433.

Lichtor JL. Psychological preparation and preoperative medication. In: Miller RD, ed. *Anesthesia*. Vol. 1. 3rd ed. New York, NY: Churchill Livingstone; 1990:896–928.

Lingam VR, Lazarus LW, Groves L, et al. Methylphenidate in treating post-stroke depression. *J Clin Psychiatry*. 1988;49:151–153.

Lipper S, Bermanzohn P. Electroconvulsive therapy in patients with parkinsonism [letter]. *Am Psychiatry*. 1975;132:457.

Lipsey JR, Robinson RG, Pearlson GD. Nortryptiline treatment of post-stroke depression: a double-blind study. *Lancet*. 1984;1:297–300.

Lisanby SH, Maddox JH, Prudic J, et al. The effects of electroconvulsive therapy on memory of autobiographical and public events. *Arch Gen Psychiatry*. 2000;57:581–590.

Loo H, Galinowski A, DeCarvalho W, et al. Use of maintenance ECT for elderly depressed patients [letter]. *Am J Psychiatry*. 1991;148:810.

Magni G, Fisman M, Helmes E. Clinical correlates of ECT-resistant depression in the elderly. *J Clin Psychiatry*. 1988;49:406–407.

Malcolm K. Patient's perceptions and knowledge of electroconvulsive therapy. *Psychiatr Bull*. 1989;13:161–165.

Malek-Ahmadi P, Sedler RR. Electroconvulsive therapy and asymptomatic meningioma. *Convuls Ther*. 1989;5:168–170.

Malla AK. Characteristics of patients who receive electroconvulsive therapy. *Can J Psychiatry*. 1988;33:696–701.

Maltbie AA, Wingfield MS, Volow MR, et al. Electroconvulsive therapy in the presence of brain tumor. *J Nerv Ment Dis*. 1980;168:400–405.

Mander AJ, Withfield A, Keen DM, et al. Cerebral and brain stem changes after ECT revealed by nuclear magnetic resonance imaging. *Br J Psychiatry*. 1987;151:69–71.

Manly DT, Oakley SP, Bloch RM. Electroconvulsive therapy in old-old patients. *Am J Psychiatry*. 2000;8:232–236.

Manly DT, Swartz CS. Asymmetric bilateral right frontotemporal left frontal stimulus electrode placement: comparisons with bifrontotemporal and unilateral placements. *Convuls Ther*. 1994;10:267–270.

Markowitz J, Brown R, Sweeney J, et al. Reduced length and cost of hospital stay for major depression in patients treated with ECT. *Am J Psychiatry*. 1987;144:1026–1029.

Martin M, Figiel G, Mattingly G, et al. ECT-induced interictal delirium in patients with a history of CVA. *J Geriatr Psychiatry Neurol*. 1992;5:149–155.

McCall W, Farah B, Reboussin D, et al. Comparison of the efficacy of titrated, moderate dose and fixed, high-dose right unilateral ECT in elderly patients. *Am J Geriatr Psychiatry*. 1995;3:317–324.

McCall WV. Cardiovascular risk during ECT: managing the managers [editorial]. *Convuls Ther*. 1997;13:123–124.

McCall WV, Dunn A, Rosenquist PB, Hughes D. Markedly suprathreshold right unilateral ECT versus minimally suprathreshold bilateral ECT: antidepressant and memory effects. *J ECT*. 2002;18:126–129.

McCall WV, Reboussin DM, Weiner RD, et al. Titrated, moderately suprathreshold versus fixed, high dose RUL ECT: acute antidepressant and cognitive effects. *Arch Gen Psychiatry*. 2000;57:438–444.

McDonald WM, Phillips VL, Figiel GS, et al. Cost-effective maintenance treatment of resistant geriatric depression. *Psychiatr Ann.* 1998;28:47–52.

McElhiney MC, Moody BJ, Steif BL, et al. Autobiographical memory and mood: effects of electroconvulsive therapy. *Neuropsychology.* 1995;9:501–517.

McKinney PA, Beale MD, Kellner CH. Electroconvulsive therapy in a patient with a cerebellar meningioma. *J ECT.* 1998;14:49–52.

Mendels J. Electroconvulsive therapy and depression. I. The prognostic significance of clinical factors. *Br J Psychiatry.* 1965;111:676–681.

Messina AG, Paranicas M, Katz B, et al. Effect of electroconvulsive therapy on the electrocardiogram and echocardiogram. *Anesth Analg.* 1992;75:511–514.

Meyers BS, Greenberg R. Late-life delusional depression. *J Affect Disord.* 1986;11:133–137.

Meyers BS, Mei-Tal V. Empirical study on an inpatient psychogeriatric unit: biological treatment in patients with depressive illness. *Int J Psychiatry Med.* 1985–1986;15:111–124.

Miller ME, Siris SG, Gabriel AN. Treatment delays in the course of electroconvulsive therapy. *Hosp Community Psychiatry.* 1986;37:826–827.

Miller RD, Savarese JJ. Pharmacology of muscle relaxants and their antagonists. In: Miller RD, ed. *Anesthesia.* Vol 1. 3rd ed. New York, NY: Churchill Livingstone; 1990:389–435.

Milstein V, Small JG, Klapper MH, et al. Uni- versus bilateral ECT in the treatment of mania. *Convuls Ther.* 1987;3:1–9.

Monroe RR. Maintenance electroconvulsive therapy. *Psychiatr Clin North Am.* 1991;14:947–960.

Mukherjee S. Mechanisms of the antimanic effects of electroconvulsive therapy. *Convuls Ther.* 1988;4:74–80.

Mukherjee S, Sackeim HA, Lee C. Unilateral ECT in the treatment of manic episodes. *Convuls Ther.* 1988;4:74–80.

Mukherjee S, Sackeim HA, Schnur DB. Electroconvulsive therapy of acute manic episodes: a review of 50 years' experience. *Am J Psychiatry.* 1994;151:169–176.

Mulsant BH, Rosen J, Thornton JE, et al. A prospective naturalistic study of electroconvulsive therapy in late-life depression. *J Geriatr Psychiatry Neurol.* 1991;4:3–13.

Murray GB, Shea V, Conn DK. Electroconvulsive therapy for post-stroke depression. *J Clin Psychiatry.* 1986;47:258–260.

Nelson JP, Benjamin L. Efficacy and safety of combined ECT and tricyclic antidepressant drugs in the treatment of depressed geriatric patients. *Convuls Ther.* 1989;5:321–329.

Nelson JP, Rosenberg DR. ECT treatment of demented elderly patients with major depression: a retrospective study of safety and efficacy. *Convuls Ther.* 1991;7:157–165.

Nobler MS, Sackeim HA, Prohovnik I, et al. regional cerebral blood flow in mood disorders. III. Treatment and clinical response. *Arch Gen Psychiatry.* 1994;51:884–897.

Nobler MS, Sackeim HA, Solomou M, et al. EEG manifestations during ECT: effects of electrode placement and stimulus intensity. *Biol Psychiatry.* 1993;34:321–330.

Nymeyer L, Grossberg GT. Delirium in a 76-year-old woman receiving ECT and levo-dopa. *Convuls Ther.* 1997;13:114–116.

O'Connor MK, Knapp R, Husain M, et al. The influence of age on the response of major depression to electroconvulsive therapy: a C.O.R.E. report. *Am J Psychiatry.* 2001;9:382–390.

Oh JJ, Rummans TA, O'Conner MK, et al. Cognitive impairment after ECT in patients with Parkinson's disease and psychiatric illness [letter]. *Am J Psychiatry.* 1992;149: 271.

O'Leary D, Gill D, Gregory S, et al. Which depressed patients respond to ECT? The Nottingham results. *J Affect Disord.* 1995;33:246–250.

Olfson M, Marcus S, Sackeim HA, et al. Use of ECT for the treatment of recurrent major depression. *Am J Psychiatry.* 1998;155:22–29.

Ottoson JO. Experimental studies of the mode of action of electroconvulsive therapy. *Acta Psychiatr Scand Suppl.* 1960;145:1–141.

Oztas B, Kaya M, Camurcu S. Age related changes in the effect of electroconvulsive shock on the blood brain barrier permeability in rats. *Mech Ageing Dev.* 1990;51: 149–155.

Pande AC, Grunhaus LJ, Haskett RF, et al. Electroconvulsive therapy in delusional and non-delusional depressive disorder. *J Affect Disord.* 1990;19:216–219.

Papakostas Y, Fink M, Lee J, et al. Neuroendocrine measures in psychiatric patients: course and outcome with ECT. *Psychiatry Res.* 1981;4:56–64.

Petrides G, Fink M, Husain M, et al. ECT remission rates in psychotic versus nonpsy-chotic depressed patients: a report from CORE. *J ECT.* 2001;17:244–253.

Pettinati HM, Mathisen KS, Rosenberg J, et al. Meta-analytical approach to reconciling discrepancies in efficacy between bilateral and unilateral electroconvulsive therapy. *Convuls Ther.* 1986;2:7–17.

Philbert RA, Richards L, Lynch CF, et al. Effect of ECT on mortality and clinical out-come in geriatric unipolar depression. *J Clin Psychiatry.* 1995;56:390–394.

Post RM. Transduction of psychosocial stress into the neurobiology of recurrent affec-tive disorder. *Am J Psychiatry.* 1992;149:999–1010.

Pratt RTC, Warrington EK, Halliday AM. Unilateral ECT as a test for cerebral domi-nance, with a strategy for treating left-handers. *Br J Psychiatry.* 1971;119:79–83.

Price TRP, McAllister TW. Safety and efficacy of ECT in depressed patients with demen-tia: a review of clinical experience. *Convuls Ther.* 1989;5:61–74.

Prien R, Kupfer D. Continuation drug therapy for major depressive episodes: how long should it be maintained? *Am J Psychiatry.* 1986;143:18–23.

Prohovnik I, Sackeim HA, Decina P, et al. Acute reductions of regional cerebral blood flow following electroconvulsive therapy: interactions with modality and time. *Ann N Y Acad Sci.* 1986;462:249–262.

Prudic J, Haskett RF, Mulsant B, et al. Resistance to antidepressant medications and short-term clinical response to ECT. *Am J Psychiatry.* 1996;153:986–992.

Prudic J, Peyser S, Sackeim HA. Subjective memory complaints: a review of patient self-assessment of memory after electroconvulsive therapy. *J ECT.* 2000;16:121–132.

Prudic J, Sackeim HA, Decina P, et al. Acute effects of ECT on cardiovascular functioning: relations to patient and treatment variables. *Acta Psychiatr Scand.* 1987;75: 344–351.

Prudic J, Sackeim, HA, Devanand DP. Medication resistance and clinical response to electroconvulsive therapy. *Psychiatry Res.* 1990;31:287–296.

Prudic J, Sackeim HA, Spicknall K. Potential pharmacologic agents for the cognitive effects of electroconvulsive treatment. *Psychiatr Ann.* 1998;28:40–46.

Rasmussen K, Abrams R. Treatment of Parkinson's disease with electroconvulsive therapy. *Psychiatr Clin North Am.* 1991;14:926–933.

Rayburn BK. Electroconvulsive therapy in patients with heart failure or valvular disease. *Convuls Ther.* 1997;13:146–156.

Reynolds CF, Perel JM, Kupfer DJ, et al. Open-trial response to antidepressant treatment in elderly patients with mixed depression and cognitive impairment. *Psychiatry Res.* 1987;21:111–122.

Rice EH, Sombrotto LB, Markowitz JC, et al. Cardiovascular morbidity in high-risk patients during ECT. *Am J Psychiatry.* 1994;151:1637–1641.

Rich CL, Spiker DG, Jewell SW, et al. *DSM-III*, RDC, and ECT: depressive subtypes and immediate response. *J Clin Psychiatry.* 1984a;45:14–18.

Rich CL, Spiker DG, Jewell SW, et al. The efficacy of ECT. I. Response rates in depressive episodes. *Psychiatry Res.* 1984b;11:167–176.

Rich CL, Spiker DG, Jewell SW, et al. ECT response in psychotic versus nonpsychotic unipolar depressives. *J Clin Psychiatry.* 1986;47:123–125.

Roberts JM. Prognostic factors in the electroshock treatment of depressive states. I. Clinical features from history and examination. *J Ment Sci.* 1959;105:693–702.

Robinson RG, Price TR. Post-stroke depressive disorders: a follow-up study of 103 patients. *Stroke.* 1982;13:636–641.

Rosenberg R, Vostrup S, Andersen A, et al. Effect of ECT on cerebral blood flow in melancholia assessed with SPECT. *Convuls Ther.* 1988;4:62–73.

Roth S, Mukherjee S, Sackeim H. Electroconvulsive therapy in a patient with mania, parkinsonism and tardive dyskinesia. *Convuls Ther.* 1988;4:92–97.

Rubin EH, Kinsoherf DA, Wehrman SA. Response to treatment of depression in the old and very old. *J Geriatr Neurol.* 1991;4:66–70.

Rummans TA, Lauterbach EC, Coffey CE, et al. Pharmacologic efficacy in neuropsychiatry: a review of placebo-controlled treatment trials—a report of the ANPA Committee on Research. *J Neuropsychiatry Clin Neurosci.* 1999;11:176–189.

Sackeim HA. Are ECT devices underpowered [editorial]? *Convuls Ther.* 1991;7:233–236.

Sackeim HA. Continuation therapy following ECT: directions for future research. *Psychopharmacol Bull.* 1994;30:501–521.

Sackeim HA. The use of electroconvulsive therapy in late-life depression. In: Salzman C, ed. *Geriatric Psychopharmacology.* 3rd ed. Baltimore, MD: Williams and Wilkins; 1998:262–309.

Sackeim HA. Memory and ECT: from polarization to reconciliation. *J ECT.* 2000;16: 87–96.

Sackeim HA, Decina P, Kanzler M, et al. Effects of electrode placement on the efficacy of titrated, low-dose ECT. *Am J Psychiatry.* 1987;144:1449–1455.

Sackeim HA, Decina P, Prohovnik I, et al. Anticonvulsant and antidepressant properties of electroconvulsive therapy: a proposed mechanism of action. *Biol Psychiatry*. 1983;18:1301–1310.

Sackeim HA, Devanand DP, Prudic J. Stimulus intensity, seizure threshold, and seizure duration: impact on the efficacy and safety of electroconvulsive therapy. *Psychiatr Clin North Am*. 1991;14:803–843.

Sackeim HA, Haskett RF, Mulsant BH, et al. Continuation pharmacotherapy in the prevention of relapse following electroconvulsive therapy: a randomized controlled trial. *JAMA*. 2001;285:1299–1307.

Sackeim HA, Prudic J, Devanand DP, et al. The impact of medication resistance and continuation pharmacotherapy on relapse following response to electroconvulsive therapy in major depression. *J Clin Psychopharmacol*. 1990;10:96–104.

Sackeim HA, Prudic J, Devanand DP, et al. Effects of stimulus intensity and electrode placement on the efficacy and cognitive effects of electroconvulsive therapy. *N Engl J Med*. 1993;328:839–846.

Sackeim HA, Prudic J, Devanand DP, et al. A prospective, randomized, double-blind comparison of bilateral and right unilateral ECT at different stimulus intensities. *Arch Gen Psychiatry*. 2000;57:426–434.

Salzman C. Electroconvulsive therapy in the elderly patient. *Psychiatr Clin North Am*. 1982;5:191–197.

Scott AI, Dougall N, Ross M, et al. Short-term effects of electroconvulsive treatment on the uptake of ^{99m}Tc-exametazime into brain in major depression shown with single photon emission tomography. *J Affect Disord*. 1994;30:27–34.

Scott AI, Douglas RH, Whitfield A, et al. Time course of cerebral magnetic resonance changes after electroconvulsive therapy. *Br J Psychiatry*. 1990;156:551–553.

Seager CP, Bird RL. Imipramine with electrical treatment in depression: a controlled trial. *J Ment Sci*. 1962;108:704–707.

Segman RH, Shapira B, Gorfine M, et al. Onset and time course of antidepressant action: psychopharmacological implications of a controlled trial of electroconvulsive therapy. *Psychopharmacology (Berlin)*. 1995;119:440–448.

Shapira B, Gorfine M, Lerer B. A prospective study of lithium continuation therapy in depressed patients who have responded to electroconvulsive therapy. *Convuls Ther*. 1995;11:80–85.

Shapira B, Lerer B. Speed of response to bilateral ECT: an examination of possible predictors in two controlled trials. *J ECT*. 1999;15:202–206.

Shettar MS, Grunhaus L, Pande AC, et al. Protective effects of intramuscular glycopyrrolate on cardiac conduction during ECT. *Convuls Ther*. 1989;5:349–352.

Slawson P. Psychiatric malpractice: the electroconvulsive therapy experience. *Convuls Ther*. 1985;1:196–203.

Small JG, Klapper MH, Kellams JJ, et al. ECT compared with lithium in the management of manic states. *Arch Gen Psychiatry*. 1988;45:727–732.

Small JG, Milstein V, Small IF. Electroconvulsive therapy for mania. *Psychiatr Clin North Am*. 1991;14:887–903.

Sobin C, Prudic J, Devanand DP, et al. Who responds to electroconvulsive therapy? *Br J Psychiatry*. 1995;169:322–328.

Sobin C, Sackeim HA, Prudic J, et al.: Predictors of retrograde amnesia following ECT. *Am J Psychiatry*. 1995;152:7.

Solan WJ, Khan A, Avery DH, et al. Psychotic and nonpsychotic depression: comparison of response to ECT. *J Clin Psychiatry.* 1988;49:97–99.

Staton RD. Electroencephalographic recording during bitemporal and unilateral nondominant hemisphere (Lancaster position) electroconvulsive therapy. *J Clin Psychiatry.* 1981;42:264–269.

Steffens DC, Krystal AD, Sibert TE, et al. Cost effectiveness of maintenance ECT [letter]. *Convuls Ther.* 1995;11:283–284.

Stoudemire A, Hill CD, Morris R, et al. Improvement in depression-related cognitive dysfunction following ECT. *J Neuropsychiatry Clin Neurosci.* 1995;7:31–34.

Stoudemire A, Knos G, Gladson M, et al. Labetalol in the control of cardiovascular responses to electroconvulsive therapy in high-risk depressed medical patients. *J Clin Psychiatry.* 1990;51:508–512.

Strömgren LS. Unilateral versus bilateral electroconvulsive therapy: investigations in to the therapeutic effect in endogenous depression. *Acta Psychiatr Scand Suppl.* 1973; 240:8–65.

Strömgren LS, Christensen AL, Fromholt P. The effects of unilateral brief-interval ECT on memory. *Acta Psychiatr Scand.* 1976;54:336–346.

Sullivan MO, Ward NG, Laxton A. The woman who wanted electroconvulsive therapy and do-not-resuscitate status. *Gen Hosp Psychiatry.* 1992;14:204–209.

Swartz CM. Clinical and laboratory predictors of ECT response. In: Coffey CE, ed. *The Clinical Science of Electroconvulsive Therapy.* Washington, DC: American Psychiatric Press; 1993:53–71.

Tew JD, Mulsant BH, Haskett RF, et al. Acute efficacy of ECT in the treatment of major depression in the old-old. *Am J Psychiatry.* 1999;156:1866–1870.

Tew JD Jr, Mulsant BH, Haskett RF, et al. A randomized comparison of high-charge right unilateral electroconvulsive therapy and bilateral electroconvulsive therapy in older depressed patients who failed to respond to 5 to 8 moderate-charge right unilateral treatments. *J Clin Psychiatry.* 2002;63:1102–1105.

Thienhaus OJ, Margletta S, Bennett JA. A study of the clinical efficacy of maintenance ECT. *J Clin Psychiatry.* 1990;51:141–144.

Thompson JW, Weiner RD, Myers CP. Use of ECT in the United States in 1975, 1980, and 1986. *Am J Psychiatry.* 1994;151:1657–1661.

Tomac TA, Rummans TA, Pileggi TS, et al. safety and efficacy of electroconvulsive therapy in patients over age 85. *Am J Geriatr Psychiatry.* 1997;5:126–130.

Volkow ND, Bellar S, Mullani N, et al. Effects of electroconvulsive therapy on brain glucose metabolism: a preliminary study. *Convuls Ther.* 1988;4:199–205.

Ward C, Stern GM, Pratt R, et al. Electroconvulsive therapy in parkinsonian patients with the "on-off" syndrome. *J Neural Transm.* 1980;49:133–135.

Webb MC, Coffey CE, Saunders WR, et al. Cardiovascular response to unilateral electroconvulsive therapy. *Biol Psychiatry.* 1990;28:758–766.

Weiner RD. Does ECT cause brain damage? *Behav Brain Sci.* 1984;7:1–53.

Weiner RD, Coffey CE. Indications for use of electroconvulsive therapy. In: Frances AJ, Hales RE, eds. *American Psychiatric Press Review of Psychiatry.* Vol. 7. Washington, DC: American Psychiatric Press; 1988:458–481.

Weiner RD, Coffey CE, Krystal AD. Electroconvulsive therapy in the medical and neurological patient. In: Stoudemire A, Fogel B, Greenberg D, eds. *Psychiatric Care of the Medical Patient.* 2nd ed. New York, NY: Oxford University Press; 2000:419–428.

Weiner RD, Krystal AD. EEG monitoring of ECT seizures. In: Coffey CE, ed. *The Clinical Science of Electroconvulsive Therapy.* Washington, DC: American Psychiatric Press; 1993:93–109.

Weiner RD, Rogers HJ, Davidson JRT, et al. Effects of stimulus parameters on cognitive side effects. *Ann N Y Acad Sci.* 1986;462:316–325.

Weiner RD, Whanger AD, Erwin CW, et al. Prolonged confusional state and EEG seizure following concurrent ECT and lithium use. *Am J Psychiatry.* 1980;137:1452–1453.

Weintraub D, Lippmann SB. ECT for major depression and mania with advanced dementia. *J ECT.* 2001;17:66–67.

Weisberg LA, Elliott D, Mielke D. Intracerebral hemorrhage following electroconvulsive therapy. *Neurology.* 1991;41:1849.

Welch CA. ECT in medically ill patients. In: Coffey CE, ed. *The Clinical Science of Electroconvulsive Therapy.* Washington, DC: American Psychiatric Press; 1993:167–182.

Welch CA, Drop LJ. Cardiovascular effects of ECT. *Convuls Ther.* 1989;5:36–43.

Wengel SP, Burke WJ, Pfeiffer RF, et al. Maintenance electroconvulsive therapy for intractable Parkinson's disease. *Am J Geriatr Psychiatr.* 1998;6:263–269.

Wesner RB. Prolonged T-wave inversion associated with electroconvulsive therapy. *Convuls Ther.* 1986;2:203–206.

Wesner RB, Winokur G. The influence of age on the natural history of unipolar depression when treated with electroconvulsive therapy. *Eur Arch Psychiatry Neurol Sci.* 1989;238:149–154.

Wilkinson AM, Anderson DN, Peters S. Age and the effects of ECT. *Int J Geriatr Psychiatry.* 1993;8:401–406.

Young R, Alexopoulos G, Shamoian A. Dissociation of motor response from mood and cognition in a parkinsonian patient treated with ECT. *Biol Psychiatry.* 1985;20:566–569.

Yudofsky SC. Parkinson's disease, depression and electroconvulsive therapy: a clinical and neurobiologic synthesis. *Compr Psychiatry.* 1979;20:579–581.

Zervas IM, Calev A, Jandorf L, et al. Age-dependent effects of electroconvulsive therapy on memory. *Convuls Ther.* 1993;9:39–42.

Zervas IM, Fink M. ECT for refractory Parkinson's disease. *Convuls Ther.* 1991;7:222–223.

Zibrak JG, Jensen WA, Bloomingdale K. Aspiration pneumonitis following electroconvulsive therapy in patients with gastroparesis. *Biol Psychiatry.* 1988;24:812–814.

Zielinski RJ, Roose SP, Devanand DP, et al. Cardiovascular complications of ECT in depressed patients with cardiac disease. *Am J Psychiatry.* 1993;150:904–909.

Zink M, Sartorius A, Lederbogen F, Henn FA. Electroconvulsive therapy in a patient receiving rivastigmine. *J ECT.* 2002;18:162–164.

Zorumski CF, Rubin EH, Burke WJ. Electroconvulsive therapy for the elderly. *Hosp Community Psychiatry.* 1988;39:643–647.

Zubenko GS, Mulsant BH, Rifai AH, et al. Impact of acute psychiatric inpatient treatment on major depression in late life and prediction of response. *Am J Psychiatry.* 1994;151:987–994.

Zvara DA, Brooker RF, McCall WV, et al. The effects of esmolol on ST-segment depression and arrhythmias after electroconvulsive therapy. *Convuls Ther.* 1997;13:166–174.

Zwill A, McAllister TW, Price TRP. Safety and efficacy of ECT in depressed patients with organic brain disease: review of a clinical experience. *Convuls Ther.* 1992;8:103–109.

30

Psychopharmacology

Barnett S. Meyers, MD
Robert C. Young, MD

INTRODUCTION

Growth of our knowledge base in geriatric psychopharmacology is reflected by textbooks devoted to this topic (Jenike, 1985a; Nelson, Atillasoy, et al., 1998; Sadavoy, 2004; Salzman, 1998), the inclusion of chapters in general textbooks of psychopharmacology (Bloom & Kupfer, 1995; Schatzberg & Nemeroff, 1998), and the frequency with which review articles are published. Clinicians can rely increasingly on information derived from prospective, controlled trials conducted in elderly samples rather than case reports and retrospective reviews alone. Increased attention to geriatric psychopharmacology results both from industries seeking Food and Drug Administration (FDA) approval of new "geriatric indications" for medications previously approved for use in general populations and from investigator-initiated research supported by governmental agencies such as the National Institute of Mental Health (NIMH). The increased emphasis on effectiveness research (NIMH, 1999) that focuses on treatment outcomes in the more heterogeneous patients encountered in "real-world" settings is consistent with the geriatric psychiatrist's focus on patients with comorbid medical and cognitive disorders.

This chapter is organized around classes of treatments, rather than disorders, because particular agents are prescribed for a number of disorders. Emphasis is given to the following important principles:

- A thorough knowledge of the patient is required for safe and effective pharmacotherapy.
- An accurate psychiatric diagnosis is necessary, but not sufficient; the clinician must understand the patient's physical health status, including comorbid illnesses, and the potential for related drug-drug interactions.
- Differences in the health and physiological functioning of geriatric patients necessitates knowledge of pharmacokinetics and pharmacodynamics so that treatment may be individualized; the injunction to "start low and go slow" is neither sufficiently precise nor informed. Rather, the speed of upward dosage titration and the ultimate target dose should be dictated by the characteristics of a particular patient, including factors expected to influence pharmacological processes, and not an individual's chronological age alone.

Treatment of the cognitive deficits and behavioral complications of neurodegenerative/structural brain disorders has increasingly become a focus of geriatric psychopharmacology. Therefore, this chapter includes a review of the use of cholinesterase inhibitors and other new pharmacological treatments for patients with dementia.

The use of standard pharmacotherapies to treat the psychiatric complications of dementia is reviewed in sections that discuss the various classes of these medications. The importance of appropriately treating both the cognitive and psychiatric features of dementia has been underscored by findings from the epidemiological literature. Among persons residing in long-term care facilities, 80% suffer from dementia; in addition, 50% of these individuals demonstrate clinically significant psychopathology, with disturbances in this domain resulting in excess disability (Rovner et al., 1990). Studies that demonstrated a dose-dependent association between treatment with conventional psychotropic medications and untoward events such as hip fractures (Ray et al., 1980, 1987) led Congress to pass the Nursing Home Reform Amendments to the Omnibus Budget Reconciliation Act of 1987 (OBRA 87). As described in Chapter 34, OBRA 87 created guidelines designed to regulate the use of psychotropic medications in long-term care settings.

Despite its many limitations, the OBRA initiative has resulted in four major benefits:

- Geriatric psychiatrists have been brought into the nursing home to consult on the care of elderly residents with primary psychiatric disturbances and both the cognitive and behavioral features of dementia.
- The use of psychotropic agents decreased generally (Rovner et al., 1992; Schorr et al., 1994), including a 26.7% decrease in antipsychotic drug use; compliance with most guidelines now exceeds 70% (Llorent et al., 1998).
- Increased attention has been given to delineating specific psychopatho-

logical states and determining the efficacy and safety of psychotropic medications through randomized controlled trials. The latter initiative led to the development of consensus criteria for the psychosis associated with Alzheimer's disease (Jeste & Finkel, 2000), which the FDA has accepted as a new indication for antipsychotic treatment (Division of Neuropharmacological Drug Products, 2000).

PRINCIPLES OF CLINICAL PHARMACOLOGY IN ELDERLY PATIENTS

Pharmacokinetics

Pharmacokinetics can be described as the "effect of a patient on a drug," which includes the processes of absorption, distribution, and elimination. Elimination includes the metabolism of drugs to a water-soluble form and their excretion in the urine. An understanding of pharmacokinetics, which translates into the concentration of a drug and its availability in active or unbound form, allows the clinician to anticipate the amount of active medication that will be available for therapeutic activity or adverse effects. The pharmacokinetic effects of physiological changes that accompany aging are described in Table 30-1.

ABSORPTION Psychotropic drugs are generally well absorbed from the gastrointestinal tract. Age-related changes might be expected to decrease drug absorption and may result in a lower rate of absorption for certain medications. Nevertheless, available evidence indicates that the bioavailability of an orally ad-

TABLE 30-1. Pharmacokinetic components, age effects, and examples of consequences

Component	Age effect	Consequence
Absorption	Decreased gastric pH, motility, surface transport	Slows absorption, without clinical significance
Metabolism	Decrease in some microsomal enzyme activities	Higher tertiary amine TCA plasma levels/dose
Distribution	Increased ratio of fat to water	Decreased levels/dose and clearance of fat-soluble drugs; increased levels/dose and clearance of hydrophilic drugs
	Increased serum AAG/decreased albumin	May alter interpretation of total drug levels
Excretion	Decreased renal clearance	Increased levels/dose of lithium and water-soluble drug metabolites

AAG, alpha acid glycoprotein; TCA, tricyclic antidepressant.

ministered dose of medication is not significantly affected by aging in the absence of gastrointestinal disease (Israili & Wenger, 1981; von Moltke et al., 1998).

METABOLISM   The liver is the principal site for metabolic transformation of lipid-soluble psychotropic medications. Phase I metabolic processes are mediated by the P450 enzyme system and include demethylation, ring hydroxylation, and sulfoxidation, depending on the compound. Phase I metabolism produces metabolites that may be pharmacologically active or inactive. For example, temazapam and oxazepam are metabolites of diazepam that presumably contribute to clinical effects. Similarly, norfluoxetine is an active metabolite of fluoxetine that has a longer half-life than fluoxetine. Phase I metabolism is followed by the Phase II processes of conjugation or glucuronidation, which generate largely inactive, water-soluble compounds that are excreted in the urine. Some compounds do not require Phase I metabolism for inactivation or excretion.

Most psychotropic drugs undergo hepatic metabolism. They may also act as inhibitors or inducers of the metabolism of other medications (Cozza & Armstrong, 2001). As P450 substrates, pharmacotherapeutic agents may have their own metabolism affected by other medications a patient may be taking. Potential effects of aging and concomitant medications on P450 enzymes that metabolize psychotropic medications are listed in Table 30-2. These effects

TABLE 30-2.   Examples of effects of concomitant nonpsychiatric medications on P450-mediated metabolism of psychotropics

	1A2	2C9/19	2D6*	3A4
Inhibitor	Ciproflaxicin	Valproic acid Omeprazole Ritonavir	Valproic acid Opiates Quinidine Cimetidine Ritonavir	Grapefruit juice Ketoconazole Nifedipine Erythromycin Clarithromycin
Inducer	Carbamazapine Cigarette smoking Caffeine	Phenytoin, barbiturates	Carbamazepine	Carbamazepine Barbiturates Phenytoin
Substrate	Clozapine Fluvoxamine Olanzapine Tertiary amine TCAs	Tertiary amine TCAs Fluvoxamine Diazepam	Fluoxetine Haloperidol Paroxetine Perphenazine Risperidone Venlafaxine Secondary TCAs	Alprazolam Triazolam Tertiary TCAs Fluvoxamine Nefazodone Quetiapine Ziprasidone

*Polymorphisms for deficient 2D6 metabolism occur in 3% of Caucasians, 6% of some African populations, and 10%–25% of Asians.
TCA, tricyclic antidepressant.

could lead to blood concentrations that are either higher or lower than expected. For psychotropic medications with a narrow therapeutic window or a high potential for toxicity, such as the tertiary amine tricyclic antidepressants (TCAs) and long-acting benzodiazepines, P450 inhibition by concomitant medications can lead to clinically significant adverse reactions.

Table 30-3 describes potentially important effects of psychotropic agents on the activity of P450 hepatic enzymes that metabolize psychotropics and other classes of medications. Elevated plasma levels of other classes of medication can similarly be associated with increase in, and prolongation of, their effects.

Despite the decreases in hepatic blood flow and mass and in total content of P450 enzymes that occur with aging (Sontaniemi et al., 1997; Vestal et al., 1975), there is limited evidence for clinically significant age-related decreases in P450 activity. Nevertheless, age-related decreases in P450 enzymes have been postulated to contribute to the decreases in the metabolism of TCAs or other medications that have a demethylation step in their metabolism (DeVane & Pollock, 1999); for example, the ratio of plasma imipramine to desmethylimipramine is greater with increased age. P450 3A4, which is involved in demethylation of various pharmacotherapeutic medications, including diazepam, is decreased in postmenopausal women (DeVane & Pollock, 1999). There is evidence that estrogen inhibits 1A2 metabolism, in that clearance of caffeine, a

TABLE 30-3. Enzyme inhibition by psychotropics and examples of substrates

	1A2	2c9/19	2D6	3A4
Inhibitors	Fluvoxamine	Fluoxetine Sertraline (minor) Fluvoxamine	Fluoxetine (potent) Paroxetine (potent) Haloperidol Perphenazine TCAs Sertraline	Fluvoxamine Nefazodone
Substrates	Caffeine Phenacetin Tacrine Theophylline	Barbiturates Moclobemide Phenytoin Tolbutamide Warfarin	Codeine opiates Dextromethorphan Metroprolol Propranolol Timolol Verapamil	Astemizole Carbamazepine Cortisol Cyclosporine Diltiazem Estradiol Erythromycin Lidocaine Nifedipine Quinidine Tamoxifen Verapramil

TCA, tricyclic antidepressant.

1A2 substrate, is reduced by estrogen replacement therapy (Nagler & Pollock, 2000).

DISTRIBUTION Drugs are distributed throughout the body in three compartments: fat tissue, body water, and bound to plasma proteins. The *volume of distribution* indicates how widely a particular drug is distributed.

Drug distribution is determined in part by lipid solubility. Most psychotropic drugs are highly lipid soluble; the notable exception is lithium, which is a hydrophilic ion. The ratio of body fat to water increases with age (Hollister, 1981), which results in an increased volume of distribution and prolonged clearance of lipid-soluble psychotropic agents (Table 30-1).

Psychotropic drugs, with the exception of lithium, are bound to plasma proteins. Basic drugs such as polycyclic antidepressants are bound extensively to α-acid glycoprotein, whereas benzodiazepines and acidic compounds, such as valproate, are bound predominantly to albumin (Curry, 1981). Although only unbound drug is available for pharmacodynamic activity and subject to pharmacokinetic processes, standard methods of therapeutic monitoring measure both bound and unbound forms of the drug. Aging or age-associated factors can change concentrations of binding proteins, which will affect total drug concentrations measured in routine therapeutic monitoring (von Moltke et al., 1998).

Knowledge of these processes can make sense of otherwise misleading plasma levels. For example, elevation in α-acid glycoprotein levels in association with an acute inflammatory process may increase the total level of a medication bound to this protein (e.g., a TCA), resulting in an elevated plasma concentration without increasing the availability of active drug. Similarly, displacement of warfarin from its protein binding site by sertraline or another medication may result in a small increase in free warfarin and a patient's prothrombin time without changing the plasma concentration of the psychotropic medication.

EXCRETION Psychotropic drugs are eliminated mainly by the kidneys. Renal excretion of lipid-soluble drugs occurs mainly as hydrophilic metabolites. The decrease in glomerular filtration that is associated with aging (Rowe, 1980) accounts for part of the increased accumulation of hydrophilic metabolites in some elderly patients (Nelson, Mazure, et al., 1988; Potter et al., 1984; Young et al., 1984). Diminished renal function accounts for the decreased clearance of lithium in elderly patients (Chapron et al., 1982; Hardy et al., 1987).

CLEARANCE *Clearance* refers to the volume of blood from which all drug is removed per unit of time. The *half-life* of a drug is the time required for half of an amount of drug to be eliminated; the half-life is directly proportional to the volume of distribution and inversely proportional to clearance.

Steady-state concentrations are achieved when the amount of drug entering plasma on repeat administration balances its clearance. Such concentrations are directly proportional to dose, at a given dosing interval, and they are inversely proportional to clearance. Steady-state concentrations occur after five or six half-lives of repeated administration. Age-related prolongation of the half-life of certain drugs increases the time required to reach steady-state concentrations.

DRUG-DRUG INTERACTION AT THE PHARMACOKINETIC LEVEL   Tables 30-2 and 30-3 provide guidance for considering dosing and identifying potential drug-drug interactions at the hepatic level. As such, they underscore important principles and summarize available information. These tables are not exhaustive, but describe major known effects from an evolving literature. Additional information is provided in the descriptions of specific medications, including other levels of interaction, such as excretion. Many psychotropic agents are metabolized through multiple pathways. For these medications, such as sertraline, the availability of alternative enzyme systems limits increases in drug concentrations when a primary metabolic enzyme is inhibited.

The 3A4 pathway has received attention because of the association between elevated concentrations of drugs metabolized by this system and the occurrence of potentially fatal torsades de pointes arrhythmias. Such interactions led to the removal of cisapride and terfenadine from the market by the FDA. Because other commonly used medications, such as clarithromycin, erythromycin, and specific antihistamines metabolized by 3A4, have also been implicated in the prolongation of QT_c intervals (Haverkamp et al., 2000), such medications must be used cautiously with potent 3A4 inhibitors such as nefazodone.

DISEASE EFFECTS ON PHARMACOKINETICS   Illnesses can alter pharmacokinetics. They can decrease absorption, increase or decrease the concentration of plasma proteins, slow hepatic metabolism, or diminish renal clearance (Table 30-4). Important examples are described in sections dealing with specific drugs.

Pharmacodynamics and Aging

In addition to differing in pharmacokinetic characteristics, individuals may differ in tissue response to a given concentration of drug, that is, *pharmacodynamics*. Age-associated changes occur in both peripheral and central neurobiology (Pomara et al., 1998; Sunderland, 1998), and these changes may contribute to altered therapeutic and toxic effects of a drug at a given concentration.

Age effects on responses to acute administration of drugs, including psychotropic agents, have been reported. These effects include blunted prolactin response to neuroleptic medications, presumably related to altered dopaminergic neurotransmission (Rolandi et al., 1982); decreased response of

TABLE 30-4. Components of pharmacokinetics: examples of medical disorders and consequences

Component	Medical disorder	Consequence
Absorption	Gastric or small bowel resection; heart failure; use of antacids	Decreased absorption
Metabolism	Severe liver disease; heart failure	Decreased metabolism
	Inflammatory states	Increased alpha acid glycoprotein level; increased total plasma antidepressant concentration
	Malnutrition; chronic illness; liver disease	Decreased binding proteins (albumin and alpha acid glycoprotein); deceased metabolism
Excretion	Renal failure; heart failure	Decreased clearance of lithium and hydrophilic metabolites; increased alpha acid glycoprotein level

peripheral β-adrenergic receptors to agonist drugs (Vestal et al., 1979); and decreased noradrenergic response to desipramine administration (Sunderland, 1998).

Pharmacodynamic considerations are complex. Most psychotropic drugs interact with many neurotransmitter systems, and these neurotransmitter systems themselves interact. Biological consequences of drug action also change over time during chronic administration.

The concept that older persons have increased sensitivity to toxic effects of conventional doses of psychotropic drugs is based largely on reports; systematic studies of this question are limited. Increased sensitivity of elderly patients to cognitive effects of diazepam has been reported (Pomara et al., 1984; Reidenberg et al., 1978). Similarly, clinical lore that therapeutic effects of psychotropic drugs occur at lower doses or concentrations in elderly patients has not been supported by empirical studies. It is not known whether elderly patients treated with a broad range of plasma concentrations have the same concentration-response relationship as younger adults. Nevertheless, it does appear that the window between toxic and therapeutic doses is smaller for elderly patients than for young adults.

Pharmacodynamic interactions with age-related physiological changes contribute to the increased risk of falls in older patients receiving psychotropic agents. Falls can be mediated through orthostatic hypotension, extrapyramidal side effects, ataxia, and impaired cognition. The public health importance of falls in older patients is supported by data demonstrating that approximately 5% of falls in older individuals result in fractures (Tinetti, 1987). Falls are the most frequent cause of death by injury in late life (Baker & Harvey, 1985); they contribute to more than one third of admissions to nursing homes (Wild et al., 1980). An increased incidence of falls has been associated with use of pharmacotherapeutic agents, including antidepressants, antipsychotics, and benzodiazepines, among older outpatients (Tinetti, 1987) and residents of nursing homes (Tinetti et al., 1988). Epidemiological data have indicated a dose-response relationship between the incidence of hip fractures and use of psychotropics in residents of long-term care facilities (Ray et al., 1987).

DISEASE EFFECT ON PHARMACODYNAMICS   Brain disorders in the elderly, such as Parkinson's disease, cerebrovascular disease, and primary degenerative dementia, are associated with additional neuronal changes that may influence drug effects. Evidence for central disruption of biogenic amine and acetylcholine neurotransmitter systems by these disorders has been summarized (Addonizio, 1987). Patients with Parkinson's disease have increased sensitivity to neuroleptic-induced exacerbation of motor dysfunction and to anticholinergic delirium (Figiel et al., 1989) and are sensitive to the sedative effects of these agents (Sunderland & Silver, 1988). Prescription of a conventional antipsychotic medication to treat psychosis in a patient with Parkinson's disease can aggravate neuromuscular impairment. Alternative approaches, such as lowering the dosage of an antiparkinsonian medication that could be causing the psychiatric symptoms or using an atypical antipsychotic medication, should be considered.

DRUG-DRUG INTERACTIONS AT THE PHARMACODYNAMIC LEVEL   Drugs for medical or neurological disorders can interact with psychotropic agents at the pharmacodynamic level. Examples of common additive interactions that increase side effects are provided in Table 30-5.

TABLE 30-5.   Examples of pharmacodynamic interactions

Drug interaction	Consequence
Tricyclics, neuroleptics or benzodiazepines with other sedative drugs	Increased sedative effect
α or β-blockers and TCAs or low-potency neuroleptics	Increased vulnerability to orthostatic hypotension
Cimetidine or other antihistamines with a TCA	Increased anticholinergic side effects
SSRI and MAOI	Life-threatening hyperthermia
Lithium with neuroleptics	Increased extrapyramidal side effects
Tricyclics with quinidine	Increased quinidinelike effects (e.g., slowing of intracardiac conduction)

MAOI, monoamine oxidase inhibitor; SSRI, selective serotonin reuptake inhibitor; TCA, tricyclic antidepressant.

ANTIDEPRESSANT DRUGS

Improved recognition of depression and the development of better-tolerated medications have been accompanied by increased use of antidepressants in both mental health and primary care settings (Pincus et al., 1998). Although there has been greater use of selective serotonin reuptake inhibitor (SSRI) antidepressants and decreased use of TCAs in older adults (Mandani et al., 2000), this pattern has not necessarily led to greater frequency of treatment that is adequate in dose and duration. Thus, elderly enrollees of a health maintenance organization received increased depression-specific treatment between 1989 and 1993, but there was a persistent tendency for underrecognition and undertreatment (Unutzer et al., 2000). Also, socioeconomic disparities exist, such that poorer, less-educated Medicare recipients are less likely to receive new-generation antidepressants than those of higher socioeconomic status (Sabamoorthi et al., 2003).

Types

The secondary amine TCAs and the SSRIs have been intensively studied and are widely used to treat geriatric depression. Venlafaxine, which acts as a serotonin reuptake inhibitor, also inhibits norepinephrine reuptake at higher doses. Monoamine oxidase inhibitors (MAOIs) have been systematically studied in elderly patients. Although clinicians remain wary of their use, the efficacy of MAOIs for the treatment of geriatric major depression is well established. Other antidepressants, including bupropion, maprotoline, mirtazapine, nefazadone, and trazadone, are efficacious as well.

Although existing literature does not demonstrate that a particular medication or class of FDA-approved medications has superior efficacy, clinicians should be guided by the quantity and quality of published studies demonstrating that specific antidepressants are both efficacious and well tolerated by older depressed patients. The selection of a particular class of antidepressants, or agents within a class, should be based on this knowledge and on the clinical characteristics of individual patients. A review (Flint, 1998) and results from a meta-analysis assessing trials using more than one active compound (Mittmann et al., 1997) support the conclusion that antidepressants within a particular class or across different classes have comparable efficacy for the treatment of geriatric depression.

Primary Indication: Major Depression

Antidepressants are approved for the acute treatment of both unipolar and bipolar major depression, and they are appropriate for continuation and maintenance treatment. Because continuation treatment is recommended for nearly

all patients following recovery from a major depression and because maintenance treatment appears to be appropriate for at least 50% of patients, it is
reasonable to continue the medication associated with an initial response for 6
to 12 additional months. The duration of continuation and maintenance treatment should be contingent on the frequency and severity of previous episodes,
and lifelong prophylactic treatment is recommended for some patients (Alexopoulos et al., 2001). Antidepressants are generally effective for treating the
anxiety symptoms associated with late-life depression. Although evidence for
the efficacy for anxiety is greatest for the SSRIs that have been approved for
the treatment of specific anxiety disorders, older studies and clinical experience
indicate that TCAs are also effective for generalized anxiety.

Tricyclic Antidepressants

Evidence for the efficacy and tolerability of secondary amine TCAs, and for
the adverse pharmacological properties of tertiary amine TCAs, has led to a
consensus that secondary amine agents are preferred in this class. The extensive experience with their use frames management issues that pertain to all
antidepressants.

EFFICACY   Rockwell and coworkers (1988) reviewed 17 controlled, acute treatment studies of polycyclic antidepressants in patients older than 60 years. Of
the studies, 12 involved TCAs; the 6 that were placebo controlled (Branconn-
nier et al., 1982; Cohn 1984; Georgotas et al., 1989; Gerner, et al., 1980;
Meredith et al., 1984; Wakelin, 1986) demonstrated efficacy of the TCAs.
Georgotas et al. (1986) demonstrated the efficacy and safety of nortriptyline in
older adults at plasma concentrations of 50 to 150 ng/mL. The remission rate
of more than 60% was comparable to that achieved with phenelzine. Elderly
patients with melancholic depression require and respond to desipramine levels
comparable to those effective in younger adults (Nelson et al., 1985). Furthermore, Reynolds, Frank, Kupfer, and colleagues (1996) demonstrated that 78.4%
of elderly patients treated openly with therapeutic concentrations of nortriptyline (80–120 ng/mL) plus interpersonal psychotherapy achieved remission with
only 12.2% discontinuing treatment.

Nortriptyline and desipramine are preferable to their parent tertiary amine
compounds amitriptyline and imipramine in elderly depressed patients. Increased age does not decrease the metabolism of secondary amine agents by
the P450 microenzyme system (Mulsant et al., 1999). Lower concentrations
are required for efficacy compared to tertiary amines. Lower antagonism of
muscarinic, histamine, and α-adrenergic receptors are associated with more tolerable side effect profiles (Richelson, 1982). The side effect profile of clomipramine is problematic, as is that of doxepin. Protriptyline is no longer used
commonly because of its prolonged half-life and adverse side effect profile. The

lack of clear concentration-response relationships as well as other properties that cause adverse effects for amitriptyline, doxepin, and protriptyline also limit their use.

It has been suggested that TCAs have a greater efficacy than SSRIs for melancholic depression. Among elderly melancholic patients with cardiac disease, the response rate to fluoxetine was significantly lower than that in a matched historical control group treated with nortriptyline (Roose et al., 1994). Similarly, the Danish University Antidepressant Group reported greater response rates among patients with "endogenous" depression who were treated with clomipramine compared to those treated with either citalopram (Danish University Antidepressant Group, 1986) or paroxetine (Danish University Antidepressant Group, 1990). A comparison of paroxetine to nortriptyline in elderly patients treated for 6 weeks found comparable response rates overall that were somewhat higher in the melancholic subsample treated with nortriptyline (62% vs. 43%) (Mulsant et al., 1999). Additional data about the comparative efficacy of these two classes of medications among elderly patients with more severe and melancholic depression are needed, particularly in light of the poorer overall tolerability of nortriptyline and its risks in cardiac patients (see below).

Limited data are available on the treatment of the older-old. Efficacy data from studies that included and identified patients 75 years and older have been reviewed (Salzman et al., 1993). Among 171 patients, some demonstrated only a modest therapeutic benefit from standard antidepressant treatment. In a placebo-controlled antidepressant trial in frail elderly patients without dementia living in residential care facilities, 58% of the 12 nortriptyline completers met criteria for response compared to only 1 of 11 completers (9%) randomized to placebo (Katz et al., 1991). The 33% dropout rate among nortriptyline subjects in this carefully conducted trial speaks to the poor tolerability to a secondary amine TCA among the frail elderly. The demonstration that adverse medical events during the acute nortriptyline trial were associated with increased mortality at follow-up demonstrates that the physical frailty contributing to TCA intolerance in elderly patients may be a marker for increased vulnerability to mortality (Katz et al., 1994).

Continuation treatment is intended to prevent relapse during the period following symptom resolution. Only 17% of older patients treated with nortriptyline at an average dose of 80 mg per day suffered a recurrence in the initial 4 months following remission (Georgotas et al., 1988). Another study found that only 6.1% of the 119 elderly subjects who had achieved remission with nortriptyline plus interpersonal psychotherapy relapsed during continuation therapy (Reynolds, Frank, Perel, et al., 1996). In contrast to the study of Georgotas and coworkers, subjects studied by Reynolds and coworkers were older, had higher nortriptyline levels, and received monthly psychotherapy sessions throughout the continuation phase.

Maintenance treatment is defined as the use of medication beyond the continuation interval to prevent a new episode or recurrence. A 1-year study found a recurrence rate of 13.3% for phenelzine and more than 50% for nortriptyline at levels of 50 to 150 ng/mL; the nortriptyline relapse rate did not differ from that with placebo (Georgotas et al., 1989). Analyses of additional unpublished data from the work of Georgotas and colleagues indicated prophylactic efficacy among individuals maintained on nortriptyline (Meyers et al., 1997).

Prophylactic effectiveness with higher levels of nortriptyline had been reported in 1989 in an open study conducted by Reynolds and colleagues in which the 3-year recurrence rate was only 14.7%. In a placebo-controlled maintenance study, during the 4 to 6 weeks of antidepressant tapering, 24% of patients randomized to placebo suffered recurrences compared to none among the 24 who remained on nortriptyline (Reynolds et al., 1992). Other data demonstrated the prophylactic efficacy of nortriptyline for geriatric depression and suggested that the efficacy of medication without concomitant psychotherapy is weaker among the older-old (Reynolds et al., 1999). Patients aged 70 years and older in that 3-year placebo-controlled maintenance study had a significantly increased overall rate of recurrence, with the frequency highest among patients who received pharmacotherapy alone. These data speak to the instability of recovery in the older-old and the potential need for adjunctive psychotherapy to prevent recurrences in these patients.

TOXICITY

Cardiac Effects. Elderly patients with cardiac disease have an increased risk of orthostatic hypotension during TCA treatment. Orthostatic hypotension is not correlated with age (Glassman et al., 1979), but it can be more severe and can have serious consequences in patients with congestive heart failure (Glassman et al., 1983). Although orthostatic hypotension is more severe in patients treated with imipramine than nortriptyline (Roose et al., 1981), it may occur with either agent, particularly in the presence of left ventricular dysfunction (Roose et al., 1986). The association between orthostatic hypotension and cardiac disease presumably results from an abnormal hemodynamic response to postural change because of decreased left ventricular function or the effects of medications such as β-blockers and diuretics.

TCA treatment can increase heart rate. The increase is usually small and is only weakly correlated with plasma TCA concentrations (Glassman & Bigger, 1981). Patients with ischemic heart disease are susceptible to developing a clinically significant sinus tachycardia, however (Roose et al., 1998). Furthermore, among patients with an underlying conduction abnormality, the quinidine-like type I antiarrhythmic effects of TCAs can lead to heart block (Roose et al., 1987). This prolongation of conduction peaks after 3 or 4 weeks of treatment (Glassman & Bigger, 1981). Therefore, cardiac conduction should be assessed prior to treatment, and electrocardiograms (ECGs) should be repeated weekly for the first 4 weeks of TCA therapy in patients with marginal cardiac conduction before treatment. The conduction effects of TCAs are dependent on plasma drug concentrations in elderly and young adult patients (Glassman & Bigger, 1981). Increased plasma concentrations of hydroxylated metabolites can contribute to such effects when they occur in elderly patients (Kutcher et al., 1986; Schneider et al., 1988; Young et al., 1985).

Although the antiarrhythmic effects of TCAs were thought to be beneficial, evidence of an association between taking type I antiarrhythmic medications and increased mortality in patients with ischemic heart disease (Echt et al., 1991) led to a reconsideration of this suggestion (Glassman et al., 1993). Data from a randomized trial of nortriptyline and paroxetine in patients with major depression and ischemic disease demonstrated an association between nortriptyline and significant increase in heart rate (11% from baseline), decreased heart rate variability, and an 18% incidence of adverse cardiac events (Roose et al., 1998). Despite the comparable overall efficacy, subjects taking nortriptyline were more likely to discontinue because of adverse cardiac events (Nelson et al., 1999).

Among psychiatric patients, age older than 65 years and taking a TCA are both independent predictors for prolonged QT_c intervals (>456 ms), a potentially life-threatening conduction delay (Reilly et al., 2000). Therefore, secondary amine TCAs may be valuable for the acute treatment of the more severely depressed geriatric patient, but their use does expose older patients to an increased risk of untoward cardiac events. This risk may be especially relevant in patients with recurrent depression, who may suffer new cardiac disease during extended maintenance therapy.

Cognitive Effects.   Adverse effects on cognitive performance have been reported at high plasma TCA concentrations in adults in a mixed-age group (Preskorn & Simpson, 1982) and are concentration dependent in elderly patients treated with nortriptyline (Young et al., 1991). However, TCA-induced delirium occurs infrequently in elderly patients and is usually associated with extremely high plasma levels (Meyers, 1991). A discontinuation study demonstrated that patients required more trials on a list-learning task during nortriptyline treatment than during placebo treatment without having an objectively assessed difference in memory (Young et al., 1991). These data suggest that the anticholinergic properties of TCAs may interfere with memory consolidation sufficiently to be noticeable to patients without being objectively detectable.

PRACTICAL GUIDELINES

Pretreatment Assessment/Clinical Monitoring.   History concerning previous successful or unsuccessful drug trials can guide selection of particular agents. Adequacy of prior treatment efforts should be assessed by noting drug dose, duration of administration, and drug blood levels. Therapeutic response should be judged, and any treatment-limiting side effects should be noted.

Clinicians can make use of psychopathology rating scales to help monitor change during treatment. For example, the Hamilton Depression Rating Scale

(HDRS) (Hamilton, 1960) is applicable for rating depressive signs and symptoms in cognitively intact patients. The Cornell Scale (Alexopoulos et al., 1988) is useful for elderly patients with cognitive impairment. The 30- and 15-item versions of the Geriatric Depression Rating Scale (Yesavage et al., 1983) self-report instruments have established reliability and validity.

Cognitive function should be evaluated before and during treatment. The Mini-Mental State Examination (MMSE) (Folstein et al., 1975) is a convenient and widely used instrument for screening, although it has limited sensitivity. Instruments that are more sensitive and detailed are available, such as the Dementia Rating Scale (Mattis, 1988).

The importance of the initial medical and cognitive assessments derives in part from the fact that side effects may be related to illness state. It is critical to compare physical complaints during treatment with those before treatment to judge whether these complaints represent drug toxicity. Blood pressure assessment before treatment should include determination of orthostatic change. Pretreatment orthostatic blood pressure changes can predict changes that occur during antidepressant treatment (Glassman et al., 1979). Assessment prior to initiating a TCA should also include an electrocardiogram. Evidence for ischemic heart disease, current dysrhythmia, or conduction abnormalities should be considered in choosing from among available antidepressants.

Pharmacokinetics, Dosing, and Drug-Drug Interactions. Treatment is initiated at a low dose that is increased more gradually than in young adults. Nevertheless, the target dose of nortriptyline or desipramine can be achieved within 1 to 2 weeks in most cases. A dose of 50 mg/day of nortriptyline could be achieved within 1 week, followed by an assessment for early therapeutic response. Among patients who appear to be improving, further increases may be unnecessary; in others, a steady-state plasma concentration should be obtained 1 week after reaching the dose of 50 mg/day, followed by an increase to 75 mg/day the following day. Dosing through gradual increments allows patients to become accustomed to side effects and may increase compliance. The half-lives of TCAs allows for once-daily dosing. A single nighttime dose is generally well tolerated and improves sleep.

Therapeutic drug monitoring (TDM) has several roles in TCA use. Low or nondetectable concentrations of steady-state dosing can indicate poor adherence or rapid metabolism. Genetically determined poor metabolism occurs in 3% of whites, 15% to 25% of Asians, and 6% of some African populations (Meyer et al., 1996; Pollock, 1994). In addition, there is a subpopulation with genetically determined rapid 2D6 metabolism that interferes with achieving therapeutic levels using standard doses. Thus, very low or nondetectable steady-state dosing can indicate poor adherence or rapid metabolism. TDM can help minimize the risk of toxicity among poor metabolizers.

Increased plasma ratios of 10-hydroxynortriptyline to nortriptyline (Young et al., 1984) and plasma ratios of 2-hydroxy-desipramine to desipramine (Kitanaka et al., 1981; Nelson, Mazure, et al., 1988) have been reported in elderly patients. Although these compounds have pharmacodynamic activity that may influence efficacy and tolerability (Nelson, Mazure, et al., 1988; Young et al., 1987, 1991), assays for these secondary amine metabolite levels are not widely available, and their general clinical relevance has not been elucidated.

Although the optimal TCA concentrations for elderly patients have not been well delineated, older patients respond to doses and steady-state plasma levels of nortriptyline and desipramine that are comparable to those effective in younger adults. Target concentrations of nortriptyline between 80 and 120 ng/mL are recommended, particularly if a response is unsatisfactory. Also, maintenance studies in young adults have demonstrated that reducing the dose used in acute treatment is associated with a loss of prophylactic benefit (Frank et al., 1990), leading to the maxim that the dose associated with response is the one that maintains wellness. Also, clinicians should not "treat" the plasma levels of patients who recover at concentrations below the usual therapeutic range.

Monoamine Oxidase Inhibitors

The MAOIs can be divided into selective and nonselective types. Selective MAOIs inhibit either MAO-A, the enzyme that metabolizes epinephrine, norepinephrine, serotonin, and tyramine, or MAO-B, the enzyme that metabolizes phenethylamine. Dopamine is metabolized by both MAO-A and MAO-B. The two MAOI antidepressants available in the United States (phenelzine and tranylcypromine) are nonselective; that is, they inhibit both enzymes. Because the binding of these medications to MAO is irreversible, their duration of action is dependent on the synthesis of new MAO rather than the half-life of the drug antidepressant. Trends include developing MAOIs that are more pharmacologically selective against MAO-A or MAO-B and therefore produce differential augmentation of the neurotransmitters metabolized by these enzymes. Also, MAOIs that are cleared more rapidly, called reversible MAOIs (RIMAs, e.g., moclobemide), are available outside the United States.

EFFICACY   Experience with MAOIs in elderly patients has been reviewed (Rockwell et al., 1988). The acute efficacy of phenelzine in ambulatory elderly patients with an "endogenous" symptom profile who are experiencing major depression was found superior to placebo and comparable to nortriptyline (Georgotas et al., 1986). Phenelzine was associated with remission in 64% of elderly patients who had failed an initial trial of therapeutic concentrations of nortriptyline (Flint & Rifat, 1996). Other MAOIs available in the United States have not received randomized controlled study in older depressed patients. Despite the need for special caution in using MAOIs, based on studies in young adults, MAOIs may have a special role in the treatment of severe and bipolar depression and for patients who have not responded to standard treatment.

Moclobemide, a RIMA in widespread use outside the United States, has specificity for MAO-A (Freeman, 1993). Moclobemide primarily inhibits noradrenaline and serotonin oxidative metabolism and, to a lesser extent, tyramine and dopamine oxidative metabolism. In the acute treatment of geriatric depressed patients, moclobemide has been reported equally effective compared to maprotiline (DeVanna et al., 1990) and miansarin (Mangoni et al., 1991); in one study, it was associated with a better outcome than fluvoxamine (Bocksberger et al., 1993).

Selegiline (l-deprenyl) selectively inhibits MAO-B activity at the doses of 5 to 10 mg/day used to treat Parkinson's disease. Oxidative metabolism of benzylamine and phenylethylamine, and to lesser extent dopamine and tyramine, is inhibited; oxidative metabolism of noradrenaline and serotonin is not inhibited. The absence of tyramine reaction at doses of selegiline that selectively inhibit MAO-B is consistent with the lack of involvement of MAO-B in the gastrointestinal metabolism of tyramine.

Although antidepressant effects of selegiline have been reported primarily at nonselective doses of 20 to 40 mg/day in young adults with major depression, they may occur at doses that inhibit MAO-B selectively in patient subgroups (Mann et al., 1989). Sunderland and colleagues (1994) demonstrated improvement during acute treatment with selegiline at nonselective doses in geriatric patients with depression who had previously failed at least two trials of adequate pharmacotherapy. Nevertheless, the effectiveness of selegiline at higher nonselective doses, which would require standard MAOI dietary precautions, has not been studied systematically.

Georgotas and associates reported on the effectiveness of an average dose of 54 mg/day of phenelzine during 4 months of continuation treatment (Georgotas et al., 1988). Also, the 13% recurrence rate during 1 year of subsequent maintenance treatment was significantly lower than the recurrence rate with placebo or nortriptyline (Georgotas et al., 1989).

TOXICITY Nonselective MAOIs have weak anticholinergic activity and do not have quinidine-like effects. Their principal side effect, orthostatic hypotension, emerges more slowly than with TCAs, but is more profound (Kronig et al., 1983). Pedal edema and paresthesia may also complicate treatment, but whether this adverse reaction is more common in elderly patients than in young adults is not clear.

Toxicity associated with selective MAO inhibition is relatively low in the elderly. Neither acute nor subchronic moclobemide administration produced detectable effects on cognitive function or psychomotor performance in normal elderly volunteers (Kerr et al., 1992). Moclobemide side effects can include nausea and sleep disturbance (Freeman, 1993; Mongoni et al., 1991). The reversible characteristics of moclobemide's pharmacological activity have potential advantage in discontinuation in the event of toxicity. Selegiline monotherapy appears to be well tolerated in geriatric patients (Agnoli et al., 1992;

Foley et al., 1992). Tariot and colleagues (1988) reported that tranylcypromine produced orthostatic hypotension in geriatric patients who had tolerated selegiline well.

PRACTICAL GUIDELINES

Pretreatment Assessment/Clinical Monitoring. Determination of a patient's ability and willingness to adhere to an MAOI diet is critical in assessing patients prior to initiating treatment. Cognitively impaired elderly persons who live in unsupervised environments and have a propensity for taking over-the-counter medications are at greatest risk for developing a tyramine reaction. Nevertheless, MAOIs have been well studied in the elderly and can be both safe and effective in this population when administered with the proper dietary and drug interaction instructions. It is helpful to have patients who take MAOIs carry a card or wristband indicating this fact.

Pharmacokinetics, Dosing, and Drug-Drug Interactions. Monitoring of blood levels or degree of MAO inhibition is not clinically applicable to nonselective MAOIs. Although body weight has been suggested as a guideline for phenelzine dosing (1 mg/kg; Robinson et al., 1978), a dosage range between 45 and 60 mg is generally used. Although the inhibition of platelet MAO activity by at least 80% from baseline is associated with better therapeutic response to phenelzine, this measurement is not readily available to clinicians.

Although plasma levels of phenelzine may be higher in elderly compared to younger patients receiving equivalent doses (Robinson, 1981), the clinical significance of this is not known. Maguire and associates (1991) reported similar single-dose pharmacokinetics of moclobemide in geriatric patients with depression, compared with younger patients, suggesting that clinicians can expect to use similar doses across the age spectrum. Therapeutic response to phenelzine in elderly patients with depression occurs at doses comparable to those used with younger depressed patients (Georgotas et al., 1986).

Special concerns with nonselective MAOIs such as phenelzine and tranylcypromine include the need for dietary restriction of foods rich in tyramine and avoidance of drug-drug interactions, particularly with sympathomimetic agents and meperidine. Analysis of the tyramine content of commonly prohibited foods suggests the lists usually given to patients are overrestrictive, however (McCabe & Tsuang, 1982; Shulman et al., 1989; Sullivan & Shulman, 1984). The availability of clear, easy-to-follow guidelines is especially relevant to treatment of elderly patients, who frequently depend on others for shopping or food preparation.

It appears that selective MAOIs and RIMAs have a reduced risk of tyramine pressor response and less need for dietary restriction. Also, there appears to be a lower rate of drug-drug interactions associated with the use of selective MAOIs (Freeman, 1993).

Selective Serotonin Reuptake Inhibitors

The SSRIs, which comprise an increasing proportion of antidepressant prescriptions to older patients, have contributed to the dramatic increased use of antidepressants to treat geriatric depression (Mandani et al., 2000). Consideration of the efficacy of SSRIs and other newer classes of antidepressants must take into account changes in the ways antidepressants are studied and receive FDA approval. Ethical concerns and the need to justify payment for inpatient days generally preclude study of inpatients in placebo-controlled trials. Therefore, the knowledge of the efficacy of new antidepressants is based primarily on studies of outpatients with less-severe and nonmelancholic forms of depression. Nevertheless, the treatment of geriatric depression is informed increasingly by trials that specifically target elderly patients, including studies of the older-old and medically frail.

EFFICACY Five selective SSRIs (fluoxetine, sertraline, paroxetine, citalopram, and escitalopram) have been approved for treatment of major depression in the United States. Fluvoxamine, which is approved as an antidepressant in Europe, has been used in this country for young adults. There is no clear evidence that the SSRIs differ in efficacy, speed of action, or tolerability.

Fluoxetine remains the only antidepressant with a specific indication for the treatment of geriatric depression. Approval was based on a 6-week, placebo-controlled study of 771 older patients with major depression. A significantly greater proportion of subjects treated with a target dose of 20 mg/day of fluoxetine than those allocated to placebo achieved response criteria of a 50% improvement in HDRS scores and remission end point scores of 8 or less (McCabe & Tsuang, 1982). Although the overall response rates were not robust, with fewer than 50% of fluoxetine patients meeting response or remission criteria, the 6-week trial may have been too brief to demonstrate maximal response rates (Georgotas & McCue, 1989; Meyers, 1999; Schweizer et al., 1990).

An 8-week, placebo-controlled fluoxetine trial among medically hospitalized elderly patients, of whom 50% had MMSE scores of 23 or less, supported the efficacy and tolerability of SSRIs in the frail medical elderly (Evans et al., 1997). The results were also consistent with extending trials beyond 6 weeks; 55% of patients treated for a minimum of 3 weeks and 67% who completed the trial met response criteria. Furthermore, fluoxetine, but not placebo, response rates increased significantly between weeks 5 and 8. A 6-week, placebo-controlled study of citalopram in frail older patients with depressive symptoms with and without dementia demonstrated the efficacy and tolerability of this SSRI as well (Nyth et al., 1992); superiority of citalopram was noted in the 74% of subjects who met criteria for major depression.

Fluoxetine has comparable efficacy and greater tolerability compared to tertiary amine agents such as doxepin (Feighner & Cohn, 1985) and amitriptyline (Altamura et al., 1989). Nevertheless, such studies are less informative because the tertiary amine comparators are not appropriate for the treatment of geriatric depression. Studies demonstrating comparable efficacy for sertraline (Cohn et al., 1990) and paroxetine (Dunner et al., 1992) as compared to a tertiary amine TCA suffer from the same limitation.

Two studies of sertraline and paroxetine have demonstrated comparable efficacy to that of nortriptyline. A 12-week comparison of sertraline to nortriptyline found similar remission rates and time to response, with 75% of improvement in depression scores occurring by week 6 (Bondareff et al., 2000). Although plasma nortriptyline levels were not controlled, the majority of subjects treated with nortriptyline had therapeutic concentrations, and lower levels were not associated with diminished response. Sertraline was more effective in the patients aged 70 years and older, suggesting that it may be more useful in the older-old if nortriptyline levels are not controlled. A double-blind comparison of nortriptyline and paroxetine in elderly patients, which maintained nortriptyline levels in the therapeutic range, demonstrated comparable efficacy for the two antidepressants (Mulsant et al., 1999). Response rates were somewhat higher for nortriptyline in the total sample and in the hospitalized and melancholic subgroups; of the subjects who completed the full 6-week trial, 66% of paroxetine-treated subjects and 78% of nortriptyline-treated subjects achieved full remission.

Roose and Suthers (1998) reviewed studies comparing nortriptyline with the SSRIs fluoxetine and sertraline in geriatric patients. Although statistically significant separation did not occur in any of the trials, nortriptyline was superior to the SSRI in each. These data are consistent with considering nortriptyline as the best-studied and probably most efficacious antidepressant for the treatment of late-life depression, particularly in severely depressed patients. Nevertheless, the possible superiority of nortriptyline in efficacy must be balanced against the diminished tolerability and potential for cardiovascular complications that are associated with TCA treatment.

There are few direct comparisons between SSRIs in elderly patients with depression. A 6-week comparison of fluoxetine to paroxetine in geriatric patients with major depression found the two SSRIs comparable in efficacy and frequency of adverse events (Schone & Ludwig, 1993). Although escitalopram, the isomer of citalopram, which accounts for its antidepressant activity, appears to have greater efficacy than racemic citalopram in young adults with depression (Burke et al., 2002), comparisons in older adults are not available. A 12-week comparison of sertraline to fluoxetine demonstrated comparable effectiveness for the two SSRIs (Finkel et al., 1999). Average depression scores continued to decrease, and the proportion of patients responding continued to increase beyond 6 weeks.

These data add to the controversy as to whether elderly subjects require longer to respond, particularly if treated with an SSRI. A naturalistic study that pooled data for outpatients treated with various classes of antidepressants reported that patients treated with TCAs or MAOIs achieved the depression rating scale cutoff for response significantly earlier than patients treated with SSRIs (Mittmann et al., 1999).

Venlafaxine is discussed within the SSRI class because it acts primarily on serotonin in the low-dose range generally utilized in geriatric patients. Nevertheless, venlafaxine also blocks the reuptake of norepinephrine, particularly when used at higher doses. Data on the efficacy of venlafaxine for geriatric depression are limited. Results from an open trial of 68 elderly patients with depression demonstrated effectiveness of venlafaxine at average doses of 114 ± 59 mg/day (Kahn et al., 1995). A controlled comparison with dothiepin, a TCA widely used in the United Kingdom, revealed comparable efficacy and tolerability with each at doses up to 150 mg/day (Mahapatra & Hackett, 1997). Among patients of various ages, a dose-response relationship to venlafaxine has been reported, with doses exceeding 200 mg/day associated with greater effectiveness (Mendels et al., 1993). Data on the efficacy or tolerability of this dose range of venlafaxine for older patients are not available.

Studies in young adults have demonstrated the efficacy of maintenance therapy with SSRIs for the prevention of recurrences. Available data indicate that these medications are similarly effective for preventing recurrences in older patients. An open geriatric trial with paroxetine demonstrated high prophylactic efficacy that was comparable to that of nortriptyline (Walters et al., 1999). Similarly, 80% of 28 geriatric patients with recurrent major depression who achieved remission during venlafaxine treatment at doses averaging 112.5 mg/day remained well for 2 years of ongoing treatment (Amore et al., 1997). Paroxetine was also reported to have greater efficacy than imipramine in preventing relapses among severely depressed older patients who recovered following electroconvulsive therapy (ECT) (Lauritzen et al., 1996). A placebo-controlled maintenance study conducted in geriatric outpatients demonstrated the effectiveness of citalopram for preventing recurrences (Klysener et al., 2002).

SSRIs have been found to be effective in the treatment of a variety of anxiety disorders. Based on studies in young adults, some have received FDA approval for specific forms of anxiety disorders. SSRI trials designed specifically for older patients with anxiety disorders are not available. A secondary analysis of data from geriatric patients who had participated in placebo-controlled, flexible-dose trials of extended-release venlafaxine for generalized anxiety disorder did demonstrate that efficacy and tolerability in patients aged 60 years and older were comparable to the response in younger adults (Katz et al., 2002). In the absence of specific studies of late-life anxiety disorders, the benefits established in studies of young adults and the side effects noted in studies of geriatric depression should be considered when treating the older patient with an anxiety disorder.

TOXICITY SSRIs have low propensity for cardiovascular and anticholinergic side effects. An acute trial with paroxetine failed to demonstrate adverse cognitive effects despite the anticholinergic activity of this antidepressant (Kerr et al., 1992). An extended trial comparing paroxetine with fluoxetine among older depressed patients without cognitive impairment demonstrated comparable tolerability, with performance on most cognitive measures improving over the 1-year trial period (Cassano et al., 2002). Among elderly depressed patients with mild cognitive impairment treated with sertraline, clinical response was associated with improvement in attention and a measure of executive function (Devanand et al., 2003). Thus, existing studies of SSRIs indicated that these agents do not decrease memory in older patients, but may be associated with improvement in measures of cognition that are adversely affected by depression.

SSRI treatment has been associated with development of the syndrome of inappropriate antidiuretic hormone secretion, which may lead to hyponatremia (Druckenbrod & Mulsant, 1994). Case report literature suggesting that the elderly may be at increased risk for this reaction, particularly at higher SSRI doses (Pillans & Coulter, 1994), have been augmented by a large pharmacy database study. The odds ratio for hospital admission for hyponatremia was fourfold higher among SSRI users than in community controls (5% vs. 1%), with the incidence appearing to occur within 2 weeks of the initiation of treatment (Movig et al., 2002).

Drug-induced parkinsonism has been reported in middle-aged adults in association with SSRI treatment (Bouchard et al., 1989; Broud, 1989). Although an open prospective study did not find worsening of symptoms among patients with Parkinson's disease treated with a variety of SSRIs (Dell'Agnello et al., 2001), results from a case-control study demonstrated that patients treated with SSRIs had a greater rate of having their antiparkinsonian medications increased than either patients who did not receive antidepressants or those who received TCAs (van de Vijver et al., 2002). Further clarification of the relationship between SSRI treatment and worsening of motor symptoms in patients with Parkinson's disease will require a prospective randomized trial comparison with an antidepressant from another class.

Sertraline, but not paroxetine, has been associated with an increase in body sway (Laghrissi-Thode et al., 1995). Whether this finding has clinical significance is uncertain. The association between hip fractures and SSRI treatment reported in epidemiological studies of nursing home residents (Thapa et al., 1998) and both falls and hip fractures among 8,000 elders in a health service database (Liu et al., 1998) did not distinguish among the various SSRIs. These cross-sectional data do not address whether these associations are because of direct effects of SSRIs on postural stability or an increased risk of falls associated with the diagnosis of depression (Whooley et al., 2001). Alternatively, it is likely that frail elders who are at greatest risk for falling are "channeled" to receive SSRI antidepressant treatment (Avorn, 1998).

Case reports have implicated SSRIs in the occurrence of purpura and prolongation of bleeding time (Ottervanger et al., 1994; Yaryra-Tobias et al., 1991). This adverse effect occurs in the absence of concurrent warfarin treatment and results from the inhibition of platelet aggregation by SSRIs (Alderman et al., 1996). Platelet function is lower in depressed patients with ischemic heart disease than in nondepressed controls (Laghrissi-Thode et al., 1997), and paroxetine but not nortriptyline inhibits platelet function in this population (Pollock et al., 2000). A case registry study found that use of SSRIs was associated with a 3.6 times increase in upper gastrointestinal bleeding; antidepressants without serotonin activity did not increase the risk compared to control patients (Dalton et al., 2003). Combined use with a nonsteroidal antiinflammatory or low doses of aspirin increased the risk further; the elevated risk disappeared among individuals who had discontinued SSRI treatment. Additional data are needed to determine the risks versus benefits of possible SSRI effects on platelet functioning so that clinical practice can be informed appropriately.

Both venlafaxine and paroxetine should be discontinued through gradual tapering because of the occurrence of a "discontinuation syndrome" with these agents that may be associated with malaise, increased anxiety, sleep disturbance, and gastrointestinal upset. Fluoxetine and sertraline have active metabolites with longer half-lives, which may explain the absence of discontinuation syndromes with these agents. Discontinuation syndromes with citalopram are also quite rare, perhaps because of the longer half-life of this SSRI.

PRACTICAL GUIDELINES

Pretreatment Assessment. Because adverse medical events are infrequent with SSRI treatment, a pretreatment medical workup is not required. Some patients have difficulty tolerating this class of medications because of the development of increased anxiety or a syndrome of akathisia. Patients who have had such a reaction in response to an SSRI previously should be treated with an alternative antidepressant class.

Because hyponatremia is an infrequent side effect, pretreatment electrolyte levels are not required. An alternative class of medication should be considered for patients who have developed water intoxication during antidepressant treatment previously.

Venlafaxine has been associated with increases in systolic blood pressure that may reach clinically significant levels (Thase, 1998). This infrequent side effect, which occurs primarily at doses over 200 mg/day, may result from the mixed noradrenergic and serotonin activity of higher venlafaxine doses. Baseline hypertension does not predict subsequent blood pressure elevations, and taking an antihypertensive for preexisting hypertension appears to decrease the risk of developing elevated blood pressure during treatment (Feighner, 1994). Nevertheless, assessing blood pressure would be appropriate before exceeding 150 mg/day, particularly in patients who are not under treatment for hypertension.

Pharmacokinetics, Dosing, and Drug-Drug Interactions. The SSRIs are metabolized primarily by the hepatic P450 system. The specific pathways by which SSRIs are metabolized and the relationships between these pathways and both aging and drug-drug interactions have been extensively reviewed (DeVane & Pollock, 1999; Greenblatt et al., 1998; Nemeroff et al., 1996; Preskorn, 1997). Aging has no effects to minimal effects on the metabolism of the different SSRIs; furthermore, modest variations in plasma levels of SSRIs are not related to clinical efficacy or tolerability.

Fluoxetine has a longer half-life than sertraline or paroxetine (Meredith et al., 1984). Norfluoxetine, the major active metabolite of fluoxetine, has a half-life several times longer than that of fluoxetine. Limited data indicate that metabolism of fluoxetine appears to be unaffected by aging (Bergstrom et al., 1988; Lemberger et al., 1985).

Sertraline has a longer half-life than paroxetine. It has a demethylated metabolite that is a less potent serotonin reuptake inhibitor than sertraline and has a half-life that is several times longer than that of sertraline. Increased plasma steady-state sertraline concentration/dose ratios in elderly patients have been reported (Moleman et al., 1986), but the clinical significance of this age effect is uncertain.

Paroxetine has no major metabolites. Steady-state plasma paroxetine concentrations have been reported as higher in elderly patients compared to young adults at doses of 30 mg to 40 mg per day, but not at doses of 20 mg per day (Hebenstreit et al., 1989).

Both citalopram and escitalopram are metabolized to monodesmethylated and didesmethyl metabolites. These metabolites have limited pharmacodynamic activity at the concentrations produced by humans. These medications have similar metabolic pathways and have a half-life longer than 1 day. Discontinuation is not associated with rebound symptoms. As with many SSRIs, the concentration/dose ratio of citalopram and escitalopram increases modestly with age.

Venlafaxine metabolism is not affected by aging. Both venlafaxine and its less-active o-desmethylated metabolite are eliminated through renal excretion, and clearance is decreased in association with renal impairment.

SSRIs can be administered in once-daily dosing and require minimal to no upward dose titration. Some elderly patients develop nausea or anxiety early in treatment, with tolerance developing within a few days. In these individuals, the initial dose should be lowered and then increased to the full dose within a week. If the less-common side effects of intolerable anxiety or akathisia develop, a different class of antidepressants should be selected. Although most SSRIs are given in the morning because of their potential for causing insomnia, some patients find these agents mildly sedating and prefer taking them before bed. Most elderly depressed patients respond to target doses of 10 mg of escitalopram; 20 to 40 mg/day of citalopram, fluoxetine, and paroxetine; and 50 to 100 mg/day of sertraline. The appropriate target doses of sertraline and venlafaxine are somewhat wider and may reach 150 to 200 mg/day of sertraline and 225 to 300 mg/day of venlafaxine in patients with more severe depression and melancholia.

Although existing data indicate that older patients both tolerate and respond to doses that are generally used to treat young adults, clinical experience suggests that older patients may require slower initial dose titration, particularly if side effects such as restlessness, anxiety, or nausea are troublesome. Thus, treatment with fluoxetine, which is particularly activating, may require initial doses of 5 to 10 mg/day. Similarly, older patients may require initiation of venlafaxine at 37.5 mg/day to minimize the severity of nausea.

Both paroxetine and venlafaxine are available in extended-release forms, which may reduce the risk of discontinuation syndromes with these agents.

Drug-Drug Interactions. As substrates for the P450 isoenzymes, SSRI concentrations may be influenced by the P450-inhibiting or P450-inducing effects of other medications a patient may be taking, although such interactions do not have clinical significance generally. Most of the SSRIs inhibit P450 pathways and thereby increase concentrations of other medications; this effect is more likely to be clinical relevant. Fluoxetine and paroxetine are strong 2D6 inhibitors, and they can significantly increase plasma TCA, risperidone, and conventional antipsychotic levels and levels of opiates and other drugs metabolized by this system (van Harten, 1993).

Sertraline is metabolized by multiple P450 pathways and particularly by 3A4 (Preskorn, 1997). Sertraline is a weaker inhibitor of 2D6 and 3A4 than paroxetine and fluoxetine (von Moltke et al., 1995). Sertraline has been found to have an inhibitory effect in vitro (Nelson et al., 1991), but both an in vitro study (Crewe et al., 1992) and in vivo research (von Moltke et al., 1995) have demonstrated that sertraline has a weaker effect on inhibiting desipramine hydroxylation by 2D6 than either fluoxetine or paroxetine. Thus, desipramine concentrations increased by only 30% after extended combination treatment with sertraline (Preskorn et al., 1994).

Venlafaxine is also metabolized by 2D6, but does not significantly inhibit this isoenzyme (Greenblatt et al., 1998). Also, venlafaxine concentrations do not rise significantly if a patient is taking a 2D6 inhibitor. Similarly, citalopram does not significantly inhibit P450 isoenzymes (Greenblatt et al., 1998).

The possibility that concurrent use of psychiatric medication will increase the prothrombin times of patients taking warfarin is of potential concern. SSRIs are highly bound to plasma proteins. Sertraline may modestly increase prothrombin times by displacing warfarin from its protein binding sites (Apseloff et al., 1997). Although this small kinetic effect is unlikely to have clinical significance (Preskorn, 1997), it does warrant monitoring of the prothrombin time after starting an SSRI in such a patient.

There is a potentially lethal interaction between MAOIs and SSRIs, including venlafaxine, in addition to meperidine and indirect-acting catecholamine drugs.

Bupropion

EFFICACY Bupropion has been assessed in controlled studies of older patients with depression. Two studies of older outpatients found that both low-dose (150 mg/day) and high-dose (450 mg/day) bupropion were equivalent in antidepressant efficacy to 150 mg/day of imipramine (Branconnier et al., 1983; Kane et al., 1983).

Older subjects may have greater difficulty tolerating the activating properties and possible neurological side effects associated with higher doses of bupropion. The sustained-release bupropion appears to be better tolerated by elderly patients. A controlled comparison of 100 to 300 mg/day sustained-release bupropion with 10 to 40 mg/day of paroxetine for geriatric depression found the antidepressants to have comparable efficacy and excellent tolerability (Weihs et al., 2000). Thus, sustained-release bupropion is an addition to the therapeutic arsenal of geriatric psychiatrists. Because of the absence of pharmacokinetic and pharmacodynamic interactions with SSRIs, bupropion has been used to augment the antidepressant effects of these antidepressants. Nevertheless, controlled data supporting this use of bupropion is lacking.

TOXICITY The relative absence of anticholinergic, antihistaminic, and cardiovascular side effects make bupropion potentially suitable for use with geriatric patients. Bupropion has been associated with the development of seizures, particularly at doses exceeding 450 mg/day. A history of seizures, but not age, may increase the occurrence of seizures in patients treated with bupropion (Davidson, 1989). Although clinical experience and uncontrolled data suggest that bupropion may be associated with an increased risk for falling in some elderly patients, the incidence of neurological side effects among older adults treated with this antidepressant has not been studied systematically.

PRACTICAL GUIDELINES

Pretreatment Evaluation, Clinical Monitoring. Other than obtaining information about a history of prior seizures, no specific evaluations are required prior to treatment with bupropion.

Pharmacokinetics, Dosing, and Drug-Drug Interactions. There are no dose recommendations specific for use with elderly patients. Multiple dosing of both short-acting and sustained-release bupropion should be separated by 6 hours. The short-acting form should not be administered after midafternoon because activation associated with peak blood levels may cause insomnia. Because older patients may be more sensitive to developing anxiety or motor restlessness at higher doses or after rapid dose titration, it is recommended that bupropion dosing begin at 75 mg of short-acting bupropion twice a day and 100 mg of sustained-release bupropion daily. Maximum doses of 450 mg of short-acting forms and 200 to 300 mg of sustained-release forms may be used if a patient does not respond to lower doses in 2 to 3 weeks.

Bupropion has several active metabolites, including a hydroxylated form, that are present in plasma in higher concentrations than the parent compound. These metabolites have been implicated in clinical effects (Golden et al., 1988; Pollock et al., 1993). Pollock and colleagues (1993) noted higher plasma concentrations of bupropion metabolite in geriatric patients with depression who did not respond to bupropion compared to those who responded.

Trazodone and Nefazodone

EFFICACY Trazodone, a triazolopyridine, has minimal anticholinergic activity. An early placebo-controlled trial in older depressed outpatients demonstrated a robust response among study completers treated with an average of 305 mg/day. Nevertheless, older patients had difficulty tolerating the sedative effects of such high doses, and less than 30% of subjects allocated to trazodone completed the study. The introduction of an SSRI, nefazodone, and other forms of better tolerated antidepressants led to the common use of the sedative properties of trazodone at 50 to 100 mg before bed for hypnotic effects.

Nefazodone, which is chemically related to trazodone, blocks serotonin reuptake and acts as a $5-HT_2$ receptor antagonist. The antidepressant efficacy of nefazodone has been found comparable to that of imipramine in adults of mixed ages (Fontaine et al., 1975; Rickels et al., 1994). Blockade of the $5HT_2$ receptor may give nefazodone a mild anxiolytic effect that may benefit anxious depressed patients. Although patients up to 81 years of age have been included in nefazodone studies (Goldberg, 1997), separate analyses of elderly subgroups and studies of purely geriatric samples are not available. The FDA has issued a black box warning about potential liver failure associated with nefazodone, and it has been withdrawn from the market by manufacturers in some jurisdictions such as Canada.

TOXICITY Although clinically significant ECG effects were not identified in early studies of healthy older outpatients (Hayes et al., 1983), trazadone has been associated with ventricular ectopy (Janowsky et al., 1983). Excessive sedation has been noted, and orthostatic hypotension with syncope can occur (Nambudiri et al., 1989; Spivak et al., 1989), presumably mediated through competitive blockade at the α_1-adrenergic receptor. Clinicians must therefore consider the patient's baseline cardiovascular status and risks versus potential benefits prior to prescribing this antidepressant.

Nefazodone is associated with weak α_1-adrenergic receptor blockade; this may explain the low frequency of orthostatic hypotension in treatment studies. Nevertheless, higher doses of nefazodone are also associated with sedative side effects. In contrast to most classes of antidepressants, nefazodone does not adversely affect sleep architecture and is not associated with sexual dysfunction (Preskorn, 1995).

Pretreatment Assessment. A baseline electrocardiogram may be useful before treating patients with antidepressant doses of trazodone because of the reported association between this medication and ventricular ectopy. There are no specific assessments required prior to instituting treatment with nefazodone, although a careful review of concurrent medication use is particularly relevant because of the potent inhibitory effects of nefazodone on the 3A4 metabolism of medications associated with prolongation of the QT_c interval.

Pharmacokinetics, Dosing, and Drug-Drug Interactions. Trazodone clearance is decreased in elderly patients (Greenblatt et al., 1982). One fixed-dose study suggested better response at a steady-state trazodone concentration above 650 ng/mL (Monteleone & Gnocch, 1990). Trazodone's one active metabolite, *m*-chlorophenylpiperazine, is a serotonin receptor agonist.

Dose-response relationships in depressive patients of mixed ages have been demonstrated for nefazodone (Fontaine et al., 1975). Also, nefazodone is metabolized through 3A4. An age-related decrease in activity of this isoenzyme in women may explain the higher nefazodone levels found with increased age. Thus, dosage should be increased gradually over a period of weeks, beginning at 50 to 100 mg twice a day as tolerated. Although tolerability to higher doses among adults has not been established, peak target doses of 200 to 400 mg/day appear to be appropriate.

Concurrent use of nefazodone with medications metabolized by the 3A4 system, such as astemizole, hisminal, cyclosporine, triazolam, and alprazolam, may increase concentrations and the effects of these agents. Loratadine is also partially metabolized by the 3A4 system, and both loratadine concentration and QT_c intervals have been noted to increase when this antihistamine is used in combination with nefazodone (Abernathy et al., 2001). Combining alprazolam with nefazodone to treat anxious depression effectively increases the alprazolam dose by 30% to 50%, which may lead to rebound anxiety when alprazolam levels decrease after nefazodone is discontinued.

Mirtazapine

The antidepressant effects of mirtazapine are mediated in part by blockade of the presynaptic α_2-autoreceptors and stimulation of presynaptic α_1-receptors on serotonin neurons (DeBoer, 1996). Mediation of both noradrenergic and serotonergic activity is proposed to result in both antidepressant and anxiolytic activity; blockade of postsynaptic $5HT_2$ and $5HT_3$ receptors may prevent the occurrence of nausea or insomnia (Goodnick et al., 1999).

EFFICACY A 6-week, placebo-controlled study of older patients with moderate to severe major depression using an average mirtazapine dose approximating 20 mg/day and 200 mg/day of trazodone found comparable improvement with the two agents (Halikas, 2001). Both antidepressants were associated with significantly greater sedation and dry mouth than placebo. A multicenter comparison of mirtazapine to amitriptyline for geriatric major depression utilized higher mirtazapine doses, averaging 37.3 mg/day, and relatively low amitriptyline doses of 73.8 mg/day (Heyberg et al., 1997). Comparable improvement was found for the two treatment groups. A large-scale comparison of mirtazapine to paroxetine for the treatment of geriatric depression found the antidepressant had comparable efficacy and tolerability (Schatzberg et al., 2001).

TOXICITY   Sedation and weight gain are common side effects of mirtazapine that presumably result from the antihistaminic effects of this antidepressant (Preskorn, 1997). These side effects have been applied to improve weight loss and sleep in frail nursing home residents with dementia and depression. Paradoxically, the incidence of sedation appears lower when mirtazapine is used at the higher end of the recommended dose range (Stimmer et al., 1997).

PHARMACOKINETICS, DOSING, AND DRUG-DRUG INTERACTIONS   Mirtazapine is generally instituted at a dose of 15 mg/day given before bed. Increasing the dose to a target range of 30 to 45 mg/day reduces sedative side effects. Mirtazapine has only weak effects as an inhibitor of P450 isoenzymes (Delbressine & Voss, 1997). Use with MAOIs is contraindicated.

Stimulants

EFFICACY   Psychostimulants include dextroamphetamine, methylphenidate, and pemoline. Despite the numerous reports that stimulants can reverse fatigue, apathy, and anergic symptoms, particularly when occurring in association with dementia (Galynker et al., 1997; Maletta & Weingarden, 1993) or debilitating physical illness (Chiarello & Cole, 1987), controlled studies in patients of mixed ages with major depression have not demonstrated a greater antidepressant efficacy with stimulants than with placebo (Satel & Nelson, 1989).

For example, methylphenidate improved, without improving HDRS scores, "negative symptoms" in patients with dementia without a depressive disorder (Galynker et al., 1997). An open trial demonstrated that combining target doses of 5 mg methylphenidate twice a day with citalopram was associated with a remission in 8 of 10 elderly patients with major depression over 4 to 8 weeks (Lavretsky & Kumar, 2001). Of the subjects, 50% achieved remission by the end of week 2. These provocative results require replication in a larger controlled trial.

Treatment Resistance

Most patients fail to respond to treatment because they have not received an adequate dose or duration of treatment (Lydiard, 1985). The presence of undiagnosed medical conditions (e.g., hypothyroidism; Lydiard, 1985) presenting as depression must be reconsidered in nonresponders. Although treatment resistance has been defined as lack of response to adequate blood levels for at least 4 to 6 weeks in young adults, a longer duration may be appropriate for this definition in elderly patients.

For example, open data have demonstrated a late response among a subset of older patients treated with nortriptyline (Georgotas et al., 1986), which led to the suggestion that some older patients may require 9 weeks or longer for symptom resolution (Georgotas et al., 1989). In a post hoc comparison study, older patients treated with nortriptyline took significantly longer to achieve remission than a younger sample treated with imipramine (Reynolds, Frank, Kupfer, et al., 1996).

The question of time to full response, which may require 12 weeks, must be distinguished from the question of whether the absence of improvement early in treatment predicts ultimate nonresponse. In both young adult (Nierenberg et al., 2000) and elderly patients with major depression (Jarvik & Mintz, 1987), improvement during the first weeks of treatment has predicted eventual response, suggesting that early improvement may provide a guide for whether a change in medication or augmentation is appropriate. Most clinicians will consider an alternative medication or augmentation if noticeable improvement does not occur within 2 to 4 weeks of achieving a target dose. Reviews of approaches to resistance to adequate acute treatment in young adult (Extein, 1989) and elderly patients with depression (Goff & Jenike, 1986) are available, but systematic data that support a specific algorithm are not. The ongoing NIMH STAR-D study of treatment resistance of depression will provide clinicians with guidelines.

LITHIUM AUGMENTATION   The use of lithium augmentation is supported by empirical studies in younger adults. Early evidence for the efficacy of lithium augmentation of a TCA (Joffe et al., 1993) has been supplemented by a meta-analysis of placebo-controlled studies demonstrating a greater than threefold increased odds of responding when lithium is added to a variety of antidepressants (Bauer et al., 2000). Although these analyses suggested a minimum of 2 weeks at lithium levels of 0.5 mEq/L or higher, many older patients may not tolerate or require this lithium concentration.

Data concerning the risk-benefit ratio of lithium augmentation in geriatric major depression are limited. Van Marwijk and associates (1990) reported a therapeutic benefit in 33 of 51 geriatric patients, although serious side effects occurred in 20%. Zimmer and coworkers (1991) also noted side effects and found only equivocal benefit. Flint and Rifat (1994) found that 60% of elderly patients suffering from nondelusional depression who had not responded to intensive antidepressant treatment achieved partial (38%) or full (24%) remission at lithium levels averaging 0.67 ± 0.17 mmol/L. Older patients were more likely to develop side effects. In the absence of clear data on sensitivity to neurological side effects among elderly patients, lithium augmentation should be targeted initially to concentrations of 0.6 mEq/L or less prior to using higher concentrations.

Potentiation of response to TCA by adding triiodothyronine (T_3) has been demonstrated in adults of mixed ages (Joffe et al., 1993). The appropriateness of this strategy for treatment-resistant geriatric depression is unclear. Increasing heart rate and cardiac work can cause coronary insufficiency in patients with marginal cardiac status; consultation with the patient's internist or cardiologist prior to instituting thyroid augmentation is recommended.

Combination of SSRIs with standard TCAs may augment efficacy (Crewe et al., 1992; Nelson et al., 1991; von Moltke et al., 1995; Weilburg et al., 1989). Clinicians should be aware of the drug-drug interactions discussed above. Dosage adjustment and therapeutic drug monitoring is needed when combining these classes of medication.

Following effective augmentation, clinicians must consider whether to taper the augmenting agent during continuation therapy. Reynolds, Frank, Kupfer, and colleagues (1996) noted that 52% of elderly subjects suffered a relapse following discontinuation of an augmenting medication, compared to a relapse of 6.1% in subjects who had responded to nortriptyline alone. This report was unable to clarify whether patients who required augmentation had a more unstable remission generally or whether relapses occurred only when the augmenting agent was discontinued. Controlled discontinuation studies in adults in a mixed-aged group (Bauer & Dopfmer, 1999) and elderly patients (Wilkinson et al., 2002) further support the importance of continuing lithium augmentation; patients randomized to placebo following successful lithium augmentation of a heterocyclic drug or SSRI in these studies were more likely to relapse than those who remained on lithium.

Data from neuroimaging and neuropsychological studies demonstrated that aging-related brain changes may diminish treatment response in some older patients with major depression. Naturalistic studies indicated that both chronicity of depression and poor response to antidepressants are associated with subcortical hyperintensities on magnetic resonance imaging (Coffey et al., 1989; Hickie et al., 1995). These prefrontal areas are involved in executive functioning, and patients with deficits in executive function also have limitation of acute treatment response (Kalayam & Alexopoulos, 1999; Simpson et al., 1997). Evidence indicates that patients with microstructural abnormalities in these areas have a poorer antidepressant response than patients without evidence of such disrupted white matter integrity (Alexopoulos et al., 2002).

Results from continuation and maintenance studies demonstrated that executive dysfunction is also associated with a more brittle course with more frequent relapses during nortriptyline continuation therapy and more frequent recurrences on nortriptyline or, particularly, following randomization to placebo (Alexopoulos et al., 2000). The association between prefrontal deficits and poor antidepressant responses may explain why the time to recovery for late-onset depression, which is more likely to occur secondary to acquired structural deficits, is longer than for age-matched patients with onset of depression in earlier life (Alexopoulos et al., 1996). The next frontier of research into the relationship between prefrontal lesions and treatment resistance will require identification of pharmacological strategies to optimize treatment response in this population.

Minor Depression and Dysthymia

Increasing attention is being given to the recognition and treatment of both dysthymia and depressive syndromes that do not meet full criteria for a diagnosis of major depression, particularly in primary care. A comparison of paroxetine and problem-solving psychotherapy to placebo in primary care demonstrated superiority of paroxetine over both placebo and the brief therapy on measures of depression and global functioning, particularly in the patients with dysthymia and more severe minor depression (Williams et al., 2000).

Additional Clinical Situations

Antidepressants are also approved for major depression that is associated with delusions or that occurs following cerebrovascular accidents or in the context of dementia. In addition, antidepressants have been used to treat depressive symptoms in dementia and for poststroke pathological crying, both of which are unapproved or "off-label" uses. In this section, we describe evidence for the efficacy of antidepressants for these forms of major depression and depressive syndromes. In light of the limited data or clear evidence that one class of antidepressants is superior to others, antidepressants are discussed according to the specific form of depression rather than by class.

LATE-LIFE DELUSIONAL DEPRESSION Delusional symptoms are relatively common among elderly patients with major depression. Adults of mixed ages with delusional depression respond less well to intensive TCA monotherapy than do nondelusional patients (Glassman et al., 1975). A combination of high doses of both the conventional neuroleptic perphenazine and the tertiary amine TCA amitriptyline was effective in 78% of young adults with delusional depression (Spiker et al., 1985). Among geriatric patients with delusional depression, the response rates to combined perphenazine and nortriptyline and to nortriptyline monotherapy were comparably low (Mulsant et al., 2001). The inability of older patients to tolerate the high doses of conventional antipsychotics found effective in young adults (Nelson et al., 1986) may have contributed to the negative results. Thus, an effective pharmacotherapy for late-life delusional depression has not been identified.

European studies using double-blind, parallel group controlled designs have indicated that various SSRIs are associated with remission in young patients (Zanardi et al., 1996, 2000). These studies suggested differential efficacy in that sertraline was statistically significantly better compared to paroxetine, and venlafaxine was significantly better compared to imipramine. Although these studies utilized standard diagnostic criteria and outcome measures, they have been criticized on methodological grounds, particularly because of the possible misclassification of patients with either body dysmorphic or obsessive-compulsive disorder associated with depression as suffering from delusional depression (Rothschild & Phillips, 1999). Determination of the efficacy of high doses of specific SSRIs for late-life delusional depression must await systematically conducted trials.

DEPRESSION ASSOCIATED WITH ALZHEIMER'S DISEASE   Approximately 20% of patients with Alzheimer's disease meet criteria for a comorbid major depression, particularly early in the course of the dementia (Rovner et al., 1987). Studies have demonstrated statistically significant improvement in major depression in association with the TCAs imipramine (Reifler et al., 1989) and clomipramine (Petracca et al., 1996). Interpretation of these studies is confounded by the improvement that occurred with placebo, but the clomipramine study did suggest greater improvement during antidepressant treatment. Cognitive decline was not associated with allocation to active medication in either of these studies using antidepressants with anticholinergic activity. In the study of Reifler and colleagues (1989), significant improvement on the Mattis Dementia Rating Scale (Mattis, 1988) occurred in imipramine-treated patients with depression. These finding are consistent with an earlier study by Reynolds and coworkers (1987), which demonstrated a correlation between improvement in depression and improvement in dementia rating scores among elderly depressives with comorbid cognitive impairment following treatment with nortriptyline or ECT.

The instability of mood symptoms in the major depression of Alzheimer's disease may contribute to a large placebo response and the absence of drug-placebo differences in most studies (Petracca et al., 2001; Reifler et al., 1989). Nortriptyline studies of major depression in cognitively impaired patients have suggested that this population can respond to concentrations below the standard therapeutic range (Streim et al., 1997; Young et al., 1991), complicating the interpretation of studies using standard TCA target concentrations in this population.

Placebo-controlled studies for patients with depressive syndromes or major depression with or without cognitive decline or dementia have been conducted using citalopram (Nyth et al., 1992) and the RIMA moclobomide (Roth et al., 1996). Interpretation of these studies is confounded by the mixing of patients who were heterogeneous for the presence of Alzheimer's disease and major depression without having adequate numbers of subjects with both disorders to determine the efficacy of these agents when both major depression and Alzheimer's disease are present. Interpretation of a trial comparing paroxetine to imipramine, which found improvement with both antidepressants (Katona et al., 1998), is further confounded by the absence of a placebo group to control for the improvement usually noted in depressed patients with dementia. A placebo-controlled sertraline trial (Lyketsos et al., 2000) that required subjects to have both major depression and Alzheimer's disease demonstrated that an average dose of 81 mg/day of sertraline was associated with significantly greater improvement than placebo on a scale for rating depression in dementia (Alexopoulos et al., 1988) and in global response. The development of consensus criteria for depression of Alzheimer's disease (Olin et al., 2001) that parallels the criteria for the psychosis of Alzheimer's disease (Jeste & Finkel, 2000) will provide a target for future studies.

POSTSTROKE MAJOR DEPRESSION AND PATHOLOGICAL CRYING   Between 20% and 30% of patients who have cerebrovascular accidents develop a subsequent major depression. Some, but not all, studies indicated that lesion location is a predictor of this complication (Carson et al., 2000; Robinson et al., 1983). An early study demonstrated the efficacy of nortriptyline for poststroke depression despite the occurrence of complications because of orthostatic hypotension in a minority (Lipsey et al., 1984). A trial again demonstrated the efficacy of nortriptyline, with a significantly higher proportion (77%) of subjects receiving nortriptyline demonstrating a 50% reduction in Hamilton Depression Scale scores than patients treated with fluoxetine or placebo (Robinson et al., 2000); there were no dropouts or significant cardiovascular side effects reported in the nortriptyline-treated patients, indicating that it can be a safe and effective treatment for patients with major depression following a stroke. Although fluoxetine was not more beneficial than placebo in this study, other studies have demonstrated the efficacy of SSRIs, including fluoxetine (Wiart et al., 2000) and citalopram (Andersen et al., 1994).

Emotional lability, including the syndrome of pathological crying, is a well-described consequence of brain injuries, including strokes (Starkstein et al., 1991). Both crossover studies (Andersen et al., 1993) and controlled studies using TCAs (Schiffer et al., 1985) and SSRIs (Burns et al., 1999) have demonstrated that antidepressants can decrease poststroke pathological crying that occurs in the absence of major depression.

BEHAVIORAL DISTURBANCES ASSOCIATED WITH DEMENTIA   MAOIs and SSRIs decrease behavioral disturbances in patients with dementia. Use of selegiline in patients with Alzheimers disease has been associated with improvement in behavioral disturbances (Agnoli et al., 1992; Foley et al., 1992; Tariot et al., 1987). Selegiline may also potentiate the effects of cholinomimetic treatment (Schart et al., 1988). A placebo-controlled study found an association between citalopram and reduction in emotional and behavioral disturbances among patients with dementia without concomitant depression (Nyth & Gottfries, 1990). An open citalopram trial reported decreases in both behavioral disturbances and psychotic symptoms (Pollock et al., 1997).

A double-blind comparison of citalopram, perphenazine, and placebo documented the potential of SSRIs to treat multiple psychiatric complications of dementia (Pollock et al., 2002). Patients treated with both active medications demonstrated significant improvement on several domains of a rating scale used to assess psychiatric and behavioral pathology. Citalopram-treated subjects had greater improvement overall and more improvement on agitation/aggression and lability/tension factor scores. The last finding may result from the mood-stabilizing property of the SSRI.

The use of MAOIs in depressive syndromes in demented patients has not received systematic study. The increase in MAO activity in brain and platelets in patients with senile dementia of the Alzheimer (SDAT) type suggests a particular rationale for use of MAOIs in this context. Case reports have demonstrated that MAOIs can be used safely and effectively in SDAT patients (Jenike, 1985b). Use of selegiline in patients with SDAT has been associated with improvement in behavioral disturbance (Agnoli et al., 1992; Foley et al., 1992; Patel et al., 1987). In Parkinson's disease, selegiline at selective doses has been reported to improve motor and cognitive performance and delay need for L-dopa when used alone (Allain et al., 1993; Myllyla et al., 1993); it may also potentiate the therapeutic and toxic effects of L-dopa or L-dopa/carbidopa. Allain and coworkers (1993) noted that depressed mood was improved by selegiline.

MOOD STABILIZERS AND ANTIMANIC AGENTS

Lithium salts and divalproex are first-line antimanic agents for patients of all ages. A number of other anticonvulsants, including carbamazepine, gabapentin, lamotrigine, and topiramate are used widely, generally to augment lithium or divalproex. Nevertheless, these agents have not received FDA approval for the treatment of mania, and reports of their effectiveness in geriatric patients are limited. One atypical antipsychotic, olanzapine, has received FDA approval as an antimanic agent.

Lithium Salts

Lithium salts have been a mainstay of treatment of acute mania and bipolar and related disorders in young adult patients. Elixir and sustained-release formulations are available.

The mechanisms of action of lithium are not understood. Lithium can alter catecholamine and other neurotransmitter systems, and important effects on intracellular signal transduction pathways are being delineated (Manji et al., 1996).

INDICATIONS The primary indications for lithium salts in elderly patients are acute mania or hypomania (Mirchandani & Young, 1993; Shulman & Herrmann, 1999). Additional indications are bipolar depression, potentiation of acute antidepressant therapy in unipolar major depression, and in management of bipolar schizoaffective disorders. Lithium salts are also efficacious for continuation and maintenance treatment.

EFFICACY Response to lithium in acute mania has not been compared with placebo in geriatric patients, partly because of ethical concerns. However, limited literature in elderly patients indicates that lithium can often be effective (Chen et al., 1999; Schaffer & Garvey, 1984; Wylie et al., 1999; Young, 1996).

Whether aged patients with manic disorder respond less well than younger patients has received limited study. Van der Velde (1970) noted a significantly poorer acute therapeutic benefit with age in an early report of a mixed-age group of patients; blood levels and neurocognitive features were not stated, and the measure used was a global clinical categorization. A prospective study of naturalistic lithium treatment also indicated negative age effect in a mixed-age group of patients, but the sample included few elderly patients (Young & Falk, 1989).

Studies of pharmacotherapy of geriatric bipolar depression are lacking. Optimized mood stabilizer dosing is considered an important first approach to bipolar patients presenting with depressive syndrome (Sachs, 2001).

Data from adult patients in a mixed age range indicate possible antisuicide effects of mood stabilizer treatment in patients with mood disorders; these effects may be independent of the effect on mood (Baldessarini et al., 2001). Suicide risk, although not well defined in geriatric bipolar disorder, is substantial in bipolar disorder among a mixed-age group (Perris, 1966; Taschev, 1974; Tsuang et al., 1979).

The efficacy of lithium for continuation or maintenance treatment has also received little study in elderly bipolar patients. Abou-Saleh and Coppen (1983) observed no difference in affective morbidity over an average of 5 years in elderly compared to younger patients maintained on comparable lithium levels. In a mixed-age prospective study, Murray and colleagues (1983) observed greater manic psychopathology, although more frequent hospitalizations were not noted among older patients. Both studies used maintenance levels between 0.6 and 1.0 mEq/L. Bipolar illness apparently does not "burn out" (Goodwin & Jamison, 1990), and lithium prophylaxis can continue to play a crucial role as patients with bipolar illness age.

Neurocognitive impairment and extrapyramidal dysfunction, rather than age, may predict poor outcomes (Himmelhoch et al., 1980). Whether age at onset affects treatment outcomes in geriatric mania is not clear (Wylie et al., 1999; Young & Klerman, 1992).

TOXICITY Data are limited on whether geriatric patients develop lithium side effects at lower levels than younger patients. Although elderly patients may be more likely to present fine tremor compared to younger patients treated with equivalent lithium levels, polyuria and polydipsia apparently do not increase with age (Murray et al., 1983).

Effects of acute lithium toxicity include tremor, ataxia, gastrointestinal distress, cognitive impairment, and severe polyuria. Roose, Bone and colleagues (1979) reported more instances of toxicity in elderly compared with younger bipolar outpatients in a maintenance treatment program. Lithium-associated sick sinus syndrome (Roose, Nurnberger, et al., 1979) may be encountered at therapeutic levels of lithium in older patients if the sinus node has been compromised by coronary disease.

Lithium-related neurocognitive toxicity during acute treatment has been linked to preexisting extrapyramidal syndromes and dementia (Himmelhoch et al., 1980). Lithium levels were not specified in that study, however.

Concern about long-term adverse reactions to lithium includes impact on renal function. A small number of patients treated with lithium have been identified who developed impaired renal concentrating ability (DePaulo et al., 1986) or diminished glomerular function, which may progress to insufficiency. Diminished glomerular function may be more likely after repeated exposures to toxic lithium levels (Gitlin, 1993). Nevertheless, the presence of renal disease does not preclude use of lithium when dosage is decreased to adjust for diminished creatinine clearance.

Antagonism of thyroid gland function by lithium, in combination with the diminished thyroid reserve that accompanies aging (Sawin et al., 1985), may make the elderly population particularly vulnerable to developing hypothyroidism during lithium treatment. A high proportion (32%) of geriatric patients treated with lithium receive thyroxine replacement or have elevated thyroid stimulating hormone (TSH) levels (Head & Dening, 1998).

PRACTICAL GUIDELINES

Pretreatment Assessment and Monitoring. A baseline ECG to assess sinus function is indicated prior to use of lithium salts because of the risk of sick sinus syndrome (Roose, Nurnberger, et al., 1979). Serum creatinine is adequate to screen for normal renal functioning, but it is not a sensitive index of change. Patients with renal insufficiency who require careful monitoring and for whom collection of 24-hour urine output is not feasible can have creatinine clearance approximated using the Cockroft-Gault equation: Clearance in mL/minute = $(140 - \text{Age}) \times \text{Body weight}/(\text{Serum creatinine} \times 72) \times 0.85$ if female (Friedman et al., 1989). Conservative management includes twice-yearly monitoring of renal function.

Thyroid function should be assessed annually, especially if there is a change in the course of the affective illness or symptoms develop that are consistent with hypothyroidism. Increase in thyroid-stimulating hormone can be managed with thyroid hormone replacement.

Pharmacokinetics, Dosing, and Drug-Drug Interactions. The half-life for lithium approximates 24 hours in patients older than 70 years without renal disease (Chapron et al., 1982; Hardy et al., 1987). The lithium dose necessary to achieve a particular plasma level is therefore usually one half to two thirds of that required in younger adults (Hardy et al., 1987). This is consistent with beginning at low doses, in the range of 300 mg to 600 mg per day, and increasing in small increments while monitoring plasma levels. The plasma level obtained 5 days after a patient has started a specific dose of lithium is relatively stable unless medical illness or use of medications that influence lithium excretion supervene.

The relationship between specific plasma concentrations and therapeutic response in elderly patients is not well delineated despite clinical lore suggesting increased sensitivity. Case reports (Schaffer & Garvey, 1984) have suggested that geriatric patients with mania may respond at lower levels (e.g., 0.4–0.8 mEq/L) than the usual targets in adults of mixed ages. On the other hand, one naturalistic study suggested better responses to higher lithium levels in both geriatric patients and young adults (Young et al., 1992). A retrospective study similarly suggested better outcomes among elderly patients treated with levels above 0.8 mEq/L (Chen et al., 1999).

Important pharmacokinetic drug-drug interactions have been described for lithium. Thiazide diuretics block reabsorption of sodium in the distal tubule, leading to increased proximal reabsorption of sodium and lithium and a 33% increase in lithium plasma levels (Jefferson & Greist, 1979). Potassium-sparing diuretics may have a similar, although less profound, effect. Furosemide, a loop diuretic, is not associated with significant increase in lithium level (Crabtree et al., 1991). Dietary salt restriction can also increase renal reabsorption of lithium and can raise plasma levels (Jefferson & Greist, 1979). Some nonsteroidal antiinflammatory medications diminish renal clearance of lithium by nearly 50% (Jefferson et al., 1981). Availability of over-the-counter forms of these agents (e.g., ibuprofen) makes it necessary for the psychiatrist to instruct elderly patients not to begin a new medication without discussion.

Clinicians should monitor lithium levels carefully when an angiotensin-converting enzyme inhibitor is added to a patient's lithium regime because these agents may increase lithium levels. However, a study of lithium combined with enalapril in 10 healthy young volunteers failed to find a robust effect of the angiotensin-converting enzyme inhibitor; 1 subject did have a 31% increased lithium level (Das Gupta et al., 1992). The conservative approach of reassessing lithium levels 1 week after a medication that may affect renal clearance (such as an angiotensin-converting enzyme or loop diuretic) is therefore recommended, even though a consistent effect of these agents on lithium clearance has not been demonstrated. If patients are placed on current thiazide or potassium-sparing diuretics or nonsteroidal antiinflammatory medications known to decrease lithium clearance, a 50% reduction in lithium dosage, followed by repeated steady-state lithium is strongly recommended.

Treatment Resistance. Adequate concentration and duration of treatment trials in geriatric patients are not defined. This limits discussion of management of partial response and nonresponse. Systematic studies of combination therapy, or of differential efficacy of monotherapies, are also lacking (Goldberg et al., 2000).

Black and coworkers (1988) reported that "complicated" manias (i.e., those with coexisting nonaffective psychiatric illness or with serious medical illness) had poorer immediate response to lithium treatment. Shukla and associates (1987) also reported that mixed-age patients with "secondary" manias had a poor acute response. Similarly, geriatric manic patients with neurocognitive impairments (i.e., dementia and extrapyramidal disease) have a poorer acute therapeutic response to lithium (Himmelhoch, 1980).

Divalproex Sodium

Divalproex sodium was the first agent to be FDA approved for acute mania besides lithium salts. It is increasingly prescribed for elderly patients (Shulman et al., 2003). The mechanism of action of divalproex and other anticonvulsant mood stabilizers is not understood. Although some effects on neurotransmitters are similar to those of lithium (Post, 1989), as with lithium, mediation of intracellular signal transduction is considered relevant to the mechanism of action (Manji et al., 1999).

EFFICACY There are no placebo-controlled studies of the efficacy of anticonvulsant monotherapy in geriatric patients with acute mania. Placebo-controlled studies of acute treatment in mixed-age populations supported the efficacy of divalproex in mania (Ball, 1992; Pope et al., 1991). Further, many reports indicated that divalproex can be useful in geriatric manic patients (Chen et al., 1999; Gnam & Flint, 1993; Kando et al., 1996; McFarland et al., 1990; Mordecai et al., 1999; Noagiul et al., 1998; Puryear et al., 1995; Risinger et al., 1994; Wylie et al., 1999).

There are no published randomized comparisons of divalproex to lithium in acute treatment of elderly patients. One retrospective study (Chen et al., 1999) suggested that divalproex was less effective than lithium, at least in those patients lacking mixed features.

Younger, female geriatric patients had better outcomes with divalproex in one series (Neidermeyer & Nasrallah, 1998). Experience in young patients indicates that divalproex monotherapy may be useful for patients who did poorly with lithium (Bowden, 1995; Swan et al., 2000) and patients with mixed bipolar states (Swann, 1995). Combination treatment with divalproex and lithium can be useful in patients who are only partially responsive to lithium salts or in rapid-cycling geriatric bipolar patients (Goldberg et al., 2000). Data are available to support the efficacy of divalproex in continuation-maintenance treatment of bipolar disorder in mixed-age populations (Bowden et al., 2000).

TOXICITY Divalproex is generally well tolerated in elderly patients (Bowden et al., 1994). Divalproex has a different side effect profile from lithium salts (Chen et al., 1999; Wylie et al., 1999). It may have a lower side effect profile than carbamazepine, including less sedative and anticholinergic effects, although direct comparisons are needed in elderly patients. Absence of cognitive toxicity on neuropsychological testing was reported (Craig & Tallis, 1994) in a series of geriatric patients with seizure disorder. Nevertheless, patients with dementia are sensitive to developing sedation during rapid dose titration and at high doses of divalproex.

Divalproex can inhibit platelet production; furthermore, platelet function may be impaired despite a normal platelet count. It can produce hepatic enzyme elevations, which are usually mild. Elevated serum ammonia levels without hepatic enzyme elevations have been reported in patients with lethargy (Eze et al., 1998; Raby, 1997). Reversal of this toxicity by carnitine administration has been reported (Raby, 1997). Divalproex may rarely be associated with pancreatitis.

PRACTICAL GUIDELINES

Pretreatment Assessment and Clinical Monitoring. Patients treated with divalproex should undergo pretreatment hematologic assessment and liver function tests.

Pharmacokinetics, Dosing, and Drug-Drug Interactions. Divalproex is extensively bound to albumin in plasma in a concentration-dependent manner. This binding decreases with increased age. Aspirin and diazepam coadministration can decrease valproate binding.

Valproate is hepatically metabolized by mitochondrial B oxidation and by glucuronide conjugation. Numerous metabolites are generated, some of which are pharmacologically active, but their plasma concentrations are low (Sugimoto et al., 1996). Although metabolism of unbound divalproex is linear, the compound is highly protein bound, and linear kinetics do not occur until protein binding is saturated. As with other protein-bound pharmacotherapeutic agents, therapeutic monitoring of total concentrations reflects both bound and unbound medication.

Optimal dosing with divalproex has not been established in geriatric patients. Relationships between total valproate plasma concentrations and antimanic response are not well delineated in any age group. Bowden (1998) recommended concentration ranges from 50 to 120 μg/mL. Chen and coworkers observed poorer response outside the range 60 to 90 μg/mL in a retrospective study. The clinical significance of differences in nonbound concentrations is not known.

Because divalproex is an inhibitor of cytochrome P450 enzymes, it can increase plasma levels of some concurrently used medications. These include nortriptyline and lamotrigine.

Treatment Resistance. The categories of rapid cycling mania and treatment resistance developed initially to describe patients with frequent cycles during lithium treatment or who failed to respond to this medication. Therefore, it is not surprising that lithium-resistant patients may respond preferentially to divalproex. Of further interest, studies have suggested that divalproex may be more effective for the treatment and prevention of mixed depressive episodes and the prevention of future depression (Bowden, 1995; Bowden et al., 2000; Swann et al., 2000).

ADDITIONAL CLINICAL SITUATIONS   Use of divalproex in geriatric unipolar depression and schizoaffective disorders remains to be studied.

Other Anticonvulsants and Novel Approaches

Carbamazepine, although not FDA approved for bipolar disorder, has been widely used clinically for many years. In the past several years, gabapentin, lamotrigine, and other anticonvulsants have become available. In addition to other new anticonvulsants such as topiramate, the geriatrician should be aware of other novel agents under study in preliminary trials. These include cholinomimetic agents, inositol monophosphate inhibitors, and dietary manipulations, including omega–fatty acid administration.

EFFICACY   Carbamazepine can have therapeutic effects in geriatric manic patients (Kellner & Neher, 1991). It was reportedly adequately tolerated.

Gabapentin and lamotgrigene have been reported to be effective in studies of young patients with bipolar disorder (Post, 1989). Lamotrigine may have particular benefits in the treatment of depression associated with bipolar I disorder (Calabrese et al., 1999) and in patients with rapid cycling bipolar disorder (Bowden et al., 1999). These drugs remain unstudied in the elderly.

TOXICITY   Carbamazepine can cause sedation, confusion, ataxia, and sialorrhea (Gleason & Schneider, 1990; Patterson, 1988). Central nervous system side effects generally are dose dependent, and they occur most frequently at the high end of the anticonvulsive concentration range (Schneider & Sobin, 1991). Carbamazepine also has quinidine-like properties and can cause prolongation of cardiac conduction. Hepatic enzyme elevations, usually small and transient, can occur. Reduction in leukocyte count and platelet count occurs frequently; agranulocytosis is rare.

Lamotrigine can produce dermatitis in 5% to 10% of cases. The more serious and potentially life-threatening Stevens-Johnson syndrome occurs far less frequently, in approximately 0.03% of cases.

Gabapentin side effects include sedation, ataxia, and nystagmus. Topiramate is less well studied, but is associated with weight loss and the side effects of sedation and ataxia.

Pretreatment Assessment and Clinical Monitoring. An ECG, baseline complete blood count (CBC), and liver function tests should be obtained for patients under consideration for carbamazepine treatment. Serum creatinine should be reviewed prior to initiation of gabapentin. An ECG, CBC, and liver function tests should be repeated during carbamazepine treatment.

Pharmacokinetics, Dose, and Drug-Drug Interactions. Carbamazepine is hepatically metabolized through the cytochrome 3A4 system and is a potent inducer of this enzyme system. An active 10,11-epoxide metabolite is generated.

Lamotrigine is primarily metabolized hepatically to an inactive N-glucuronide conjugate.

Gabapentin is primarily excreted without hepatic metabolism through renal clearance. Therefore, concentration/dose ratios can be increased in older persons because of diminished glomerular functioning.

Lamotrigine doses should be increased gradually to minimize the risk of Stevens-Johnson syndrome. Increments of 50 mg/week have been recommended; furthermore, because divalproex inhibits lamotrigine metabolism and raises levels significantly, dose increments should be even lower when these two anticonvulsants are administered concurrently.

Relationships between plasma concentrations of these agents and clinical responses are not well delineated in any age group. Anticonvulsant concentrations (6–12 μg/mL) are typically used as a guideline for carbamazepine treatment.

Carbamazepine is a substrate for P450 3A4 and induces P450 metabolism of medications metabolized through multiple P450 pathways. Carbamazepine use can, therefore, decrease concentration/dose ratios of drugs, including valproate and lamotrigine, clozapine, haloperidol, and alprazolam.

Additional Clinical Situations

Anticonvulsants have been used as adjuncts to treatment of unipolar major depression (see above).

Antimanic Treatment in Patients with Brain Disease

Manic states in dementia have not been well characterized, but aspects of mania may be prevalent in demented populations (Folstein, 1999). Use of mood stabilizers in dementia for manic symptoms has received limited attention, although the overlap between forms of agitation and mania has been discussed.

Poor outcomes of lithium treatment in demented elderly manic patients compared to nondemented elderly manic patients were noted (Himmelhoch et al., 1980).

A placebo-controlled trial (Alda, 1999) of divalproex in demented patients with agitation supported its efficacy; treatment was generally well tolerated. This is consistent with observation of others (Grossman, 1998), although side effects such as sedation are more likely to occur at full anticonvulsant doses in patients with dementia.

Carbamazepine has been used successfully to control agitated, aggressive behaviors in patients with organic brain disease (Patterson, 1987, 1988). The literature consists only of case reports, however. Gleason and Schneider (1990) reported that hostility and irritability were the features most improved in an open study of patients with a probable Alzheimer's disease diagnosis. Chambers and colleagues (1982) observed toxicity, but no benefit, in 19 patients with dementia, however.

A case report suggested that gabapentin can be useful in demented patients with agitation (Roane et al., 2000).

Preclinical studies have suggested that lithium and some other mood stabilizers may have neuroprotective effects (Manji et al., 1999) in animal models. Ongoing research will evaluate whether these are clinically relevant.

Therapeutic effects of cholinomimetic effects on psychopathology in dementia is an active area of investigation (Cummings, 1998). Cholinesterase inhibitors may reduce manic symptoms in demented patients (Cummings, 2000).

ANTIPSYCHOTICS

Types

Antipsychotic drugs are discussed using the categories conventional and atypical. Typical or classical agents are often ranked on a spectrum from low potency (e.g., chlorpromazine) to high potency (e.g., haloperidol and fluphenazine). Atypical compounds include aripiprazole, risperidone, olanzapine, quetiapine, ziprasidone, and clozapine.

Indications

Antipsychotic drugs are first-line agents for managing psychotic symptoms in elderly patients. Conventional antipsychotic drugs have been used to treat elders with schizophrenia (Tran-Johnson et al., 1992) and late-onset chronic psychoses (Post, 1966). They also have a role in the management of manic states, of psychotic depression, and of behavioral disturbance in the context of brain disease. Because of their side effect profile, atypical antipsychotics are now drugs of first choice for these same indications.

Efficacy

SCHIZOPHRENIAS

Conventional Antipsychotics. In late-life psychoses, antipsychotic treatment has proven more effective than placebo (Post, 1962) or no treatment

(Myllyla et al., 1993). In elderly patients with schizophrenia (Raskind et al., 1979) depot fluphenazine was more effective than oral haloperidol in outpatient management, presumably by increasing compliance.

Atypical Agents. Negative symptoms are noted in geriatric patients with chronic psychosis. In young patients, atypical antipsychotics may improve negative symptoms more than conventional antipsychotics (Jeste et al., 1999). The mechanisms responsible for such differences between classes of antipsychotics remain an active area of research; interactions with serotonergic receptors or differences in speed of dissociation from dopamine receptors (Kapur & Seeman, 2001) are those currently discussed.

These drugs are beginning to move beyond case reports into more systematic studies in subgroups of geriatric patients. Evidence for the effectiveness of risperidone (Kiraly et al., 1998; Madhusoodanan et al., 1999; Zarate & Tohen, 1996) and olanzapine (Madhusoodanan et al., 2000) has been published. The introduction of quetiapine (Arvanitis & Miller, 1997; Solomons & Geiger, 2000) has also been followed by reports of its effectiveness in late-life psychotic disorders (McManus et al., 1999).

Ziprasidone has most recently been approved as an antipsychotic (Daniel et al., 1999; Keck et al., 2001), but studies of the efficacy and tolerability of this agent in specific syndromes among geriatric patients remain to be elucidated. The newest approved antipsychotic, aripiprazole, shows promise for use in elders.

As in young adults, clozapine can be an effective medication for geriatric patients who are refractory to other neuroleptic medications (Bajulaiye & Addonizio, 1992; Ball, 1992; Frankenburg & Kalunian, 1994; Oberholzer et al., 1992; Salzman et al., 1995).

MANIC DISORDERS

Conventional Agents. Antipsychotic medications are useful adjuncts in acute management of manic episodes in the young adult population and have not been systematically studied in geriatric mania. Consideration of their side effects and the possibly increased risk of tardive dyskinesia in patients with mood disorder and in the aged suggest that the use of conventional antipsychotics should be minimized. The use of conventional drugs in young adult patients with bipolar disorder for maintenance treatment has not been investigated systematically, including among patients who were psychotic during their manic episode.

Atypical Agents. Atypical drugs have been increasingly used in young adult patients with mania. Benefit from risperidone as an adjunct to mood stabilizer treatment has been described in an open-label study (Tohen et al., 1996). Olanzapine has been found superior to placebo for the treatment of bipolar mania (Tohen et al., 2000) and is FDA approved for this indication. The risks and benefits of risperidone, olanzapine (Beyer et al., 2001), quetiapine (Sajatovic 2002), clozapine (Frye et al., 1996; Shulman et al., 1997), and other antipsychotic agents in elderly manic patients remains to be evaluated systematically.

Toxicity

CENTRAL NERVOUS SYSTEM TOXICITY

Conventional Agents. Low-potency drugs, such as chlorpromazine, have greater affinity as receptor antagonists at muscarinic and other receptors (e.g., α-adrenergic and histaminic). Their propensity for causing sedation appears greater than that of high-potency agents such as haloperidol and fluphenazine.

The high-potency agents are more selective for dopamine D_2 receptor blockade compared to low-potency drugs, and they produce greater parkinsonian side effects; whether they carry greater risk of tardive dyskinesia or neuroleptic malignant syndrome compared to low-potency agents has been unclear.

Vulnerability to parkinsonian side effects may increase with age. On the other hand, vulnerability to acute dystonic reactions may decrease; akathisia may occur at similar rates across the life span (Caligiuri et al., 2000).

Anticholinergic drugs, such as benzotropine, can reduce antipsychotic-induced rigidity, but they are largely ineffective for tremor and akathisia (Shader & DiMascio, 1970). They can cause central anticholinergic toxicity, and they may increase the risk for tardive dyskinesia or worsen existing dyskinesia (Jeste & Wyatt, 1987).

Elderly patients receiving antipsychotic medications are at increased risk for falls and related morbidity (Ray et al., 1987). Drug-induced parkinsonism may be one of the mechanisms for this adverse outcome.

Aged patients are at increased risk for tardive dyskinesia (Jeste & Wyatt, 1987). Prevalence estimates exceed 40% in patients older than 60 years, and late-life tardive dyskinesia is reported to be more severe and less likely to remit spontaneously (Smith & Baldessarini, 1980). In patients older than 55 years treated with antipsychotic drugs for the first time, a cumulative incidence of 31% after 43 weeks was reported (Saltz et al., 1991).

Although female patients (Woerner et al., 1991) and those with affective disorders (Gardos & Casey, 1984; Kane et al. 1983; Woerner et al., 1991; Yassa et al., 1992) may be at increased risk for tardive dyskinesia, this is controversial (Jeste & Wyatt, 1987; Kane et al., 1983). Additional risk factors may include late initiation of treatment, alcohol abuse, early extrapyramidal side effects, and cumulative exposure (Jeste & Finkel, 2000; Woerner et al., 1998). An association of facial dyskinesia with cognitive impairment has been noted (Byne et al., 1998).

Akathisia occurs across a broad range of ages, including the aged. The behavioral manifestations of this adverse reaction are thought to result from an internal sense of restlessness induced by the antipsychotic agent (Crane & Naranjo, 1971).

The neuroleptic malignant syndrome can occur in elderly patients (Addonizio, 1987). It is characterized by development of severe muscle rigidity and elevated temperature associated with use of neuroleptic medication and is accompanied by two or more of the following: diaphoresis, dysphagia, tremor, incontinence, change in level of consciousness, mutism, tachycardia, elevated or labile blood pressure, leukocytosis, and laboratory evidence of muscle injury (according to the *Diagnostic and Statistical Manual of Mental Disorders, Fourth Edition* [*DSM-IV*], American Psychiatric Association, 1994). It is possible that age masks the phenomenology of the syndrome and that dementia confounds diagnosis.

Treatment with these agents can impair cognitive performance (Devanand et al., 1989; Perlick et al., 1986). The pharmacological mechanisms may involve anticholinergic effects and dopaminergic receptor blockade.

Because excess use of conventional neuroleptics in institutional settings has been suggested, controlled studies of drug withdrawal have been conducted; symptomatology has not increased, but a decrease in extrapyramidal side effects has been noted (Harris et al., 1997). One study noted improved executive function (Cohen-Mansfield et al., 1999).

Atypical Agents. Atypical drugs all have reduced liability for acute motor side effects compared to conventional agents (Caligiuri et al., 1999; Collaborative Working Group, 1998; Massand 2000; Systematic Assessment of Geriatric Drug Use, 2000). Also, atypical antipsychotics are associated with lower risk of tardive dyskinesia than conventional agents (Llorent et al., 1998).

Sedative effects of some atypical agents, especially clozapine and olanzapine (Ball, 1992), may interfere with cognition in the elderly, and dosing must take this into account. The incidence of agranulocytosis during clozapine therapy is greater in geriatric patients (Alvir et al., 1993; Barak et al., 1999; Ma Jose et al., 1993). Agranulocytosis may occur in elders at a rate as high as or higher than in younger patients at doses above 100 mg/day (Salzman et al., 1995). Clinicians therefore must monitor leukocyte counts frequently (i.e., weekly during the first 6 months). Fever or leukocyte counts less than 3,500 require more frequent monitoring. Leukocyte counts less than 3,000 or absolute neutrophil counts less than 1,500 require interruption of clozaril treatment. Respiratory problems, including respiratory arrest, should be kept in mind at doses of clozaril above 100 mg/day (Pitner et al., 1995).

There is evolving and inconsistent literature on the benefits and possible adverse effects of atypical antipsychotic medications on cognitive processes in young adults with schizophrenia. Whether the studies of effects on working memory in this population are generalizable to elderly patients, including those with dementia, is uncertain. In young adults with schizophrenia, atypical antipsychotics may even benefit aspects of cognition; anticholinergic properties of atypical agents such as olanzapine and clozapine might theoretically antagonize cognitive function. Evidence for this effect in geriatric patients is lacking, and enhancement of acetylcholine release by these agents has been postulated as well (Byerly et al., 2001).

CARDIOVASCULAR EFFECTS

Conventional Agents. Low-potency conventional neuroleptics have receptor antagonist effects that may contribute to cardiovascular side effects. They have greater anticholinergic effects, perhaps mediated by muscarinic receptor antagonism, compared to high-potency agents. Their greater α_1-adrenergic receptor antagonism compared to high-potency agents may contribute to liability for orthostatic hypotension (Richelson, 1982), which may contribute to increased risk of falls associated with antipsychotic treatment.

Prolonged intracardiac conduction, specifically the QT interval (QT_c), has been associated with antipsychotic treatment; this can represent a vulnerability to life-threatening arrhythmia. Thioridazine and butyrophenones have been particularly implicated in prolongation of QT_c (Reilly et al., 2000; Welch & Chue, 2000) and the FDA requires special labeling of thioridazine for this side effect.

Atypical Agents. Prolonged intracardiac conduction (QT_c) has also been a concern with atypical agents. The risk for this effect differs among atypical agents and is greater for olanzapine and ziprasidone (Haverkamp et al., 2000; Welch & Chue, 2000). It is particularly important to obtain a baseline ECG before beginning ziprasidone in an elderly patient because of the association of use of this agent with arrhythmias associated with prolonged QT_c intervals. Patients with prolonged ventricular conduction at baseline, those vulnerable to hypokalemia and hypomagnesemia, and patients with histories of significant cardiac disease should be considered at increased risk for developing the life-threatening arrhthymia of torsades de pointes during ziprasidone therapy.

OTHER EFFECTS

Conventional Agents. Peripheral anticholinergic effects may occur. These can be a function of potency, as noted above. However, these effects can be dose dependent. Hepatotoxicity is unusual.

Atypical Agents. Atypical antipsychotics can cause or exacerbate glucose intolerance and hyperlipidemia. The evidence has been strongest for clozapine (Collaborative Working Group, 1998). As described in a review by Haupt and Newcomer (2001), mechanisms may include direct effects on insulin secretion activity and the development of insulin intolerance. Despite the increased incidence of diabetes and hyperlipidemia associated with aging, retrospective data suggest that increased age is associated with a diminished rather than increased occurrence of these metabolic abnormalities (Meyer, 2002).

Risk of corneal opacities has been linked to atypical as well as conventional neuroleptics. Among atypical agents, an association between cataracts and quetiapine use has been noted in dogs. As a result, it is recommended that elderly patients receive a slit lamp examination or other suitable opthalmological assessment prior to beginning quetiapine treatment and periodically thereafter, particularly because of the inherent increased incidence of cataracts associated with aging.

Clozapine can produce hepatic and hematologic changes. In elders, poor tolerance of clozapine was described in case series (Ball, 1992; Salzman et al., 1995).

Practical Guidelines

PRETREATMENT ASSESSMENT AND CLINICAL MONITORING

Conventional Agents. Administration of antipsychotic drugs should be preceded by assessment of neuromotor states. This approach enables the clinician to identify the drug-induced extrapyramidal side effects of parkinsonism and tardive dyskinesia. Elderly patients have increased vulnerability to both forms of adverse reactions (Ayd, 1976; Jeste & Wyatt, 1987). A simple screening instrument, such as the Abnormal Involuntary Movement Scale (AIMS; Whittier, 1969) can be useful. Pretreatment orthostatic blood pressure measures and ECG should be obtained and fasting blood sugar when atypical antipsychotics are being used. A complete blood count should be obtained, especially in patients for whom clozapine is under consideration.

Orthostatic blood pressure changes should be monitored. ECG should be repeated. In patients receiving clozapine, complete blood count is repeated and blood sugar is followed in patients taking atypical antipsychotics. Therapeutic drug monitoring may assist assessment of treatment adherence or metabolism in selected cases. A limited database concerning concentration-effect relationships in the elderly restricts the routine utility of these measures.

PHARMACOKINETICS, DOSING, AND DRUG-DRUG INTERACTIONS

Conventional Agents. Increase in steady-state concentration-dose ratios with age have been reported for chlorpromazine (Aoba et al., 1996; Rosenblatt et al., 1981) and thioridazine (Axelsson, 1976). Such differences have not been found consistently for haloperidol. Perphenazine concentration/dose ratios are higher in slow CYP2D6 metabolizers (Linnet & Wiborg, 1996).

Less information on dose-response relationships is available for antipsychotic drugs than for antidepressants and mood stabilizers. Neuroleptics should be prescribed empirically, in the lowest effective dose.

Differences in dose-effect relationships in patient subgroups have not received systematic study. Based on open trials (Jeste et al., 1982), it was suggested that patients with late-onset schizophrenia may respond to lower doses of antipsychotics than individuals with geriatric early onset.

Some studies that have included elderly patients have noted associations between relatively high antipsychotic concentration/dose ratios and tardive dyskinesia (Jeste et al., 1982; Yesavage et al., 1983). Other studies have been negative (McCreadie et al., 1992; Nelson et al., 1983).

Mazure and coworkers (1998) noted that use of higher doses did not increase the rate of therapeutic response, but did increase side effects; they suggested that therapeutic effects may require longer treatment in older than in young patients.

Pharmacokinetic drug interactions involving conventional antipsychotics can involve hepatic metabolism. Antidepressant elimination can be retarded by concomitant antipsychotic administration. For example, nortriptyline concentrations can be higher in patients treated with conventional antipsychotics (Meyers et al., 1999; Sweet et al., 1998).

Pharmacodynamic interactions, sometimes used for therapeutic benefit, include enhanced sedative effects of other agents, such as benzodiazepines combined with antipsychotics. An example related to toxicity is the enhancement of neuroleptic-induced extrapyramidal side effects by lithium (Miller et al., 1986).

Atypical Agents. Risperidone has a pharmacologically active 9-hydroxylated metabolite. Age-related increase in elimination half-life of both risperidone and its hydroxylation metabolite are reported; their accumulation may contribute to greater clinical effects at low doses in the elderly.

The elimination half-life of olanzapine increases with age. Single-dose pharmacokinetics of quetiapine suggested minimal impact of hepatic or renal impairment on pharmacokinetics (Thyrum et al., 2000).

Ziprasidone pharmacokinetics are reportedly little affected by age (Wilner et al., 2000) or by hepatic or renal disease (Aweeka et al., 2000). Clozapine plasma concentration/dose ratios may be higher in elderly patients compared to younger patients (Haring et al., 1990). It has been suggested that lower doses of atypical agents are useful in elderly compared to younger patients. These issues await systematic study.

Available reports describe clozapine treatment in geriatric psychiatric patients at doses ranging from 75 to 350 mg per day. Clozapine has an active demethylated metabolite, norclozapine, that can contribute to toxicity. A relationship between plasma drug concentrations and therapeutic response has been observed for clozapine in patients of varying ages (Perry et al., 1991), but has not been described in elderly patients.

Drug-drug interactions involving antipsychotics can occur. SSRI treatment can increase clozapine concentration/dose ratios (Centurrino et al., 1994; Jerling et al., 1994).

Patients with Brain Disease

DEMENTIAS Treatment of behavioral disturbances and psychosis accompanying dementia is receiving increasing attention (Schneider et al., 1990; Sunderland & Silver, 1988). Among patients with dementia who reside in the community, approximately 70% demonstrated disturbed behavior, and approximately 50% had psychotic symptoms (Rabins et al., 1982). The severity of the dementia may be correlated with the number and type of behavioral problems (Teri et al., 1988); 82% of mildly impaired patients with Alzheimer's disease reported behavior problems compared to 96% of patients with severe cognitive dysfunction; 38% of patients with severe dementia had agitation compared with 10% with mild impairment; the rates for hallucinations were 30% and 10%, respectively. This issue has special public health relevance because persistently unmanageable and disruptive behavior is the principal reason reported by caregivers for seeking institutionalization (Ferris et al., 1985). Cohen-Mansfield (1986) found that 73% of nursing home residents demonstrated a minimum of one agitated behavior at a frequency of several times a day; 56% of these individuals were receiving neuroleptics.

Conventional Agents. Conventional antipsychotics are superior to placebo in controlling agitation and psychosis in patients with dementia, but do not abolish behavioral disturbance and produce only modest improvement (Raskind et al., 1998; Schneider et al., 1990; Sunderland & Silver, 1988; Wragg, 1988). Barnes and coworkers (1982) noted improved functioning in a mixed sample with Alzheimer's and multiinfarct dementia who received loxapine or thioridazine compared to placebo. However, review of thioridazine treatment studies in dementia concluded that it had equal or greater side effects compared to alternative drugs without clear advantage in efficacy for psychopathology in dementia (Kirchner et al., 2000).

Efficacy of antipsychotic drugs appears to be proportional to the degree of disturbance. There is no evidence for the superiority of one conventional agent over another (Tune et al., 1991).

Although controversy persists (Moleman et al., 1986), patients with dementia (Peabody et al., 1998) probably have an increased vulnerability to extrapyramidal reactions during neuroleptic drug treatment. More than 50% of geriatric patients who receive these agents have parkinsonian side effects (Ayd, 1976; Salzman et al., 1992). These side effects may be aggravated by higher plasma levels of neuroleptic medications and increase with duration of drug exposure (Wragg, 1988). Haloperidol doses that decrease agitation are associated with greater extrapyramidal side effects (Devanand et al., 1989). Neuroleptic drug side effects can emerge over several months of treatment (Tune et al., 1991).

The diminished ability of demented patients to vocalize their sensations could lead to underdiagnosis of akathisia in this population (Wragg, 1988). A cycle of motor restlessness that leads to increasing doses of neuroleptic medication can ensue. Suspecting "agitated behavior" may be an expression of akathisia can lead to trials of decreased dosage.

Devanand and colleagues (1989) examined 19 subjects with probable Alzheimer's disease who manifested psychosis or behavioral disturbance. Higher doses of haloperidol, close to 5 mg/day, were associated with greater improvement in behavior, but worsened cognitive performance, compared to doses in the range of 1 mg/day. Blood levels of haloperidol were more strongly associated with symptomatic improvement and with severity of extrapyramidal features than dose. Further work by this group has suggested a curvilinear relationship between plasma levels and benefit (Pelton et al., 2003).

Dysken and colleagues (1990) studied haloperidol plasma concentrations in 18 patients with primary degenerative dementia. A "good response" was seen between 0.3 and 2.5 ng/mL, a range of concentrations in which many commercial laboratories could not detect plasma haloperidol. There was no significant linear or curvilinear relationship between response and plasma levels of haloperidol and reduced haloperidol.

Atypical Agents. Relatively early clinical experience supports a role for these drugs in treatment of behavioral disturbances and psychosis associated with dementia. A placebo-controlled trial of risperidone indicated efficacy (Katz et al., 1999). Doses of 1 and 2 mg of risperidone were associated with greater improvement in psychosis and agitation than 0.5 mg and placebo, but subjects treated with 2 mg had increased extrapyramidal side effects. Therefore, standard target doses for agitation or psychotic symptoms in dementia should be 1 to 1.5 mg. A case report noted that dystonia can be associated with antipsychotic treatment in dementia, including use of risperidone (Magnuson et al., 2000).

In a placebo-controlled, randomized trial of olanzapine in patients with Alzheimer's dementia complicated by behavioral disturbance of psychotic symptoms, Street and associates (2000) demonstrated the superiority of 5 and 10 mg/day to both placebo and doses of 15 mg/day. The drug was generally well tolerated, although sedation and gait disturbances were noted in some patients.

MOVEMENT DISORDERS

Conventional Agents. Use of typical antipsychotic drugs can be problematic in those patients with Parkinson's disease who require treatment for psychosis. Exacerbation of baseline motor abnormalities and peripheral autonomic dysregulation leading to hypotension can limit treatment. Typical agents are now second-line drugs in Parkinson's disease.

Atypical Agents. In Parkinson's disease, atypical agents can be beneficial without marked aggravation of motor dysfunction. Case reports have supported the use of clozapine (Scholz & Dichgans, 1985; Wolters et al., 1990). Encouraging experience with quetiapine has been described (Targum & Abbott, 2000). Controlled studies are needed.

SEDATIVES AND HYPNOTICS

Sedatives and hypnotics are the most commonly prescribed psychotropic agents. Patients use anxiolytic agents chronically despite absence of long-term efficacy data and the potential risk of dependence.

The primary anxiolytic agents in clinical use are the benzodiazepines. Buspirone is structurally and pharmacologically distinct from benzodiazepines; it interacts with serotonin and dopamine receptors (Zimmer & Gershon, 1991). The anxiolytic class also includes antihistamines, antidepressants, and β-blockers.

Drugs used as hypnotics have included benzodiazepines and barbiturates. The newer agents zolpidem and zaleplon both interact selectively with the GABA$_A$ receptor omega-1 subtype.

Indications

A comprehensive text on anxiety and anxiolytics in the elderly is available (Salzman & Lebowitz, 1991). The indications for anxiolytic use appear to be narrow; in cognitively intact elderly patients without dementia, they are analogous to those in younger adults. The main indications for anxiolytic use include generalized anxiety and panic disorder. They are also used cautiously as adjuncts for treatment of anxiety in depression and dementia. They have also been used in management of psychosis.

Meprobamate should be avoided as an anxiolytic because it greatly induces the metabolism of other medications, has a narrow therapeutic index, and is associated with dependence and fatality on overdose. Some states now require special prescriptions for benzodiazepines, which may lead to increased use of agents that carry greater risk but are less restricted.

Benzodiazepines and related agents have utility in the short-term management of sleep disturbance. Barbiturates are not recommended for insomnia because of their potential risk of respiratory suppression in high dosage or overdose and their potential for dependency and for drug-drug interactions. Glutethamide, methaqualone, and ethylchlorvynol should also be avoided as hypnotics for the same reasons.

Efficacy

ANXIETY   Studies of aged patients generally involve small samples. The clinician therefore should be skeptical regarding findings for any specific drug. The acute efficacy of anxiolytic agents has received limited investigation in the elderly. Anxiolytic efficacy has been demonstrated in placebo-controlled studies of oxazepam (Koepke et al., 1982) and alprazolam (Cohn, 1984; Krishnan & McDonald, 1993). Anxiety can be associated with depression after middle age; nearly one third of older depressed patients continue to report anxiety more than a year after discharge from hospital treatment (Blazer et al., 1989).

Buspirone treatment, in open studies, reduced Hamilton Anxiety Rating Scale scores in elderly patients (Levine et al., 1989; Napoliello, 1986; Robinson & Napoliello, 1988). The samples studied were clinically quite heterogeneous.

INSOMNIA The same limitations as for anxiolytic use in elders pertain to sedative use in sleep disturbance. A study of temazepam and behavioral management found both effective; the benefits of behavioral management were more persistent on follow-up (Morin et al., 1999). Reports support efficacy of zolpidem (Declerck & Smits, 1999) and zaleplon (Hedner et al., 2000) in elders with insomnia.

SCHIZOPHRENIA AND MANIC DISORDERS Benzodiazepines have been used in mixed-age schizophrenia populations to reduce neuroleptic dose requirement. They may also ameliorate neuroleptic side effects, including akathisia and tardive dyskinesia. Benzodiazepines such as lorazepam (Lenox et al., 1992) and clonazepam (Bradwejn et al., 1990; Chouinard, 1987) have been used primarily as adjuncts in the management of manic states in mixed-age populations.

The potential for increased risks of benzodiazepine use in elderly patients needs to be weighed against potential benefit. Alternative strategies need thorough consideration, and more data specific to the elderly are needed.

Toxicity

"Therapeutic" doses of benzodiazepines can decrease memory consolidation in the elderly (Jenike, 1985a; Murphy, 1983; Rickels et al., 1987). There are apparent pharmacodynamic differences among benzodiazapines. For example, impairment of cognitive performance was less frequent with lorazepam and alprazolam compared to diazepam in acute studies (Pomara et al., 1998); on the other hand, even the short-acting compounds caused greater impairment than placebo. Triazolam has a propensity to cause anterograde amnesia (Schart et al., 1988) and has been delisted in Britain. Effects on memory of benzodiazepines are dose dependent (Hanlon et al., 1998).

A pharmacodynamic component to the sensitivity of some elders to anxiolytics has also been described (Murphy, 1983; Reidenberg et al., 1978). Sedative use not only can reduce cognitive performance on neuropsychologic tests, but also can potentially increase disability in geriatric patients. Two studies have found that benzodiazepine treatment is associated with further functional decline (Reid et al., 1998; Sarkisian et al., 2000).

Increased postural sway, which can lead to falls, can be caused by benzodiazepines. This has been noted even with compounds with short half-lives (Passaro et al., 2000). Femur fractures during benzodiazepine treatment are dose dependent and are a particular risk among older patients within the geriatric population (Sgadari et al., 2000). The greatest risk is in the first 2 weeks after prescription.

"Paradoxical" reactions to benzodiazepines may occur (Murphy, 1983). These can involve increased irritability, agitation, and loss of behavioral control. The triazolo-benzodiazepines may have greater potential for this response, which generally occurs during the first week of treatment. Whether aged patients have greater vulnerability to such reactions is not known.

Tolerance to the effects of benzodiazepines can occur, and dependence can become a problem with long-term use. Dependence and toxicity are of sufficient concern that therapeutic trials should be initiated with careful monitoring and on a time-limited basis.

The side effect profile of buspirone differs from that of benzodiazepines in that it may be associated with less sedative and cognitive toxicity (Hart et al., 1991; Lawlor et al., 1992). It produces less euphoria than benzodiazepines and may have less potential for dependence and abuse. It can produce dizziness, headache, sleep disturbances, and gastrointestinal complaints in elderly patients. Tardive dyskinesia has been reported (Strauss, 1988). The toxicity profiles of zolpidem and zaleplon appear to overlap with those of benzodiazepines.

Given the potential adverse effects of benzodiazepines and their extensive use, studies have addressed whether systematic withdrawal of these agents can reduce toxicity without worsening clinical state. Withdrawal of benzodiazepines can be accomplished without increase in symptoms, but with resultant cognitive improvement (Cohen-Mansfield et al., 1999; Petrovic et al., 1999). Clinicians should bear in mind that physiological dependence will develop in several weeks of chronic treatment, and that patients are at risk for withdrawal syndrome and rebound effects. Tapering off benzodiazepines in the elderly, as in younger patients, therefore can be difficult.

Practical Guidelines

PRETREATMENT ASSESSMENT AND CLINICAL MONITORING   In documenting treatment history when considering use of benzodiazepines and related drugs, it is essential to assess for any prior history of substance abuse and dependence.

PHARMACOKINETICS, DOSING, AND DRUG-DRUG INTERACTIONS   Pharmacokinetic concomitants of aging make some older patients especially vulnerable to toxic effects of benzodiazepines. Some benzodiazepines, predominantly longer acting agents, are metabolized through the P450 3A4 cytochrome system.

There is a two- to threefold increase in the half-life of long-acting benzodiazepines with active metabolites (i.e., diazepam, chlordiazepoxide, and flurazepam) over short-acting compounds (i.e., lorazepam, oxazepam, temazepam, and triazolam) in elderly patients compared to young adults (Greenblatt et al., 1982; Salzman et al., 1983). This argues for the use of the latter group of medications in elderly patients to avoid drug accumulation. An exception is ultrashort-acting agents like triazolam that often produce next-day amnestic symptoms and should be avoided. Alprazolam concentration/dose ratios increase with age (Kaplan et al., 1998).

Buspirone is metabolized by the cytochrome P450 system; it has a short half-life, and it lacks pharmacologically active metabolites. The hypnotics zolpidem and zaleplon each have short elimination half-lives and have no active metabolites. Benzodiazepines and buspirone are extensively protein bound, primarily to albumin, in the vascular compartment. Zaleplon has relatively low plasma protein binding.

Benzodiazepines have potential for pharmacokinetic interactions involving cytochrome 3A4 metabolism. Concomitant use of nefazadone can lead to prolonged half-life of some benzodiazepines, such as diazepam, alprazolam, clonazepam, and triazolam. Pharmacodynamic interactions include potentiation of sedative effects of antidepressants and antipsychotics. Buspirone does not interact pharmacodynamically with alcohol, but does with haloperidol; concomitant use of MAO inhibitors with buspirone should be avoided. Zaleplon metabolism has minimal involvement of the 3A4 cytochrome P450 system, which may lessen potential for some drug-drug interactions.

Additional Clinical Situations

Alprazolam may have antidepressant properties, although panic disorder is its primary indication. Weissman and coworkers (1992) compared alprazolam, imipramine, and placebo in geriatric outpatients older than 60 years with major depression who also received weekly interpersonal psychotherapy. Alprazolam treatment was associated with greater decreases in depression and anxiety ratings after 2 weeks, but the differences between drug treatment groups disappeared by week 6; this may be because of benefits from psychotherapy. Thus, alprazolam may contribute to improvement in geriatric depression, but the antidepressant efficacy of alprazolam monotherapy remains to be demonstrated.

Benzodiazepines have been used in conjunction with antidepressant treatment of major depression to reduce anxiety prior to the onset of effects of the antidepressant. A study of clonazepam use during initial fluoxetine treatment indicated benefits from clonazepam compared to placebo augmentation (Smith et al., 1998).

Anxiolytics also have a limited place in the management of demented patients. In a comparison with thioridazine, diazepam was found more calming, but was associated with less improvement of behavioral disturbance (Kirven & Montero, 1973). Salzman (Salzman, 1998; Salzman & Lebowitz, 1991) and others (Sizaret et al., 1974), however, noted that lorazepam was effective in reducing agitation and restlessness in demented patients. Also, a randomized comparison of oxazepam with haloperidol and diphenhydramine found all three agents comparably effective in reducing dementia-related agitation (Coccaro et al., 1990). Buspirone has also been reported as beneficial (Tariot et al., 1997); in an open trial, agitation decreased by 22% using an average dose of 35 mg/day in demented patients (Sakauye et al., 1993).

Benzodiazepines can increase agitation in some demented patients in association with worsening cognitive impairment, however. Discontinuation of benzodiazepines has been found to improve cognitive performance in nursing home patients with dementia (Salzman et al., 1992).

MEDICATIONS FOR ALZHEIMER'S DISEASE

The demonstration that degeneration of neurons in the cholinergic system is fundamental to the neuropathology of Alzheimer's disease and is correlated with accompanying cognitive deficits (Coyle et al., 1983; Perry et al., 1978; Whitehouse et al., 1981) provided the conceptual basis for contemporary pharmacotherapies for this disorder (Bartus et al., 1982). Prior to the introduction of medications designed to enhance cholinergic function, a heterogeneous group of agents, many of which were called *nootropics* because of their novel mechanisms of action, had been studied with limited success to treat patients with Alzheimer's disease and other forms of dementia. Dihydroergotoxine (Hydergine), which was thought to act as a weak vasodilator or an MAOI, received FDA approval for the treatment of the nonspecific syndrome of "senile mental decline." Nevertheless, benefits from dihydroergotoxine were slight and demonstrated on less-sensitive instruments than those used in current dementia trials (Hollister & Yesavage, 1984). It is likely that any benefits observed resulted indirectly through the mild beneficial effects of the compound on mood and attention.

Initially, therapies were designed to increase available acetylcholine (ACh), the neurotransmitter released by cholinergic neurons, by providing its precursor, choline, or by directly stimulating cholinergic neurons with drugs such as arecholine. Both approaches failed. The use of ACh precursors has been limited by the difficulty of making adequate doses of choline available with the central nervous system. Furthermore, providing cholinergic agonists could not stimulate postsynaptic neurons in a pattern consistent with normal physiological function. The alternative approach of maximizing the effect of ACh released by cholinergic neurons that remain functional by inhibiting ACh metabolism at the synaptic cleft has proved more fruitful. Scholarly reviews, which describe the history, rationale, and effects of cholinesterase inhibitor treatments, are available (Cummings, 2000; Farlow, 2002; Parnetti et al., 1997). This section discusses the use of available cholinesterase inhibitors, followed by a brief discussion of other pharmacological approaches for the treatment of cognitive deficits associated with Alzheimer's disease.

Cholinesterase Inhibitors

Tacrine, donepezil, galantamine, and rivastigmine are the cholinesterase inhibitors approved currently in the United States for the treatment of Alzheimer's disease. The efficacy of each has been documented for the treatment of cognition and general clinical functioning. The Alzheimer's Disease Assessment Scale (ADAS; Rosen et al., 1984) has become the standard instrument for assessing cognitive functioning. General improvement is assessed using structured interviews that are administered to caregivers.

Despite the documented efficacy of these agents, benefits are modest. Only

50% of treated patients demonstrated improvement in most studies (Parnetti et al., 1997), and the overall separation from placebo on the Cognitive subscale of the ADAS (ADAS-Cog) is limited. Thus, studies using currently available agents have demonstrated a 3- to 5-point difference favoring cholinesterase inhibitors (improvement) in ADAS-Cog scores compared to placebo during 6 months of treatment.

Data from the donepezil trial (Rogers et al., 1998) are representative for the pattern of change found in placebo-controlled trials of cholinesterase inhibitors: Compared to subjects assigned randomly to placebo, those treated with donepezil demonstrated greater initial improvement. As a result of the progressive deterioration that is inherent to Alzheimer's disease, both groups demonstrated cognitive decline during the course of the trial, but the ADAS-Cog scores of subjects who had received donepezil remained significantly better in 6 months than scores of subjects in the placebo group. Progression of the disease led ADAS-Cog scores to return to their pretreatment levels in approximately 6 months (Rogers et al., 1998).

Thus, cholinesterase treatment can be thought of as providing mild initial improvement and as turning back the clock of decline for up 6 months. The "buying time" rationale has been extended to consider other possible indications. Other domains of benefit that are under exploration include (1) the treatment of cognition in patients with "pre-Alzheimer's disease" mild cognitive impairment (MCI) or for other forms of dementia; (2) to improve psychiatric symptoms that develop in association with Alzheimer's disease; and (3) to slow the rate of progression of Alzheimer's disease by decreasing the rate of cholinergic cell loss.

EFFICACY   Although the four approved agents of this class inhibit brain acetylcholinesterase, differences between their mode of action have been identified. As summarized by Farlow (2002), published data from 6-month studies of cognitive effects demonstrated somewhat greater effect sizes for rivastigmine (2.4–4.9) and galantamine (2.9–3.6) than for donepezil (1.5–3.1), but overlap exists. The suggestion of greater potency for rivastigmine and galantamine must be balanced against the tolerability and easy dosing schedule of donepezil. Finally, the studies cited used different patient populations and somewhat different methodologies, including a larger number of monthly dosage increases with galantamine and rivastigmine, limiting the value of these results for assessing relative efficacy. Head-to-head comparisons are required to determine whether an approved agent has superior efficacy for a specific target population.

Mechanisms and sites of action of the various cholinesterase inhibitors are summarized in Table 30-6. Representative data on efficacy and tolerability are provided in Table 30-7. Donepezil has been thought to have the advantage of acting by inhibiting the activity of central acetylcholinesterase only, without affecting butyrylcholinesterase. Inhibition of central acetylcholinesterase without affecting peripheral enzymes was thought to explain the high tolerability associated with donepezil treatment. Butyrylcholinesterase, which is located

TABLE 30-6.   Properties of approved cholinesterase inhibitors

Cholinesterase inhibitor	Tacrine	Donepezil	Rivastigmine	Galantamine
Brain versus peripheral selectivity	No	Yes	Yes	No
Type of cholinesterase inhibited	Acetyl and butyryl	Acetyl	Acetyl and butyryl	Acetyl
Reversible inhibition	Rapidly reversible	Rapidly reversible	Slowly reversible	Rapidly reversible
Dosing schedule: monthly increments to maximize tolerability	10 mg four times daily up to 30–40 mg four times daily, between meals if possible	5 mg daily to 10 mg daily	1.5 mg twice daily up to 6 mg twice daily with meals	4 mg twice daily up to 12 mg twice daily with meals

TABLE 30-7.   Efficacy and tolerability of approved cholinesterase inhibitors

Cholinesterase inhibitor	Tacrine	Donepezil	Rivastigmine	Galantamine
Improvement on ADAS-Cog scores in 6-month studies	2.2 (Knapp et al., 1994)	2.9 (Rogers et al., 1998)	4.9 (Corey-Bloom et al., 1998)	3.9 (Raskind et al., 2000)
Patients improving or not worsening in 6 months	Approximately 67%	81%	56%	72%
Patients not completing trial	73%	32%	35%	31%
Representative side effects*				
Elevated transaminase	29%	+	+	+
Nausea	28%	19%	47%	17%
Vomiting	28%	8%	31%	10%
Diarrhea	16%	15%	9%	+
Dizziness	12%	+	21%	+
Muscle cramps	+	8%	+	+
Insomnia	6%	14%	9%	

Source: Adapted from Sramek et al. (2001).

ADAS-Cog, Alzheimer's Disease Assessment Scale, Cognitive subscale.

+ Indicates side effects are reported to occur infrequently or rarely.

*Adapted from *Physician's Desk Reference* (2002).

primarily in the periphery, was thought to contribute to specific side effects such as diarrhea and increases in pulse that may occur with cholinesterase inhibitors without benefiting cognition. This argument that central inhibition of acetylcholinesterase but not butyrylcholinesterase by donepezil provides an advantage has been questioned (Farlow, 2002).

Evidence indicates that butyrylcholinesterase is present in cholinergic systems centrally and increases relative to acetylcholinesterase as Alzheimer's disease progresses (Arendt et al., 1992). Data indicating that rivastigmine is particularly effective in patients with more rapidly progressive illness (Farlow, 2002) is consistent with the possible advantage of inhibiting butyrylcholinesterase in addition to acetylcholinesterase for patients with more severe illness or a more rapid decline. Data suggesting that the inhibition of both acetylcholinesterase and butyrylcholinesterase provides benefits over the inhibition of acetylcholinesterase alone, including effects on the neuropathology and course of Alzheimer's disease, is provided in a review (Grieg et al., 2002). Also, it has been argued that the binding of galantamine to nicotinic receptors modulates their function, which may enhance ACh release (Lilienfeld & Kurtz, 2002).

Most of the arguments favoring one or another of the available cholinesterase inhibitors are based on theoretical extensions of findings from in vitro studies, secondary analyses of pivotal trials conducted to obtain FDA approval, and data from phase IV (postmarketing) studies supported by manufacturers of specific agents. The situation is not different from choosing among different SSRIs. Theoretical reasons for selecting one SSRI over another are available, but superiority in efficacy or tolerability cannot be determined without head-to-head prospective comparisons in specified patient groups.

Limitations in efficacy must be balanced against the progressive nature of Alzheimer's disease. Any improvement that does not change the underlying pathophysiology must be time limited. Therefore, the clinician cannot conclude that a medication is not working because cognition has not improved or cognitive decline has progressed. Discontinuation of cholinesterase inhibitor treatment following completion of a placebo-controlled trial has been associated with rapid deterioration in cognition (Rogers et al., 1998), a "rebound effect."

Therefore, uncertainty about whether a particular patient is benefiting from a specific treatment may be addressed by instituting a trial of gradual discontinuation to determine whether cognitive deterioration appears to be worsening. Rapid discontinuation to assess for a rebound has the potential for causing a devastating increase in symptoms. Nevertheless, this problem cannot be addressed easily. Deterioration following discontinuation of a cholinesterase inhibitor may be because of a change in the course of the disease. Also, declines that result from delaying the initiation of treatment may not be "made up" after the drug is initiated (Farlow et al., 2000).

Resolving whether patients who fail to respond to one cholinesterase inhibitor may respond to another also requires systematic study. Rasmusen and coworkers (2001) demonstrated that 53% of patients who had not responded to donepezil demonstrated improved cognition when switched to galantamine. Similar results were found among patients who were switched from donepezil to rivastigmine because of lack of effectiveness or poor tolerability (Auriacombe et al., 2002).

One option is to begin treatment with the medication a patient tolerates best, particularly in mild cases. Patients whose disease progresses may require dosage augmentation to the limits of tolerability or effectiveness, followed by switching to a cholinesterase inhibitor with a somewhat different mode of action. The suggestion that dual cholinesterase inhibition provides greater benefit and that providing this treatment early may slow the progression of dementia (Farlow, 2002) would argue for more aggressive treatment earlier in the course.

CHOLINESTERASE INHIBITORS FOR OTHER FORMS OF DEMENTIA   Trials of cholinesterase inhibitors for the treatment of vascular dementia and mixed vascular-Alzheimer's dementia have generated promising results. A large-scale, placebo-controlled trial of donepezil for probable vascular dementia demonstrated significant improvement on the ADAS-Cog (Pratt & Perdomo, 2002b). A subgroup of 10 patients with definite vascular dementia demonstrated cognitive improvement on MMSE scores compared to untreated patients, who demonstrated cognitive decline (Pratt & Perdomo, 2002a). Additional support comes from a secondary analysis of an Alzheimer's disease data set. Patients with Alzheimer's disease who had vascular risk factors demonstrated greater improvement on rivastigmine over placebo than patients without these risk factors (Kumar et al., 2000). Also, the efficacy of galantamine compared to placebo has been demonstrated in patients with mixed dementia, but a significant benefit was not found in the subgroup diagnosed with pure vascular dementia (Erkinjuntti et al., 2002).

Lewy body dementia is associated with a greater loss of central cholinergic activity than occurs in pure Alzheimer's disease (McKeith & O'Brien, 1999). Open trials with donepezil (Samuel et al., 2000; Shea et al., 1998) and a placebo-controlled trial with rivastigmine (McKeith et al., 2000) both demonstrated benefits of cholinesterase inhibitors in these patients. Data are also available supporting the use of cholinesterase inhibitors to treat dementia in patients with Parkinson's disease, despite the theoretical expectation that increasing cholinergic function would worsen motor symptoms. Results from a trial of adding tacrine or donepezil to standard medications for Parkinson's disease (Werber & Rabey, 2001) resulted in cognitive improvement. Also, results from a controlled trial demonstrated that patients who were randomly placed in a donepezil treatment group demonstrated improved cognition compared to those who received a placebo (Aarsland et al., 2002).

CHOLINESTERASE INHIBITOR TREATMENT OF NEUROPSYCHIATRIC DISTURBANCES ASSOCIATED WITH DEMENTIA   Increasing evidence exists that cholinesterase inhibitors are psychoactive compounds that may improve the behavioral and psychiatric symptoms associated with dementia (Cummings, 2000). Evidence from open trials (Kaufer et al., 1998) and secondary analyses of placebo-controlled data (Mega et al., 1999) using tacrine and donepezil have been extended to studies of other agents. Although apathy and visual hallucinations may be most likely to respond (Cummings, 2000), improvement has been noted on multiple domains of the Neuropsychiatric Inventory (Cummings et al., 1994), including items assessing mood, apathy, and behavioral and psychotic symptoms (Mega et al., 1999). Results from a meta-analysis of 29 controlled trials (Trinh et al., 2003) indicated that improvement in neuropsychiatric symptoms in association with cholinesterase treatment occurs across different medications of this class.

Although a theoretical link to diminished central cholinergic function has been suggested (Cummings, 1998; Mega, 2000), the relationships between improvement in attention, cognition, and psychiatric symptoms that occur with cholinesterase inhibition have not been fully established. Nevertheless, broadening the role of cholinesterase inhibitors to the treatment of neuropsychiatric disturbances and of patients with more severe cognitive impairment can be expected to counteract the tendency to consider cholinesterase inhibitor treatment as an ineffective and inefficient use of health care resources in long-term care settings.

PRACTICAL GUIDELINES

Pretreatment Assessment and Clinical Monitoring. Recently introduced cholinesterase inhibitors are generally well tolerated. Tacrine has a direct hepatotoxic effect, with 30% of patients treated with this medication developing a more than threefold increase in transaminase levels. Plasma monitoring of hepatic functioning and other ongoing physiological assessments are not required for other agents of this class. Although cholinesterase inhibitors vary in potential for peripheral effects (Table 30-6), all of these agents may cause bradycardia, worsening of pulmonary obstructive disease, or increased gastric acid secretion by enhancing cholinergic tone. Although these adverse reactions were not a problem in published trials with these agents, patients with preexisting diseases that affect these vulnerable systems were generally excluded. Therefore, clinicians should consider a patient's comorbid clinical conditions, such as peptic ulcer disease or sick sinus syndrome, before prescribing a cholinesterase inhibitor. Clinical monitoring should assess for changes in cognitive functioning. The absence of improvement in cognition or the rate of decline should suggest an absence of clinical benefit and lead to consideration of a cholinesterase inhibitor with a somewhat different mode of action.

Pharmacokinetics, Dosing, and Drug-Drug Interactions. Although cholinesterase inhibitors are metabolized through the P450 hepatic microsomal enzyme system, their presence does not affect the metabolism of other drugs metabolized through this pathway. Theoretically, inhibition of enzymes that metabolize cholinesterase inhibitors would result in increases in plasma levels, but adverse reactions attributable to such interactions have not been reported.

The possibility of synergistic cholinergic action when cholinesterase inhibitors are provided in combination with other cholinergic medications such as succinylcholine and bethanechol should be considered when these medications are coadministered. Conversely, cholinesterase inhibitors would be expected to counteract effects of anticholinergic compounds used to treat comorbid medical problems.

Dosing of cholinesterase inhibitors should take the half-life of the particular agent and reversibility of binding to the cholinesterase inhibitor into account (Table 30-7). Thus, donepezil, an irreversible inhibitor with a half-life of nearly 3 days, is administered only once daily, generally in the evening. Selectivity of donepezil for central acetylcholinesterase inhibition may explain the increase in insomnia and reports of disturbed sleep because of vivid dreaming that has been associated with its use. Patients who develop sleep-related symptoms during donepezil treatment may benefit from administering the once-daily dose in the morning.

Attention to side effects is required to maximize tolerability and adherence. Nausea is common to each of these agents and appears to result from increases in brain ACh levels that result in increased dopamine release (Farlow, 2002). Evidence that centrally acting antiemetics reduce nausea and vomiting in patients treated with rivastigmine (Jhee et al., 2002) is consistent with a central mechanism for this effect. Monthly upward dose titration should be used for all cholinesterase inhibitors to provide time to develop tolerance to the effects of increased central cholinergic activity and minimize gastrointestinal side effects.

Despite evidence for a central mechanism, the experience with tacrine in this regard is illuminating: Unlike other cholinesterase inhibitors, the absorption of tacrine is markedly diminished when taken with meals. Despite this, it is recommended that tacrine should be taken with meals if significant gastrointestinal symptoms occur (*Physician's Desk Reference*, 2002). It is also suggested that galantamine and rivastigmine should be taken with meals.

N-Methyl-D-Aspartate (NDMA) Receptor Antagonists: Memantine

Glutamate, an excitatory neurotransmitter, is released by damaged neurons. Excessive release of glutamate results in further toxicity to nerve cells, a process considered to contribute to neuronal loss in degenerative diseases (Lipton & Rosenberg, 1994). Results from a placebo-controlled study indicated that memantine, an antagonist of the NMDA glycine receptor, may slow the rate of decline of Alzheimer's disease in patients who are moderately to severely impaired (Reisberg et al., 2003). Memantine was superior to placebo on global measures of functioning, on activities of daily living scores, and on a cognitive assessment instrument used in severely impaired patients. The ADAS-Cog was not used because of the severity of cognitive impairment in this sample with average baseline MMSE scores less than 8. Preliminary results of a placebo-controlled trial of combining memantine plus donepezil produced similar results: The combination was superior to donepezil plus placebo on these cognitive and functional outcome measures (Tariot et al., 2002).

Although memantine is not approved currently by the FDA, these trials underscore the importance of exploring methods to slow the decline associated with Alzheimer's disease beyond enhancing ACh neurotransmission. Furthermore, combining approaches that use different mechanisms is a reasonable approach until the cause of and cure for progressive neurodegeneration is identified.

SUMMARY

Major advances in geriatric psychopharmacology have occurred since the last edition of this textbook. Antidepressant studies have contributed to our understanding of the patterns of response of geriatric patients. Findings from acute and maintenance studies of the older old have become available. Broadening eligibility criteria for participation, which is consistent with studying the effectiveness of medications in real world populations, has provided data on how aging-related comorbid conditions affect antidepressant responsiveness. Syndromes such as vascular and executive dysfunction depression have been delineated, contributing to our understanding of why some elderly patients respond poorly to standard antidepressant treatments.

Expansion of our knowledge base about the responsiveness of a broad population of elderly patients to standard medications has occurred in parallel with the development of new classes of medications and new medications within classes. The introduction of atypical antipsychotic medications has provided agents with a lower risk of the neuromuscular side effects that develop during treatment using conventional agents. Studies using agents of this class will continue to delineate the appropriate use of these medications for older patients and the effect of aging on efficacy and tolerability. Geriatric psychiatry has borrowed data on treatment with mood stabilizers from studies of mixed-age patients, but much remains to be learned about the use of these medications in older adults. Geriatric syndromes such as the psychosis of dementia and the depression of dementia have been described, providing targets for focused studies of the effectiveness of psychopharmacological approaches to reduce the symptoms, excess suffering, and disabilities that are associated with these complications.

We can expect that the "aging imperative" will lead to further advances in geriatric psychopharmacology. New classes of medications are needed to treat patients who do not respond to or cannot tolerate agents that are available currently. For progressive disorders such as Alzheimer's disease, improved understanding will lead to treatments that interrupt the disease process, an advance over current agents that only modestly slow the rate of deterioration.

Synergy between studies conducted by investigators from the domains of basic science, drug development, and clinical trials research can be expected to enhance our understanding of mechanisms that underlie the psychiatric disorders of later life and their optimal pharmacological treatment.

REFERENCES

Aarsland A, Laake K, Larsen JP, Janvin C. Donepezil for cognitive impairment in Parkinson's disease: a randomized controlled study. *J Psychiatry Neurol Neurosurg Psychiatry*. 2000;72:708–712.

Abernathy DR, Barbey JT, Franc J, et al. Loratidine and terfenadine interaction with nefazodone. Both antihistamines are associated with QTc prolongation. *Clin Pharmacol*. 2001;69:96–103.

Abou-Saleh MT, Coppen A. Prognosis of depression in old age: the case for lithium therapy. *Br J Psychiatry*. 1983;143:527–528.

Addonizio G. Neuroleptic malignant syndrome in elderly patients. *J Am Geriatr Soc.* 1987;35:1011–1012.

Agnoli A, Fabbrini G, Fioravanti M, et al. CBF and cognitive evaluation of Alzheimer type patients before and after IMAO-B treatment: a pilot study. *Eur Neuropsychopharmacol*. 1992;2:31–35.

Alda M. Pharmacogenetics of lithium response in bipolar disorder. *J Psychiatry Neurosci*. 1999;24:154–158.

Alderman CP, Seshadri P, Ben-Tovim DI. Effects of serotonin reuptake inhibitors on hemostasis. *Ann Pharmacother*. 1996;30:1231–1234.

Alexopoulos GS, Abrams RC, Young RC, et al. Cornell Scale for depression in dementia. *Biol Psychiatry*. 1988;23:271–284.

Alexopoulos GS, Katz IR, Reynolds CF III, Carpenter D, Docherty JP. The Expert Consensus Series: pharmacotherapy of depressive disorders in older adults. *Postgrad Med*. 2001:1–86.

Alexopoulos GS, Kiosses DN, Choi SJ, Murphy CF, Lim KO. Frontal white matter microstructure and treatment responses of late-life depression: a preliminary study. *Am J Psychiatry*. 2002;159:1929–1932.

Alexopoulos GS, Meyers BS, Young RC, et al. Executive dysfunction worsens the long-term outcome of geriatric depression. *Arch Gen Psychiatry*. 2000;57:285–290.

Alexopoulos GS, Meyers BS, Young RC, et al. Recovery in geriatric depression. *Arch Gen Psychiatry*. 1996;53:305–312.

Allain H, Pollak P, Neukirch HC. Symptomatic effect of selegiline in de novo parkinsonian patients: the French selegiline multicenter trial. *Mov Disord*. 1993;8(Suppl): S36–S40.

Altamura AC, Percudani M, Guercetti G, et al. Efficacy and tolerability of fluoxetine in the elderly: a double blind study vs amitriptyline. *Int Clin Psychopharmacol*. 1989; 4:103–106.

Alvir JY, MA J, Lieerman JA, et al. Clozapine-induced agranulocytosis. *N Engl J Med*. 1993;329:162–167.

American Psychiatric Association. *Diagnostic and Statistical Manual of Mental Disorders*. 4th ed. Washington, DC: American Psychiatric Association; 1994.

Amore M, Ricci M, Zanardi R, et al. Long-term treatment of geropsychiatric depressed patients with venlafaxine. *J Affect Disord.* 1997;46:292–296.

Andersen G, Vestergaard K, Lauritzen L. Effective treatment of poststroke depression with the selective serotonin reuptake inhibitor citalopram. *Stroke.* 1994;25:1099–1104.

Andersen G, Vestergaard K, Riis JO. Citalopram for post-stroke pathological crying. *Lancet.* 1993;342:837–839.

Aoba A, Yamaguchi N, Shedo M. Plasma neuroleptic levels in age patients on various neuroleptic. In: Kitani K, ed. *Liver and Aging.* New York, NY: Elsevier; 1996: 115–126.

Apseloff G, Wilner KD, Gerber N, Tremaine LM. Effect of sertraline on protein binding of warfarin. *Clin Pharmacol.* 1997;32(Suppl 1):37–42.

Arendt T, Bruckner MK, Lange M, Bigl V. Changes in acetylcholinesterase and butyrylcholinesterase in Alzheimer's disease resemble embryonic development—a study of molecular forms. *Neurochem Int.* 1992;21:381–396.

Arvanitis LA, Miller BG. Multiple fixed doses of Seroquel (quetiapine) in patients with acute exacerbation of schizophrenia: a comparison with haloperidol and placebo. *Biol Psychiatry.* 1997;15:233–246.

Auriacombe S, Pere JJ, Loria-Kanza Y, Vellas B. Efficacy and safety of rivastigmine in patients with Alzheimer's disease who failed to benefit from treatment with donepezil. *Curr Med Res Opin.* 2002;18:129–138.

Avorn J. Depression in the elderly-falls and pitfalls. *N Engl J Med.* 1998;339:918–920.

Aweeka F, Jayesekara D, Horton M, et al. The pharmacokinetics of ziprasidone in subjects with normal and impaired renal functions. *Br J Clin Pharmacol.* 2000; 49(Suppl 1):27S–33S.

Axelsson R. On the pharmacokinetics of thioridazine in psychiatric patients. In: *Antipsychotic Drugs: Pharmacodynamics and Pharmacokinetics.* New York, NY: Pergamon Press; 1976:353–358.

Ayd FJ. A survey of drug-induced extrapyramidal reactions. *JAMA.* 1976;175:1045–1060.

Bajulaiye R, Addonizio G. Clozapine in the treatment of psychosis in an 82 year old woman with tardive dyskinesia. *J Clin Psychopharmacol.* 1992;12:364–365.

Baker SP, Harvey AH. Fall injuries in the elderly. *Clin Geriatr Med.* 1985;1:501–512.

Baldessarini RJ, Tondo L, Hennen J. Treating the suicidal patient with bipolar disorder. Reducing risk with lithium. *Ann N Y Acad Sci.* 2001;932:24–38.

Ball CJ. The use of clozapine in older people. *Int J Geriatr Psychiatry.* 1992;7:689–692.

Barak Y, Wittenberg N, Naor S, et al. Clozapine in elderly psychiatric patients: tolerability, safety, and efficacy. *Compr Psychiatry.* 1999;40:320–325.

Barnes R, Veith R, Okimoto J, et al. Efficacy of antipsychotic medications in behaviorally disturbed dementia patients. *Am J Psychiatry.* 1982;139:1170–1174.

Bartus RT, Dean RL, Beer B, Lippa AS. The cholinergic hypothesis of geriatric memory dysfunction. *Science.* 1982;217:408–417.

Bauer M, Bschor T, Kunz D, et al. Double blind placebo-controlled trial of the use of lithium augment antidepressant medication in continuation treatment of unipolar major depression. *Am J Psychiatry.* 2000;157:1429–1435.

Bauer M, Dopfmer S. Lithium augmentation in treatment-resistant depression: meta-analysis of placebo-controlled studies. *J Clin Psychopharmacol.* 1999;19:427–434.

Bergstrom RF, Lemberger L, Farid NA, et al. Clinical pharmacology and pharmacokinetics of fluoxetine: a review. *Br J Psychiatry.* 1988;153(Suppl):47–50.

Beyer J, Siegal A, Kennedy J, et al. Olanzapine, divalproex and placebo treatment non-head-to-head comparisons of older adult acute mania. Abstract. *Int Psychogeriatr Assoc.* 2001.

Black DW, Winokus G, Bell S, et al. Complicated mania. *Arch Gen Psychiatry.* 1988; 45:232–236.

Blazer D, Hughes DC, Fowler N. Anxiety as an outcome symptom of depression in elderly and middle-aged adults. *Int J Geriatr Psychiatry.* 1989;4:273–278.

Bloom F, Kupfer DJ. *Psychopharmacology—The 4th Generation of Progress.* New York, NY: Raven Press; 1995.

Bocksberger JP, Gachoud JP, Richard J, et al. Comparison of the efficacy of moclobemide and fluvoxamine in elderly patients with a severe depressive episode. *Eur Psychiatry.* 1993;8:319–324.

Bondareff W, Alpert M, Friedlhoff AJ, et al. Comparison of sertraline and nortriptyline in the treatment of major depressive disorder in late life. *Am J Psychiatry.* 2000; 157:729–736.

Bouchard RH, Pourcher E, Vincent P. Fluoxetine and extrapyramidal side effects. *Am J Psychiatry.* 1989;146:1352–1353.

Bowden CL. Anticonvulsants in bipolar elderly. In: Nelson JC, ed. *Geriatric Psychopharmacology.* New York, NY: Marcel Dekker; 1998:285–299.

Bowden CL. Predictors of response to divalproex and lithium. *J Clin Psychiatry.* 1995; 56:25–30.

Bowden CL, Brugger AM, Swann AC, et al. Efficacy of divalproex vs lithium and placebo in the treatment of mania. *JAMA.* 1994;271:918–923.

Bowden CL, Calabrese JR, McElroy SL, et al. A randomized, placebo-controlled 12-month trial of divalproex in treatment of outpatients with bipolar 1 disorder. Divalproex Maintenance Study Group. *Arch Gen Psychiatry.* 2000;57:481–489.

Bowden CL, Calabrese JR, McElroy SL, et al. The efficacy of lamotrigine in rapid cycling and non-rapid cycling patients with bipolar disorder. *Biol Psychiatry.* 1999;46: 1711–1712.

Bradwejn J, Shriqui C, Koszycki D, et al. Double-blind comparison of the effects of clonazepam and lorazepam in acute mania. *J Clin Psychopharmacol.* 1990;10:403–408.

Branconnier RJ, Cole JO, Ghazvinian S, et al. Clinical pharmacology of bupropion and imipramine in elderly depressives. *J Clin Psychiatry.* 1983;44:130–133.

Branconnier RJ, Cole JO, Ghazvinian S, et al. Treating the depressed elderly patient: the comparative behavioral pharmacology of mianserin and amitriptyline. In: Costa E, Racagni G, eds. *Typical and Atypical Antidepressants: Clinical Practice.* New York, NY: Raven; 1982.

Broud TM. Fluoxetine and extrapyramidal side effects [letter]. *Am J Psychiatry.* 1989; 146:1353.

Burke WG, Gurgel I, Bose A. Fixed-dose trial of the single isomer SSRI escitalopram in depressed outpatients. *J Clin Psychiatry.* 2002;63:331–336.

Burns A, Russell E, Stratton-Powell H, et al. Sertraline in stoke-associated lability of mood. *Int J Geriatr Psychiatry.* 1999;14:681–685.

Byerly MJ, Weber MT, Brook DL, et al. Antipsychotic medications and the elderly: effect on cognition and implications for use. *Drugs Aging.* 2001;18:45–61.

Byne W, White L, Parella M, et al. Tardive dyskinesia in a chronically institutionalized population of elderly schizophrenic patients: prevalence and association with cognitive impairment. *Int J Geriatr Psychiatry.* 1998;13:473–479.

Calabrese JR, Bowden CL, McElroy SL, et al. A double-blind placebo-controlled study of lamotrigine in rapid cycling and non-rapid cycling patients with bipolar disorder. *J Clin Psychiatry.* 1999;60:79–88.

Caligiuri M, Jeste DV, Lacro JP. Antipsychotic induced movement disorders in the elderly: epidemiology and treatment recommendations. *Drugs Aging.* 2000;17:363–384.

Caligiuri MP, Lacro JP, Jeste DV. Incidence and predictors of drug-induced parkinsonism in older psychiatric patients treated with very low doses of neuroleptics. *J Clin Psychopharmacol.* 1999;19:322–328.

Carson AJ, MacHale S, Allen K, et al. Depression after stroke and lesion location: a systemic review. *Lancet.* 2000;356:122–126.

Cassano GB, Puca F, Scapicchio PL, Trabucchi M, Italian Study Group on Depression in Elderly Patients. Paroxetine and fluoxetine effects on mood and cognitive functions in depressed nondemented elderly patients. *J Clin Psychiatry.* 2002;63:396–402.

Centurrino F, Baldessarini RJ, Kando JC, et al. Clozapine and metabolites: concentrations in serum and clinical findings during treatment of chronically psychotic patients. *J Clin Psychopharmacol.* 1994;14:119–125.

Chambers CA, Bain BJ, Rosbottom R, et al. Carbamazepine in senile dementia and overactivity: a placebo controlled double blind trial. *IRCS Med Sci.* 1982;10:505–506.

Chapron DJ, Cameron IR, White, LB, et al. Observations on lithium disposition in the elderly. *J Am Geriatr Soc.* 1982;30:651–655.

Chen ST, Altshuler LL, Melnyk KA, et al. Efficacy of lithium vs valproate in the treatment of mania in the elderly: a retrospective study. *J Clin Psychiatry.* 1999;60:181–185.

Chiarello RJ, Cole JO. The use of psychostimulants in general psychiatry. *Arch Gen Psychiatry.* 1987;44:286–295.

Chouinard G. Clonazepam in the acute and maintenance treatment of bipolar affective disorder. *J Clin Psychiatry.* 1987;48:29–36.

Coccaro EF, Kramer E, Zemishlany Z, et al. Pharmacologic treatment of noncognitive behavioral disturbances in elderly demented patients. *Am J Psychiatry.* 1990;137:1640–1645.

Coffey CD, Figiel GS, Djang WT, et al. White matter hyperintensity on magnetic resonance imaging: clinical and neuroanatomic correlates in the depressed elderly. *J Neuropsychiatry.* 1989;1:135–144.

Cohen-Mansfield J. Agitated behaviors in the elderly. II. Preliminary results in the cognitively deteriorated. *J Am Geriatr Soc.* 1986;34:722–727.

Cohen-Mansfield J, Sipson S, Werner P, et al. Withdrawal of haloperidol, thioridazine, and lorazepam in the nursing home: a controlled, double-blind study. *Arch Intern Med.* 1999;159:1733–1740.

Cohn CK, Shrivastava R, Mendels J, et al. Double-blind, multicenter comparison of sertraline and amitriptyline in elderly depressed patients. *J Clin Psychiatry.* 1990;51(Suppl 12):28–33.

Cohn JB. Double-blind safety and efficacy comparison of alprazolam and placebo in the treatment of anxiety in geriatric patients. *J Clin Psychiatry.* 1984; 45:104–107.

Collaborative Working Group on Clinical Trial Evaluations. Adverse effects of the atypical antipsychotics. *J Clin Psychiatry.* 1998;59:17–22.

Corey-Bloom J, Anand R, Veach J, for the ENA-713 (rivastigmine tartare) B352 Study Group. A randomized trial evaluation the efficacy and safety of ENA-713, a new acetylcholinesterase inhibitor in patients with mild to moderately severe Alzheimer's disease. *Int J Geriatr Psychopharmacol.* 1998;1:55–66.

Coyle JS, Price DL, DeLong MR. Alzheimer's disease: a disorder of cortical cholinergic innervation. *Science.* 1983;219:1184–1190.

Cozza KL, Armstrong SC. Concise guide to the cytochrome P450 system. In: Cozza KL, Armstrong SC, Cole MA, Oesterheld, JR, eds. *Drug Interaction Principles for Medical Practice.* Washington, DC: American Psychiatric Publishing; 2001.

Crabtree BL, Mack JE, Johnson CD, et al. Comparison of hydrochlorthiazide and furosemide on lithium disposition. *Am J Psychiatry.* 1991;148:1060–1063.

Craig I, Tallis R. Impact of valproate and phenytoin on cognitive function in elderly patients: results of a single-blind randomized comparative study. *Epilepsia.* 1994; 35:381–390.

Crane GE, Naranjo ER. Motor disturbances induced by neuroleptics. *Arch Gen Psychiatry.* 1971;24:179–184.

Crewe HK, Lennard MS, Tucker GT, et al. The effect of selective serotonin re-uptake inhibitors on cytochrome P450 6 (CYP-6) activity in human liver microsomes. *Br J Clin Pharmacol.* 1992;34:262–265.

Cummings JL. Cholinesterase inhibitors: a new class of psychotropic compounds. *Am J Psychiatry.* 2000;157:4–15.

Cummings JL, Back C. The cholinergic hypothesis of neuropsychiatric symptoms in Alzheimer's disease. *Am J Geriatr Psychiatry.* 1998;6(Suppl 1):S64–S78.

Cummings JL, Mega MS, Gray K, Rosenberg-Thompson S, Carursi DA, Gornbein J. The neuropsychiatric inventory. *Neurology.* 1994;44:2308–2314.

Curry SH. Binding of psychotropic drugs to plasma protein and its influence on drug disposition. In: Usdin E, ed. *Clinical Pharmacology in Psychiatry.* New York, NY: Elsevier; 1981:213–223.

Dalton SO, Johansen C, Mellemkjaer L, Norgard B, Sorensen HT, Olsen JH. Use of selective serotonin reuptake inhibitors and risk of upper gastrointestinal bleeding: a population-based cohort study. *Arch Intern Med.* 2003;163:59–64.

Daniel DG, Zimbroff DL, Potkin SG, et al. Ziprasidone 80 mg/day and 160 mg/day in the acute exacerbation of schizophrenia and schizoaffective disorder: a 6 week placebo controlled trial. *Neuropsychopharmacology.* 1999;20:491–505.

Danish University Antidepressant Group. Paroxetine: a selective serotonin reuptake inhibitor showing better tolerance but weaker antidepressant effect than clomipramine in a controlled multicenter study. *J Affect Disord.* 1990;18:289–299.

Danish University Antidepressant Group. Citalopram: clinical effect profile in comparison with clomipramine: a controlled multicenter study. *Psychopharmacology (Berlin).* 1986;90:131–138.

Das Gupta K, Jefferson JW, Kobak KA, et al. The effect of enalapril on serum lithium levels in healthy men. *J Clin Psychiatry.* 1992;53:398–400.

Davidson J. Seizures and bupropion: a review. *J Clin Psychiatry.* 1989;50:256–261.

DeBoer T. The pharmacologic profile of mirtazapine. *J Clin Psychiatry.* 1996;57(Suppl 4):19–25.

Declerck A, Smits M. Zolipem a valuable alternative to benzodiazepine hypnotics for chronic insomnia. *J Int Med Res.* 1999;27:253–263.

Delbressine LPC, Voss RME. The clinical relevance of preclinical data: mirtazapine, a model compound. *J Clin Psychol.* 1997;17(Suppl 1):29s–34s.

Dell'Agnello G, Ceravolo R, Nuti A, et al. SSRIs do not worsen Parkinson's disease: evidence from an open-label, prospective study. *Clin Neuropharmacol.* 2001;24: 221–227.

DePaulo J Jr, Correa EI, Sapir DG. Renal function and lithium: a longitudinal study. *Am J Psychiatry.* 1986;143:892–895.

Devanand D, Sackeim H, Brown R, et al. A pilot study of haloperidol treatment of psychosis and behavioral disturbances in Alzheimer's disease. *Arch Neurol.* 1989; 46:854–857.

Devanand DP, Pelton GH, Maston K, et al. Sertraline treatment of elderly patients with depression and cognitive impairment. *Int J Geriatr Psychiatry.* 2003;18:123–130.

DeVane CL, Pollock BG. Pharmacokinetic considerations of antidepressant use in the elderly. *J Clin Psychiatry.* 1999;60(Suppl 20):38–44.

DeVanna M, Kummer J, Agnoli A, et al. Moclobemide compared with second-generation antidepressants in elderly people. *Acta Psychiatr Scand.* 1990;S360:64–66.

Division of Neuropharmacological Drug Products of FDA. Position Paper. FDA; 2000.

Druckenbrod R, Mulsant BH. Fluoxetine induced syndrome of inappropriate antidiuretic hormone section: a geriatric case report and a review of the literature. *J Geriatr Psychiatry Neurol.* 1994;7:255–258.

Dunner DL, Cohn JB, Walshe T, et al. Two combined, multicenter double-blind studies of paroxetine and doxepin in geriatric patients with major depression. *J Clin Psychiatry.* 1992;53:57–60.

Dysken MW, Johnson SB, Holden L, et al. Haloperidol concentrations in patients with Alzheimer's dementia. *Clin Pharmacol Ther.* 1990;47:162.

Echt DS, Liebson PR, Mitchell LB, et al. Mortality and morbidity in patients receiving encainaide, flecainide or placebo. *N Engl J Med.* 1991;324:781–788.

Erkinjuntti A, Kurz S, Gauthier R, Bollock S, Lilienfeld S, Damaraju CV. Efficacy of galantamine in probable vascular dementia and Alzheimer's disease combined with cerebrovascular disease: a randomized trial. *Lancet.* 2002;359:1283–1290.

Evans M, Hammon M, Wison K, et al. Placebo-controlled treatment trial of depression in elderly physically ill patients. *Int J Geriatr Psychiatry.* 1997;12:817–924.

Extein I. *Treatment of Tricyclic-Resistant Depression.* Washington, DC: American Psychiatric Association; 1989:51–79.

Eze E, Workman M, Donley B. Hyperammonemia and coma developed by a woman treated with valproic acid for affective disorder. *Psychiatr Serv.* 1998;49:1358–1359.

Farlow M. A clinical overview of cholinesterase inhibitors in Alzheimer's disease. *Int Psychogeriatr.* 2002;14(Suppl 1):93–126.

Farlow M, Anand R, Messina J Jr, Hartmann R, Veach J. A 52 week study of the efficacy of rivastigmine in patients with mild to moderately severe Alzheimer's disease. *Eur J Neurol.* 2000;44:236–241.

Feighner JP. The role of venlafaxine in rational antidepressant therapy. *J Clin Psychiatry.* 1994;55(Suppl A):62–68.

Feighner JP, Cohn JB. Double-blind comparative trials of fluoxetine and doxepin in geriatric patients with major depressive disorder. *J Clin Psychiatry.* 1985;46:20–25.

Ferris SH, Steinberg G, Shulman E, et al. Institutionalization of Alzheimer's patients: reducing precipitating factors through family counseling. *Arch Found Thanatol.* 1985;12:7.

Figiel GS, Krishnan KRR, Breitner JC, et al. Radiologic correlates of antidepressant-induced delirium: the possible significance of basal-ganglia lesions. *J Neuropsychiatry.* 1989;1:188–190.

Finkel SF, Richter EM, Clary CM, et al. Comparative efficacy of sertraline vs fluoxetine in patients age 70 or over with major depression. *Am J Geriatr Psychiatry.* 1999; 7:221–227.

Flint A. A risk-benefit assessment of available agents. *Age Aging.* 1998;13:269–280.

Flint AJ, Rifat SL. A prospective study of lithium augmentation in antidepressant-resistant geriatric depression. *J Clin Psychopharmacol.* 1994;14:353–356.

Flint AJ, Rifat SL. The effect of sequential antidepressant treatment on geriatric depression. *J Affect Disord.* 1996;36, 95–105.

Foley DJ, Ostfeld AM, Branch LG, et al. The risk of nursing home admission in three communities. *J Aging Health.* 1992;4:155–173.

Folstein M. Mania agitation and Alzheimer's disease. *Abstract AAGP.* 1999.

Folstein MF, Folstein SE, McHugh PR. Mini-Mental State: a practical method for grading the cognitive state of patients for the clinician. *J Psychiatry Res.* 1975;12:189–198.

Fontaine R, Ontiveros A, Elie R, et al. A double-blind comparison of nefazodone, imipramine and placebo in major depression. *J Clin Psychiatry.* 1975;55:234–241.

Frank E, Kupfer DJ, Perel TM, et al. Three-year outcomes for maintenance therapies in recurrent depression. *Arch Gen Psychiatry.* 1990;47:1093–1099.

Frankenburg FR, Kalunian D. Clozapine in the elderly. *J Geriatr Psychiatry Neurol.* 1994;7:129–132.

Freeman H. Moclobemide. *Lancet.* 1993;342:1528–1532.

Friedman JR, Norman DC, Yoshikawa TT. Correlation of estimated renal function parameters vs 24 hour creatinine clearance in ambulatory elderly. *J Am Geriatr Soc.* 1989;37:145–149.

Frye MA, Altshuler LL, Bitran JA. Clozapine in rapid cycling bipolar disorder (letter). *Clin Psychopharm.* 1996;16:87–90.

Galynker I, Ieronimo C, Miner C, et al. Methylphenidate treatment of negative symptoms in patients with dementia. *J Neuropsychol Clin Neurosci.* 1997;9:231–239.

Gardos G, Casey D. *Tardive Dyskinesia and Affective Disorders.* Washington, DC: American Psychiatric Publishing; 1984.

Georgotas A, McCue RE. The additional benefit of extending an antidepressant trial past seven weeks in the depressed elderly. *Int J Geriatr Psychiatry.* 1989;4:191–195.

Georgotas A, McCue RE, Cooper TB. A placebo-controlled comparison of nortriptyline and phenelzine in maintenance therapy of elderly depressed patients. *Arch Gen Psychiatry.* 1989;46:783–786.

Georgotas A, McCue RE, Cooper TB, et al. How safe and effective is continuation therapy in elderly depressed patients? *Arch Gen Psychiatry.* 1988;45:929–936.

Georgotas A, McCue RE, Hapworth W, et al. Comparative efficacy and safety of MAOIs versus TCAs in treating depression in the elderly. *Biol Psychiatry.* 1986; 21:1155–1166.

Gerner R, Estabrook W, Steuer J. Treatment of geriatric depression with trazodone, imipramine and placebo: a double-blind study. *J Clin Psychiatry.* 1980;41:216–220.

Gitlin MJ. Lithium-induced renal insufficiency. *J Clin Psychopharmacol.* 1993;132:276–279.

Glassman AH, Bigger JT Jr. Cardiovascular effects of therapeutic doses of the tricyclic antidepressants: a review. *Arch Gen Psychiatry.* 1981;38:815–820.

Glassman AH, Bigger JT Jr, Giardina EV, et al. Clinical characteristics of imipramine-induced orthostatic hypotension. *Lancet.* 1979;1:468–472.

Glassman AH, Kantor SJ, Shostak M. Depression, delusions, and drug response. *Am J Psychiatry.* 1975;132:716–719.

Glassman AH, Johnson GG, Giardina EG, et al. The use of imipramine in depressed patients with congestive heart failure. *JAMA.* 1983;280:1987–2001.

Glassman AH, Roose SP, Bigger JT Jr. The safety of tricyclic antidepressants in cardiac patients: risk-benefit reconsidered (commentary). *JAMA.* 1993;269:2673–2675.

Gleason RP, Schneider LS. Carbamazepine treatment of agitation in Alzheimer's outpatients refractory to neuroleptic. *J Clin Psychiatry.* 1990;51:115–118.

Gnam W, Flint AJ. New onset rapid cycling bipolar disorder in an 87 year old woman. *Can J Psychiatry.* 1993;38:324–326.

Goff DC, Jenike MA. Treatment resistant depression in the elderly. *J Am Geriatr Soc.* 1986;34:63–70.

Goldberg JF, Sachs MH, Kocsis JH. Low-dose lithium augmentation of divalproex in geriatric mania. *J Clin Psychiatry.* 2000;61:304.

Goldberg RD. Antidepressant use in the elderly. Current status of nefazadone, venlafaxine and moclebide. *Drugs Aging.* 1997;11(Suppl 2):119–131.

Golden RN, DeVane CL, Laizure SC, et al. Bupropion in depression. II. The role of metabolites in clinical outcome. *Arch Gen Psychiatry.* 1988;45:145–149.

Goodnick PJ, Puig A, DeVane CL, et al. Mirtzapine in major depression with comorbid generalized anxiety disorder. *J Clin Psychiatry.* 1999;60:446–448.

Goodwin FK, Jamison R. *Manic Depressive Illness.* New York, NY: Oxford University Press; 1990.

Greenblatt DJ, Sellers EM, Shader RI. Drug disposition in old age. *N Engl J Med.* 1982;306:1081–1088.

Greenblatt DJ, von Moltke LL, Harmatz JA, et al. Drug interactions with newer antidepressants: role of human cytochromes P450. *J Clin Psychiatry.* 1998;59(Suppl 15):19–27.

Greig NH, Lahiri DK, Sambamurti K. Butyrylcholinesterase: an important new target in Alzheimer's disease therapy. *Int Psychogeriatr.* 2002;14(Suppl 1):77–91.

Grossman F. A review of anticonvulsants in treating agitated demented elderly patients. *Pharmacotherapy.* 1998;18:600–606.

Halikas JA. Org 3770 (Mirtazapine) versus trazodone: a placebo-controlled trial in depressed elderly patients. *Hum Psychopharmacol.* 2001;10(Suppl):125–133.

Hamilton M. A rating scale for depression. *Neurol Neurosurg Psychiatry.* 1960;23:56–62.

Hanlon JT, Horner D, Schmader KE, et al. Benzodiazepine use and cognitive function among community-dwelling elderly. *Clin Pharmacol Ther.* 1998;64:684–692.

Hardy BG, Shulman KI, Mackenzie SE. Pharmacokinetics of lithium in the elderly. *J Clin Psychopharmacol.* 1987;7:153.

Haring C, Meise U, Humpel C, et al. Influence of patient-related variables on clozapine plasma levels. *Am J Psychiatry.* 1990;147:1471–1475.

Harris MJ, Heaton RK, Schalz A, et al. Neuroleptic dose reduction in older psychotic patients. *Schizophr Res.* 1997;27:241–248.

Hart RP, Colenda CC, Hamer RM. Effects of buspirone and alprazolam on the cognitive performance of normal elderly subjects. *Am J Psychiatry.* 1991;148:73–77.

Haupt DW, Newcomer JW. Hyperglycemia and antipsychotic medications. *J Clin Psychiatry.* 2001;62(Suppl 27):15–26.

Haverkamp W, Breithardt G, Camm AJ, et al. The potential for t prolongation and proarrhythmia by non-antiarrhythmic drugs: clinical and regulatory implications. *Eur Heart J.* 2000;21:1216–1231.

Hayes RL, Gerner RH, Fairbands L, et al. EKG findings in geriatric depressives given trazodone, placebo or imipramine. *J Clin Psychiatry.* 1983;44:180–183.

Head L, Dening T. Lithium in the over-65s: who is taking it and who is monitoring it? A survey of older adults on lithium in the Cambridge Mental Health Services catchment area. *Int J Geriatr Psychiatry.* 1998;13:164–171.

Hebenstreit GF, Fellerer K, Zochling R, et al. A pharmacokinetic dose titration study in elderly depressed patients. *Acta Psychiatr Scand Suppl.* 1989;350:81–84.

Hedner J, Yaeche R, Emilien G, et al. Zalipem shortens subjective sleep latency and improves subjective sleep quality in elderly patients with insomnia. *Int J Geriatr Psychiatry.* 2000;15:704–712.

Heyberg OJ, Maragakis B, Mullin J, et al. A double-blind multicenter comparison of mirtazapine and amitriptyline in elderly depressed patients. *Acta Psychiatr Scand.* 1997;93:184–190.

Hickie I, Scott E, Mitchell P, et al. Subcortical hyperintensities on magnetic resonance imaging: clinical correlates and prognostic significance in patients with severe depression. *Soc Biol Psychiatry.* 1995;37:151–160.

Himmelhoch J, Neil JR, May SJ, et al. Age, dementia, dyskinesias, and lithium response. *Am J Psychiatry.* 1980;137:941–945.

Hollister LE. General principles of treating the elderly with drugs. In: Jarvik LF, Greenblatt D, Harman E, eds. *Clinical Pharmacology and the Aged Patient.* New York, NY: Raven; 1981:1–9.

Hollister LE, Yesavage J. Ergoloid mesylates for senile dementias: unanswered questions. *Ann Intern Med.* 1984;100:894–898.

Israili ZH, Wenger J. Aging, gastrointestinal disease, and response to drugs. In: Jarvik LF, Greenblatt D, Harman E, eds. *Clinical Pharmacology and the Aged Patient.* New York, NY: Raven; 1981;131–155.

Janowsky D, Curtis G, Zisook S, et al. Ventricular arrhythmias possibly aggravated by trazodone. *Am J Psychiatry.* 1983;140:796–797.

Jarvik L, Mintz J. In: Awad AG, Durost HMHMR, et al., eds. *Treatment of Depression.* New York, NY: Pergamon; 1987;51–57.

Jefferson JW, Greist JH. Lithium: interactions with other drugs. In: David JM, Greenblatt D, eds. *Psychopharmacology Update.* New York, NY: Grune & Stratton; 1979;81–104.

Jefferson JW, Greist JH, Baudhuin M. Lithium: interactions with other drugs. *J Clin Psychopharmacol.* 1981;1:124–131.

Jenike, MA. *Handbook of Geriatric Psychopharmacology.* Littleton, CO: PSG; 1985a.

Jenike MA. Monoamine oxidase inhibitors as treatment for depressed patients with primary degenerative dementia (Alzheimer's disease). *Am J Psychiatry*. 1985b;142: 763–764.

Jerling M, Lindstrom L, Bondesson U, et al. Fluvoxamine inhibition and carbamazepine induction of the metabolism of clozapine: evidence from a therapeutic drug monitoring service. *Ther Drug Monit*. 1994;16:368–374.

Jeste DV, Finkel SI. Psychosis of Alzheimer's disease and related dementias: diagnostic criteria for a distinct syndrome. *Am J Geriatr Psychiatry*. 2000;8:29–34.

Jeste DV, Linnoila M, Wagner RL, et al. Serum neuroleptic concentrations and tardive dyskinesia. *Psychopharmacology*. 1982;76:377–380.

Jeste DV, Rockwell E, Harris MJ, et al. Conventional versus newer antipsychotics in elderly patients. *Am J Ger Psychiatry*. 1999;7:70.

Jeste DV, Wyatt RJ. Aging and tardive dyskinesia. In: Miller NE, Cohen GD, eds. *Schizophrenia and Aging: Schizophrenia, Paranoia, and Schizophreniform Disorders in Later Life*. New York, NY: Guilford; 1987.

Jhee SS, Shiovitz T, Harman RD, et al. Centrally acting antiemetics mitigate nausea and vomiting in patients with Alzheimer's disease who receive rivastigmine. *Clin Neuropharmacol*. 2002;25:122–128.

Joffe RT, Singer W, Levitt AJ, et al. A placebo controlled comparison of lithium and triiodothyronine augmentation of tricyclic antidepressants in unipolar refractory depression. *Arch Gen Psychiatry*. 1993;50:387–393.

Kahn A, Fabre LF, Rudolph R. Venlafaxine in depressed geriatric outpatients: an open label clinical study. *Psychopharmacol Bull*. 1995;3:753–758.

Kalayam B, Alexopoulos GS. Prefrontal dysfunction and treatment response in geriatric depression. *Arch Gen Psychiatry*. 1999;56:713–718.

Kando JC, Tohen M, Castillo J, et al. The use of valproate in an elderly population with affective symptoms. *J Clin Psychiatry*. 1996;57:238–240.

Kane JM, Cole K, Sarantakos S, et al. Safety and efficacy of bupropion in elderly patients: preliminary observations. *J Clin Psychiatry*. 1983;44:134–136.

Kaplan GB, Greenblatt DJ, Ehrenberg BL, et al. Single-dose pharmacokinetics and pharmacodynamics of alprazolam in elderly and young subjects. *J Clin Pharmacol*. 1998;38:14–21.

Kapur S, Seeman P. Does fast dissociation from the dopamine d(2) receptor explain the action of atypical antipsychotics? A new hypothesis. *Am J Psychiatry*. 2001;158: 360–369.

Katona CLE, Hunter BN, Bray J. A double-blind comparison of the efficacy and safety of paroxetine and imipramine in the treatment of depression with dementia. *Int J Geriatr Psychiatry*. 1998;13:100–108.

Katz IR, Jeste DV, Mintzer JE, et al. Comparison of risperidone and placebo for psychosis and behavioral disturbances associated with dementia: a randomized, double-blind trial. *J Clin Psychiatry*. 1999;60:107–115.

Katz IR, Parmaelee PA, Beaston-Wimmer P, et al. Association of antidepressants and other medications with mortality in the residential care elderly. *J Geriatr Psychiatry Neurol*. 1994;7:221–226.

Katz IR, Reynold CR III, Alexopoulos GS, Hackett D. Venlafaxine ER as a treatment for generalized anxiety disorder in older adults: pooled analysis of five randomized placebo-controlled clinical trials. *J Am Geriatr Soc*. 2002;18–25.

Katz IR, Simpson GM, Curlick SM, et al. Pharmacological treatment of major depression for elderly patients in residential care settings. *J Clin Psychiatry.* 1991; 51(Suppl):41–47.

Kaufer D, Cummings JL, Christine D. Differential neuropsychiatric symptom responses to tacrine in Alzheimer's disease: relationship to dementia severity. *J Neuropsychiatry Clin Neurosci.* 1998;10:55–63.

Keck P, Buffenstein A, Ferguson J, et al. Ziprasidone 40 and 120 mg/day in the acute exacerbation of schizophrenia and schizoaffective disorder: a week placebo controlled trial. *Psychopharmacology.* 2001;140:173–184.

Kellner MB, Neher F. A first episode of mania after age 80. *Can J Psychiatry.* 1991;36: 607–608.

Kerr JS, Fairweather DB, Mahendran R, et al. The effects of paroxetine alone and in combination with alcohol on psychomotor performance and cognitive function in the elderly. *Int Clin Psychopharm.* 1992;7:101–108.

Kiraly SJ, Gibson RE, Ancill RJ, et al. Risperidone: treatment response in adult and geriatric patients. *Int J Psychiatr Med.* 1998;28:255–263.

Kirchner V, Kely CA, Harvey RJ. Thioridazine for dementia. *Cochrane Database Syst Rev.* 2000;2:CD000464.

Kirven LE, Montero EF. Comparison of thioridazine and diazepam in the control of nonpsychotic symptoms associated with senility: double blind control study. *J Am Geriatr Soc.* 1973;21:545–551.

Kitanaka I, Aavadil AP, Cutler NR, et al. Altered hydroxydesipramine concentrations in the elderly. *Clin Pharmacol Ther.* 1981;29:258.

Klysener R, Bent-Hasnen J, Hansen HL, et al. Efficacy of citalopram in the prevention of recurrent depression in elderly patients: placebo-controlled study of maintenance therapy. *Br J Psychiatry.* 2002;181:29–35.

Knapp MR, Knopman DS, Solomon PR, et al., for the Tacrine Study Group. A 30-week randomized controlled trial of high-dose tacrine in patients with Alzheimer's disease. *JAMA.* 1994;271:985–991.

Koepke HH, Golde RL, Linden ME, et al. Multicenter controlled study of oxazepam in anxious elderly patients. *Psychosomatics.* 1982;23:641–645.

Krishnan KRR, McDonald WM. Magnetic resonance morphometry: image analysis methodology development for affective disorder. *Depression.* 1993;1:159–171.

Kronig MH, Roose SP, Walsh BP, et al. Blood pressure effects of phenelzine. *J Clin Psychopharmacol.* 1983;3:307–310.

Kumar V, Anand R, Messina J, Hartman R, Veach J. An efficacy and safety analysis of Exelon (rivastigmine) in Alzheimer's disease patients with concurrent vascular risk factors. *Eur J Neurol.* 2000;7:159–169.

Kutcher SP, Reid K, Dubb JD, et al. Electrocardiogram changes and therapeutic desipramine and 2-hydroxydesipramine concentrations in elderly depressives. *Br J Psychiatry.* 1986;148:676–679.

Laghrissi-Thode F, Pollock BG, Miller et al. Comparative effects of sertraline and nortriptyline on body sway in older depressed patients. *Am J Geriatr Psychiatry.* 1995; 3:217–228.

Laghrissi-Thode F, Wagner WR, Pollock BG, et al. Elevated platelet factor 4 and b-thromboglobulin plasma levels in depressed patients with ischemic heart disease. *Biol Psychiatry* 1997;42:290–295.

Lauritzen L, Odgaard K, Clemmesen L, et al. Relapse prevention by means of paroxetine in ECT-treated patients with major depression: a comparison with imipramine and placebo in medium-term continuation therapy. *Acta Psychiatr Scand.* 1996;94: 241–251.

Lavretsky H, Kumar A. Methylphenidate augmentation of citalopram in elderly depressed patients. *Am J Geriatr Psychiatry.* 2001;9:298–303.

Lawlor BA, Hill JL, Radcliffe JL. Single oral dose challenge of buspirone does not affect memory processes in older volunteers. *Biol Psychiatry.* 1992;32:101–103.

Lemberger L, Bergstrom RF, Wolen RF, et al. Fluoxetine: a clinical pharmacology and psychologic disposition. *J Clin Psychiatry.* 1985;46:14–19.

Lenox RH, Newhouse PA, Creelman WL, et al. Adjunctive treatment of manic agitation with lorazepam versus haloperidol: a double-blind study. *J Clin Psychiatry.* 1992; 53:47–52.

Levine S, Napoliello MJ, Domantay AG. Open study of buspirone in octogenarians with anxiety. *Hum Psychopharmacol.* 1989;4:51–53.

Lilienfeld S, Kurz A. Broad therapeutic benefits in patients with probably vascular dementia or Alzheimer's disease with cerebrovascular disease treated with galantamine. *Ann N Y Acad Sci.* 2002;977:487–492.

Linnet K, Wiborg O. Steady-state serum concentrations of the neuroleptic perphenazine in relation to CYP2D6 genetic polymorphism. *Clin Pharmacol Ther.* 1996;60:41–47.

Lipsey JR, Robinson RG, Pearlson GD. Nortriptyline treatment of poststroke depression: a double blind study. *Lancet.* 1984;1:297–300.

Lipton SA, Rosenberg PA. Excitatory amino acids as a final common pathway for neurologic disorders. *N Engl J Med.* 1994;330:613–622.

Liu B, Anderson G, Mittman N, et al. Use of selective serotonin-reuptake inhibitors or tricyclic antidepressants and risk of hip fractures in elderly people. *Lancet.* 1998; 351:1303–1307.

Llorent MD, Olsen EJ, Leyva O, et al. Use of antipsychotic drugs in nursing homes: current compliance with OBRA regulations. *J Am Geriatr Soc.* 1998;46:198–201.

Lydiard BR. Tricyclic resistant depression: treatment resistance or inadequate treatment? *J Clin Psychiatry.* 1985;46:412–417.

Lyketsos CG, Sheppard JM, Steele CD, et al. Randomized, placebo-controlled, double-blind clinical trial of sertraline in the treatment of depression complicating Alzheimer's disease: initial results from the depression in Alzheimer's disease study. *Am J Psychiatry.* 2000;157:1686–1689.

Madhusoodanan S, Brecher M, Brenner R, et al. Risperidone in the treatment of elderly patients with psychotic disorders. *Am J Geriatr Psychiatry.* 1999;7:132–138.

Madhusoodanan S, Brenner R, Suresh P, et al. Efficacy and tolerability of olanzapine in elderly patients with psychotic disorders: a prospective study. *Ann Clin Psychiatry.* 2000;12:11–18.

Magnuson TM, Roccaforte WH, Wengel SP, et al. Medication induced dystonias in nine patients with dementia. *J Neuropsychiatr Clin Neurosci.* 2000;12:219–225.

Maguire K, Pereira A, Tiller J. Moclobemide pharmacokinetics in depressed patients: lack of age effect. *Hum Psychopharmacol.* 1991;6:249–252.

Mahapatra SN, Hackett D. A randomized double blind parallel group comparison of venlafaxine and dothiepin in geriatric patients with major depression. *Int J Clin Pract.* 1997;51:209–213.

Ma Jose J, Alvin PH, Lieberman JA, et al. Clozapine-induced agranulocytosis: incidence and risk factors in the United States. *JAMA.* 1993;329:162–167.

Maletta GJ, Weingarden T. Reversal of anorexia by methylphenidate in apathetic, severely demented nursing home patients. *Am J Psychiatry.* 1993;1:243.

Mandani MM, Parikh SV, Austin PC, et al. Use of antidepressants among elderly subjects: trends and contributing factors. *Am J Psychiatry.* 2000;157:36-367.

Mangoni A, Grassi MP, Frattola L, et al. Effects of MAO-B inhibitor in the treatment of Alzheimer's disease. *Eur Neurol.* 1991;31:100-107.

Manji HK, Chen G, Hsiao JK, et al. Regulation of signal transduction pathways by mood stabilizing agents: implications for the delayed onset of therapeutic efficacy. *J Clin Psychiatry.* 1996;57(Suppl 13):34-46.

Manji HK, Moore GJ, Chen G. Lithium at 50: have the neuroprotective effects of this unique medication been overlooked? *Biol Psychiatry.* 1999;46:929-940.

Mann JJ, Aarons SF, Wilner PJ, et al. A controlled study of the antidepressant efficacy and side effects of deprenyl: a selective monoamine oxidase inhibitor. *Arch Gen Psychiatry.* 1989;46:45-50.

Massand PS. Side effects of antipsychotics in the elderly. *J Clin Psychiatry.* 2000;61:43-49.

Mattis S. *Dementia Rating Scale.* Psychological Assessment Resource; 1988.

Mazure CM, Nelson JC, Jatlow PI, et al. Acute neuroleptic treatment in elderly patients without dementia. *Am J Ger Psychiatry.* 1998;6:221-229.

McCabe B, Tsuang MT. Dietary consideration in MAO inhibitor regimens. *J Clin Psychiatry.* 1982;43:178-181.

McCreadie RG, Robertson LJ, Wiles D. The Nithsdale Schizophrenia Survey, IX: Akathisia, parkinsonism and tardive dyskinesia and plasma neuroleptic levels. *Br J Psychiatry.* 1992;161:793-799.

McFarland BH, Miller MR, Straumfjord AA. Valproate use in the older manic patient. *J Clin Psychiatry.* 1990;51:479-481.

McKeith I, Del Ser T, Spano PF, et al. Efficacy of rivastigmine in dementia with Lewy bodies: a randomized double-blind, placebo-controlled international study. *Lancet.* 2000;356:2031-2036.

McKeith I, O'Brien J. Dementia with Lewy body. *Aust N Z J Psychiatry.* 1999;33:800-808.

McManus DQ, Arvanitis LA, Kowalcyk BB. Quetiapine, a novel antipsychotic: experience in elderly patients with psychotic disorders. Seroquel Trial 48 Study Group. *J Clin Psychiatry.* 1999;60:292-298.

Mega MS. The cholinergic deficit in Alzheimer's disease: impact on cognition, behavior and function. *Int J Neuropsychopharmacol.* 2000;3(Suppl 2):s3-s12.

Mega MS, Masterman DM, O'Connor SM, Barclay TR, Cummings JL. The spectrum of behavioral responses to cholinesterase inhibitor therapy in Alzheimer's disease. *Arch Neurol.* 1999;56:1388-1391.

Mendels J, Johnson R, Mattes J, et al. Efficacy of bid doses of venlafaxine in a dose response study. *Psychopharmacol Bull.* 1993;29:169-174.

Meredith CH, Feighner JP, Hendrickson G. A double-blind comparative evaluation of the efficacy and safety of nomifensine, imipramine, and placebo in depressed geriatric outpatients. *J Clin Psychiatry.* 1984;45:73-77.

Meyer JM. A retrospective comparison of weight, lipid, and glucose changes between risperidone- and olanzapine-treated inpatients: metabolic outcomes after one year. *J Clin Psychiatry.* 2002;63:425-433.

Meyer UA, Amrein R, Balant LP, et al. Antidepressants and drug-metabolizing enzymes—expert group report. *Acta Psychiatrica Scand.* 1996;93:71–79.

Meyers BS. Adverse cognitive effects of tricyclic antidepressants in the treatment of geriatric depression: fact or fiction. In: Shamoian CA, ed. *Psychopharmacological Side Effects of Psychotropics in the Elderly.* Washington, DC: American Psychiatric Publishing; 1991;1–16.

Meyers BS. Time to response of geriatric depression. *Abstract NCDEU.* May 1999.

Meyers BS, Kakuma T, Ippolito L, et al. Nortriptyline maintenance for geriatric depression: an expansion of the Georgotas studies. *Abstract NCDEU.* May 1997.

Meyers BS, Klimstra S, Kakuma T, et al. Continuation treatment of delusional depression in older adults. *Abstract ACNP Annual Meeting.* 1999.

Miller F, Menninger J, Whitchup SM. Lithium neuroleptic neurotoxicity in the elderly bipolar patient. *J Clin Psychopharmacol.* 1986;6:176–178.

Mirchandani IC, Young RC. Management of mania in the elderly: an update. *Ann Clin Psychiatry.* 1993;5:67–71.

Mittmann N, Herrmann N, Einarson TR, et al. The efficacy, safety and tolerability of antidepressants in late life depression: a meta-analysis. *J Affect Disord.* 1997;46: 191–217.

Mittmann N, Herrmann N, Shulman KI, et al. The effectiveness of antidepressants in elderly depressed outpatients: a prospective case series study. *J Clin Psychiatry.* 1999;60:690–697.

Moleman P, Janzen G, vonBargen BA, et al. Relationship between age and incidence of Parkinsonism in psychiatric patients treated with haloperidol. *Am J Psychiatry.* 1986;143:232–234.

Monteleone P, Gnocch G. Evidence for a linear relationship between plasma trazodone levels and clinical response in depression in the elderly. *Clin Neuropharmacol.* 1990;14:s84–s89.

Mordecai DJ, Sheikh JI, Glick ID. Divalproex for the treatment of geriatric bipolar disorder. *Int J Geriatr Psychiatry.* 1999;14:494–496.

Morin CM, Colecchi C, Stone J, et al. Behavioral and pharmacological therapies for late-life insomnia: a randomized controlled trial. *JAMA.* 1999;281:991–999.

Movig KL, Leufkens HG, Lendrerink AW, Egberts AC. Serotonergic antidepressants associated with an increased risk for hyonatremia in the elderly. *Eur J Clin Pharmacol.* 2002;58:143–148.

Mulsant BH, Pollock BG, Nebes D, et al. A double-blind randomized comparison of nortriptyline and paroxetine in the treatment of late-life depression: 6 week outcome. *J Clin Psychiatry.* 1999;60(Suppl 20):16–20.

Mulsant BH, Sweet BA, Rosen J, et al. A randomized double blind comparison of nortriptyline plus perphenazine vs nortriptyline plus placebo in the treatment of psychotic depression in late life. *J Clin Psychiatry.* 2001;62:597–604.

Murphy E. The prognosis of depression in old age. *Br J Psychiatry.* 1983;142:111–119.

Murray E, Hopwood S, Balfour JK. The influence of age on lithium efficacy and side effects in outpatients. *Psychol Med.* 1983;13:53–60.

Myllyla VV, Sotaniemi KA, Vuorinen JA, et al. Selegiline in de novo parkinsonian patients: the Finnish study. *Mov Disord.* 1993;8:s41–s44.

Nagler RM, Pollack S. Sjorgren's syndrome induced by estrogen therapy. *Semin Arthritis Rheum.* 2000;30:209–214.

Nambudiri DE, Mirchandani IC, Young RC. Two more cases of trazodone-related syncope in the elderly. *Int Geriatr Psychiatry Neurol*. 1989;2:225.

Napoliello MJ. An interim multicentre report on 677 anxious geriatric out patients treated with buspirone. *Br J Clin Pract*. 1986;71–73.

National Institute of Mental Health. National Advisory Mental Health Council. Bridging Science and Service. *NIMH*. 1999;99–4353:1–64.

Nelson CG, Kennedy JS, Pollock BG, et al. Treatment of major depression with nortriptyline and paroxetine in patients with ischemic heart disease. *Am J Psychiatry*. 1999;156:1024–1028.

Nelson JC. *Geriatric Psychopharmacology*. New York, NY: Marcel Dekker; 1998.

Nelson JC, Atillasoy E, Mazure C, et al. Hydroxydesipramine in the elderly. *J Clin Psychopharmacol*. 1988;8:428–433.

Nelson JC, Bock JL, Jatlow PI. Clinical implications of 2-hydroxydesipramine concentrations in the elderly. *Clin Pharmacol Ther*. 1983;33:183–189.

Nelson JC, Jatlow P, Mazure C. Desipramine plasma levels and response in elderly melancholic patients. *J Clin Psychopharmacol*. 1985;5:217–220.

Nelson JC, Mazure C, Bowers MB, et al. A preliminary open study of the combination of fluoxetine and desipramine for rapid treatment of major depression. *Arch Gen Psychiatry*. 1991;48:303–307.

Nelson JC, Mazure C, Jatlow PI. Antidepressant activity of 2-hydroxydesipramine. *Clin Pharmacol Ther*. 1988;44:283–288.

Nelson JC, Price LH, Jatlow PI. Neuroleptic dose and desipramine concentrations during combined treatment of delusional depression. *Am J Psychiatry*. 1986;143:1151–1154.

Nemeroff CB, DeVane CL, Pollock BG. Newer antidepressants and the cyctochrome P450 system. *Am J Psychiatry*. 1996;153:311–320.

Niedermier JA, Nasrallah HA. Clinical correlates of response to valproate in geriatric inpatients. *Ann Clin Psychiatry*. 1998;10:165–168.

Nierenberg AA, Farabaugh AH, Alpert JE, et al. Timing of onset of antidepressant response with fluoxetine treatment. *Am J Psychiatry*. 2000;157:1423–1428.

Noagiul S, Narayan M, Nelson CJ. Divalproex treatment of mania in elderly patients. *Am J Geriatr Psychiatry*. 1998;6:257–262.

Nyth AL, Gottfries CG. The clinical efficacy of citalopram in the treatment of emotional disturbances in dementia disorders. *Br J Psychiatry*. 1990;157:894–901.

Nyth AL, Gottfries CG, Lyby K, et al. A controlled multicenter clinical study of citalopram and placebo in elderly depressed patients with and without concomitant dementia. *Acta Psychiatr Scand*. 1992;86:138–145.

Oberholzer AF, Hendricksen C, Monsch AU, et al. Safety and effectiveness of low-dose clozapine in psychogeriatric patients: a preliminary study. *Int Psychogeriatr*. 1992;4:187–195.

Olin JT, Katz IR, Meyers BS, Schneider LS, Lebowitz BD. Provisional diagnostic criteria for depression of Alzheimer's disease: rationale and background. *Am J Geriatr Psychiatry*. 2002;10:129–141. Erratum in: *Am J Geriatr Psychiatry*. 2002;10:264.

Omnibus Reconciliation Act of 1987. 101, 100–203; 1987.

Ottervanger JP, Striker BH, Weeds JN. Bleeding attributed to the intake of paroxetine. *Am J Psychiatry*. 1994;25:243–250.

Parnetti L, Senin U, Mcocci P. Cognitive enhancement therapy for Alzheimer's disease: the way forward. *Drugs*. 1997;53(S5):752–768.

Passaro A, Volpato S, Romagnoni F, et al. Benzodiazepines with different half-life and falling in hospitalized population. *J Clin Epidemiol.* 2000;53:1222–1229.

Patel A, Young RC, Klein R, et al. Alpha acid glycoprotein in psychiatric inpatients. *Soc Neurosci.* 1987;151:11.

Patterson JF. A preliminary study of carbamazepine in the treatment of assaultive patients with dementia. *J Geriatr Psychiatry Neurol.* 1988;1:21–23.

Peabody CA, Warner D, Whiteford HA, et al. Neuroleptics and the elderly. *J Am Geriatr Soc.* 1998;35:233–238.

Pelton GH, Devanand DP, Bell K, et al. Utility of plasma haloperidol levels in Alzheimer's patients with psychosis and behavioral dyscontrol [abstract]. Proceedings of the 11th Annual Meeting, American Association for Geriatric Psychiatry. 2003:120–121.

Perlick D, Stastny P, Katz I, et al. Memory deficits and anticholinergic levels in chronic schizophrenia. *Am J Psychiatry.* 1986;143:230–232.

Perris C. The course of depressive psychoses. *Acta Psychiatr Scand.* 1966;44:238–248.

Perry EK, Tomlinson BE, Blessed G, et al. Correlation of cholinergic abnormalities with senile plaques and mental test scores in senile dementia. *BMJ.* 1978;2:1457–1459.

Perry P, Miller D, Arndt SV, et al. Clozapine and norclozapine concentrations and clinical response in treatment refractory schizophrenic patients. *Am J Psychiatry.* 1991;148:231–235.

Petracca G, Teson A, Cherminski E, et al. A double-blind placebo controlled study of clomipramine in depressed patients with Alzheimer's disease. *J Neuropsychiatr Clin Neurosci.* 1996;8:270–275.

Petracca GM, Chemerinski E, Starkstein SE. A double-blind, placebo-controlled study of fluoxetine in depressed patients with Alzheimer's disease. *Int Psychogeriatr.* 2001;13:233–240.

Petrovic M, Pevernagie D, VanDen Noortgate N, et al. A program for short-term withdrawal from benzodiazepines in geriatric hospital inpatients: success rate and effect on subjective sleep quality, *Int J Geriatr Psychiatry.* 1999;14:754–760.

Physician's Desk Reference. 56th ed. Medical Economics; 2002.

Pillans PI, Coulter DM. Fluoxetine and hyponatraemia: a potential hazard in the elderly. *N Z Med J.* 1994;107:85–86.

Pincus HA, Tanielain TL, Marcus SC, et al. Prescribing trends in psychotropic medications: primary care, psychiatry, and other medical specialties. *JAMA.* 1998;279:526–531.

Pitner, JK, Mintzer, JE, Pennypacker, LC, Jackson CW. Efficacy and adverse effects of clozapine in four elderly psychotic patients. *J Clin Psychiatry.* 1995;56:180–185.

Pollack BR. Recent developments in drug metabolism of relevance to psychiatrists. *Harvard Rev Psychiatry.* 1994;2:204–213.

Pollock BG, Lagrissi-Thode F, Wagner WR. Evaluation of platelet activity in depressed patients with ischemic heart disease after paroxetine or nortriptyline treatment. *J Clin Psychopharmacol.* 2000;20:137–140.

Pollock BG, Mulsant BH, Rosen J, et al. Comparison of citalopram, perphenazine, and placebo for the acute treatment of psychosis and behavioral disturbances in hospitalized, demented patients. *Am J Psychiatry.* 2002;159:460–465.

Pollock BG, Mulsant BH, Sweet RA, et al. An open pilot study of citalopram for behavioral disturbances of dementia: plasma levels and real time observations. *Am J Geriatr Psychiatry.* 1997;5:770–788.

Pollock BG, Perel JM, Wright B. Bupropion: need for hydroxymetabolite monitoring in the elderly depressed [abstract 18]. *Ther Drug Monit.* 1993;15:162.

Pollock BG, Wylie M, Stack JA, et al. Inhibition of caffeine metabolism by estrogen replacement therapy in postmenopausal women. *J Clin Pharmacol.* 1999;39:936–940.

Pomara N, Stanley B, Block R, et al. Adverse effects of single therapeutic doses of diazepam on performance in normal geriatric subjects: relationship to plasma concentrations. *Psychopharmacology.* 1984;84:342–346.

Pomara N, Tun H, DaSilva D, et al. The acute and chronic performance effects of alprazolam and lorazepam in the elderly: relationship to duration of treatment and self-rated sedation. *Psychopharmacol Bull.* 1998;34:139–153.

Pope HG, McElroy SL, Keck PE, et al. Valproate in the treatment of acute mania: a placebo controlled study. *Arch Gen Psychiatry.* 1991;48:62–68.

Post F. The impact of modern drug treatment on old age schizophrenia. *Gerontol Clin.* 1962;4:137–146.

Post F. *Persistent Persecutory States of the Elderly.* Oxford, UK: Pergamon; 1966.

Post RM. Introduction: emerging perspectives on valproate in affective disorders. *J Clin Psychiatry.* 1989;50(3):3–9.

Potter WZ, Rudorfer MF, Lane EA. Active metabolites of antidepressants: pharmacodynamics and relevant pharmacokinetics. In: Usdin E, ed. *Frontiers in Biochemical and Pharmacological Research in Depression.* New York, NY: Raven Press; 1984; 373–390.

Pratt RD, Perdomo CA. Donepezil-treated patients with probable vascular dementia demonstrate cognitive benefits. *Ann N Y Acad Sci.* 2002a;977:513–522.

Pratt RD, Perdomo CA. Donepezil treatment of vascular dementia. *Ann N Y Acad Sci.* 2002b;977:548–586.

Preskorn SH. Comparison of the tolerability of bupropion, fluoxetine, imipramine, nefazodone, paroxetine, sertraline and venlafaxine. Review. *J Clin Psychiatry.* 1995; 56(Suppl 6):12–21.

Preskorn SH. Clinically relevant pharmacology of selective serotonin reuptake inhibitors. *Clin Pharmacokinet.* 1997;32(Suppl 1):1–21.

Preskorn SH, Alderman J, Chung M, et al. Pharmacokinetics of desipramine coadministered with sertraline or fluoxetine. *J Clin Psychopharmacol.* 1994;90:98.

Preskorn SH, Simpson S. Tricyclic antidepressant induced delirium and plasma drug concentrations. *Am J Psychiatry.* 1982;139:822–823.

Puryear LJ, Kunik ME, Workman R. Tolerability of divalproex sodium in elderly psychiatric patients with mixed diagnoses. *J Geriatr Psychiatry Neurol.* 1995;8:234–237.

Rabins PV, Mace NL, Lucas MJ. The impact of dementia on the family. *JAMA.* 1982; 248:333–335.

Raby WL. Carnitine for valproic acid-induced hyperammonemia [letter]. *Am J Psychiatry.* 1997;154:1168–1169.

Raskind MA, Alvarez C, Herlin S. Fluphenazine enanthate in the outpatient treatment of late paraphrenia. *J Am Geriatr Soc.* 1979;27:459–469.

Raskind MA, Peskind RE, Wessel T, Uuan W, for the Galantimine USA-1 Study Group. Galantamine in AD: a six-month randomized placebo-controlled trial with a six-month extension. *Neurology.* 2000;54:2261–2268.

Raskind MA, Risse SC, Lampe TH. Dementia and antipsychotic drugs. *J Clin Psychiatry.* 1998;48:,s16–s18.

Rasmusen L, Yan B, Robillard A, Dunbar F. Effects of washout and dose-escalation periods on the efficacy, safety, and tolerability of galantamine in patients previously treated with donepezil: ongoing clinical trials. *Clin Ther.* 2001;23(Suppl A):A25-A30.

Ray WA, Federspiel CF, Schaffner W. A study of antipsychotic drug use in nursing homes: epidemiologic evidence suggesting misuse. *Am J Public Health.* 1980;70: 485-491.

Ray WA, Griffin MR, Schaffner W, et al. Psychotropic drug use and the risk of hip fracture. *N Engl J Med.* 1987;316:363-369.

Reid LD, Johnson RE, Gettman DA. Benzodiazepine exposure and functional status of older people. *J Am Geriatr Soc.* 1998;46:71-76.

Reidenberg MM, Levy M, Warner H, et al. Relationship between diazepam dose, plasma level, age, and central nervous system depression. *Clin Pharmacol Ther.* 1978;23: 371-374.

Reifler BV, Teri L, Raskind M, et al. Double blind trial of imipramine in Alzheimer's disease in patients with and without depression. *Am J Psychiatry.* 1989;146:45-49.

Reilly JG, Ayis SA, Ferrier IN, et al. QT-interval abnormalities and psychotropic drug therapy in psychiatric patients. *Lancet.* 2000;355:1048-1052.

Reisberg B, Doody R, Stoffler A, Schmitt F, Gerris S, Mobius HJ, for the Memantine Study Group. Memantine in moderate to severe Alzheimer's disease. *N Engl J Med.* 2003;348:1333-1341.

Reynolds CF, Frank E, Kupfer DJ, et al. Treatment outcome in recurrent major depression: a post hoc comparison of elderly (young old) and midlife patients. *Am J Psychiatry.* 1996;153:1288-1292.

Reynolds CF, Frank E, Perel JM, et al. Combined pharmacotherapy and psychotherapy in the acute and continuation treatment of elderly patients with recurrent major depression: a preliminary report. *Am J Psychiatry.* 1992;149:1687-1692.

Reynolds CF, Frank E, Perel JM, et al. High relapse rates after discontinuation of adjunctive medication for elderly patients with recurrent major depression. *Am J Psychiatry.* 1996;1418-1422.

Reynolds CF, Frank E, Perel JM, et al. Nortriptyline and interpersonal psychotherapy as maintenance therapies for recurrent major depression: a randomized controlled trial in patients older than 59 years. *JAMA.* 1999;281:39-45.

Reynolds CF, Perel JM, Frank E. Open-trial maintenance pharmacotherapy in late life depression: survival analysis. *Psychiatry Res.* 1989;27:225-231.

Reynolds CF, Perel JM, Kupfer DJ, et al. Open-trial response to antidepressant treatment in elderly patients with mixed depression and cognitive impairment. *Psychiatry Res.* 1987;21:111-122.

Richelson E. Pharmacology of antidepressants in use in the US. *J Clin Psychiatry.* 1982; 43:4-13.

Rickels K, Schweizer E, Clary C, et al. Nefazodone and imipramine in major depression: a placebo controlled trial. *Br J Psychiatry.* 1994;164:802-895.

Rickels K, Schweizer E, Lucki I. *Benzodiazepine Side Effects.* Washington, DC: American Psychiatric Association; 1987.

Risinger RC, Risby ED, Risch SC. Safety and efficacy of divalproex sodium in elderly bipolar patients. *J Clin Psychiatry.* 1994;55:215.

Roane DM, Feinberg TE, Mekler L, et al. Treatment of dementia-associated agitation with gabapentin. *J Neuropsychiatr Clin Neurosci.* 2000;12:40-43.

Robinson D. Monoamine oxidase inhibitors and the elderly. In: Raskin A, Robinson DS, Levine J, eds. *Age and the Pharmacology of Psychoactive Drugs.* New York, NY: Elsevier; 1982:149–161.

Robinson D, Napoliello MJ. The safety and usefulness of buspirone as an anxiolytic in elderly versus young patients. *Clin Ther.* 1988;10:740–746.

Robinson D, Nies A, Ravaris L, et al. Clinical pharmacology of phenelzine. *Arch Gen Psychiatry.* 1978;35:29–635.

Robinson RG, Kubos KL, Starr LB, et al. Mood changes in stroke patients: relationship to lesion location. *Compr Psychiatry.* 1983;24:555–566.

Robinson RG, Schultz SK, Castillo C, et al. Nortriptyline vs. fluoxetine in the treatment of depression and short-term recovery after stroke: a placebo-controlled, double-blind study. *Am J Psychiatry.* 2000;157:351–359.

Rockwell E, Lam RW, Zisook S. Antidepressant drug studies in the elderly. *Psychiatr Clin North Am.* 1988;11:215–233.

Rogers SL, Farlow MR, Doody RS, Mohs R, Friedhoff LT. A 24-week double-blind placebo-controlled trial of donepezil in patients with Alzheimer's disease. *Neurology.* 1998;50:136–145.

Rolandi E, Magnani G, Sannia A, et al. Evaluation of Prl secretion in elderly subjects. *Acta Endocrinol.* 1982;42:148–151.

Roose SP, Bone S, Haidorfer C, et al. Lithium treatment in older patients. *Am J Psychiatry.* 1979;136:843–844.

Roose SP, Glassman AH, Attia E, et al. Comparative efficacy of selective serotonin reuptake inhibitors and tricyclics in the treatment of melancholia. *Am J Psychiatry.* 1994;151:1735–1739.

Roose SP, Glassman AH, Giardina EG, et al. Tricyclic antidepressants in patients with cardiac conduction disease. *Arch Gen Psychiatry.* 1987;44:273–275.

Roose SP, Glassman AH, Giardina EGV, et al. Nortriptyline in depressed patients with left ventricular impairment. *JAMA.* 1986;256:3253–3257.

Roose SP, Glassman AH, Siris SG. Comparison of imipramine and nortriptyline-induced orthostatic hypotension: a meaningful difference. *J Clin Psychopharmacol.*, 1981; 1:316–319.

Roose SP, Laghrissi-Thode F, Kennedy JS, et al. Comparison of paroxetine and nortriptyline in depressed patients with ischemic heart disease. *JAMA.* 1998;27:287–291.

Roose SP, Nurnberger J, Dunner D, et al. Cardiac sinus mode dysfunction during lithium treatment. *Am J Psychiatry.* 1979;136:804–806.

Roose SP, Suthers KM. *J Clin Psychiatry.* 1998;59(S10):4–8.

Rosen WG, Mohs RC, Davis KL. A new rating scale for Alzheimer's disease. *Am J Psychiatry.* 1984;141:1356–1364.

Rosenblatt JE, Pary RJ, Bigelow LB, et al. Measurement of serum neuroleptic concentrations by radioreceptor assay: concurrent assessment of clinical response and toxicity. In: Usdin E, Bunney WE, Davis JM, eds. *Neuroreceptors—Basic and Clinical Aspects.* New York, NY: Wiley; 1981:165–188.

Roth M, Mountjoy CQ, Amrein R. Moclobemide in elderly patients with cognitive decline and depression: an international double-blind, placebo-controlled trial. *Br J Psychiatry.* 1996;168:149–157.

Rothschild AJ, Phillips KA. Selective serotonin reuptake inhibitors and delusion depression. *Am J Psychiatry.* 1999;156:977–978.

Rovner BW, Broadhead J, Spencer M, et al. Depression and Alzheimer's disease. *Am J Psychiatry*. 1987;146:350–356.

Rovner BW, Edelman BA, Cox MP, et al. The impact of antipsychotic drug regulations on psychotropic prescribing practices in nursing homes. *Am J Psychiatry*. 1992; 1390–1392.

Rovner BW, German PS, Broadhead J, et al. The prevalence and management of dementia and other psychiatric disorders in nursing homes. *Int Psychogeriatr*. 1990;2: 13–36.

Rowe JW. Aging and renal function. *Annu Rev Gerontol Geriatr*. 1980;1:161–179.

Sambamoorthi U, Olfson M, Walkup JT, Crystal S. Diffusion of new generation antidepressant treatment among elderly diagnosed with depression. *Med Care*. 2003;41: 180–194.

Sachs G. Systematic treatment enhancement program for bipolar disorder. *NCDEU Annu Mtg*. 2001.

Sadavoy J. *Psychotropic Drugs and the Elderly: Fast Facts*. New York, NY: Norton; 2004.

Sajatovic M. Treatment of bipolar disorder in older adults. *Int J Geriatr Psychiatry*. 2002;17:865–873.

Sakauye KM, Camp CJ, Ford PA. Effects of buspirone on agitation associated with dementia. *Am J Ger Psychiatry*. 1993;1:82–84.

Saltz BL, Woerner MG, Kane JM. Prospective study of tardive dyskinesia incidence in the elderly. *JAMA*. 1991;266:2402–2406.

Salzman C. *Clinical Geriatric Psychopharmacology*. 3rd ed. New York, NY; 1998.

Salzman C, Fisher J, Nobel K, et al. Cognitive improvement following benzodiazepine discontinuation in elderly nursing home residents. *Int J Geriatr Psychiatry*. 1992;7: 89–93.

Salzman C, Lebowitz B. *Anxiety in the Elderly: Treatment and Research*. New York, NY: Springer; 1991.

Salzman C, Schneider L, Lebowitz B. Antidepressant treatment of very old patients. *Am J Geriatr Psychiatry*. 1993;1:21–29.

Salzman C, Shader RI, Greenblatt DJ, et al. Long versus half-life benzodiazepines in the elderly: kinetics and clinical effects of diazepam and oxazepam. *Arch Gen Psychiatry*. 1983;40:293–297.

Salzman C, Vaccaro B, Leiff J, et al. Clozapine in older patients with psychosis and behavioral disruption. *Am J Geriatr Psychiatry*. 1995;3:26–33.

Sambamoorthi U, Olfson M, Walkup JT, Crystal S. Diffusion of new generation antidepressant treatment among elderly diagnosed with depression. *Med Care*. 2003;41: 180–194.

Samuel W, Caligiuri M, Galasko D, et al. Better cognitive and psychopathological response to donepezil in patients prospectively diagnosed as dementia with Lewy bodies: a preliminary study. *Int J Geriatr Psychiatry*. 2000;15:794–802.

Sarkisian CA, Liu H, Gutierrez PR, et al. Modifiable risk factors predict functional decline among older women: a prospectively validated clinical prediction tool. The study of osteoporotic fractures research group. *J Am Geriatr Soc*. 2000;48:170–178.

Satel SL, Nelson JC. Stimulants in the treatment of depression: a critical overview. *J Clin Psychiatry*. 1989;50:241–249.

Sawin CT, Castelli WP, Hershman JM, et al. The thyroid: thyroid deficiency in the Framingham study. *Arch Intern Med*. 1985;145:1386–1388.

Schaffer CB, Garvey MJ. Use of lithium in acutely manic elderly patients. *Clin Gerontol.* 1984;3:58.

Schart MB, Fletcher K, Graham JP. Comparative amnestic effects of benzodiazepine hypnotic agents. *J Clin Psychiatry.* 1988;49:134–137.

Schatzberg A, Kremer C, Rodrigues H. Mirtzapine versus paroxetine in elderly depressed patients. Poster presented at: AAGP Annual Meeting; 2001.

Schatzberg A, Nemeroff CB. *American Psychiatric Press Textbook of Pharmacology.* 2nd ed. Washington, DC: APPI; 1998.

Schatzberg AF, Kremer C, Rodrigues HE, Murphy GM Jr. Mirtazapine vs. paroxetine study group: double-blind, randomized comparison of mirtazapine and paroxetine in elderly depressed patients. *Am J Geriatr Psychiatry.* 2002;10:541–550.

Schiffer RB, Herndon RM, Rudick RA. Treatment of pathological laughing and weeping with amitriptyline. *N Engl J Med.* 1985;312:1480–1482.

Schneider LS, Cooper TB, Severson JA, et al. Electrocardiographic changes with nortriptyline and 10-hydroxynortriptyline in elderly depressed outpatients. *J Clin Psychopharmacol.* 1988;8:402–408.

Schneider LS, Pollock VE, Lyness SA. A metaanalysis of controlled trials of neuroleptic treatment in dementia. *J Am Geriatr Soc.* 1990;38:553–563.

Schneider LS, Sobin PB. Non neuroleptic medications in the management of agitation in Alzheimer's disease and other dementias. *Int J Geriatr Psychiatry.* 1991;6:691–708.

Scholz E, Dichgans J. Treatment of drug-induced exogenous psychosis in parkinsonism with clozapine and fluperlapine. *Eur Arch Psychiatr Clin Neurol.* 1985;235:60–64.

Schone W, Ludwig M. A double blind study of paroxetine compared with fluoxetine in geriatric patients with major depression. *J Clin Psychopharmacol.* 1993;13(Suppl 2):34s–39s.

Schorr RI, Fought RL, Ray WA. Changes in antipsychotic drug use in nursing homes during implementation of OBRA-87 regulations. *JAMA.* 1994;271:358–362.

Schweizer E, Rickels K, Amsterdam JD, et al. What constitutes an adequate antidepressant trial for fluoxetine? *J Clin Psychiatry.* 1990;51:8–11.

Sgadari A, Lapane KL, Mor V, et al. Oxidative and nonoxidative benzodiazepines and the risk of femur fracture. The Systematic Assessment of Geriatric Drug Use Via Epidemiology Study Group, *J Clin Psychopharmacol.* 2000;20:234–239.

Shader R, DiMascio A. *Clinical Handbook of Psychopharmacology.* New York, NY: Science House; 1970.

Sharma V, Persad E. Augmentation of valproate with lithium in a case of rapid cycling affective disorder. *Can J Psychiatry.* 1992;37:584–585.

Shea GC, MacKnight C, Rockwood K. Donepezil for treatment of dementia with Lewy bodies: a case series of nine patients. *Int Psychogeriatr.* 1998;10:229–238.

Shukla S, Hoff A, Aaronson T, et al. *Treatment Outcome in Organic Mania.* Washington, DC: American Psychiatric Association; 1987.

Shulman KI, Herrmann N. The nature and management of mania in old age. *Psychiatr Clin North Am.* 1999;22:649–665.

Shulman KI, Rochon P, Sykora K, et al. Changing prescription patterns for lithium and divalproex in old age: shifting without evidence. *Br Med J.* 2003;326:960–961.

Shulman KI, Walker SE, MacKenzie S. Dietary restrictions, tyramine and the use of monoamine oxidase inhibitors. *J Clin Psychopharmacol.* 1989;9:397–402.

Shulman RW, Singh A, Shulman KI. Treatment of elderly institutionalized bipolar patients with clozapine. *Psychopharmacol Bull.* 1997;33:113–118.

Simpson SW, Jackson RC, Baldwin RC, et al. Subcortical hyperintensities in late-life depression: acute response to treatment and neuropsychological impairment. *Int Psychogeriatr*. 1997;9:257–296.

Sizaret P, Versavel M C, Engel G, et al. Clinical investigation of lorazepam. *Psychol Med*. 1974;6:591–598.

Smith JM, Baldessarini RJ. Changes in prevalence, severity, and recovery in tardive dyskinesia with age. *Arch Gen Psychiatry*. 1980;37:1368–1375.

Smith WT, Londborg PD, Glaudin V, et al. Short term augmentation of fluoxetine with clonazepam in the treatment of depression: a double-blind study. *Am J Psychiatry*. 1998;155:1339–1345.

Solomons K, Geiger O. Olanzapine use in the elderly: a retrospective analysis. *Can J Psychiatry*. 2000;45:151–155.

Sotaniemi EA, Arranto AF, Pelkonen O, et al. Age and cytochrome P450 linked drug metabolism in humans: an analysis of 226 subjects with equal histopathological condition. *Clin Pharmacol Ther*. 1997;61:331–339.

Spiker DG, Stein J, Rich CL. Delusional depression and electroconvulsive therapy: one year later. *Convuls Ther*. 1985;1:167–182.

Spivak B, Radvan M, Meltzer M. Side effects of trazodone in a geriatric population. *J Clin Psychopharmacol*. 1989;9:62–63.

Sramek JJ, Alexander MS, Cutler NR. Acetylcholinesterase inhibitors for the treatment of Alzheimer's disease. *Ann Long-Term Care*. 2001;9:15–22.

Starkstein SE, Federoff P, Berthier ML, et al. Manic depressive and pure manic states after brain lesions. *Biol Psychiatry*. 1991;29:773–782.

Stimmer GL, Dopheide JA, Stahl SM. Mirtzapine: an antidepressant with noradrenergic and specific serotonergic effects. *Pharmacotherapy*. 1997;17:10–21.

Strauss A. Oral dyskinesia associated with buspirone use in an elderly woman. *J Clin Psychiatry*. 1988;39:322–323.

Street JS, Clark WS, Gannon KS, et al. Olanzapine treatment of psychotic and behavioral symptoms in patients with Alzheimer's disease in nursing care facilities: a double-blind, randomized, placebo-controlled trial. *Arch Gen Psychiatry*. 2000;57:968–976.

Streim JE, Oslin DO, DiFilippo S, et al. Inverse nortriptyline dose-response, relationships in dementia. Abstract, APA; 1997.

Sugimoto T, Muro H, Woo M, et al. Metabolite profiles in patients on high-dose valproate monotherapy. *Epilepsy*. 1996;25:107–112.

Sullivan EA, Shulman KI. Diet and monoamine oxidase inhibitors: a reexamination. *Can J Psychiatry*. 1984;29:707–711.

Sunderland T. Neurotransmission in the aging central nervous system. In: Salzman C, ed. *Clinical Geriatric Psychopharmacology*. Baltimore, MD: Williams and Wilkins; 1998.

Sunderland T, Cohen RM, Molchan S, et al. High dose selegiline in treatment-resistant older depressive patients. *Arch Gen Psychiatry*. 1994;51:607–615.

Sunderland T, Silver MA. Neuroleptic in the treatment of dementia. *Int J Geriatr Psychiatry*. 1988;3:79–88.

Swann AC. Mixed or dysphoric manic states: psychopathology and treatment. *J Clin Psychiatry*. 1995;56:6–10.

Swann AC, Bowden CL, Calabrese JR, et al. Mania: differential effects of previous depressive and manic episodes on response to treatment. *Acta Psychiatr Scand*. 2000; 101:444–451.

Sweet R, Akil M, Mulsant BH, et al. Determinants of spontaneous extrapyradmidal symptoms in elderly psychiatric inpatients diagnosed with Alzheimer's disease, major depressive disorder, or psychotic disorders. *J Neuropsychiatr Clin Neurol.* 1998; 10:68–77.

Systematic Assessment of Geriatric Drug Use Via Epidemiology Study Group. Oxidative and nonoxidative benzodiazepines and the risk of femur fracture. *J Clin Psychopharmacol.* 2000;20:234–239.

Targum SD, Abbott JL. Efficacy of quetiapine in Parkinson's patients with psychosis. *J Clin Psychopharmacol.* 2000;20:54–60.

Tariot PN, Cohen RM, Sunderland T, et al. Deprenyl in Alzheimer's disease: preliminary evidence for behavioral change with monoamine oxidase B inhibition. *Arch Gen Psychiatry.* 1987;44:427–433.

Tariot PN, Farlow MR, Grossberg G, Gergel I, Graham S, Jin J. Memantine/donepezil dual-therapy is superior to placebo/donepezil therapy for treatment of moderate to severe Alzheimer's disease. Poster presented at: American College of Neuropharmacology Meeting; December 8–12, 2002; San Juan, PR.

Tariot PN, Gaile SE, Castelli NA, et al. Treatment of agitation in dementia. *New Dir Ment Health Serv.* 1997;109–123.

Tariot PN, Sunderland T, Cohen RM, et al. Tranylcypromine compared with l-deprenyl in Alzheimer's disease. *J Clin Psychopharmacol.* 1988;8:23–27.

Taschev T. The course and prognosis of depression on the basis of 652 patients deceased. In: Angst J, ed. *Classification and Prediction of Outcome of Depression.* New York, NY: F. K. Schattauer Verlag; 1974.

Teri L, Larson EB, Reifler BV. Behavioral disturbances in dementia of the Alzheimer's type. *J Am Geriatr Soc.* 1988;36:1–6.

Thapa PB, Gideon P, Cost TW, et al. Antidepressants and the risk of falls among nursing home residents. *N Engl J Med.* 1998;339:875–882.

Thase ME. Effects of venlafaxine on blood pressure: a meta-analysis of original data from 3,744 depressed patients. *J Clin Psychiatry.* 1998;59:502–508.

Thyrum PT, Wong YW, Yeh C. Single-dose pharmacokinetics of quetiapine in subjects with renal or hepatic impairment. *Prog Neuropsychopharmacol Biol Psychiatry.* 2000;24:521–533.

Tinetti ME. Factors associated with serious injury during falls by ambulatory nursing home residents. *J Am Geriatr Soc.* 1987;35:644–648.

Tinetti ME, Speechley M, Ginter SF. Risk factors for falls among elderly persons living in the community. *N Engl J Med.* 1988;319:1701–1707.

Tohen M, Jacobs RG, Grundyh SL, et al. Efficacy of olanzapine in acute bipolar mania: a double-blind placebo-controlled study. The Olanzapine HGGW Study Group. *Arch Gen Psychiatry.* 2000;57:841–849.

Tohen M, Zarate CA, Centorrino F, et al. Risperidone in the treatment of mania. *J Clin Psychiatry.* 1996;57:249–253.

Tran-Johnson TK, Krull AJ, Jeste DV. Late life schizophrenia and its treatment: pharmacologic issues in older schizophrenic patients. *Clin Geriatr Med.* 1992;8:401–410.

Trinh NH, Hoblyn J, Mohanty S, Yaffe K. Efficacy of cholinesterase inhibitors in the treatment of symptoms and functional impairment in Alzheimer's disease. *JAMA.* 2003;289:210–216.

Tsuang MT, Woolson RF, Fleming JA. Long term outcome of major psychosis. 1.

Schizophrenia and affective disorders compared with psychiatrically symptom-free surgical conditions. *Arch Gen Psychiatry.* 1979;36:1295–1301.

Tune LE, Steele C, Cooper T. Neuroleptic drugs in the management of behavioral symptoms of Alzheimer's disease. *Psychiatr Clin North Am.* 1991;14:353–373.

Unutzer J, Simon G, Belin TR, et al. Care for depression in HMO patients aged 65 and older. *J Am Geriatr Soc.* 2000;48:871–878.

van de Vijver DA, Roos RA, Jansen PA, Porsius AJ, de Boer A. Start of a selective serotonin reuptake inhibitor (SSRI) and increase of antiparkinsonian drug treatment in patients on levodopa. *Br J Clin Pharmacol.* 2002;54:168–170.

van der Velde CD. Effectiveness of lithium carbonate in the treatment of manic-depressive illness. *Am J Psychiatry.* 1970;123:345–351.

van Harten J. Clinical pharmacokinetics of selective serotonin reuptake inhibitors. *Clin Pharmacokinet.* 1993;14:203–220.

van Marwijk HW, Bekker FM, Nolen WA, et al. Lithium augmentation in geriatric depression. *J Affect Disord.* 1990;20:217–223.

Vestal RE, Norris AH, Tobin JD, et al. Antipyrine metabolism in man: influence of age, alcohol caffeine and smoking. *Clin Pharmacol Ther.* 1975;18:425–432.

Vestal RE, Wood AJ, Shand DG. Reduced beta adrenergic receptor sensitivity in the elderly. *Clin Pharmacol.* 1979;26:181–186.

von Moltke L, Greenblatt DJ, Court MH, et al. Inhibition of alprazolam and desipramine hydroxylation in vitro by paroxetine and fluvoxamine: comparison with other serotonin reuptake inhibitors. *J Clin Psychopharmacol.* 1995;15:125–131.

von Moltke LL, Abernathy DR, Greenblatt DJ. Kinetics and dynamics of psychotropic drugs in the elderly. In: Salzman C, ed. *Clinical Geriatric Psychopharmacology.* Baltimore, MD: Williams and Wilkins; 1998.

Wakelin JS. Fluvoxamine in the treatment of the older depressed patient: double-blind, placebo-controlled data. *Int Clin Psychopharmacol.* 1986;1:221–220.

Walters G, Reynolds CF, Mulsant BH, et al. Continuation and maintenance pharmacotherapy in geriatric depression: an open trial comparison of paroxetine and nortriptyline in patients older than 70 years. *J Clin Psychiatry.* 1999;60(Suppl 20):21–25.

Weihs KL, Settle EC Jr, Batey SR, Houser TL, Donahue RM, Ascher JA. Bupropion sustained release versus paroxetine for the treatment of depression in the elderly. *J Clin Psychiatry.* 2000;61:196–202.

Weilburg JB, Rosenbaum JF, Biederman J. Fluoxetine added to non-MAOI antidepressants converts nonresponders to responders: a preliminary report. *J Clin Psychiatry.* 1989;50:447–449.

Weissman MM, Prusoff B, Sholomskas AJ. A double-blind clinical trial of alprazolam, imipramine, or placebo in the depressed elderly. *J Clin Psychopharmacol.* 1992;12: 175–182.

Welch R, Chue P. Antipsychotic agents and QT changes. *Rev Psychiatr Neurosci.* 2000; 25:154–160.

Werber EA, Rabey JM. The beneficial effect of cholinesterase inhibitors on patients suffering from Parkinson's disease and dementia. *J Neural Transm.* 2001;108:1319–1325.

Whitehouse PJ, Price DL, Clark AW, et al. Alzheimer's disease: evidence for selective loss of cholinergic neurons in the nucleus basalis. *Ann Neurol.* 1981;10:122–126.

Whittier JR. *Psychotropic Drugs and Dysfunctions of the Basal Ganglia.* Washington, DC: US Public Health; 1969.

Whooley MA, Kip KE, Cauley JA, et al. Depression, falls and risk of fracture in older women. *Arch Intern Med.* 2001;159:484–490.

Wiart L, Petit H, Joseph PA, et al. Fluoxetine in yearly poststroke depression: a double-blind placebo-controlled study. *Stroke.* 2000;31:1829–1832.

Wild D, Nayak USL, Isaacs B. Characteristics of old people who fall at home. *J Clin Exp Gerontol.* 1980;2:271–287.

Wilkinson D, Holmes C, Wooldford J, Stammers S, North J. Prophylactic theraphy with lithium in elderly patients with unipolar major depression. *Int J Geriatr Psychiatry.* 2002;17:619–622.

Williams JW, Barrett J, Oxman T, et al. Treatment of dysthymia and minor depression in primary care: a randomized controlled trial in older adults. *JAMA.* 2000;284:1519–1526.

Wilner KD, Tensfeldt TG, Baris B, et al. Single and multiple dose pharmacokinetics of ziprasodine in healthy young and elderly volunteers. *Br J Clin Pharmacol.* 2000;49(Suppl 1):15s–20s.

Woerner MG, Alvir JM, Saltz BL, Lieberman JA, Kane JM. Prospective study of tardive dyskinesia in the elderly: rates and risk factors. *Am J Psychiatry.* 1998;155:1521–1528.

Woerner MG, Kane JM, Lieerman JA, et al. The prevalence of tardive dyskinesia. *J Clin Psychopharmacol.* 1991;11:34–42.

Wolters EC, Hurwitz TA, Mak E, et al. Clozapine in the treatment of parkinsonian patients with dopaminomimetic psychoses. *Neurology.* 1990;40:832–834.

Wragg RE. Neuroleptic and alternative treatments: management of behavioral symptoms and psychosis in Alzheimer's disease and related conditions. *Psychiatr Clin North Am.* 1988;11:195–213.

Wylie ME, Mulsant BH, Pollock B, et al. Age at onset in geriatric bipolar disorder. *Am J Geriatr Psychiatry.* 1999;7:77–83.

Yaryra-Tobias JA, Kirschen H, Ninvan P, et al. Fluoxetine and bleeding in obsessive-compulsive disorder. *Am J Psychiatry.* 1991;148:949.

Yassa R, Nastase C, Dupont D. Tardive dyskinesia in elderly psychiatric patients: a 5 year study. *Am J Psychiatry.* 1992;149:1206–1211.

Yesavage JA, Brink TL, Rose TL, et al. The geriatric depression rating scale: comparison with other self report and psychiatric rating scales. In: Crook T, Ferris S, Bartus R, eds. *Assessment in Geriatric Psychopharmacology.* New Canaan, CT: Mark Powley Associates; 1983:153–163.

Young RC. Lithium in geriatric bipolar disorder. *Geriatr Psychopharmacol.* 1996.

Young RC, Alexopoulos GS, Kent E, et al. Plasma 10-hydroxynortriptyline and ECG changes in elderly depressed patients. *Am J Psychiatry.* 1985;142:866–868.

Young RC, Alexopoulos G, Shamoian CA, et al. Plasma 10-hydroxynortriptyline in elderly depressed patients. *Clin Pharmacol Ther.* 1984;35:540–544.

Young RC, Alexopoulos GS, Shamoian CA, et al. Hydroxylated metabolites of tricyclic antidepressants in the elderly. *Br J Psychiatry.* 1987;150:131–132.

Young RC, Falk JR. Age, manic psychopathology and treatment response. *Int J Geriatr Psychiatry.* 1989;4:73–78.

Young RC, Kalayam B, Tsuboyama G, et al. Mania: response to lithium across the age spectrum. *Soc Neurosci.* 1992;18:669.

Young RC, Klerman GL. Mania in late-life: focus on age at onset. *Am J Psychiatry.* 1992;149:867–876.

Young RC, Mattis S, Alexopoulos GS, Meyers BS, Shindledecker RD, Dhar AK. Verbal memory and plasma drug concentrations in elderly depressives treated with nortriptyline. *Psychopharmacol Bull.* 1991;27:291–294.

Zanardi R, Franchini L, Gasperine M, et al. Double-blind controlled trial of sertraline versus paroxetine in the treatment of delusional depression. *Am J Psychiatry.* 1996; 153:1631–1633.

Zanardi R, Franchini L, Serretti A, et al. Venlafaxine versus fluvoxamine in the treatment of delusional depression: a pilot double blind controlled study. *J Clin Psychiatry.* 2000;61:26–29.

Zarate CA, Tohen M. Outcome of mania in adults. In: Shulman K, Tohen M, Kutcher SP, eds. *Mood Disorders Across the Life Scan.* New York, NY: Wiley-Liss; 1996: 281–297.

Zimmer B, Gershon S. The ideal late life anxiolytic. In: Salzman C, Levowitz B, eds. *Anxiety in the Elderly: Treatment Research.* New York, NY: Springer; 1991:277–303.

Zimmer B, Rosen J, Thornton JE, et al. Adjunctive lithium carbonate in nortriptyline resistant elderly depressed patients. *J Clin Psychopharmacol.* 1991;11:254–256.

31

Individual Psychotherapy

Joel Sadavoy, MD, FRCP(C)
Lawrence W. Lazarus, MD, FAPA

Accumulated evidence supports the efficacy of psychotherapies for geriatric patients, although clear superiority of one modality over another has not emerged (Arean & Cook, 2002; Scogin & McElreath, 1994). Cognitive-behavioral therapy (CBT) and interpersonal psychotherapy (IPT) may show some superiority (Karel & Hinrichsen, 2000). Psychotherapy has been demonstrated to be as effective for the elderly as for younger populations, that no approach is necessarily better than any other (Thompson et al., 1987), and that psychotherapy can be used as both a primary and an adjunctive method of treatment, depending on the patient and the presenting problem.

The data on geriatric psychotherapy are based increasingly on empirical data available for specific areas, such as CBT (Gallagher & Thompson, 1982; Thompson et al., 1991); IPT (Miller et al., 1998, 2003; Scocco et al., 2002); dialectical behavior therapy (Lynch et al., 2003); behavioral, group, and milieu therapies (Sadavoy & Robinson, 1989); institutional treatment (Goldfarb & Turner, 1953); and brief psychotherapy (Lazarus et al., 1987; Silberschatz & Curtis, 1991); goal-focused group psychotherapy (Klausner et al., 1998); and problem-solving treatment (Mynors-Wallis, 1996). A seminal comparative study of treatments in old age remains that of Gallagher and Thompson. Gallagher and Thompson (1983) compared cognitive-behavior and brief relational and insight therapies in 30 patients with depression (15 endogenous and 15 nonendogenous). All three modalities produced positive results that were comparable to studies of tricyclic antidepressants in similar populations.

Data continue to confirm that age per se defines neither indications nor contraindications for specific therapies (Hollon, 2003; Myers, 1984; Nemiroff & Colarusso, 1985; Rechtschaffen, 1959; Sadavoy & Leszcz, 1987; Steuer, 1982; Yesavage & Karasu, 1982). The utility of psychotherapy for patients in their ninth and tenth decades has been reported (Settlage, 1996; Strauss, 1996). For example, some patients in their seventh or later decade may be candidates for psychodynamically oriented therapy. Reviews of various modalities consistently show effectiveness for a range of interventions (Arean & Cook, 2002; Gatz et al., 1998).

Psychotherapeutic goals, indications, techniques, and process are best defined based on a functional, rather than chronological, perspective. Function in old age may be conceptualized as a continuum between two poles, with normative aging at one extreme and physical and mental frailty at the other (Kahana, 1979). Influencing the adjustment of elderly individuals to the aging process is a variety of life stressors, some presenting as crises and others as chronic strain (Figure 31-1).

As with young adults, individual psychotherapy of older persons must consider the more psychodynamic and less empirically studied approaches in addition to the more structured and frequently manualized contemporary treatments, such as cognitive, interpersonal, and problem-solving therapies. Even within the psychodynamic treatments, therapies emphasize different conceptual modes, ranging from that derived from classical psychoanalysis to treatments based on object relations theory and self-esteem regulation. The last approach is relevant to the treatment of older adults because of the assumption that the narcissistic wounds associated with aging are particularly pertinent to this age group (Lazarus, 1988).

Other approaches, briefer and often manualized, have been subject to more empirical scrutiny in both young adult and elderly patients (e.g., Gallagher & Thompson, 1981). Nevertheless, because these modalities have been designed and studied for the treatment of specific Axis I disorders, particularly

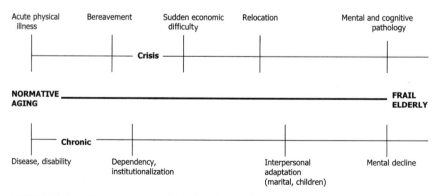

FIGURE 31-1. The continuum of functioning in old age.

major depression, their empirically validated relevance to clinical practice is limited. Little information is available regarding the effectiveness of structured short-term psychotherapies for adjustment disorders, maladaptive personality traits, or diagnosable personality disorders. Moreover, these treatments are not included in the professional education of many psychiatrists, and those who are trained may resist adherence to a manualized treatment that is used primarily for research—even if it is effective.

This chapter provides a general overview of a range of psychotherapeutic approaches, including psychodynamic therapies that emphasize different theoretical perspectives.

BARRIERS TO PSYCHOTHERAPY

Societal attitudes and biases toward the elderly probably influence the willingness of practitioners to recommend and use psychotherapy, and negative biases have persisted despite dramatic changes in our understanding of human development and psychiatric disorders of old age (Alvidrez & Arean, 2002; Olfson et al., 2002; Orbach, 1994; Sonderegger & Seigel, 1995). Among clinical psychology trainees, positive attitudes toward psychotherapy with elders may be improving (Lee et al., 2003).

Raised in an era when shame and embarrassment were associated with seeing a psychiatrist, older people may shun such intervention and become indignant when a family member or personal physician suggests it. Negative beliefs about psychiatry, common to their age cohort; sociocultural stereotypes regarding psychiatry; and geographic inaccessibility reinforce this hesitation. Some aging individuals believe that depression and anxiety are expected with aging or attribute the symptoms to medical rather than psychiatric causes. Moreover, the psychiatric problems themselves (e.g., depression with its associated helplessness and apathy) are often deterrents to treatment.

Additional barriers include such practical problems as arranging transportation and interruptions of therapy because of illness. Adult children of aging parents may harbor the same negative, stereotypical attitudes about psychiatry held by their parents, and they may minimize or deny their parents' psychiatric symptoms. The family may fear their parents' disapproval and anger if treatment were suggested. Conscious and unconscious resentment or ambivalence toward an aging parent or concerns about assuming financial responsibility may act as additional deterrents to adequate psychiatric care.

Primary care physicians may question the value of psychiatric intervention for frail, debilitated, elderly patients and may believe that their shortened life span renders them unsuitable for psychotherapy. Difficulty convincing elderly patients and their families of the usefulness of psychiatric treatment may be another deterrent. Elderly patients seem to prefer treatment by their family physicians (Klausner & Alexopoulos, 1999), and it is probably true that family physicians are the primary triage agents in assigning patients for psychotherapy.

However, this poses an important barrier for elderly patients seeking care because family physicians may selectively prescribe psychotherapy less readily to elders than to younger patients (Mackenzie et al., 1999). Beyond age-specific barriers, elders from minority cultures face additional barriers to seeking mental health care, including psychotherapy. Stigma and associated feelings of shame are major deterrents, as are instrumental matters such as language and cultural interpretation, location of services, and general availability of appropriate resources (Sadavoy et al., in press).

GENERAL PRINCIPLES OF INDIVIDUAL PSYCHOTHERAPY

The therapist of the elderly patient must individualize interventions in a flexible manner (Blau & Berezin, 1975; Yesavage & Karasu, 1982) and take into account the possible need to change to another therapeutic approach because of crises, health changes, family conflicts, and so on. The therapist should use psychotherapy when appropriate, either as a primary or as an adjunctive treatment, in combination with medications, social and environmental manipulation, and patient advocacy. No single technique, principle, or rule of psychotherapy adequately addresses the heterogeneous geriatric population.

The complex interplay of medical, psychological, and sociocultural problems confronting frail elderly individuals requires flexibility and ingenuity on the part of the therapist. The therapist may need to function in different roles with the same patient; these may include family therapist, psychopharmacotherapist, primary care physician, and at times, coordinator of the patient's treatment team. The psychiatrist is also concerned about previously undiagnosed medical problems and medication side effects that may be masquerading as, or aggravating, a psychiatric disorder.

The initial office visit usually requires more than an hour to complete a comprehensive assessment of biopsychosocial factors and, when indicated, to obtain information from, and an assessment of, the patient's family. For a somatically oriented patient, beginning an initial interview in a medically oriented manner may provide the advantage of familiarity for the patient and place him or her at ease. There also is a rich interplay between the psychological inner world of the aging patient and Axis I disorders. Personality and developmental factors are closely associated with depressive, anxiety, and somatization disorders, impacting therapeutic efficiency and prognosis (Sadavoy, 1999). Evidence is beginning to emerge that, under these circumstances, therapy is likely to be more effective when psychotherapeutic interventions are combined with biological ones (Cornes et al., 1994; Keller et al., 2000; Miller et al., 1998). A study by Reynolds and coworkers (1992) gave some support for the superiority of combined psychotherapy and pharmacotherapy (nortriptylene plus interpersonal psychotherapy) over reported success rates with antidepressant medication alone. The benefit of psychotherapy was particularly pronounced in patients aged 70 years and older.

Therapists must be aware of concurrent physical problems that may accompany psychiatric symptoms and must ensure that psychotherapy or any other treatment has been preceded by a thorough medical workup. Families often may have to be involved so the clinician can obtain important collateral information not attainable from the patient and gain the family's support and cooperation with the treatment plan, particularly when dealing with frail elderly individuals. However, the therapist should take care to respect the competent patient's wishes regarding confidentiality and other issues. Setting realistic psychotherapeutic goals helps both patient and therapist avoid mutual frustration and a sense of failure.

The identified elderly patient is usually first interviewed alone to convey respect for confidentiality and the patient's individuality and to elicit information that may not be obtainable in the family's presence. Some elderly patients are apprehensive about seeing a psychiatrist, so careful exploration of reactions and resistances to therapy should precede empathic explanations and realistic reassurances. When the patient or family is highly anxious, hopeless, or resistant to treatment, the therapist should adopt an active stance in working through patient and family resistances to therapy, demonstrate a willingness to help, and aid the patient and family to experience benefits from the very first interview.

INDICATIONS FOR INDIVIDUAL PSYCHOTHERAPY

Insight-oriented, intensive psychotherapy is indicated most frequently for the normative-aging cohort and is most productive if the patient is motivated; has a capacity for self-observation, insight, and mourning; is able to tolerate painful affects without excessive regression; and has demonstrated a capacity for productive work, intimacy, and pleasure (Pollock, 1987). Older patients who have benefited from exploratory psychotherapy previously sometimes resume this treatment in later life to address unresolved issues that are now pressing or new manifestations of long-standing conflicts that have arisen because of aging-related factors.

Psychotherapy, and perhaps pharmacological intervention, may be necessary for bereaved patients who are identified as having a poor prognosis. For women, transition to the state of widowhood is challenging and is an indication for psychotherapy when risk factors are high (Crose, 1999). Specific risk factors include an intense initial symptom response, absence of perceived or actual social support, suddenness of the loss, and the presence of multiple concurrent stressful life events (Windholz et al., 1985).

Adaptation to the stresses and losses associated with aging can be accompanied by a variety of conflicts that may be indications for individual psychotherapy directed toward structural change. These issues include adaptation to loss; conflicts over feared or actual sexual decline; loss of identity and the accompanying narcissistic gratification as a productive worker; marital conflict;

fears of dependency; failure to achieve goals that often arose from an idealized self-perception; and coming to grips with mortality and the imminence of death (King, 1980).

As aging progresses, crises often become the entree to therapy, and crisis intervention techniques may be helpful. Supportive therapy is generally indicated until the patient's defenses and adaptive capacities can be reconstituted. Psychotherapy in these circumstances is often an adjunct to medical, pharmacological, and environmental support (Kahana, 1987b). Although brief psychotherapy and cognitive therapy are particularly useful, long-term therapy may follow in selected cases. However, caution is necessary because defenses should not be challenged by interpretative therapy unless the patient has the capacity to replace long-standing maladaptive defenses with new, adaptive, and fulfilling mechanisms for bolstering narcissistic supplies, protecting against damaged self-esteem, and replacing selfobject relationships (Yesavage & Karasu, 1982).

Neugarten (1979) suggested that expectable and age-appropriate crises are handled more easily than crises that are temporally out of phase with an individual's life; for example, coming to terms with the death of a middle-aged child may be exceedingly difficult because it is out of phase with the normal chronology of expected life events. Psychotherapy is indicated when the individual is unable to master and adapt to the psychological impact of the crisis. Vulnerability is enhanced if there is a history of serious early life deprivation; long-standing reliance on rigid or primitive defenses; overreliance on the selfobject component of intimate relationships; previous unmourned losses; multiple or unbearably intense assaults on the individual's life circumstance, such as may occur during war or severe deprivation; breakdown of ego capacities because of physical or emotional abnormality; and inability of caregivers, especially family, to tolerate the elderly family member's decline and disability.

Frailty usually interferes with the capacity to tolerate intensive psychotherapy and, in general, severely restricts or contraindicates its use. However, even in frail elderly individuals, focal therapy focused on specific, here-and-now issues can use techniques of insight and interpretation (Rosenthal, 1985) in conjunction with cognitive, supportive, and educational techniques. Psychotherapy combined with rehabilitation significantly improved outcome in one cohort of patients with mild vascular dementia (Kruglov, 2003). Anecdotal case reports suggest that psychotherapy specifically adapted to frail and institutionalized elderly person (Aronson, 1958; Goldfarb, 1956; Sadavoy & Dorian, 1983; Sadavoy & Robinson, 1989) has been used successfully. The more limited and frail the patient, the greater the indication for problem-oriented interventions such as behavioral therapies and environmental manipulation.

Often, the frail patient welcomes a more familiar relationship with the therapist (e.g., sitting closer, physical contact, use of first names). However, this wish for closeness is not universal among geriatric patients and can be experienced as unprofessional or disturbing, especially by those in the normative-aging end of the spectrum. The therapist should be extremely careful to individualize his or her approach.

THEMES AND ISSUES DISCUSSED IN PSYCHOTHERAPY

One of the most common issues discussed by elderly patients is loss. Many psychotherapists believe that a major developmental task for the aging individual is to find restitution for the myriad biopsychosocial losses associated with this stage of the life cycle (Cath, 1976; Meissner, 1975). The significance of a particular loss is often associated with the amount of self-esteem invested in the lost function (e.g., the effect of arthritis on a concert pianist). What appears to be very devastating for some elderly persons is the rapidity and cumulative effect of repeated losses before sufficient time has passed to allow for mourning and resolution.

Erikson (1968) conceptualized the last phase of life as the struggle to attain and maintain ego integrity, with failure to do so leading to a state of despair and disgust. Cath (1976) characterized the middle and later years as a balance between factors that support a person's self-esteem, such as wisdom derived from life experience, attainment of a satisfying philosophical and religious worldview, and past accomplishments, versus factors that lead to emotional depletion, such as failing health and cognitive impairment. Cath asserts that, given adequate ego resources and a sustaining environment, most elderly people master the challenges of later life. Cohen has articulated his human potential theory, which describes four phases of life development.

Atchley (1982), a sociologist, stated that persons who lose self-esteem in late life do so because they have lost a feeling of control over their environment to such a degree that they feel defenseless, because self-esteem had previously been too dependent on work or social roles, or because physical deterioration had become so extensive that the person must accept a less-desirable self-image. Elderly individuals, according to Atchley, defend themselves against a negative self-image by interacting with people who provide a positive egosyntonic experience, refusing to apply negative societal myths about aging to themselves, discounting messages that do not fit with their existing self-image, and focusing on past successes. Although continuity theory suggests that individuals age in a typical fashion (Atchley, 1989), others emphasize the ability of elders to change as they transcend the assaults of old age (Tornstam, 1996).

Elderly individuals, especially the very old, do not seem to express much death anxiety (Berezin, 1972, 1987; Pollock, 1987; Weisman & Hackett, 1967). Indeed, death-related anxiety and conflict may be much more a phenomenon of earlier adult life (Jacques, 1965; Yalom, 1980). Elderly individuals who are confronting illness, decline, or death often tend to be more concerned with fears of pain, disability, abandonment, and dependency than with fear of death.

Transference

The literature on geriatric psychotherapy generally endorses the premise of the timelessness of the unconscious that leads to the persistence of unconscious attitudes and fantasies from early life (Berezin, 1972). Transference processes are acknowledged to be as persistent and vibrant in old age as in youth (Newton & Jacobowitz, 1999). These factors determine much of the content of the transference. Little clinical evidence strongly supports the concept of a highly age-specific transference, although the stressors inherent in old age tend to mobilize certain reactions more often than others. Furthermore, developmental theory suggests that the transference not only derives from unconscious ties to significant childhood figures, but also contains elements of significant object relationships acquired (internalized) during adult life (e.g., spousal, child [or filial], and peer transferences) (Nemiroff & Colarusso, 1985). Table 31-1 summarizes some of the age-related conflicts that tend to be associated with certain transferences that arise in therapy.

Frail elderly individuals, struggling with various fears and conflicts (including abandonment to institutions by their adult children and helpless reliance on caregivers), easily develop parental transferences with hopes for an idealized, magical protector and savior. The self in the transference constellation is experienced as weak and helpless, whereas the other (e.g., physician or nurse)

TABLE 31-1.   Age-related conflicts associated with transference

Age-related conflicts	Developmental stage	Type of transference
Giving up of ideal goals (Kahana, 1987a)	Normative	Sibling rivalry; envy; jealousy; peer; mirror transference
Sexual decline/unavailability	Normative	Erotic
Loss of roles	Normative	Sibling rivalry; idealized, filial, or peer
Conflict over death and mortality (Segal, 1958)	Entire spectrum	Idealized protector, negative filial, or parental
Conflicts with adult children (Meerloo, 1955; Myers, 1984)	Entire spectrum	Filial
Bereavement (Levin, 1965b)	Normative/crisis	Spousal, erotic, or peer
Narcissistic assaults (Grunes, 1987; Lazarus, 1980, 1988)	Normative/frail	Mirror, idealized, or peer; rivalry; envy
Dependency/abandonment (Levin, 1965a)	Frail/crisis	Parental
Vulnerability/helplessness (Goldfarb, 1956)	Frail/crisis	Idealized; magical savior
Pain, illness, lost capacity to adapt (Gitelson, 1981)	Frail/crisis	Parental, idealized, or filial

is powerful and protective. At times, the patient, especially when disappointed, may angrily reject the therapist and relate to the therapist as an abandoning parent, child, or spouse.

Narcissistic assaults inherent in lost beauty, power, and physical prowess often promote an idealizing or mirror transference to the therapist (Lazarus, 1980). To cope with narcissistic assaults on the self, the patient may experience himself or herself as a powerful, admired person, just as he or she perceives the therapist as powerful and admired. The patient unconsciously believes that the therapist is admiring and beneficent to him or her and basks in the fantasized approval of the therapist. Frail patients, who are often institutionalized and coping with pain, illness, and lost capacity, are prone to these idealizing transference constellations. This tendency for frail patients to develop an idealized type of transference can be useful therapeutically, as discussed in the section on psychotherapy with cognitively impaired individuals.

Bereavement and grief, especially for a lost spouse, may cause the patient to turn unconsciously to the therapist as a wished-for replacement, leading to spousal or "lover" transference that may be eroticized. The patient may identify with a much more youthful self-image and see himself or herself as sexually appropriate for the therapist (Crusey, 1985). Similar eroticized transference may be mobilized as the patient becomes aware of his or her sexual decline and the unavailability of sexual objects. This normative stage of self-awareness may also lead to intense negative feelings toward the therapist, who may be perceived as unable or unwilling to restore the patient's lost youth and sexuality. Beneath the anger lies depressive loss of self-esteem.

Classic oedipal conflicts also arise in the transference, leading the patient to experience libidinal, aggressive, and competitive feelings toward the therapist. These feelings are associated with anxiety and neurotic behavior generated by the unconscious neurotic conflict.

The normative giving up of one's occupation through retirement can lead to loss of self-esteem and an angry or depressive sibling rivalry transference. The patient may begin to feel like the devalued, unloved child and perceive the therapist as the successful, valued child. Conscious or unconscious conflicts over death and mortality may cause the patient to view the therapist as an idealized, magical protector with parental, filial, or spousal qualities who will ward off the inevitability of death. The realistic inability of the therapist to provide the needed comfort and protection may then induce negative, angry feelings toward the perceived, disappointing parental, spousal, or filial transference figure.

Geriatric patients may develop "apparent" transference resistances to therapy in which they challenge the therapist, for example, as being too young and inexperienced and therefore incapable of understanding an elderly person. This defensive stance, however, often is the patient's initial defense against deeper fears of lost self-esteem. In this version of the so-called reverse transference (Grotjahn, 1955; Levin, 1965a; Myers, 1984), the patient adopts the "old-experienced" self-perception, whereas the therapist is seen as young and therefore in need of help and education. Another version of the reverse transference may be evident when the patient adopts a kindly, parental stance. However, beneath the surface interaction, whether positive or negative, often lurk feelings of helplessness and inferiority and fears of decline.

Countertransference

Therapists may not advise or think of psychotherapy for elderly individuals (Ford & Sbordone, 1980). Countertransference reactions may account for much of this apparent avoidance (Butler & Lewis, 1977). Reactions include feeling that elderly individuals are unattractive, unproductive, close to death, chronic, unchangeable, and unrewarding. These ideas about therapy with elderly individuals are not supported by clinical experience.

Frail elderly individuals, especially those who are institutionalized, are more likely to mobilize the therapist's unresolved conflicts about aging, including unconscious fears of illness, decline, and death (Nemiroff & Colarusso, 1985; Yesavage & Karasu, 1982). Therapists may become anxious about a patient's apparent helplessness and dependency; this anxiety in turn promotes fears of engulfment and can lead to withdrawal from or rejection of the patient. Conversely, in the face of the patient's decline, therapists may act on a grandiose need to conquer the forces of aging (Myers, 1984). The therapist's narcissism is easily at risk in these circumstances, and he or she may experience depression or unreasonable anger when efforts to rescue the patient fail (Nemiroff & Colarusso, 1985).

When the therapist overidentifies with the patient's problems, feelings of pity and sadness may arise (Hiatt, 1971) that block accurate empathy and realistic exploration of the possibilities for change. Conversely, the therapist may unconsciously avoid the pain of accurately empathizing with the patient's loneliness and loss. If overwhelmed by the patient's problems, the therapist may avoid termination of therapy because of the conviction that he or she is keeping the patient alive, so that continuing therapy becomes a defense to ward off the patient's death (King, 1980).

With geriatric patients, especially in the normative-aging group, therapists (particularly those who are younger and inexperienced) may be shocked or repelled by the patient's eroticized transference toward them or by their erotic countertransference feelings. Belief in the asexuality of elderly individuals (Meerloo, 1953) can act as a defense against unresolved conflicts over parental sexuality or oedipal conflicts (Myers, 1984; Nemiroff & Colarusso, 1985; Zinberg & Kaufman, 1963).

More readily than with younger patients, therapy with older patients may mobilize countertransference feelings associated with unresolved conflicts with parents (King, 1980; Myers, 1986). For example, unresolved hostility toward a parent may lead the therapist to a defensive idealization of the patient or inappropriate reliance on superficial, supportive modes of intervention; either way, avoidance of deeper areas of psychological conflict results (Grotjahn, 1955; Lazarus & Weinberg, 1980). Similar feelings may lead to an unconscious wish to dominate the patient (parent) and promote an overmedicalized or controlling stance. The younger therapist can easily impose the perspectives of youth on the older patient, thereby obscuring the elder's preferences and needs (Malamud, 1996).

Use of Defenses

In general, the dramatic defensive maneuvers of youth (e.g., promiscuity), self-destructive actions (e.g., self-mutilation), and antisocial behaviors seem to abate in old age (Sadavoy & Fogel, 1992), although long-term follow-up and study of elderly individuals with regard to these behaviors has not yet been done. Frail elderly individuals are more likely to use defenses of withdrawal, infirmity, and physical preoccupation to deal with intrapsychic conflict and anxieties. Patients may use these defenses to avoid therapy, claiming illness or immobility, or they may take refuge in past accomplishments, overusing reminiscence and avoiding the present, including the transference. The normative group demonstrates a fuller range of defenses, however, that take on an age-related coloration (e.g., denial of aging by attempts at youthful dress, seductiveness, or physical activity). In crises or periods of decline, regression may be intense.

Defenses and other unconscious material are expressed in a variety of forms, including dreams (Myers, 1984) and acting out (Kahana, 1987a, 1987b; Miller, 1987; Nemiroff & Colarusso, 1985; Sadavoy & Leszcz, 1987). For example, a 65-year-old executive dealt with anxiety over illness, loss of physical energy, and sexual potency by canceling therapy sessions to take up white water rafting despite his problems with chronic asthma and morbid obesity.

CULTURAL AWARENESS AND PSYCHOTHERAPY

The prudent psychotherapist will begin the process of therapy with every geriatric individual (and their related important others, such as family members) with the knowledge that there will be a gap between the culture of the therapist and the culture of the patient. Even with individuals who belong to the same ethnic, racial, or cultural group, no assumptions should be made about the experiences or understanding of the individual patient. After all, therapists are inherently from different cultures than their patients. This is relevant not only to differences that arise from ethnicity, but also more subtly to other factors such as age differences (e.g., a younger psychiatrist treating an older patient who is part of a different birth cohort and has developed in the cultural reality of that cohort). Thus, it is difficult to know the experiences of growing up during World War II or the Great Depression without having lived them as a child. This reality is an accepted "truth" about psychotherapy and should be remembered when treating patients from different cultures, including different birth cohorts, whose childhood experiences occurred in a vastly different reality.

Aging patients often enter therapy with some feeling of vulnerability. Their age, per se, may lead them to feel devalued by society, and they often harbor questions of whether they are actually wanted by the therapist. The uncertainty with which the geriatric patient arrives into the therapeutic situation is compounded in therapy situations in which the therapist and patient are from different cultural backgrounds. The first contacts are colored by culturally determined expectations on both sides and can be uncomfortable for the uninitiated therapist.

The study of modes of communication among cultural groups highlights the importance of nonverbal communication, which is especially potent in conveying meaning. There are cultural determinants of communication in four spheres: (1) proxemics (the perception and use of personal space); (2) kinesics (bodily movements); (3) paralanguage (vocal cues such as loudness of voice or inflections); and (4) high/low-context communication (overt, low context, intellectualized communication in which the words convey the true meaning) versus high-context subtle or hidden communication).

To deal with culturally determined behaviors and self-perceptions, the therapist must be an archaeologist and social anthropologist in attitude and practice. This does not mean knowing everything, but it does mean having as much knowledge of the context of the individual as possible. Although no one can hope to know all about every culture, a basic ingredient here is the therapist's recognition that elderly patients struggle with culturally determined issues, including uncertainty and mistrust of the dominant culture, but have often felt that they have had no right to speak about them in mainstream society or even within their families. They may feel uncertain about how safe it is to reveal feelings such as anger and may view the therapist as a symbol of the very oppression and loss that they have suffered.

Early in the therapy, therefore, it is useful to indicate clear acceptance of patients' uncertainty and actively open the issues for discussion, not forcing patients to speak, but rather letting them know that the therapist is aware of their possible feelings and understands their difficulty with being candid. This can be reinforced in the first assessment, when the therapist can ask about patients' feelings about traditional beliefs; experiences with the mainstream, including racism; the difference between their private thoughts and their public beliefs; their sense of belonging in society and, by implication, in the therapy. But beware, because there are widely differing beliefs about the expression of feelings and the nature of relationships. For example, Tang (1997) offered a concise primer on the influences of worldviews and child-rearing practices on psychological development of Chinese and other Confucian-influenced societies, such as those of Vietnam, Korea, and Japan.

A result is to create a climate in which the therapeutic principles of the

West, especially psychodynamics, are often in direct conflict with the culturally determined beliefs of individuals. Encouraging expression of feelings, expecting a reciprocal equal relationship, and delving into the past as a cause of current emotional states are all likely to be initially foreign to the traditional Chinese patient. More familiar will be the idea that their emotional pain must be born in silence with fortitude, and that their innermost secrets should never be revealed.

The task here is to understand clearly the ways in which elderly patients understand themselves and their world and to use that understanding in the therapeutic context. Any evidence from the therapist of dismissal of the validity of patients' beliefs will produce immediate alienation. The therapist is helpful when he or she understands that patients who speak a second language fluently do not always use that language effectively for emotional expression. Frequently, for example, elderly patients say that they cannot fully express their emotional state in English when this is their second language, but rather they can only get the true meaning when they revert to their language of origin. This issue becomes increasingly relevant with advancing age, especially in dementia, if language skills begin to decline slightly.

The therapist will be most effective if he or she is able to take a truly inquiring attitude with the patient; that is, the therapist is open to the patient's explicit attempts to educate the therapist. In so doing, the therapist must also take care that the patient is not taking refuge in cultural differences to explain away all emotional reactions. It is an easy matter for geriatric patients to experience the therapist as distant, remote, or lacking understanding and thus to say that this must be because the therapist does not know their background. Because the therapist may already be uncertain in this area, he or she will begin to question and perhaps doubt his or her ability with the patient. However, it is important for the therapist not to draw away under these circumstances. Another important capacity of the therapist is the ability to gauge accurately the degree of closeness and distance required by the patient.

The effective therapist who treats elderly patients from another culture will have the capacity to match the nature of the therapy to the level of belief and sophistication about Western methods that the patient holds. That is, the therapist has the ability to pull various perspectives together and to integrate the patient's beliefs with more "scientific" interventions. For example, the ideas that there are social and interpersonal origins for feelings or that early life experience affects later life development are not held in many cultures.

APPROACHES TO ASSESSMENT

Especially when dealing with culturally diverse elders, it may be necessary for therapists to relinquish a degree of reliance on empiricism and linear cause-and-effect thinking. Traditional perceptions of self and other often rely much more on matters of faith, religious doctrine, concepts of the flow of energy, awareness of matters of balance within nature and harmony within the self, and methods of intervention that have not emerged from careful scientific study.

The Family

Considering the deep involvement that children have with elders in many cultures and the sense of obligation and perhaps guilt that is attached to this phase of life, the family is an inextricably bound component of the therapy (Lee, 1997). This is particularly true for immigrants who came to a country under sponsorship of children who emigrated earlier. The culturally focused assessment of family dynamics takes into account the internal family system (the so-called microculture), understanding the individuals and the relationships, particularly parental and grandparental life-cycle issues, hierarchy and leadership issues, and power dynamics. It must also take into account external factors, which include the impact of racism, and various environmental stressors, such as economics and housing.

Level of Acculturation

It is apparent that the older the individual, the more difficult and complex is the acculturation process following migration. Past exposure to Western culture also can aid the process, although elderly immigrants from Eastern cultures often have had very limited contact with the concepts and assumptions of Western culture, especially regarding medicine. Moreover, for some, such contact may have strong negative connotations because it may have been in the context of colonialism and devaluation of the traditional culture.

Attitudes to professional confidentiality are another reflection of acculturation. For example, the individual's confidentiality is not routinely valued in mainland Chinese professional psychiatric practice because there is a different sense of boundaries and of roles of such others as family members.

Immigration Experience

A key component in treating patients from diverse cultures is consideration of the immigration experience. Often associated with immigration is a history of trauma. In elders, these traumatic experiences may remain hidden. It is important to explore the issues, but to follow the patient's lead and allow the material to come out at a pace the patient can tolerate.

Friendship Networks

Isolation from friendship networks and spiritual life, so profoundly important to many traditional elders from other cultures, is important to assess. Failure to understand the nature of the isolation that the patient is experiencing and the internal struggles overlaid on the problems of simple aging will lead to distance and impaired therapeutic alliances.

Dependency Issues

Elders' roles within their family systems under the impact of migration are often characterized by new dependent and helpless relationships. However, shame about family relations of this type may be profound, and there are taboos about exposing family matters publicly. These issues often present to therapists in an indirect fashion, couched symbolically as physical complaints, which have meanings the front-line practitioners easily miss.

TERMINATION

Brief therapy approaches that have a defined end are effective for some aging patients. For them, termination is both appropriate and necessary. However, for others, especially frail elderly with multiple major issues to deal with and frequent recurrent crises, a more open-ended therapeutic relationship is often necessary. Patients feel very reassured when the therapist expresses concern and availability if problems occur in the future. The therapist can ease the appropriate return to therapy by anticipating with the patient the potential resistances that may inhibit reinstituting therapy, such as fear of dependency or admission of failure because of recurrent symptoms.

The process of termination often mobilizes conflicts associated with issues such as the remaining life span and mortality, loneliness, abandonment, and dependency, as well as recurrence of the same issues and symptoms that led to the initiation of therapy. However, the older patient with good interpersonal supports and ego strengths often will be able to work through termination and other disengagement conflicts (Cath, 1975).

SPECIALIZED APPROACHES TO PSYCHOTHERAPY WITH ELDERLY INDIVIDUALS

Psychotherapy With Cognitively Impaired Individuals

Psychodynamic issues remain important in cognitively impaired individuals and influence interpersonal relationships, behavior expression, and response to treatment (Cohen, 1989). Psychotherapeutic interventions with this group address the remaining reflective capacity of the individual patient and at the same time use psychodynamic understanding to intervene at the level of environmental manipulation and family and caregiver education and support. Often, therapy is directed at minimizing excess disability (Brody et al., 1971; Kahn, 1965). For example, correcting hearing and other sensory deficits, reducing isolation and withdrawal, maximizing independent function, treating concomitant depression, and improving medical status can significantly improve the patient's overall functioning.

A wide variety of psychotherapeutic techniques has been employed with these patients, most often in institutions. Cognitive-behavioral techniques often focus on changing specific target behaviors. Goals of therapy include increasing the patient's level of participation in activities of daily living, enhancing social interest and interaction, and improving skills in communication and such concrete tasks as toileting, bathing, ambulation, and feeding (Hussian, 1984). Studies suggest that behavior therapies are most effective when integrated with milieu and other individual techniques (Sadavoy & Robinson, 1989; Tobin, 1989). Similar results have been shown for reality orientation techniques—that is, the more interactive and "person centered" the interventions, the greater the improvement (Hanley et al., 1981).

Psychotherapy may be useful for cognitively impaired individuals if employed judiciously and with well-defined goals (Cohen, 1989; Kruglov, 2003; Sadavoy & Robinson, 1989), although no controlled studies are yet available. The therapist should empathically communicate his or her understanding of the patient's distress over the loss of cognitive abilities, with sensitivity to the patient's sense of damaged self and propensity to shame. Because the patient's emotions, compared with his or her cognitive functioning, may remain relatively intact and can be understood by observing posture and facial gestures, sensitivity to the patient's emotional state may help establish contact and relieve loneliness and isolation. A touch on the patient's shoulder at the appropriate moment may augment verbal expressions of concern, particularly when aphasia interferes with communication. The interviewer should refrain from asking stress-inducing questions, such as those that assess cognition, until rapport is established.

The tendency of a patient with dementia to reminisce about the past not only may represent a way to stave off depression and represent relatively unimpaired neurological functioning, but also may remind the patient of a time when he or she felt worthwhile, vital, and competent. In addition to encouraging constructive reminiscing, the therapist supports the patient's mastery of those current activities and interests from which he or she can still derive self-esteem and satisfaction. Occasional references to intensive psychotherapy are made in the literature (Grotjahn, 1940; Hollos & Ferenczi, 1925; Sadavoy & Robinson, 1989), but these efforts are best viewed as investigative rather than of general practical value.

Communication with the cognitively impaired patient begins with basic understanding and knowledge of the patient's behavior as well as its psychodynamic underpinnings. Behavior and verbal expression may be otherwise unintelligible to the uninformed caregiver (Cohen, 1989; Sadavoy, 1991; Sadavoy & Robinson, 1989). Because the patient with moderate to severe dementia cannot convey his or her life story and achievements, uninformed staff in long-term care institutions have no way of understanding the patient's utterances and behavior. Cohen (1989) advocates that family members, health care professionals, and others knowledgeable about the patient convey the patient's personal history to the staff in various ways (e.g., by conveying brief verbal histories or bringing memorabilia) to increase the staff's understanding, interest, and involvement. The more advanced the cognitive decline, the greater the patient's need to interact on a nonverbal level (for example, through activity, movement, or music). Duffy (1997) emphasizes the importance of using nonverbal language to establish and maintain therapeutic contact with demented patients. Some of the guidelines emphasized include maintaining clinical attachment; working to discover the "person" behind the dementia; approaching versus avoiding the patient; attending to subvocal and paralinguistic signals such as tone, inflections, and breathing; and using touch as a medium of communication.

Frequently, cognitive impairment is accompanied by delusions. Gentle redirection of the patient's attention to another focus or simple distraction of the patient's attention may be helpful (Cohen, 1989). Aggressive reality orientation can exacerbate psychosis or increase the patient's agitation. For example, confronting a patient who has the delusion that his or her long-deceased parent has recently visited may precipitate agitation and depression. Instead, the therapist can refocus the patient's attention on real interactions with living family members. (For illuminating case reports of the effectiveness of this approach, the reader is directed to Cohen's 1989 work.)

The therapist is most helpful if he or she is able to tolerate the often ambiguous, impoverished, repetitive, and sometimes bizarre verbal interactions with these patients. Such patients frequently have a need to idealize the therapist, who must be able to tolerate the idealization despite his or her knowledge of therapeutic limitations.

Reminiscence or Life Review Therapy

To varying degrees, most patients in therapy, including elderly individuals, reminisce about the past, seek meaning for their life, and strive for some resolution of interpersonal and intrapsychic conflicts. Reminiscence and life review are useful in both individual and group therapy (Butler, 1963; Molinari, 1999). The purpose of life review therapy is to enhance this process and make it more conscious and deliberate. Lewis and Butler (1974) reported that this technique helps to resolve old problems; increases tolerance of conflict; relieves guilt and fears; and enhances creativity, generosity, and acceptance of the present. Empirical evidence for the effectiveness of reminiscence therapy is still equivocal and requires further study (Hsieh & Wang, 2003).

Brief Psychodynamic Psychotherapy

A brief psychodynamic therapy approach can be considered for elderly patients with clearly defined, circumscribed problems that can be expected to resolve within a limited time. Examples of problems amenable to brief psychotherapy include adjustment disorder, grief reaction, and traumatic stress disorder that has not become chronic and entrenched. Setting a time limit on therapy reinforces the patient's confidence in personal ability to resolve the problem, focuses and accelerates the therapeutic process, diminishes the patient's fear of protracted dependency on the therapist, and considers the patient's limited finances (Lazarus et al., 1987).

In one preliminary, uncontrolled study of the process and outcome of brief psychodynamic psychotherapy with eight elderly outpatients (four men and four women) ranging in age from 63 to 77 years, individually constructed outcome scales were used for each patient (Lazarus et al., 1987). Most outpatients met the criteria of the *Diagnostic and Statistical Manual of Mental Disorders, Third Edition* (*DSM-III*; American Psychiatric Association, 1980) for an adjustment disorder with depressed mood, and one patient had a panic disorder.

Assessment of the process of therapy with these elderly outpatients suggested that patients often used the therapeutic relationship to reestablish a positive sense of self over time or to consolidate diverse and disparate aspects of the self into a more positive sense of self. The therapist was used by the patient for validation of competency and normalcy and for restoration of feelings of mastery and self-esteem. The generalizability of this preliminary study to other elderly outpatients is limited by the small sample size and reliance on unvalidated, individualized scales.

Silberschatz (1986) and Silberschatz and Curtis (1986, 1991) studied extensively the process and outcome of time-limited psychotherapy with older outpatients and found that patients entered treatment with specific conscious and unconscious goals essential for the therapist to understand. These goals sometimes included a wish for the therapist (1) to help the patient overcome initial resistances to treatment (often based on ageist attitudes and myths) and guilt feelings over surviving or being successful, while others (family and friends) died or became disabled; and (2) to provide support for overcoming negative attitudes and beliefs about the self. These investigators believed that what is most predictive of successful therapy is the ability of the therapist to ascertain and respond appropriately to the patient's goals for therapy and to help the patient disconfirm pathogenic beliefs about the self. It is likely that these researchers carefully selected patients who could articulately explore their presenting problems and were capable of an insight-oriented approach to therapy; therefore, the generalizability of their findings may be restricted to this patient cohort. Nevertheless, longstanding ageist biases that contend that most elderly patients require supportive rather than insight-oriented therapy may underestimate patients' abilities and provide a watered-down approach to therapy.

Cognitive-Behavioral Psychotherapy

Cognitive psychotherapy (Beck et al., 1979) is a brief therapy approach that uses interpretations, explanations, and practical information to correct the depressed patient's stereotypical, self-defeating thoughts and dysfunctional attitudes. In adults, indications for CBT are very broad. The best evidence in elders is still for depressive disorders, and CBT has been shown to be effective for depression associated with physical problems such as stroke (Lincoln & Flannaghan, 2003). The goal is to promote integration of positive perceptions and thinking patterns and thereby diminish depression. Effectiveness of CBT requires the patient's full participation in the process. Elders often cope with issues that may interfere with the efficacy of CBT. Hence, careful evaluation can be helpful for determining the suitability of patients for this form of intervention. Assessment includes information on cognitive skills, role conflicts and demands on energy and time, attitudes to psychotherapy, comorbid mood disturbances, impact of medical conditions, presence of acute life-threatening or otherwise risky issues such as suicidality, and substance abuse history (Coon et al., 1999; Thompson et al., 1991).

As with most forms of psychotherapy for the elderly, techniques of CBT are largely similar to those used for patients of any age. However, modifications of cognitive therapy have been suggested to address the special problems of elderly patients with depression (Coon et al., 1999; Gallagher & Thompson, 1982; Thompson et al., 1991). These modifications include the following:

- Acclimatizing patients for therapy (e.g., presenting therapy as a way to learn to adjust to the stress of life and encouraging active participation in the therapeutic process)
- Enhancing learning capabilities (e.g., by empathically understanding the patient's hesitation to try therapeutic suggestions)
- Terminating therapy gradually (e.g., anticipating future problems and leaving the door open for the patient to return)
- Extending treatment to 30 to 40 sessions, instead of the usual 15 to 20, for patients with chronic depression or a depressive episode superimposed on a dysthymic disorder

Additional modifications include greater flexibility and activity on the part of the therapist, keeping the patient focused on the "here and now," proceeding at a slower pace, and adopting the patient's own language when addressing certain issues. Compliance with homework has been shown to improve outcome of treatment of mild to moderate depression (Coon & Thompson, 2003). For patients with cognitive slowing or sensory deficits, it is helpful to present important information in several sensory modalities, such as repeating important themes or concepts, having the patient take notes, providing a tape recording of the interview for review between sessions, and giving specific work assignments between sessions. Several strategies may help reluctant patients overcome resistance to therapy. If patients complain they are "too old to change," the therapist may respond, "Perhaps it is true that you cannot learn new ways of thinking about your problems, but how will you know this for certain unless you try?" If the patient complains that the therapist is "too young to help," the therapist can encourage temporary suspension of this belief so that a trial of therapy can proceed.

Therapy is aided when the therapist is sensitive to elders' concerns about doing "homework," educational or sensory limitations on carrying out instructions, overly broad or ambitious goals, and hopelessness about their perceived overwhelming circumstances. Instructions for taking goal-centered action (behavioral interventions) must be tailored to match the patient's capacities.

When CBT was used for treating depression in aging patients, age was not a predictor of outcome; very elderly patients responded as well as younger elderly patients to CBT, IPT, and brief dynamic psychotherapy. Patients with major depression who were less responsive to all three treatment modalities had many endogenous signs, a concomitant personality disorder, and low expectations of improvement (Thompson et al., 1988, 1991). Patients with comorbid personality disorders or severe major depressive, melancholic disorders often require more prolonged courses of therapy (Thompson et al., 1991), and medication is required for severe major depression.

Pinkston and Linsk (1984) utilized behavioral therapy methods to teach 21 separate families at-home care for an impaired elderly relative. Although the elderly patients had a variety of psychiatric diagnoses, they all had severe mental and physical impairment. Also, their caregivers were willing to undergo rigorous study procedures involving assessment and training derived from operant and social learning theories of behavioral intervention. Impressive results were obtained. There was improvement in 73% of all behaviors (e.g., excessive negative verbalizations and self-care deficits) by the end of the study, and at 6-month follow-up, the improvement was maintained in 78% of previously targeted behaviors that had improved. Also, at the end of the study most of the caregivers personal health status was self-rated as unchanged or improved. However, the high motivation of these caregivers (e.g., their resources, wherewithal, and willingness to engage in a comprehensive and time-consuming teaching program) limits the generalizability of these results.

PERSONALITY DISORDERS

Elderly patients with a Cluster B personality disorder (DSM-IV) (American Psychiatric Association, 1994) tend to be excessively demanding, extremely sensitive, emotionally labile, and impulsive, and they may engage in destructive, acting-out behavior. They often have few or inadequate support systems because of their propensity for unstable relationships. Therapists may become frustrated because of the preponderance of demands and expectations.

The signs and symptoms present in the elderly patient with personality disorder are similar to those present in the younger adult, but with modifications brought on by age-relevant factors, such as confinement in a nursing home and physical infirmities. These elderly patients, because of impaired motoric behavior and generalized "slowing down," are less likely than their younger counterparts to flagrantly act out with criminal or promiscuous behavior (see Chapter 24). Passive-dependent behavior, social withdrawal, apathy, and vulnerability to depression may be prominent, and previous personality traits may become accentuated with cognitive and other health impairments. There is also a significant impact of personality disorders on Axis I disorders (Sadavoy, 1999). Whereas the elderly patient without significant character abnormality shows some resiliency and flexibility in dealing with change and trauma associated with aging, the patient with a personality disorder remains rigid, overwhelmed, and unable to adapt to age-related stresses.

Presentation

The elderly patient with a personality disorder in the dramatic, Cluster B spectrum carries psychopathology established in early stages of intrapsychic development. Sadavoy (1987) pointed to five unresolved intrapsychic maldevelopments that affect the elderly patient with a personality disorder: (1) fear of abandonment or loneliness; (2) real or fantasized narcissistic injury to self-esteem and failure of self and selfobject relationships; (3) impaired affect tolerance; (4) failure in the development of modulators of rage, which in turn leads to increased use of splitting; and (5) loss of self-cohesion induced by age-associated stressors, which may be so extreme as to cause brief psychotic episodes.

Dysfunction of intrapsychic structure can impair mourning and ability to cope with grief. This issue is a particularly familiar and difficult one to address in geriatric treatment because elderly patients are routinely faced with the task of coping with losses.

Like similar patients at other ages, these geriatric patients express personality disorders in many ways. Most frequent is their pathological way of relating to family and other caregivers. The patient may become increasingly helpless (Breslau, 1987) and exhibit panicky behavior (e.g., calling family members for unreasonable reassurances). Patients may make incessant demands on caregivers that interfere with other obligations, expecting that others will change plans and cancel activities to respond to their requests. Such behavior eventually angers and frustrates family, caregivers, or staff. Treatment of concomitant anxiety can often lessen the patient's demands and acting out. Another common presentation consists of exaggerated somatic complaints that cannot be alleviated by reassurance.

Patients with depressive withdrawal may exhibit anhedonia, apathy, anorexia, and loss of the will to live. In these cases, life-threatening depressions may be superimposed on the personality disorder and require vigorous treatment. The therapist should be careful not to ascribe an Axis II personality disorder diagnosis without careful assessment for an Axis I diagnosis that may have a favorable prognosis. Treatable depressions and psychoses may be masked by readily apparent disruptive signs of a personality disorder.

Treatment

In developing a treatment plan, consideration is given to the patient's pathological behavior, to the stresses on the family and health care team, and to the patient's ability to engage in individual psychotherapy. Various treatment strategies have been suggested, although no formal studies of effectiveness have been undertaken to date.

Sadavoy and Dorian (1983) described a psychodynamic approach that incorporates behavioral techniques for use in a long-term care setting. They enlist the help of the family or other caregivers in preparing a written statement of expected behavior from the patient. This approach takes into account the patient's underlying psychodynamics—as evident, for example, in his or her need for a sense of control—and recognizes the limitations of the staff's tolerance of the patient's unreasonable demands, acting out, and other disturbing behaviors. The staff sets nonpunitive limits on verbal and physical acting out, specific requirements for participation in prescribed activities, adherence to medication schedules, and conditions for privileges. With a clearly spelled out contract, a working alliance may be established that includes family and caregivers, who work together to strive for mutually established goals.

In individual therapy with these patients, the therapist should adjust the frequency of sessions, titrating the intensity of therapy against the patient's sensitivity to rejection and forestalling the patient's feeling of overwhelming rage and anxiety. Therapy focuses on helping the patient to connect feelings to causal events, thus promoting maintenance of self-esteem and self-cohesion. Developmental history is largely used for understanding the patient's needs and actions. Sadavoy and Dorian (1983) limited the emphasis on past unresolvable losses and mourning during the earlier phases of treatment, focusing instead on current, here-and-now issues. This technique employs clarification and confrontation instead of deeper interpretations. In some cases, as a working alliance develops, a measure of working through of unresolved mourning may be attempted.

Gabbard (1989) addressed the issue of splitting, a common defense of the adult patient with a personality disorder that is also found in elderly patients. The reality of the caregiver's efforts is distorted by the disordered intrapsychic self of the patient. The caregiver is perceived as either good or bad, as defined by split-off, internal representations from the patient's past. For example, the patient may willingly accept medication from one caregiver, but not from another. Thus, the same situation provokes either compliant or negativistic reaction, depending on the patient's intrapsychic assessment of a particular caregiver, despite the fact that each caregiver may behave toward the patient in a similar fashion. The psychotherapist deals with the internal world of the patient by using explanations, clarifications, and sometimes interpretations, with the goal of minimizing splitting of internal self and object representations. Staff intervention addresses the integration and moderation of the external world of the patient.

INTEGRATING PSYCHOTHERAPEUTIC
TREATMENT MODALITIES

Three basic psychotherapy interventions (individual psychodynamic, cognitive-behavioral, and interpersonal) have been effective and may be productively combined (Sadavoy, 1994). To utilize these therapies rationally, an organized assessment process is important and includes a tripartite evaluation at three levels: psychodynamic, interpersonal, and cognitive-behavioral. The assessment attends not only to the analysis of the patient's current crisis, but also to the history of the patient's adult roles and relationships as well as his or her earlier developmental history. (It is important to note that the developmental history frequently is left out of geriatric assessments, perhaps because of the immediacy and importance of evaluating the more recent events in the patient's life.) The therapist determines the patient's strengths and weaknesses of function; the nature of his or her response to stresses throughout life, particularly during adult years; defense mechanisms and habitual modes of behavior; and earlier life trauma, whether in childhood or adulthood. This last issue is particularly relevant in ethnocultural communities of elderly persons, whose histories often include significant early trauma such as war experience, immigration, torture, assault, or accidents. Such events often lead to chronic symptoms of posttraumatic stress that may emerge with greater intensity in old age (Sadavoy, 1987).

The assessment of interpersonal factors is of special relevance in old age because this is a period of transition in several interpersonal areas and includes conflicts over increased dependency, loss, and bereavement. The vicissitudes of aging may lead to stressors that uncover preexisting and perhaps long-standing deficiencies in interpersonal relationships. For example, individuals who have relied on defensive personality styles that require activity, intensity, and environmental control may have difficulty adapting to old age and its requirements for relinquishing appropriate control to others. Interpersonal conflicts or rebellious avoidance of using necessary support systems will sometimes emerge. Such individuals may experience strong longings for closeness and at the same time fear rejection or engulfment. Intolerance of imposed intimate relationships may develop because of declining capacities and dependency on others.

As noted, cognitive-behavioral assessment is relevant in elderly individuals, who are easily prone to cognitive distortions and vulnerable to developing inaccurate perceptions of their roles and place in the world; their value to others; and fears of real or imagined assault from threatening forces and catastrophic images of decline, infirmity, pain, and abandonment. This element of inquiry focuses on the central themes of aging, particularly the evaluation of the patient's belief system, the presence of distortions, and concomitant affective responses.

In deciding on treatment interventions, the therapist of the geriatric patient is often placed in the position of having to make a triage decision—that is, evaluating the individual patient's capacity to utilize psychotherapy and, if so, at which level. Moreover, limited resources may force therapists into the position of deciding where to concentrate their efforts. It is important that this choice be made actively, based on the therapist's knowledge of a variety of therapeutic modalities. Unfortunately, often the therapist's preference for a particular therapy or his or her narrow range of expertise may determine the treatment choice. In making a triage decision, the therapist is faced with three decision points:

1. *The accessibility of the patient to therapy* (i.e., Is the patient able to attend? Does the patient have the mental and sensory capacity, or are there other barriers?).
2. *Assessment of need* (i.e., Does the patient require an active intervention, or does he or she have the psychological strength and supports to reconstitute without formal intervention? Will the natural course of the disorder lead to improvement over time without active psychotherapy?).
3. *Which of the therapeutic modalities is most likely to be effective and whether it is available.* To make this decision, the therapist must be familiar with the indications for the three main therapeutic modalities. Parenthetically, geriatric psychiatry training programs may not adequately address the need to train geriatric psychiatrists in the indications for and implementation of a range of psychotherapeutic modalities.

Use of these treatments with patients in institutions is highly vulnerable to triage decisions because the patients may be deemed inaccessible (i.e., too impaired in cognition or function to be reachable). More important, treatment, particularly psychotherapy treatment, is often unavailable.

SUMMARY

Many clinical reports and a limited number of outcome studies support the contention that elderly patients are very responsive to various modalities of psychotherapy. Individual psychotherapy with elderly individuals is distinguished from that with younger adults by (1) greater attention to specific developmental tasks and challenges associated with aging; (2) the need for especially active therapeutic intervention to overcome patient, family, and health care system barriers to treatment; (3) the nature of the transference and countertransference reactions and resistances; and (4) the need to employ specialized psychotherapeutic approaches for patients who are frail or have dementia or personality disorders. The therapist of the elderly patient must maintain a flexible approach because the patient's changing clinical status may require a shift from one treatment approach to another.

REFERENCES

Alvidrez J, Arean P. Physician willingness to refer older depressed patients for psychotherapy. *Int J Psychiatry Med.* 2002;32:21–35.
American Psychiatric Association. *Diagnostic and Statistical Manual of Mental Disorders.* 3rd ed. Washington, DC: American Psychiatric Association; 1980.

American Psychiatric Association. *Diagnostic and Statistical Manual of Mental Disorders*. 4th ed. Washington, DC: American Psychiatric Association; 1994.

Arean P, Cook B. Psychotherapy and combined psychotherapy/pharmacotherapy for late life depression. *Biol Psychiatry*. 2002;52:293–303.

Aronson MI. Psychotherapy in a home for the aged. *Arch Neurol Psychiatry*. 1958;79: 671–674, 1958.

Atchley RC. The aging self. *Psychother Theory Res Pract*. 1982;9:338–396.

Atchley RC. A continuity theory of normal aging. *Gerontologist*. 1989;29:183–190.

Beck A, Rush J, Shaw BF, et al. *Cognitive Therapy of Depression*. New York, NY: Guilford; 1979.

Berezin M. Psychodynamic considerations of aging and the aged: an overview. *Am J Psychiatry*. 1972;128:12, 33–41.

Berezin M. Reflections on psychotherapy with the elderly. In: Sadavoy J, Leszcz M, eds. *Treating the Elderly With Psychotherapy: The Scope for Change in Later Life*. Madison, CT: International Universities Press; 1987:45–63.

Blau D, Berezin MA. Neurosis and character disorders. In: Howells JG, ed. *Modern Perspectives in the Psychiatry of Old Age*. New York, NY: Brunner/Mazel; 1975: 201–233.

Breslau L. Exaggerated helplessness syndrome. In: Sadavoy J, Leszcz M, eds. *Treating the Elderly With Psychotherapy: The Scope for Change in Later Life*. Madison, CT: International Universities Press; 1987:157–173.

Brody E, Kleban MH, Lawton MP, et al. Excess disabilities of mentally impaired aged: impact of individualized treatment. *Gerontologist*. 1971;11:133.

Butler RN. The life review: an interpretation of reminiscence in the aged. *Psychiatry*. 1963;26:65–70.

Butler RN, Lewis MI. *Aging and Mental Health: Positive Psychosocial Approaches*. St. Louis, MO: Mosby; 1977.

Cath SH. Some dynamics of middle and later years: a study in depletion and restitution. In Berezin MA, Cath SH, eds. *Geriatric Psychiatry: Grief, Loss, and Emotional Disorders in the Aging Process*. New York, NY: International Universities Press; 1975:21–72.

Cath SH. Functional disorders: an organismic view and attempt at reclassification. In: Bellak L, Karasu TB, eds. *Geriatric Psychiatry*. New York, NY: Grune and Stratton; 1976.

Cohen GD. Psychodynamic perspectives in the clinical approach to brain disease in the elderly. In: Conn D, Grek A, Sadavoy J, eds. *Psychiatric Consequences of Brain Disease in the Elderly*. New York, NY: Plenum Press; 1989:85–99.

Coon D, Thompson L. The relationship between homework compliance and treatment outcomes among older adult outpatients with mild-to-moderate depression. *Am J Geriatr Psychiatry*. 2003;11:53–61.

Coon DW, Rider K, Gallagher-Thompson D, Thompson L. Cognitive behavioural therapy for the treatment of late life distress. In: Duffy M, ed. *Handbook of Counseling and Psychotherapy With Older Adults*. New York, NY: John Wiley and Sons; 1999:57–76.

Cornes C, Silberman R, Ehrenpries LS, Zaltman J, Malloy J, Reynolds CF. Applying interpersonal psychotherapy to bereavement-related depression following loss of a spouse in late life. *J Psychother Pract Res*. 1994;3:149–162.

Crose RG. Addressing late life developmental issues for women: body image, sexuality and intimacy. In: Duffy M, ed. *Handbook of Counseling and Psychotherapy with Older Adults.* New York, NY: John Wiley and Sons; 1999:57–76.

Crusey J. Short-term psychodynamic psychotherapy with a sixty-two-year-old man. In: Nemiroff RA, Colarusso CA, eds. *The Race Against Time.* New York, NY: Plenum; 1985:147–170.

Duffy M. Individual therapy in longterm care institutions. In: Molinari V, ed. *Professional Psychology in Long Term Care.* New York, NY: Hatherleigh; 1997.

Erikson EH. The human life cycle. In: Sills DL, ed. *International Encyclopedia of the Social Sciences.* New York, NY: Macmillan; 1968:286–292.

Ford CV, Sbordone RT. Attitudes of psychiatrists toward elderly patients. *Am J Psychiatry.* 1980;137:571–575.

Gabbard GO. Splitting in hospital treatment. *Am J Psychiatry.* 1989;146:444–451.

Gallagher DE, Thompson LW. *Depression in the Elderly: A Behavioral Treatment Manual.* Los Angeles: University of Southern California Press; 1981.

Gallagher DE, Thompson LW. Differential effectiveness of psychotherapies for the treatment of major depressive disorders in older adult patients. *Psychother Theory Res Pract.* 1982;19:482–490.

Gallagher DE, Thompson LW. Effectiveness of psychotherapy for both endogenous and non-endogenous depression in older adult outpatients. *J Gerontol.* 1983;38:707–712.

Gatz M, Fiske A, Fox LS, Kaskie B, Kasl-Godley JE, McCallum TJ, et al. Empirically validated psychological treatments for older adults. *J Ment Health Aging.* 1988;4: 9–46.

Goldfarb AI. Psychotherapy of the aged: the use and value of an adaptational frame of reference. *Psychoanal Rev.* 1956;43:168–181.

Goldfarb AI, Turner H. Psychotherapy of aged persons. II. Utilization and effectiveness of "brief" therapy. *Am J Psychiatry.* 1953;109:916–921.

Grotjahn JM. Psychoanalytic investigation of a 71-year-old man with senile dementia. *Psychoanal Q.* 1940;9:80–97.

Grotjahn M. Analytic psychotherapy with the elderly. *Psychoanal Rev.* 1955;42:419–427.

Hanley IG, McGuire RJ, Boyd WD. Reality orientation and dementia: a controlled trial of two approaches. *Br J Psychiatry.* 1981;138:10–14.

Hiatt H. Dynamic psychotherapy with the aging patient. *Am J Psychother.* 1971;25: 591–600.

Hollon S. Psychotherapy research with older populations. *Am J Geriatr Psychiatry.* 2003;11:7–8.

Hollos S, Ferenczi S. *Psychoanalysis and the Psychic Disorder of General Paresis.* New York, NY: Nervous and Mental Disease; 1925.

Hsieh H, Wang J. Effect of reminiscence therapy on depression in older adults: a systematic review. *Int J Nursing Studies.* 2003;40:335–345.

Hussian RA. *Behavioral Geriatrics: Progress in Behavior Modification.* Vol. 16. New York, NY: Academic Press; 1984:159–183.

Jacques E. Death and the mid-life crisis. *Int J Psychoanal.* 1965;46:502–514.

Kahana R. Strategies of dynamic psychotherapy with the wide range of older individuals. *J Geriatr Psychiatry.* 1979;12:71–100.

Kahana R. Discussion: the Oedipus complex and rejuvenation fantasies in the analysis of a seventy-year-old woman. *J Geriatr Psychiatry.* 1987a;20:53–60.

Kahana R. Geriatric psychotherapy: beyond crisis management. In: Sadavoy J, Leszcz M, eds. *Treating the Elderly With Psychotherapy: The Scope for Change in Later Life.* Madison, CT: International Universities Press; 1987b:233–263.

Kahn RS. Comments. In: *Proceedings of the York House Institute on the Mentally Impaired Aged.* Philadelphia, PA: Philadelphia Geriatric Center, 1965.

Karel MJ, Hinrichsen G. Treatment of depression in late life—Psychotherapeutic interventions. *Clin Psychol Rev.* 2000;20:707–729.

Keller MB, McCullough JP, Klein DM, et al. A comparison of nefazodone, the cognitive behavioral-analysis system of pychotherapy, and their combination for the treatment of chronic depression. *N Engl J Med.* 2000;342:1462–1470.

King PMH. The life cycle as indicated by the nature of the transference in the psychoanalysis of the middle-aged and elderly. *Int J Psychoanal.* 1980;61:153–159.

Klausner EJ, Alexopoulos GS. The future of psychosocial treatments for elderly patients. *Psychiatr Serv.* 1999;50:1198–1204.

Klausner EJ, Clarkin JF, Spielman L, Pupu C, Abrams R, Alexopoulos GS. Late life depression and functional disability—The role of goal-focused group psychotherapy. *Int J Geriatr Psychiatry.* 1988;13:707–716.

Kruglov L. The early stage of vascular dementia: significance of a complete therapeutic program. *Int J Geriatr Psychiatry.* 2003;18:402–406.

Lazarus LW. Self-psychology and psychotherapy with the elderly: theory and practice. *J Geriatr Psychiatry.* 1980;13:69–88, 1980.

Lazarus LW. Self-psychology: its application to brief psychotherapy with the elderly. *J Geriatr Psychiatry.* 1988;21:109–125.

Lazarus LW, Groves L, Guttman D, et al. Brief psychotherapy with the elderly: a study of process and outcome. In: Sadavoy J, Leszcz M, eds. *Treating the Elderly With Psychotherapy: The Scope for Change in Later Life.* Madison, CT: International Universities Press; 1987:265–293.

Lazarus LW, Weinberg J. Treatment in the ambulatory-care setting. In: Busse EW, Blazer DG, eds. *Handbook of Geriatric Psychiatry.* New York, NY: Van Nostrand Reinhold; 1980:427–452.

Lee E. Chinese American families. In: Lee E, ed. *Working With Asian Americans.* New York, NY: Guilford Press; 1997:46–77.

Lee, K, Volans P, Gregory N. Attitudes towards psychotherapy with older people among trainee clinical psychologists. *Aging Ment Health.* 2003;7:133–141.

Levin S. Some comments on the distribution of narcissistic and object libido in the aged. *Int J Psychoanal.* 1965b;46:200–208.

Lewis MI, Butler RN. Life-review therapy: putting memories to work in individual and group psychotherapy. *Geriatrics.* 1974;29:165–169, 172–173.

Lincoln N, Flannaghan T. Cognitive behavioral psychotherapy for depression following stroke: a randomized controlled trial. *Stroke.* 2003;34:111–115.

Lynch T, Morse J, Mendelson T, Robins C. Dialectical behavior therapy for depressed older adults: a randomized pilot study. *Am J Geriatr Psychiatry.* 2003;11:33–45.

Mackenzie CS, Gekoski WL, Knox VJ. Do family physicians treat older patients with mental disorders differently from younger patients? *Can Fam Physician.* 1999;45:1219–1224.

Malamud WI. Countertransference issues with elderly patients. *J Geriatr Psychiatry.* 1996;29:33–41.

Meerloo JAM. Contribution of psychoanalysis to the problem of the aged. In: Hermann

M, ed. *Psychoanalysis and Social Work*. New York, NY: International Universities Press; 1953:321–337.

Meissner WW. Normal psychology of the aging process revisited. I. Discussion. Paper presented at: Annual Scientific Meeting of the Boston Society of Gerontologic Psychiatry; 1975; Boston, MA.

Miller E. The Oedipus complex and rejuvenation fantasies in the analysis of a seventy-year-old woman. *J Geriatr Psychiatry*. 1987;20:29–51.

Miller M, Frank E, Cornes C, Houck P, Reynolds C. The value of maintenance interpersonal psychotherapy (IPT) in older adults with different IPT foci. *Am J Geriatr Psychiatry*. 2003;11:97–102.

Miller MD, Wolfson L, Frank E, et al. Using interpersonal psychotherapy in a combined psychotherapy/medication research protocol with depressed elders. *J Psychother Pract Res*. 1998;7:47–55.

Molinari V. Using reminiscence and life review as natural therapeutic strategies in group therapy. In: Duffy M, ed. *Handbook of Counseling and Psychotherapy with Older Adults*. New York, NY: John Wiley and Sons; 1999:57–76.

Myers WA. *Dynamic Therapy of the Older Patient*. New York, NY: Jason Aronson; 1984:6.

Myers WA. Transference and countertransference issues in treatments involving older patients and younger therapists. *J Geriatr Psychiatry*. 1986;19:221–239.

Mynors-Wallis, L. Problem-solving treatment—Evidence for effectiveness and feasibility in primary care. *Int J Psychiatry Med*. 1966;26:249–262.

Nemiroff RA, Colarusso CA. The literature on psychotherapy and psychoanalysis in the second half of life. In: Nemiroff RA, Colarusso CA, eds. *The Race Against Time*. New York, NY: Plenum; 1985:25–43.

Neugarten B. Time, age and the life-cycle. *Am J Psychiatry*. 1979;136:887–894.

Newton NA, Jacobowitz J. Transferential and countertransferential processes in therapy with older adults. In: Duffy M, ed. *Handbook of Counseling and Psychotherapy With Older Adults*. New York, NY: John Wiley and Sons; 1999:21–40.

Olfson M, Marcus S, Druss B, Pincus H. National trends in the use of outpatient psychotherapy. *Am J Psychiatry*. 2002;159:1914–1920.

Orbach A. Psychotherapy in the third age. *Br J Psychotherapy*. 1994;11:171–231.

Pinkston EM, Linsk NL. Behavioral family intervention with the impaired elder. *Gerontogist*. 1984;26:576–583.

Pollock GH. The mourning-liberation process: ideas on the inner life of the older adult. In: Sadavoy J, Leszcz M, eds. *Treating the Elderly With Psychotherapy: The Scope for Change in Later Life*. Madison, CT: International Universities Press; 1987:3–29.

Rechtschaffen A. Psychotherapy with geriatric patients: a review of the literature. *J Gerontol*. 1959;14:73–84.

Reynolds CF, Frank E, Perel JM, et al. Combined pharmacotherapy and psychotherapy in the acute and continuation treatment of elderly patients with recurrent major depression: a preliminary report. *Am J Psychiatry*. 1992;149:1687–1692.

Rosenthal HM. The use of psychoanalytic principles in the treatment of older people. *Am J Psychoanal*. 1985;45:119–134.

Sadavoy J. Character disorders in the elderly: an overview. In: Sadavoy J, Leszcz M, eds. *Treating the Elderly With Psychotherapy: The Scope for Change in Later Life*. Madison, CT: International Universities Press; 1987:175–229.

Sadavoy J. Psychodynamic perspectives on dementia: Alzheimer's disease and the individual. *Am J Alzheimer's Care Res.* 1991;6:12–20.

Sadavoy J. Integrated psychotherapy for the elderly. *Can J Psychiatry.* 1994;39(Suppl 1):519–526.

Sadavoy J. The effect of personality disorders on Axis I disorders in the elderly. In: Duffy M, ed. *Handbook of Counseling and Psychotherapy with Older Adults.* New York, NY: John Wiley and Sons; 1999:397–414.

Sadavoy J, Dorian B. Treatment of the elderly characterologically disturbed patient in the chronic care institution. *J Geriatr Psychiatry.* 1983;16:223–240.

Sadavoy J, Fogel B. Personality disorders in old age. In: Birren J, Slane RB, Cohen GD, eds. *Handbook of Mental Health and Aging.* 2nd ed. San Diego, CA: Academic Press; 1992:433–462.

Sadavoy J, Leszcz M, eds. *Treating the Elderly With Psychotherapy: The Scope for Change in Later Life.* Madison, CT: International Universities Press; 1987.

Sadavoy J, Meier R, Ong A. Barriers to access to mental health care in ethnocultural seniors: the Toronto Study. *Can J Psychiatry.* In press.

Sadavoy J, Robinson A. Psychotherapy and the cognitively impaired elderly. In: Conn D, Grek A, Sadavoy J, eds. *Psychiatric Consequences of Brain Disease in the Elderly.* New York, NY: Plenum; 1989:101–135.

Scocco, P, Frank E. Interpersonal psychotherapy as agumentation treatment in depressed elderly responding poorly to antidepressant drugs: a case series. *Psychother Psychosom.* 2002;71:357–361.

Scogin F, McElreath L. Efficacy of psychosocial treatments for geriatric depression: a quantitative review. *J Consult Clin Psychol.* 1994;62:64–97.

Settlage CF. Transcending old age: creativity, development and psychoanalysis in the life of a centenarian. *Int J Psychoanal.* 1996;77:549–564.

Silberschatz G. Testing pathogenic beliefs. In: Weiss J, Sampson H, eds. *The Psychoanalytic Process: Theory, Clinical Observation, and Empirical Research.* New York, NY: Guilford Press; 1986:256–266.

Silberschatz G, Curtis JT. Clinical implications on research on brief dynamic psychotherapy. II. How the therapist helps or hinders therapeutic progress. *Psychoanal Psychol.* 1986;3:27–37.

Silberschatz G, Curtis JT. Time-limited psychodynamic therapy with older adults. In: Myers W, ed. *New Techniques in the Psychotherapy of Older Patients.* Washington, DC: American Psychiatric Press; 1991:95–110.

Sonderegger TB, Seigel R J. Conflicts in care: later years of the lifespan. In: Rave EJ, Larsen CC, eds. *Ethical Decision-Making in Therapy: Feminist Perspectives.* New York, NY: Guilford Press; 1995:223–246.

Steuer J. Psychotherapy with the elderly. *Psychiatr Clin North Am.* 1982;5:199–213.

Strauss HM. Working as an elder analyst. In: Gerson B, ed. *The Therapist as Person: Life Crisis Life Choices, Life Experiences, and Their Effect on Treatment.* Hillsdale, NJ: Analytic Press; 1996:277–294.

Tang NM. Psychoanalytic psychotherapy with Chinese Americans. In: Lee E, ed. *Working With Asian Americans.* New York, NY: Guilford Press; 1997:323–341.

Thompson LW, Frank G, Florsheim M, et al. Cognitive-behavioral therapy for affective disorders. In: Myers WA, ed. *New Techniques in the Psychotherapy of Older Patients.* Washington, DC: American Psychiatric Press; 1991:3–19.

Thompson LW, Gallagher D, Breckenridge JS. Comparative effectiveness of psychotherapies for depressed elders. *J Consult Clin Psychol.* 1987;55:385–390.

Thompson LW, Gallagher D, Czirr R. Personality disorder and outcome in the treatment of late-life depression. *J Geriatr Psychiatry.* 1988;21:133–153.

Tobin SS. Issues of care in long-term settings. In: Conn D, Grek A, Sadavoy J, eds. *Psychiatric Consequences of Brain Disease in the Elderly.* New York, NY: Plenum; 1989:163–187.

Tornstam L. Gerotranscendence: a theory about maturing into old age. *J Aging Identity.* 1996;1:37–50.

Weisman AD, Hackett TP. Denial as a social act. In: Levin S, Kahana RJ, eds. *Psychodynamic Studies on Aging, Creativity, Reminiscing, and Dying.* New York, NY: International Universities Press; 1967:79–110.

Windholz MJ, Marmar CR, Horowitz MJ. A review of the research on conjugal bereavement: impact on health and efficacy of intervention. *Compr Psychiatry.* 1985;26:433–477.

Yalom I. *Existential Psychotherapy.* New York, NY: Basic Books; 1980.

Yesavage JA, Karasu TB. Psychotherapy with elderly patients. *Am J Psychother.* 1982;36:41–55.

Zinberg NE, Kaufman I. Cultural and personality factors associated with aging: an introduction. In: Zinberg NE, Kaufman I, eds. *Normal Psychology of the Aging Process.* New York, NY: International Universities Press; 1963:17–71.

32

Group Therapy

Molyn Leszcz, MD

OVERVIEW

Group psychotherapy interventions are emerging as an important component of comprehensive treatment of the elderly, reflecting the value of group therapy with regard to both effectiveness and resource efficiency (Clemens et al., 2000). Group and individual therapy appear largely equivalent in comparative studies (Toseland, 1995). Both specific and nonspecific therapeutic factors contribute to positive outcomes (Leszcz, 1997). What links all effective group approaches is the creation of a context for interpersonal engagement between and among a number of patients and a therapist that operates according to certain structures and group norms and aims to achieve a degree of group cohesiveness that is reflected in feelings of mutual interest, attachment, and task effectiveness. Recognition of specific needs, attributes, and concerns of the elderly underscores the recognition that the elderly are a heterogeneous population warranting a broad range of group interventions. In general, however, the attributes of the group therapies and requirements of the elderly are well matched.

Table 32-1 lists the types of group therapy currently employed with geriatric patients. Many foci exist. These include the treatment of specific functional disorders (commonly, mood disorders); the psychotherapeutic treatment of developmental and transitional phenomena and the impact of these life events on self-esteem, self-worth, and the individual's underlying personality; the pursuit

TABLE 32-1. Group therapy approaches for the elderly

Verbal-centered groups for the cognitively intact:
  Cognitive-behavioral groups
  Psychodynamic psychotherapy groups
  Reminiscence groups
  Homogeneous groups (e.g., bereavement, postretirement, substance abuse)
  Burdened caregivers groups
Verbal-centered groups for the cognitively impaired:
  Resocialization and remotivation groups
  Reality orientation groups
Creativity- and activity-centered groups:
  Dance-movement therapy groups
  Project groups
  Nutrition groups
  Drama, art, or poetry groups
Service and advocacy groups:
  Self-help groups
  Self-actualization groups
Settings:
  Ambulatory groups
  Day hospital and partial hospitalization groups
  Acute hospital groups
  Institutional settings (i.e., hospital groups, nursing home groups)

of growth, creativity, and self-expression; remediation of organic deficits in the cognitive and physical domains; and the provision of support, education, and assistance in coping with caregiver burden. Toseland (1995) also adds service/ advocacy groups as a group format, in which the group leader coordinates and facilitates group members to achieve an expressed social or even political task.

A key concept in this chapter is the requirement that the therapist be flexible in conducting the group. Differences between supportive and expressive groups and between depth and nondepth groups are frequently blurred. Many geriatric patients in fact are treated in some modified group that contains both insight-oriented and supportive approaches commingled. In many instances, the therapist's awareness of both psychodynamic and process considerations, as well as structured techniques of cognitive-behavioral skill acquisition, enhances therapeutic efficacy. Throughout, realistic therapeutic perspective that recognizes the scope for growth or restoration of lost interpersonal, emotional, and cognitive capacities is essential.

This chapter addresses these considerations by examining the indications for group therapy, the contemporary range of group therapy approaches, technical considerations for the therapist, and the effectiveness and outcome of these treatments.

INDICATIONS FOR GROUP THERAPY

A review by Klausner and Alexopoulous (1999) underscored the need to provide meaningful psychosocial treatment for the elderly, ideally integrated within the primary care setting to facilitate access. Psychosocial interventions, of which group therapy is a central element, generally may reduce psychological and physical morbidity through both the impact of direct treatment and enhanced compliance with other treatments, reducing excess disability. Failure to understand the psychological underpinnings of common patient concerns is a problem for patients and primary care practitioners that reduces utilization of effective services (Radley et al., 1997)

Social isolation, interpersonal alienation, maladaptive interpersonal skills, diminished self-worth, depressive disengagement, and withdrawal are common presenting features, and group therapy offers an opportunity for addressing these difficulties, promoting social engagement and the development of social networks (Wong, 1991). Group therapy may be employed as the sole treatment or be adjunctive to pharmacotherapy or individual therapy.

The need for provision of effective psychosocial interventions is evident in the large number of elderly reporting mood and anxiety disturbances. Gurland (1996) noted an incidence of 2%–4% for depressive disorders diagnosable according to the DSM-IV (*Diagnostic and Statistical Manual of Mental Disorders, Fourth Edition*, American Psychiatric Association, 1994) in community samples older than 65 years. This increases to 10%–15% if clinically significant depressive symptoms are included, mounting even higher within institutional settings. The common occurrence of bereavement in the elderly also poses a large risk for affective and psychosocial morbidity (Reynolds et al., 1999).

Because depression in the elderly is often a chronic, relapsing disorder with a high prevalence, even with initially effective pharmacological treatment (Murphy, 1983) the importance of the psychosocial therapies is underscored. This was noted by the 1997 National Institutes of Health (NIH) Consensus Development Update on the Diagnosis and Treatment of Depression in Late Life (Lebowitz et al., 1997), which recognized the need to evaluate psychosocial therapies in the acute, continuation, and maintenance process of treatment.

Although it remains unclear whether social isolation and lack of social supports cause depression or whether depression-induced loss of social skills results in isolation, it is clear that the depressed elderly are indeed more likely to have both diminished social supports and diminished social skills (Gallagher, 1981; Grant et al., 1988). What is cause and what is effect is often unclear, but this self-perpetuating, reverberating cycle can be interrupted at either point. Enhanced social integration improves outcome in depression (Sherbourne et al., 1995), and social integration and social support are important mediators of well-being and buffers against stress (Gurland, 1996).

Group therapy may be more acceptable and less anxiety provoking than individual therapy due to the collaborative sharing of concerns and mutual helpfulness. It provides direct support and fosters opportunities to develop interpersonal awareness and skills. Regressive feelings of dependency may also be diminished by participation in the group. In addition, the concrete opportunity for behavioral change and practice that occurs in all groups may hold special appeal for those older persons who may be less able to deal with abstract psychological issues. The current population of elderly is increasingly likely to have had earlier psychotherapy, increasing their understanding of and appreciation for psychosocial interventions.

In some instances, these objectives can be met entirely by the manifest content of the interaction around group activities. In other instances, these benefits can be accessed only by addressing the process of the group and effectively working through the patients' resistances to engagement. The ideal treatment setting offers the broadest range of group modalities—a form of therapeutic "buffet," phasing and tailoring groups to patients, ideally with graded levels of intensity and depth (Thompson et al., 2000). Resistance to engagement and the severity of presenting symptoms often determine the relative indications for verbal-centered or activity-centered groups. Depression is unlikely to be treated effectively by an activity-centered or creativity-centered group alone, and the resistive, devaluing patient is unlikely to connect effectively in such a setting. Activity-centered groups serve useful maintenance and prophylactic functions, and for the highly motivated individual, participation in such groups may be all that is required to maintain psychological integration. Referral to these groups should be linked to the special interests, talents, and concerns of the patient. The more depressed or functionally impaired patient may use activity-centered groups to good effect, in an ongoing fashion, following a period of more intensive treatment.

Group composition should be homogeneous for level of ego function, intellect, and degree of cognitive functioning. Chronological age generally is not a determining factor. In fact, the active elderly may be treated effectively in psychotherapy groups with younger patients. Such groups provide a rich opportunity to work through issues of feeling old and inadequate in a youthful society. On the other hand, even in homogeneous geriatric settings, mixing cognitively intact and impaired patients can result in the former feeling an aversion and unwillingness to engage and the latter being unable to sustain engagement.

Homogeneous groups generally become cohesive quickly and generally are more supportive (Salvendy, 1993). Feelings of universality are enhanced, but there is a risk that excessive homogeneity will result in a lack of contrasting perspective that can diminish the range of potential problem solving. In general, the importance to group members of being able to identify positively with one another should be recognized in the selection and composition of groups. Individuals who are significantly deviant from the group norm are more likely to be early dropouts (Yalom, 1995).

Group therapy is contraindicated for patients who are in acute crisis or who are suicidal; patients with active drug or alcohol abuse, unless the group is specific to that concern; paranoid or violently aggressive patients; patients with persistent inability to attend to the process of the group because of severe cognitive impairment, sedation, irremediable hearing loss, or differences in language; and difficult, characterologically disturbed patients who persistently attack and devalue others in maladaptive efforts to bolster their own self-esteem. These contraindications are relative and are intended to serve as guidelines to maintain the viability and effectiveness of the group and to avoid negative outcomes to any individual patient, such as group rejection or extrusion. A strong, well-established, and mature group is better able to contain a difficult patient than is a beginning, developmentally immature group. The group therapist needs to evaluate whether a particular group and a particular patient can benefit from one another at a particular time. Unlike the individual setting, in the group setting the therapist's selection of patients not only commits the therapist to the patient, but also commits each of the other group members to a relationship with that patient.

Preparation and pretraining of patients prior to entry into group therapy has not been specifically researched with the elderly, but the evidence for its usefulness in other patient populations, as reviewed in detail by Yalom (1995), is quite substantial. Preparation and pretraining are incorporated in virtually all cognitive and behavioral group treatments (Thompson et al., 1991). Preparation may emphasize provision of information alone or may directly aim at initiating therapeutic engagement by involving the client in role play or simulations (Thompson et al., 2000). Explaining the rationale of psychotherapy demystifies an otherwise anxiety-provoking situation, and preparation helps establish a therapeutic alliance and sets group norms regarding regular attendance, confidentiality, and extra group socialization. Preparation also should encompass clear setting of goals collaboratively, including specific foci and objectives. Effective pretraining results in enhanced group tenure, task adherence, increased hopefulness, reduced anxiety, and increased interaction and self-disclosure, thereby increasing the prospects for successful treatment (Yalom, 1995).

Dropout rates for group therapy with younger patients range between 10% and 50% (Yalom, 1995), and with the elderly the frequency rate is at least the same (Steuer et al., 1984). The likelihood of a premature dropout is increased further with the severity of depression, presence of severe physical illness, and a characterological style that devalues, externalizes, and blames. Patients' ability to choose the intervention confers a greater likelihood for completion of treatment (Rokke et al., 1999–2000).

In institutional settings, group therapy is further indicated to provide a forum to deal with the imposed accommodations to changes in life situation and the reduced feelings of autonomy. Loss of identity, isolation, and loneliness are also common complaints, notwithstanding the presence of others in the

TABLE 32-2.   Themes in group therapy

Loss of significant relationships
Loss of physical and cognitive capacities
Loss of functions and tasks
Loss of self-worth and self-esteem
Loneliness and isolation
Depression, demoralization, and shame
Dependency-autonomy conflicts
Interpersonal conflict with spouse and family
Hopelessness, helplessness, and purposelessness
Wish for restoration of a sense of competence, mastery, and identity
Engaging and negotiating the contemporary world

milieu. The opportunity to work through and reconcile interpersonal difficulties in institutional relationships may enhance the quality of life of residents in institutions. In addition, some settings have a heavy preponderance of female residents and staff, and group therapy may provide an opportunity for the relatively few men in the institution to meet, stimulating models of identification with male figures in the matriarchal environment typical of many nursing homes (Leszcz et al., 1985).

Examination of the themes that emerge in group therapy (see Table 32-2) illustrates that many of the psychological concerns of the elderly are generated by age-induced losses and changes and the patient's difficulty in negotiating the late-life developmental challenge of maintaining a sense of self that is continuous in the present with the past (Leszcz, 1987). Aging may necessitate a shift over the life span from a perspective of primary control, in which a person affects the environment to remove obstructions to his or her needs, to a perspective of secondary control, in which beliefs and attitudes must be realigned to encompass these obstructions. Failure to do so may lead to intense self-criticalness about personal competence (Heckhausen & Schultz, 1995). These themes shape the overall objectives of group therapies with the elderly (see Table 32-3).

TABLE 32-3.   Objectives of treatment

Restoration of a sense of self-esteem and self-worth
Reduction of isolation and promotion of interpersonal engagement
Symptom reduction and mastery
Acquisition of coping skills and interpersonal skills
Grieving and adaptation to loss
Appropriate acceptance of dependency and rational utilization of available resources
Enhanced compliance with medical care
Improved cognitive and behavioral function

GROUP THERAPY MODELS AND APPLICATION

Psychodynamic Group Psychotherapy

As reported by Tross and Blum (1988), a range of psychodynamic group approaches has been effectively employed. Kohut's (1984) conceptualization of narcissism and self-psychology has greatly influenced the conduct of individual and group psychotherapy with the elderly because of the understanding it provides of the internal and subjective experience of the elderly individual (Lazarus, 1980). This conceptualization is particularly relevant to the individual faced with the challenge of maintaining a sense of self in the face of the narcissistic injuries of aging and the loss of central functions, capacities, and self-object relationships. This conceptualization augments and facilitates the use of the interpersonal and interactive group therapeutic mechanisms described by Yalom (1995).

Group therapy provides a self-esteem, self-sustaining treatment matrix in which the narcissistic injuries to the self may be addressed and restored through the feeling of group cohesion and the provision of relationships that serve necessary self-object functions in addition to providing real objects for relatedness and support (Baker & Baker, 1993; Schwartzman, 1984). A central premise is that the self is at the center of the individual's psychosocial universe. It is the organizer and initiator of experience, shaped both by the individual's unique talents, achievements, resources, and capacities and by the relationships the individual maintains with self-objects (Baker & Baker, 1993).

Self-objects are interpersonal relationships that are experienced as being part of the individual's internal world—and not as distinct, separate relationship objects. The self-object relationship sustains, enhances, and completes the individual's sense of self. Through maturation, most of these self-object, mirroring, and soothing functions become internalized, but the independence of the individual from these relationships is relative and never absolute. The consequences of aging, for some, may increase the need for these narcissistic supplies to offset feelings of loss, depletion, and diminishment. The self-object transference may be to the other individuals, the group as a whole, or the therapist, and it serves to restore a sense of self-stability and vitality by providing one or more of four central elements (Baker & Baker, 1993): (1) mirroring self-objects, which value, praise, and admire the individual; (2) idealized self-objects, in whose presence the individual feels safe, protected, and worthwhile; (3) alter ego or twinning self-objects with whom the individual can feel an essential alikeness and resonance through the process of pairing with another person (Lothstein & Zimet, 1988); and (4) adversarial self-objects, with whom robust and vital engagement can be sustained, maintaining both autonomous opposition and empathic connectedness (Wolf, 1988).

The emphasis on empathic recognition of the subjective experience of the elderly in the group deepens the therapist's understanding of the processes of relationships, interactions, and resistances in the group and the importance of feeling "human amongst humans" (Kohut, 1984). With a self-psychology perspective, it becomes more possible to understand empathically the interpersonal phenomena of defensive withdrawal, haughty devaluation, grandiose exhibitionism, monopolization, idealization, and the pursuit of special relatedness as attempts to protect or stabilize the vulnerable sense of self (Stone & Whitman, 1977). Disruptive and alienating behavior that could threaten group cohesiveness can thereby be better contained, facilitating further opportunities for interpersonal engagement and interpersonal learning rather than leading to rebuke and condemnation, furthering the individual's despair about being understood or valued and fueling negative interpersonal cycles (Leszcz, 1992). In addition to the considerations of the individual's sense of self, group therapy also is well suited to address other psychodynamic considerations of individual member's core concerns and conflicts through the interpersonal articulation and feedback within the social microcosm of the group.

Reminiscence Group Therapy

The process of reminiscing, or life review (Butler, 1974; Poulton & Strassberg, 1986), has been employed in a variety of ways in psychotherapy groups. Conceptualized as a developmentally appropriate and natural process of review through which the elderly person can organize and evaluate his or her life, it has been used to promote reintegration of an individual's sense of self by having the person reconnect to what he or she was, fostering (in Eriksonian terms) the predominance of ego integrity over despair (Erikson, 1950). Although often used interchangeably, Burnside (1991) clarifies the distinction between the more comprehensive life review approaches that emphasize uncovering, exploration, and working through and the more narrow reminiscence approaches that emphasize ego support and aim to avoid generating anxiety.

Reminiscence has been used as a technique to enhance the development of cohesion in beginning groups and groups experiencing demoralization in the face of group developmental difficulties (Leszcz, 1997). In addition, it has been used effectively as an organizing anchor in group psychotherapy for more impaired patients (Lesser et al., 1981), creating a clear and achievable focus that enhances self-esteem. It may rekindle a desire for vital engagement again. These processes may emerge spontaneously or follow a prescribed, chronological format (Goldwasser et al., 1982; Kavanagh & Burnside, 1992). Only positive events may be addressed, milestoning (Lowenthal & Marrazzo, 1990), or the life review may be more complete to promote the individual's mourning and acceptance of life as it indeed was.

In practice, the process of reminiscing may be used adaptively or maladaptively, correlated with the way it is experienced by the group members and managed by the group therapist. At its best, the reminiscing process fleshes out individuals within the group and makes them three-dimensional people rather than one-dimensional objects of projection for one another. It restores feelings of worth, stature, and competence through the articulation of past successes and the recollection of prior credentials and, through the mutual reverberations and identifications, promotes feelings of affiliation and much needed social support (Wong, 1991).

What has been of greatest importance to any individual often cannot be assumed without confirmation, and subjective valuation may be very different from objective valuation. Reminiscing about previous challenges that have been mastered often helps to soothe the apprehension about facing the unknown future. Further, appropriate grieving and conflict resolution may be facilitated, promoting better engagement in the current environment.

However, with profoundly depressed or withdrawn patients, reminiscing may result in a further preoccupation with the past; guilt over irreparable errors; and a heightened, morbid self-absorption that results in social alienation. In such instances, group cohesion can be seriously undermined, and the therapist needs to determine if the reminiscing is serving the intended purpose of deepening the group members' understanding of one another, strengthening feelings of group cohesion and universality, and promoting both a sense of mastery and willingness to engage.

Benefits can be maximized and risks reduced if the therapist establishes a group norm that all reminiscing, and the experience of talking about, listening to, and sharing, be brought back centripetally into the here and now of the group and examined at the interpersonal level (Poulton & Strassberg, 1986). This structuring of the reminiscing process plays a critical role in the effectiveness of this approach (Bachar et al., 1991).

Cognitive-Behavioral Group Therapy

Cognitive-behavioral group therapy emphasizes conscious cognition and learning, adapting behavioral strategies and the cognitive therapy model to the group setting. It is well suited to address disturbances in mood and is certainly the modality that has been best researched and evaluated in terms of effectiveness in the realm of geriatric group therapy (Thompson et al., 2000). From a cognitive perspective, depression is the product of faulty information processing, impacting on and shaped by negative schemas—beliefs about oneself in relationship to the world—and resulting in the prototypical negative cognitive triad (Thompson et al., 2000). The treatment aims to restore self-efficacy.

Three overarching elements define the group cognitive-behavioral therapy (CBT) model: (1) mood monitoring, (2) increasing pleasurable activities, and (3) monitoring dysfunctional thoughts and attitudes. Each area requires a process of logging and recording mood, thoughts, and behaviors to identify the links between domains (Thompson et al., 2000). With geriatric patients, a modified thought record, identified as the Daily Record of Unhelpful Thoughts (DRUT), has been employed (Thompson et al., 2000) to facilitate tracking the interconnection between thoughts, feelings, and behaviors.

Treatment aims to (1) help patients identify and monitor their reactions in particular situations; (2) confront and correct distortions by realignment of the attributions of meaning made by the individual; (3) determine the basic assumptions and themes that shape these reactions; (4) practice alternative cognitive and behavioral responses to anticipated stresses by encouraging patients to tackle ever-increasing challenges; and (5) achieve mastery and maintenance of positive affects that breed alternative and more correct and objective assumptions (Beck, 1995). A wide range of cognitive errors and associated thought processes are illuminated and corrected, including defocusing; depersonalizing; challenging the assumption that thoughts are facts; reducing dichotomous, all-or-nothing thinking; and reframing and focusing attention on partial positive outcomes as a way to counteract cognitive distortions (Steinmetz et al., 1985; Thompson et al., 1991).

In this model, repetitive, maladaptive, depressogenic behaviors and cognitions are viewed as automatic. They reflect a form of learned behavior that is blind to other options. Psychodynamic considerations and questions of motivation are viewed as irrelevant, and process phenomena within the group are generally not a focus of intervention unless the process issues are interfering with group functioning.

Social isolation and the lack of alternative input exacerbate negative, self-devaluing, and self-blaming assumptions and make some elderly individuals particularly prone to distortions in attributing meaning (Parham et al., 1982). The exchange and feedback that occur in a group are particularly well suited to confronting such assumptions and distortions. Treatment promotes the realignment and objectification of cognitive assumptions and the attribution of meaning to events and experiences. The emphasis placed on collaborative acquisition of improved coping is also less likely to contribute to a sense of devaluation or stigmatization.

More focused behavioral approaches (Gallagher, 1981; Lewinsohn et al., 1985) employ modeling, role playing, didactic discussions, and feedback about each group member's efforts in using skills required to reengage with pleasurable experiences. The focus is on external and observable behavior only. The aim of treatment is to break the vicious cycle of depressed mood, resulting in reduced interaction and reduced stimulation of positive interpersonal reinforcement, further social withdrawal, and the consequent erosion of social skills.

Lewinsohn and colleagues (Lewinsohn, 1974; Lewinsohn et al., 1985), emphasizing the centrality of interpersonal interaction, explained depression in behavioral terms as a reduction of social reinforcement obtained by the depressed individual from the environment as a reflection of diminished skills or diminished availability of reinforcement due to loss or to an excess of aversive experiences. Individual predispositions, attributions, and consequent interactional processes increase vulnerability or resilience. Common elements of CBT approaches for the treatment of depression emphasize the principles that the patient can control and modify behavior; that treatment provides skills to do so, in a patient-congruent fashion; that these skills are the patient's and not the treater's; and that these skills directly affect mood (Lewinsohn et al., 1985).

Relaxation techniques and problem-solving skills, as well as time management, self-assertion and self-expression, may also be taught. Meditation, relaxation, and visual imagery techniques can also be utilized with the elderly (Abraham et al., 1992).

The format of CBT groups often is structured to set an agenda each session regarding a focus on particular skills or techniques, set time aside to review and to assign homework assignments, and to conclude each session with a summary. Regular evaluation of progress is essential, with elaboration of the obstructions to task completion or compliance. This provides group members with the opportunity to problem solve, reflect on their experiences, or support and reinforce each other. Homework assignments should be viewed as skill-building opportunities, and as the group matures, even over the relatively brief course of 10 to 12 sessions, a breadth of tailored homework may be assigned (Thompson et al., 2000).

Integrated Verbal-Centered Group Therapy

In clinical practice, the three models—psychodynamic, life review, and cognitive-behavioral—may be effectively integrated into an approach that capitalizes on the strengths of each. This reflects a growing move within psychotherapy to integrate models seriously and meaningfully through the construction of overarching models of theoretical understanding (Wachtel, 1991). Norcross (1995) noted that the move to psychotherapy integration reflects the pursuit of improved efficacy, efficiency, and applicability. Limitations of monomodal approaches, and the reports of equivalence in some comparative trials (Albeniz & Holmes, 1996), have also fueled this movement.

Focusing on the elaboration of affect and self-disclosure is useful to gain an understanding of the individual, and the life review further fleshes out this understanding. However, patients require and highly value skill acquisition (Thompson et al., 2000). Skill acquisition aids in mastery, restoration of competence, and generalization of gains and amplifies the very important therapeutic factor of group cohesion by virtue of the feeling of shared achievement in the group. On the other hand, disregard for the group process or the subjective experience of the individual can result in the assumption of an unempathetic, alienating, superficial, "pick yourself up by the bootstraps" orientation by the group.

Depth understanding of the subjective internal experience of interpersonal behavior maximizes the opportunities for behavioral prescriptions (Kiesler, 1996). Augmenting the documented effectiveness of "cold processing," role playing, simulations, and modeling to illuminate maladaptive interpersonal skills and interpersonal distortions with the direct, in vivo, "hot processing" of a more interactive group that focuses on the actual interpersonal relationships created in the here and now of the group may generate additional benefit, particularly for patients with comorbid personality disturbance, who may have blind spots about their interpersonal process (Leszcz, 1992; Safran & Segal, 1990).

In an integrated model, individuals in the group have the opportunity, for example, of examining their experience of isolation and loneliness, exploring what they do that minimizes and maximizes their isolation and loneliness, and practicing new skills and risk taking. A productive and logically consistent synthesis is formed of the patients' subjective experiences and the specific importance of their interpersonal relatedness, the historical context of the individuals and their relationships, coupled with challenging of cognitive and interpersonal distortions and direct behavioral practice of successful relating. This model emphasizes the individual's authorship of his or her relational world, building on the social microcosm of the treatment experience to foster, actively and at times prescriptively, an adaptive spiral from the group into the larger environment in the services of the restoration of a more stable sense of self.

Schmid and Rouslin (1992) described another dimension to integrated group therapy, actively linking a predischarge hospitalized psychiatric patients' group with an aftercare group. This group includes significant family members along with the identified patients, facilitating both reentry to the community and continuity of care. Patient-caregiver issues can be addressed, and this approach also provides a forum for provision to the family members of clarification of active treatment issues.

Homogeneous Groups

There is a broad range of homogeneous groups, which generally meet for a short-term contract of 8 to 20 sessions. Their composition is generally determined by a particular common problem, characteristic, or developmental issue. A relevant model is that of postretirement groups (Salvendy, 1989), which may emphasize mutual support to counter the isolation and the loss of self-esteem induced by loss of employment status. Also prominent are groups for the recently bereaved (Lund & Caserta, 1992). The latter may be led professionally or may use a self-help model. Group interventions have also been employed to treat substance abuse and dependence in the elderly (Segal et al., 1996). In these models, mutual identification fosters rapid cohesion within the group, providing opportunities to examine shared developmental concerns and shared areas of distress.

Self-Help Groups

A range of community-based groups that operate with and without professional input are also important and provide support, advocacy, and opportunities for growth and normalize adaptational challenges (Lieberman & Gourash-Bliwise, 1985; Toseland et al., 1995). Their role and scope are likely to increase in the future (Klausner & Alexopoulous, 1999), reflecting the growth of self-help groups across all ages.

The interface with professional leadership and training is complex. Lieberman and Gourash-Bliwise (1985) noted the risk of impairing the therapeutic effectiveness of peer-led groups by providing limited training, such that the peer leaders may be neither full-fledged peers nor well-trained leaders, introducing countertherapeutic elements of hierarchy and diminished client control.

Groups for Burdened Caregivers

Caregiver groups have developed in response to the increasing number of frail or cognitively impaired and dementing individuals cared for at home by their families (Kahan et al., 1985; Saul, 1988). Stone (1991) estimated that over 2 million individuals in the United States provide intensive primary care to family members, while an additional 2 million provide assistance with more instrumental elements of daily living.

The rationale for these groups stems from the recognition that caregivers often are highly burdened, isolated, exhausted, and depressed (Baldwin et al., 1989; Thompson et al., 2000). The absence of social supports exacerbates the caregivers' strain (Zarit et al., 1980). A central psychological issue is the working through of the pain of providing care for a loved one who may have lost the capacity not only to express gratitude, but also to recognize the caregiver or whose intermittent periods of recognition and lucidity may confuse and frustrate the caregiver. The declining cognitive capacities appear to be most stressful to many caregivers, even beyond the physical decline (Toseland, 1995). Prominent issues relate to coping with the intense dependence the impaired individual has on the caregiver. Hence, providing this validation within the group is highly valued by participants. Homogeneity of situation promotes rapidly cohesive groups with much self-disclosure and mutual support. Extragroup contact is endorsed, and the self-help nature of the group is supported as well.

Objectives of these groups include (1) education about the dementing or illness process and available resources, as well as learning ways of interacting with the patient and providing care; (2) working through loss and grief by providing opportunities for ventilation, promoting appropriate disengagement, and promoting realistic decisions about placement, if necessary; (3) acquiring skills in problem solving and stress reduction; (4) normalizing and legitimizing the needs of the caregiver, thereby promoting self-care and self-regard, to counter isolation and self-neglect; (5) working through relationships with health care professionals, including how to advocate effectively; (6) validating and affirming the efforts of the caregiver; and (7) less commonly, helping individuals work through anger and guilt. An overarching focus that centers on the caregiver directly relates to self-management skills, recognizing the understandable strains the caregiver experiences in situations that are not easily managed or avoided. In some cognitive-behavioral frameworks, this is the central focus of the group intervention, with active use of psychoeducation, role playing, and simulations (Thompson et al., 2000). The more charged affective aspects of caregiving are not always readily accessed in a very highly focused and time-limited group treatment, and added treatment may be required (Toseland, 1995; Toseland et al., 1989).

VERBAL-CENTERED GROUPS FOR THE COGNITIVELY IMPAIRED

Resocialization and Remotivation Groups

Since Linden's pioneering group work (1953), there has been growing recognition of the need to develop and evaluate psychosocial, nonpharmacological interventions for the treatment of late-life dementias, as noted in contemporary practice guidelines (American Psychiatric Association, 1997). Group therapy aims at stimulation and reengagement through leader-originated or patient-originated discussion and interaction, melded with the provision of as much sensory stimulation as possible to engage reality.

These groups focus on members' strengths and fundamental humanness and, although highly structured, do have a group process that needs to be attended to and understood by the therapist. The groups achieve interpersonal engagement more through the structure and content of the group than through the process. Patient engagement is both prompted and reinforced by the therapist repeatedly.

The array of content stimuli offered should be broad to maximize opportunities for effective activation and engagement. The leader may increase or decrease the amount of attention placed on process or activity according to patient needs, but throughout must be accepting and encouraging of patient communication. Reinforcement of interaction and cohesive, group-valuing comments need to be provided. Cognitive exercises, activity and word games, life review, discussions, and participation in music, art, baking, and physical exercise are all components of these groups. The range is virtually limitless, but in each instance, the emphasis should be on sensory stimulation, improved ego function, reality orientation, memory, judgment, problem solving, and interaction (Burnside, 1978; Saul, 1988; Toseland, 1995). Groups of 6 to 10 participants work best in this format as group size must be small enough to engage all members regularly.

Reality Orientation Groups

Objectives of reality orientation groups (Drummond et al., 1978) are the reversal of social and verbal disengagement and of the diminished use of cognitive functions by continual stimulation and reorientation in an interactive environment. There is substantial overlap between reality orientation groups and resocialization and remotivation groups. Reality orientation occurs in two modes. The chief mode is a 24-hour milieu approach to provide consistent and persistent orientation of the individual, making the milieu as rational and knowable as possible. The second mode is classroom or group reality orientation. The reality orientation group room contains a full array of multisensory stimuli. Every opportunity is utilized to elucidate and remind individual patients of the who, where, what, and why of what is going on in a firm, friendly, nondemanding fashion, repeatedly bringing the patient back to the immediate present.

Reinforcement for successful reorientation can be interpersonal or behavioral (Miller, 1977) and can be linked to all activities of daily living. Reality orientation therapy may be utilized effectively to prepare for further resocialization therapy or reminiscence therapy because prior reality orientation therapy has a significant, priming impact on the effective utilization of subsequent therapeutic interventions (Baines et al., 1987). Small group reality orientation enhances the 24-hour program, but appears to be of less use in the absence of the more comprehensive milieu approach. Furthermore, without active therapeutic input and reinforcement, no generalization occurs, and learning is readily extinguished.

Some preliminary efforts are also being made in the utilization of cognitive and behavioral approaches in the treatment of depressed patients with Alzheimer's disease to decrease excess disability. The involvement of family members is essential to organize and coordinate the treatment program for their cognitively impaired relative (Teri & Gallagher-Thompson, 1991). It is imperative to ensure that the reality orientation approach is applied in a humane and dignified fashion as it is likely that the key ingredient in any possible effectiveness emerges from human interaction and not behavioral contingencies (Toseland, 1995).

Validation techniques (Feil, 1983) provide a modified form of reality orientation to more impaired individuals who do not respond well to reality orientation. Validation therapy posits that each expression or action put forward by the cognitively impaired individual reflects a compromised, but meaningful, effort at communication. Conferring meaning rather than dismissing the communication as irrelevant is a central aspect of this intervention (Feil, 1983). The group leader maintains a very high level of verbal and nonverbal engagement with each group member, responding, mirroring, and rephrasing consistently and repeatedly.

Integrative group psychotherapy employing wellness principles of relaxation techniques, sensory awareness, and guided imagery has been utilized with cognitively impaired institutionalized elderly individuals; its aim was to improve self-awareness, health promotion, and self-integrity (Lantz et al., 1997). Weekly sessions of an hour, over a minimum period of 10 weeks, improved patients' agitation and behavioral disruption.

CREATIVITY-CENTERED
AND ACTIVITY-CENTERED GROUPS

There is a broad range of activity-centered and creativity-centered groups, with substantial interplay among them (MacLennan et al., 1988). These groups provide opportunities for patients whose verbal skills may be diminished to express and rekindle a sense of self through the artistic or creative process, which is enhanced through working together with others. Both pleasure and mastery may be stimulated, challenging self-denigration and constricting distortions about the self. In many instances, the nonverbal expression may be of even greater psychological depth than the verbal expression. The objective is not only to experience art, but also to create it. These modalities are also important vehicles to retain a sense of self in the midst of institutional life, with its tendency toward homogenization and the blurring of individual differences. Creative expression is used as a form of engagement with the world and with others, as well as an expression of self.

Dance movement therapy focuses on the integration of the self through reconnection of the individual with his or her body (Samberg, 1988). It is not task oriented like physical exercise, but rather is process oriented, promoting the opportunity to study the relationship among mood, movement, and physical sensations. In a conceptual fashion analogous to the way that cognitive therapy challenges cognitive distortions and may treat depression by altering the way in which a person thinks about himself or herself, dance movement therapy aims at ameliorating depression and demoralization by evoking positive and pleasurable bodily expressions. This therapy involves challenging negative or depressive assumptions of the physical self, its restrictions, and its limitations and increasing a person's sense of physical mastery.

TECHNICAL APPLICATIONS OF GROUP THERAPY

General Considerations

The objectives and indications of the various geriatric group therapies necessitate certain adaptations in therapist technique. The elderly are often resistant to engaging in group psychotherapy and, especially when depressed, behave in ways that interfere with the development of group cohesion. Withdrawal, devaluing self and others, blaming, and hopelessness generally are not conducive to group cohesion.

It is striking that, regardless of the model of group therapy used, the recommended therapist posture and attitude is the same (Gallagher, 1981). In their review of the effectiveness of group therapy with the elderly, Tross and Blum (1988) concluded that the therapist's posture of respect, hopefulness, genuine warmth, and empathy appears to be as important as the therapist's theoretical rationale. In fact, Williams-Barnard and Lindell (1992) confirmed this intuitive truth in their study of the significant and powerful impact on patients' self-concept of the direct effect of the degree to which rated group leaders demonstrated attitudes and behaviors toward group members that reflected the Rogerian concept of *prizing*—unconditional positive reward.

Advances in psychotherapy research have demonstrated the value of clarity in model and application, adding specificity to the nonspecific elements of psychotherapy. Some interventions have been written in the form of therapy manuals to afford easy replicability and mechanisms to monitor therapist model adherence (Thompson et al., 2000).

In general, the group leader carries a greater burden of responsibility to initiate and activate a geriatric group than is the case for groups of younger patients (Thompson et al., 1991). The group leader anchors the group, ensuring the psychological integrity of each individual and the logistical and functional integrity of the group as a whole. Determining a set and inviolate time for the group in an inviolate and comfortable location, free from time conflicts with other appointments, is essential. The format of the intervention should also reflect ethnic competence (Henderson et al., 1993) in that it is culturally attuned and respectful of cultural diversity and the unique beliefs, customs, and attitudes of the identified population.

Active outreach by the group leaders to reduce fluctuations in composition of the group is a prerequisite for effective treatment. A cohesive group may not form spontaneously, and waiting for the group to activate itself is likely to result in a contagion of demoralization and group dropouts. Within institutional settings, cohesion may be fostered by the therapist functioning as a gatekeeper, pacing the entry of new members so that a sense of stability and reliability is achieved within the group. Absences, and even deaths, must be addressed, staying alert to the burden of affect generated.

In view of the difficulty that some elderly persons have in getting started in the morning and the requirements of arranging transportation, it may be preferable to select a late morning or midafternoon time for the group. Normally, such a time would foredoom a younger person's group, but with the elderly it may be ideal as it also promotes the opportunity for extragroup contact around lunch and coffee. In younger persons' groups, extragroup contact is generally prohibited because it often leads to subgrouping and, ultimately, to fragmentation in the group. In the geriatric population, however, extragroup contact may be fostered, with the goal of providing opportunities for real relatedness because the elderly do experience a realistic reduction in opportunities for such engagement. Furthermore, in institutional settings, extragroup contacts are a fact of life. The key to successful management of this extragroup contact or subgrouping is to diminish the boundary of secretiveness around the relationships and to bring these interactions into the purview of the group, even if it is only to endorse and not to interpret them (Lothstein & Zimet,

1988). Extragroup contact can be a rich source of feedback about the individuals in the group, reducing treatment blind spots while providing an opportunity to practice interpersonal skills learned in the group proper.

While drawing attention to certain parameters that may be useful in conducting group therapy with the elderly, it is important also to recognize that excessive focus on the patients' limits and vulnerabilities may emphasize deficits and underplay patients' strengths, resources, and capacity to tolerate the process of working through. The patient's readiness for change, growth, and resolution of long-standing concerns and psychological conflicts may be quite substantial. Pollock contends that the elderly are essentially dealing with forces and events that must be dealt with by all individuals across the entire life span. He describes the process of mourning the loss of what was, to facilitate the liberation of what will be, as a lifelong process, often resulting in creativity and regeneration (Pollock, 1987). Hence, the therapist must be alert to potential sources of ageism or countertransference that would tend to emphasize supportive interventions when expressive interventions would be better indicated (Leszcz, 1987). At the same time, it is also essential not to overload the group members with affect, ensuring a tolerable pace and affect load to challenge the patient's premise that demoralization is a necessary or fixed state of aging (Leszcz, 1999).

In situations in which both pharmacotherapy and psychotherapy are employed concurrently, successful treatment is facilitated by bilateral respect for each treatment's contribution, with alertness for devaluation of the subjective meaning or importance of either modality.

Verbal-Centered Groups

Verbal-centered groups function best with 6 to 10 patients and generally will meet weekly in ambulatory settings or as frequently as daily in partial hospitalization and day hospital institutional settings. Groups with larger membership appear to be less useful psychotherapeutically (Gorey & Cryns, 1991). However, activity-centered and creativity-centered groups may function quite well with much larger numbers and may benefit from multiple leaders. The cognitively intact patients may participate in the group meeting for 1 to 1.5 hours, whereas cognitively impaired patients generally make better use of briefer time frames (45 minutes) in light of their reduced attention and concentration. Duration of treatment is often focused for 12 to16 weeks. There is growing awareness, however, of the need to provide longer exposure to treatment through a continuation and maintenance phase, which employs intermittent booster sessions and meets less frequently, perhaps monthly for an open-ended period (Reynolds et al., 1999).

The group therapist should ensure that the therapy is an esteem-enhancing and nonfailure experience for each member. A related task is that of protecting the group from fragmentation and rupture, a function more easily achieved when the therapist empathically recognizes the subjective experience of each group member. Awareness of what is subjectively important to each individual provides the therapist with a direction for the treatment and safeguards against the individual's loss of identity through group homogenization. Supporting even small gains and steps toward self-assertion and self-expression are essential.

Face-to-face interaction, direct contact, mutual support, and interaction in the here and now of the group will need to be reinforced repeatedly by the therapist, as should any pro-group cohesive interaction or feedback. The initial perspective articulated by Yalom and Terrazas (1967) of "ego enhancement" continues to be pivotal. They recommended that therapists always search for the central vulnerability, interpersonal core, or adaptive focus in every interchange. Externalization of blame for failures of the self and projection, devaluation, and denigration pose particular therapeutic challenges as these defenses are often quite ego-syntonic and valued by the patient (Lazarus & Groves, 1987). The therapist who focuses on inviting desired behavior rather than only rebuffing what is undesirable enhances group cohesion and the opportunities for the group to feel effective without damaging its members through hostile confrontation. For example, the therapist's efforts at accessing the loneliness that resides beneath manifest hostility may make an off-putting member of the group more approachable and comprehensible to his or her peers.

The relevance of each patient's comments and communications should be noted. The group language and metaphors should be familiar and resonant to the group members and voiced in a culturally acceptable form. Diversity will need to be endorsed actively and viewed as an opportunity for learning from one another, challenging prejudices as self-limiting attitudes (Toseland, 1995). The group may move at a slower pace than with younger adults, and the therapist may need to reframe, integrate, translate, summarize, and underscore, ideally in a fashion that is not excessively gratifying of dependency needs but that continues respectfully to insist on patients being accountable for themselves.

In those instances when sensory impairment is prominent, the use of audio aids such as FM (frequency modulation) amplifying systems is an additional consideration, but this will be of little use if the hearing impairment is used defensively to maintain isolation and disengagement. Specific accommodations must be made in response to the patient who is hearing impaired. These may include speaking more slowly or clearly, with appropriate pauses; reducing crosstalk; eliminating background room noise; and repeating and restating to ensure that the communication has been understood (Toseland, 1995).

When skill acquisition and homework assignments are a prominent aspect of the treatment, enlisting a reliable family member to prompt and support the patient between sessions can be invaluable. Other modifications that are required in administering CBT group interventions with the elderly include simplification of the thought records and mood and pleasurable activities logs. A slower pace, with greater repetition, and provision of ample time for registration and consolidation of techniques is also helpful. Manuals for the elderly patient's personal use also need revision to ensure access and clarity (Yost et al., 1986).

Psychoeducational groups aim to provide information and foster mastery through enhanced knowledge and improved individual competence and compliance with positive health behaviors. Models for group therapy that employ telephone conference calls are also emerging, building on the experience reported with the blind and the physically disabled (Kaslyn, 1999). These models recognize that at times logistical impediments to physical attendance are insurmountable, and the phone conference is the only viable alternative for housebound individuals. Technological advances will likely make this model even more accessible in the future. The absence of visual nonverbal cues and face-to-face interaction will understandably place a much greater burden on the therapist to attend to language, inflection, volume, and other sound cues as a way of understanding group process and individual concerns. Practitioners of this model note that, in contrast to the manifest difficulties, telephone group work offers advantages related to access, convenience, and anonymity that reduce inhibitions about stigma and judgment. These groups appear to function best with fewer participants, around 4, as it becomes progressively more difficult to keep track of one another in a larger telephone group conference call (Kaslyn, 1999).

Activity-Centered Groups

Activity-centered groups and verbal groups for the cognitively impaired also require substantial therapist activity. Structured exercises and activities cannot be prescribed without the therapist's active and genuine participation to safeguard against the group feeling patronized. In resocialization and remotivation groups, patient initiative and responsibility enhance the group functions, and such groups are experienced as more cohesive than leader-dependent groups in which there is little patient initiation.

SPECIAL PROBLEMS

A broad range of countertransferential reactions may emerge in the treatment of the elderly, as noted elsewhere in this volume, including existential anxiety about confronting personal limits in the face of evident decline, isolation, and mortality (Yalom, 1980). Along with the countertransferential issues faced by the individual therapist due to the therapist's exposure within the group, because of group pressures, the group therapist is more vulnerable to a complementary response to the group's depressive demoralization and feelings of futility. The demoralization expressed and experienced by group members, coupled with skepticism or a dismissive posture toward a much younger therapist, may generate a sense of being therapeutically de-skilled (Toseland, 1995). Warning signs include the therapist's boredom, lateness, or even cancellation of meetings with the rationalization that the group members will not notice the missed meeting (Leszcz, 1987). In fact, the opposite appears true. Geriatric groups can be exquisitely sensitive to feeling devalued and diminished, although their reaction and protest may be more silent and isolative than angry.

Conversely, the therapist may be an idealized object, the recipient of patients' projections of lost successes, health, and competence. The idealization is contained by the therapist more readily if the therapist can recognize its transferential, self-object roots and not feel personally overstimulated (Leszcz et al., 1985). Alternately, if the idealization fails to strengthen and comfort group members, but leaves them feeling bereft of any personal power or efficacy, it needs to be confronted actively.

Resistances to engagement, dependence on authority, and, frequently, inexperience in verbalization may slow the group work and make it more arduous than group work with younger patients. The therapist may feel devalued in identification with patients who devalue themselves. Group members may resist joining or affiliating if participation stimulates negative identification with illness and decline. Searching for common ground without excessive homogenization is important in this area (Kelly, 1999). Consultation, supervision, and cotherapy serve to diminish these potential countertransferential difficulties by diluting their intensity and providing an opportunity for their recognition and exploration. The burden of activating the group and engaging resistant patients is decreased by sharing the responsibility among coleaders. In addition, cotherapy ensures that the group meets regularly despite therapists' vacations or illnesses and thereby reduces threats to the group's integrity.

In institutional settings, it is useful if at least one of the coleaders is a regular team member of the ward or floor staff to facilitate exchange of information and treatment planning. Cotherapy also may provide more engagement with impaired individuals, who require direct and specific input, and at times containment, to make their continued participation tenable (Toseland, 1995). The group program should be experienced as an integrated and integral part of the overall treatment. Without administrative and institutional support, logistical obstacles to attendance emerge. Furthermore, both depth and nondepth approaches need to be valued; otherwise, interdisciplinary rivalries produce subtle devaluation of various parts of the group treatment, which can be detected by the patients and lead to their reluctance to participate. A strong alliance between treaters and administrators is essential (Klausner & Alexopoulous, 1999).

The general psychology of the milieu exerts significant influence on the actual group treatments (Astrachan et al., 1968). Group therapy both influences and is influenced by its setting, and generally staff morale is enhanced on wards where there is an opportunity for active psychological treatment (Reichenfeld et al., 1973).

An additional challenge in group therapy with the elderly is the presence of physical illness, notwithstanding the fact that real deficits may become the focus of specific skill acquisition, problem solving, and cognitive interventions. Physical impairment requires some adaptations of techniques in recognition of limitations placed on certain behavioral interventions by an individual's physical impairment (Gallagher, 1981). Physical impairment interferes logistically with attendance and participation in the group and may result in group attrition. Steuer and Hammen (1983) similarly commented on the slower pace of cognitive approaches with elderly patients, who have a tendency to be more concrete and less abstract than younger patients.

The interplay among real and excess disability, true restriction, and treatment resistance is complex and requires diligence and patience to sort out. The group is vulnerable to demoralization because of physical illness and impairment, but if contained effectively, the presence of real illness and real physical threats provides an opportunity for group members to address issues of quality of life, death, and dying.

Termination issues may present both challenges and opportunities. When successful, the group may be viewed as one of the most meaningful encounters of the week for certain individuals. Hence, from the outset, encouragement of the transfer of gains and skills into the larger world is critical. Although booster sessions that are less frequent may reduce some of the feelings of loss, mourning and reengagement within the group itself can be a useful bridge to the world at large. Demonstrating to group participants that they have achieved meaningful engagement with one another, after beginning as strangers, sets the stage for further transferal of skills from the present to the future.

OUTCOME OF GROUP THERAPY

Early research tended to employ small sample sizes, brief time frames, and the study of nonpatient populations; had a lack of consensus on outcome measures; and utilized patients receiving more than one form of treatment at a time. Ethical difficulties in maintaining a nontreatment control group have hampered evaluation of the outcome of group treatments (Parham et al., 1982; Steuer et al., 1984). More recent research, particularly with geriatric depression, has demonstrated significant effectiveness. In a fashion that mirrors the finding with nongeriatric patients, group and individual therapy appear equally effective, pointing to the added benefit of group therapy's efficiency with regard to therapist resources and time (Arean & Miranda, 1996). By combining multiple studies, meta-analyses have overcome the limits of determining effectiveness in small studies. Scogin and McElreath (1994) concluded that psychosocial interventions, among which group therapies are prominent, achieve a robust effect size, and they noted substantial impact. There is sufficient outcome research to point with optimism to a number of conclusions about the usefulness, efficacy, and practical considerations of group therapies with the elderly.

Cognitively Intact Patients

Group psychotherapy is significantly superior to no treatment (Tross & Blum, 1988), although group therapy alone is probably less effective than psycho-pharmacotherapy in the treatment of severe depression in the elderly (Gorey & Cryns, 1991; Steuer & Hammen, 1983). Group therapy can play a strong ad-junctive role, and in some instances, psychotherapy may be the only treatment patients can tolerate medically. Combined psychotherapy and pharmacother-apy increase tenure in treatment as each modality affects a different set of con-cerns (Gallagher-Thompson & Thompson, 1995; Reynolds et al., 1999). There is evidence that, across all ages, cognitive therapy is more effective at reducing relapse rates of depression in follow-up than antidepressant medication alone (Gloaguen et al., 1998).

The strongest and most methodologically sound efficacy data for group therapy of geriatric major depression is based on cognitive-behavioral approaches, underscoring the importance of the acquisition of specific coping skills (Rokke et al., 1999–2000). However, there is evidence for the significant effectiveness of other coherent and rational models of group therapy, including the psycho-dynamic approaches, in reducing symptoms of depression, improving interper-sonal and social functioning, and bolstering self-esteem (Gallagher et al., 1982; Steuer et al., 1984; Sweet et al., 1989; Thompson et al., 1991). Much of the comparative research underscores similar and significant rates of effectiveness in the comparison of cognitive, behavioral, and psychodynamic psychotherapy in the treatment of geriatric depression, with substantial durability of gains at 2-year follow-up (Gallagher-Thompson et al., 1990). All treatment should fos-ter a sense of improved self-efficacy and acquisition of coping skills to improve resilience. Skill acquisition confers greater posttreatment durability of positive outcomes achieved (Gloaguen et al., 1998; Rokke et al., 1999–2000).

Structured reminiscing group therapy is significantly superior to unstruc-tured group therapy in the treatment of elderly depressed inpatients in terms of effectiveness, patient participation, and subjective valuation, and the poten-tial exists for patient deterioration in unstructured and undirected group treat-ments (Bachar et al., 1991). The effectiveness of reminiscence approaches, such as a structured autobiographical group, is reflected in significant improvements in measures of self-acceptance and feelings of validation of personal efforts in life (Botella & Feixas, 1992–1993). Beyond structured reminiscing therapy, skills achieved by social problem-solving groups confer greater gains in geriat-ric depression than reminiscence alone.

In general, improvements in psychological well-being correlate signifi-cantly with both the amount of each individual's interpersonal engagement and interaction within the group (Rattenbury & Stones, 1989) and with the experi-ence of interpersonal effectiveness and competence within the group (Moran & Gatz, 1987). The patient's choice of intervention, as opposed to prescription, confers greater tenure in treatment and reduces early noncompletion (Rokke et al., 1999–2000). Group therapy decreases anxiety and enhances group members' ability to deal with emotions verbally and to use the present more than the past to sustain self-esteem (Lieberman & Gaurash, 1979). Cognitive-behavioral group intervention also reduces symptoms of anxiety associated with social avoidance and cognitive symptoms of anxiety (Radley et al., 1997). Group cognitive therapy appears to be a modality that will draw much attention in the future due to its significant effectiveness and its ready description and guide for treaters that lends itself to more widespread and reliable clinical application (Thompson et al., 2000; Yost et al., 1986).

Some interesting questions regarding specific treatment benefits are also raised regarding the role of group therapy for the spousally bereaved. Participants are generally consistent in their report of high satisfaction and positive valuation of the group experience, both for peer-led and leader-led groups, particularly regarding the provision of social and emotional support (Lieberman & Yalom, 1992; Lund & Caserta, 1992). However, Lieberman and Yalom (1992) concluded that, in their sample of midlife and late-life bereaved spouses treated in a brief group therapy, there were no significant treatment benefits at 1-year follow-up. Regardless of the degree of initial distress, all bereaved individuals improved, leaving open for further scrutiny the role of psychological interventions in spousal bereavement.

Perhaps answers to this and related questions reside in the need to determine what is an effective dosage of psychotherapeutic intervention in terms of duration and intensity, along with improved assessment of who requires treatment and of treatment matching (Lund & Caserta, 1992). Bereavement groups are more helpful for those with lesser psychological resources (Caserta & Lund, 1993). In contrast, individuals with more psychological resources may not find such groups helpful because the focus on loss may impede development (Caserta & Lund, 1993).

Outcome research on groups for burdened caregivers indicates that participants in these groups value the groups highly, but the complexities of measurement of subjective and objective burden, reflecting both what is objectively demanded and subjectively experienced by the caregiver and the common situation of the progressive functional deterioration of the care receiver may translate into a lack of measurably significant intervention impact on measures of burden (Kosberg et al., 1990; Toseland et al., 1989; Zarit et al., 1980).

Much of the assistance offered to burdened caregivers is provided in time-limited groups of 6 to 12 weekly sessions. However, longer term maintenance treatment, once monthly for an additional 10 months, may sustain and broaden treatment effects, significantly reducing the subjective experience of burden and even improving the caregiver's evaluation of the ill relative's health status (Labrecque et al., 1992). Although most participants value very highly the group and peer support, some severely distressed caregivers may require individual professional assistance (Toseland et al., 1989).

Research on groups employing CBT and psychoeducational models has also demonstrated effectiveness in reducing stress, anxiety, and depression (Thompson et al., 2000). Comprehensive psychosocial interventions, encompassing individual counseling, family counseling, and peer support groups that provide specific and tailored assistance, can significantly reduce institutionalization by 50% compared to routine support (Mittelman et al., 1993). In addition to reducing economic burden, the psychosocial burden on caregivers can also be reduced. This mirrors the benefits achieved using cognitive-behavioral family interventions (Marriott et al., 2000). However, it is important to note that meta-analysis of controlled interventions for distressed caregivers documented that group interventions in general have only a small, but positive, effect on caregiver burden and dysphoria (Knight et al., 1993), notwithstanding the participants' subjectively high valuation of all groups.

Significant and durable treatment benefits to the caregivers include improved feelings of mastery, self-directedness, and problem-solving ability; increased ability to consider appropriate alternatives to care for the family member; relationship improvement with the care receiver; increased capacity to grieve; and, quite importantly, an increased capacity to care for themselves (Kahan et al., 1985; Perkins & Poynton, 1990; Toseland et al., 1989). Both professionally led and peer-led groups show significant effects, although the former emphasize provision of information and problem solving, whereas the latter emphasize peer support and social networking (Toseland et al., 1989).

Successful outcome in geriatric group therapy is linked to sufficient tenure in treatment (Arean & Miranda, 1996); therefore, therapeutic strategies to facilitate treatment maintenance, as described above, are essential. There is good evidence for the value of continuation-and-maintenance phase treatment for depression employing pharmacotherapy (Reynolds et al., 1999). Combined pharmacotherapy and psychotherapy confer a greater likelihood of completed treatment (Reynolds et al., 1999), and compliance may be improved with pharmacotherapy.

Although severe physical illness and chronicity of depression are negatively correlated with successful outcome (Gallagher, 1981; Parham, 1982; Steuer et al., 1984), it is also evident that depressed older persons with medical and disabling illnesses can in fact benefit significantly from active treatment, as reflected in improved mood scores (Arean & Miranda, 1996) and functional ability (Kemp et al., 1991–1992). However, unlike the depressed elderly who are physically well and who may demonstrate even further gains in longer term follow-up, the physically disabled depressed elderly plateau or fail to retain their gains (Kemp et al., 1991–1992). Further and ongoing physical difficulties are likely one mediator of this result, and ongoing or maintenance treatment would appear to be indicated. In addition, physical disabilities, if not adequately encompassed psychotherapeutically, may interfere with or obstruct in-group participation and practice of homework assignments between group sessions (Brand & Clingempeel, 1992).

Cognitively Impaired Patients

Evaluation of outcome effectiveness of group approaches with the cognitively impaired elderly is hampered by a lack of consistency in measures utilized to determine improvements in cognition, behavior, and orientation. In addition, in many instances the underlying dementing disorder is progressive. Hence, evaluation of outcome must compare well-matched control and treated subjects over time. The literature demonstrates a broad range of creative approaches that blend elements of structured reality orientation, resocialization, and structured reminiscence therapy. Greater precision and description of the models employed will facilitate generalizability and better testing of the efficacy of particular models.

Early outcome studies (Linden, 1953; Reichenfeld et al., 1973) based on populations of institutionalized, chronic, psychogeriatric patients documented statistically significant increases in hospital discharge rates and reductions in behavioral deterioration, although those who were physically more ill or more cognitively impaired at the outset improved less. Although improvements in verbal orientation and socially appropriate behavior may be produced by group interventions (Bower, 1967), gains in orientation are often rapidly extinguished without ongoing staff and family reinforcement (Gerber et al., 1991). However, some behavioral improvement may endure beyond the active treatment phase and be readily reactivated by treatment resumption, as evidenced by one of the few controlled studies in this area (Baines et al., 1987).

A recent review of randomized controlled trials that employed reality orientation in the form of regular group sessions for 30 to 60 minutes demonstrated a significant effect on both cognitive and behavioral measures, substantially slowing decline and deterioration. Both specific and nonspecific factors, such as behavioral and reinforcement factors, are essential (Spector et al., 2000).

Structured reminiscence group therapy has produced significant, albeit short-lived, improvements in patient mood and depression scores (Goldwasser et al., 1982). Preliminary reports of significant improvement in cognitive functioning effected by focused visual imagery group therapy and cognitive therapy warrant further study and replication (Abraham et al., 1992). Validation therapy has been shown to be effective in reducing physical aggression, but was not helpful in reducing the need for pharmacotherapy or restraints (Toseland et al., 1997).

It remains unclear how much of the improvements effected are linked not only to the specifics of reality orientation techniques, but also to the social engagement and behavioral reinforcement of more adaptive social functioning. Indeed, it remains unclear what, if any, are the active ingredients of treatment beyond social stimulation and interaction (Baines et al., 1987; Toseland et al., 1997). Exposure to reality orientation techniques is insufficient without actual interaction, encouragement, and consistent reinforcement by the staff. The staff's enthusiasm, realistic hopefulness, and behaviorally consistent responses are essential ingredients of effective treatment (Katz, 1976). The staff's broadened intervention repertoire and greater involvement with their patients, fostering utilization of the techniques employed in the group within their individual contact with patients, may be an important mediator of therapeutic impact (Lantz et al., 1997). Clearly, staff morale is an important mediator of the quality of patient experience in institutional life. Specific interventions employed by staff may mediate some of their impact through the nonspecific variable of increased staff feelings of self-efficacy and competence.

REFERENCES

Abraham IL, Neundorfer MM, Currie LJ. Effects of group interventions on cognition on depression in nursing home residents. *Nurs Res.* 1992;41:196–202.

Albeniz A, Holmes J. Psychotherapy integration: its implications for psychiatry. *Br J Psychiatry.* 1996;169:563–570.

American Psychiatric Association. *Diagnostic and Statistical Manual of Mental Disorders.* 4th ed. Washington, DC: American Psychiatric Association; 1994.

American Psychiatric Association. Practice guidelines for the treatment of patients with Alzheimer's disease and other dementias of later life. *Am J Psychiatry.* 1997; 154(supp).

Arean P, Miranda J. The treatment of depression in elderly primary care patients: a naturalistic study. *J Clin Geropsychol.* 1996;2:153–160.

Arean PA, Perri MG, Nezu AM, Scheir RL, Christophe F, Joseph TX. Comparative effectiveness of social problem-solving therapy and reminiscence therapy as treatments for depression in older adults. *J Consult Clin Psychol.* 1993;61:1003–1010.

Astrachan BM, Harrow M, Flynn HR. Influence of the value system of a psychiatric setting on behaviour in group therapy meetings. *Soc Psychiatry.* 1968;3:165–172.

Bachar E, Kindler S, Schoflar G, et al. Reminiscing as a technique in the group psychotherapy of depression: a comparative study. *Br J Clin Psychol.* 1991;30:375–377.

Baines S, Saxby P, Ehlert K. Reality orientation and reminiscence therapy. *Br J Psychiatry.* 1987;151:222–231.

Baker MN, Baker HS. In: Alonso A, Swiller MI, eds. *Self-Psychological Contributions to the Theory and Practice of Group Psychotherapy.* Washington, DC: American Psychiatric Press; 1993:49–68.

Baldwin BA, Kleeman KM, Stevens GL, et al. Family caregiver stress: clinical assessment and management. *Int Psychogeriatr.* 1989;1:185–193.

Beck J. *Cognitive Therapy: Basics and Beyond.* New York, NY: Guilford Press; 1995.

Botella L, Feixas G. The autobiographical group: a tool for the reconstruction of past life experience with the aged. *Int J Aging Hum Dev.* 1992–1993;36:303–319.

Bower HM. Sensory stimulation and the treatment of senile dementia. *Med J Aust.* 1967; 22:1113–1119.

Brand E, Clingempeel WG. Group behavioural therapy with depressed geriatric inpatients: an assessment of incremental efficacy. *Behav Ther.* 1992;23:475–482.

Bruce ML, Kim K, Leaf PJ, Jacobs S. Depression episodes and dysphoria resulting from conjugal bereavement in a prospective community sample. *Am J Psychiatry.* 1990; 147:608–610.

Burnside IM. Reminiscence: an independent nursing intervention for the elderly. *Issues Ment Health Nurs.* 1991;11:33–48.

Burnside IM. *Working With the Elderly: Group Process and Techniques.* North Scituate, MA: Duxbury Press; 1978.

Butler R. Successful aging and the role of the life review. *J Am Geriatr Soc.* 1974;22: 529–535.

Caserta MS, Lund PA. Intrapersonal resources and the effectiveness of self-help groups for bereaved older adults. *Gerontologist.* 1993;33(5):619–629.

Clemens NA, MacKenzie KR, Griffith J, Markowitcz J. Psychotherapy by psychiatrists in a managed care environment: must it be an oxymoron. *J Psychother Pract Res.* 2000;10:53–62.

Drummond L, Kirschhoff L, Scarbrough DR. A practical guide to reality orientation: a treatment approach for confusion and disorientation. *Gerontologist.* 1978;18: 568–573.

Erikson EH. *Childhood and Society.* New York, NY: Norton; 1950.

Feil N. Group work with disoriented nursing home residents. In: Saul S, ed. *Group Work With the Frail Elderly.* Binghamton, NY: Haworth Press; 1983:57–63.

Gallagher DE. Behavioural group therapy with elderly depressives: an experimental study. In: Upper D, Ross SM, eds. *Behavioural Group Therapy.* Champaign, IL: Research Press; 1981.

Gallagher DE, Thompson LW. Treatment of major depressive disorder in older adult outpatients with brief psychotherapies. *Psychother Theory Res Pract.* 1982;19: 482–490.

Gallagher-Thompson D, Hanley-Peterson P, Thompson LW. Maintenance of gains versus relapse following brief psychotherapy for depression. *J Consult Clin Psychol.* 1990;58:371–374.

Gallagher-Thompson D, Thompson LW. Psychotherapy with older adults in theory and practice. In: Bongar B, Boulter LE, eds. *Comprehensive Textbook of Psychotherapy Theory and Practice.* New York, NY: Oxford University Press; 1995:359–379.

Gerber GJ, Prince PN, Snider MC, et al. Group activity and cognitive improvement among patients with Alzheimer's disease. *Hosp Community Psychiatry.* 1991;42: 843–845.

Gloaguen V, Cottraux J, Cucherat M, Blackburn IM. A meta-analysis of the effects of cognitive therapy in depressed patients. *J Affect Disord.* 1998;49:59–72.

Goldwasser AN, Averbach SM, Harkins SW. Cognitive, affective and behavioural effects of reminiscence group therapy on demented elderly. *Int J Aging Hum Dev.* 1982; 25:209–222.

Gorey KM, Cryns AG. Group work as interventive modality with the older depressed client: a meta-analytic review. *J Gerontol Soc Work.* 1991;16:137–157.

Grant I, Patterson TL, Yager JC. Social supports in relation to physical health and symptoms of depression in the elderly. *Am J Psychiatry.* 1988;145:1254–1258.

Gurland B. Epidemiology of psychiatric disorders. In: Sadavoy J, Lazarus LW, Jarvik LF, Grossberg GT, eds. *Comprehensive Review of Geriatric Psychiatry.* 2nd ed. Washington, DC: American Psychiatric Press; 1996:3–47.

Heckhausen J, Schultz R. A life-span theory of control. *Psychol Rev.* 1995;102:284.

Henderson JN, Gutierrez-Mayka M, Garcia J, et al. A model for Alzheimer's disease support group development in African-American and Hispanic populations. *Gerontologist.* 1993;33:409–414.

Kahan J, Kemp B, Staples RF, et al. Decreasing the burden in families caring for a relative with a dementing illness: a controlled study. *J Am Geriatr Soc.* 1985;33: 664–670.

Kaslyn M. Telephone group work: challenges for practice. *Soc Work Groups.* 1999;22: 63–72.

Katz MM. Behavioural change in the chronicity pattern of dementia in the institutional geriatric resident. *J Am Geriatr Soc.* 1976;11:522–528.

Kavanagh B, Burnside J. Reminiscing and life review. Conducting the processes. *J Gerontol Nurs.* 1992;18:37–42.

Kelly TB. Mutual aid groups with mentally ill older adults. *Soc Work Groups.* 1999;21: 63–80.

Kemp BJ, Corgiat M, Gill C. Effects of brief cognitive-behavioural group psychotherapy on older persons with or without disabling illness. *Behav Health Aging.* 1991–1992;2:21–28.

Kiesler DJ. *Contemporary Interpersonal Theory and Research.* New York, NY: Guilford Press; 1996.

Klausner EJ, Alexopoulous GS. The future of psychosocial treatments for elderly patients. *Psychiatr Serv.* 1999;50:1198–1204.

Knight BG, Lutzky SM, Macofsky-Urban F. A meta-analytic review of interventions for caregiver distress: recommendations for future research. *Gerontologist.* 1993;33: 240–243.

Kohut H. *How Does Analysis Cure?* Chicago, IL: University of Chicago Press; 1984.

Kosberg JI, Cairl RE, Keller DM. Components of burden: intervention implications. *Gerontologist.* 1990;30:236–242.

Labrecque MS, Peak T, Toseland RW. Long-term effectiveness of a group program for caregivers of frail elderly veterans. *Am J Orthopsychiatr.* 1992;62:575–588.

Lantz MS, Buchalter E, McRea L. The wellness group: a novel intervention for coping with disruptive behaviour in elderly nursing home residents. *Gerontologist.* 1997; 37:551–556.

Lazarus LW. Self-psychology and psychotherapy with the elderly: theory and practice. *J Geriatr Psychiatry.* 1980;13:69–88.

Lazarus LW, Groves L. Brief psychotherapy with the elderly: a study of process and outcome. In: Sadavoy J, Leszcz M, eds. *Treating the Elderly With Psychotherapy: The Scope for Change in Later Life.* Madison, CT: International Universities Press; 1987:265–294.

Lebowitz BD, Pearson JL, Schneider LS, et al. Diagnosis and treatment of depression in late life: consensus statement and update. *JAMA.* 1997;278:1186–1190.

Lesser J, Frankel R, Havasy S. Reminiscence group therapy with psychotic geriatric inpatients. *Gerontologist.* 1981;21:291–296.

Leszcz M. Geriatric group therapy. In: Kaplan HI, Sadock BJ, eds. *Comprehensive Textbook of Psychiatry.* Vol. 7. New York, NY: Williams & Wilkins; 1999:1327–1331.

Leszcz M. Group psychotherapy with the elderly. In: Sadavoy J, Leszcz M, eds. *Treating the Elderly With Psychotherapy: The Scope for Change in Later Life.* Madison, CT: International Universities Press; 1987:325–349.

Leszcz M. Integrated group psychotherapy for the treatment of depression in the elderly. *Group.* 1997;21:89–107.

Leszcz M. The interpersonal approach to group psychotherapy. *Int J Group Psychother.* 1992;42:37–62.

Leszcz M, Feigenbaum E, Sadavoy J, et al. A men's group: psychotherapy of elderly men. *Int J Group Psychother.* 1985;35:177–196.

Lewinsohn PM. A behavioural approach to depression. In: Friedman R, Katz M, eds. *The Psychology of Depression.* New York, NY: Wiley; 1974:157–176.

Lewinsohn PM, Hoberman H, Teri L, Hautzinger M. An integrated theory of depression. In: Reiss S, Bootzin R, eds. *Theoretical Issues in Behaviour Therapy.* New York, NY: Academic Press; 1985:331–359.

Lieberman MA, Gaurash N. Evaluating the effects of group changes on the elderly. *Int J Group Psychother.* 1979;29:283–304.

Lieberman MA, Gaurash-Bliwise N. Comparison among peer and professionally directed group for the elderly: implications for the development of self-help groups. *Int J Group Psychother.* 1985;35:155–175.

Lieberman MA, Yalom ID. Brief group psychotherapy for the spousally bereaved: a controlled study. *Int J Group Psychother.* 1992;42:117–132.

Linden M. Group psychotherapy with institutionalized senile women: study in gerontologic human relations. *Int J Group Psychother.* 1953;3:150–170.

Lothstein LM, Zimet G. Twinship and alter ego self-object transferences in group therapy with the elderly: a reanalysis of the pairing phenomenon. *Int J Group Psychother.* 1988;38:303–317.

Lowenthal RI, Marrazzo RA. Milestoning, evoking memories for resocialization through group reminiscence. *Gerontologist.* 1990;30:269–272.

Lund DA, Caserta MS. Older bereaved spouses' participation in self-help groups. *Omega.* 1992;25:47–61.

MacLennan BW, Saul S, Weiner MB. *Group Psychotherapies for the Elderly.* Madison, CT: International Universities Press; 1988. American Group Psychotherapy Association Monograph 5.

Marriott A, Donaldson C, Tarrier N, Burns A. Effectiveness of cognitive-behavioural family intervention in reducing the burden of care in carers of patients with Alzheimer's disease. *Br J Psychiatry.* 2000;176:557–562.

Miller E. The management of dementia: a review of some possibilities. *Br J Soc Clin Psychol.* 1977;16:77–83.

Mittelman MS, Ferris SH, Steinberg G, et al. An intervention that delays institutionalization of Alzheimer's disease patients: treatment of spouse caregivers. *Gerontologist.* 1993;33:730–740.

Moran JA, Gatz M. Group therapies for nursing home adults: an evaluation of two treatment approaches. *Gerontologist.* 1987;27:588–591.

Murphy E. The prognosis of depression in old age. *Br J Psychiatry.* 1983;142:111–117.

Norcross, JC. A roundtable on psychotherapy integration: common factors, technical eclecticism and psychotherapy research. *J Psychother Pract Res.* 1995;4:248–249.

Parham JA, Priddy MJ, McGovern TU, et al. Group psychotherapy with the elderly: problems and prospects. *Psychother Theory Res Pract.* 1982;19:437–447.

Perkins RE, Poynton CF. Group counselling for relatives of hospitalized presenile dementia patients: a controlled study. *Br J Clin Psychol.* 1990;29:287–295.

Pollock GH. The mourning-liberation process: ideas in the inner life of the older adult. In: Sadavoy J, Leszcz M, eds. *Treating the Elderly With Psychotherapy.* Madison, CT: International Universities Press; 1987:3–30.

Poulton JL, Strassberg DS. The therapeutic use of reminiscence. *Int J Group Psychother.* 1986;36:381–398.

Radley M, Redston C, Bates F, Pontefracts M. Effectiveness of group anxiety management with elderly clients of a community psychogeriatric team. *Int J Geriatr Psychiatry.* 1997;12:79–84.

Rattenbury C, Stones MJ. A controlled evaluation of reminiscence and current topics discussion groups in a nursing home context. *Gerontologist.* 1989;29:768–771.

Reichenfeld HF, Csapo KG, Carriere L, et al. Evaluating the effect of activity programs on a geriatric ward. *Gerontologist.* 1973;13:305–310.

Reynolds C, Miller M, Pasternak R, et al. Treatment of bereavement-related major depressive episodes in later life: a controlled study of acute and continuation treatment with nortriptyline and interpersonal psychotherapy. *Am J Psychiatry.* 1999; 156:202–208.

Rokke PD, Greving-Trunkhill C, Nicola J. Cognitive-behavioural therapy for older adults: current states and issues in the treatment of depression. *Adv Med Psychother.* 210:13–23, 1999–2000.

Rush AJ. Cognitive therapy of depression. *Psychiatric Clin N Am.* 1983;6:105–127.

Safran JO, Segal ZV. *Interpersonal Processes in Cognitive Therapy.* New York, NY: Basic Books; 1990.

Salvendy JT. Brief group psychotherapy at retirement. *Group.* 1989;13:43–52.

Salvendy JT. Selection and preparations of patients and organizations of the group. In: Kaplan HI, Sadock BJ, eds. *Comprehensive Group Therapy.* 3rd ed. Baltimore, MD: Williams & Wilkins; 1993:72–84.

Samberg S. Dance therapy groups for the elderly. In: MacLennan BW, Saul S, Bakur Weiner M, eds. *Group Psychotherapies for the Elderly.* Madison, CT: International Universities Press; 1988:233–244. American Group Psychotherapy Association Monograph 5.

Saul SR. Group therapy with confused and disoriented people. In: MacLennan BW, Saul S, Bakur Weiner M, eds. *Group Psychotherapies for the Elderly.* Madison, CT: International Universities Press; 1988:199–208. American Group Psychotherapy Association Monograph 5.

Schmid AH, Rouslin M. Integrative outpatient group therapy for discharged elderly psychiatric inpatients. *Gerontologist.* 1992;32:558–560.

Schwartzman G. The use of the group as self-object. *Int J Group Psychother.* 1984;34: 229–242.

Scogin F, McElreath L. Efficacy of psychosocial treatments for geriatric depression: a quantitative review. *J Consult Clin Psychol.* 1994;62:69–74.

Segal DI, Van Hasselt VB, Hersen M, King C. Treatment of substance abuse in older adults. In: Cautela JR, Ishag W, eds. *Contemporary Issues in Behaviour Therapy.* New York, NY: Plenum Press; 1996:69–85.

Sherbourne CD, Hays RD, Wells KB. Personal and psychosocial risk factors for physical and mental health outcomes and course of depression among depressed patients. *J Consult Clin Psychol.* 1995;63:345–355.

Spector A, Davies S, Woods B, Orrell M. Reality orientation for dementia: a systematic review of the evidence for effectiveness from randomized controlled trials. *Gerontologist.* 2000;40:206–212.

Steinmetz-Breckenridge J, Thompson LW, Breckenridge JN, et al. Behavioural group therapy with the elderly. In: Upper D, Rose S, eds. *Handbook of Behavioural Group Therapy.* New York, NY: Plenum Press; 1985:275–302.

Steuer JL, Hammen CL. Cognitive-behavioural group therapy for the depressed elderly: issues and adaptations. *Cogn Ther Res.* 1983;7:285–296.

Steuer JL, Mintz J, Hammen CL, et al. Cognitive-behavioural and psychodynamic group psychotherapy in treatment of geriatric depression. *J Consult Clin Psychol.* 1984; 52:80–89.

Stone R. Defining family caregivers of the elderly: implications for research and social policy. *Gerontologist.* 1991;31:724–725.

Stone WN, Whitman RM. Contributions of the psychology of self to group process and group therapy. *Int J Group Psychother.* 1977;27:343–359.

Sweet M, Stoler N, Kelter R, et al. A community of builders: support groups for veterans forced into early retirement. *Hosp Community Psychiatry.* 1989;40:172–176.

Teri L, Gallagher-Thomson D. Cognitive-behavioural interventions for treatment of depression in Alzheimer's patients. *Gerontologist.* 1991;31:413–416.

Thompson LW, Gantz F, Florsheim M, et al. Cognitive-behavioural therapy in affective disorders in the elderly. In: Myers WA, ed. *New Techniques in the Psychotherapy of Older Patients.* Washington, DC: American Psychiatric Press; 1991:3–19.

Thompson LW, Powers DP, Coon DW, Takagi K, McKibbin C, Gallagher-Thompson D. Older adults. In: White JR, Freeman AS, eds. *Cognitive-Behavioural Group Therapy for Specific Problems and Populations.* Washington, DC: American Psychological Association; 2000:235–262.

Toseland RW. *Group Work With the Elderly and Family Caregivers.* New York, NY: Springer; 1995.

Toseland RW, Diehl M, Freeman K, Manzanares T, Naleppa M, McCallion P. The impact of validation group therapy on nursing home residents with dementia. *J Appl Gerontol.* 1997;16:31–50.

Toseland RW, Rossiter CM, Labrecque M. The effectiveness of three group intervention strategies to support family caregivers. *Am J Orthopsychiatry.* 1989;59:420–429.

Tross S, Blum JE. A review of group therapy with the older adult: practice and research. In: MacLennan BW, Saul S, Bakur Weiner M, eds. *Group Psychotherapies for the Elderly.* Madison, CT: International Universities Press; 1988:3–29. American Group Psychotherapy Association Monograph 5.

Wachtel PL. From eclecticism to synthesis: toward a more seamless psychotherapeutic integration. *J Psychother Integration.* 1991;1:43–54.

Williams-Barnard CL, Lindell AR. Therapeutic use of "prizing" and its effect on self-concept of elderly clients in nursing homes and group homes. *Issues Ment Health Nurs.* 1992;13:1–17.

Wolf E. *Treating the Self: Elements of Clinical Self Psychology.* New York, NY: Guilford Press; 1988.

Wong P. Social support functions of group reminiscence. *Can J Community Ment Health.* 1991;10:151–161.

Yalom ID. *Existential Psychotherapy.* New York, NY: Basic Books, 1980.

Yalom ID. *The Theory and Practice of Group Psychotherapy.* 4th ed. New York, NY: Basic Books; 1995.

Yalom ID, Terrazas F. Group therapy for psychotic elderly patients. *Am J Nurs.* 1967; 68:1690–1694.

Yost EB, Beutler LE, Corbishley MA, et al. *Group Cognitive Therapy: A Treatment Approach for Depressed Older Adults.* Oxford, UK: Pergamon Press; 1986.

Zarit SH, Reever KE, Bach-Peterson J. Relatives of the impaired elderly: correlates of feelings of burden. *Gerontology.* 1980;6:649–655.

33

Family Issues in Mental Disorders of Late Life

Jacobo Mintzer, MD
Barry Lebowitz, PhD
Jason T. Olin, PhD
Kristen Miller, MD
Robert H. Payne, MD

INTRODUCTION

The belief that clinicians should concentrate solely on patients and disregard families is one of the most common misconceptions in the field of geriatric psychiatry. This misconception can be traced to the 1965 report of the Committee on Aging of the Group for Advancement of Psychiatry (GAP, 1968) and amplified in an important 1968 Research Report of the American Psychiatric Association (Simon & Epstein, 1968). In these reports, families were seen as geographically and emotionally distant, distracted by issues of employment and mobility, disintegrated, reduced in size, and generally indifferent to the concerns of the older generation.

At roughly the same time, a different conclusion was building from the social and behavioral science literature. The works of Blenkner (1965), Brody (1966), Shanas and Streib (1965), and others were establishing a framework for what later came to be called *caregiving*. A large study of service use (Comptroller General, 1977) documented the important contributions of family members to the ongoing care and support of disabled older persons in the community. Today, the critical role of the family in the care of elderly persons suffering from mental disorders has been well established (Lefley & Hatfield, 1999; Zarit et al., 1986; Zarit & Teri, 1991).

The goal of this chapter is to highlight the critical importance of understanding the family when treating mental health disorders of late life. Furthermore, this chapter aims to provide the rationale for the need to incorporate this understanding in the treatment of chronically mentally ill elderly. The available empirical literature is vast in some areas and limited in others. This chapter does not review this literature, but it aims to provide, based on empirical information and clinical experience, a road map that can aid the clinician in the task of providing adequate treatment to the families of the chronically mentally ill elderly patient.

UNDERSTANDING THE PATIENT AND THE FAMILY

Recognizing the Importance of the Family

The landmark 1981 publication of *The 36-Hour Day* (Mace & Rabins, 1981), now in its third edition, dramatically altered our understanding of family issues. The family was now more properly seen as the fundamental structure providing care to its older members. The title of Brody's 1984 Kent Award Lecture, "Parent Care as Normative Family Stress" (Brody, 1985) summarized the new conceptualization of the centrality of the family. Other authors have developed books and articles that further discuss the importance of the family in the life of the elderly (e.g., Berman & Shulman, 2001; Jarvik & Small, 1988); the role of clinicians in engaging families in geriatric care (Hamrick & Blazer, 1980); and family counseling (Herr & Weakland, 1979b; Knight & McCallum, 1998; Qualls, 1996; Shields, 1992).

Living Arrangements of Older People and Their Families

Most of the elderly in the United States live with family members. The demographics are clear: In 1997, two thirds of the noninstitutionalized population older than 65 years lived either with a spouse or with other relatives.

In addition, some significant differences exist by age and sex. The proportion of older people living alone rises with age, especially in elders 85 years of age or older. The proportion of elders 85 years of age and older living alone is about double the proportion of those aged 65 to 74 years. At all ages, women are about twice as likely to be living alone as men. These factors combine to produce the reality that approximately 60% of women over the age of 85 years are living alone, a population that has been seen as being at particularly high risk for a variety of negative outcomes (e.g., greater vulnerability to crime) (Commonwealth Fund, 1993).

Race and ethnicity also enter into this picture. At any age, African American and Hispanic women are more likely to live with other relatives than non-Hispanic white women. On the other hand, older African American men are considerably more likely to live alone than other men.

Importance of the Patient's Age at the Time of Disease Onset

The evaluation of the relationship between the family and the elderly patient suffering from a mental disorder requires an early differentiation between two groups. The first group involves patients who develop a mental disorder early in life (Ory et al., 1999). Because of the early onset of the disease, many of these patients do not have the opportunity to develop a nuclear family. Their parents usually care for them. Examples of this group of elderly patients are those suffering from early-onset schizophrenia. The second is a group of patients that develop a mental disorder in late life. These patients often have the opportunity to form a nuclear family. The spouse is usually the primary care provider. Patients suffering from dementia or late-onset depression belong to this group.

ELDERLY PATIENTS SUFFERING FROM A CHRONIC EARLY-ONSET MENTAL DISORDER   More than one third of chronic mentally ill patients live with their families (Lefley, 1987). Large proportions of these patients live with aging parents. As the patients and their caregivers age, the burden to the extended family increases. With time, the possibility that patients will outlive their aging caregivers often becomes a reality. The burden of patient care is then shifted to the surviving family members. Frequently, the lack of ability or willingness of the surviving family members to carry on with the caregiving tasks puts the patient at risk for housing disruption and traumatic institutionalization (Lefley & Hatfield, 1999).

Caregiver variables also appear to play a role in determining the willingness and ability of family members to provide care for elderly patients suffering from a chronic mental illness. A specific example is a study by Given and collaborators (1999). They compared family caregivers facing high numbers of new demands for patient care with caregivers facing similar burdens of care in the absence of new demands. They found that the presence of new demands rather than the level of preexisting burden was associated with increased caregiver burden and depression. As a result, it was suggested that stabilizing the patient's symptoms could be important in preserving family caregiving. Preventing acute exacerbations through effective treatment can be an important tool in preserving family involvement in the care of the chronic mentally ill elderly patient.

These findings are also consistent with data comparing the characteristics of elderly patients with schizophrenia and those with bipolar disorder living in a nursing home with those living in the community. In their study, Bartels and associates (1997) found that nursing home residency was associated with more severe overall symptom ratings. Marital status (single, never married), cognitive impairment, functional impairment, and the presence of aggressive behaviors were strongly associated with nursing home placement.

In summary, families of elderly patients suffering from early-onset chronic mental illness provide a large proportion of patient care. Traditionally, parents have provided the majority of this care. However, as patients and their parents age, the responsibility of care changes from parents to the family at large. Families as an entity can now be considered the caregivers. A number of family and patient variables can moderate the relationship between patients and their caregiving families. An understanding of these variables is crucial to develop interventions aimed to preserve the family/patient caregiving relationship.

ELDERLY PATIENTS SUFFERING FROM A LATE-ONSET MENTAL ILLNESS   Families of demented elderly patients, as a rule, take responsibility for a wide range of caregiving tasks, such as transportation, nutrition, personal care, and finances (Marin et al., 2000). Spouses and daughters usually assume a leading role in providing this care (Sparks et al., 1998). The onset of behavioral symptoms in patients with dementia is one of the most difficult issues families have to confront. Indeed, the onset of these symptoms is usually associated with caregiver burden and patient institutionalization (Hurley & Volicer, 2002). Impairment in activities of daily living also appears to be one of the most difficult issues facing caregivers of demented patients (Hurley & Volicer, 2002).

Above all, this group of caregivers has to confront the emotional toll of witnessing the constant deterioration of their loved one and having to adapt the quality of the relationship to the progression of the disease (Hurley & Volicer, 2002). In our experience, a reluctance to accept the ongoing process of deterioration often ensues and is one of the distinct landmarks of caring for patients with dementia.

Family Consequences of Providing Care for the Mentally Impaired Elder

Family caregiving for an elderly chronic mentally ill patient can have serious consequences (Butcher et al., 2001). For example, family caregivers of demented patients manifest medical morbidity, including deterioration in immune functions (Wu et al., 1999); psychosocial morbidity such as decrease in social activities, private time; deterioration of family relations and work-related performance (Cohen, 2000).

Zarit and colleagues (1986) referred to these negative consequences of caregiving as *subjective burden*. In contrast, they used the term *objective burden* to refer to the patient's needs and deficits that could affect caregiving practices. A number of patient characteristics can affect objective burden, such as the degree of cognitive impairment, functional dependency, medical burden, and the presence of psychiatric symptoms (Clyburn et al., 2000).

The relationship between subjective and objective burden has been a productive area of research (Stuckey et al., 1996; Zarit et al., 1986). For example, Coen and colleagues (1997) studied predictors of caregiver burden among patients diagnosed with Alzheimer's disease (AD) and found that daughters who were primary caregivers were particularly prone to suffer from high levels of burden (as defined by Zarit and colleagues; see above). In this study, neither cognitive nor functional status of the patient predicted caregiver burden. Behavioral disturbances and the lack of availability of informal social support, however, were independent predictors of caregiver burden.

Families who provide care for patients who live in the community are not the only ones who experience burden. For example, Crispi and colleagues (1997) found that there was significant burden for adult children of patients with dementia, even after the parent had been institutionalized.

Cultural and ethnic background also appears to influence caregiver burden. For example, Harwood and collaborators (1998) studied the prevalence of depressive symptoms among white Hispanic (WH) and white non-Hispanic (WNH) first-degree family caregivers of patients with Alzheimer's disease who were treated in a memory disorders clinic. The collaborators evaluated depression using the Center for Epidemiological Studies–Depression Scale (CES-D) and found that symptoms of depression were common in both groups (with higher prevalence rates [45%] among WH than among WNH [36%] caregivers). Further, risk factors for caregiver depression differed by ethnic group. Increased patient level of cognitive impairment was a risk factor for depression among WH spouses and children. The presence of psychiatric symptoms in a demented patient predicted caregiver depression only among WNH caregivers. Female gender was a good predictor of depression among all groups except WH children.

However, the relationship between the elderly chronically ill patient and his or her caregiver can sometimes be mutually satisfactory and enriching (MacPhail, 1993). Patient behavior and personality traits appear to be important determinants of successful relationships between caregiver and care receiver. Comjs and collaborators (1999) evaluated the association between patient personality and mistreatment. They identified elderly victims of chronic verbal aggression, physical aggression, and financial abuse and compared these subjects to an equal number of controls. They found that victims of chronic verbal aggression had a strong tendency to respond with aggression when feeling angry or frustrated. Physical aggression toward a victim was associated with a victim's tendency to be passive and avoidant. Finally, financial mistreatment was associated with the victim's tendency to have negative attitudes toward self-efficacy. Moreover, a history of aggressive behavior by the patient toward the caregiver was a strong predictor of caregiver's negative attitudes (Graftstrom et al., 1993).

In summary, the role of the family as caregivers is full of challenges (Lebowitz, 1985; Light et al., 1994). The correlations of the burden of caregiving with psychosocial and medical disorders are clinically significant (Schulz et al., 1995). However, this relationship does not always result in burden. Exploration of variables that promote the perception of burden as well as those enhancing relationships will aid clinicians in developing successful interventions.

ASSESSMENT

The circumstances and the course of a psychiatric/emotional illness can vary over the lifetime of an individual and his or her family. Therefore, we strongly recommend performing a new patient/family assessment as new circumstances emerge even if the clinician has had prior contact with the patient or the family. Based on our experience, we recommend including the areas discussed next in the patient and family assessments.

Patient Assessment

The mental status examination should include the timing of the first appearance of the symptoms as well as the presence and the duration of remissions as they relate to significant family events:

- Patient's previous level of functioning within the family
- History of patient-family relations before and after the onset of illness
- Patient's marital history

Family Assessment

There is a shortage of literature providing empirical information to guide the clinician on a specific approach to evaluate the family of the chronically mentally ill elderly patient. In our experience, however, the clinician should include the information listed below about the patient's immediate (nuclear) family as well as his or her siblings, parents, and grandchildren.

Such a three-generation view offers a broad perspective on the family emotional system in operation (Kerr & Bowen, 1988). We suggest that the clinician collect some of the following information from the extended family whenever possible:

- Documentation of the efforts (helpful or not) the family has made to address the problems in the past
- Degree of functional impairment associated with the symptoms and the nature of the adjustments that the family has made to compensate for the patient's functional impairments
- Identify which members are and which members are not involved with the identified patient
- Frequency and quality of family contacts
- Additional relevant information, which may include presence of pets, births and deaths, marriages, divorces, criminal behavior, or natural disasters

Some clinicians also recommend documenting the quality of emotional "connectedness" among family members. This is often very difficult information to obtain because it requires facts not only about the frequency of family contacts, but also about their quality and the extent to which the family can tolerate open, honest communication. In addition, an understanding of how much each person is permitted to be himself or herself in the context of this family relationship system can be critical in assessing the family's flexibility and adaptiveness to stress.

INTERVENTIONS

Useful Ideas for a Practical Approach

Early interventions with families can prevent the onset of major symptoms. Specifically, in our experience, if the psychiatric impairment is recent, the clinician has an opportunity to assist the family in lowering or blunting the emotional reactions associated with the illness and perhaps prevent the onset of psychosocial and medical disorders in the patient's family members.

Strong emotional reactions can be expected. For example, the diagnosis of dementia in a family matriarch who has always been the central figure and has provided support for others will threaten the family's stability far more than an illness that develops in a more peripheral person. A gradual loss of functioning allows the family time to stabilize and "transition time" for a new family leader to move into place. For example, a sudden dementia associated with a major vascular event may require early involvement of a family therapist. Such involvement may aid in establishing new leadership (if the patient is a dominant, supportive, or authoritative figure).

All families are not equally equipped to handle burden. Clinicians may indeed encounter significant variables in families' coping skills. Clinicians may find that, for some families, an early supportive intervention is enough. In other cases, however, prolonged family therapy with the intervention of a trained family therapist may be necessary. The most common family intervention is to provide the family with some information about the illness. The following are some key areas on which information should be provided to families (Hurley & Volicer, 2002):

- The diagnosis (Drickamer & Lachs, 1992) and nature of the disease (Hurley et al., 1996) should be discussed. Potentially lifesaving safety issues such as driving (Berger & Rosner, 2000) have to be addressed early in the course of the disease.
- Clinicians should initiate discussions about selecting a health care proxy and informing the proxy about future treatment preferences because, at different stages of the disease, patients may or may not have the capacity for making complex decisions (Rempusheski & Hurley, 2000).
- Many families are unfamiliar with the dying process. The topic merits discussion with families of patients suffering from Alzheimer's disease or other progressive mental disorders. When feasible, the patient should also be involved (e.g., early in the course of dementia with patients who

wish to be involved). Family members may find themselves in the role of proxy decision makers and need support from knowledgeable clinicians as they make some of the most difficult decisions of their lives— selecting life-prolonging treatments that may also increase discomfort or choosing care that would provide comfort, but may be seen as hastening death (Robinson, 2000; Robinson et al., 1998).

- Understanding the progression of the disease is critical. For example, AD can be characterized by slow and progressive cognitive deterioration and the onset of behavioral and functional decline; schizophrenia or depression will be characterized by acute episodes and remissions with different degrees of functional deterioration. Health teaching should target the patient's current problems, symptoms likely to occur soon, and symptoms for which caregivers should be prepared.

- The importance of accessing available community services and funding resources to provide adequate care should also be addressed.

- Further, the family should be aware of institutional placement options. There often comes a time when the family has to relinquish home care because of the inability to manage problematic patient behaviors (Spector et al., 2000) or because they lack the resources to provide care (Gaugler et al., 2000) and must seek institutionalized care. Information about nursing homes, community living facilities, and state-supported institutions should be provided.

In most cases, however, if the clinician can make contact with well-functioning family members (who may be the patient's sibling or adult child), it may be desirable to move beyond a symptom focus. The clinician can assist such persons in developing a clear direction for redefining themselves in relation to the elder member and the family system.

Another therapeutic target is decreasing emotional "cutoff" in the family by establishing viable emotional contact between the patient and as many family members as possible. Other goals may include developing person-to-person relationships, encouraging active involvement in caregiving, and supporting the establishment of boundaries in the family systems.

Finally, the clinician can provide ongoing long-term family treatment through individual interactions with one or more family members. The clinician can encourage high-functioning members to manage controversial issues without taking sides. The clinician can also foster the development of potentially beneficial family processes. For example, the clinician can aid family members in identifying their beliefs and principles and developing "I positions" consistent with them in the context of the family interactions. When one family member is able to say, "This is what I believe," or "This is what I will do" and sticks to it despite the pressure from other family members to stop or change, a family is often able to pull itself up around that person and gain stability.

Clinicians who work with families should be aware of the occasional presence of opposing family units of power. At times of elevated anxiety, these opposing units are active and visible in the family. There is increased pressure on the clinician to take sides in a family disagreement even though doing so can decrease his or her value as a family resource. By communicating appreciation of the various alignments and allegiances within the family, the clinician demonstrates the ability to maintain neutrality.

This is not to say the clinician has no opinion; rather, the emphasis is on leaving it to the family to resolve the differences. Families may resolve differences if they have a "concerned outsider" to whom they can communicate their thoughts and feelings without judgment or criticism. According to some theories (Bowen, 1978), the effort by the therapist aimed at keeping the relation within the family, rather than between the family and the therapist, can be crucial. With the latter, there is more unfinished emotional business than the family can ever fully resolve, and nothing is gained by encouraging unrealistic expectations or projections onto the therapist.

These transference elements will be present to some degree simply by virtue of the position of the clinician/therapist. Transference is magnified or intensified by clinicians who appear to have answers for the family or who act as if they can save the family from themselves. Clinicians should convey to the family the conviction that the family is capable of dealing with the challenges it faces, and that the best the clinician can do is assist them by providing information about human emotional functioning as it applies to their specific issues.

Bowen, one of the relatively few psychiatrists with an early interest in family therapy, postulated that interconnected triangles within the nuclear (mother, father, children) family and beyond (aunts, uncles, grandparents) form the basic building blocks of the human relationship system. They operate as circuits for the spread of anxiety. Extremes of this process are posited to impair the family's ability to deal successfully with a chronic mental illness, especially when the illness is expressed in one of the weaker members, such as the frail, chronically mentally ill elder. This three-person interconnectedness provides stability and is a means for anxiety to be shifted or managed as levels of anxiety rise and fall.

Clinicians can help the family by being a nonanxious presence. Maintaining an emotional connection with the patient or family is essential, and this skill is difficult to learn. It does not mean the clinician knows or understands everything the family says or experiences. It does not mean the clinician has to "feel their pain" or must have gone through the same experience as the family. Making the judgment on when to provide an empathetic comment, when to provide information, and when to make statements as part of defining the self of the clinician is one of the most difficult challenges the clinician is likely to confront.

In summary, families can either be a source of additional pathology or an important therapeutic resource for the treatment of the mentally ill elder.

Through the understanding of basic principles of family systems, clinicians can improve the likelihood that families play a positive and rewarding role in the treatment of the mentally ill elder.

Specific Family Interventions

FAMILY SUPPORT AND EDUCATION   The focus on family education has been a long-held tradition in geriatric psychiatry. Further, this tradition is well grounded on empirical evidence. Literature reviews have summarized the research on psychoeducational, psychotherapeutic, and self-help interventions for family caregivers of patients with dementia (Teri & McCurry, 1994; Zarit & Teri, 1991). A review of this literature showed evidence that professional therapeutic brief individual or group psychotherapy treatment of family caregivers of demented patients can lead to reductions in self-reports of caregiver distress.

For example, Greene and Monahan (1989) found that significant reductions in caregivers' anxiety, depression, and burden were observed after 8 weeks of group counseling that contained educational and relaxation components. Further, a nurse-administered psychoeducational intervention decreased caregiver depression (Buckwalter et al., 1999), and a long-term family intervention program led to significant delays in nursing home placement (Montgomery & Karner, 1996).

The efficacy of caregiver training programs to reduce stress in caregivers of dementia patients was also shown by Brodaty and Gresham (1989). In their program, caregivers providing care for patients at home had educational sessions on how to cope with difficult behaviors and other complexities of dementia care while patients received memory training. At 12 months, caregivers enrolled in the training program had lower psychological stress than family caregivers on a waiting list. A number of other researchers found comparable results when treating dementia caregivers using similar types of educational interventions (Hosaka & Sugiyama, 1999).

Confirming these findings, Mittelman and collaborators (1996) evaluated the effects of a multidimensional intervention that used a combination of caregiver support and education to treat caregivers of Alzheimer's patients. Specifically, the intervention consisted of six sessions of individual and family counseling, support group attendance, and ongoing counselor availability. This randomized study enrolled 206 spouse caregivers of Alzheimer patients during a 3.5-year period and found statistically significant differences in caregiver depression between the intervention and the control groups. Further, time from baseline to nursing home placement of AD patients was 329 days longer in the intervention group than in the control group. Treatment had the greatest effect on risk of placement for patients who were mildly and moderately impaired.

DELIVERY OF SPECIFIC SERVICES   In another line of investigation, researchers have attempted to decrease family burden through provision of in-home respite to family caregivers. For example, Gitlin and collaborators (2001) studied the short-term effects of a home environmental intervention on self-efficacy and upset in caregivers and daily function of dementia patients. They also studied if treatment effect varied by caregiver gender, race, and relationship to patient.

Briefly, the authors (Gitlin et al., 2001) randomly placed 171 families of dementia patients in an intervention or usual care. The intervention involved five 90-minute home visits by occupational therapists, which provided the caregiver with education on physical and social environmental modifications useful in the care of demented patients. When compared with controls, intervention caregivers reported fewer declines in patients' instrumental activities of daily living, fewer declines in self-care, and fewer behavior problems 3 months post-test. Also, intervention spouses reported "reduced upset." Women reported enhanced self-efficacy in managing behaviors. Women and minority caregivers reported enhanced self-efficacy in managing functional dependency.

COGNITIVE-BEHAVIORAL INTERVENTIONS   A number of cognitive-behavioral interventions have been used for the treatment of depression in caregivers of demented patients (Brown & Lewinsohn, 1984; Teri, 1994; Teri et al., 1997; Teri & Gallagher-Thompson, 1991; Teri & Logsdon, 1990; Teri & Wagner, 1992). The most comprehensive study to evaluate the efficacy of these techniques was performed by Teri and collaborators (1997). The study evaluated the efficacy of a behavior therapy–problem-solving approach and a behavioral care pleasant event approach with two control situations, a typical care control and a wait list control. They found that behavioral treatment significantly reduced caregiver depression in both behavioral treatment groups when compared with control situations. Interestingly, caregivers who suffered from the most severe symptoms of depression were the most likely to benefit.

CONCLUSION

Families play a critical role in the treatment of the elderly who suffer from mental disorders. This role has a high cost. Members of caregiving families suffer from severe physical and mental problems that can be attributed to their caregiving role. Fortunately, a growing body of information suggests that interventions can be helpful. It is the role of the geriatric clinician to be knowledgeable concerning these techniques and ensure appropriate access to care for the patient and his or her family.

REFERENCES

Bartels SJ, Mueser KT, Miles KM. A comparative study of elderly patients with schizophrenia and bipolar disorder in nursing homes and the community. *Schizophr Res.* 1997; 27:181–190.

Berger JT, Rosner F. Ethical challenges posed by dementia and driving. *J Clin Ethics.* 2000;11:304–308.

Berman R, Shulman BH. *How to Survive Your Aging Parents*. Chicago, IL: Surrey Books; 2001.

Blenkner M. Social work and family relationships in later life with some thoughts on filial maturity. In: Shanas E, Streib G, eds. *Social Structure and the Family: Generational Relations*. Englewood Cliffs, NJ: Prentice-Hall; 1965:379–391.

Bowen M. *Family Therapy in Clinical Practice*. Washington, DC: Jason Aronson; 1978.

Brodaty H, Gresham M. Effect of a training programme to reduce stress in carers of patients with dementia. *BMJ*. 1989;299:1375–1379.

Brody EM. The aging family. *Gerontologist*. 1966;6:201–206.

Brody EM. Parent care as a normative family stress. The Donald P. Kent Memorial Lecture. *Gerontologist*. 1985;25:19–29.

Brown RA, Lewinsohn PM. A psychoeducational approach to the treatment of depression: comparison of group, individual, and minimal contact procedures. *J Consult Clin Psychol*. 1984;52:774–783.

Buckwalter KC, Gerdner L, Kohout F, et al. A nursing intervention to decrease depression in family caregivers of persons with dementia. *Arch Psychiatr Nurs*. 1999; 13(2):80–88.

Butcher HK, Holkup PA, Buckwalter KC. The experience of caring for a family member with Alzheimer's disease. *West J Nurs Res*. 2001;23:33–55.

Clyburn LD, Stones MJ, Hadjistavropoulos T, Tuokko H. Predicting caregiver burden and depression in Alzheimer's disease. *J Gerontol B Psychol Sci Soc Sci*. 2000;55: S2–S13.

Coen RF, Swanwick GR, O'Boyle CA, Coakley D. Behavior disturbance and other predictors of carer burden in Alzheimer's disease. *Int J Geriatr Psychiatry*. 1997;12: 331–336.

Cohen D. Caregivers for persons with Alzheimer's disease. *Curr Psychiatry Rep*. 2000; 2:32–39.

Comijs HC, Jonker C, van Tilburg W, et al. Hostility and coping capacity as risk factors of elder mistreatment. *Soc Psychiatry Psychiatr Epidemiol*. 1999;34:48–52.

Commonwealth Fund. *The Unfinished Agenda: Improving the Well-Being of Elderly People Living Alone*. New York, NY: Commonwealth Fund; 1993.

Comptroller General of the United States. *Report to Congress on Home Health—The Need for a National Policy to Better Provide for the Elderly*. Washington, DC: US General Accounting Office; 1977. HRD-78-19.

Crispi EL, Schiaffino K, Berman WH. The contribution of attachment to burden in adult children of institutionalized parents with dementia. *Gerontologist*. 1997;37:52–60.

Drickamer MA, Lachs MS. Should patients with Alzheimer's disease be told their diagnosis. *N Engl J Med*. 1992;326:947–951.

Gaugler JE, Edwards AB, Femia EE, et al. Predictors of institutionalization of cognitively impaired elders: family help and the timing of placement. *J Gerontol B Psychol Sci Soc Sci*. 2000;55:P247–P255.

Gitlin LN, Corcoran M, Winter L, Boyce A, Hauck WW. A randomized, controlled trial of a home environmental intervention: effect on efficacy and upset in caregivers and on daily function of persons with dementia. *J Consult Clin Psychol*. 2001;41:4–14.

Given CW, Given BA, Stommel M, et al. The impact of new demands for assistance on caregiver depression tests using an inception cohort. *Gerontologist*. 1999;39: 76–85.

Graftstrom M, Norberg A, Hagberg B. Relationships between demented elderly people and their families: a follow-up study of caregivers who had previously reported abuse when caring for their spouses and parents. *J Adv Nurs.* 1993;18:1747–1757.

Greene VL, Monahan DJ. The effect of a support and educational program on stress and burden among family caregivers to frail elderly persons. *Gerontologist.* 1989; 29:472–477.

Group for the Advancement of Psychiatry. *Psychiatry and the Aged: An Introductory Approach.* Washington, DC: American Psychological Association, 1968.

Hamrick K, Blazer D. Older adults and their families in a community mental health center: strategies for interventions. *Hosp Community Psychiatry.* 1980;31:332–335.

Harwood DG, Barker WW, Cantillon M, et al. Depressive symptomatology in first-degree family caregivers of Alzheimer disease patients: a cross-ethnic comparison. *Alzheimer Dis Assoc Disord.* 1998;12:340–346.

Herr J, Weakland J. Communication within family systems: growing older within and with the double bind. In: Ragan PK, ed. *Aging Parents.* Los Angeles: University of Southern California Press; 1979a.

Herr J, Weakland J. *Counseling Elders and Their Families: Practical Techniques for Applied Gerontology.* New York, NY: Springer; 1979b.

Hosaka T, Sugiyama Y. A structured intervention for family caregivers of dementia patients: a pilot study. *Tokai J Exp Clin Med.* 1999;24:35–39.

Hurley A, Volicer L. Alzheimer disease: it's okay, Mama, if you want to go, it's okay. *JAMA.* 2002;288:2324–2331.

Hurley A, Volicer L, Mahoney E. Progression of Alzheimer's disease and symptom management. *Fed Pract.* 1996;13(suppl):16–22.

Jarvik LF, Small GW. *Parentcare: A Commonsense Guide for Adult Children.* New York, NY: Crown; 1988.

Kerr M, Bowen M. *Family Evaluation: An Approach Based on Bowen Therapy.* New York, NY: Norton; 1988.

Knight B, McCallum TJ. Interventions in nursing homes and other alternative living settings. In: Nordhus IH, ed. *Clinical Geropsychology.* Washington, DC: American Psychological Association; 1998.

Lebowitz BD. Family caregiving in old age. *Hosp Community Psychiatry.* 1985;36:457–458.

Lefley HP. Aging parents as caregivers of mentally ill adult children: an emerging social problem. *Hosp Community Psychiatry.* 1987;38:1063–1070.

Lefley HP, Hatfield AB. Helping parental caregivers and mental health consumers cope parental aging and loss. *Psychiatry Serv.* 1999;50:369–375.

Light E, Niederehe G, Lebowitz BD, eds. *Stress Effects on Family Caregivers in Alzheimer's Patients.* New York, NY: Springer; 1994.

Mace NL, Rabins PV. *The 36-Hour Day.* Baltimore, MD: Johns Hopkins University Press; 1981.

MacPhail J. Intergenerational caring in professional and family life. *Geriatr Nurse.* 1993; 14:104–107.

Marin DB, Dugue M, Schmeidler J, et al. The Caregiver Activity Survey (CAS): longitudinal validation of an instrument that measures time spent caregiving for individuals with Alzheimer's disease. *Int J Geriatr Psychiatry.* 2000;15:680–686.

Mittelman MS, Ferris SH, Shulman E, et al. A family intervention to delay nursing home placement of patients with Alzheimer's disease: a randomized, controlled trial. *JAMA.* 1996;276:1725–1731.

Montgomery JV, Karner TX. *Strategies for the Future: White Paper for Respite Care Issues Forum.* Chicago, IL: Alzheimer's Association; 1996:10–13.

Ory MG, Hoffman RR 3rd, Yee JL, Tennstedt S, Schultz R. Prevalence and impact of caregiving: a detailed comparison between dementia and nondementia caregivers. *Gerontologist.* 1999; 39:177–185.

Qualls S. Family therapy with aging families. In: Zarit SH, Knight BG, eds. *A Guide to Psychotherapy and Aging: Effective Interventions in a Life-Stage Context.* Washington, DC: American Psychological Association; 1996:121–138.

Rempusheski VF, Hurley AC. Advance directives and dementia. *J Gerontol Nurs.* 2000; 26:27–34.

Robinson EM. Wives' struggle in living through treatment decisions for husbands with advanced Alzheimer' disease. *J Nurs Law.* 2000;7:21–39.

Robinson EM, Hurley AC, Volicer L. Advanced proxy planning in patients who become incompetent. *Fed Pract.* 1998;15:26–42.

Schulz R, O'Brien AT, Bookwala J, Fleissner K. Psychiatric and physical morbidity effects of dementia caregiving: prevalence, correlates, and causes. *Gerontologist.* 1995;35:771–791.

Shanas E, Streib GF, eds. *Social Structure and the Family: Intergenerational Relations.* Englewood Cliffs, NJ: Prentice-Hall; 1965.

Shields CG. Family interaction and caregivers of Alzheimer's disease patients: correlates of depression. *Fam Process.* 1992;31:19–33.

Simon A, Epstein LJ. *Aging in Modern Society.* Psychiatric Research Report 23. Washington, DC: American Psychiatric Association; 1968.

Sparks MB, Farran CJ, Donner E, Keane-Hagerty E. Wives, husbands, and daughters of dementia patients: predictors of caregivers' mental and physical health. *Sch Inq Nurs Pract.* 1998;12:221–234.

Spector WD, Fleishman JA, Pezzin LE, Spillman BC. *The Characteristics of Long-Term Care Users.* Washington, DC: US Dept of Health and Human Services; 2000.

Stuckey JC, Neundorfer MM, Smyth KA. Burden and well-being: the same coin or related currency. *Gerontologist.* 1996;36:686–693.

Teri L. Behavioral treatment of depression in patients with dementia. *Alzheimer Dis Assoc Disord.* 1994;8(suppl 3):66–74.

Teri L, Gallagher-Thompson D. Cognitive-behavioral interventions for treatment of depression in Alzheimer's patients. *Gerontologist.* 1991;31:413–416.

Terri L, Logsdon R. Assessment and management of behavioral disturbances in Alzheimer's disease. *Compr Ther.* 1990;16(5):36–42.

Teri L, Logsdon RG, Uomoto J, McCurry SM. Behavioral treatment of depression in dementia patients: a controlled clinical trial. *J Gerontol B Psychol Sci Soc Sci.* 1997; 52:P159–P166.

Teri L, McCurry SM. Psychological therapies. In: Coffey CE, Cummings JL, eds. *Textbook of Geriatric Neuropsychiatry.* Washington, DC: American Psychiatric Press; 1994:662–682.

Teri L, Wagner A. Alzheimer's disease and depression. Review. *J Consult Clin Psychol.* 1992;60:379–391.

Wu H, Wang J, Cacioppo JT, Glaser R, Kiecolt-Glaser JK, Malarkey WB. Chronic stress associated with spousal caregiving of patients with Alzheimer's dementia is associated with down regulation of B-lymphocyte GH mRNA. *J Gerontol A Biol Sci Medi Sci.* 1999;54:M212–M215.

Zarit SH, Teri L. Interventions and services for family caregivers. *Ann Rev Gerontol Geriatr.* 1991;11:241–265.

Zarit SH, Todd PA, Zarit JM. Subjective burden of husbands and wives as caregivers: a longitudinal study. *Gerontologist.* 1986;26:260–266.

34

Psychiatric Aspects of Long-Term Care

Joel E. Streim, MD
Ira R. Katz, MD, PhD

SPECTRUM OF LONG-TERM CARE

Long-term care refers to a wide range of medical, nursing, and rehabilitative services required by older adults who have chronic illnesses and disabilities that interfere with their ability to care for themselves. Long-term care has expanded to include a spectrum of health services provided in an array of settings that offer various levels of care. As the lengths of stay have shortened in hospitals providing acute care, the settings that traditionally provide long-term care have evolved to include care provided over intervals of weeks or months. This can entail subacute, step-down, or convalescent care for patients recovering from illness after discharge from an acute care hospital, rehabilitation after illness or injury, and palliative care for patients with incurable or terminal illness, in addition to lifelong care for those with irreversible disability.

These services are provided in an expanding variety of settings for delivery of health care, such as home, day care centers, partial hospital programs, assisted-living facilities, and nursing homes. More diverse forms of residential care have become available, with various models of assisted living providing multiple levels of personal and nursing care. Nursing homes provide short-stay subacute care as well as special care units (SCUs) for ventilator-dependent patients and for patients with dementia. Accreditation standards have been developed for some long-term care settings, such as nursing homes, that provide long-term, subacute rehabilitative, and dementia care.

This spectrum of long-term care options has evolved in the context of the aging of the population in the United States and the resulting increase in the number of older adults with chronic illnesses and disabilities. The prevalence of dependency in performing self-care tasks (activities of daily living, ADLs) is 3.5% for adults who are 65 to 74 years of age; this figure increases 10-fold to 35% for those who are 85 years of age and older (Krauss & Altman, 1998). It is estimated that 43% of those who turned 65 years old in 1990 will enter a nursing home at some time (Rhoades & Krauss, 1999), although only half of these will have a total lifetime use of at least 1 year, and only 21% will have a total lifetime use of 5 years or more.

In fact, most long-term care is provided in settings other than nursing homes. The majority of older patients with self-care deficits live in the community, and their long-term care is usually provided at home (Hobbs & Damon, 1996), much of this in the form of informal assistance from family members. The proliferation of community-based, in-home health care services has enabled many disabled older adults to remain at home longer; for others, the emergence of assisted-living facilities has provided an alternative to nursing homes for those whose disability requires residential care.

From the mid-1980s to the mid-1990s, there was a decline in the proportion of older adults residing in nursing homes. Between 1985 and 1995, there was an 18% increase in the population over 65 years of age, but only a 3.8% increase in the number of nursing home residents during that time. Thus, the ratio of nursing home residents to the general population over age 65 decreased from approximately 46.2 per 1,000 in 1985 to 41.3 per 1,000 in 1995 (Gabrel & Jones, 2000). Some of this may be attributable to the growth of alternative forms of long-term care in combination with a trend toward healthier aging.

Despite the diversity of available long-term care options and settings and the decline in the proportion of older adults residing in nursing homes, nursing homes remain the most important residential care setting for the oldest and most disabled patients. Also, the major advances in scientific knowledge about the mental health aspects of long-term care are mostly from studies conducted in nursing homes. This chapter therefore focuses primarily on psychiatry in the nursing home setting.

DEMOGRAPHICS

Characteristics of this population are summarized in Table 34-1. Substantially higher rates of disability were reported from the Medical Expenditure Panel Survey (MEPS), which found in 1996 that 13.9% required assistance with one to two ADLs, and 83.3% needed help with three or more (Krauss & Altman, 1998; Rhoades & Krauss 1999). The proportion of residents requiring assistance with three or more ADLs was 15% higher in 1996 than in 1987. During the same period, the mean age of residents increased by 0.9 year, and the proportion aged 85 years or older increased from 49% to 56% for women and

TABLE 34-1.   Characteristics of the nursing home population in the United States

Age distribution	65–74 yrs old	13%
	75–84 yrs old	36%
	85+ yrs old	51%
Gender	Male	25%
	Female	75%
Race	Caucasian	90%
	African American	9%
	Other	1%
Marital status	Single, never married	12%
	Married	16%
	Divorced or separated	6%
	Widowed	66%
Sensory deficits	Visual impairment	27%
	Hearing impairment	23%
Impaired mobility	Dependent for ambulation	30%
	Dependent for transfers	24%
Dependence in ADLs	Bathing	96%
	Dressing	86%
	Toileting	57%
	Feeding	45%
Incontinence	Any bladder + bowel	43%

Source: Data from the 1995 National Nursing Home Survey (Strahan, 1997; Dey 1997).

ADLs, activities of daily living.

29% to 33% for men. Thus, the population of nursing home residents is characterized by extreme old age and high levels of disability.

Data from the 1995 National Nursing Home Survey also reflect the heterogeneity of US nursing homes (Dey, 1997). Of the estimated 16,700 nursing homes, 66% were for profit, 26% were nonprofit, and 8% were government owned; 54% belonged to management or ownership chains. Three quarters of nursing homes in the survey had between 50 and 199 beds. Nearly all were certified by either Medicare or Medicaid; 70% were certified by both. Approximately 58% of nursing home costs were paid by Medicaid; half of the Medicaid costs are funded by the federal government, half by the states.

EPIDEMIOLOGY AND CLINICAL CHARACTERISTICS OF PSYCHIATRIC DISORDERS IN THE NURSING HOME

In the early 1960s, the prevalence of psychiatric disorders in nursing homes was estimated at greater than 80%. Since then, epidemiological studies using rigorous methods have consistently demonstrated similar high rates. Rovner and coworkers found a prevalence of 80.2% among new admissions to a proprietary chain of nursing homes (Rovner, German, et al., 1990). Parmelee and colleagues surveyed the residents of a single large urban nursing home, confirmed diagnoses by clinical evaluation, and found psychiatric disorders according to the *Diagnostic and Statistical Manual of Mental Disorders, Third Edition, Revised* (*DSM-III-R*; American Psychiatric Association [APA], 1987) in 91% of the residents. Other studies, based on psychiatric interviews of randomly selected samples and using established diagnostic criteria (APA, 1980, 1987), detected prevalence rates as high as 94% (Chandler & Chandler, 1988; Rovner et al., 1986; Tariot et al., 1993). Other studies have reported lower rates, but used less-rigorous methods or sampled only selected subpopulations of nursing home residents (Burns et al., 1988; Custer et al., 1984; German et al., 1986; National Center for Health Statistics, 1987; Teeter et al., 1976).

Findings from this earlier research describe a profile of psychiatric disorders (Rovner, German, et al., 1990): 67.4% of residents had dementia, with approximately two thirds of these cases attributable to Alzheimer's disease; 10.4% had depression; and 2.4% had schizophrenia and other psychotic disorders. Data from the MEPS revealed that 70% to 80% of residents have cognitive impairment, and 20% have a diagnosis of a depressive disorder. These data support the previous findings and even suggest that the rates of depression and dementia have increased in comparison to prevalence rates found in nursing home studies conducted a decade earlier.

Dementia

In all epidemiological studies, the most common psychiatric disorder is dementia, with prevalence rates from one half to three quarters of residents (Chandler & Chandler, 1988; Parmelee et al., 1989; Rovner et al., 1986; Rovner, German, et al., 1990; Tariot et al., 1993; Teeter et al., 1976). The Epidemiologic Catchment Area (ECA) study reported a lower prevalence of cognitive impairment, but the more severely impaired residents who could not complete testing procedures were excluded (German et al., 1986). The Nursing Home Component of the MEPS reported a 48% prevalence of dementia diagnoses in US nursing home residents (Kraus & Altman, 1998). However, these data from both the ECA and MEPS probably underestimated the actual prevalence. As noted above, other MEPS data support previous findings of higher prevalence rates of cognitive disorders, demonstrating approximately 70% of residents with memory problems, 73% with orientation problems, and 80% with impaired decision-making capacity.

Among nursing home cases of dementia, Alzheimer's disease accounts for 50% to 60% of cases and vascular dementia for 25% to 30% (Barnes & Raskind, 1980; Rovner et al., 1986; Rovner, German, et al., 1990). Other causes of dementia are reported with lower prevalence and greater variability across sites. The prevalence of dementia with Lewy bodies has not been ascertained specifically in nursing home populations.

Approximately 40% of residents with dementia have other psychiatric syndromes complicating their illness, most commonly delirium, psychosis, and depression. These patients, who have associated psychiatric complications, are most likely to exhibit behavioral disturbances as well as excess cognitive and functional disability.

The rates of delirium detected in epidemiological studies are in the range of 6% to 7% (Barnes & Raskind, 1980; Rovner et al., 1986), with delirium superimposed in 10% of patients with dementia (Rovner, Lucas-Blaustein, et al., 1990). This probably underestimates the number of patients with reversible components to their cognitive impairment. One study found that 52 (47%) of 111 cognitively impaired residents had potentially reversible conditions (Sabin et al., 1982). Katz and colleagues (1991) found that 6% to 12% of residential care patients with dementia improved in cognitive performance over the course of 1 year. In the nursing home, as well as other settings, the most common cause of cognitive impairment may be cognitive toxicity from drugs used to treat medical and psychiatric conditions.

Psychotic symptoms have been reported in 13% to 50% of nursing home residents with dementia (Berrios & Brook, 1985; Chandler & Chandler, 1988; Rovner et al., 1986; Rovner, Lucas-Blaustein, et al., 1990; Teeter et al., 1976). Clinically significant depression is reported in about 6% to 25% of patients with dementia. Approximately one third of these individuals have symptoms of major depression (Parmelee et al., 1989). Depression may also account for some of the reversible cognitive impairment seen in patients with dementia.

Behavioral Disturbances in the Nursing Home

Behavioral disturbances may be present in up to three fourths of nursing home residents, with multiple behavior problems in at least one half (Chandler & Chandler, 1988; Cohen-Mansfield, 1986; National Center for Health Statistics, 1979; Rovner et al., 1986; Rovner, Lucas-Blaustein, et al., 1990; Tariot et al., 1993; Zimmer et al., 1984). MEPS data indicate that approximately 30% of residents have behavioral problems, with 11.8% exhibiting verbal abuse, 9.1% physical abuse, 14.5% socially inappropriate behavior, 12.5% resistance to care, and 9.4% wandering.

These reported rates are substantially lower than rates found in previous studies. This is likely to reflect different methods of case ascertainment rather than improved management leading to decreased prevalence. Nevertheless, the range of reported rates of behavioral disturbances (approximately 30%–75%) indicates that this is a major problem in caring for older adults in nursing homes.

Disturbances of behavior and impaired ability to perform ADLs have been identified as the most common reasons that patients with dementia are admitted to nursing homes (Steele et al., 1990), and disruptive behaviors frequently complicate care after admission (Cohen-Mansfield et al., 1989; Teeter et al., 1976; Zimmer et al., 1984). Most psychiatric consultations in the nursing home are for evaluation and treatment of behavioral disturbances, mostly in patients with dementia (Loebel et al., 1991).

Risk factors for behavioral disturbances include both dementia and psychoses. Among patients with dementia, the association of psychosis and behavioral disturbance remains even after controlling for the level of cognitive impairment (Rovner, Lucas-Blaustein, et al., 1990). Other causes of agitated behavior may include depression, delirium, sensory deprivation or overload, occult physical illness, pain, constipation, urinary urgency or retention, and adverse drug effects (Cohen-Mansfield & Billig, 1986).

Cohen-Mansfield and coworkers (1989) made substantial contributions to the characterization and measurement of agitation and related behavioral disturbances occurring in nursing home residents, emphasizing that agitation is a nonspecific symptom, not a specific diagnosis. As such, agitation requires evaluation to identify causal, contributing, or aggravating factors that are targets for specific treatment strategies. Factor analysis has identified three categories of agitation that are common in nursing home residents: verbally agitated behavior, nonaggressive physical behavior, and aggressive behavior. These investigators found that verbal agitation that occurs frequently in the nursing home setting includes constant requests for attention, negativism, repetitious phrases and questions, screaming, and complaining. The physically nonaggressive agitated behaviors observed most frequently were pacing, inappropriate dressing/disrobing, trying to get to a different place, handling things inappropriately, general restlessness, and inappropriate mannerisms.

Depression

Depression is the second most common psychiatric diagnosis among nursing home residents. Most studies report a 15% to 50% prevalence rate, a range that reflects differences in the population studied and the instruments used, whether major depression or depressive symptoms are reported, and whether primary depression and depression occurring secondary to dementia are considered together or separately (Baker & Miller, 1991; Chandler & Chandler, 1988; Hyer & Blazer, 1982; Katz, Lesher, et al., 1989; Lesher, 1986; Parmelee et al., 1989; Rovner et al., 1986, 1991; Tariot et al., 1993; Teeter et al., 1976). Studies from other countries have reported similar rates (Ames, 1991; Ames et al., 1988; Harrison et al., 1990; Horiguchi & Inami, 1991; Mann et al., 1984; Snowdon, 1986; Snowdon & Donnelly, 1986; Spangoli et al., 1986; Trichard et al., 1982).

The risk of depressive disorder is significantly higher in nursing home residents than in elderly persons residing in the community (Blazer & Williams,

1980; Kramer et al., 1985). Approximately 6% to 10% of all nursing home residents and 20% to 25% of the subgroup who are not demented meet *DSM-III* (APA, 1980) or *DSM-III-R* (APA, 1987) criteria for major depression. The prevalence of less-severe, but clinically significant, depression (i.e., minor depression or depressive symptoms or "subsyndromes" that do not meet diagnostic criteria for major depression) is even higher.

Little information is available on the incidence of new episodes of depression in the nursing home setting. In a study by Parmelee and colleagues (1992b), residents who were euthymic at baseline had a 1-year incidence of 7.4% for minor depression. Those with minor or no depression at baseline had a 1-year incidence of major depression of 9.4%, with greater risk in those who began with minor depression. Other, smaller scale, studies reported comparable rates (Foster et al., 1991; Katz, Lesher, et al., 1989). Thus, minor depression in nursing home residents appears to be a risk factor for major depression, suggesting that treatment of these disorders represents an opportunity for prevention as well as symptom relief.

Depression among nursing home residents tends to be persistent. Although one study showed a decrease in self-rated depression as a function of time elapsed since admission to the nursing home (Snowden & Donnelly, 1986), other investigators found that only 17% of surviving patients with depression had recovered at follow-up after an average of 3.6 years (Ames et al., 1988).

In nursing home populations, evidence for morbidity associated with depression comes from studies that show an increase in pain complaints (Parmelee et al., 1991) and an association between depression and biochemical markers of subnutrition (Katz et al., 1993). The association of depression with pain in this population may reflect an amplification of pain because of comorbid medical illness rather than unfounded somatic complaining. The association of depression and nutritional deficits in this population suggests a physiological response akin to "failure to thrive" in frail older adults as conceptualized by Braun and colleagues (1988). Depression is also associated with increased disability.

Although the direction of cause and effect is not always clear, it is likely that the relationship between depression and disability is reciprocal; that is, depression contributes to disability, and disability contributes to depression. Thus, depression may represent a treatable source of distress and disability, even in nursing home residents with other irreversible disabling diseases.

In addition to causing morbidity and disability, depression in nursing home residents is also associated with increased mortality, with studies finding effect sizes that ranged from 1.6 to 3 (Ashby et al., 1991; Katz, Lesher, et al., 1989; Parmelee et al., 1992a; Rovner et al., 1991). Rovner and coworkers (1991) reported that the increase in mortality remained even after controlling for medical diagnoses and level of disability. However, Parmelee and colleagues (1992a) found that mortality was attributable to the interrelationships among depression, medical illness, and disability. Thus, there is an unresolved contro-

versy about whether nursing home patients with depression are dying because
they are depressed or depressed because they are dying; the mechanism by
which mortality is increased in depressed nursing home residents has yet to be
elucidated.

NURSING HOME PROBLEMS AND REFORMS

Despite the extent of psychiatric disorders in US nursing homes and the high
prevalence of dementia and its attendant psychiatric and behavioral complications, most nursing homes chartered during the second half of the 20th century
were designed, staffed, and operated under the premise that the individuals
served are cognitively intact and behaviorally stable (Streim & Katz, 1994).
Most proprietors and nursing home administrators did not originally intend to
manage patients with mental illness. Individuals applying for nursing home
staff jobs were not expected or trained to care for patients with cognitive impairment or other psychiatric symptoms. Similarly, activities and medical consultative services were not created with this population in mind.

Studies in the 1980s revealed that as many as two thirds of nursing home
residents with psychiatric disorders were improperly diagnosed (German et al.,
1986; Sabin et al., 1982). Lack of diagnosis and misdiagnosis was, and still is,
of grave concern when considering the prevalence rates, the numbers of patients involved, the risks of excess disability, and the impact on humane treatment and quality of life. Inadequate and improper diagnostic assessment has
also been associated with inadequate and inappropriate treatment, including
the misuse of psychotropic drugs. One study reported that only 15% of residents receiving psychotropic drugs had received a psychiatric consultation
(Zimmer et al., 1984). Others reported that mental health services were available to less than 5% of those with a known psychiatric illness, and that 21%
of patients with no psychiatric diagnosis received psychotropic medication
(Burns et al., 1988), that physician characteristics (rather than those of patients) predicted drug dosage (Ray et al., 1980), and that psychotropic drugs
were often prescribed in the absence of any charted reference to patients' mental status (Avorn et al., 1989).

There has been a history of widespread concern regarding the overuse of
psychotropic drugs in treatment of nursing home residents. In particular, patient advocacy groups such as the National Citizens' Coalition for Nursing
Home Reform and the Alzheimer's Association publicized the excessive prescription of drugs originally developed for use as psychotherapeutic medications that were instead misused as "chemical restraints" to control patient
behaviors. Studies in the 1970s and 1980s revealed that about 50% of nursing
home residents had orders for psychotropic medications, with 20% to 40%
taking antipsychotic drugs, 10% to 40% taking anxiolytics or hypnotics,
and 5% to 10% taking antidepressants (Avorn et al., 1989; Beers et al.,
1988; Buck, 1988; Burns et al., 1988; Cohen-Mansfield, 1986; Custer et al.,

1984; DeLeo et al., 1989; Ray et al., 1980; Teeter et al., 1976; Zimmer et al., 1984).

Although concerns in the 1970s and 1980s tended to focus on the over-prescribing of tranquilizing drugs, a report of the Institute of Medicine (1986) highlighted both problems of overuse of antipsychotic drugs and the underuse of antidepressants for treatment of affective disorders in nursing homes. A re-view of epidemiological studies on the use of psychotropic drugs in nursing homes also noted that antidepressants were underutilized and that much of the major depression in this setting went untreated (Murphy, 1989).

Another major area of concern has been the use of physical restraints for control of behavior in nursing home residents. A 1977 survey of US nursing homes found that 25% of 1.3 million people were restrained by geriatric chairs, vests, cuffs, belts, or similar devices (National Center for Health Statistics, 1979). Other surveys have reported prevalence rates as high as 85%. Patient factors predicting use of restraints in nursing homes include age, cognitive impairment, risk of injury to self (e.g., from falls) or others (e.g., from combative behavior), physical frailty, presence of monitoring or treatment devices, and the need to promote body alignment. Institutional and system factors include pressure to avoid litigation, staff attitudes and expectations, insufficient staffing, and the availability of restraint devices. Mechanical restraints are frequently used to control disruptive behavior or behavior that is perceived by staff as problematic, socially unacceptable, or simply inconvenient. However, it has been shown that restraint use is often ineffective and is not without significant risks.

Although restraints are often used in response to agitation, they do not significantly decrease behavioral disturbances (Werner et al., 1989). Potential adverse effects of restraint use include falls, injuries, skin breakdown, functional decline, physiological effects of immobilization stress, disorganized behavior, and emotional desolation. Cross-national studies have shown that it is possible to manage nursing home residents without restraints (Cape, 1983; Evans & Strumpf, 1989; Innes & Turman, 1983).

Avoidance of restraints often requires that mental health professionals be involved in evaluating behavioral disturbances and formulating treatment interventions. It is important for mental health professionals who work in this setting to be knowledgeable about the physical and social environment of the nursing facility, as well as about the behavioral disorders of elderly individuals (Evans & Strumpf, 1989).

The concerns cited by consumer advocacy groups and the 1986 Institute of Medicine report regarding the inappropriate use of physical and chemical restraints in nursing homes were major factors prompting Congress to enact nursing home reform legislation. In addition, the General Accounting Office recognized that states had a strong incentive to place patients with psychiatric problems in Medicaid-certified nursing facilities, thereby shifting a substantial portion of the costs of their care from the states to the federal government.

In 1987, the Congressional House Committee on the Budget ascertained that substantial numbers of mentally retarded and mentally ill residents were inappropriately placed at Medicaid expense in nursing homes, where they usually did not receive the active psychiatric treatment or services that they needed.

Thus, it was a combination of fiscal concerns and clinical issues related to inadequate, inappropriate, and even inhumane care that prompted Congress to approve the sweeping Nursing Home Reform Amendments as part of the Omnibus Budget Reconciliation Act of 1987 (OBRA '87; Public Law 100–203). This legislation transformed nursing homes into one of the most highly regulated environments for health care delivery in the United States, providing for government oversight of most aspects of the operation of nursing facilities and of the care that they provide (Elon & Pawlson, 1992).

The laws enacted by Congress directed the Health Care Financing Administration (HCFA, subsequently renamed the Centers for Medicre and Medicaid Services [CMS]), the agency that administers Medicare and Medicaid, to issue regulations designed to make the laws operational (HCFA, 1991). States were charged with responsibility for enforcing these regulations by conducting periodic surveys of nursing facilities. To assist state surveyors in determining whether nursing facilities were in compliance with the regulations, HCFA developed a set of interpretive guidelines keyed to specific sections of the regulations (HCFA, 1992c). These guidelines have been revised over the past 10 years to reflect changes in health care practice and policy. Facilities that are out of compliance are required to submit remediation plans and are subject to penalties, including withholding of Medicare and Medicaid funds, for failure to comply.

The federal regulations cover nearly all aspects of nursing home operation, including administration (e.g., licensure, staff qualifications, record keeping, quality assurance); physical environment (e.g., space, equipment, safety); infection control; and specialized services (e.g., nursing, dietary, dental, rehabilitation, pharmacy). The Nursing Home Reform Amendments hold nursing facilities, rather than physicians, responsible for compliance. However, the regulations affect numerous aspects of medical and mental health practice. Mental health screening, evaluation, care planning, and treatment are addressed under sections of the regulations that pertain to resident assessment, resident rights, facility practices, and quality of care.

The OBRA regulations mandate Preadmission Screening and Annual Resident Review (PASARR) to identify patients with psychiatric disorders and ensure that they are not placed in nursing homes if there is a need for acute psychiatric care (e.g., inpatient psychiatric admission) that precludes adequate treatment in the nursing home setting (HCFA, 1992a). However, patients who have a primary diagnosis of dementia are considered eligible for nursing home admission regardless of psychiatric complications or comorbid conditions. After admission to a nursing facility, all patients are required to undergo periodic comprehensive assessments using the Minimum Data Set (MDS). This is a standardized instrument that includes several areas relevant to mental health, including mood, cognition, communication, behavior patterns, activities, functional status, psychosocial well-being, oral/nutritional status, comorbid disease, medications, and other treatments (HCFA, 1992b).

Responses on the MDS that indicate deficits or changes in the resident's health status trigger second-stage assessments with Resident Assessment Protocols (RAPs). These are assessment tools that furnish nursing staff with prompts to look for signs and symptoms of potential clinical problems; differential diagnoses of common problems; algorithms to direct further evaluations; and guidelines for treatment planning. RAP problem areas related to mental health include delirium, cognitive loss/dementia, psychosocial well-being, mood state, behavior problems, psychotropic drug use, and physical restraints. The OBRA regulations hold facilities responsible for ensuring that the MDS is completed on time and the RAPs are followed. Although physicians have no mandated role in this process, physician involvement is necessary for proper diagnosis and treatment of conditions covered by the RAPs (Elon & Pawlson, 1992). Psychiatric consultation may be needed when RAPs indicate a need for evaluation of problems related to mental health.

The OBRA regulations include provisions that affect psychiatric treatment in the nursing home. Sections of the regulations related to resident rights and facility practices restrict the use of physical restraints and psychotropic drugs when they are "administered for purposes of discipline or convenience and not required to treat the resident's medical symptoms" or promote improved functioning (HCFA, 1991, p. 48875).

Regulations related to quality of care also require that residents do not receive *unnecessary drugs*, defined as any drug when used (1) in excessive dose, (2) for excessive duration, (3) without adequate monitoring, (4) without adequate indications for its use, (5) in the presence of adverse effects indicating that it should be reduced or discontinued, or (6) any combination of these factors (HCFA, 1991). The regulations specifically target antipsychotic drugs, stating that they may not be given "unless these are necessary to treat a specific condition as diagnosed and documented in the clinical record" (p. 48910). The interpretive guidelines that accompany these regulations also limit the use of anxiolytic agents and drugs used as sedative hypnotics, as well as antipsychotics; but not antidepressants (HCFA, 1992c). For each of these classes, the guidelines provide a list of acceptable indications as well as specific agents that are prohibited; daily dose limits, which if exceeded, require documentation that the benefits justify the risks; requirements for monitoring treatment and adverse effects; and time frames for attempting dose reductions and discontinuation. These guidelines were updated in 2000 to reflect new clinical knowledge and accepted practice and to include new drugs approved by the US Food and Drug Administration (FDA).

To minimize concerns about federal interference with medical practice and the provision of appropriate individualized patient care, the current guidelines include qualifying statements that recognize cases in which strict adherence to prescribing limits is "clinically contraindicated." Although the emphasis remains on limiting the inappropriate use of psychotropic drugs, the guidelines acknowledge that appropriate treatment sometimes must depart from these limits. The guidelines instruct surveyors to allow nursing facilities the opportunity to present a rationale for the use of drugs prescribed contrary to the guidelines and to explain why such use is in the best interest of the resident before finding that the facility is not in compliance with the regulations on unnecessary drugs.

Thus, the physician's options for treating nursing home residents need not be restricted by the regulations as long as the clinical reasoning process demonstrates that the benefits to the patient (in terms of symptom relief, improved health status, or improved functioning) outweigh the risks, and the justification is clearly documented in the clinical record. Although the facility is accountable for compliance with these regulations, the physician's clinical reasoning and judgment still play a critical role in the process of ensuring quality care.

In addition to addressing the use of psychotropic drugs, the interpretive guidelines also outline conditions for the use of physical restraints. The guidelines state that restraints may not be used unless there is documentation that (1) efforts were made to identify and correct preventable or treatable factors that cause or contribute to the problem; (2) that prior attempts to use less-restrictive measures failed; and (3) that use of restraints enables the resident to achieve or maintain the highest practicable level of function. Physical or occupational therapists must be consulted if restraints are deemed necessary to enhance body positioning or improve mobility.

Although many sections of the federal regulations emphasize the need to limit inappropriate treatment, there are also provisions that require recognition and provision of appropriate treatment for mental health problems in nursing home patients. Sections of the regulations related to quality of care state that "the facility must ensure that a resident who displays mental or psychosocial adjustment difficulties receives appropriate services to correct the assessed problem" (HCFA, 1991, p. 48896). Together with the requirements for screening and assessment, these regulations clearly assign responsibility for both case finding and treatment of mental disorders. In addition, the regulations require that "a facility must care for its residents in a manner and in an environment that promotes maintenance or enhancement of each resident's quality of life" (p. 48910), with specific attention to issues that are important for promoting and maintaining mental health: dignity, individuality, and self-determination; participation in social, religious, and community activities; availability of ongoing activities in programs designed in accordance with the resident's interests and well-being; and delivery of all services in a manner that reasonably accommodates the individual needs and preferences of the resident.

In 1999, HCFA introduced quality indicators (QIs), derived from the MDS, to enable surveyors to compare individual facilities within the same state (Clark, 1999). There are 24 QIs within 11 different domains, including behavior/emotional problems, cognitive patterns, and psychotropic drug use. Behavioral/emotional patterns cover the prevalence of behavioral symptoms affecting others (e.g., verbally or physically abusive, socially inappropriate, or disruptive behavior); prevalence of symptoms of depression; and prevalence of depression without antidepressant therapy. The cognitive pattern domain examines the incidence of cognitive impairment when consecutive MDS assessments reveal new onset of impairments in short-term memory or decision-making capacity. The psychotropic drug use domain includes the prevalence of antipsychotic use for patients without psychotic conditions, the prevalence of anxiolytic/hypnotic use, and the prevalence of hypnotic use more than twice in a 7-day period. QIs that are indirectly related to mental disorders and their treatment include the use of nine or more different medications and the prevalence of falls, weight loss, daily application of physical restraints, and little or no activity.

Whenever a review in any of these areas results in a citation of deficiency, a plan of correction must be developed and submitted for approval. This system is a first step in monitoring quality of care, although the face validity of some of the quality indicators has been questioned, and the results of quality surveys may be difficult to interpret. Nevertheless, the results from every nursing home surveyed are available for public inspection, and consumers of nursing home services (and their families) are beginning to pay attention to the QI reports.

IMPACT OF NURSING HOME REFORM

In the decade after the implementation of the Nursing Home Reform Amendments contained in OBRA '87, substantial changes occurred in the delivery of nursing home care, including mental health care. Although multiple factors are likely to have contributed, many of the observed changes may be attributable to the federal regulations and dissemination of information about the regulatory requirements, as well as education regarding good clinical practice.

Soon after the regulations were implemented, several investigators developed and evaluated educational programs designed to reduce excessive use of medications in nursing homes. Ray and colleagues (1993) tested an educational intervention aimed at physicians and nursing staff; the intervention was based on a model of care that included evaluations of patients for reversible medical or psychosocial causes of behavioral disorders, nonpharmacological techniques for prevention and management, use of low-dose antipsychotics for serious behavioral disorders, and gradual withdrawal of antipsychotic drugs when possible. In nursing homes receiving the intervention, a 72% reduction in antipsychotic use was observed, compared with only 13% in control nursing homes. In a subsequent randomized controlled trial of their educational intervention in 12 nursing homes that had continued high rates of antipsychotic use even after OBRA implementation, this group of investigators showed a 23% reduction in antipsychotic drug use in homes with the educational intervention relative to control homes, suggesting that focused provider education programs may facilitate reduction of antipsychotic drug use above and beyond that attributable to the effects of regulatory changes alone (Meador et al., 1997).

Avorn and coworkers (1992) also evaluated the efficacy of an educational program in geriatric psychopharmacology that was aimed at physicians, nurses, and aides. Scores on an index of psychotropic drug use, measuring both the magnitude and the probable inappropriateness of medication use, declined significantly in the experimental nursing homes compared to control facilities.

Rovner and colleagues (1992) evaluated changes in psychotropic prescribing and quality assurance data in 17 corporately owned nursing homes in which a pharmacy service provided educational materials about medication use and OBRA regulations to medical directors, primary care physicians, and directors of nursing. Over 6 months, there was a 36% reduction in antipsychotic drug use, with no increase in use of sedative-hypnotics or anxiolytics. Similarly, Schnelle and colleagues (1992) evaluated management procedures designed to improve staff adherence to federal regulations regarding physical restraints; they found that a simple strategy of cues to remind staff about acceptable approaches was effective in increasing compliance.

Research on psychotropic drug prescriptions during the early 1990s after OBRA implementation showed evidence of substantial reductions in antipsychotic drug use and increases in antidepressant use (Lantz et al., 1996). Shorr and coworkers (1994) conducted a longitudinal study of 9,432 elderly Tennessee Medicaid enrollees and found a 26.7% decline in antipsychotic drug use without a concomitant increase in other psychotropic drug use. Of interest, the extent of antipsychotic reduction was positively correlated with third-shift staffing levels. Although this decrease may be consistent with an improvement in the quality of nursing home care, this study did not examine effects of reduced antipsychotic drug use on resident outcomes.

Siegler and colleagues (1997) examined the effect of OBRA regulations on appropriateness of antipsychotic use and found the percentage of residents on antipsychotics who lacked an OBRA-approved indication declined from 21.3% to 14.6%. A retrospective study in a single nursing facility described attempts to discontinue or lower the dose of antipsychotic drugs in 75% of subjects studied and found that residents with appropriate indications for antipsychotic use according to the federal regulations were significantly less likely to have their antipsychotic agent stopped (Semla et al., 1994). Nevertheless, 20% of residents whose antipsychotic was discontinued or reduced in dose subsequently had the agent resumed or its dose increased. This is consistent with earlier discontinuation studies and suggests that the finding of a reduction in overall rates of antipsychotic use cannot be interpreted as an indication of "across-the-board" improvement in the quality of care for all residents.

A study of pharmacy records in eight nursing homes found that, of the 17.7% of residents receiving antipsychotic medications, 70.9% had an OBRA-approved diagnostic indication, 90.4% had documentation of appropriate target symptoms, and 90.1% were on doses within recommended limits stipulated in the HCFA guidelines, suggesting relatively high rates of compliance with the OBRA regulations (Llorente et al., 1998). In general, however, pharmacoepidemiological studies have not adequately examined the impact of compliance with the federal guidelines for medication use or discontinuation on symptom control, functional status, quality of life, and other relevant health care outcome measures.

Since the mid-1990s, there has been evidence of shifting trends in psychotropic drug use. It has been estimated that the use of psychotherapeutic medications in US nursing homes increased from 21.7% in 1991 to 46.1% in 1997 (HCFA, 1998). This was the net result of a 52% decrease in the use of antipsychotic medications from 33.7% to 16.1% and a 97% increase in the use of antidepressants from 12.6% to 24.9%. Likely determinants of these shifts in medication use include federal regulations, cumulative effects of professional education, availability of new drugs, and advances in scientific knowledge.

A somewhat different picture emerged from a retrospective chart review of psychiatric referrals in seven Massachusetts nursing homes during 1995–1996 (Lasser & Sunderland, 1998). These authors reported that 42% of nursing home patients were taking antipsychotic drugs, with more than 30% of these treated with risperidone. This represents a higher rate of prescribing antipsychotic drugs compared to rates reported by HCFA, but is based on a smaller regional sample of patients referred to a geriatric psychiatry service who had been treated mostly by primary care physicians. It nevertheless suggests that another shift in prescribing may have begun during this period, which could be explained by the availability of new medications with better tolerability and safety profiles.

More impressive is the finding that 61% of patients in this sample were taking antidepressants, with 53% taking serotonin reuptake inhibitors (SRIs; Lasser & Sunderland, 1998). In a study of 5 Pennsylvania nursing homes, Datto and colleagues (2002) found that 47% of residents were taking antidepressants. Both the Massachusetts and Pennsylvania studies and the data reported by HCFA represent an extraordinary change in the pattern of drug utilization in a population that has traditionally received inadequate pharmacotherapy for depression. Before 1990, fewer than 15% of residents with a known diagnosis of depression were receiving antidepressant medication (Heston et al., 1992). The dramatic increase in antidepressant prescriptions is probably due in part to the wide availability of newer antidepressants that are thought to be well tolerated by elderly nursing home residents with medical-psychiatric comorbidity. Aggressive marketing to primary care physicians may also play a role. With current antidepressant drug utilization rates that appear comparable to or greater than the estimated prevalence of depression in nursing homes, it might appear that the previous problems of undertreatment of depression in nursing homes have been remedied. However, Brown and co-workers (2002) have shown that, of nursing home residents known to be depressed and receiving antidepressants, 32% were on doses less than the manu-facturers' recommended minimum effective dose. The study by Datto and coworkers revealed that, of the 47% of nursing home residents taking antide-pressants, nearly half were still depressed. Although more residents are receiv-ing antidepressant treatment, many may not be getting follow-up care that is sufficient to achieve remission.

Despite the concerns about the interpretation of trends in psychotropic drug use, most investigators agree that the impact of the federal regulations with respect to restraint use has been positive; several studies showed signifi-cant reductions in the use of physical restraints. One study found restraint use rates of 37.4% in 1990 (before OBRA implementation) and 28.1% in 1993 (after introduction of the standardized Resident Assessment Instrument, which is part of the MDS required by OBRA) (Hawes et al., 1997).

Siegler and coworkers (1997) enlisted three nursing homes in a clinical trial of educational and consultation interventions to support OBRA man-dates to reduce physical restraint use. They found that restraint use declined significantly in the home that received the combined educational/consultation program, and none of the interventions was associated with an increase in antipsychotic or benzodiazepine use.

A more controversial issue has been the utility of the PASARR (Snow-den & Roy-Byrne, 1998). Concern has been expressed that some patients who require nursing home services have been denied admission because PASARR identifies them as having a mental illness even if they are determined not to need acute psychiatric care (Colenda et al., 1999). Borson and associates (1997) examined a sample of 510 patients referred for psychiatric assessment as part of their required preadmission screening. They found a primary mental illness, evenly divided between psychoses and mood disorders, in 60% of those re-ferred for assessment and a psychiatric disorder associated with dementia or mental retardation in 25%. In this sample, 88% were appropriately placed based on their care needs, and 55% had unmet mental health services needs. The authors found that the PASARR is efficient for identifying patients with schizophrenia; but the exemption from assessment for dementia results in underrepresentation of patients with psychiatric disturbances secondary to de-mentia. Because a majority of nursing home residents have dementia, and pa-tients with schizophrenia represent only a small minority, the PASARR process is inadequate as a mechanism for identifying nursing home candidates who require mental health services, and PASARR results cannot be used to estimate mental health service needs in nursing homes.

The high prevalence of psychiatric problems and the federal mandate to ensure quality of care together define a need for geriatric mental health services in nursing homes (Smith et al., 1990). Although the OBRA regulations have resulted in measurable improvements in patient care, it has not been shown that the federal requirements for assessment and treatment of mental disorders have led to improved access to mental health care. In a survey conducted by

Reichman and coworkers (1998) of nursing homes across six states, 47.6% of 899 respondents indicated that the frequency of on-site psychiatric consultation was inadequate. Directors of nursing judged that 38% of their residents needed a psychiatric evaluation, but more than one fourth of respondents in rural homes and over one fifth of those in small homes reported that no psychiatric consultant was available to them. Thus, there is evidence that the OBRA requirement for patients to receive services to "attain or maintain the highest practicable physical, mental, and psychosocial well-being" (p. 48910) has not resulted in sufficient access to mental health services in US nursing homes (Colenda et al., 1999).

TREATMENT OF PSYCHIATRIC DISORDERS IN THE NURSING HOME

As described above, the available evidence suggests that, over the past 15 years, the high levels of psychiatric morbidity in nursing home residents have not diminished, and the distribution of disorders has remained the same. However, during the same period, there has been significant progress in developing and evaluating treatments for psychiatric disorders in nursing homes. An appreciation of the unique characteristics of nursing home populations—particularly the extremes of old age and frailty and the high prevalence of cognitive impairment, psychiatric-medical comorbidity, and disability, all in the context of residential long-term care institutions—has led to increased recognition that results of treatment efficacy studies conducted in general adult outpatient populations may not be readily generalizable to nursing home residents. This points to the need for studies of the effectiveness of psychiatric treatment conducted specifically in nursing home patients. Although the number of randomized, controlled studies is limited, there is a growing body of literature on treatment outcomes in the nursing home.

Research has demonstrated the effectiveness of several nonpharmacological interventions for managing behavioral disturbances associated with dementia in the nursing home setting. One promising approach combined augmented activities, guidelines for psychotropic medication use, and educational rounds for nursing home staff (Rovner et al., 1996). In a randomized clinical trial, it was effective in reducing the prevalence of problem behaviors and the use of both antipsychotic drugs and physical restraints. Individualized consultation for staff nurses about the management of patients with dementia has also been demonstrated to reduce the use of physical restraints (Evans et al., 1997). Other programs rely on modification of the physical environment to decrease behavioral difficulties. Research on individualized behavioral interventions for patients with behavioral disturbances of dementia has been limited to case series and small-scale controlled trials that are often difficult to replicate, although some of the findings are promising (Allen-Burge et al., 1999).

Although the growing evidence for the efficacy of psychotherapy in other settings suggests that it may be of value for those patients whose cognitive abilities allow them to participate, there have been only a small number of controlled studies of the effectiveness of specific psychotherapy modalities, individual or group, for elderly nursing home residents. Controlled research on psychotherapy interventions has included studies of task-oriented versus insight-oriented therapy (Moran & Gatz, 1987); reality orientation (Baines et al., 1987); reminiscence groups (Baines et al., 1987; Goldwasser et al., 1987; McMurdo & Rennie, 1993; Orten et al., 1989; Rattenburg & Stones, 1989; Youssef, 1990); exercise, activity, and progressive relaxation groups (Bensink et al., 1992; McMurdo & Rennie, 1993); supportive group psychotherapy (Goldwasser et al., 1987; Williams-Barnard & Lindell, 1992); and cognitive or cognitive-behavioral group therapies (Abraham et al., 1992; Zerhusen et al., 1991). With the exception of the investigation by Abraham, most of these studies did not select patients based on specific psychiatric symptoms or syndromes; rather, they selected on the basis of age, cognitive status, or mobility. Some of these studies reported improvement on measures of communication, behavior, cognitive performance, mood, social withdrawal, physical function, somatic preoccupation, self-esteem, perceived locus of control, and life satisfaction. There are also case reports and demonstration projects by experienced clinicians that have documented the value of psychotherapy in the treatment of depressed nursing home residents (Leszcz et al., 1985; Sadavoy, 1991).

Overall, there remains a critical lack of research to evaluate the outcomes of specific psychotherapies—modalities with proven efficacy in other settings for treating mental disorders of aging—in nursing home residents who have well-characterized psychiatric disorders. Nevertheless, the available evidence from nursing home research, considered together with outcomes of psychotherapy for older adults in other clinical settings, suggests that psychotherapy should be regarded as an important component of mental health treatment for the more cognitively intact nursing home residents with depression.

Pharmacological treatments are commonly used in nursing homes to treat dementia and its psychiatric and behavioral complications and to treat depression. Prior to 1990, there were few randomized controlled clinical trials of psychotropic drugs conducted specifically in nursing home populations. Some of these earlier studies provided evidence for the efficacy of antipsychotic drugs in managing agitation and related symptoms in nursing home residents with dementia, but the effect sizes were often modest, and high placebo response rates were common (Barnes et al., 1982; Schneider et al., 1990).

Two multicenter, randomized, double-blind, placebo-controlled clinical trials demonstrated the efficacy of risperidone (an atypical antipsychotic agent) for the treatment of psychotic symptoms and agitated behavior in nursing home residents with dementia (DeDeyn et al., 1999; Katz et al., 1999). The results showed that it has antipsychotic effects and independent effects on aggression or agitation. The study by DeDeyn et al. included a comparison group treated with haloperidol. Follow-up studies suggested that risperidone may cause less tardive dyskinesia than typical antipsychotic agents (Jeste et al., 2000). A randomized clinical trial of olanzepine versus placebo in nursing home residents showed efficacy similar to that of risperidone (Street et al., 2000). A multicenter, randomized , placebo-controlled trial of aripiprazole found significant improvement in agitation and depression, but not psychosis, in residents of nursing homes and assisted living facilities with dementia (Streim, 2003). Findings from a nursing home study examining the effects of quetiapine are expected soon.

These controlled clinical trials have examined only the acute effects of treatment, typically for 6 to 12 weeks of treatment, and little is known about the effectiveness of treatment for longer periods. However, there is evidence to suggest that the need for and benefit from antipsychotic drug treatment changes over the course of months in nursing home patients with dementia. Two double-blind, placebo-controlled studies of antipsychotic drug discontinuation demonstrated that the majority of patients who have been receiving longer term treatment can be withdrawn from these agents without reemergence of psychosis or agitated behaviors (Bridges-Parlet et al., 1997; Cohen-Mansfield et al., 1999). This is consistent with findings from previous discontinuation studies (Barton & Hurst, 1966; Risse et al., 1987). Thus, it is important to reevaluate the need for continuing antipsychotic drug treatment on a regular basis.

Two randomized clinical trials evaluated the efficacy of mood-stabilizing anticonvulsant drugs for the treatment of agitation and aggression in nursing home residents. The first was a study of carbamazepine that showed it is effective for agitation, hostility, and aggression, but not for psychotic symptoms such as delusions and hallucinations (Tariot et al., 1998). In this study, nursing reports indicated that less staff time was required for patient care in the group treated with carbamazepine. Another placebo-controlled study evaluated divalproex and found evidence for efficacy in reducing agitated behavior (Porsteinsson et al., 2001), although sedation and diminished oral intake may be problems in elderly nursing home residents with dementia.

Acetylcholinesterase inhibitors have been shown to be efficacious for delaying the decline in cognitive function in patients with mild-to-moderate Alzheimer's disease. However, little is known about the effects of these agents in patients with more advanced disease, as is commonly found in nursing home populations. One randomized clinical trial of donepezil in nursing home residents showed effects on cognitive performance that were comparable to those observed in less-impaired outpatients (Tariot et al., 2001). Some studies examined the effects of acetylcholinesterase inhibitors on behavioral disturbances, usually as a secondary outcome measure in outpatients, and some findings suggest these agents may be useful for this purpose (Kaufer et al., 1998; Morris et al., 1998). Prospective trials need to evaluate the effects on behavioral disturbances in nursing home populations.

Two randomized clinical trials evaluated the effects of antidepressants in nursing home residents; both trials used nortriptyline. The earlier study, which was placebo controlled, confirmed the validity of the diagnosis of major depression among nursing home residents despite potential confounds from medical, environmental, and existential factors that might have otherwise explained the occurrence of depressive symptoms in this setting (Katz et al., 1990). This study also found that patients with major depression associated with low levels of serum albumin and high levels of disability (impaired ADL function) were less likely to respond to treatment. It was suggested that patients with this clinical profile were "failing to thrive" and might benefit from early hospitalization and evaluation of the need for electroconvulsive therapy. In the second study, patients were randomly assigned to receive regular versus low-dose nortriptyline, and significant plasma level-response relationships were demonstrated in cognitively intact patients (Streim et al., 2000). This again confirmed the validity of the diagnosis of depression in nursing home residents in the context of significant medical comorbidity and disability. However, in patients with dementia, the plasma level-response relationship was significantly different, suggesting that the depression of dementia might be a treatment-relevant subtype of depression or a distinct disorder.

Although the SRIs might be expected to be well tolerated by frail elderly nursing home patients because their side effect profile is less noxious appearing, there is evidence that they can cause serious adverse events in this population. Thapa and associates (1998) demonstrated that SRI use is associated with a nearly two-fold increase in the risk of falls in nursing home residents, comparable to the risk found with tricyclic antidepressant drugs. Available open-label studies of the efficacy of SRIs in nursing home residents with depression had mixed results, with some findings suggesting that they may be less effective for depression in those with dementia compared to those who are cognitively intact (Magai et al., 2000; Oslin et al., 2000; Rosen et al., 2000; Trappler & Cohen, 1996, 1998). There is some evidence that methylphenidate may be useful in demented patients with symptoms of apathy and withdrawal (Galynker et al., 1997; Kaplitz, 1975).

SPECIAL CARE UNITS

Beyond the modification of individual environmental factors to help manage nursing home residents with dementia, special care units (SCUs) have evolved to address the needs of this patient population. Encouraged by both consumer demand and other market forces, 10% of all US nursing homes had established a special care unit by 1991. It is now estimated that 22% of nursing homes have designated SCUs for patients with dementia. Research on SCUs has been hampered by the heterogeneity of these facilities (Ohta & Ohta, 1988).

In an effort to characterize the population served by these units, Holmes and coworkers (1990) reported that SCU patients had more severe cognitive, behavioral, and functional deficits than non-SCU patients with dementia who lived in the same nursing home. More than 90% of residents on SCUs have behavior problems (Wagner et al., 1995). Some studies indicated that the facilities, services, and programs offered by SCUs may not be significantly superior to those available on conventional nursing home units. Gold and colleagues (1991) found that SCUs were associated with higher quality care than were traditional units, although the quality of SCUs was not uniformly outstanding. A study of Minnesota nursing homes described unit and facility characteristics, noting that the designation of SCU did not necessarily translate into richer or more tailored services for dementia compared with units without the designation. However, some dementia-specific features were less likely to be found in regular units of nursing homes with designated SCUs (Grant et al., 1995). This sample of SCUs had a higher proportion of residents with dementia and fewer residents with acute problems.

A case-control study of 625 patients on 31 SCUs and 32 traditional units found that residence in an SCU was associated with reduced use of physical restraints, but not with less "pharmacological restraint" use (Sloane et al., 1991). A study that included data on more than 1,100 residents in 48 SCUs reported that restraint use was not different, and likelihood of psychotropic medication use was greater for patients on SCUs compared to their counterparts on traditional units (Phillips et al., 2000). These authors suggested that residents of SCUs might even receive a poorer quality of care compared to that provided to similar residents in traditional units.

Earlier research suggested that residence in SCUs might be associated with a trend toward increased hospital admission rates, usually for hip fractures; and greater cognitive decline after these hospitalizations (Coleman et al., 1990). Rather than indicating poorer quality of care, these findings might be interpreted as a manifestation of SCU policy to support more independence in ambulation in a population with increased risk of falls because of cognitive impairment, with a resultant increase in the rate of falls and fractures. Although there is evidence that mobility may be maintained longer (Saxton et al., 1998), others have found that the rate of decline in ADL function is not significantly slower for residents of SCUs (Phillips et al., 1997).

Studies that showed benefits for behavioral disturbances are limited (Leon & Ory, 1999), and randomized clinical trials that reported positive outcomes have been limited to catastrophic reactions (Swanson et al., 1993). Some studies have demonstrated psychological benefits not only for patients (Lawton et al., 1998), but also for caregivers (Kutner et al., 1999; Wells & Jorm, 1987), with evidence of increased family involvement (Hansen et al., 1988).

Sloane and colleagues (1998) also examined the extent to which agitation is associated with aspects of the treatment environment on SCUs. Independent correlates of low agitation levels on these units included favorable scores on measures of physical environment and unit activities, low rates of physical restraint use, a high proportion of residents in bed during the day, small unit size, fewer comorbid conditions, and low levels of functional dependency.

Despite the efforts of these investigators, there is still insufficient knowledge about the essential elements of treatment in SCUs. Evidence for the effectiveness of these units has not been adequately demonstrated.

Although the development of special care units has focused on the specific needs of patients with dementia, other nursing home residents also have unique problems of aging, comorbidity, and disability, and they, too, have "special" needs. For both demented and cognitively intact residents, it has been established that both quality of life and health outcomes are improved when the environment is designed to foster the resident's sense of autonomy and control.

Lawton and colleagues (1994, 1998) emphasized the need for attention to the fit between individual residents and the care environment. In their model of aging and adaptation, the demands presented by the environment must match the resident's capabilities and competencies. Maximal *performance* is elicited when the demands and challenges from the environment slightly exceed the level that would match the resident's current abilities, a condition that may be most appropriate for a rehabilitation program. Maximal *comfort* can be achieved when the environmental pressure is slightly below the resident's current abilities, a condition that may be most appropriate during recovery from acute illness or during a terminal illness.

According to the model of Lawton and colleagues, affective or behavioral disorders can result when environmental demands exceed the zone of maximal performance (causing the resident to become overwhelmed) or when they fall below the zone of maximal comfort (leaving unmet needs and causing the resident to experience a state of deprivation). The key to engineering the nursing home environment for optimal mental health and functioning is to modify the demands that the environment places on the resident. This usually requires the input of mental health professionals, who can assist nursing home staff in evaluating and managing the complexities presented by nursing home residents.

ROLES OF THE PSYCHIATRIST IN THE NURSING HOME

Psychiatrists have begun to play an important role in promoting the goals of nursing home reform and translating research findings into clinical practice in the nursing home setting. With the substantial advances in our knowledge about mental health and long-term care, improvement in the quality of mental health care in nursing homes is attainable.

In addition to traditional direct patient care activities, such as clinical evaluation and treatment, psychiatrists also provide consultation-liaison services, staff education, and administrative consultation (Bienenfeld & Wheeler, 1989; Borson et al., 1987; Grossberg et al., 1990; Liptzin, 1983; Sakauye & Camp, 1992; Streim & Katz, 1995). Often, a combination of these functions is required to meet the needs of patients, families, nursing home staff, and administrators. In working within nursing homes, psychiatrists often function as part of an interdisciplinary team that may include the primary care physician or the facility medical director, nurses, aides, social worker, rehabilitation therapists, activities staff, dietitian, pharmacist, and administrators (Cohn & Smyer, 1988; Sakauye & Camp, 1992). In response to variations in facility staffing and operating characteristics, as well as individual work styles, the psychiatrist may, for example, adopt the role of team member, consultant to the team or individual team members, or supervisor of other clinicians who are direct providers of mental health services.

Although Medicare Part B and other health insurance generally limits payment to those services rendered directly to the patient, consultation that focuses on helping nursing home staff is an important component of nursing home psychiatry; payment for the time spent delivering staff consultation can sometimes be negotiated with nursing home administrators who appreciate the value of this service. Many programs have been described in which nurses and aides rely on consulting psychiatrists to provide guidance in assessing, understanding, and managing patients with psychiatric symptoms and behavioral disturbances (Colthart, 1974; Liptzin, 1983; Loebel et al., 1991; Sakauye & Camp, 1992; Tourigny-Rivard & Drury, 1987). In collaborative practice, the psychiatrist also relies on the staff, who have numerous opportunities to participate in the psychiatric assessment by making observations of clinical signs and symptoms, the context in which behavior problems occur, and the patient's involvement in social, recreational, and therapeutic activities.

Staff consultation can also be helpful in developing the role of nursing home staff in mental health treatment. Direct daily care provides numerous opportunities for negative as well as positive interactions between staff and patients, and the frequency and intensity of staff-patient contact can either be an important factor in the pathogenesis of behavior problems or a key component in their treatment. Through staff consultation, the psychiatrist can promote therapeutic staff-patient interactions and can guide staff in reducing maladaptive responses and supporting adaptive behaviors and more independent functioning in nursing home residents (APA, 1989; Moses, 1982). The psychiatric consultant can also instruct staff to make observations regarding treatment outcomes.

Thus, staff consultation is a vehicle by which the consulting psychiatrist can improve psychiatric assessment and management by facilitating clinical observations and therapeutic interventions during the many hours of direct contact between staff and residents. In this model, the psychiatrist functions as an on-site professional consultant who is "extrinsic" to the nursing facility, and the staff function as agents of direct mental health care who are part of the "intrinsic" nursing home system (Streim & Katz, 1996).

Another role for the psychiatrist in the nursing home is to provide staff education (Herst & Moulton, 1985). Useful formats include case-oriented staff consultation, case conferences, workshops, and seminars for in-service training (Liptzin, 1983; Sakauye & Camp, 1992; Smith et al., 1990; Westlake & Rubano, 1983). The goals of these educational efforts are to enhance staff knowledge and skills in recognizing psychiatric symptoms, knowing when to request consultation, managing behavioral disturbances, tracking treatment response, and monitoring for adverse effects of treatment. Disruptive or dangerous behaviors are usually apparent to staff and are likely to prompt requests for psychiatric consultation (Birkett, 1991; Loebel et al., 1991). However, education is crucial to help staff recognize the importance of less-dramatic presentations of psychiatric disorders with "silent" symptoms such as withdrawal, decreased initiative, diminished activity, or decline in functional capacity (APA, 1989).

The psychiatrist can also serve in the role of mental health consultant for administrative matters such as policy formulation, program development, and environmental design. Because the high prevalence of psychiatric disorders can be a source of significant distress for nursing home staff, most of whom do not have specific training in mental health, other goals of administrative consultation may be to improve staff effectiveness and job satisfaction, reduce absenteeism and staff turnover (Cohn & Smyer, 1988), and recognize and prevent abuse of nursing home residents. In SCUs, where patients are usually admitted because of disability resulting from a psychiatric disorder, the physicians with the training and experience to best perform the administrative role of medical director may well be geriatric psychiatrists (Streim & Katz, 1995).

REFERENCES

Abraham IL, Neundorfer MM, Currie LJ. Effects of group interventions on cognition and depression in nursing home residents. *Nurs Res.* 1992;41:196–202.

Allen-Burge R, Stevens AB, Burgio LD. Effective behavioral interventions for decreasing dementia-related challenging behavior in nursing homes. *Int J Geriatr Psychiatry.* 1999;14:213–228.

American Psychiatric Association. *Nursing Homes and the Mentally Ill Elderly.* Washington, DC: American Psychiatric Association; 1989. Task Force Report 28.

American Psychiatric Association. *Diagnostic and Statistical Manual of Mental Disorders.* 3rd ed. Washington, DC: American Psychiatric Association; 1980.

American Psychiatric Association. *Diagnostic and Statistical Manual of Mental Disorders.* 3rd ed., rev. Washington, DC: American Psychiatric Association; 1987.

Ames D. Epidemiological studies of depression among the elderly in residential and nursing homes. *Int J Geriatr Psychiatry.* 1991;6:347–354.

Ames D, Ashby D, Mann AH, et al. Psychiatric illness in elderly residents of Part III homes in one London borough: prognosis and review. *Age Aging.* 1988;17:249–256.

Ashby D, Ames D, West CR, et al. Psychiatric morbidity as prediction of mortality for residents of local authority homes for the elderly. *Int J Geriatr Psychiatry.* 1991;6:567–575.

Avorn J, Dreyer P, Connelly K, et al. Use of psychoactive medication and the quality of care in rest homes. *N Engl J Med.* 1989;320:227–232.

Avorn J, Soumerai SD, Everitt DE, et al. A randomized trial of a program to reduce the use of psychoactive drugs in nursing homes. *N Engl J Med.* 1992;327:168–173.

Baines S, Saxby P, Ehlert K. Reality orientation and reminiscence therapy. *Br J Psychiatry.* 1987;151:222–231.

Baker FM, Miller CL. Screening a skilled nursing home population for depression. *J Geriatr Psychiatry Neurol.* 1991;4:218–221.

Barnes R, Veith R, Okimoto J, et al. Efficacy of antipsychotic medications in behaviorally disturbed dementia patients. *Am J Psychiatry.* 1982;139:1170–1174.

Barnes RF, Raskind, MA. *DSM-III* criteria and the clinical diagnosis of dementia: a nursing home study. *J Gerontol.* 1980;36:20–27.

Barton R, Hurst L. Unnecessary use of tranquilizers in elderly patients. *Br J Psychiatry.* 1966;112:989–990.

Beers M, Avon J, Soumerai SB, et al. Psychoactive medication use in intermediate-care facility residents. *JAMA.* 1988;260:3016–3020.

Bensink GW, Godbey KL, Marshall MJ, et al. Institutionalized elderly: relaxation, locus of control, self-esteem. *J Gerontol Nurs.* 1993;18:30–36.

Berrios GE, Brook P. Delusions and psychopathology of the elderly with dementia. *Acta Psychiatr Scand.* 1985;75:296–301.

Bienenfeld D, Wheeler BG. Psychiatric services to nursing homes: a liaison model. *Hosp Community Psychiatry.* 1989;40:793–794.

Birkett PD. *Psychiatry in the Nursing Home.* Binghamton, NY: Haworth Press; 1991.

Blazer D, Williams CD. Epidemiology of dysphoria and depression in an elderly population. *Am J Psychiatry.* 1980;137:439–444.

Borson S, Liptzin B, Nininger J, et al. Psychiatry and the nursing home. *Am J Psychiatry.* 1987;144:1412–1418.

Borson S, Loebel JP, Kitchell M, Domoto S, Hyde T. Psychiatric assessments of nursing home residents under OBRA-87: should PASARR be reformed? Pre-admission screening and annual review. *J Am Geriatr Soc.* 1997;45:1173–1181.

Braun JV, Wykle MH, Cowling WR. Failure to thrive in older persons: a concept derived. *Gerontologist.* 1988;28:809–812.

Bridges-Parlet S, Knopman D, Steffes S. Withdrawal of neuroleptic medications from institutionalized dementia patients: results of a double-blind, baseline-treatment-controlled pilot study. *J Geriatr Psychiatry Neurol.* 1997;10:119–126.

Buck JA. Psychotropic drug practice in nursing homes. *J Am Geriatr Soc.* 1988;36:409–418.

Burns BJ, Larson DB, Goldstrom ID, et al. Mental disorder among nursing home patients: preliminary findings from the national nursing home survey pretest. *Int J Geriatr Psychiatry.* 1988;3:27–35.

Cape RD. Freedom from restraint. *Gerontologist.* 1983;23(special issue):217.

Chandler JD, Chandler JE. The prevalence of neuropsychiatric disorders in a nursing home population. *J Geriatr Psychiatry Neurol.* 1988;1:71–76.

Clark TR, ed. *Nursing Home Survey Procedures and Interpretive Guidelines. A Resource for the Consultant Pharmacist.* Alexandria, VA: American Society of Consultant Pharmacists; 1999:section 3, pp. 1–8.

Cohen-Mansfield J. Agitated behaviors in the elderly: preliminary results in the cognitively deteriorated. *J Am Geriatr Soc.* 1986;34:722–727.

Cohen-Mansfield J, Billig N. Agitated behaviors in the elderly: a conceptual review. *J Am Geriatr Soc.* 1986;34:711–721.

Cohen-Mansfield J, Lipson S, Werner P, et al. Withdrawal of haloperidol, thioridazine, and lorazepam in the nursing home: a controlled, double-blind study. *Arch Intern Med.* 1999;159:1733–1740.

Cohen-Mansfield J, Marx MS, Rosenthal AS. A description of agitation in a nursing home. *J Gerontol.* 1989;44:M77–M84.

Cohn MD, Smyer MA. Mental health consultation: process, professions, and models. In: Smyer MA, Cohn MD, Brannon D, eds. *Mental Health Consultation in Nursing Homes.* New York, NY: New York University Press; 1988:47–63.

Coleman EA, Barbaccia JC, Croughan-Minihane MS. Hospitalization rates in nursing home residents with dementia: a pilot study of the impact of a special care unit. *J Am Geriatr Soc.* 1990;38:108–112.

Colenda CC, Streim JE, Greene JA, Meyers N, Beckwith E, Rabins P. The impact of the Omnibus Budget Reconciliation Act of 1987 (OBRA'87) on psychiatric services in nursing homes. *Am J Geriatr Psychiatry.* 1999;7:12–17.

Colthart SM. A mental health unit in a skilled nursing facility. *J Am Geriatr Soc.* 1974; 22:453–456.

Custer RL, Davis JE, Gee SC. Psychiatric drug usage in VA nursing home care units. *Psychiatr Ann.* 1984;14:285–292.

Datto CJ, Oslin DW, Streim JE, Scheinthal SM, DiFilippo S, Katz IR. Pharmacological treatment of depression in nursing home residents: a mental health services perspective. *J Geriatr Psychiatry Neurol.* 2002;15:141–146.

De Deyn PP, Rabheru K, Rasmussen A, et al. A randomized trial of risperidone, placebo, and haloperidol for behavioral symptoms of dementia. *Neurology.* 1999;53:946–955.

DeLeo D, Stella AG, Spagnoli A. Prescription of psychotropic drugs in geriatric institutions. *Int J Geriatr Psychiatry.* 1989;4:11–16.

Dey AN. *Characteristics of Elderly Nursing Home Residents: Data From the 1995 National Nursing Home Survey.* Hyattsville, MD: National Center for Health Statistics; 1997. Advance Data from Vital and Health Statistics, No. 289. Available at: http://www.cdc.gov/nchs/data/ad/ad289.pdf. Accessed July 16, 2003.

Elon R, Pawlson LG. The impact of OBRA on medical practice within nursing facilities. *J Am Geriatr Soc.* 1992;40:958–963.

Evans LK, Strumpf NE. Tying down the elderly: a review of the literature on physical restraint. *J Am Geriatr Soc.* 1989;37:65–74.

Evans LK, Strumpf NE, Allen-Taylor SL, et al. A clinical trial to reduce restraints in nursing homes. *J Am Geriatr Soc.* 1997;45:675–681.

Foster JR, Cataldo JK, Boksay IJE. Incidence of depression in a medical long-term care facility: findings from a restricted sample of new admissions. *Int J Geriatr Psychiatry.* 1991;6:13–20.

Gabrel C, Jones A. The National Nursing Home Survey: 1995 summary. *Vital Health Stat.* 2000;13:1–83. Available at: http://www.cdc.gov/nchs/data/series/sr_13/sr13_146.pdf. Accessed July 16, 2003.

Galynker I, Iexonimo C, Miner C, Rosenblum J, Vilkas N, Rosenthal R. Methylphenidate treatment of negative symptoms in patients with dementia. *J Neuropsychiatry Clin Neurosci.* 1997;9:231–239.

German PS, Shapiro S, Kramer M. Cognitive impairment in the nursing home. In: Harper MS, Lebowitz BD, eds. *Mental Illness in Nursing Homes: Agenda for Research.* Rockville, MD: National Institute of Mental Health; 1986:27–40.

Gold DT, Sloane PD, Matthew LJ, et al. Special care units: a typology of care settings for memory impaired older adults. *Gerontologist*. 1991;31:467–475.

Goldwasser AN, Auerbach SM, Harkins SW. Cognitive, affective, and behavioral effects of reminiscence group therapy of demented elderly. *Int J Aging Hum Dev*. 1987; 25:209–222.

Grant LA, Kane RA, Stark AJ. Beyond labels: nursing home care for Alzheimer's disease in and out of special care units. *J Am Geriatr Soc*. 1995;43:569–576.

Grossberg GT, Rakhshanda H, Szwabo PA, et al. Psychiatric problems in the nursing home. *J Am Geriatr Soc*. 1990;38:907–917.

Hansen SS, Patterson MA, Wilson RW. Family involvement on a dementia unit: the Resident Enrichment and Activity Program. *Gerontologist*. 1988;28:508–514.

Harrison R, Savla N, Kafetz K. Dementia, depression, and physical disability in a London borough: a survey of elderly people in and out of residential care and implications for future developments. *Age Aging*. 1990;19:97–103.

Hawes C, Mor V, Phillips CD, et al. The OBRA-87 nursing home regulations and implementation of the Resident Assessment Instrument: effects on process quality. *J Am Geriatr Soc*. 1997;45:997–985.

Health Care Financing Administration. Medicare and Medicaid; requirements for long term care facilities, final regulations. 56 *Federal Register* 48865–48921 (1991).

Health Care Financing Administration. Medicare and Medicaid Programs; preadmission screening and annual resident review. 57 *Federal Register* 56450–56504 1992a.

Health Care Financing Administration. Medicare and Medicaid; resident assessment in long term care facilities. 57 *Federal Register* 61614–61733 1992b.

Health Care Financing Administration. *State Operations Manual: Provider Certification, Transmittal No. 250*. Washington, DC: US Government Printing Office; April 1992c.

Health Care Financing Administration. A Report to Congress, Study of Private Accreditation (Deeming) of Nursing Homes, Regulatory Incentives and Non-Regulatory Incentives, and Effectiveness of the Survey and Certification System. Available at http://cms.hhs.gov/medicaid/reports.htm. Accessed July 16, 2003.

Herst L, Moulton P. Psychiatry in the nursing home. *Psychiatr Clin North Am*. 1985;8: 551–561.

Heston LL, Garrard J, Makris L, et al. Inadequate treatment of depressed nursing home elderly. *J Am Geriatr Soc*. 1992;40:1117–1122.

Hobbs BF, Damon BL. 65+ in the United States. In: *United States Bureau of the Census: Current Population Reports, Special Studies*. Washington, DC: US Government Printing Office; April 1996:23–190. Available at: http://www.census.gov/prod/1/pop/p23-190/pdf. Accessed July 16, 2003.

Holmes D, Teresi J, Weiner A, et al. Impact associated with special care units in long term care facilities. *Gerontologist*. 1990;30:178–181.

Horiguchi J, Inami Y. A survey of the living conditions and psychological states of elderly people admitted to nursing homes in Japan. *Acta Psychiatr Scand*. 1991;83: 338–341.

Hyer L, Blazer D. Depressive symptoms: impact and problems in long term care facilities. *Int J Behav Gerontol*. 1982;1:33–44.

Innes EM, Turman WG. Evolution of patient falls. *QRB*. 1983;9:30–35.

Institute of Medicine, Committee on Nursing Home Regulation. *Improving the Quality of Care in Nursing Homes*. Washington, DC: National Academy Press; 1986.

Jeste DV, Okamoto A, Napolitano, et al. Low incidence of persistent tardive dyskinesia in elderly patients with dementia treated with risperidone. *Am J Psychiatry.* 2000; 157:1150–1155.

Kaplitz SE. Withdrawn, apathetic geriatric patients responsive to methylphenidate. *J Am Geriatr Soc.* 1975;23:271–276.

Katz IR, Beaston-Wimmer P, Parmelee PA, et al. Failure to thrive in the elderly: exploration of the concept and delineation of psychiatric components. *J Geriatr Psychiatry Neurol.* 1993;6:161–169.

Katz IR, Jeste DV, Mintzer JE, et al. Comparison of risperidone and placebo for psychosis and behavioral disturbances associated with dementia: a randomized, double-blind trial. *J Clin Psychiatry.* 1999;60:107–115.

Katz IR, Lesher E, Kleban M, et al. Clinical features of depression in the nursing home. *Int Psychogeriatr.* 1989;1:5–15.

Katz IR, Parmelee PA. Depression in the residential care elderly. In: Schneider LS, Reynolds CF, Lebowitz BD, Friedhoff A, eds. *Diagnosis and Treatment of Depression in Late Life: Results of the NIH Consensus Development Conference.* Washington, DC: American Psychiatric Press; 1993:437–461.

Katz IR, Parmelee PA, Brubaker K. Toxic and metabolic encephalopathies in long term care patients. *Int Psychogeriatr.* 1991;3:337–347.

Katz IR, Simpson GM, Curlik SM, et al. Pharmacological treatment of major depression for elderly patients in residential care settings. *J Clin Psychiatry.* 1990;51(7 Suppl): 41–47.

Katz IR, Simpson GM, Jethanandani V, et al. Steady state pharmacokinetics of nortriptyline. *Neuropsychopharmacology.* 1989;2:229–236.

Kaufer D, Cummings JL, Christine D. Differential neuropsychiatric symptom responses to tacrine in Alzheimer's disease: relationship to dementia severity. *J Neuropsychiatry Clin Neurosci.* 1998;10:55–63.

Kramer M, German PS, Anthony JC, et al. Patterns of mental disorders among the elderly residents of eastern Baltimore. *J Am Geriatr Soc.* 1985;33:236–245.

Krauss NA, Altman BM. *Characteristics of Nursing Home Residents—1996.* Rockville, MD: Agency for Health Care Policy and Research; 1998; MEPS Research Findings No. 5, AHCPR Pub. No. 99–0006.

Kutner N, Mistretta E, Barnhart H, et al. Family members' perceptions of quality of life change in dementia SCU residents. *J Appl Gerontol.* 1999;18:423–439.

Lantz MS, Giambanco V, Buchalter EN. A ten-year review of the effect of OBRA-87 on psychotropic prescribing practices in an academic nursing home. *Psychiatr Serv.* 1996;47:951–955.

Lasser RA, Sunderland T. Newer psychotropic medication use in nursing home residents. *J Am Geriatr Soc.* 1998;46:202–207.

Lawton MP, Van Haitsma K, Kapper M. A balanced stimulation and retreat program for a special care dementia unit. *Alzheimer's Dis Assoc.* 1994;8(suppl 1):S133.

Lawton MP, Van Haitsma K, Klapper J, et al. A stimulation-retreat special care unit for elders with dementing illness. *Int Psychogeriatr.* 1998;10:379–395.

Leon J, Ory M. Effectiveness of special care unit (SCU) placements in reducing physically aggressive behaviors in recently admitted dementia nursing home residents. *Am J Alzheimer's Dis.* 1999;14:270–277.

Lesher E. Validation of the Geriatric Depression Scale among nursing home residents. *Clin Gerontol.* 1986;4:21–28.

Leszcz M, Sadavoy J, Feigenbaum E, et al. A men's group psychotherapy of elderly men. *Int J Group Psychother.* 1985;33:177–196.

Liptzin B. The geriatric psychiatrist's role as consultant. *J Geriatr Psychiatry.* 1983;16: 103–112.

Llorente MD, Olsen EJ, Leyva O, Silverman MA, Lewis JE, Rivero J. Use of antipsychotic drugs in nursing homes: current compliance with OBRA regulations. *J Am Geriatr Soc.* 1998;46:198–201.

Loebel JP, Borson S, Hyde T, et al. Relationships between requests for psychiatric consultations and psychiatric diagnoses in long term care facilities. *Am J Psychiatry.* 1991;148:898–903.

Magai C, Kennedy G, Cohen CI, et al. A controlled clinical trial of sertraline in the treatment of depression in nursing home patients with late-stage Alzheimer's disease. *Am J Geriatr Psychiatry.* 2000;8:66–74.

Mann AH, Graham N, Ashby D. Psychiatric illness in residential homes for the elderly: a survey in one London borough. *Age Ageing.* 1984;13:257–265.

McMurdo MET, Rennie L. A controlled trial of exercise by residents of old people's homes. *Age Ageing.* 1993;22:11–15.

Meador KG, Taylor JA, Thapa PB, Fought RL, Ray WA. Predictors of antipsychotic withdrawal or dose reduction in a randomized controlled trial of provider education. *J Am Geriatr Soc.* 1997;45:207–210.

Moran JA, Gatz M. Group therapies for nursing home adults: an evaluation of two treatment approaches. *Gerontologist.* 1987;27:588–591.

Morris JG, Cyrus PS, Orazem J, et al. Metrifonate benefits cognitive, behavioral, and global function in patients with Alzheimer's disease. *Neurology.* 1998;50:1222–1230.

Moses J. New role for hands-on caregivers: part-time mental health technicians. *J Am Health Care Assoc.* 1982;8:19–22.

Murphy E. The use of psychotropic drugs in long-term care (editorial). *Int J Geriatr Psychiatry.* 1989;4:1–2.

National Center for Health Statistics. *The National Nursing Home Survey.* Washington, DC: US Government Printing Office; 1979. DHEW Publication PHS 79–1794.

National Center for Health Statistics. *Use of Nursing Homes by the Elderly: Preliminary Data from the 1985 National Nursing Home Survey.* Hyattsville, MD: Public Health Service; 1987. DHHS Publication (PHS) 87–1250.

Ohta RJ, Ohta BM. Special units for Alzheimer's disease patients: a critical look. *Gerontologist.* 1988;28:803–808.

Orten JD, Allen M, Cook J. Reminiscence groups with confused nursing center residents: an experimental study. *Soc Work Health Care.* 1989;14:73–86.

Oslin DW, Streim JE, Katz IR, et al. Heuristic comparison of sertraline with nortriptyline for the treatment of depression in frail elderly patients. *Am J Geriatr Psychiatry.* 2000;8:141–149.

Parmelee PA, Katz IR, Lawton MP. Depression among institutionalized aged: assessment and prevalence estimation. *J Gerontol.* 1989;44:M22–M29.

Parmelee PA, Katz IR, Lawton MP. The relation of pain to depression among institutionalized aged. *J Gerontol Psychol Sci.* 1991;46:15–21.

Parmelee PA, Katz IR, Lawton MP. Depression and mortality among institutionalized aged. *J Gerontol Psychol Sci.* 1992a;47:P3–P10.

Parmelee PA, Katz IR, Lawton MP. Incidence of depression in long term care settings. *J Gerontol Med Sci.* 1992b;47(6):M189–M196.

Phillips CD, Sloane PD, Hawes C, et al. Effects of residence in Alzheimer's disease special care units on functional outcomes. *JAMA*. 1997;278:1340–1344.

Phillips CD, Spry KM, Sloane PD, Hawes C. Use of physical restraints and psychotropic medications in Alzheimer special care units in nursing homes. *Am J Public Health*. 2000;90:92–96.

Porsteinsson AP, Tariot PN, Erb R, et al. Placebo-controlled study of divalproex sodium for agitation in dementia. *Am J Geriatr Psychiatry*. 2001;9(1):58–66.

Rattenburg C, Stones MJ. A controlled evaluation of reminiscence and current topics discussion groups in a nursing home context. *Gerontologist*. 1989;29:768–771.

Ray WA, Federspiel CF, Schaffner W. A study of antipsychotic drug use in nursing homes: epidemiologic evidence suggesting misuse. *Am J Public Health*. 1980;70: 485–491.

Ray WA, Taylor JA, Meador KG, et al. Reducing antipsychotic drug use in nursing homes. A controlled trial of provider education. *Arch Intern Med*. 1993;153(6): 71–721.

Reichman WE, Coyne AC, Borson S, et al. Psychiatric consultation in the nursing home: a survey of six states. *Am J Geriatr Psychiatry*. 1998;6:320–327.

Rhoades J, Krauss N. *Nursing Home Trends, 1987 and 1996*. Rockville, MD: Agency for Health Care Policy and Research; 1999. MEPS Chartbook No. 3. AHCPR Publication 99–0032.

Risse SC, Cubberley L, Lampe TH, et al. Acute effects of neuroleptic withdrawal in elderly dementia patients. *J Geriatr Drug Ther*. 1987;2:65–77.

Rosen J, Mulsant BH, Pollock BG. Sertraline in the treatment of minor depression in nursing home residents: a pilot study. *Int J Geriatr Psychiatry*. 2000;15:177–180.

Rovner BW, Edelman BA, Cox MP, Shmuely Y. The impact of antipsychotic drug regulations (OBRA 1987) on psychotropic prescribing practices in nursing homes. *Am J Psychiatry*. 1992;149:1390–1392.

Rovner BW, German PS, Brant LJ, et al. Depression and mortality in nursing homes. *JAMA*. 1991;265:993–996.

Rovner BW, German PS, Broadhead J, et al. The prevalence and management of dementia and other psychiatric disorders in nursing homes. *Int Psychogeriatr*. 1990;2: 13–24.

Rovner BW, Kafonek S, Filipp L, et al. Prevalence of mental illness in a community nursing home. *Am J Psychiatry*. 1986;143:1446–1449.

Rovner BW, Lucas-Blaustein J, Folstein MF, et al. Stability over one year in patients admitted to a nursing home dementia unit. *Int J Geriatr Psychiatry*. 1990;5:77–82.

Rovner BW, Steele CD, Shmuely Y, et al. A randomized trial of dementia care in nursing homes. *J Am Geriatr Soc*. 1996;44:7–13.

Sabin TD, Vitug AJ, Mark VH. Are nursing home diagnosis and treatment inadequate? *JAMA*. 1982;248:321–322.

Sadavoy J. Psychotherapy for the institutionalized elderly. In: Conn DK, Herrman N, Kaye A, et al., eds. *Practical Psychiatry in the Nursing Home: A Handbook for Staff*. Toronto, Ontario, Canada: Hogrefe and Huber; 1991:217–236.

Sakauye KM, Camp CJ. Introducing psychiatric care in to nursing homes. *Gerontologist*. 1992;32:849–852.

Saxton J, Silverman M, Ricci E, et al. Maintenance of mobility in residents of an Alzheimer's special care facility. *Int Psychogeriatr*. 1998;10:213–224.

Schneider L, Pollock VE, Liness SA. A metaanalysis of controlled trials of neuroleptic treatment in dementia. *J Am Geriatr Soc.* 1990;38:553–563.

Schnelle JF, Wood S, Schnelle ER, Simmons SF. Measurement sensitivity and the Minimum Data Set depression quality indicator. *Gerontologist.* 2001;41:401–405.

Semla TP, Palla K, Poddig B, Brauner DJ. Effect of the Omnibus Reconciliation Act 1987 on antipsychotic prescribing in nursing home residents. *J Am Geriatr Soc.* 1994;42:648–652.

Shorr RI, Fought RL, Ray WA. Changes in antipsychotic drug use in nursing homes during implementation of the OBRA-87 regulations. *JAMA.* 1994;271:358–362.

Siegler EL, Capezuti E, Maislin G, Baumgarten M, Evans L, Strumpf N. Effects of a restraint reduction intervention and OBRA '87 regulations on psychoactive drug use in nursing homes. *J Am Geriatr Soc.* 1997;45:791–796.

Sloane PD, Mathew LS, Scarborough M, Desai JR, Koch GG, Tangen C. Physical and pharmacologic restraint of nursing home patients with dementia: impact of specialized units. *JAMA.* 1991;265:1278–1282.

Sloane PD, Mitchell CM, Preisser JS, Phillips C, Commander C, Burker E. Environmental correlates of resident agitation in Alzheimer's disease special care units. *J Am Geriatr Soc.* 1998;46:862–869.

Smith M, Buckwalter KC, Albanese M. Geropsychiatric education programs: providing skills and understanding. *J Psychosoc Nurs Ment Health Serv.* 1990;28:8–12.

Snowden M, Roy-Byrne P. Mental illness and nursing home reform: OBRA-87 ten years later. Omnibus Budget Reconciliation Act. *Psychiatr Serv.* 1998;49:229–233.

Snowdon J. Dementia, depression, and life satisfaction in nursing homes. *Int J Geriatr Psychiatry.* 1986;1:85–91.

Snowdon J, Donnelly N. A study of depression in nursing homes. *J Psychiatr Res.* 1986; 20:327–333.

Spagnoli A, Forester G, MacDonald A, et al. Dementia and depression in Italian geriatric institutions. *Int J Geriatr Psychiatry.* 1986;1:15–23.

Steele C, Rovner BW, Chase GA, Folstein MF. Psychiatric symptoms and nursing home placement in Alzheimer's disease. *Am J Psychiatry.* 1990;147:1049–1051.

Strahan GW. *An Overview of Nursing Homes and Their Current Residents: Data From the 1995 National Nursing Home Survey.* Hyattsville, MD: National Center for Health Statistics; 1997. Advance Data From Vital and Health Statistics, No. 280. Available at: http://www.cdc.gov/nchs/data/ad/ad280.pdf. Accessed July 16, 2003.

Street JS, Clark WS, Gannon KS, et al. Olanzepine treatment of psychotic and behavioral symptoms in patients with Alzheimer disease in nursing care facilities, a double-blind, randomized, placebo-controlled trial. *Arch Gen Psychiatry.* 2000;57:968–976.

Streim JE. New findings from clinical trials in Europe and the United States: aripiprazole for the treatment of psychiatric symptoms associated with dementia. Presented at the 11th International Congress of the International Psychogeriatric Association, Chicago, Illinois, August 19, 2003.

Streim JE, Katz IR. Federal regulations and the care of patients with dementia in the nursing home. *Med Clin North Am.* 1994;78:895–909.

Streim JE, Katz IR. The psychiatrist in the nursing home, part II: consultation, primary care, and leadership. *Psychiatr Serv.* 1995;46:339–341.

Streim JE, Katz IR. Clinical psychiatry in the nursing home. In: Busse EW, Blazer DG, eds. *Textbook of Geriatric Psychiatry*. 2nd ed. Washington, DC: American Psychiatric Press; 1996:413–427.

Streim JE, Oslin DW, Katz IR, et al. Drug treatment of depression in frail elderly nursing home residents. *Am J Geriatr Psychiatry*. 2000;8:150–159.

Swanson E, Maas M, Buckwalter K. Catastrophic reactions and other behaviors of Alzheimer's residents: special unit compared with traditional units. *Arch Psychiatr Nurs*. 1993;7:292–299.

Tariot PN, Cumming JL, Katz IR, et al. A randomized, double-blind, placebo-controlled study of the efficacy and safety of donepezil in patients with Alzheimer's disease in the nursing home setting. *J Am Geriatr Soc*. 2001;49:1590–1599.

Tariot PN, Erb R, Podgorski CA, et al. Efficacy and tolerability of carbamazepine for agitation and aggression in dementia. *Am J Psychiatry*. 1998;155:54–61.

Tariot PN, Podgorske CA, Blazina L, et al. Mental disorders in the nursing home: another perspective. *Am J Psychiatry*. 1993;150:1063–1069.

Teeter RB, Garetz FK, Miller WR, et al. Psychiatric disturbances of aged patients in skilled nursing homes. *Am J Psychiatry*. 1976;133:1430–1434.

Thapa PB, Gideon P, Cost CW, Milam AD, Ray WA. Antidepressants and the risk of falls among nursing home residents. *N Engl J Med*. 1998;339:875.

Tourigny-Rivard MF, Drury M. The effects of monthly psychiatric consultation in a nursing home. *Gerontologist*. 1987;27:363–366.

Trappler B, Cohen CI. Using fluoxetine in "very old" depressed nursing home residents. *Am J Geriatr Psychiatry*. 1996;4:258–262.

Trappler B, Cohen CI. Use of SSRIs in "very old" depressed nursing home residents. *Am J Geriatr Psychiatry*. 1998;6:83–89.

Trichard L, Zabow A, Gillis LS. Elderly persons in old age homes: a medical, psychiatric and social investigation. *S Afr Med J*. 1982;61:624–627.

Wagner AW, Teri L, Orr-Rainey N. Behavior problems of residents with dementia in special care units. *Alzheimer's Dis Assoc Disord*. 1995;9:121–127.

Wells Y, Jorm FA. Evaluation of a special nursing home unit for dementia suffers: a randomized controlled comparison with community care. *Aust N Z J Psychiatry*. 1987;21:524–531.

Werner P, Cohen-Masfield J, Braun J, et al. Physical restraint and agitation in nursing home residents. *J Am Geriatr Soc*. 1989;37:1122–1126.

Westlake RJ, Rubano GL. Psychogeriatric seminars for nursing home nurses. *Hosp Community Psychiatry*. 1983;34:1056–1058.

Williams-Barnard CL, Lindell AR. Therapeutic use of "prizing" and its effect on self-concept of elderly clients in nursing homes and group homes. *Issues Ment Health Nurs*. 1992;13:1–17.

Youssef FA. The impact of group reminiscence counseling on a depressed elderly population. *Nurse Pract*. 1990;15:32–38.

Zerhusen JD, Boyle K, Wilson W. Out of the darkness: group cognitive therapy for depressed elderly. *J Psychol Nurs*. 1991;29:16–21.

Zimmer JG, Watson N, Treat A. Behavioral problems among patients in skilled nursing facilities. *Am J Pub Health*. 1984;74:1118–1121.

35

Psychogeriatric Programs: Inpatient Hospital Units and Partial Hospital Programs

Rona E. Pasternak, MD
Barry W. Rovner, MD

OVERVIEW

This chapter reviews current published knowledge on the assessment and treatment of older patients admitted to inpatient and partial hospital programs. For clinical descriptions of geriatric psychiatry inpatient units, Tourigny-Rivard and Potoczny's chapter in the second edition of the *Comprehensive Review of Geriatric Psychiatry* and Rovner and Folstein's chapter in *Modern Hospital Psychiatry* provide useful reviews.

Inpatient and partial hospitalization programs are increasingly important in the care of older persons; they parallel the rapid growth of the elderly population, increasing rates of psychiatric and comorbid medical problems, and declining social supports and financial resources for many older persons. Because older patients' psychiatric, medical, functional, and social problems are complex and interrelated, specialized multidisciplinary inpatient care is often necessary for optimal assessment and treatment.

Treatment begins with the comprehensive evaluation of patients' symptoms and their caregivers' ability to continue care at home. Common clinical symptoms include behavioral problems (e.g., combativeness, agitation, wandering), affective symptoms (depression, mania), anxiety (somatic and psychological), and psychotic symptoms (hallucinations, delusions). There is careful attention to comorbid medical problems, nutrition, education of family members, identification of discharge needs, and opportunities to promote functional independence and socialization. Discharge planning includes developing information on patients' families, social supports, and availability of community resources, all recruited to maintain the patient in the least restrictive setting. Unfortunately, contraction of health care resources for inpatient care has required addressing these complexities in fewer than 2 weeks of hospital stay. In response, partial hospital programs have grown to complement inpatient care.

DEMOGRAPHIC CHARACTERISTICS

Research reports on the demographic characteristics and psychiatric diagnoses of older persons admitted to psychiatric inpatient care began to appear in the late 1980s and early 1990s. Conwell et al. (1989) reported on 168 older patients admitted to a general hospital psychiatry unit; they found that 76% had a primary affective disorder, of which 85% were unipolar and 15% bipolar. Dementia was the second most common diagnosis, complicated by co-occurring depression, delusions, or delirium. Outcome measures showed a favorable response to treatment in 75% of patients, suggesting that the general hospital psychiatry inpatient setting was well suited to care for the combined medical and mental illnesses of elderly patients. Rubin and Kinscherf (1991) and Greene et al. (1994) described assessment and treatment protocols on specialty geriatric psychiatry inpatient units and emphasized the value of routine assessment of mood, cognition, behavior, and function.

Zubenko et al. (1997) described the high level of medical comorbidity in this population. Their multidisciplinary diagnostic evaluation of 868 inpatients revealed that 46% met the criteria of the *Diagnostic and Statistical Manual of Mental Disorders, Third Edition, Revised* (DSM-III-R; American Psychiatric Association [APA], 1987) for dementia, 38% for mood disorder, and 10% for psychotic disorder. The patients had an average of 5.6 (SD 3.1) active medical problems. This level of medical comorbidity was significantly greater than that of older psychiatric outpatients and comparable to that of older patients on general medical units.

Perry et al. (1995) conducted a 6-month prospective study of 72 admissions to an old-age psychiatry unit in Great Britain. Defining *significant illness* as a condition that was life threatening or required urgent medical or surgical intervention to prevent further deterioration, they found that 24 (34%) had such a significant physical illness that was unsuspected at the time of admission. In 5 of these 24 patients, the physical problem alone accounted for the psychiatric presentation, and in 14 patients, the physical illness probably contributed to the psychiatric presentation. Patients with an "organic psychotic diagnosis" were somewhat more likely to suffer a significant illness compared with patients with a "functional" diagnosis. The investigators noted that almost two thirds of the physical disorder diagnoses were made by a combination of common clinical evaluations and blood tests such as complete blood count, fecal occult blood tests, thyroid function studies, and chest x-rays.

Among the most frequent medical diagnoses were infections, cancer, and anemias.

Weintraub and Mazour (2000) described changes over the prior 10 years in the clinical and demographic characteristics of patients admitted to geriatric psychiatry units. Patients at the time of the study were older and were more likely to be demented, have psychotic symptoms or agitation, stay fewer days in the hospital, receive more psychotropic medications, and more likely discharged to a nursing home. Pasternak et al. (1998) reported that their psychiatric symptoms and medical problems were more severe than community-residing or homebound psychiatric patients. Many inpatients come from nursing homes, where the majority of residents have mental or behavioral disorders and where access to geriatric psychiatry services, adequately trained staff, and therapeutic activity programs are limited. These limitations often necessitate admission to more highly developed psychiatric services and confirm that psychogeriatric inpatient units are important adjuncts to nursing home care, especially for patients with dementia.

As noted, length of stay has markedly decreased. Conwell and coworkers' (1989) article cited an average length of stay of 53.3 days; in 1994, Greene et al. reported a 9.5-day average length of stay. Few studies have investigated factors influencing length of stay. Draper and Luscombe (1998) found that major depression and high levels of caregiver stress accounted for almost 25% of variance in length of stay. This indicates the need to develop strong contacts with intensive outpatient or partial hospital programs for subsequent depression care and with respite care and other supports for overwhelmed caregivers.

Snowden et al. (2000) reported the median length of stay for older patients on a general unit was 18 days; although the older patients' psychiatric symptoms were less severe than those of younger patients, their length of stay was longer (18 vs. 13 days) because of comorbid medical illness. However, Sager et al. (1996) found that older persons improved functionally after acute psychiatric admission, in contrast to the functional decline frequently associated with medical hospitalizations.

TREATMENT OF DEPRESSION

Zubenko et al. (1994) described the treatment responses of 205 inpatients consecutively admitted to the Western Psychiatric Institute and Clinic, Pittsburgh, Pennsylvania, who met *DSM-III-R* criteria for major depression. The patients were treated with a combination of somatic and psychotherapeutic interventions. Despite considerable medical and psychiatric comorbidity, patients responded well to treatment, as reflected by a 50% reduction in Hamilton Depression Rating Scale scores and a 50% remission rate. Black race, better cognitive performance, lower medical burden, treatment with electroconvulsive therapy (ECT), and shorter hospitalization independently contributed to positive clinical response. The investigators concluded that short-term psychiatric hospitalization effectively treats severe or complicated cases of major depression in the elderly.

Rubin et al. (1991) described the treatment responses of 101 depressed patients hospitalized on a geriatric psychiatry unit, of whom 46% received ECT. They found that advanced age was not associated with poor outcome, and that ECT was the most important variable predicting response to treatment. In a second study from this program, Allen-Burge et al. (1994) found that the Geriatric Depression Scale (GDS) and the Beck Depression Inventory were less effective in identifying depressed men than women in 191 geriatric psychiatry inpatients with major depression. Their data supported the need for separate cutoff scores for older men and women on depression screening instruments in this population.

Oslin et al. (2000) examined the relationship between functional disability and improvement in late-life depression after acute inpatient treatment. The sample was 2,572 older persons hospitalized in 1 of 71 inpatient geriatric psychiatry treatment programs in the southwestern United States. The programs were nonacademic units of general hospitals that were participating in a quality management program. Depressive symptoms were measured using the GDS; disability was measured using an instrumental activities of daily living (IADL) scale and the Medical Outcomes SF-36. Depressive symptoms improved in the majority of patients; the improvement was significantly related to improvement in IADLs and to health-related quality of life. The data suggest that treatment of depression can lead to significant improvements in functional disability in older patients. In a subsequent analysis, Oslin et al. (2002) found that arthritis, circulatory problems, a speech disorder, or a skin problem, but not other general medical conditions, were related to worse outcome with respect to depression. The effect of each of these conditions was mediated by the residual disability after treatment.

We gathered data on 2,663 older patients admitted to the Jefferson Geriatric Psychiatry Unit at Wills Eye Hospital, Philadelphia, from 1991 to 2000. Most suffered from chronic age-related psychiatric, medical, and neurological conditions, such as major depression (39.7%), primary degenerative or vascular dementia with noncognitive psychiatric complications (33.3%), or psychotic conditions (3%). The majority were women (69.6%), white (90.4%), and widowed, divorced, or single (66.5%). The average age was 78.3 years, and the average length of stay in 2000 was 14 (SD 9.4) days; in 1991–1992, the average length of stay was 26.6 (SD 19.4) days.

Research on this unit explored the longitudinal associations among depression, physical health, function, and family relationships in a sample of patients with major depression ($N = 207$). Table 35-1 shows the demographic and selected medical characteristics, including average Mini-Mental State Examination (MMSE) and Cumulative Illness Rating Scale (CIRS) scores, which approximate severity of cognitive impairment and comorbid medical disorders, respectively.

TABLE 35-1. Characteristics of depressed inpatients (N = 207)

	Mean	SD
Age	77.4	6.9
Years of eduction	11.8	2.8
Admission MMSE	25.7	3.4
Admission CIRS (without the psychiatry item)	10.4	5.2

	N	%
Female	147	70.7
White	200	96.6
Married	66	32.0
Widowed/single/divorced	140	68.0
Number of medical conditions	3.5	2.0
Received ECT	92	45.3
Number of ECT treatments (mean, SD)	6.7	2.6

CIRS, Cumulative Illness Rating Scale; ECT, electroconvulsive therapy; MMSE, Mini-Mental State Examination.

Figure 35-1 shows the proportion of the subjects with GDS score of 5 or higher over 1 year. It reveals substantial improvement for the majority of GDS-positive patients from admission to discharge, although slightly over one third remained depressed at discharge.

Of the 79 subjects for whom there were GDS data at four time waves (admission, discharge, 3 and 12 months postdischarge), 45 (57%) were classified as "remitted" (e.g., GDS ≥ 5 on admission, but GDS < 5 at months 3 and

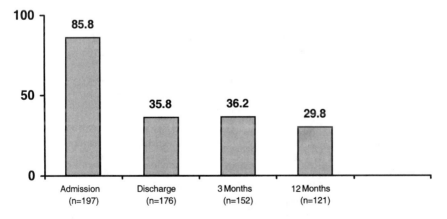

FIGURE 35-1. Percentage of inpatients with Geriatric Depression Scale scores of 5 or above at four time points.

12 postdischarge); 24 (30.4%) were classified as "relapsed/recurrent" (e.g., GDS < 5 on discharge, but GDS ≥ 5 at either months 3 or 12); and 10 (12.7%) were classified as "continuous depressed" (e.g., GDS ≥ 5 at all four times). The data indicate further that the admission characteristics of elevated GDS scores, worse IADL functioning, poor self-rated health, and high levels of pain intensity predict poor outcome in this population and suggest that intensive treatment be devoted to patients with these characteristics.

Figure 35-2 illustrates the shift from higher to lower levels of disability as GDS scores decline; it demonstrates the global adverse effects of major depression on health-related quality of life and the effectiveness of multidisciplinary inpatient treatment to produce improvements in all relevant domains.

Casten et al. (2000) examined whether self-perceptions of function improved and were maintained as depression resolved. A subsample of 64 inpatients with major depression were asked to evaluate their function (e.g., "How much do your health problems limit your everyday physical activities?") on admission and then again 3 months postdischarge. Subjects' caregivers also rated patients' usual level of function at the same points. Self-perceptions improved over time, while caregivers' perceptions remained stable, suggesting that patients' perceptions of functioning came to resemble the more objective caregiver assess-

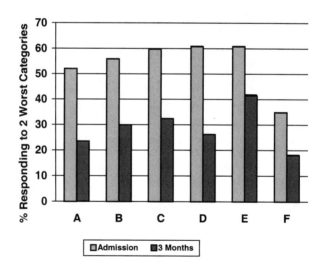

FIGURE 35-2. Medical Outcome Study-6 responses at admission and 3 months postdischarge: (A) How much do your health problems limit your everyday physical activities? (quite a bit/extremely). (B) How hard has it been to do your daily work due to physical health or emotional problems? (quite a bit/could not do). (C) How much have your social activities been limited due to physical or emotional problems? (quite a bit/extremely). (D) How much have you been bothered by emotional problems lately? (quite a bit/ extremely). (E) Overall, how would you rate your current health? (fair/poor). (F) If you had physical pain, how intense has it been? (severe/very severe).

ments with resolution of depression. The implication is that patients' self-perceptions are more accurate when they are not depressed, demonstrating that reporting bias changes in response to the successful treatment of depression.

Casten et al. (1999) investigated the importance of caregivers' beliefs as
predictors of recovery from major depression. Caregivers rated whether they
thought each of the 12 depressive symptoms that comprise the DSM-IV (APA,
1994) criteria for major depression was or was not within the control of their
patient or relative. The "symptom control score" was the number of symptoms
thought to be within the patient's control. At discharge, 64.7% of patients
were "remitted," and 35.3% were "not remitted" based on a GDS less than 5.
Multivariate analysis indicated that having a lower symptom control score,
receiving ECT, and female sex predicted depression remission at discharge.
These data indicate that patients whose caregivers believe that the former can
"control" depressive symptoms are less likely to recover during the hospitalization; caregivers possibly blame patients for symptoms over which they have
diminished control and thereby intensify their guilt and deplete their sense of
emotional support. These data emphasize the importance of addressing caregivers' beliefs as important factors related to recovery from depression.

DEMENTIA

Zubenko et al. (1992) evaluated 120 consecutive inpatients with Alzheimer's
disease to examine the clinical utility of the four DSM-III-R subtypes of primary degenerative dementia (i.e., with delirium, delusions, depression, or uncomplicated). Each behavioral subtype responded in expected ways to inpatient
treatment, as reflected by improvements in cognitive impairment, psychiatric
symptom severity, and level of functioning. They noted that the uncomplicated
subtype designation did not accurately reflect the burden of behavioral symptoms that these patients exhibited. Half of all patients admitted from their
homes and two thirds of those with depression returned home following discharge. Although many patients required institutional care, psychiatric hospitalization effectively reduced the need for institutionalization for many
patients.

Edell and Tunis (2001) examined the Mental Health Outcomes Quality
Management Program data (see Oslin et al., 2000) for 2,747 patients with a
DSM-IV diagnosis of dementia who were admitted to participating psychiatric
inpatient units from 1996 to 1998. Two thirds (65.7%) of the patients were
female, with an average age of 81 (56–108) years. The most common dementia
diagnosis was Alzheimer's disease (65.4%), followed by vascular dementia
(15.8%), dementia not otherwise specified (NOS) (12.4%), and dementia due
to a general medical condition (6.4%). The average MMSE score was 11.6.

Edell and Tunis (2001) used the Psychogeriatric Dependency Rating Scale
(PGDRS) to define the Behavioral and Psychological Symptoms of Dementia
(BPSD). To compare treatment outcomes with respect to specific antipsychotic

medication therapy, patients were identified who were treated with a single antipsychotic medication (e.g., haloperidol, olanzapine, risperidone). A total of 998 patients (36.6% of the dementia disorder cohort) were identified as receiving antipsychotic "monotherapy." Of these 998 patients, 500 (50.1%) were treated with risperidone, 289 (29%) with haloperidol, and 209 (20.9%) with olanzapine. There were no significant differences among the three groups on the majority of patient characteristics examined. All three antipsychotic agents were associated with clinical improvement. Patients taking olanzapine experienced a significantly greater improvement in overall PDGRS score (mean change = 5.0) compared with those taking haloperidol (mean change = 3.1; $P < .1$) or risperidone (mean change = 2.8; $P < .001$).

Kunik et al. (1996) specifically examined the treatment responses of nursing home residents admitted to a geriatric psychiatry inpatient unit. Using standardized clinical measures, the investigators reported significant decreases in general psychiatric symptoms, depression, and agitation, with significant improvement in global functioning. These data demonstrate the value of psychiatric hospitalization for nursing patients, enabling many residents to continue care in long-term care facilities and reducing the burden of their psychiatric symptoms in this setting.

Koponen et al. (1989) studied 70 elderly patients (mean age 75 years) admitted to a geriatric psychiatry inpatient unit with delirium most commonly caused by stroke, infections, and metabolic disorders. Of these individuals, 81% had a predisposing central nervous system(CNS) disease (e.g., Alzheimer's disease, Parkinson's disease, vascular dementia). During the hospitalization, cognitive function improved significantly (MMSE scores 9.7 [SD 6.6] on admission and 13.9 [SD 7.2] at discharge; $P < .001$). The 1-year follow-up showed progression of cognitive and functional decline in patients with Alzheimer's disease and vascular dementia, however.

PSYCHOSIS

Webster and Grossberg (1998) conducted a chart review of over 1700 admissions to the geriatric psychiatry service at St. Louis University Hospital in Missouri from 1988 to 1995. Most psychotic symptoms (64%) were delusions, usually persecutory or paranoid. Almost one third (29%) were hallucinations, most often visual. The etiologies of psychosis included dementia (40%), depression (33%), medical/toxic causes (7%), delirium (7%), bipolar disorder (5%), and primary psychotic disorders (4%). These data demonstrate the nonspecific nature of psychotic symptoms, especially in the elderly, and the need for both medical and psychiatric evaluation to avoid misdiagnosis and suboptimal treatment.

Tunis et al. (2000) also examined the Mental Health Outcomes Quality Management Program data on 514 geriatric psychiatry inpatients with schizophrenia or schizoaffective disorder. The patients' mean age was 70 years; 72%

were female, and 81% were white. Most patients had behavioral problems secondary to delusions or hallucinations or serious impairment in communication or judgment. The study assessed the burden of illness and prescribing patterns for psychotropic medication. Many patients required help with activities of daily living, and only 22% were able to take medications unassisted. There was a high rate of comorbid affective symptoms: 41% were treated with antidepressants, 31% with mood stabilizers, and 23% with anxiolytics. Over half (56%) were treated with a second-generation antipsychotic, and 33% were treated with a conventional agent. At discharge, 30% were treated with olanzapine, 21% with risperidone, 3% with quetiapine, and 2% with clozapine. This research documents the substantial illness burden experienced by older patients with schizophrenia and describes the prescribing practices for psychotropic medications in this setting.

Verma et al. (2001) demonstrated the effectiveness of the atypical antipsychotic medications risperidone and olanzapine to treat psychotic symptoms and agitation in 34 patients admitted to a Veterans Affairs (VA) medical center geriatric inpatient unit. The drugs were equally efficacious as measured by outcome scores in the Cohen-Mansfield Agitation Inventory (CMAI) and the Positive and Negative Syndrome Scale (PANSS) score for schizophrenia. There were no differences in side effects or length of stay, although the daily cost of risperdal was one third as much as for olanzapine.

PERSONALITY DISORDERS

Casey and Schrodt (1989) reviewed the inpatient records of 100 patients older than 65 years of age admitted to a general psychiatry unit. They found that 7% met criteria for a personality disorder (PD), and an additional 16% had PD traits that were "dysfunctional," but did not meet diagnostic criteria. Dependent PD accounted for over half the PD diagnoses. Kunik et al. (1993) examined the effect of comorbid personality disorder on response to treatment for major depression in older inpatients. Over a 2-year study period, 24% of patients admitted with unipolar major depression met *DSM-III-R* criteria for a PD, most commonly PD NOS (32%) and dependent PD (27%). Compared to patients without PD, PD patients were more likely to have recurrent depression, earlier age of onset, and comorbid anxiety disorder. They were also more likely to (1) never marry, (2) have separated or divorced, or (3) attempted suicide. Patients with or without PD did not differ in mode or outcome of treatment or length of stay. Both groups benefited equally from inpatient treatment, with improved functioning and relief of depression, as measured by the Global Assessment Scale (GAS) and the Hamilton Depression Rating Scale (HAM-D), respectively.

Kunik et al. (1994) subsequently described rates of comorbid PD by psychiatric diagnosis in 547 elderly inpatients; 69 (13%) received a PD diagnosis. Personality disorders from the anxious cluster (33%) were the most common, followed by PD NOS (32%), PD from the odd cluster (18%), and PD from the dramatic cluster (16%). The diagnostic rate of comorbid PD varied fourfold in relation to the primary *DSM-III-R* Axis I diagnosis: 6% in patients with organic mental disorders and 24% in those with major depression. The investigators concluded that the low prevalence of comorbid PD diagnoses in geriatric inpatients may be because of its lower rate in those with dementia.

Molinari et al. (1994) completed the Structured Interview for Disorders of Personality–Revised (SIDP-R) on 100 men from a VA geropsychiatric inpatient ward and 100 women from a geropsychiatry inpatient ward of a private hospital. They found a 56.5% rate of PD in these older patients, with significantly more older men than women diagnosed with a PD; the men were more likely diagnosed with paranoid, avoidant, and multiple PD. Compared with a younger population, older subjects in general were less likely to be diagnosed with multiple PD or dramatic cluster PD and were more likely to be diagnosed with the odd/eccentric Cluster C PD. In a subsequent study, Molinari and Marmion (1995) used the SIDP-R to evaluate 24 geropsychiatric outpatients and 52 inpatients with affective disorders; 67% of the outpatients and 61.5% of the inpatients were diagnosed with PDs. They noted that these rates are higher than reported in other studies and attributed this to use of the structured clinical assessments. The investigators also found that the presence of PDs was not related to relapse among inpatients over 1 year.

Taken together, the studies on rates of PD in older psychiatric inpatients reveal a wide range (7%–61.5%), depending on the samples studied and the diagnostic methods employed. There is little consensus on the prevalence of specific PD diagnoses. However, the data dispel the notion that PD "burnout" occurs entirely with age and indicate that older patients with PDs benefit from inpatient care.

PARTIAL HOSPITAL PROGRAMS

Overview

Community-based mental health services, such as partial hospital programs, provide a sustained interdisciplinary approach to treatment more readily than can be delivered in standard outpatient clinics. For a comprehensive historical review of partial programs, see the work of Tourigny-Rivard and Potoczny (1996). Briefly, partial hospital care is a less-restrictive and less-expensive alternative to inpatient care. Medicare covers treatment costs, typically provided over 8 weeks. Partial services differ from adult day centers, which provide long-term respite-type care that is not covered by Medicare for patients with dementia.

The intent of partial hospitalization care is to improve or maintain a patient's condition and to prevent relapse or hospitalization. For most psychiatric patients, control of symptoms and maintenance of functional level is an acceptable expectation of improvement. Given this, admission criteria include (1) the patient requires inpatient psychiatric care in the absence of this service, (2) an individualized written plan of care is established, and (3) the patient is or was under the care of a physician.

Common interventions include individual and group psychotherapy, pharmacotherapy, and social intervention. Clinical services are provided by an onsite psychiatrist and nursing and other professional therapists. Typically, such programs provide 5 hours of service a day, 5 days per week. Group therapies include community group (e.g., introduction of new members, termination processes for patients discharged, setting goals for the day, discussion of previous accomplishments/problems, etc.) (see Chapter 32 for discussion of group therapy), psychoeducational groups, medication education, individual therapy, education regarding healthy lifestyles, current events, family therapy, and specialty groups such as reminiscence therapy, assertiveness training, and relaxation, art, occupational, and music therapies.

Medicare Benefits

In the late 1980s, Congress authorized a hospital-based partial hospitalization benefit as an alternative to hospitalization and expanded the benefit in 1990 to include community mental health centers (CMHCs). In 1997, Medicare issued a reimbursement policy that required a physical examination by a physician within 24 hours of admission and at least 3 hours per day and 4 days per week of intensive services.

Payment is covered at a per diem rate rather than a cost for each component of the service. The Health Care Financing Administration established a per diem Ambulatory Payment Classification (APC) rate of $208.25 per day with a $46.78 copay. Although Medicare does not limit partial hospital days, other payers do.

Medicare spending for partial hospitalization services jumped from $60 million in 1993 to $369 million in 1997, which led to greater federal scrutiny. In fact, in October 2000, a subcommittee of the House Commerce Committee closed 80 CMHC-based partial programs because they failed to provide active treatment (National Alliance for the Mentally Ill, 2000). Currently, four kinds of providers participate in Medicare partial hospital programs: hospital based, CMHC based, freestanding programs, and "storefront operations" (i.e., family-owned programs that are considered CMHCs for Medicare billing).

As an intermediate level of care, partial hospitalization programs have provided support for many thousands of older patients since their development. However, few studies have evaluated their effectiveness in research paradigms. One of the chief obstacles has been the diversity of clinical services and patients eligible for participation. Typically, many services are bundled together, making it difficult to discern the primary therapeutic elements.

The Senior Adult Growth and Enrichment (SAGE) program was a demonstration project funded by the National Institute of Mental Health (NIMH) to provide outreach and day treatment for rural elderly mentally ill persons. The median age of patients was 71 years; 20% were older than 80 years. The primary diagnoses reported were depression (36%), schizophrenia (23%), and dementia (19%). Patients were divided into a "transitional" group and a "community support" group. Patients with primary diagnoses of depression and anxiety comprised the former; the latter consisted of patients with schizophrenia, psychotic depression, bipolar disorder, and mild-to-moderate dementia.

Recognizing their differing treatment needs, the treatment team developed appropriate care approaches. Patients in the transitional group were primarily treated with cognitive-behavioral therapy that complemented psychopharmacological treatments. Treatment for the community support group focused on rehabilitation and improving quality of life in addition to psychopharmacological management. Although no data have been reported regarding the efficacy of these treatments, valuable clinical experience was developed in this model partial hospital program and is described in Atkinson and Stuck's (1991) report of the SAGE experience.

Although there are other published reports describing services and patient characteristics, few investigated program effectiveness. Boyle (1997) described a partial program that followed a biopsychosocial social work philosophy and utilized group discussion, current events groups, patient education sessions, visual arts, crafts, games, exercise, dance, music, and field trips to promote interests and social interactions. Focusing on depression primarily, patients were evaluated using the GDS and the Global Assessment of Functioning (GAF) scale.

The program described by Boyle (1997) enrolled 32 patients: 78% were female, and 82% were white; the average age was 75 years (SD 8.7). The rates of psychiatric diagnoses were as follows: dementia 56%; schizophrenia 9%; major depression 4%; dysthymia 4%; anxiety disorders 18%; and bipolar disorders 9%. Pretest GDS scores ranged from 2 to 26, with a mean of 11.2 (SD 7); posttest scores ranged from 0 to 17, with a mean of 6.0 (SD 5.9). These differences were significant and suggested the value of the intervention to reduce depressive symptoms using primarily nonpharmacological techniques in this heterogeneous group of patients.

Plotkin and Wells (1993) conducted a retrospective chart review of geriatric patients in partial treatment at the Neuropsychiatric Institute and Hospital of the University of California, Los Angeles; they abstracted data on 100 patients over 5 years. The typical patient was a widowed white woman in her 70s with a depressive disorder. Treatment was primarily group therapy that complemented ongoing psychopharmocological treatments. Of the patients, 57% improved; variables associated with favorable outcome included the diagnosis of a mood disorder (rather than a psychotic disorder), better initial functional status, greater initial social support, fewer stressful life events during treatment, and longer duration of treatment. They concluded that geriatric partial treatment can be effective, but also noted the need for further study.

Mintzer et al. (2000) described the effectiveness of a continuum of care using brief and partial hospitalization for agitated patients with dementia. Describing the evolution of an inpatient program for treating these patients, the investigators modified the inpatient program to develop an integrated continuum of care that blended inpatient and outpatient and partial hospitalization programs. Comparing 68 patients treated on the inpatient unit with 110 patients treated in the continuum of care, the investigators found a significant reduction in agitation using the Cohen-Mansfield Agitation Inventory in both groups, with no significant differences between them. Both groups showed improvement in physical aggression, verbal aggression, and nonaggressive behavior. A cost-effective analysis revealed clear advantages for the continuum-of-care program compared with the more expensive inpatient treatment.

Noting that nonattendance at psychogeriatric day programs is a major obstacle to effective treatment, Wright et al. (1995) described an administrative intervention to identify risk for nonattendance through careful scrutiny at weekly multidisciplinary staff meetings. Discussion of the multidisciplinary team focused on greater contact with caseworkers, activation of community psychiatric nurses, visits from team members to homes, and consideration of alternative treatments. They found that the intervention successfully reduced nonattendance rates by 18%, demonstrating its value to maintain patients in indicated treatment.

CONCLUSION

Despite changes in the financing of partial hospital programs, they remain important components in the continuum of care for older persons. They provide multidisciplinary assessment and care for seriously ill persons who, by merit of their partial hospital treatment, can remain in their homes.

Challenges to the field include developing uniform standards of care, quality improvement programs to evaluate variability in practice patterns and outcomes, appropriate admission and discharge criteria, and research demonstrating the effectiveness of treatment.

ACKNOWLEDGMENTS

This work was supported by the Farber Institute for Neurosciences of Thomas Jefferson University.

REFERENCES

Allen-Burge R, Storandt M, Kinscherf DA, Rubin EH. Sex differences in the sensitivity of two self-report depression scales in older depressed inpatients. *Psychol Aging.* 1994;9:443–445.

American Psychiatric Association. *Diagnostic and Statistical Manual of Mental Disorders.* 3rd ed., rev. Washington, DC: American Psychiatric Association; 1987.

American Psychiatric Association. *Diagnostic and Statistical Manual of Mental Disorders.* 4th ed. Washington, DC: American Psychiatric Association; 1994.

Atkinson VL, Stuck BM. Mental health services for the rural elderly: the SAGE experience. *Gerontologist.* 1991;31:548–551.

Boyle DP. The effect of geriatric day treatment on a measure of depression. *Clin Gerontol.* 1997;18(2):43–63.

Casey DA, Schrodt CJ. Axis II diagnoses in geriatric inpatients. *J Geriatr Psychiatry Neurol.* 1989;2:87–88.

Casten RJ, Rovner BW, Pasternak RE, Pelchat R. A comparison of self-reported function assessed before and after depression treatment among depressed geriatric inpatients. *Int J Geriatr Psychiatry.* 2000;15:813–818.

Casten RJ, Rovner BW, Shmuely-Dulitzki Y, Pasternak RE, Pelchat R, et al. Predictors of recovery from major depression among geriatric psychiatry inpatients: the importance of caregivers' beliefs. *Int Psychogeriatr.* 1999;11:149–157.

Conwell Y, Nelson JC, Kim K, et al. Elderly patients admitted to the psychiatric unit of a general hospital. *J Am Geriatr Soc.* 1989;37:35–41.

Cummings JL, Donohue JA, Brooks RL. The relationship between donepezil and behavioral disturbances in patients with Alzheimer's disease. *Am J Geriatr Psychiatry.* 2000;8:134–140.

Draper B, Luscombe G. Quantification of factors contributing to length of stay in an acute psychogeriatric ward. *Int J Geriatr Psychiatry,* 1998;13:1–7.

Edell WS, Tunis SL. Antipsychotic treatment of behavioral and psychological symptoms of dementia (BPSD) in geropsychiatric inpatients. *Am J Geriatr Psychiatry.* 2001;9: 289–297.

Greene JA, Wagner J, Johnson W. Development of a geropsychiatric unit. *South Med J.* 1994;87:392–396.

Koponen H, Senback U, Mattila E, et al. Delirium among elderly persons admitted to a psychiatric hospital: clinical course during the acute stage and one-year follow-up. *Acta Psychiatr Scand.* 1989;79:579–585.

Kunik ME, Mulsant BH, Rifai AH, et al. Personality disorders in elderly inpatients with major depression. *Am J Geriatr Psychiatry.* 1993;1:38–45.

Kunik ME, Mulsant BH, Rifai AH, Sweet RA, Pasternak R, Zubenko GS. Diagnostic rate of comorbid personality disorder in elderly psychiatric inpatients. *Am J Psychiatry.* 1994;151:603–605.

Kunik ME, Ponce H, Molinari V, et al. The benefits of psychiatric hospitalization for older nursing home residents. *J Am Geriatr Soc.* 1996;44:1062–1065.

Mintzer JE, Colenda C, Waid LR, et al. Effectiveness of a continuum of care using brief and partial hospitalization for agitated dementia patients. *Psychiatr Serv.* 1997;48: 1435–1439.

Molinari V, Ames A, Essa M. Prevalence of personality disorders in two geropsychiatric inpatient units. *J Geriatr Psychiatry Neurol.* 1994;7:209–215.

Molinari V, Marmion J. Relationships between affective disorders and axis II diagnoses in geropsychiatric patients. *J Geriatr Psychol Neurol.* 1995;8:61–64.

National Alliance for the Mentally Ill. The Medicare partial hospitalization benefit. 2000. Available at: www.nami.org.

Oslin DW, Datia CJ, Kallan MJ, Katz, IR, Edell WS, Tenhave T. Association between medical comorbidity and treatment outcomes in late-life depression. *J Am Geriatr Soc.* 2002;50:823–828.

Oslin DW, Streim J, Katz IR, et al. Change in disability follows inpatient treatment for late life depression. *J Am Geriatr Soc.* 2000;48:357–362.

Pasternak RE, Rosenzweig A, Booth B, et al. Morbidity of homebound versus inpatient elderly psychiatric patients. *Int Psychogeriatr.* 1998;10:117–125.

Perry DW, Milner E, Krishnan VHR. Physical morbidity in a group of patients referred to a psychogeriatric unit; a 6-month prospective study. *Int J Geriatr Psychiatry.* 1995;10:151–154.

Plotkin DA, Wells KB. Partial hospitalization (day treatment) for psychiatrically ill elderly patients. *Am J Psychiatry.* 1993;150:266–271.

Rovner BW, Folstein MF. The inpatient psychiatric treatment of the elderly. In: Lyon JR, Adler W, Webb W, eds. *Modern Hospital Psychiatry.* New York, NY: Norton; 1987:322–333.

Rubin EH, Kinscherf DA. Assessments on a geropsychiatry unit. *J Geriatr Psychiatry Neurol.* 1990;3:17–20.

Rubin EH, Kinscherf DA, Wehrman SA. Response to treatment of depression and the old and very old. *J Geriatr Psychiatry Neurol.* 1991;4:65–70.

Sager MA, Franke T, Inouye SK, et al. Functional outcomes of acute medical illness and hospitalization in older persons. *Arch Intern Med.* 1996;156:645–652.

Snowden M, Upadhyaya M, Russo J, et al. Medical illness, rather than discharge disposition or use of ECT, is associated with longer length of stay in geriatric patients. In: Abstracts from the AAGP 13th Annual Meeting; March 12–15, 2000; Miami Beach, FL. TP059, p. 39.

Tourigny-Rivard MF, Potoczny WM. Acute care inpatient and day hospital treatment. In: Sadavoy J, Lazarus LW, Jarvik LF, Grossberg GT, eds. *Comprehensive Review of Geriatric Psychiatry.* 2nd ed. Washington, DC: American Psychiatric Press; 1996:973–1001.

Tunis SL, Edell WS, Greenwood KL, Kennedy JS. Burden of illness and prescribing patterns for geriatric inpatients with schizophrenia. In: Abstracts from the AAGP 13th Annual Meeting; March 12–15, 2000; Miami Beach, FL. MP031, p. 42.

Verma S, Orengo CA, Kunik ME, Hale D, Molinari VA. Tolerability and effectiveness of atypical antipsychotics in male geriatric inpatients. *Int J Geriatr Psychiatry.* 2001;6:223–227.

Webster J, Grossberg G. Late-life onset of psychotic symptoms. *Am J Geriatr Psychiatry.* 1998;63:196–202.

Weintraub D, Mazour I. Clinical and demographic changes over a 10-year period on an inpatient psychogeriatric unit. In: Abstracts from the AAGP 13th Annual Meeting; March 12–15, 2000; Miami Beach, FL. TP061, p. 42.

Wright BD, Lunt B, Harris SJ, Wallace D. A prospective study in three psychogeriatric day hospitals using administrative interventions to improve non-attendance. *Int J Geriatr Psychiatry.* 1995;10:55–61.

Zubenko GS, Marino LJ, Sweet RA, et al. Medical comorbidity in elderly psychiatric inpatients. *Biol Psychiatry.* 1997;41:724–736.

Zubenko GS, Mulsant BH, Rifai AH, et al. Impact of acute psychiatric inpatient treatment on major depression in late life and prediction of response. *Am J Psychiatry.* 1994;151:987–994.

Zubenko GS, Rosen J, Sweet RA, et al. Impact of psychiatric hospitalization on behavioral complications of Alzheimer's disease. *Am J Psychiatry.* 1992;149:1484–1491.

36

Geriatric Consultation-Liaison Psychiatry

Jules Rosen, MD
Ashok J. Bharucha, MD
Stephanie S. Richards, MD

INTRODUCTION

The importance of a geriatric psychiatry consultation-liaison service in general hospitals, rehabilitation centers, and outpatient settings cannot be overstated. Typically, the work of psychiatrists occurs behind closed doors, with privacy and confidentiality protected. However, consultation-liaison is visible to other health care professionals participating in the medical care of the patient. Thus, geriatric psychiatry consultation-liaison provides the opportunity to deliver clinical service to patients while educating other health care providers on the impact of psychiatric illness, comorbidity, and social stressors on patients with medical problems. Elderly patients in particular can benefit from both the consultation and liaison functions when a comprehensive approach is used that takes into account the biological/physical changes and emotional and social challenges often experienced by the elderly.

This chapter presents various models of providing consultative services to elderly patients in medical/surgical settings. The data describing effectiveness of consultation-liaison services are presented, and specific clinical problems are discussed.

NEED FOR GERIATRIC PSYCHIATRY
CONSULTATION-LIAISON SERVICE

A specialized geriatric psychiatry consultation-liaison service is important for several reasons. Most studies show that approximately 30% of individuals who are general hospital admissions are at least 65 years of age, and approximately 40% of these inpatients will have some psychiatric disorder (Bergmann & Eastham, 1974; Lipowski, 1983; Mainprize & Rodin, 1987; Popkin et al., 1984; Schuckit et al., 1975). A study that examined consultation requests over a 10-year period showed that the demographics of the patients did not change over that period (Diefenbacher & Strain, 2002). Elderly patients in medical settings have psychiatric needs and problems that differ from the clinical problems typically addressed in young or midlife adults.

Furthermore, the emotional stress and associated fears experienced by elderly patients with medical problems differ from those of a younger person in the hospital. Especially for those patients who are physically frail or forgetful, hospitalization may reflect a loss of autonomy and control that is overwhelming in a strange, new environment, resulting in emotional distress, confusion, and behavioral disturbances. When comorbid medical problems emerge, elderly patients often exhibit symptoms of increased confusion, behavior problems, or frank delirium. This can lead to poor compliance with care in the hospital, resistance to interventions, and at times, aggression and assaultiveness. These are only some of the complex issues that underscore the need for a consultation service with expertise in geriatric psychiatry.

CONSULTATION

Consultation refers specifically to the evaluation of a patient for a particular problem. In medical settings, consultation is requested with a written order by the physician of record; however, the impetus for requesting psychiatric assistance may come from the nursing staff, social worker, family, or patient.

Lipowski (1991) described three main types of geropsychiatry consultations in medical settings. The most common scenario is a request for the patient-oriented consultation, in which the patient is the primary focus. In this model, psychiatric consultation is formally requested and ordered by the attending physician. Typically, the consulting psychiatrist will be asked to participate in the evaluation of acute mental status changes or management of behaviors that are either disruptive or interfere with care in the medical setting. In addition, patients with a history of persistent mental illness may need to be monitored carefully while being treated for acute medical problems. For example, a cardiologist who is treating an elderly patient for an acute myocardial infarction who also has a diagnosis of recurrent major depression may need consultation to help switch the patient from his or her traditional tricyclic antidepressant to one of the newer agents. Lipowski described four phases of the consultation process: (1) receipt of the consultation, (2) information gathering, (3) communication of findings, and (4) follow-up recommendations.

Receipt of Consultation

When a consultation is requested, the specific reason for this request should be specified by the attending physician. In most cases, the consultation process should begin within 24 hours of receiving the request. However, in the case of acute confusional states that are either the reason for hospital admission or are interfering with evaluation and treatment of other medical problems, emergency consultation may be requested, which requires a more rapid response. Typically, reasons for a consultation request include assistance with the evaluation process, management or treatment recommendations, or assessment of mental status to determine competency to make medical decisions.

Information Gathering

The information-gathering phase starts with a review of the medical records, frequently includes discussions with nursing staff and family, and in all cases, includes an examination of the patient. The task of information gathering can be both time consuming and arduous, but is critically important. For example, a consultation request to assist in the management of a nursing home patient admitted to the hospital for acute pneumonia may require multiple sources of information to assess the clinical problem adequately. The extent of information gathering depends on the clinical needs and availability of information.

A focused, problem-oriented consultation would address the problem of managing the patient's behavior during the inpatient treatment. For some patients, that is all that is required. However, a comprehensive consultation may be invaluable if the patient's mental health history is not clear. For example, during the information-gathering phase of the consultation on a patient with a diagnosis of Alzheimer's disease (AD), the consultant should assess how the diagnosis of AD was made and if the patient's history is consistent with that diagnosis. This might require a phone conversation with family members, previous physicians, or nursing home staff. If the history is inconsistent, a more extensive consultation is indicated, and the consultant should recommend a reevaluation of the AD diagnosis. In this case, the information gathering may include a complete review of the medical record, including laboratory assessment, vital sign reports, and nursing notes to assess sleep, appetite, and diurnal variations.

Communication of Findings

Communication of findings always includes a written report for the medical record, but may also involve conversations with the attending physician and nursing or social work staff. The written communication should include a summary of the patient's present and past psychiatric history, alcohol or drug use (including prescribed medications), mental status exam, and assessment of danger to self or others. Social history, including current living situation, is often very important. Medical problems, medications used, and laboratory findings that may have an impact on mental status should be addressed. Recommendations for additional workup should be specified and treatment or management recommendations addressed.

Follow-up

The follow-up of the patient, if needed, may include another visit by the consulting psychiatrist or recommendations for social work intervention during the hospitalization or psychiatric treatment following discharge from the hospital. In most cases, mental health follow-up is needed if psychotropic medications were initiated or if the psychiatric problems identified during the hospitalization are likely to continue after discharge. If an appointment cannot be confirmed prior to discharge, the importance of follow-up psychiatric care should be conveyed to the patient or family in the written discharge instructions.

LIAISON

The liaison component of consultation-liaison is less well defined. According to Merriam-Webster's *Collegiate Dictionary*, *liaison* means "communication for establishing and maintaining mutual understanding and cooperation." The liaison function can be conducted by a psychiatrist, nurse, psychologist, or other professional working as part of a consultation-liaison team. The contact can be formal and regular, such as weekly rounds with a medical or surgical team, or can be informal and "as needed" as part of a patient-focused consultation.

The role of formal liaison has been subject to critical review (Lipowski, 1991). Although there has been some concern that formal liaison associations may give rise to inappropriate and excessive use of psychiatric consultation, which is the "billable" component of consultation-liaison (Pauser et al., 1987), empirical evidence suggests that formal liaison work is appropriate in terms of both resource utilization and patient care. Scott and coworkers (1988) reported a positive change in referral patterns following the initiation of a formal geriatric psychiatry liaison function. Prior to the liaison service, 12% of the individuals referred had depression according to the consulting psychiatrist, and 14% were identified as having no psychiatric illness. Following initiation of the service, 28% of the patients who were seen by the consultants had depression, and only 7% had no psychiatric diagnosis.

Another study addressed the role of the consult-liaison psychiatrist in determining elderly patients' competency to sign informed consent (McKegney et al., 1992). Liaison work with the nursing staff dramatically reduced the use of psychiatric consultation for patients whose capacity for consent was "obvious" from a monthly total of 100 requests before the intervention to 15 after liaison intervention.

In another study on the impact of providing a psychogeriatric liaison team in a teaching hospital, the volume and characteristics of consults requested were relatively unchanged (Poynton, 1988). However, a recent naturalistic study that assessed the impact of introducing a liaison component to an existing psychogeriatric consultation service demonstrated a significant decline in the number of consultations requested (Baheerathan & Shah, 1999). The disparity in these reports may reflect differences in settings. A randomized study of consultation with and without a strong liaison component is needed to clarify these findings.

PREVALENCE OF GEROPSYCHIATRIC PROBLEMS
IN MEDICAL SETTINGS

Psychiatric disorders are common among the elderly in medical settings (Feldman et al., 1987). Approximately 16% of elderly inpatients have affective illness, almost one third are diagnosed with an organic disorder with cognitive deficits, and approximately 20% of elderly men are reported to have a "drinking problem." Table 36-1 presents an overview of published accounts of the psychiatric diagnoses of elderly patients seen in consultation in medical settings. Interestingly, the rate of consultation requests appears to mirror the prevalence of psychiatric problems of the elderly inpatients, with the exception of the low utilization of consultation service for alcohol-related problems. All cited reports reflect patterns of geriatric psychiatry consultation in academic medical centers. It is not known if community hospitals have similar profiles. In these studies, the proportion of elderly patients compared to all consultations requested was 15% to 50%, with the majority of the studies reporting geriatric consultation requests as more than 40%. None of those reports utilized standard research diagnostic criteria, but rather relied on the clinical impression of the various treating physicians.

EFFECTIVENESS OF CONSULTATION

Having established a high prevalence of psychiatric disorders among elderly medical/surgical inpatients, it is important to examine the data assessing the impact of psychiatric consultation in these patients in terms of clinical outcomes, length of stay in the hospital, and overall cost of care. While the medical literature is full of anecdotal reports, few randomized clinical trials assessed the effectiveness of consultation.

Cole and colleagues (1991) conducted a randomized trial of geriatric psychiatry consultation in an acute care hospital. In this study, 80 patients aged 65 years or older for whom consultation by a multidisciplinary geriatric team

TABLE 36-1. Diagnoses (percentage) of elderly inpatients referred for psychiatric consultation

Reference	Dementia/ delirium	Affective disorder	Psychosis or schizophrenia	Adjustment disorder	Anxiety disorder	Personality disorder	Other diagnosis
Rabins et al. (1983), N = 139	54	27	1	—	4	5	4
Popkin et al. (1984), N = 266	46	23	0	9	2	3	3
Ruskin (1985), N = 67	37	24	16	—	0	12	—
Mainprize and Rodin (1987), N = 70	51	17	1	17	0	14	4
Small and Fawzy (1988), N = 88	47	55	16	22	4	5	7
Levitte and Thornby (1989), N = 384	36	25	5	—	8	8	16
Grossberg et al. (1990), N = 147	36	27	2	26	3	1	1

May not total 100% as several studies listed multiple diagnoses for a single patient.

(MGT) was requested were randomly selected to receive standard MGT evaluation or MGT evaluation with additional geropsychiatric assessment. The intervention included an initial assessment and, when appropriate, weekly follow-up visits for up to 8 weeks. Of note, the members of the standard MGT included a geriatrician, occupational and recreational therapists, social worker, and others. In this relatively small study of highly selected patients, a trend toward improved clinical outcomes was noted in the group receiving additional geropsychiatric consultation. Although length of stay was no different between groups, twice as many patients receiving additional psychiatric consultation were discharged home rather than to residential care homes or nursing homes.

Another study compared the impact of psychogeriatric consultation on patients 75 years of age and older who were randomly assigned to either standard care ($N = 97$) on a 40-bed medical unit or care on a similar unit, but with the additional intervention of a multidisciplinary psychogeriatric team ($N = 140$) (Slaets et al., 1997). Measures of functional independence, mobility, and activity of daily living (ADL) status all were significantly higher for patients on the intervention unit compared to the control group, even when controlling for potentially confounding baseline characteristics. Furthermore, length of stay and readmission within 6 months were also significantly decreased for the intervention group. Finally, patients randomly assigned to psychogeriatric intervention were less likely to be discharged to a nursing home. The differences in the outcomes between the study of Slaets and colleagues compared to that of Cole and coworkers (1991) may be the comparison group of standard care. In the former study, standard care included the expertise of a multidisciplinary geriatric team, but without an identified geropsychiatrist. In the latter study, standard care was care on a typical medical unit without any additional intervention.

Several trials have addressed the impact of psychogeriatric consultation on elderly patients specifically with hip fracture. In an early study, Levitan and Kornfeld (1981) reported that patients whose care involved a liaison psychiatrist spent an average of 12 fewer days in the hospital and were less likely to be discharged to a nursing home compared to patients who did not receive this intervention. A limitation of this study included the small sample size and lack of randomization.

A time-controlled study of patients with hip fracture aged 65 years and older evaluated the cost-benefit ratio of psychogeriatric consultation (Strain et al., 1991). The subjects were 452 patients who were consecutively admitted for surgical repair of fractured hips. During a baseline year, the patients (control group) received traditional referral for psychiatric consultation. During the experimental year, the patients were screened for psychiatric consultation through a psychiatric liaison program. Treatment, if needed, was initiated. The patients who received psychiatric liaison screening had a higher consultation rate than those who received traditional consultation. They also experienced significant improvement in their Mini-Mental State Exam and Geriatric Depression Scale scores compared to the control group. The mean length of stay was reduced by approximately 2 days, resulting in reductions in hospital costs. There was no difference, however, between the 2 years in the discharge placement of patients.

Finally, the importance of identifying psychiatric illness in elderly patients with hip fractures was highlighted by Shamash and coworkers (1992). In this retrospective study, both depression and dementia were associated with a higher rate of mortality 1 year after surgery.

Inpatient Settings

There are different models of geropsychiatric consultation in medical/surgical settings. In the traditional consultation model, the attending physician formally requests a psychiatric consultation for a specific reason. The consultation typically is done within 24 hours of the request and must include a diagnosis and recommendations for further evaluation or treatment. Consultations can range from brief to complex. The consultant should always respect the patient's right to privacy and confidentiality and not gratuitously discuss sensitive information revealed by the patient with either medical professionals or family. The presence of a roommate can present additional challenges concerning confidentiality for the psychiatric consultant.

An alternative model combines the typical consultation function with a strong liaison component. Often, a psychogeriatric team, which may include a nurse with an advanced degree or social worker and a geriatric psychiatrist, provides direct patient consultation (both evaluation and follow-up) and staff education focused on the management of the particular patient. This model works particularly well for nursing home patients who are frightened by environmental changes. The liaison/education can help the nursing staff to orient the resident and work with the family to reduce agitation. The consulting role would address the medical evaluation of delirium and perhaps provide recommendation for treatment options.

A third model involves an active liaison component that functions independently from the patient-oriented consult service. An example of this model is a geriatric psychiatrist or geriatric nurse clinical specialists who attend weekly orthopedic surgery team meetings to help address the complex psychiatric and emotional needs of elderly patients undergoing hip repair. Face-to-face contact with the patient would require a specifically generated request for consultation.

Outpatient Settings

Outpatient medical clinics and primary care sites are important sites for geropsychiatric consultation and liaison. Implementation of practice guidelines for the diagnosis and treatment of depression in particular can positively influence both the process of care and clinical outcomes in primary care (Mulsant et al.,

2001). However, evidence suggests that traditional educational efforts are insufficient to produce marked and sustained change in physician behavior, especially given the time constraints of current primary care practice (Katon et al., 1995). The collaborative care model (CCM) has been developed to overcome both the limitations in traditional approaches to physician education and time constraints. In the CCM, depressed patients are managed conjointly by their primary care provider (PCP) and by a mental health specialist (i.e., a psychiatrist, a psychologist, a psychiatric nurse, or a social worker) (Katon et al., 1999).

Several studies of collaborative care have been conducted among younger and middle-aged adults. Katon and colleagues showed that the treatment of depression in a large primary care clinic could be improved by the implementation of such a collaborative care model. In these studies, midlife patients with depression treated with an antidepressant or psychotherapy had higher adherence to treatment and better symptomatic outcomes when they were seen collaboratively by their PCP and by a psychiatrist or a psychologist than when they received usual care from their PCP only (Katon et al., 1995, 1996, 1997, 1999). To our knowledge, there are not yet any published results from studies of the collaborative care model in older depressed patients. However, several such studies are ongoing (Mulsant et al., 2001; Unutzer, 2002).

GENERAL PRINCIPLES OF GERIATRIC PSYCHIATRY IN CONSULTATION SETTINGS

Beyond the skills of most general psychiatrists, knowledge of geriatric psychopharmacology, knowledge of end-of-life issues (including suicide), and an understanding of disposition planning are essential for providing geriatric consultation (Lipowski, 1983). In addition, the consultant must understand the concepts of competency and capacity to make decisions.

Pharmacology

Elderly patients commonly experience serious adverse reactions to medications or experience drug interactions that lead to serious medical complications (Pollock, 2000). Often, these drug reactions lead to mental status changes, such as delirium or depression. Furthermore, not uncommonly, psychotropic medications are involved in these adverse reactions. Although only 3% of all hospital admissions are attributed to adverse drug reactions for people younger than 70 years old, 18% of hospitalized patients over the age of 70 years experience adverse drug reactions that are believed to contribute to the need for admission (Beard, 1992; Benrimoj et al., 1995; Stewart & Cooper, 1994).

There are several explanations for this wide disparity. Although people over the age of 65 years represent approximately 13% of the US population, they receive more than one third of all medications prescribed. Furthermore, the typical older American uses eight medications regularly, four by prescription and four over the counter. Therefore, with all else equal, more older Americans are exposed to more medications and more combinations of medications. Common offenders for adverse drug reactions involving psychotropic medications include cardiovascular drugs, anticholinergics, and anti-inflammatory drugs (Beard, 1992; Hallas et al., 1990; Hinderling, 1988). In addition to the numerous drugs prescribed, the pharmacokinetic and pharmacodynamic considerations described in Chapter 30 magnify the potential for adverse drug reactions.

End-of-Life Issues and Suicide

Thoughts of death and feeling ready to die are not indicators of psychiatric illness by themselves in the elderly, especially if the patient is challenged with life-threatening medical problems. In clinical practice, patients are frequently encountered who willingly admit that they are ready to die "if the Lord is ready" to take them. Although this may reflect a depressive illness, it may also reflect a sense of spiritual comfort with their station in life. If the death wish is accompanied by withdrawal from family or other pleasurable activities, intense hopelessness, or other symptoms of depression, consideration of treatment should be discussed with the patient. Treatment may include pastoral and hospice care in addition to supportive therapy and medications.

Increasing age and physical illness are two of the factors associated with successful suicide. In particular, hospitalized elderly men experiencing additional stressors, such as spousal bereavement, are at high risk for suicide (Conwell, Caine, et al., 1990; Conwell, Rotenberg, et al., 1990; Conwell et al., 1991). A recent study of suicidal ideation in cognitively capable, medically ill inpatients admitted to geriatric medicine wards reported that more than one third endorsed suicidal ideation at the time of admission, and almost 20% remained suicidal 6 months later (Shah et al., 2000). The symptom of hopelessness should be carefully assessed in medically ill elders as, even in the absence of other indicators of depression, this trait alone is a risk factor for suicide (Rifai et al., 1993).

Functional Assessment and Disposition Planning

The consulting geriatric psychiatrist can be extremely helpful in planning disposition following hospitalization. In addition to a referral for ongoing psychiatric follow-up if needed, the geropsychiatric team will have an appreciation of the different levels of supportive care in the community, which range from in-home services to nursing facilities that will meet the needs of the elderly inpatients with functional impairment (Sadavoy & Reiman-Sheldon, 1983). Occupational and physical therapy assessments may be essential to understand the level of functional impairment and prognosis for rehabilitation.

For example, an elderly depressed patient, living alone, who became in-

creasingly frail and was hospitalized for pneumonia may be severely functionally impaired. Appropriate discharge plans for this patient might be in-home
services and outpatient psychiatric treatment. A patient with similar social situation and functional impairment but with Alzheimer's disease may require
nursing home placement because the reason for the increased frailty is due to
an irreversible process in this case (Brown et al., 1995; Raphael et al., 1995).
Effective psychogeriatric consultation coordinates all the medical, psychiatric,
functional, and social information so that disposition planning can be optimized for an individual patient (Harris et al., 1988).

Assessment of Competence and Capacity to Make Informed Decisions

A frequent reason for consultation requests is to determine if a patient is competent to make informed decisions regarding medical treatment. It is important
to note that the diagnosis of dementia does not necessarily mean a patient is incompetent to make a specific decision. It is up to the consultant to determine
if a legal adjudication of incompetence for specific decisions is indicated.

Consultation-liaison psychiatrists do not decide that a patient is incompetent. Rather, they render their opinion if a judicial determination of competency is warranted (Appelbaum & Roth, 1981). To do this, the consultant must
specify for which decisions a patient's competence is questioned. Family involvement, when possible, is essential in determining if a patient's decision is consistent with his or her general outlook on life, even if the family does not agree.

According to Appelbaum and Grisso (1988), four basic categories must be
assessed to make a determination of competency.

1. Can the patient communicate choices? For example, a patient may verbalize that there is an option for a regular or low-salt diet. On the other
   hand, the patient may not be able to verbalize that there are two
   choices for cancer treatment, radiation alone or in combination with
   chemotherapy.
2. Does the patient understand the information given? The patient must
   remember the information long enough to repeat it to the examiner.
   The patient should be able to reconstitute the choices in his or her own
   words, demonstrating that the concepts discussed are understood. For
   example, the patient must be able to explain what it means if a procedure has a 50–50 chance of success. Finally, the patient must be asked
   to explain the purpose of the consent process and who, in his or her
   mind, is making this decision.
3. Does the patient understand the situation and its consequences? The
   patient should acknowledge the illness and verbalize repercussions of
   refusing treatment. If financial competency is questioned, the patient
   must be able to verbalize the consequence of failure to pay rent.
4. Can the patient manipulate the information rationally? The patient

should be able to logically follow the expressed information and describe how this information leads to choices. The final decision must
be rationally linked to the starting premises. For example, a patient
who acknowledges having terminal cancer and insists that "everything
possible be done, no matter what" cannot refuse a statistically better
treatment of radiation and chemotherapy in combination (compared to
radiation alone) because the patient does not want to lose his or her
hair. In this case, the starting premises and final decisions are not logically connected.

CLINICAL SYNDROMES

Delirium

Delirium (see Chapter 18 for a detailed discussion), also known as metabolic
encephalopathy, acute confusional state, intensive care unit (ICU) psychosis,
and sundowning, is the most common reason for psychiatric consultation
among elderly inpatients in the general hospital. Psychiatric consultation is
usually obtained for delirious patients who are demonstrating disturbing or
dangerous behavior or patients who are not cooperative with their medical
treatment.

The cost of delirium is high in terms of both patient outcome and health
care expenditures. Delirium is associated with significant morbidity, including
increased complications, limited recovery, longer hospital stays, and poor long-
term outcome. Mortality rates increase, with an estimated 22% to 76% dying
during the index hospitalization and another 25% dying within 6 months
(Cameron et al., 1987; Rabins et al., 1983; Rabins & Folstein, 1982; Trzepacz
et al., 1985).

One of the major barriers to treatment of delirium in hospital settings is
inadequate detection (Inouye et al., 1993). Medical and surgical teams should
maintain a high index of suspicion for delirium, particularly in patients with
multiple predisposing factors on admission and more than one precipitating
factor during the hospital course. Due to the fluctuating nature of the symptoms, a brief morning visit by the medical team may not reveal the scope of
the attentional or cognitive deficits, and the perceptual disturbances need specific queries to be detected (Lipowski, 1967).

Input from nursing, direct care, and ancillary staff is necessary to obtain
an accurate picture of the patient over time. Families can also provide valuable
information about changes in the patient's mental status and behavior. Because
symptoms tend to fluctuate widely, it is imperative to obtain collateral information from direct care staff and families who see the patient at different times.
Onset of symptoms is generally abrupt over a short period of time, but depending on the cause, may be chronic and steady over weeks, months, or even years.

Evaluation in the hospital includes monitoring for safety issues such as threats to self and others. Assessment of risk of pulling out intravenous lines, central lines, or Foley catheters; falling out of bed; and walking unassisted as well as for threats to direct care staff in the form of aggressive or violent behaviors is conducted. Evaluation of psychological issues such as personality traits may help promote an understanding of the patient's reaction to the environment and assist in alleviating potential conflicts. Family dynamics and the sociocultural environment of the patient may also help to explain reactions or behaviors and elucidate contributing environmental factors.

In the acute care setting, unexplained delirium may reflect a medical emergency. The medical team should be made aware of the increased morbidity and mortality associated with delirium. Once potential medical etiologies are determined, all treatable contributing factors should be addressed and all nonessential medications discontinued. Patients should receive close monitoring of vital signs, input and output, and oxygenation.

Maintaining safety is a priority. Restraints should be avoided, if possible, as they can contribute to increased agitation and carry a risk for injury. An alternative is a sitter who stays with the patient and provides redirection if safety is threatened. Often, family members can serve this role, particularly at night when delirious patients are most confused and disoriented.

Other nonpharmacological interventions include education for family and staff members about delirium so that they can interact more appropriately with the patient. The patient needs constant reassurance and reorientation. Orientation cues such as calendars and clocks should be provided. Communication should be clear and simple, with concrete statements and one-step commands. Familiar objects brought from home can minimize confusion and disorientation in an unfamiliar environment. Family visits and overnight stays can be very helpful. Adequate lighting and noise reduction, as well as optimizing sensory input by providing glasses and hearing aids when needed, are also helpful (Wengel et al., 1998).

Postdelirium management includes monitoring for resolution of symptoms and cognitive impairment as well as providing emotional support. Many patients have vivid and frightening memories of perceptions and experiences while delirious. In some cases, actual posttraumatic stress disorder (PTSD) can emerge. It is often difficult for patients to recognize or accept that these experiences were unreal. Providing education about delirium, its apparent causes, and the psychotic processes that can occur during delirium may be helpful. Sometimes, psychotherapy is indicated for working through the experiences of the delirium.

Depressive Disorders

CLINICAL EPIDEMIOLOGY   Depressive disorders in the elderly often emerge or are exacerbated in the context of a medical illness. According to the National Hospital Discharge Survey (Hall & Owings 2002), the five most common discharge diagnoses among persons 65 years of age and older from nonfederal short-stay hospitals were heart disease, stroke, malignant neoplasms, pneumonia/bronchitis, and fractures, respectively. The prevalence rates of depressive disorders specifically for those over the age of 65 years suffering from these medical conditions are not known, but are alarmingly high in the general population (Table 36-2). Methodological limitations such as the variability in instruments and cutoff scores used to measure major depression, the lack of a standard definition of minor depression, and the heterogeneity of the medical conditions themselves contribute to the wide prevalence range of depressive disorders (Borson et al., 1986; Evans et al., 1999; Gonzalez et al., 1996; Lesprance & Frasure-Smith, 2000; Lieberman et al., 1999; McDaniel et al., 1995; Robinson et al., 1998; Van Ede et al., 1999).

A review of the prevalence studies performed in Veterans Affairs hospitals in the United States suggested that 5% to 45% of hospitalized elders (Kitchell et al., 1982; Koenig et al., 1988, 1991; Koenig & Blazer, 1992; Rapp, Parisi, et al., 1988) and 10% to 31% of outpatients (Borson et al., 1986; Norris et al., 1987; Okimoto et al., 1982) suffer from major depression. Subsequent studies from the medical inpatient services of a university teaching hospital, however, reported a 10% to 21% rate of major depression and 14% to 25% rate of minor depression (Koenig, George, Peterson, et al., 1997), still substantially higher than the 1-month prevalence of less than 1% reported for community-dwelling elders (Regier et al., 1988). Despite the high prevalence rates and the potentially reversible nature of depression, it is thought to be detected in less than 10% of elderly medical inpatients by non-psychiatric physicians (Rapp, Walsh, et al., 1988), leading to myriad adverse consequences—noncompliance with medical treatment (Stoudemire & Thompson, 1983; Strain, 1978), prolonged hospitalization (Fulop et al., 1987; Verbosky et al., 1993), slower recovery from illness (Mossey et al., 1990), persistent impairments in daily functioning (Parikh et al., 1990), and premature mortality (Lesprance & Frasure-Smith, 2000).

TABLE 36-2.   Prevalence rates of major and minor depression in the top five medical inpatient discharge diagnoses for individuals older than 65 years

	Major depression, %	Minor depression, %
Coronary artery disease	15–25	15–25
Cerebrovascular disease	13–20	20
Malignancy	24	25
Chronic obstructive pulmonary disease	20	6–28
Fracture (mostly hip)	16–20	15–20

DIAGNOSIS The diagnosis of depression in medically ill older persons is challenging because of the difficulties in disentangling symptoms stemming from the aging process from those of the medical illness and its treatment and the neurovegetative symptoms of depression (Kurlowicz & Streim, 1998). The *Diagnostic and Statistical Manual of Mental Disorders, Fourth Edition* (*DSM-IV*; American Psychiatric Association, 1994), for example, advises that a symptom be counted toward the diagnosis of depression if it is felt not to be "due to a general medical condition," an imprecise matter left to the rater's clinical judgment. Morrison and Kastenberg (1997) complicated matters further by asserting that some depressive symptoms are clearly attributable to the underlying pathophysiological processes of the medical condition (i.e., secondary depression). Moreover, it is far from clear which features distinguish an expectable psychological reaction to a medical illness from a clinically significant mood disorder.

Several diagnostic approaches have been proposed to minimize the misattribution of somatic symptoms and hence improve the proper recognition of depression. In the inclusive approach, a symptom is counted toward a diagnosis of depression regardless of the presumed cause, whereas in the etiologic approach employed by the *DSM-IV*, a symptom is attributed to depression only if the clinician believes it is not due to a general medical condition. The exclusive approach (Bukberg et al., 1984) reduces the nine *DSM-IV* criteria symptoms to seven by eliminating anorexia and fatigue, which are ubiquitous in medical illness. Likewise, Endicott's (1984) substitutive approach replaces the more somatic neurovegetative symptoms of depression with those that are primarily cognitive or affective—irritability, tearfulness, feeling punished, and social withdrawal.

Koenig, George, Peterson, and colleagues (1997) examined the impact of these diagnostic schemes (inclusive, etiologic, exclusive-inclusive, exclusive-etiologic, substitutive-inclusive, and substitutive-etiologic) on the detection rates of depression, its correlates, and longitudinal course of symptoms (median follow-up time 47 weeks) in cognitively unimpaired elders (aged 60 years or older) admitted to the inpatient medical services of Duke Hospital, Durham, North Carolina. In summarizing the findings, Koenig et al. reported a 10% to 21% rate of major depression and 14% to 25% rate of minor depression, depending on the diagnostic scheme. Although the exclusive-etiologic approach identified the most severe and persistent major depressive episodes, it did not detect 49% of patients with major depression who were captured by the inclusive strategy, 60% of whom remained depressed 9 weeks postdischarge. The sensitivity and reliability of the inclusive approach may lead to a more false positives. The *DSM-IV* approach yielded prevalence rates of major depression between those of the inclusive and exclusive-etiologic schemes, encompassing most individuals with high levels of impairment and persistence of depressive symptoms.

The inpatient medical setting offers an opportunity not only to detect depressive symptoms that may reach syndromal level in the context of an acute medical illness, but also to identify and evaluate the nature of the coexisting cognitive impairment that is so prevalent in the depressed elderly, sometimes referred to as *pseudodementia*. Cognitive dysfunction is thought to accompany 10% to over 20% of depressive episodes (Garcia et al., 1981; Jeste et al., 1990; Marsden & Harrison, 1972; Nott & Fleminger, 1975; Reynolds et al., 1988) and raises a challenging diagnostic dilemma because there are no pathognomonic clinical features that distinguish cognitive changes associated with depression from those of Alzheimer's disease or vascular dementia with depressed mood.

Lockwood and colleagues (2000), however, reported some progress in characterizing cognitive impairment in depressed older adults. In their investigation of the cognitive profiles of 104 older adults with major depression, three distinct patterns of cognitive impairment emerged. All three subgroups suffered from memory deficits, while one third of subjects experienced either executive dysfunction or attentional deficits. Notably, the group with executive impairments exhibited greater behavioral disability.

The subtyping of cognitive deficits in older adults may not only shed light on the mechanisms of late-life depression and the pathophysiology of antidepressant response as the authors suggested, but also may help identify a subgroup particularly vulnerable to subsequent development of a progressive dementia. Indeed, longitudinal studies of cognitive loss with depression reported an alarming 38% to 50% rate of subsequent degenerative dementia (Alexopoulos et al., 1987; Bulbena & Berrios, 1986; Reding et al., 1985), although refuting findings also exist (Pearlson et al., 1989; Rabins et al., 1984; Sachdev et al., 1990).

A meta-analysis by Jorm (2000) also supported an association between depression and subsequent development of dementia in both case-control and prospective studies. The high rates of depressive symptomatology and cognitive dysfunction in Linka and coworkers' (2000) study of elderly medical inpatients highlighted the importance of psychiatric consultation in this setting.

OUTCOME   What is the course and outcome of depression in elderly medical inpatients postdischarge? Some insight was offered by Cole and Bellavance's (1997) meta-analysis of original research studies published in English or French that focused on depressed medical inpatients age 60 years and older; in these studies affective state was reported as an outcome. In the eight studies (265 patients) that met these inclusion criteria, only 19% of patients were well at 12 months, with 29% persistently depressed and 53% dead. Diagnostic scheme (symptom rating scales vs. formal diagnostic criteria, inclusive vs. etiologic approach) had no impact on specific outcomes. Poor prognostic factors included more severe depression in two studies (Fenton et al., 1997; Pomerant et al., 1992); presence of dysthymia before admission in one study (Fenton et al., 1997); and more severe medical illness in the study of Rapp and coworkers (1991), but not in that of Koenig and colleagues (1992). In contrast, the highest

1-year recovery rate of 39% was reported by Evans and Lye (1992), whose depressed patients all received fluoxetine and follow-up.

Koenig and Kuchibhatla (1999) examined the use of health services over a median postdischarge follow-up of 47 weeks by 160 depressed and 171 non-depressed patients aged 60 years and older admitted to the cardiology, neurology, or general medicine inpatient services of Duke Hospital. Even after controlling for the physical health status, depressed patients made more outpatient physician visits, were rehospitalized at higher rates, and spent more days in the nursing home. Notably, however, there was no difference in the utilization of mental health services by those who remained depressed and physically disabled compared to those whose depression and disability improved at follow-up. Koenig and George (1998) also demonstrated via time series analyses that depression and disability tend to track together, with the first 6 months postdischarge the critical window of greatest improvement. Of the elderly in this cohort, however, 52% still remained depressed at 6 months after hospital discharge. Lower recovery rate from depression was associated with a prior history of depression, more medical diagnoses, and greater severity of the index episode of depression.

Despite the high prevalence and disabling adverse outcomes of depressive disorders in elderly medical inpatients, underdiagnosis and undertreatment remain the rule, even after the primary treatment team is informed by a mental health specialist of the presence of depression (Koenig & Blazer, 1992; Koenig, George, & Meador, 1997; Rapp, Walsh, et al., 1988; Rapp et al., 1991). In the minority of cases for which depression is recognized, treatment is often characterized by subtherapeutic doses and duration of antidepressant therapy, lack of psychotherapy, and undue reliance on benzodiazepines for symptomatic relief (Koenig et al., 1989, 1992; Koenig, George, & Meador, 1997).

A study by Koenig, George, Peterson, and colleagues (1997) highlighted this challenge. Using a structured psychiatric interview by a geropsychiatrist, 153 elderly medical inpatients at Duke Hospital were identified as suffering from major or minor depression; of these individuals, only 13% were referred for psychiatric consultation. An antidepressant was prescribed by the medical team for 40.5% of these patients during the hospitalization or subsequently in the follow-up period of almost a year, with nearly half of the cohort receiving amitriptyline, a highly anticholinergic antidepressant, at a subtherapeutic average dose of 49 mg/day. Of the 59.5% of patients whose depression was not treated before or during the hospitalization, only 11% subsequently received an antidepressant postdischarge. Factors predicting greater intensity of depression treatment included a prior psychiatric history, higher income, and most important, the patient's perception of the severity of his or her symptoms. Formal classification of major and minor depression and severity of medical burden did not predict the intensity of treatment received. Alarmingly, benzodiazepines were dispensed to 25.5% of the cohort.

These findings are particularly disturbing in light of the fact that evidence exists that points to the effectiveness of psychiatric consultation and treatment in curbing depressive symptoms and their negative impact on medical outcomes and health care resource utilization (Borson et al., 1992; Evans, 1993; Evans & Lye, 1992; Hengeveld et al., 1988; Kemp et al., 1991; Lesprance & Frasure-Smith, 2000; Masand et al., 1991; Miranda & Munoz, 1994; Schwartz et al., 1988). In summary, an elderly individual with the following profile may be at the greatest risk of persistent depression after hospital discharge (Koenig & George, 1998): history of dysthymia or depression, stressful life events in the year prior to the index admission, greater number of active medical diagnoses, and very importantly, the patient's perception of his or her depression severity.

Future research on depression in the medically ill hospitalized elderly should focus on (1) identifying baseline demographic, psychosocial, and clinical characteristics that confer vulnerability to persistent depression (or, alternatively, protection from depression); (2) the efficacy and safety of the newer serotonergic and serotonin-norepinephrine combination antidepressants; (3) characterizing depressive syndromes based on differential response to antidepressants or psychotherapy; (4) tracking depression/disability interactions postdischarge, particularly in the first 6 months; (5) implementing educational and collaborative interventions to recognize and treat depression for both primary care physicians and patients; and (6) subclassifying cognitive deficits associated with depression in this setting to identify those at greatest risk of dementia or behavioral impairment.

Alcoholism and Substance Abuse

Interestingly, the prevalence of alcohol or other substance abuse diagnoses was very low across all the studies cited in Table 36-1. However, alcoholism has been described as one of the most underrecognized and poorly understood public health problems in elderly persons. This belief is supported by data showing that 9% of more than 300 elderly men admitted to the hospital were classified as "problem drinkers" compared to 0% of women admitted during the same time period (Bristow & Clare, 1992). Analysis of Medicare data shows that alcohol-related admissions to medical hospitals for elderly people are similar to those for myocardial infarction (Adams et al., 1993). One can only speculate that the low rate of alcoholism as a reason for consultation request cited in the prevalence studies was due to the fact that alcohol-related problems are handled by the internist or PCP without additional psychiatric consultation or that the psychiatric comorbidity of depression, delirium, or dementia associated with alcoholism were secondary diagnoses and thus were not recorded. Nonetheless, geriatric psychiatrists should be aware of the high prevalence of problem drinking in the hospitalized elderly and the risks of acute withdrawal.

Similarly, the epidemiological studies did not find high rates of benzodiazepine-related psychiatric consultation requests despite the high prevalence of the use of these drugs in the elderly population.

CONCLUSION

Psychiatry consultation and liaison work with geriatric patients requires special skills and knowledge. Improved quality of care, reduced burden on medical staff, enhanced understanding by families, and reduced health care costs are all possible favorable outcomes.

REFERENCES

Adams WL, Yuan Z, Barboriak JJ, Rimm AA. Alcohol-related hospitalizations of elderly people: prevalence and geographic variation in the United States. *JAMA*. 1993;270: 1222–1225.

Alexopoulos GS, Young RC, Lieberman KW, et al. Platelet MAO activity in geriatric patients with depression and dementia. *Am J Psychiatry*. 1987;144:488–492.

Appelbaum PS, Grisso T. Assessing patients' capacities to consent to treatment. *N Engl J Med*. 1988;319:1635–1638.

Appelbaum PS, Roth LH. Clinical issues in the assessment of competency. *Am J Psychiatry*. 1981;138:1462–1467.

Baheerathan M, Shah A. The impact of two changes in service delivery on a geriatric psychiatry liaison service. *Int J Geriatr Psychiatry*. 1999;14:767–775.

Beard K. Adverse reactions as a cause of hospital admission in the aged. *Drugs Aging*. 1992;2:356–367.

Benrimoj SI, Langford JH, Bowden MG, Triggs EJ. Switching drug availability from prescription only to over-the-counter status: are elderly patients at increased risk? *Drugs Aging*. 1995;7:255.

Bergmann K, Eastham JH. Psychogeriatric ascertainment and assessment for treatment in an acute medical ward setting. *Age Ageing*. 1974;3:174–188.

Borson S, Barnes RF, Kukull WA. Symptomatic depression in elderly medical outpatients. I. Prevalence, demography and health service utilization. *J Am Geriatr Soc*. 1986;34:341–347.

Borson S, McDonald GJ, Gayle T, et al. Improvement in mood, physical symptoms, and function with nortriptyline for depression in patients with chronic obstructive pulmonary disease. *Psychosomatics*. 1992;33:190–201.

Bristow MF, Clare AW. Prevalence and characteristics of at-risk drinkers among elderly acute medical in-patients. *Br J Addict*. 1992;87:291–294.

Brown I, Renwick R, Raphael D. Frailty: constructing a common meaning, definition, and conceptual framework. *Int J Rehabil Res*. 1995;18:93–102.

Bukberg J, Penman D, Holland J. Depression in hospitalized cancer patients. *Psychosom Med*. 1984;46:199–212.

Bulbena A, Berrios G. Pseudodementia: facts and figures. *Br J Psychiatry*. 1986;148: 87–94.

Cameron DJ, Thomas RI, Mulvihill MBH. Delirium: a test of the *Diagnostic and Statistical Manual III* criteria on medical inpatients. *J Am Geriatr Soc*. 1987;35:1007–1010.

Cole MG, Bellavance F. Depression in elderly medical inpatients: a meta-analysis of outcomes. *Can Med Assoc J*. 1997;157:1055–1060.

Cole MG, Fenton FR, Engelsmann F, Mansouri I. Effectiveness of geriatric psychiatry consultation in an acute care hospital: a randomized clinical trail. *J Am Geriatr Soc.* 1991;39:1183–1188.

Conwell Y, Caine ED, Olsen K. Suicide and cancer in late life. *Hosp Community Psychiatry.* 1990;41:1334–1339.

Conwell Y, Olsen K, Caine ED, Flannery C. Suicide in later life: psychological autopsy findings. *Int Psychogeriatr.* 1991;3:59–66.

Conwell Y, Rotenberg M, Caine ED. Completed suicide at age 50 and over. *J Am Geriatr Soc.* 1990;38:640–644.

Diefenbacher A, Strain JJ. Consultation-liaison psychiatry: stability and change over a 10-year period. *Gen Hosp Psychiatry.* 2002;24:249–256.

Endicott J. Measurement of depression in patients with cancer. *Cancer.* 1984;53:2243–2249.

Evans DL, Staab JP, Petitto JM, et al. Depression in the medical setting: biopsychological interactions and treatment considerations. *J Clin Psychiatry.* 1999;60:40–55.

Evans ME. Depression in elderly physically ill in-patients: a 12-month prospective study. *Int Clin Psychopharmacol.* 1993;8:333–336.

Evans ME, Lye M. Depression in the elderly physically ill: an open study of treatment with the 5-HT reuptake inhibitor fluoxetine. *Exp Gerontol.* 1992;14:297–307.

Feldman E, Mayou R, Hawton K, Ardern M, Smith EB. Psychiatric disorder in medical in-patients. *Q J Med New Ser.* 1987;63:405–412.

Fenton FR, Cole MG, Engelsmann F, et al. Depression in older medical inpatients: one-year course and outcome. *Int J Geriatr Psychiatry.* 1997;12:389–394.

Fulop G, Strain J, Vita J, et al. Impact of psychiatric comorbidity on length of hospital stay for medical/surgical patients: a preliminary report. *Am J Psychiatry.* 1987;144:878–881.

Garcia CA, Reding MJ, Blass JP. Overdiagnosis of dementia. *J Am Geriatr Soc.* 1981;29:407–410.

Gonzalez MB, Snyderman T.B., Colket JT, et al. Depression in patients with coronary artery disease. *Depression.* 1996;4:57–62.

Grossberg GT, Zimny GH, Nakra BRS. Clinical practice and service development: geriatric psychiatry consultations in a university hospital. *Int Psychogeriatr.* 1990;2:161–168.

Hall JM, Owings MF. *Vital Health Statistics.* Atlanta, GA: Division of Health Care Statistics, Centers for Disease Control; June 19, 2002; no. 329.

Hallas J, Haghfelt T, Gram LF, Grodum E, Damsbo N. Drug related admissions to a cardiology department: frequency and avoidability. *J Intern Med.* 1990;228:379–384.

Harris RE, Mion LC, Patterson MB, Frengley JD. Severe illness in older patients: the association between depressive disorders and functional dependency during the recovery phase. *J Am Geriatr Soc.* 1988;36:896.

Hengeveld MW, Ancion FA, Rooijmans H. Psychiatric consultations with depressed medical inpatients: a randomized controlled cost-effectiveness study. *Int J Psychiatry Med.* 1988;18:33–43.

Hinderling PH. Detection of populations at risk and problem drugs during drug development and in pharmacotherapy. *Ther Drug Monit.* 1988;10:245–249.

Inouye SK, Viscoli CM, Horwitz RI, Hurst LD, Tinetti ME. A predictive model for delirium in hospitalized elderly medical patients based on admission characteristics. *Ann Intern Med.* 1993;119:474–481.

Jeste DV, Gierz M, Harris MJ. Pseudodementia: myths and realities. *Psychiatr Ann.* 1990;20:71–79.

Jorm AF. Is depression a risk factor for dementia or cognitive decline? *Gerontology.* 2000;46:219–227.

Katon W, Robinson P, VonKorff M, et al. A multifaceted intervention to improve treatment of depression in primary care. *Arch Gen Psychiatry.* 1996;53:924–932.

Katon W, VonKorff M, Lin E, et al. Collaborative management to achieve depression treatment guidelines. *J Clin Psychiatry.* 1997;58:20–23.

Katon W, Von Korff M, Lin E, et al. Stepped collaborative care for primary care patients with persistent symptoms of depression: a randomized trial. *Arch Gen Psychiatry.* 1999;56:1109–1115.

Katon W, VonKorff M, Lin E, et al. Collaborative management to achieve treatment guidelines. *JAMA.* 1995;273:1026–1031.

Kemp BJ, Corgiat M, Catherine G. Effects of brief cognitive-behavioral group psychotherapy on older persons with and without disabling illness. *Behav Health Aging.* 1991;2:21–28.

Kitchell MA, Barnes RF, Veith RC, et al. Screening for depression in hospitalized geriatric patients. *J Am Geriatr Soc.* 1982;30:174–177.

Koenig HG, Blazer DG. Epidemiology of geriatric affective disorders. *Clin Geriatr Med.* 1992;8:235–251.

Koenig HG, George LK. Depression and physical disability outcomes in depressed medically ill hospitalized older adults. *Am J Geriatr Psychiatry.* 1998;6:247.

Koenig HG, George LK, Meador KG. Use of antidepressants by nonpsychiatrists in the treatment of medially ill hospitalized depressed elderly patients. *Am J Psychiatry.* 1997;154:1369–1375.

Koenig HG, George LK, Peterson BL, et al. Depression in medically ill hospitalized older adults: prevalence, characteristics, and course of symptoms according to six diagnostic schemes. *Am J Psychiatry.* 1997;154:1376–1383.

Koenig HG, Goli V, Shelp F. Major depression in hospitalized medically ill older men: documentation, management, and outcome. *Int J Geriatr Psychiatry.* 1992;7:25–34.

Koenig HG, Goli V, Shelp F, et al. Antidepressant use in older medically ill inpatients. *J Gen Intern Med.* 1989;4:498–505.

Koenig HG, Kuchibhatla M. Use of health services by medically ill depressed elderly patients after hospital discharge. *Am J Geriatr Psychiatry.* 1999;7:48–56.

Koenig HG, Meador KG, Cohen HJ, Blazer DG. Depression in elderly hospitalized patients with medical illness. *Arch Intern Med.* 1988;148:1929–1936.

Koenig HG, Meador KG, Shelp F, et al. Major depressive disorder in hospitalized medically ill patients: an examination of young and elderly male veterans. *J Am Geriatr Soc.* 1991;39:881–890.

Kurlowicz LH, Streim JE. Measuring depression in hospitalized, medically ill, older adults. *Arch Psychiatr Nurs.* 1998;12:209–218.

Lesprance F, Frasure-Smith N. Depression in patients with cardiac disease: a practical review. *J Psychosom Res.* 2000;48:379–391.

Levitan SJ, Kornfeld DS. Clinical and cost benefits of liaison psychiatry. *Am J Psychiatry.* 1981;138:790–793.

Levitte SS, Thornby JI. Geriatric and nongeriatric psychiatry consultation. A comparison study. *Gen Hosp Psychiatry.* 1989;11:339–344.

Lieberman D, Galinsky D, Fried V, et al. Geriatric Depression Screening Scale (GDS) in patients hospitalized for physical rehabilitation. *Int J Geriatr Psychiatry.* 1999;14: 549–555.

Linka E, Bartko G, Agardi T, et al. Dementia and depression in elderly medical inpatients. *Int Psychogeriatr.* 2000;12:67–75.

Lipowski ZJ. Delirium, clouding of consciousness and confusion. *J Nerv Ment Dis.* 1967;145:227–255.

Lipowski ZJ. The need to integrate liaison psychiatry and geropsychiatry. *Am J Psychiatry.* 1983;140:1003–1005.

Lipowski ZJ. Consultation-liaison psychiatry 1990. *Psychother Psychsom.* 1991;55: 62–68.

Lockwood KA, Alexopoulos GS, Kakuma T, et al. Subtype of cognitive impairment in depressed older adults. *Am J Geriatr Psychiatry.* 2000;8:201–208.

Mainprize E, Rodin G. Geriatric referrals to a psychiatric consultation-liaison service. *Can J Psychiatry.* 1987;32:5–9.

Marsden CD, Harrison MJ. Outcome of investigation of patients with presenile dementia. *Br Med J.* 1972;2:249–252.

Masand P, Pickett P, Muray GB. Psycho-stimulants for secondary depression in medical illness. *Psychosomatics.* 1991;32:203–208.

McDaniel JS, Musselman DL, Porter MR, et al. Depression in patients with cancer: diagnosis, biology, and treatment. *Arch Gen Psychiatry.* 1995;52:89–99.

McKegney FP, Schwartz BJ, O'Dowd MA. Reducing unnecessary psychiatric consultations for informed consent by liaison with administration. *Gen Hosp Psychiatry.* 1992;14:15–19.

Miranda J, Munoz RF. Intervention for minor depression in primary care patients. *Psychosom Med.* 1994;56:136–141.

Morrison MF, Kastenberg JS. Differentiation of secondary from primary mood disorders: controversies and consensus. *Sem Clin Neuropsychiatry.* 1997;2:232–243.

Mossey J, Knott K, Craik R. The effects of persistent depressive symptoms on hip fracture recovery. *J Gerontol.* 1990;45:M163–M168.

Mulsant BH, Alexopoulos GS, Reynolds CF, et al. Pharmacologic treatment of depression in elderly primary care patients: the PROSPECT algorithm. *Int J Geriatr Psychiatry.* 2001;16:585–592.

Norris JT, Gallagher D, Wilson A, et al. Assessment of depression in geriatric medical outpatients: the validity of two screening measures. *J Am Geriatr Soc.* 1987;35: 989–995.

Nott PN, Fleminger JJ. Presenile dementia: the difficulties of early diagnosis. *Acta Psychiatr Scand.* 1975;51:210–217.

Okimoto JT, Barnes RF, Veith RC, et al. Screening for depression in geriatric medical patients. *Am J Psychiatry.* 1982;139:799–802.

Parikh RM, Robinson RG, Lipsey JR, Starkstein SE. The impact of post stroke depression in recovery in activities of daily living over a two year follow up. *Arch Neurol.* 1990;47:785–789.

Pauser H, Bergstrom B, Walinder J. 294 psychiatric consultations involving in-patients above 70 years of age in somatic departments in a university hospital. *Acta Psychiatr Scand.* 1987;76:152–157.

Pearlson GD, Rabins PV, Kim WS, et al. Structural brain CT changes and cognitive deficits in elderly depressives with and without reversible dementia ("pseudodementia"). *Psychol Med.* 1989;19:573–584.

Pollock BG. Psychopharmacology: general principles. In: Sadock BJ, Sadock VA, eds. *Comprehensive Textbook of Psychiatry.* Vol. 2. 7th ed. New York, NY: Lippincott, Williams & Wilkins; 2000:3086–3090.

Pomerant AS, deNesnera A, West AN. Resolution of depressive symptoms in medical inpatients after discharge. *Int J Psychiatry Med.* 1992;22:281–289.

Popkin MK, Mackenzie TB, Callies AL. Psychiatric consultation to geriatric medically ill inpatients in a university hospital. *Arch Gen Psychiatry.* 1984;41:703–707.

Poynton AM. Psychiatric liaison referrals of elderly in-patients in a teaching hospital. *Br J Psychiatry.* 1988;152:45–47.

Rabins P, Lucas MJ, Teitelbaum ML, Mark SR, Folstein M. Utilization of psychiatric consultation for elderly patients. *J Am Geriatr Soc.* 1983;31:581–585.

Rabins PV, Folstein MF. Delirium and dementia: diagnostic criteria and fatality rates. *Br J Psychiatry.* 1982;140:149–153.

Rabins PV, Mace NL, Lucas MJ. The impact of dementia on the family. *JAMA.* 1982; 248:333–335.

Rabins PV, Merchant A, Nestadt G. Criteria for diagnosing reversible dementia caused by depression: validation by 2-year followup. *Br J Psychiatry.* 1984;144:488–492.

Raphael D, Cava M, Brown I, et al. Frailty: a public health perspective. *Can J Public Health.* 1995;86:224–227.

Rapp SR, Parisi SA, Wallace CE. Comorbid psychiatric disorders in elderly medical patients: a 1-year prospective study. *J Am Geriatr Soc.* 1991;39:124–131.

Rapp SR, Parisi SA, Walsh DA. Psychological dysfunction and physical health among elderly medical inpatients. *J Consult Clin Psychol.* 1988;56:851–855.

Rapp SR, Walsh DA, Parisi SA, et al. Detecting depression in elderly medical inpatients. *J Consult Clin Psychol.* 1988;56:509–513.

Reding M, Haycrox J, Blass J. Depression in patients referred to a dementia clinic. *Arch Neurol.* 1985;42:894–896.

Regier DA, Boyd JH, Burke JD, et al. One-month prevalence of mental disorders in the United States: based on five epidemiologic catchment area sites. *Arch Gen Psychiatry.* 1988;45:977–986.

Reynolds CF III, Hoch CC, Kupfer DJ, et al. Bedside differentiation of depressive pseudodementia from dementia. *Am J Psychiatry.* 1988;145:1099–1103.

Rifai AH, Mulsant BH, Sweet RA, Pasternak RE, Rosen J, Zubenko GS. A study of elderly suicide attempters admitted to an inpatient psychiatric unit. *Am J Geriatr Psychiatry.* 1993;1:126–135.

Robinson RG, Schultz SK, Paradiso S. Treatment of post-stroke psychiatric disorders. In: Nelson JC, ed. *Geriatric Psychopharmacology.* New York, NY: Marcel Dekker; 1998:161–185.

Ruskin PE. Geropsychiatric consultation in a university hospital: a report on 67 referrals. *Am J Psychiatry.* 1985;142:333–336.

Sachdev PS, Smith JS, Angus-Lepan H, et al. Pseudodementia twelve years on. *J Neurol Neurosurg Psychiatry.* 1990;199:254–259.

Sadavoy J, Reiman-Sheldon E. General hospital geriatric psychiatric treatments: a follow-up study. *J Am Geriatr Soc.* 1983;31:200–205.

Schuckit MA, Miller PL, Hahlbohm D. Unrecognized psychiatric illness in elderly medical-surgical patients. *J Gerontol.* 1975;30:655–660.

Schwartz J, Speed N, Clavier E. Antidepressant side effects in the medically ill: the value of psychiatric consultation. *Int J Psychiatry Med.* 1988;18:235–241.

Scott J, Fairbairn A, Woodhouse K. Referrals to a psychogeriatric consultation-liaison service. *Int J Geriat Psychiatry.* 1988;3:131–135.

Shah A, Hoxey K, Mayadunne V. Suicidal ideation in acutely medically ill elderly inpatients: prevalence, correlates and longitudinal stability. *Int J Geriatr Psychiatry.* 2000;15:162–169.

Shamash K, O'Connell K, Lowy MM, et al. Psychiatric morbidity and outcome in elderly patients undergoing emergency hip surgery: a one year follow-up study. *Int J Geriatr Psychiatry.* 1992;7:505–509.

Slaets JPJ, Kauffmann RH, Duivenvoorden HJ, Pelemans W, Schudel WJ. A randomized trial of geriatric liaison intervention in elderly medical inpatients. *Psychosom Med.* 1997;59:585–591.

Small GW, Fawzy I. Psychiatric consultation for the medically ill elderly in the general hospital: need for a collaborative model of care. *Psychosomatics.* 1988;29:94–103.

Stewart RB, Cooper JW. Polypharmacy in the aged. *Drugs Aging.* 1994;4:449.

Stoudemire A, Thompson TL. Medication noncompliance: systematic approaches to evaluation and intervention. *Gen Hosp Psychiatry.* 1983;5:233–239.

Strain JJ. *Psychological Interventions in Medical Practice.* New York, NY: Appleton-Century-Crofts; 1978:91–104.

Strain JJ, Lyons JS, Hammer JS, et al. Cost offset from a psychiatric consultation-liaison intervention with elderly hip fracture patients. *Am J Psychiatry.* 1991;148:1044–1049.

Trzepacz PT, Teague G, Lipowski Z. Delirium and other organic mental disorders in a general hospital. *Gen Hosp Psychiatry.* 1985;7:101–106.

Unutzer J. Diagnosis and treatment of older adults with depression in primary care. *Biol Psychiatry.* 2002;52:285–292.

Van Ede L, Yzermans CJ, Brouwer HJ. Prevalence of depression in patients with chronic obstructive pulmonary disease: a systematic review. *Thorax.* 1999;54:688–692.

Verbosky LA, Franco KN, Zrull JP. The relationship between depression and length of stay in the general hospital patient. *J Clin Psychiatry.* 1993;54:177–181.

Wengel SP, Roccaforte WH, Burke WJ. Donepezil improves symptoms of delirium in dementia: implications for future research. *J Geriatr Psychiatry Neurol.* 1998;11:159–161.

37

Integrated Community Services

Carl I. Cohen, MD
Mihaela Boran, MD

It is paradigmatic that geropsychiatric practice cannot be conducted in isolation, and that the practitioner must assist patients and families to access community resources. At times, the psychiatrist may be called on to orchestrate the various components of the treatment plan. Even if the psychiatrist does not assume a coordinating role, it is nevertheless important for the psychiatrist to become familiar with the range and content of the principal elements of community care. Indeed, a dramatic expansion of community services and housing options for older persons has been spurred by the growth of the aging population as well as by demands for programs to fill the gap between independent community living and nursing homes. The broadening of medical benefits through managed care, supplemental private health insurance, or long-term care policies in tandem with the increased number of wealthy aging consumers have encouraged private entrepreneurs to broaden the options available to seniors. These changes have occurred while the public sector has remained relatively quiescent, with only minimal modifications of existing statutes.

This chapter has a twofold purpose: (1) to provide geropsychiatrists with an overview of the relevant legislation and essential elements of the community service network for seniors and (2) to provide practitioners with basic information necessary to educate patients, families, and other health professionals about the types of support services available in the community.

Gerontological practitioners, planners, and researchers are frequently required to impose some order on the myriad services and facilities available to community-dwelling elderly individuals (Golant & McCaslen, 1979). Although there is no consensus or well-accepted rationale for any existing classification schema, Table 37-1 represents a synthesis of a classification schema proposed by Golant and McCaslen (1979) and Cantor and Little (1985). (The items listed in Table 37-1 are described in the chapter.)

On the vertical axis of the table is a measure of independence and self-functioning (mental and physical) divided into three categories: well, moderately impaired, and severely impaired. On the horizontal axis are three broad categories of needs: a basic level that consists of health needs; an intermediate level comprising self-maintenance needs such as dressing, grooming, cooking, transportation, cleaning, and handling money; and a complex level that involves social needs such as work roles, friendship, intimacy, and education. Thus, for example, a comparatively well older person who has recently lost several close friends might be helped by referrals to the social and vocational services listed in the upper right corner of Table 37-1. Similarly, a moderately impaired person with Alzheimer's disease might benefit from the self-maintenance and social services contained in the center and right middle section of Table 37-1.

Organizationally, in this chapter the hierarchical model of Table 37-1 is followed, with descriptions of items moving from those at the lowest levels of functioning to those at the highest levels. The items are placed in two broad sections: Community Services and Community Housing.

COMMUNITY SERVICES

In this section, an overview of the principal geriatric community services is provided. More detailed descriptions are available elsewhere (www.aoa.dhhs.gov; Gelfand, 1999). Note that the intensity and level of services vary between services that are primarily aimed at clinical populations (e.g., day care, nursing homes) and those that are psychosocially supportive (e.g., mutual aid groups, volunteer groups). The latter may serve a preventive function by ensuring that elderly individuals do not become socially isolated, and if disease develops, that they are already part of a network that makes clinical care accessible.

Table 37-2 summarizes the principal governmental programs and their related services and benefits. Clinicians should also be aware that a variety of private health insurance policies have emerged that may cover the costs of home care and nursing homes. Moreover, some health maintenance organizations (HMOs) may provide home and institutional care in their prepaid plans. Social health maintenance organizations (SHMOs) offer older persons prepaid long-term care, social services (e.g., homemaker, case management, day care), and prescription plans along with traditional acute health services (Skolnick & Warrick, 1985). Medicare reimburses the SHMO at a per capita rate, although participants may pay an additional premium. In a similar vein, the Program of All-Inclusive Care for Elders (PACE) is directed toward persons who are judged eligible for nursing home care by virtue of their level of disability, but who are living in the community (Kane, 1999). Medicare and Medicaid monies are pooled into a single capitated payment that allows for a combination of medical and social care. Finally, elderly veterans may be eligible for a variety of in-home and residential long-term care services (e.g., nursing home, domiciliary care) provided by the Department of Veterans Affairs.

Assistance and Protection

INFORMATION AND REFERRAL (ASSISTANCE) SERVICES   The Older Americans Act (OAA) was enacted in 1965 to assist aging individuals by providing funds to states for services, training, and resources. These activities are coordinated through the Administration on Aging (AOA), which is an independent agency in the Department of Health and Human Services. Title III of the OAA provides for each state to designate an agency for aging services. In about half the states, an independent office on aging has been established; in the remaining states, aging programs are part of a human services department. In most states, aging agencies designate smaller geographic service centers, termed area agencies on aging (AAAs), to provide local communities with information and referral services. The AAAs are forbidden to provide direct services unless absolutely necessary. In 2000, there were 660 AAAs throughout the country. A chart developed by the AOA provides a useful overview of what has been termed the "aging network" (Figure 37-1).

Whereas the AAAs are public agencies, a variety of voluntary and private resources provide information and assistance; these include family services facilities, senior centers, and mental health associations. About 85% of information and assistance programs are part of public agencies, approximately half of which are AAAs; the remainder are usually part of local social services departments (Huttman, 1985). Problems that most often require referrals are financial, social security, and transportation problems; health problems and care; housing, food and nutrition, and homemaker services; employment; consumer needs; legal problems; companionship; and nursing home care (Huttman, 1985).

Funding for information and referral programs generally comes from governmental sources, with state governments providing the largest shares. Nonprofit organizations, religious groups, and foundations are also important sources of funding. Gelfand (1999) observed that information and referral programs are used by a disproportionate number of persons already connected to the system in some way. Unfortunately, direct outreach to underserved individuals is usually too expensive for most programs.

HOW TO ACCESS SERVICES   With the dramatic expansion of geriatric services and varying eligibility requirements to obtain such services, the most expeditious way for clinicians and consumers to learn about a particular type of service in

TABLE 37-1. Types of services available to elderly individuals

Functional level	Physical and mental health needs	Self-maintenance needs	Social needs
Well elderly (60% of population)	Mutual help groups Consumer health education Health insurance Health screening	Shared housing Converted boarding homes ECHO units and "granny flats" Section 8 and Section 202 housing Elderly apartment complexes Retirement community Congregate meals program Nutrition education "Brown bag" programs	Senior center Voluntary association Retired Seniors Volunteer Program Foster parents and grandparents Senior companions Service Corps of Retired Executives Senior aides Adult education
Moderately impaired (30% of population)	Outreach services Visiting nurse Crisis intervention teams	Case management Home care services Congregate housing Foster care Vocational rehabilitation	Friendly visiting Telephone reassurance Strengthen informal social network

Severely impaired (10% of population)	Multiple help groups for family Outreach services Visiting nurses Crisis intervention teams Inpatient psychiatric and medical care	Vocational rehabilitation Assisted living Board-and-care homes Congregate housing Meals-on-wheels Transportation services Escort services Chore services Day care Respite care Home care services Hospice Nursing home Meals-on-wheels Protective services Case management	Friendly visiting Telephone reassurance Strengthen informal social support network

Source: Modified from Golant and McCaslen (1979) and Cantor and Little (1985).
ECHO, elder cottage housing opportunity.

TABLE 37-2. Principal governmental programs relevant to community services

Program	Services and benefits	Eligibility
Old Age Survivors and Disabled Insurance (OASDI) (1935)	Social Security benefits	All persons 65 years and older, disabled workers, and dependent survivors when retirees aged 62 years
Supplemental Security Income (SSI) program (1972)	Supplemental payments to bring persons up to poverty threshold; states have option to pay for residential care facilities and personal home care	Indigent persons 65 years and older, disabled, and blind
Title XVIII of the Social Security Act (1965)	Medicare, which includes hospital costs, physicians' fees, skilled nursing facility (limited), home health care, and hospice care	Persons aged 65 years and older and those younger than 65 years who receive Social Security disability payments
Title XIX of the Social Security Act (1965)	Medicaid, which includes medical services, skilled nursing care (unlimited), home health care; optional by state are adult day care, drugs, dental care, intermediate care facility	Indigent elderly, disabled, and blind
Social Services Block Grant (1981) (formerly Title XX of the Social Security Act; 1975)	Varying levels by state: chore services, congregate meals, home-delivered meals, homemaker, senior centers, protective services	Indigent persons (all ages) up to 115% of state median income
Older Americans Act (OAA) (1965), Title III	Outlines support services to be provided by states, including establishing AAAs Services vary by state: congregate meals, home-delivered meals, home health care, chore services, senior centers, friendly visiting	All persons aged 60 years and older; low-income persons are special targets

Program	Description	Eligibility
Older Americans Act (OAA) (1992), Title VII	Establishes state-level ombudsman program, a program to prevent elder abuse and neglect; an elder rights program; and an outreach, counseling, and assistance program targeted at insurance and public benefits	Persons aged 60 years and older
Older Americans Act (OAA) (1981), Title V	Community employment (e.g., senior aides, Green Thumb)	Indigent persons aged 55 years and older
Older Americans Act (OAA) (1975), Title VI	Social and nutritional programs for Native American, Alaskan, and Hawaiian natives	Tribes set age eligibility
Corporation for National and Community Service (1993)	Federal agency established to coordinate volunteer programs; includes programs for elderly persons (aged 55+ years), Foster Grandparents, RSVP, Senior Companions	Indigent persons aged 55 years and older; Some programs open only to indigent persons
Section 202 of Housing Act (1959)	Low-interest loans for construction of low-rent housing	Nonprofit sponsors
Section 8 of Housing and Community Development Act (1974)	Rent subsidies to cover difference between fair market rent and 30% of participants' income	Low-income persons
Food stamp program (1964)	Department of Agriculture program to purchase foods at lower prices	Low-income persons
Low Income Home Energy Assistance Program (1981)	Cash benefits, payments to fuel vendors, weatherization	Low-income households, renters, and owners

Sources: Gelfand (1999); Administration on Aging (www.aoa.dhhs.gov).
AAAs, area agencies on aging; RSVP, Retired Seniors Volunteer Program.

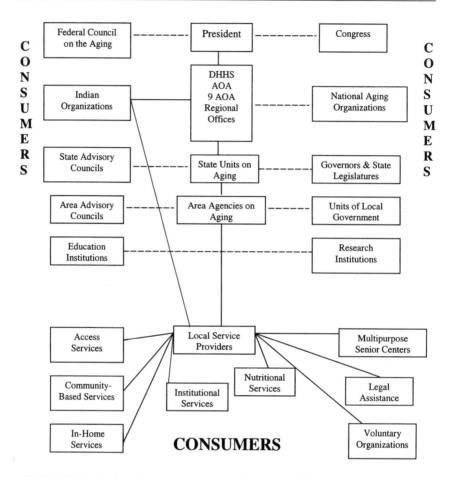

FIGURE 37-1. National Aging Services Network. (Adapted from www.aoa.dhhs.gov.)

their community is by contacting their state or local agency on aging. Senior citizen information lines are required under OAA, and they receive 3 million calls per year. Community agencies such as United Way, Family Service America, Catholic Charities, or Jewish Family Services can also assist with information and referrals.

All public and private agencies now have Web sites. The Administration on Aging Web site (www.aoa.dhhs.gov) provides the best overview of aging services as well as links to other sites. The AOA and National Institute on Aging have developed an online resource directory for laypersons and professionals that can also be accessed through the AOA Web site. Many local AAAs publish resource directories that describe services and provide toll-free numbers. The American Association of Homes for the Aging (www.aahsa.org) provides information on housing for seniors.

For those without computers, the Eldercare locator is a toll-free number (1-800-677-1116) supported by AOA that provides information on a wide variety of community resources. One of the best ways to secure services is through the local Yellow Pages, looking under appropriate headings such as "Social Services Organizations," "Home Health Services," "Senior Services," and "Nursing Services."

CASE OR CARE MANAGEMENT   The primary aim of case management is to help clients and family deal with a fragmented and complex system by locating and coordinating existing resources through a process that includes screening, assessment, case planning, linkage to services, advocacy, monitoring, and in some instances, therapeutic counseling (Huttman, 1985). Much of the growth in case management services has been spurred by the expanding need for in-home services for persons with mental or physical impairments and the variety of funding sources and eligibility requirements. Thus, various health and welfare agencies, such as public agencies, social services agencies, HMOs, health care facilities, or insurance carriers that provide services to elderly individuals, currently use case management (Westhoff, 1992). Moreover, consumers may enlist the assistance of a private case management group to obtain the appropriate mix of in-home services. Fees generally vary from $200 to $300 for an initial consultation.

Three case management approaches are commonly used to secure and coordinate services (Westhoff, 1992):

1. In the brokering model, case managers identify the appropriate service package from resources in the community; case managers do not have dollars to allocate, but negotiate and advocate with providers for various services.
2. In the service management model, the case manager authorizes both the services provided and the clients' service budget, with the funding source influencing which services can be recommended.
3. In the managed-care model, the carrier of a high-risk group of clients or a group of enrollees in a health care program prospectively pays the organization providing managed care.

White (2001) observed that the popularity and success of case management is evidenced by its proliferation in all types of health and social services settings, especially in programs serving long-term care populations. However, two major demonstration programs, the Channeling Project and the Medicare Alzheimer's Demonstration Evaluation, failed to find that the increased costs of case management interventions were offset by reduced nursing home costs, although both programs did reduce nursing home placement versus control groups (Kemper, 1988; Newcomer et al., 1999). Moreover, both projects found improved access to and use of community care and a reduction in unmet needs. Although the service system may be fragmented and confusing, Zarit and Teri (1991) noted that families are generally able to find services on their own; they speculate that case management may be more effective for older persons without involved caregivers.

ADULT PROTECTIVE SERVICES   Adult protective services (APS) serve persons who are (1) incapable of performing functions necessary to meet basic physical and health requirements, (2) incapable of managing finances, (3) dangerous to self or others, or (4) exhibiting behavior that brings them into conflict with the community. Services may be provided with an individual's consent or without consent if it is determined that guardianship is required. Such agencies may facilitate hospitalization or assist with various legal actions.

States were initially funded for these services under an amendment to the Social Security Act in 1962 and subsequently under Title XX of the Social Security Act (1974), which has now become the Social Services Block Grant Program. In general, these services have been provided by public departments of social services or under contracts with other public or private agencies (Wolf, 2001), although between states, there is some variability in agency jurisdiction based on the individual's age or whether the protective services are linked to an elder abuse program.

Congressional hearings in 1978 and various AOA initiatives helped stimulate state legislation and programs for elder abuse, neglect, or exploitation. In most states, the assessment of community dwelling for older adults is the responsibility of APS, whereas abuse, neglect, and exploitation that occur in nursing homes are the responsibility of the state ombudsman on aging (Lachs et al., 1996). If problems are verified, but cannot be handled expeditiously, APS often provides ongoing case management. All states have laws to protect elderly victims of abuse. Forty-two states require professional mandatory reporters to report even the suspicion of mistreatment (Capezuti et al., 1997). Nonmandatory reporters include family members, neighbors, clergy, utility workers, and so forth.

In states where the APS statute includes self-neglect, it is the most frequently reported type of mistreatment. Most self-neglecting elders have functional or mental impairments and poor social networks. In the 11 states that exclude self-neglecting elders, there are few options for appropriate referrals, especially during crisis situations (Capezuti et al., 1997). Cases referred to APS contain disproportionately more minority elders, lower income individuals, more women, and more persons older than 75 years (Wolf & Li, 1999).

Ironically, despite successful legislative efforts, the effectiveness of the protective casework model in use since the 1960s has been questioned (Zborowsky, 1985), and several demonstration projects were found to be no more effective than the usual community control services with respect to functional competence, institutionalization, and mortality (Blenkner et al., 1974). Earlier studies of elder abuse programs also raised questions about the ability of professionals to successfully resolve the abuse problem (Zborowsky, 1985).

Several factors have been found to affect nonreporting of elder abuse: (1) cultural differences among clients in attitudes and traditions of what is acceptable behavior; (2) a cultural imperative to preserve family harmony at the expense of individual well-being; (3) professionals who lack confidence in protective services, feel that reporting will destroy their relationships with clients, have concerns about testifying in court, express denial about the abusive situation, or lack education about elder abuse programs and interagency coordination and linkages (Thobaben, 1996; Wolf & Li, 1999). Examinations of this topic have underscored the need for physicians to become more familiar with APS referral pathways and mandatory reporting laws in their states.

Community Care

Noelker and Bass (1989) developed a useful typology to examine how community-based services affect caregivers. They delineated four patterns:

1. Complementary, in which formal and informal helpers (e.g., kin, neighbors) provide different but complementary services
2. Supplementary, in which formal services augment the efforts of the informal caregivers
3. Substitution, in which formal agencies take the place of informal helpers
4. Kin independence, in which the informal helpers provide all the assistance

The impact of formal services will vary depending on the pattern. For example, if introduction of services results in a complementary pattern, informal caregivers may feel relief that new services are being provided; however, these caregivers will be still giving the same level of assistance.

Respite Care

Respite care is provided on a short-term basis (usually several hours to several weeks) to a dependent person in the community to relieve the caregiver of responsibility for the constant care of that person (Abrahams et al., 1991). Hegeman (1989) identified five major categories: (1) in home (e.g., home companions, homemakers); (2) in the community (e.g., adult day care); (3) institutions caring for elderly individuals (e.g., adult homes, overnight stays); (4) hospitals; and (5) combination models. Religious organizations, nursing homes, home health care agencies, and voluntary agencies commonly organize these services.

IN-HOME HEALTH CARE SERVICES   In-home health care is the most commonly utilized form of respite for caregivers of elderly patients. It covers a wide array of services offered in the home; these can be grouped under three categories (Gelfand, 1999):

1. Intensive or skilled services (e.g., assistance with open wounds, catheters, or tube feedings) ordered by a physician and performed under the supervision of a nurse
2. Personal care or intermediate services, which are for medically stable individuals who require assistance with activities of daily living such as bathing, prescribed exercises, and ambulation
3. Homemaker, chore, or basic services (e.g., light housekeeping, meal preparation, or other maintenance activities), which are offered to persons who have difficulties caring for their personal environment, but who are able to do more basic activities of daily living, such as toileting or bathing

Whereas intensive services usually require visits by a physician, nurse, or physical therapist, a homemaker/home health aide generally provides services in the other two categories. Home health care services must be provided by a home health agency certified by the state health department. Five types of home health agencies exist: government-sponsored agencies (e.g., Department of Social Services), nonprofit agencies (e.g., Visiting Nurse Service), for-profit agencies, hospital-based programs, and community health centers (Gelfand, 1999). There are six ways to pay for in-home services:

1. Medicaid, which will pay for almost all costs of home health care for indigent persons.
2. Medicare, which is available to those aged 65 years and older who are confined to home and who require skilled nursing care, physical therapy, or speech therapy under a plan established by a physician. The 1997 Balanced Budget Act changed Medicare home services from a cost-based system to a prospective payment system akin to the diagnosis related group (DRG) reimbursement model used in acute care.
3. Supplemental private insurance, such as "Medigap" insurance, which covers certain home health care services and may provide supplement benefits that exceed Medicare limits.
4. Social Services Block Grants (formerly Title XX of Social Security Act), which have provided limited funds to state departments of social services to reimburse public and private home care agencies for home-based services to the indigent.
5. Title III of the OAA funnels funds to public and private agencies through local AAAs for services to persons aged 60 years and older who are generally indigent.
6. Out-of-pocket fees, which range from $8 to $18 per hour for a home-

maker/home care aide, $10 to $30 per hour for home health aides, and $85 to $90 for in-home nurses and physical therapists.

RELATED IN-HOME SERVICES There are a variety of services for homebound elderly individuals that can complement or substitute for the in-home services described in the preceding section. In most instances, these services are offered by senior centers or agencies that provide other services to elderly individuals. Such services include the following:

- *Friendly visiting.* A volunteer visits the home, usually 1 to 2 times per week, for general conversation, to inquire about needs, to help with errands, and so forth. There is usually no charge for this service, which is typically offered by a volunteer group or religious organization. However, some companions work privately and charge between $5 and $15 per hour. The usual aims of friendly visiting are to reduce social isolation, increase morale and well-being, and delay the onset of institutionalization (Korte & Gupta, 1991). The few studies that have been done are generally supportive of the effectiveness of friendly visiting (Korte & Gupta, 1991). Seniors receiving friendly visiting showed higher morale and better health, mental status, grooming, and apartment upkeep than their nonvisited counterparts (Korte & Gupta, 1991; Mulligan & Bennett, 1977).
- *Telephone reassurance.* Clients are given a number to call if they feel lonely or have a request for help. Volunteers also call to check on the client.
- *Emergency response systems.* This program provides a reliable contact by telephone or electronic device to police or rescue squads in the event of an emergency.
- *Chore services.* These services offer minor household repairs, household cleaning, and yard work. Costs range from $8 to $18 an hour, plus materials; some agencies may offer assistance at reduced costs.

ADULT DAY CARE Adult day care programs are designed for at-risk persons who are mentally, physically, or socially impaired and who need day services to maintain or improve their level of functioning so that they can remain in or return to their home. Such programs also provide some respite for families. Patients attend for 3 to 7 hours for as many as 5 days per week. In the past, day care centers could be categorized into two broad types: health oriented and social services oriented (Weissert, 1976). Although these divisions remain to some extent, some of these distinctions have become blurred.

Weissert and coworkers (1989) suggested that it is more profitable to examine programs based on their affiliations. Thus, Auspice Model 1 includes outpatient day centers affiliated with nursing homes and rehabilitation centers that cater to physically dependent older populations. Services are generally health oriented and include nursing, health assessments, social services, and physical, occupational, and speech therapies. Auspice Model 2 is situated in an outpatient unit of a general hospital or a social services or housing agency. Most patients are younger than those in Model 1 and can perform activities of daily living; more than 40% have mental disorders. Services are proportionately more social and supportive and include case management, professional counseling, transportation to and from centers, nutrition, education, and health assessment. Auspice Model 3 involves special-purpose centers that serve a single type of clientele, such as blind or mentally ill persons, those with dementia, or veterans.

All programs rely on a combination of federal, local, and private funds. Most governmental funds are provided through patients' Medicaid reimbursement, although programs may obtain additional funds through Title III and Social Services Block Grants. Medicare provides only a very small fraction of funding, usually for specific rehabilitative therapies. When not reimbursed by Medicaid, the average out-of-pocket daily cost is about $50, although this can be considerably higher if a person needs many services.

With respect to the effectiveness of the various types of respite care programs, in-home services have been found to most consistently achieve overall objectives with respect to caregivers (Zarit et al., 1999). Benefits to caregivers have included improved mood, reduced distress, and decreased time spent in caregiving activities. Some caregivers have voiced concern about home helpers who are poorly trained and unreliable. With respect to institutionalization, in-home services do not prevent nursing home placement, although they have modest effects in delaying institutionalization.

Reports of caregivers' satisfaction with adult day programs are uniformly high, but analyses of other benefits such as psychological health and care-related stressors have shown mixed results (Forster et al., 1999; Grasel, 1997; Zarit et al., 1999). Research that examined caregivers utilizing "adequate amounts" of adult day services on an ongoing basis had more positive outcomes. Adult day care has been found to have measurable impact on outcomes related to dementia patients.

There seem to be no differences in effect if patients attend a medical or a social model day program. A review of day hospital programs for medically ill older persons found that they did not differ significantly from other forms of comprehensive care with regard to death, disability, or use of resources, although persons in day hospitals had significantly better outcomes than persons who did not receive comprehensive care (Forster et al., 1999). With respect to institutionalization, rather than delaying or preventing placement, day care may be a step on the path toward institutionalization, possibly easing the transition for caregivers and making it more acceptable to turn care over to someone else. The results of studies on overnight respite have been mixed (Zarit et al., 1999). In general, overnight respite seems to reduce burden and strain on families temporarily, but levels return to baseline after the relative comes back home. Like adult day care, studies suggest that overnight respite seems to facilitate rather than delay or prevent nursing home placement by helping to break emotional bonds or overcoming apprehension about the care received in nursing homes. Despite concerns that overnight respite might be harmful to patients because of their placement in unfamiliar surroundings, studies have failed to find any deleterious effects, and patients improved in some areas, such as physical functioning.

Several well-designed research studies have examined multiple service component programs that offered caregivers an array of services that ranged from in-home care to more extensive day care (Zarit et al., 1999). A majority of these studies found that these multicomponent programs improved caregiver burden, although the effects were often modest, and there was no effect on institutionalization. Benefits to caregivers and reduced institutionalization were most likely to be found with sustained, regular use of services.

Unfortunately, caregivers often do not avail themselves of appropriate services. Indeed, a critical issue has been the extent to which eligible persons fail to use respite services after application and acceptance into such programs. One study found that significant predictors of usage included poor cognitive status of the patient and caregivers experiencing greater burden but less anxiety than nonusers (Cox, 1997).

Finally, in assessing outcome of respite services, it is important to recognize that such services are more likely to diminish those care-related stressors that have been specifically targeted by such interventions rather than broader, nonspecific dimensions such as depression or life satisfaction.

Community Mental Health Services

Government reports, special study commissions, and legislation have uniformly described older persons as unserved, underserved, or inappropriately served by community-based mental health services (Lebowitz, 2001). Rabins (1996) calculated that 63% of adults aged 65 years or older living in Baltimore, Maryland, have an unmet need for mental health care. The Community Mental Health Centers Act of 1963 was revised in 1975 to include specialized services for elderly individuals as 1 of 12 required service components; however, the Block Grant Program of 1981 eliminated elderly services as a required component (Morrissey & Goldman, 1984). Moreover, switching federal mental health funding from separate categorical funding to block grants to states allowed the states to determine the level at which mental health services to elderly individuals should be funded.

Data indicated a decline in specialized services to elderly individuals in the years immediately following the institution of block grants (Gelfand, 1999). Currently, mental health services for older persons are reimbursed through Medicare and supplemented by Medicaid if the person is indigent. Mental health centers may also receive additional funding from state and local sources.

The service system is especially ill prepared to assist older adults with se-vere and persistent mental illness (Cohen et al., 2000). Bartels and colleagues' (1999) review of the literature concluded that the ideal program for this popu-lation would include case management, general medical care, 24-hour crisis intervention, home-based mental health care, residential and family support services, caregiver training, multidisciplinary teams, active case finding and outreach, and psychosocial rehabilitation.

Lebowitz (1988) identified several factors that may enhance mental health service utilization by elderly individuals, the most critical being the existence of a unit for elderly individuals within an outpatient clinic staffed by pro-fessionals with specialized training in geriatric mental health and cooperative affiliations with local area agencies on aging. Lebowitz (2001) further recom-mended that programs be made more accessible, and that rather than relying on referrals and self-identification, programs engage in aggressive outreach. Several specialized community programs for elderly individuals are described next.

MENTAL HEALTH CRISIS INTERVENTION SERVICES   The aim of these services is to provide rapid restabilization of a person's psychiatric symptoms and social adjustment (Phipps & Liberman, 1988). Crisis services are often hospital based or tied to community mental health centers. Services may be delivered in the patient's home or at a designated place outside the home. Mobile units or home treat-ment teams may visit the home or maintain daily telephone contact (Reifler et al., 1982; Sherr et al., 1976). Alternatively, patients may receive crisis care in the hospital or emergency department or leave their homes to live in a respite home or in crisis lodging.

COMMUNITY OUTREACH   Community outreach programs have proved especially successful in meeting the mental health needs of traditionally underserved and disadvantaged populations, such as rural elderly individuals (Buckwalter et al., 1993; Raschko, 1991), homeless elderly individuals (Cohen et al., 1993), el-derly persons in public housing (Roca et al., 1990), or mentally ill older adults in suburban communities (DeRenzo et al., 1991). One comprehensive outreach program in a suburb of Baltimore addressed the mental health needs of an elderly population by dividing its program into thirds: one third of staff time is devoted to efforts in senior centers, one third to assessment and ongoing treatment in the homes of elderly individuals, and one third to services pro-vided in community mental health centers (DeRenzo et al., 1991).

A nurse-based outreach program to Baltimore seniors in public housing (the PATCH Program) found that such interventions were more effective than usual care in reducing psychiatric symptoms in persons with psychiatric disor-ders or higher levels of symptoms (Rabins et al., 2000). A rural outreach team in Iowa estimated annual costs as half those of mental health services provided by professionals in private practice (Buckwalter et al., 1993), and Parish and Landsberg (1984) found that their outreach efforts (e.g., home visits and work with family and community support networks) in a rural community reduced psychiatric hospitalization by 60%. A meta-analysis of mental health outreach programs for depressed elderly persons found a large effect size (.77) versus various control groups (Cuijpers, 1998).

Funding for outreach programs typically comes from mixes of federal, state, and local funds. Several federal and foundation studies are now under way to evaluate the effectiveness of using primary care settings to identify and treat persons for depression and suicidality (Katz & Coyne, 2000). Bartels and coworkers (1999) proposed integrating specialized psychogeriatric services with emerging systems of community-based long-term care.

PSYCHIATRIC VOCATIONAL REHABILITATION   Although psychiatric vocational rehabilitation programs underserve older patients, such programs should be considered as a treatment option for aging psychiatric patients. Two basic types of programs exist (Jacobs, 1988):

1. Sheltered employment, also known as sheltered workshops or compensated work therapy programs, provides work opportunities for individuals who are not ready for competitive employment. Workdays may be decreased, tasks simplified and structured, and on-the-job pressures reduced. Some programs are based in psychiatric treatment centers, but most are managed by nonprofit agencies such as Goodwill Industries or Jewish Vocational Services. Patients receive either piecework pay or hourly pay according to their abilities and the specific contract.
2. Transitional employment provides real-work jobs with commercial establishments that are supervised by psychiatric or rehabilitation professionals. The vocational rehabilitation program contracts with local businesses for jobs and assumes responsibility for their completion. Patients earn the same pay as regular workers. These programs are operated by various nonprofit agencies (e.g., Fountain House in New York City, and Thresholds in Chicago, Illinois).

Funding for rehabilitation programs are most often provided through special state Medicaid reimbursement rates or through funds from state offices of vocational rehabilitation; information about referrals can be obtained from the latter.

Senior Centers

In 1990, 5 to 8 million older persons, or about 15% of all seniors, were participating in 10,000 to 12,000 centers nationwide (Krout et al., 1990). Participation in senior centers is 4 to 12 times greater than reported for any other community-based service for elderly individuals (Krout et al., 1990). Thus, senior centers have high degrees of visibility, and most older persons know where they are located.

Senior centers have been conceptualized as organized around two models (Litwin, 1987). One model views the center as an informal social club or voluntary organization. The other model depicts the center as a multipurpose service provider or social services agency designed to meet a range of needs of frail elderly individuals, particularly poor and disengaged persons. Indeed, centers are often torn between efforts to serve frail individuals and the desire to attract younger, healthier, and wealthier older adults (Krout, 1995). A survey of senior center staff and participants (Gelfand et al., 1991) indicated six core programs (crafts, exercise, information and assistance, meals, opportunities for socializing, and transportation) that were thought to be essential for all centers. Five supplemental programs—arts (music, drama, painting), community college courses, health services, support groups, and trips—were considered highly desirable.

Although centers for older people can be traced to a program in New York City begun in 1943, until the 1970s most relied on nonprofit agency or local government support. An amendment to the OAA in 1973 identified "multipurpose senior centers" as a unique and separate program (Gelfand, 1999). Title III of the OAA provides for the acquisition, renovation, or construction of senior centers, as well as for their operation. Additional federal legislative support has been provided by Title XX of the Social Security Act. On average, senior centers currently receive 30% of their funding from federal sources (Krout et al., 1990).

Although considerable controversy exists about those variables that correlate with senior center participation, survey data of nearly 14,000 elderly persons from the 1984 National Health Interview Survey have provided the most reliable information to date (Krout et al., 1990). This survey indicated that higher participation was correlated with female sex, increasing age until 84 years of age, increasing education until college, lower family income, living alone, fewer difficulties with activities of daily living, and living in suburbs and rural nonfarm areas.

Contrary to some earlier findings, race was not correlated with participation. Krout and colleagues (1990) concluded that senior centers are generally used by "less advantaged" but not the "least advantaged" elderly individuals (e.g., those unable to perform activities of daily living or the very old).

Although an estimated 5% to 10% of current senior attendees are "frail" (i.e., impaired physically or mentally), there is evidence that the senior center population is increasingly becoming older and more frail (Krout, 1995). Krout argues that additional funds for modifying environments, new programs, and staff training will be needed to accommodate the increasing number of frail older people.

Social Network Interventions and Mutual Aid (Self-Help) Groups

A growing number of community mental health programs have begun to recognize the important roles that the informal social network plays in providing individuals with material and emotional assistance. The social network techniques most commonly used include (1) helping clients expand their networks, (2) assisting individuals to increase the support and exchange within existing networks, (3) identifying natural helpers and gatekeepers (e.g., clergy, letter carriers, physicians) who can assist clients, and (4) teaching service personnel to work with existing networks (Pancoast et al., 1983).

Two distinct network approaches have emerged in work with older persons. One approach involves the actual convening of members of the individual network into a "network session" in which a treatment plan is developed and sponsored by network members themselves (Garrison & Howe, 1976). A second approach (Cohen, 1991) involves the clinician utilizing the network on the client's behalf, usually by working with network members to elicit their involvement in the client's treatment. Although most reports have been descriptive and anecdotal, the more systematic studies have tended to be favorable, with several important stipulations (Cohen & Adler, 1984).

Cohen and Adler (1984) concluded that network interventions are not suitable for every problem or for every person. Transactions that have long been part of a population's cultural world are most likely to yield successful network outcomes. In other words, service workers should not expect to undertake network tasks with which clients are not already familiar. They also cautioned that natural supports should not be used to justify public policies that might result in the withholding of professional services.

Self-help or mutual help groups are one of the most popular network modalities. Self-help groups have several key attributes:

1. They are composed of members who share a common condition, situation, heritage, symptoms, or experience.
2. They are largely self-giving and emphasize self-reliance.
3. They offer a face-to-face fellowship network, available and accessible without charge.
4. They tend to be self-supporting rather than dependent on external funding (Lieberman, 1989).

Examples include informational and emotional support groups, such as Alzheimer's caregivers groups, and political action groups, such as the Gray Panthers. Self-help groups have been organized with the financial assistance of churches, community organizations, and community mental health centers. Indirect funding may come from foundations and governmental support.

Older persons appear to be underrepresented in self-help groups. The overall drop-off rate between midlife (ages 50–64 years) and older ages was about 30% for all professional psychosocial treatment, but the drop-off rate for self-help groups was 72% according to Lieberman (1989). Some of the reasons for this drop-off include the recruiting practices of self-help groups, which are typically through peers and other informal networks; the attitudes, beliefs, and needs for help among older persons; and the availability of alternative help-providing resources (e.g., widows typically find other widows within their social networks) (Lieberman, 1989).

Lieberman (1989) contended that age alone does not appear to be a valid criterion of homogeneous group component, although certain foci (e.g., retirement, grandparents of divorced children, or persons suffering death of adult children) lend themselves to more uniform age groups. However, there are few research data as to whether older persons would do better in homogeneous or heterogeneous groups.

The widespread acceptance and apparent effectiveness of self-help groups stem from commonality of experience, mutual support, receiving of help through giving it, collective willpower, information sharing, and goal-directed problem solving (Biegel et al., 1984). Self-help groups provide assistance to individuals who may have never availed themselves of professional help. Although self-help groups appear to produce beneficial effects, systematic research on outcomes that would assist in identifying which kinds of support are beneficial for which individuals under which circumstances is scarce (Maddox, 2001). The fluidity of membership and the difficulty of controlling the number of complex variables have contributed to limiting the scope of evaluative research (Lieberman & Borman, 1979).

Support groups, especially for caregivers, have evolved from a self-help modality into a more formal method of intervention, generally conducted by trained group leaders. Toseland and Rossiter (1989) have identified seven common themes found among caregiver support groups: (1) information, (2) development of the group as a support system, (3) emotional impact of caregiving, (4) self-care, (5) improving interpersonal relations and communications, (6) development of outside support systems, and (7) the improvement of home care skills. The evaluative literature on caregiver support group interventions (Biegel, 2001; Knight et al., 1993; Zarit & Teri, 1991) has indicated that self-reports of caregivers are uniformly positive; however, the changes in burden scores and other caregiver measures, using standardized instruments with control groups, have indicated a much less positive outcome. For example, Knight and coworkers' (1993) meta-analysis found respite care and psychosocial interventions had moderately strong effects on caregivers, whereas support group interventions had lesser effects.

Stewart's (1990) review found that, although empirical studies measuring self-help group members' perceptions and professionals' views indicated that even though professional interaction with self-help groups is generally perceived as desirable, professionals' lack of information concerning self-help groups and their lack of preparation for appropriate roles are perceived as barriers to such interaction. The studies showed that the indirect, nonauthoritarian role of the professional or consultant receives the most support.

Nutritional Services

In 1973, the original thrust of the National Program on Nutrition was not only to provide older persons with meals, but also to offer outreach and services such as education, counseling, and recreation. Austin (1987) argued that, because of insufficient funding, the focus over time has been primarily on serving meals, and the other goals have largely evaporated. Moreover, even the former goal has been elusive in that the average program participant receives seven meals per 10-week period—a level of participation that can barely contribute to the client's nutritional status (Austin, 1987). Beginning in 1983, budgetary cutbacks at the federal level have further weakened these programs.

HOME DELIVERY PROGRAM (MEALS ON WHEELS) Nonprofit agencies or congregate meals programs prepare, package, and deliver midday meals and occasionally cold suppers or snacks to homebound (according to accepted medical criteria) persons of any age. Funding is primarily provided by Title III of the OAA; however, United Way churches, community groups, and fees from clients are other sources of revenue. For-profit home-delivered meal services also exist. In 1995, Title III programs provided 119 million home-delivered meals to 989,000 homebound elderly people.

At-risk persons are the principal consumers of meals-on-wheels (MOW) programs. For example, Stevens and coworkers (1992) found 70% of MOW consumers had intakes below 66% of their dietary requirements, and Coulston and associates (1996) found that 74% of MOW applicants were at risk for "poor nutritional status." The former study suggested that nutritional needs are not always met by MOW, and that meals may need to be altered to meet nutritional requirements. Moreover, meals may not always be consumed or considered palatable. Both studies suggested that high-risk users should be further screened, assessed, and educated by dieticians or other clinicians (Krassie et al., 2000).

CONGREGATE MEALS PROGRAM All persons aged 60 years and older are eligible to receive inexpensive meals at nearby centers, such as churches, senior centers, and schools. Funding comes primarily from Title III of the OAA, although clients are encouraged to contribute something for the meal. The original legislation also provided for nutrition education, information and referral, social services counseling, and recreational activities.

The nutrition program is currently the largest single component in OAA funding; in 1995, the elderly nutrition program provided 242 million meals to 3.4 million people, with roughly two thirds receiving meals on site and one third receiving homebound meals. Thus, about 8% of all seniors in the country participate in the on-site congregate meal program during a given year (Krout, 1995).

A 1993 study that included congregate and homebound clients indicated that 80% to 90% of participants have incomes below 200% of the poverty level, more than twice as many live alone compared with their age peers, roughly two thirds are at risk for nutritional and health problems, and participants have twice as many physical impairments as their age peers. Some writers have proposed that meal programs be refocused more toward homebound elderly persons because they are at nearly three times greater risk for nutritional inadequacy than on-site participants, and that on-site meals have not been found to affect the nutritional status of participants appreciably (Neyman et al., 1996).

NUTRITION EDUCATION PROGRAM   Also funded under OAA, the nutrition education program is designed to provide nutrition education as part of a meal program or separately.

"BROWN BAG" PROGRAM   Various community groups provide volunteers who fill shopping bags for low-income elderly individuals, which is known as a brown bag program.

FOOD STAMP PROGRAM   Started in 1964 by the Department of Agriculture, the Food Stamp Program allows low-income Americans of all ages to purchase, at less than face value (or, if they are very indigent, obtain for free), food stamps that substitute for cash in buying specified kinds of food at grocery stores. Applications can be obtained by mail or at local Social Security offices. A large proportion of elderly individuals who are eligible do not utilize the program.

Transportation and Escort

TRANSPORTATION SERVICES   The Urban Mass Transportation Act and the OAA generally fund transportation services. Communities provide three modes of transport to assist elderly persons with physician visits and errands: subsidized taxis, minibuses, and private cars.

ESCORT SERVICES   Community agencies and police provide escorts to assist frail elderly individuals with errands and other activities.

SHOPPING ASSISTANCE   Senior centers and other senior organizations provide transport service to help elderly persons get to shopping centers.

Volunteer and Employment Programs

The proportion of persons aged 65 years and older who volunteer has increased roughly fourfold since the 1960s (Chambre, 1993). In various studies, approximately two fifths had engaged in volunteering during the year. Moreover, one in three people older than 75 years had volunteered in the past year. Differences in volunteerism among age groups have been nearly obliterated. Reasons for the surging interest in volunteerism among older persons has been the emphasis on activity in later life, the changing demographics (e.g., better education, more affluence, more native born), social factors such as the need for more volunteers as women have entered the labor force, and government and private sector initiatives for volunteers.

Most of the publicly funded volunteer programs in the country are administered under Title V of the OAA or under the Corporation for National Community Services (CNCS). This agency was created in 1993 and supersedes its predecessor, ACTION, in administering various service corps for Americans of all ages. Senior Corps, which is part of CNCS, involves three types of services:

Retired Seniors Volunteer Program (RSVP). Originated under OAA, RSVP is currently funded through CNCS. Volunteers aged 60 years or older work in hospitals, nursing homes, and senior centers. Local senior centers sponsor a variety of RSVP programs, such as friendly visiting. RSVP volunteers also work with children and juvenile delinquents.

Foster Grandparents. Subsidized through CNCS, this program provides a small stipend to low-income individuals aged 60 years or older to work with youths in need of supportive and affectionate adults; the program is conducted in schools, care centers, and hospitals.

Senior Companions. This is another CNCS-supported program that provides a stipend for low-income persons aged 60 years or older to visit other elderly individuals in nursing homes, hospitals, and private homes.

Other volunteer programs for seniors include

Service Corps of Retired Executives (SCORE). This program, sponsored by the Small Business Administration, gives retired professionals an opportunity to assist small business owners who lack funds to pay for such services.

Green Thumb. This program is funded under the Senior Community Service Employment Program (SCSEP) of OAA (Title V), which requires participants to be 55 years of age or older and have an income that is below 125% of the federal poverty line. The Green Thumb program employs retired farmers and other low-income rural elderly individuals to work part time in parks and other beautification programs.

Senior Aides. Another program of SCSEP, this offers small stipends for part-time work in community service jobs as homemakers, home health aides, and food program assistants.

In general, studies have demonstrated that older volunteers derive substantial benefit in life satisfaction, self-esteem, and mood (Cutler, 1976; Hunter & Linn, 1980–1981; Morrow-Howell et al., 2003). Stevens (1991) found four factors that predicted satisfaction and likelihood that volunteers would stay on the job longer: (1) a pattern of providing community service throughout adulthood, (2) a congruence between the volunteer's role expectations and actual experiences on the job, (3) social contact on the job, and (4) perceived recognition and appreciation for their volunteer work. Methods suggested for enhancing recruitment include making such activities meaningful alternatives to leisure activities, creating opportunities for seasonal migrants, providing transportation, offering in-home work, and providing roles that are congruent with roles acquired in later life (e.g., "grandparenting" young children).

Adult Education

There has been considerable growth in the number of specialized educational programs for older adults offered by public schools, colleges, government, industry, libraries, museums, and voluntary and religious organizations (Pearce, 1991). Increasing numbers of elderly individuals are enrolling in tuition-waiver programs in colleges, adult education courses, and elder hostel programs. The last program sponsors 1-week courses on college campuses; the participant pays the costs of transportation, tuition, and room and board.

Studies in educational gerontology have indicated that several factors correlate with increased participation: female sex, age 60 to 64 years, higher educational attainment, higher socioeconomic status, and good health (Heisel et al., 1981; Pearce, 1991). The principal motivations for attending courses are intellectual, social, and recreational interests (Heisel et al., 1981).

The few rigorous investigations of the effects of educational programs have indicated that such programs enhance personal growth and quality of life (Brady, 1983; Russ-Eft & Steel, 1980). Scanlan and Darkenwald (1984) identified six factors that deter participation in educational courses: (1) lack of confidence, (2) lack of course relevance, (3) time constraints, (4) low personal priority, (5) cost, and (6) personal problems. Peterson (2001) adumbrated three aspects concerning the future of educational programs for seniors: (1) that persons of every age will be required to expand their knowledge and skills to survive and progress; (2) that educational programs are for personal growth and development and not only for the difficulties of aging; and (3) that the content of programs will match the needs of older persons. Pearce (1991) further called for an elimination of barriers to participation, such as poor health or financial costs, to broaden and diversify participation.

COMMUNITY HOUSING

Long-Term Care Facilities

Long-term care facilities provide medical and psychosocial care to individuals who have relatively severe, chronic impairments.

NURSING HOMES Nursing homes can be divided into two broad categories: (1) skilled nursing facilities, which provide 24-hour nursing care and medical coverage for persons who require extensive care (reimbursement is provided by Medicaid and time-limited coverage by Medicare); and (2) intermediate care facilities (ICFs), which provide health-related care for persons who are more stabilized, but require some medical and nursing supervision (not full time); costs are covered by Medicaid, but at a reduced level for Medicare. Intermediate care can be provided not only in specifically designed ICFs, but also in homes for the aged, hospitals, or personal care homes. It is possible to buy long-term care insurance policies that will reimburse at part or full cost any subsequent nursing home placement. Federal regulations have given states that administer and control nursing home programs some flexibility in determining levels of care and reimbursement for services.

HOSPICES Hospices provide a setting of comfort, friendship, familiar possessions, and relief from pain in a person's last weeks of a terminal illness. Hospices may be found as (1) a hospital unit, (2) a freestanding facility, (3) an outpatient unit for counseling and medical visits, or (4) a home care program. Care averages about 1 month. Medicare provides benefits to those who are diagnosed as having 6 months or less to live. Benefits under Medicaid vary by state. Some private insurance policies also provide reimbursement.

Planned Housing

Planned housing, housing specifically targeted to older persons, has been undergoing dramatic changes since its inception in the late 1950s. About 10% of older persons live in planned housing (Lawton, 2001). In the late 1950s, the federal government inaugurated two major housing programs for senior citizens. One program, launched within the public housing sector, gave localities federal funding for the construction of housing for the poor, some of which was earmarked for older people. A second program gave assistance to nonprofit sponsors to develop senior housing, most of which was undertaken under Section 202 programs (see below). These programs were considered widely successful, with evaluation studies consistently demonstrating a favorable effect on tenants' well-being (Lawton, 2001).

However, since 1980, there has been a marked retrenchment in public funding for senior housing, with only Section 202 housing continuing at a much lower level. Along with the decline in funding, there has been increased recognition of two phenomena: aging in place, increasing frailty occurring among aging occupants of senior housing; and delayed entry, in which older persons use expanded in-home service options to delay moving to settings with more intensive care (Wilson, 1995). Thus, there is growing recognition that housing environments must be conceptualized as an inseparable component of the long-term care continuum (Lawton, 1995). This fact now drives all housing-related issues, which include new planned forms such as assisted living or retirement communities, maintenance of old forms with increased on-site services, the technology of housing design, and older persons in nonplanned housing.

Although it is intuitively logical to combine housing and services for older persons, this has not occurred naturally in the United States because of a policy that has viewed housing as independent of services for all segments of the population (Wilson, 1995). For the elderly, this division was further heightened by the passage of Medicaid and Medicare legislation that required most services to be performed by specially trained individuals in designated institutions. Consequently, states have often used board-and-care homes to house persons who did not fit federal categorical programs and were too poor to pay for services. Wealthier elders negotiated this problem by moving into continuing care communities, upscale congregate facilities, which have evolved into assisted living facilities (ALFs). Despite the lack of a cohesive federal policy, states are developing strategies to combine housing and services.

This section describes the various types of planned housing, which range from age-segregated housing for well elderly persons to facilities that provide a variety of supportive services to help persons compensate for the physical or mental decline of advanced age. The rapid changes in the senior housing field have made terminology a bit muddled. Thus, depending on jurisdiction, board and care, personal care, congregate living, homes for the aged, domiciliary care, and assisted living may refer to the same type of facility and be strictly regulated or not regulated at all.

In general, congregate housing is for persons with minimal functional impairment; board-and-care facilities are for persons with mild to moderate functional impairment; assisted living, although included under the rubric of board-and-care facilities, offers a wide range of services for persons with functional deficits that are mild to moderately severe; and nursing homes provide services for persons with severe functional deficits. The average costs for these facilities rise in tandem with the level of disability of the residents. Next, we present the most distinctive features of each (e.g., size, sponsorship, level, and types of disability).

BOARD-AND-CARE HOMES AND RESIDENTIAL CARE FACILITIES The generic terms *board-and-care homes* and *residential care facilities* (RCFs) describe various types of housing with supportive long-term services exclusive of licensed nursing homes

(Newcomer, 2001). They provide more support to residents than congregate housing or rooming houses. Board and care and RCFs are the terms used most commonly in state regulations and statutes.

Because they are regulated at the state level, each state has different definitions and names for these facilities; for instance, there are at least 30 names for these licensed facilities, and they are regulated by over 60 state agencies. Hence, these facilities also may be known as personal care homes, sheltered care, supervised care, adult congregate living facilities, homes for the aged, domiciliary care homes, and assisted living facilities. Terms like boarding home, congregate care, and group homes often refer to unlicensed board-and-care facilities (Newcomer, 2001).

Board-and-care homes and RCFs range from small "mom-and-pop" operations to larger homes operated by charitable nonprofit organizations (Kalymun, 1992); the latter typically go well beyond the standards that are set by various states (Gelfand, 1999). There are over 40,000 licensed and unlicensed homes, with over 800,000 beds (Newcomer, 2001). The numbers of residents range from 1 to more than 100. Homes typically provide three meals a day, laundry service, and 24-hour supervision; many also provide transportation services, cleaning of living areas, personal assistance, and arrangement of medical appointments (Eckert & Lyon, 1991).

The National Board and Care Reform Act (1989) required that every facility with two or more recipients of social security or Supplemental Security Income (SSI) meet minimum health and safety standards, with states allowed to control the specifics. Because these facilities are considered nonmedical, when they are licensed, it is usually by state departments of social services, and health care benefits such as Medicare or Medicaid benefits are not available to pay for stays in such facilities. However, qualified residents may receive additional reimbursement from SSI that can be used to defer the costs of accommodation.

Traditionally, board-and-care homes and RCFs have been one of three basic types (Hawes et al., 1999): (1) homes serving residents with mental retardation or developmental disabilities; (2) homes serving residents with mental illness; (3) homes serving a mixed population of physically frail elderly, cognitively impaired elderly, and persons with mental health problems. Most facilities are in the last category.

Historically, RCFs have served low-income older persons with functional disabilities whose families do not have the resources to care for them (Gelfand, 1999). Average monthly fees are between $240 and $1,150, although many of the newer assisted living facilities are considerably more expensive. Given the large number of RCFs, there have been surprisingly few evaluations of older persons in these programs. In Pennsylvania, a study of elderly participants in a domiciliary program found that they were more optimistic, engaged in more social activities, expressed greater satisfaction with living conditions, and had lower costs than a matched community control group (Vandivort et al. 1984).

ASSISTED LIVING   Assisted living constitutes a new name for a rapidly expanding sector of the traditional board-and-care housing and RCF sector (Hawes et al., 2001). Despite its tremendous growth, there is no consensus on the appropriate regulatory model, and there is considerable diversity in the types of places calling themselves assisted living. The Administration on Aging defines assisted living as facilities designed to accommodate frail elderly residents who can live independently but need assistance with activities of daily living. A *frail elderly* person is defined as an individual 62 years of age or older who is unable to perform at least three activities of daily living. The unifying philosophy among assisted living facilities is to provide a new type of long-term care that blurs the distinction between nursing home care and community-based care and reduces the chasm between receiving long-term care in one's home and in an institution (Hawes et al., 2001). Among the specific philosophical principles that distinguish assisted living are: (1) services and oversight are available 24 hours a day; (2) there are services to meet scheduled and unscheduled needs; (3) care and services are provided or arranged to promote independence; (4) there is an emphasis on consumer dignity, autonomy, and choice; (5) there is an emphasis on privacy and a homelike environment (Hawes et al., 1999).

A national survey has estimated that there are 11,459 ALFs with 611,300 beds (Hawes et al., 1999). The average number of beds was 57; two thirds of ALFs had 11 to 50 beds. The most common accommodation was a room (57%), whereas 43% were residential apartments. About 45% of ALFs were located on a multilevel campus that housed more than one residential setting and provided more than one level of care; the remainder were freestanding ALFs. The most common monthly rate was $1,582, with a range from $300 to $7,100. Typically, there are four basic service rates for residents: all inclusive, which covers all services; basic enhanced, which covers a core set of services with additional costs for extra services; fee for service, for which services are charged separately; and service levels, for which higher fees are attached to more intense service levels.

There has been considerable variability in state regulations of ALFs. In 1998, regulations had been issued by 30 states, and 22 had licensing regulations; 35 states reimbursed or planned to reimburse services in ALFs as a Medicaid covered service (Hawes et al., 1999). We can expect further regulation of this industry, especially as more facilities are developed as alternatives to nursing homes for certain segments of the frail elderly population (Wilson, 1995).

A study by Yee and colleagues (1999) of residents in 20 ALFs indicated that these residents experienced relatively independent and autonomous lives, yet many reported unmet health and long-term care needs and limited participation in meaningful activities and community life. Another study by Buelow and Fee (2000) of residents and family found positive, but not strong, satisfaction with care. Areas identified as unsatisfactory included the mealtime experience, nursing assistants, and recreational activities.

The Group for the Advancement of Psychiatry (Cohen et al., 2003) has pointed out that, as these facilities assume responsibility for persons with more severe cognitive impairment, it is essential that they address their residents' psychiatric needs, and that they identify mental health professionals as resources for on-site consultation and treatment.

CONGREGATE HOUSING   Congregate housing consists of apartment houses or group accommodations that provide limited health services and other support services (e.g., meals in a central dining room, heavy housekeeping, social services, recreational activities) to functionally impaired older persons who do not need routine nursing care. Such support services enable persons to continue an independent lifestyle. These facilities are somewhat less institutionalized than residential care facilities. As tenants grow older, facilities may opt to provide additional on-site services for frail elderly persons (Ehrlich et al., 1982).

They are usually operated by government agencies or nonprofit groups; many received funding for construction from the Section 202 federal housing program, which provides low-cost loans to develop residences that include support services (Gelfand, 1999). Costs vary widely. Ruchelin and Morris (1987) reported that monthly service costs were $563 per tenant, which they considered cost-effective in comparison to nursing home placement.

FOSTER CARE   For older persons (particularly those with chronic mental illness) in need of care and protection in a substitute family, foster care can provide socialization, stimulation, support, and protection. The number of paying residents is usually limited to four. Such programs offer a useful position on the continuum of options for frail elderly persons, an intermediate position between support and independence (Sherman, 2001).

Evaluations of foster care programs have been favorable. One study (Newman & Sherman, 1979) found that elderly participants interacted to a moderate degree with family and community, and several investigators (Braun & Rose, 1986; Kane et al., 1991; Oktay & Volland, 1987; Vandivort et al., 1984) reported generally favorable levels of well-being and use of community resources and equal improvements in activities of daily living functions in elderly foster care participants compared with nursing home patients.

Potential weaknesses include difficulties monitoring these sites, the potential to encourage premature dependency, and their inability to provide an array of organized activities (Sherman, 2001). Importantly, the annual cost of foster care is approximately $8,400 (Abrahams et al., 1991), which is substantially less than that for nursing homes.

Foster care programs are usually administered by local departments of social services using Title XX funds; therefore, they are primarily targeted to lower income elderly individuals (Gelfand, 1999).

SINGLE-ROOM OCCUPANCY HOUSING FOR OLDER PEOPLE   Single-room occupancy (SRO) housing refers to a range of building structures with various unit configurations. The Department of Housing and Urban Development definition states that these structures must have at least 12 units. The classic SRO room is about 100 square feet, with bathroom and kitchen facilities usually outside the unit and shared with other residents. SROs have been used as permanent, emergency, and transitional housing (Regnier & Culver, 1994).

Although SROs have traditionally served low-income persons who wish to maintain their independence, SRO-type housing has been used to house specific target populations, such as mentally ill persons or substance abusers. Such units often provide on-site staffing and support. The stock of SRO beds has decreased dramatically over the past 25 years, thereby increasing the probability that persons who would have found shelter in SROs will become homeless (Kovar, 2001).

ELDER COTTAGE HOUSING OPPORTUNITY Elder cottage housing opportunity (ECHO), also known as granny flats, accessory housing, and second-unit ordinances, are ancillary structures for elderly individuals (e.g., mobile minihouses or small attached units) that are permitted by special zoning variances. They are placed on land belonging to the children of these individuals, thereby enabling the older person to receive informal care and support from his or her kin (Friedman & Harris, 1991). An Andrus Foundation study found very high satisfaction levels (Hare, 1998).

CONTINUING CARE AND LIFE-CARE FACILITIES Continuing care and life-care facilities, operated by nonprofit and for-profit organizations, offer multiple levels of care, ranging in setting from one's own home to a nursing home (Friedman & Harris, 1991). These communities provide private living units with ancillary services such as meals, mail services, and health care. When there is a need for more intensive care, the resident may be transferred to a nursing home, often on the same site. In 1999, there were approximately 2,000 facilities housing about 500,000 residents (about 2% of the population older than 65 years) (Streib, 2001a).

Three levels of continuing care are available; entry fees and costs vary widely, depending on the type of health care coverage (Friedman & Harris, 1991; Streib, 2001a):

1. Unlimited or extensive care, which guarantees a full level of health and long-term care for the resident's lifetime.
2. Limited or modified care, which provides a basic level of medical care with extra health and long-term care available for additional fees.
3. Fee-for-service or pay-as-you-go care provides a living unit with meals and medical care available on a "menu" basis. There is no guarantee of future services. Entrance and monthly fees are relatively low.

Sloan and coworkers (1995) found that, after controlling for a variety of confounding factors, residents of continuing care retirement communities

(CCRCs) experienced a less-rapid decline in health, functional, and cognitive status compared to their age peers. Sherwood and colleagues (1997) found that residents of CCRCs perceived themselves in better health and had greater levels of social interaction and activities than their age peers in the community. Although CCRCs seem to address the service needs and quality-of-life issues of their residents, fewer than 25% of older Americans could afford such housing (Streib, 2001a).

RETIREMENT COMMUNITIES Retirement communities are nonlicensed, age-segregated communities of apartments or freestanding homes. Services are generally of a social nature (e.g., clubhouses, tennis courts) and do not routinely include health services. They can be divided into five categories: large-size retirement towns, medium-size retirement villages, retirement subdivisions within towns or cities (often with surrounding walls), retirement residences and apartment groupings, and continuing care centers that provide health care and support services (Hunt et al., 1984). To remain age segregated and satisfy requirements of the Fair Housing Law, these retirement communities must have at least 80% of units occupied by someone at least 55 years old, they should offer facilities and services specially designed for elderly individuals, and the age restriction must be a specific policy of the complex (Friedman & Harris, 1991). Most older Americans live in normal communities, and many consider segregation by age undesirable; however, those who move to retirement communities appear very satisfied with their chosen lifestyle (Streib, 2001b).

ELDERLY APARTMENT COMPLEXES Elderly apartment complexes include public, nonprofit, and privately owned buildings for elderly individuals; many of these complexes were built with Section 202 federal funds. They do not routinely provide health care, although the National Affordable Housing Act (1990) now requires these programs to provide a daily meal and to make available housekeeping, transportation, personal care, and chore services. There have also been demonstration grants to assess the value of also providing on-site health services. Section 8 housing allowances (i.e., a federally subsidized program administered by a local housing authority for low-income families that covers the difference in rent above 30% of the family income) have frequently provided a rent supplement to Section 202 housing.

SHARED HOUSING For shared housing ("senior matching"), a social services agency matches occupant (owner/renter) with renter or the agency buys or rents units and then rents these units to others. Results have been favorable. One study of apartment- or house-sharing elderly individuals found that two thirds of these arrangements were still functioning after 1 year (Lawton, 1981).

NATURALLY OCCURRING RETIREMENT COMMUNITIES Naturally occurring retirement communites (NORCs) are an increasingly familiar phenomenon among older persons living in nonplanned housing. NORCs refer to buildings, apartment complexes, or neighborhoods not originally developed for older persons and where, over time, the majority of residents have become elderly. The term has evolved to mean any building or neighborhood where more than 50% of the residents are older than 60 years or where a disproportionate number are older than 60 years (Bassuk, 1999). NORCs are the most common form of retirement community in the United States; that is, about 27% of elderly persons live in NORCs. NORCs typically do not include programs of social and health supports (Bassuk, 1999). Thus, when the majority of residents become elderly, the housing management is faced with problems they may not be able to handle. Innovative programs for these older persons have been established that provide social work, case management, nursing, recreation, and educational enrichment.

SUMMARY AND CONCLUSION

The expansion in community services and housing options makes it incumbent on clinicians to familiarize themselves with these developments to optimize the functioning and care of their patients. As outlined in Table 37-1, the psychiatrist should be able to match services with the patient's level of functioning and then link the patient to the appropriate services. Although assistance in securing resources is available from local area agencies on aging or from social workers and case managers, clinicians and consumers can now connect to hundreds of Web sites that provide information on virtually every service and housing option.

Even when the clinician has identified the appropriate services, patients and caregivers may still fail to access the suggested services. A variety of structural and individual barriers have been identified that may affect the utilization of services. Structural barriers thought important are inconvenient locations for services; a relative lack of services in a community; the financial cost of obtaining services; negative professional attitudes and behaviors; bureaucratic orientation of programs; and the lack of any real coordination, integration, or organization within and among agencies servicing elderly individuals (Krout, 1985; Reed, 1980).

Impediments to obtaining help at the individual patient level include fear for personal safety, poor health, lack of knowledge about the availability of services, negative attitudes toward services, and fear of becoming too dependent on such services (Krout, 1985). Impediments to obtaining help at the caregiver level include a reluctance to rely on others for assistance; feeling guilty about relinquishing care to others; a belief that their relatives have different needs than other patients; and cultural attitudes about caregiving (Neary, 1993; Zarit et al., 1999).

Finally, sources of information may play a significant role. Silverstein (1984) found that information that elderly individuals obtained through formal sources (e.g., senior centers, medical facilities) was the best predictor of service utilization. However, elderly individuals cited such formal sources much less frequently than television, newspapers, friends/relatives, and brochures as preferred channels of information (Goodman, 1992).

There has been an increase in research on community services and housing programs for older persons; however, many of the earlier deficiencies remain. Much of the evaluative research continues to be too generalized, and future research must be better at defining groups to be served and outcomes to be achieved. That is, there should be more focused outcome measures that specifically reflect the service interventions rather than generalized measures (e.g., depressed mood) that may be influenced by a variety of factors independent of the intervention. More studies are needed that identify older populations inadequately served by existing programs along with evaluations of outreach programs similar to the pioneering research conducted on the PATCH program in Baltimore (Rabins et al., 2000).

There also exists a serious shortage in mental health services and research, especially for those with severe and persistent mental illness. This problem must be addressed because the population at risk continues to grow in tandem with the aging of the population in general.

Finally, over the next several years, there will be further evolution of programs that integrate services and housing options, particularly assisted living, continuing care retirement communities, and other residential care programs that seek to fill the gap in cost and personal autonomy between community dwelling and nursing homes. With their continued development, there will be a critical need to evaluate their effects on subjective and objective measures of well-being.

Although cost-effectiveness has not always been demonstrated, community programs generally have been judged at least clinically equivalent to institutional programs and considerably more humane. However, to make the case for community care more compelling, future research will have to (1) broaden traditional economic measures to include hidden economic costs and burdens to families and society and (2) consider the economic equivalences of quality-of-life measures or at least indicate the trade-off in costs for a specified gain in quality of life. Last, community research must be conducted with the input of and in close collaboration with elderly individuals and their families for whom services are developed.

REFERENCES

Abrahams R, Bishop C, Hernandez W. Respite service delivery: learning from current programs. *Pride Inst J Long-Term Health Care* 1991;10:16–28.

Austin C. Nutrition programs. In: Maddox GL, ed. *The Encyclopedia of Aging*. New York, NY: Springer; 1987:495–496.

Bartels SJ, Levine KJ, Shea D. Community-based long-term care for older persons with severe and persistent mental illness in an era of managed care. *Psychiatr Serv.* 1999; 50:1189–1197.

Bassuk K. NORC supportive service programs: effective and innovative programs that support seniors living in the community. *Case Manage J.* 1999;1:132–137.

Biegel DE. Caregiver burden. In: Maddox GL, ed. *Encyclopedia of Aging.* 3rd ed. New York, NY: Springer; 2001:157–160.

Biegel DE, Shore BK, Gordon E. *Building Support Networks for the Elderly: Theory and Applications.* Beverly Hills, CA: Sage; 1984.

Blenkner M, Bloom M, Nielsen M, et al. *Final Report: Protective Services for Older Adults.* Cleveland, OH: Benjamin Rose Institute; 1974.

Brady EM. Personal growth and the elder hostel experience. *Lifelong Learn.* 1983;7(3): 11–26.

Braun KL, Rose CL. The Hawaii geriatric foster care experiment: impact, evaluation, and cost analysis. *Gerontologist.* 1986;26:516–524.

Buckwalter KC, Abraham IL, Smith M, et al. Nursing update: nursing outreach to rural elderly people who are mentally ill. *Hospital Community Psychiatry.* 1993;44:821–823.

Buelow JR, Fee FA. Perceptions of care and satisfaction in assisted living facilities. *Health Mark Q.* 2000;17(3):13–24.

Cantor M, Little V. Aging and social care. In: Binstock RH, Shanas E, eds. *Handbook of Aging and the Social Sciences.* 2nd ed. New York, NY: Van Nostrand Reinhold; 1985.

Capezuti E, Brush BL, Lawson WT. Reporting elder mistreatment. *J Gerontol Nurs.* 1997;24–32.

Chambre SM. Volunteerism by elders: past trends and future prospects. *Gerontologist.* 1993;33:221–228.

Cohen C, Onserud H, Monaco C. Outcomes for the mentally ill in a program for older homeless persons. *Hosp Community Psychiatry.* 1993;44:650–656.

Cohen CI. Social network therapy with inner-city elderly. In: Myers WA, ed. *New Techniques in the Psychotherapy of Older Patients.* Washington, DC: American Psychiatric Press; 1991:79–93.

Cohen CI, Adler A. Network interventions: do they work? *Gerontologist.* 1984;24: 16–22.

Cohen CI, Cohen GD, Blank K, et al. Schizophrenia and older adults. An overview: directions for research and policy. *Am J Geriatr Psychiatry.* 2000;8:19–28.

Cohen GD, Blank K, Cohen CI, et al. Mental health problems in assisted living residents. The physician's role in treatment and staff education. *Geriatrics.* 2003;58(2):44, 54–55.

Coulston AM, Craig L, Voss AC. Meals-on-wheels applicants are a population at risk for poor nutritional status. *J Am Diet Assoc.* 1996;96:570–573.

Cox C. Findings from a statewide program of respite care: a comparison of service users, stoppers, and nonusers. *Gerontologist.* 1997;37:511–517.

Cuijpers P. Psychological outreach programmes for the depressed elderly: a meta-analysis of effects and dropout. *Int J Geriatr Psychiatry.* 1998;13:41–48.

Cutler SJ. Membership in different types of voluntary associations and psychological well-being. *Gerontologist.* 1976;16:335–339.

DeRenzo EG, Byer VL, Grady HS, et al. Comprehensive community-based mental health outreach services for suburban seniors. *Gerontologist.* 1991;31:836–840.

Eckert JK, Lyon SM. Regulation of board-and-care homes: research to guide policy. *J Aging Soc Policy*. 1991;3:147–161.

Ehrlich P, Ehrlich I, Woehlke P. Congregate housing for the elderly: thirteen years later. *Gerontologist*. 1982;22:399–403.

Forster A, Young J, Langhorne P. Systematic review of day hospital care for elderly people. *BMJ*. 1999;318:837–841.

Friedman JP, Harris JC. *Keys to Buying a Retirement Home*. New York, NY: Barrons; 1991.

Garrison JE, Howe J. Community intervention with the elderly: a social network approach. *J Am Geriatr Soc*. 1976;24:329–333.

Gelfand DE. *The Aging Network Programs and Services*. 5th ed. New York, NY: Springer; 1999.

Gelfand DE, Bechill W, Chester RL. Core programs and services at senior centers. *J Gerontol Soc Work*. 1991;17:145–161.

Golant SM, McCaslen R. A functional classification of services for older people. *J Gerontol Soc Work*. 1979;1:187–209.

Goodman RI. The selection of communication channels by the elderly to obtain information. *Educ Gerontol*. 1992;18:701–714.

Grasel E. Temporary institutional respite in dementia cases: who utilizes this form of respite care and what effect does it have? *Int Psychogeriatr*. 1997;9:437–448.

Hare PH. *Accessory Apartments: The Supportive Housing Connection*. Washington, DC: National Resource and Policy Center on Housing and Long Term Care; January 1998.

Hawes C, Rose M, Phillips CD, et al. *A National Study of Assisted Living for the Frail Elderly. Results of a National Survey Facilities*. Washington, DC: US Dept of Health and Human Services/Assistant Secretary for Planning and Evaluation; December 1999.

Hegeman CR. *Geriatric Respite Care: Expanding and Improving Practice*. Albany, NY: Foundation for Long-Term Care; 1989.

Heisel MA, Darkenwald GG, Anderson RE. Participation in organized educational activities among adults age 60 and over. *Educ Gerontol*. 1981;6:227–240.

Hunt ME, Feldt AG, Marano RW, et al. *Retirement Communities: An American Original*. New York, NY: Haworth; 1984.

Hunter KI, Linn MW. Psychosocial differences between elderly volunteers and non-volunteers. *Int J Aging Hum Dev*. 1980–1981;12:205–213.

Huttman ED. *Social Services for the Elderly*. New York, NY: Free Press; 1985.

Jacobs HE. Vocational rehabilitation. In: Liberman RP, ed. *Psychiatric Rehabilitation of Chronic Mental Patients*. Washington, DC: American Psychiatric Press; 1988: 245–284.

Kalymun M. Board and care versus assisted living: ascertaining the similarities and differences. *Adult Residential Care J*. 1992;6:35–44.

Kane RA. Setting the PACE in chronic care. *Contemp Gerontol J Rev Crit Discourse*. 1999;6(2):47–50.

Kane RA, Kane RL, Illston LH, et al. Adult foster care for the elderly in Oregon: a mainstream alternative to nursing homes? *Am J Public Health*. 1991;81:1113–1120.

Katz IR, Coyne JC. The public health model for mental health care for the elderly. *JAMA*. 2000;283:2844–2845.

Kemper P. The evaluation of the nutritional long term care demonstration. 10. Overview of the findings. *Health Serv Res.* 1988;23:161–174.

Knight BG, Lutzky SM, Macotsky-Urban F. A meta-analytic review of interventions for caregiver distress: recommendations for future research. *Gerontologist.* 1993;33: 240–248.

Korte C, Gupta V. A program of friendly visitors as network builders. *Gerontologist.* 1991;31:404–407.

Kovar MG. Single room occupancy. In: Maddox GL, ed. *The Encyclopedia of Aging.* 3rd ed. New York, NY: Springer; 2001:930–931.

Krassie J, Smart C, Roberts DCK. A review of the nutritional needs of meals-on-wheels consumers and factors associated with the provision of an effective meals-on-wheels service—an Australian perspective. *Eur J Clin Nutr.* 2000;54:275–280.

Krout JA. Service awareness among the elderly. *J Gerontol Soc Work.* 1985;9:7–19.

Krout JA. Senior centers and services for the frail elderly. *J Aging Soc Policy.* 1995;7: 59–76.

Krout JA, Cutler S, Coward R. Correlates of senior center participation: a national analysis. *Gerontologist.* 1990;30:72–79.

Lachs MS, Williams C, O'Brien S, et al. Older adults: an 11-year longitudinal study of adult protective service use. *Arch Intern Med.* 1996;156:449–453.

Lawton MP. Alternative housing. *J Gerontol Soc Work.* 1981;3:61–80.

Lawton MP. Housing. In: Maddox GL, ed. *The Encyclopedia of Aging.* 3rd ed. New York, NY: Springer; 2001:510–514.

Lebowitz B. Correlates of success in community mental health programs for the elderly. *Hosp Community Psychiatry.* 1988;39:721–722.

Lebowitz B. Mental health services. In: Maddox GL, ed. *The Encyclopedia of Aging.* 3rd ed. New York, NY: Springer; 2001:682–684.

Lieberman MA. Mutual aid groups: an underutilized resource among the elderly. *Annu Rev Gerontol Geriatr.* 1989;9:285–320.

Lieberman MA, Borman L. *Self-Help Groups for Coping With Crisis.* San Francisco, CA: Jossey-Bass; 1979.

Litwin H. Administrative correlates of senior center programs. *J Appl Gerontol.* 1987; 6:201–212.

Maddox GL. Support groups. In: Maddox GL, ed. *The Encyclopedia of Aging.* 3rd ed. New York, NY: Springer; 2001:995–996.

Morrissey JP, Goldman HH. Cycles of reform in the care of the chronically mentally ill. *Hosp Community Psychiatry.* 1984;35:785–793.

Morrow-Howell N, Hinterlong J, Rozario P, et al. Effects of volunteering on the well-being of older adults. *J Gerontol Soc Sci.* 2003;58B:S137–145.

Mulligan M, Bennett R. Assessment of mental health and social problems during multiple friendly visits: the development and evaluation of a friendly visitor program for the isolated elderly. *Int J Aging Hum Dev.* 1977;8:43–65.

Neary MA. Community services in the 1990s: are they meeting the needs of caregivers. *J Community Health Nurs.* 1993;10:105–111.

Newcomer R. Board and care homes. In: Maddox GL, ed. *The Encyclopedia of Aging.* 3rd ed. New York, NY: Springer; 2001:130–131.

Newcomer R, Spitalny M, Fox P, et al. Effects of the Medicare Alzheimer's disease demonstration on the use of community-based services. *Health Serv Res.* 1999;34: 645–667.

Newman ES, Sherman SR. Community integration of the elderly in foster family care. *J Gerontol Soc Work*. 1979;1:175–186.

Neyman MR, Zidenberg-Cherr S, McDonald RB. Effect of participation in congregate-site meal programs on programs on nutritional status of the healthy elderly. *J Am Diet Assoc*. 1996;96:475–483.

Noelker LS, Bass DM. Home care for elderly persons: linkages between formal and informal caregivers. *J Gerontol Soc Serv*. 1989;44:S63–S72.

Oktay JS, Volland P. Foster homecare for the frail elderly as an alternative to nursing home care: an experimental evaluation. *Am J Public Health*. 1987;77:1505–1510.

Pancoast DL, Parker P, Froland C. *Rediscovering Self-Help*. Beverly Hills, CA: Sage; 1983.

Parish B, Landsberg G. Developing a geriatric mental health outreach unit in a rural community. *J Gerontol Soc Work*. 1984;7(3):75–82.

Pearce SD. Toward understanding the participation of older adults in continuing education. *Educ Gerontol*. 1991;17:451–464.

Peterson DA. Adult education. In: Maddox GL, ed. *The Encyclopedia of Aging*. 3rd ed. New York, NY: Springer; 2001:22–24.

Phipps C, Liberman RP. Community support. In: Liberman RP, ed. *Psychiatric Rehabilitation of Chronic Mental Patients*. Washington, DC: American Psychiatric Press; 1988:285–311.

Rabins PV. Barriers to diagnosis and treatment of depression in elderly patients. *Am J Geriatr Psychiatry*. 1996;4(suppl 1):S79–S83.

Rabins PV, Black BS, Roca R, et al. Effectiveness of a nurse-based outreach program for identifying and treating psychiatric illness in the elderly. *JAMA*. 2000;283:2802–2809.

Raschko R. Spokane community mental health center elderly services. In: Light E, Lebowitz BD, eds. *The Elderly With Chronic Mental Illness*. New York, NY: Springer; 1991:232–244.

Reed WL. Access to services by the elderly: a community research model. *J Gerontol Soc Work*. 1980;3:41–52.

Regnier V, Culver J. *Single Room Occupancy-SRO-Type Housing for Older People*. Los Angeles: National Resources and Policy Center on Housing and Long-Term Care, USC Andrus Gerontology Center; 1994.

Reifler BV, Kelhley A, O'Neill P, et al. Five-year experience of a community outreach program for the elderly. *J Am Geriatr Soc*. 1982;139:220–223.

Roca RP, Storer DJ, Robbins BM, et al. Psychogeriatric assessment and treatment in urban public housing. *Hosp Community Psychiatry*. 1990;41:916–920.

Ruchelin HS, Morris JN. The congregate housing services program: an analyses of service utilization. *Gerontologist*. 1987;27:87–91.

Russ-Eft DF, Steel LM. Contributions of education to adult quality of life. *Educ Gerontol*. 1980;5:180–209.

Scanlan CS, Darkenwald GG. Identifying deterrents to participation in continuing education. *Adult Educ Q*. 1984;34:155–166.

Sherman SR. Adult foster care. In: Maddox GL, ed. *The Encyclopedia of Aging*. 2nd ed. New York, NY: Springer; 2001:24–26.

Sherr VT, Eskridge OC, Lewis L. A mobile, mental-hospital-based team for geropsychiatric service in the community. *J Am Geriatr Soc*. 1976;24:362–365.

Sherwood S, Ruchlin HS, Sherwood CC, Morris SA. *Continuing Care Retirement Communities*. Baltimore, MD: Johns Hopkins University Press; 1997.

Silverstein NM. Informing the elderly about public services: the relationship between sources of knowledge and service utilization. *Gerontologist*. 1984;24:37–40.

Skolnick B, Warrick P. *The Right Place at the Right Time: A Guide to Long-Term Care Choices*. Washington, DC: American Association of Retired Persons; 1985.

Sloan FA, Shayne MW, Conover CJ. Continuing care retirement communities: prospects for reducing long-term care. *J Health Polit Policy Law*. 1995;20:75–97.

Stevens D, Grivetti L, McDonald R. Nutrient intake of urban and rural elderly receiving home-delivered meals. *J Am Diet Assoc*. 1992;92:714–718.

Stevens ES. Toward satisfaction and retention of senior volunteers. *J Gerontol Soc Work*. 1991;16:33–41.

Stewart MJ. Professional interface with mutual-aid self-help groups: a review. *Social Sci Med*. 1990;31:1143–1158.

Streib GF. Continuing care retirement community. In: Maddox GL, ed. *The Encyclopedia of Aging*. 3rd ed. New York, NY: Springer; 2001a:243–246.

Streib GF. Retirement communities. In: Maddox GL, ed. *The Encyclopedia of Aging*. 3rd ed. New York, NY: Springer; 2001b:890–893.

Thobaben M. Elder abuse and neglect. *Home Care Provider*. 1996;1:267–269.

Toseland RW, Rossiter CM. Group interventions to support family caregivers: a review and analysis. *Gerontologist*. 1989;29:438–448.

Vandivort R, Kurren G, Braun K. Foster family care for frail elderly: a cost-effective quality care alternative. *J Gerontol Soc Work*. 1984;7:101–114.

Weissert WG. Two models of geriatric day care findings from a comparative study. *Gerontologist*. 1976;16:420–427.

Weissert WG, Elston JM, Bolda EJ, et al. Models of adult day care: findings from a national survey. *Gerontologist*. 1989;29:640–649.

Westhoff LJ. Care management: quelling the confusion. *Health Prog*. 1992;73:43–46.

White M. Case management. In: Maddox GL, ed. *The Encyclopedia of Aging*. New York, NY: Springer; 2001:162–166.

Wilson KB. Assisted living: a residential model of long-term care. In: Maddox GL, ed. *The Encyclopedia of Aging*. New York, NY: Springer; 1995.

Wolf RS. Adult protective services. In: Maddox GL, ed. *The Encyclopedia of Aging*. 3rd ed. New York, NY: Springer; 2001:26–28.

Wolf RS, Li D. Factors affecting the rate of elder abuse reporting to a state protective services program. *Gerontologist*. 1999;39:222–228.

Yee DL, Capitman JA, Leutz WN, et al. Resident-centered care in assisted living. *J Aging Soc Policy*. 1999;10(3):7–26.

Zarit SH, Teri L. Interventions and services for family caregivers. *Annu Rev Gerontol Geriatr*. 1991;11:287–310.

Zarit SH, Gaugler JE, Jarrot SE. Useful services for families: research findings and directions. *Int J Geriatr Psychiatry*. 1999;14:165–177.

Zborowsky E. Developments in protective services: a challenge for social workers. *J Gerontol Soc Work*. 1985;8:71–83.

Medical-Legal, Ethical, and Financial Issues

38

Legal and Ethical Issues

Karen Blank, MD

G eriatric psychiatrists commonly face a wide range of ethical challenges and legal issues. While advanced age should not, in and of itself, influence the ethics of health care, many features of geropsychiatric care combine to place the elderly at special risk and make their care ethically and legally complex (Kapp, 1996). Issues of patient autonomy, beneficence, and social justice compete for dominance in clinical decisions in an ongoing and often uneasy process. These tensions are felt most acutely in the care of vulnerable elders, particularly of patients whose conditions impair their cognition and communication. This chapter focuses on the legal and ethical framework relevant to clinical decision making and research participation. Legal and ethical issues relating to end-of-life decision making are covered in the following chapter.

PRINCIPLES OF CLINICAL MEDICAL ETHICS

While ethics are distinct from law, legal requirements often embody society's consensus on important ethical issues (Kapp, 1996). Most clinical ethical values are guided by four principles: respect for autonomy, beneficence, fidelity, and justice. *Respect for autonomy* forms the moral and legal nucleus of the doctor-patient relationship. *Autonomy* has been defined as the right of a decisionally capable individual to make personal life choices voluntarily, free from external interference or unwanted intervention (Kapp, 1994). In clinical practice, autonomy is advanced through informed consent and refusal and advanced directives. Respect becomes particularly critical in the care of geriatric patients who have impaired cognitive capacity. When meaningful dialogue is lost and the patient's values and personality become less accessible, much of the interaction that normally elicits respect is absent (Hayley et al., 1996). The physician caring for such vulnerable persons must cultivate attitudes and behaviors that compensate for these changes, taking special care to exercise respect and compassion.

Beneficence addresses the obligation to do what is best for the patient. Beneficent determinations should combine the physician's medical judgment about what is best for the patient and the patient's personal perspective. Beneficent decisions contrast with paternalistic ones, by which one person makes decisions on behalf of another, as a parent would for a child.

Fidelity encompasses critical elements of the doctor-patient relationship such as trust, truthfulness, physician availability, confidentiality and the physician's fiduciary responsibility, that is, the requirement to act primarily to protect and promote the interests of the patient. The law imposes fiduciary responsibilities to rectify the vast disparity between the powerful professional and the unknowledgeable patient (Kapp, 1999). Fiduciary responsibility requires that the patient's best interests supersede the physician's self-interests, including economic interests.

The principle of *justice* addresses the equitable access and distribution of resources. Justice can be considered at the level of the individual patient, intergenerationally, the institution, and the society at large. Justice is particularly challenging to achieve and often conflicts with other ethical principles. For example, costly individual treatment may be justified from the perspective of respect for an individual's autonomous desires, but may not be the most equitable use of resources when viewed at a broader societal level.

PATIENT AUTONOMY AND INFORMED CONSENT

In clinical settings, the informed consent doctrine rests on the fundamental ethical principle of respect for personal autonomy, that a patient has the right to make informed choices about the nature and course of treatment. Unfortunately, informed consent too often becomes an empty ritual (Lidz et al., 1988). This results when physicians misperceive the informed consent process, failing to appreciate it as integral to medical practice, but rather viewing it as a mechanistic procedure with the goal of obtaining a signature on a form. In this context, psychiatrists are sometimes called in to function as informed consent technicians (Gutheil & Duckworth, 1992), solely to facilitate the process of either getting the consent or having the patient declared incompetent. Geropsychiatrists should resist this practice as it circumvents the appropriate role of the treating physician in establishing a consent dialogue. It also diminishes the psychiatrist's potential for providing therapeutic interventions for the disorders responsible for the patient's incapacity. At times, it is possible to improve capacity with interventions that target not only cognitive impairments, but also psychotic distortions, affective disturbances, and interpersonal and psychodynamic issues (Dunn & Jeste, 2001; Gutheil & Bursztajn, 1986; Schwartz & Roth, 1989).

Elements of Informed Consent

For a patient's choice to be considered valid, three essential conditions must be present: voluntariness, information, and competency.

VOLUNTARINESS   The process of decision making must be voluntary and free of coercion. Older persons commonly face multiple forces that pose risks to their ability to make voluntary decisions. Inequality in the power gradient between the infirm older patient and powerful physician or healthy family member may undermine self-determination (Kapp, 1999). Likewise, the environments in which patients are cared for often have inherently coercive features. For example, the culture of acute care hospitals is biased toward active care choices, therefore requiring deliberate dissent for patients who want to forgo such treatment.

The long-term care patient's ability to make voluntary decisions is particularly jeopardized by the institutional environment. It is difficult to maintain autonomy in an institution (often not one of the resident's choosing) in which most decisions are made by someone other than the resident. Serious diminutions of privacy and confidentiality further compromise the resident's sense of autonomy and self-determination. Roberts (2002) proposed a useful framework that organizes the influences on voluntarism into domains that include illness-related factors (e.g., pain, physical dependency), psychological issues, cultural and religious values, and external pressures.

INFORMATION   Consent given in the absence of sufficient information is not considered to be adequate consent. There are several competing standards that detail what type and how much information to disclose. Some jurisdictions have adopted the professional standard (also known as the reasonable physician or community standard). Under this standard, the sufficiency of information is judged by the amount and type of information that a reasonable health professional would reveal to the patient under similar circumstances.

Many jurisdictions support an alternative, the reasonable person (or objective) standard (Gutheil & Appelbaum, 2000; Kapp, 1999), which requires that the health care professional share the information that a reasonable person in the same situation would need to make an informed, intelligent decision (Kapp, 1999). The reasonable person standard is a halfway step between allowing physicians to determine which information is pertinent (as in the professional standard) and full disclosure. Full disclosure involves sharing all known and knowable significant and possibly pertinent information. Despite the challenges and impracticalities of full disclosure, it is advisable to attempt it, if possible, when the risks of a choice are grave.

Despite some variability in the information standards, most involve the following elements:

1. Diagnosis and nature of the condition
2. Nature and purpose of the proposed treatment
3. Risks and consequences
4. Expected benefits and probability of success
5. Available alternatives and their benefits and risks
6. Result if nothing is done and "nature takes its course"

When evaluating the decisional capacity of the patient who refuses treatment, the psychiatrist must learn what information has been disclosed to the patient. If risks and negative outcomes have been overemphasized, the patient may refuse the intervention out of fear and be deflected from needed care. Attempting to reconstruct what the patient has been told can be difficult as much of geriatric care is administered through a number of physicians and multidisciplinary teams. The patient may be dealing with multiple, conflicting items of disclosure, leading to confusion and erroneous conclusions.

COMPETENCY   Competency is one of the essential elements of the informed consent doctrine and the source of greatest confusion. Inconsistent definitions of terms are at the start of the confusion, with the terms *decisional capacity, decision-making abilities*, and *decisional competency* frequently used inconsistently and inaccurately.

Competency is a legal term; decisional capacity is a clinical determination. Every adult is presumed to be competent until something triggers a question of mental incapacity. Incompetency is determined only by a judge's express ruling, usually in probate court. Both decisional competency and decisional capacity are categorical determinations; a person either has or lacks decisional capacity to make a specific decision at that particular moment. Decisional abilities are the functional abilities necessary for decision making and are dimensional. That is, they are measurable to varying degrees (Kim et al., 2002).

Kim and colleagues (2002) further clarified that the competency evaluation is a two-step process. First, the clinician assesses the person's decisional abilities. Next, the clinician incorporates the results of this assessment with the important contextual factors, particularly the risk-benefit ratio of the options at hand, to determine the categorical judgment regarding the person's capacity or competency.

Standards of Competency.   Competency evaluations have long been hampered by disagreement over the standards of competency to be applied. There is no single test or scale of competency or capacity. This owes, in part, to the inherent characteristics of decisional capacity assessments, their specificity, their complexity, and the flexibility needed for application across a limitless range of treatment scenarios. Recently, of the numerous abilities relevant to competency described in the literature, four major elements have reached general consensus (Grisso et al., 1997):

1. The ability to *understand* relevant information
2. The ability to *reason* about the risks and benefits of options
3. The ability to *appreciate* the nature of one's situation, including the consequences of one's choices
4. The ability to *express a choice*

The presence of understanding had long been held as the most substantial element of competent decision making. However, factual understanding standards emphasize a somewhat limited, cognitive domain. These standards favor patients with good verbal skills and recall and are biased against the inarticulate, the less educated, or patients of lower intelligence (Stanley et al., 1984).

Appreciation requires a higher degree of understanding, beyond technical and intellectual comprehension of the information. Appreciation relates to forming adequate beliefs about how the given information applies to oneself (Saks et al., 2002). Appreciation brings in relevant personal and emotional components that should follow the logic of the individual's values and belief system (including minority religious beliefs) (Bursztajn et al., 1991; Drane, 1985; Saks et al., 2002). An older person might understand that selling her lifelong home means that it will no longer belong to her, but she may not appreciate the consequences of the sale—that she must find another place to live, and that her adjustment may be difficult (Gutheil & Appelbaum, 2000). Specific attention to the appreciation component should be triggered by patient choices that seem unreasonable, are high risk, or are inconsistent with long-held values (Drane, 1985). The development of valid and reliable appreciation assessments is essential, particularly to minimize evaluator subjectivity. Recently, the California Scale of Appreciation (CSA) was introduced; it attempts to make appreciation assessment operational (Saks et al., 2002).

In assessing decisional capacity, the clinician must determine which standard best applies to the clinical decision at hand. The choice of a rigorous capacity standard risks depriving some persons of their rights to make decisions or can subject patients to delays while proxies are secured or court involvement is sought. A less stringent standard, however, will fail to identify some impaired patients who should be protected from their own bad decisions. Most of the literature supports using a sliding scale model that selects capacity standards according to the risk of the decision at hand; when the net balance of benefits and risks is unfavorable, more stringent capacity standards are required (Buchanan & Brock, 1989; Drane, 1985).

Global Versus Specific Incapacities.   While some unfortunate individuals are globally incapacitated, more often incapacity is restricted to particular realms of decision making. Decisional capacity and competency are task specific; that is, they are specific to the particular situation and decision at hand. The importance of context cannot be overstated. Incapacity in one domain does not necessarily generalize to another. Incapacity to render a particular medical decision, for example, does not necessarily imply incapacity to execute a will, to drive, or to participate in certain research. It follows that capacity is not diagnosis dependent.

Although dementia and serious mental disorders are the most common reasons patients lack decisional capacity, having a psychiatric diagnosis does not imply that a patient necessarily lacks capacity. In most jurisdictions, even involuntarily committed mentally ill patients are presumed competent until proven otherwise, and they have a right to refuse treatment (although it is generally qualified). People who are psychotic can, and often do, retain significant capacities as long as psychotic defenses or serious frontal lobe impairments do not impede the awareness of their situation and specific decision-making ability.

Likewise, patients in the early and middle stages of Alzheimer's disease (AD) can retain certain decisional capacities, particularly if provided with the support and structure needed to navigate through the decision-making process (Appelbaum & Grisso, 1995; Dunn & Jeste, 2001; Grisso & Appelbaum, 1995; Grisso et al., 1995). Generally, patients with Alzheimer's disease show more decisional impairments when held to the understanding legal standard (Marson, Ingram, et al., 1995). But several studies have demonstrated that many subjects with mild to moderate Alzheimer's disease demonstrated adequate decisional abilities when legally relevant decisional standards such as choice, reasoning, appreciation, and comprehension were included in addition to the understanding standard (Kim et al., 2001; Marson, Ingram, et al., 1995; Stanley et al., 1988).

Structured Instruments and Decision-Making Abilities.   Existing neuropsychological tests can measure some of the cognitive functions found to be associated with impaired decision making. Not surprisingly, *executive cognitive functions*, defined as "those processes which orchestrate relatively simple ideas, movements, or actions into complex goal directed behavior" (Royall et al., 1992). have been identified as critically important to decisional capacity in AD (Kim et al., 2002; Marson et al., 1997). Impairments on tests such as the Executive Interview (EXIT) (Royall et al., 1992), Trails A (Bassett, 1999), tests of word fluency (Marson et al., 1996), and tests of conceptualization (Marson, Cody, et al., 1995) are often correlated with decisional incapacity.

Structured instruments to assess decision-making capacity have been created, most prominently the MacArthur Competence Assessment Tool (MacCAT-T for consent for treatment, MacCAT-CR for consent for clinical research) (Grisso et al., 1997; Grisso & Appelbaum, 1998a,b). The MacCAT assesses patient decision-making abilities in the 4 consensus areas—*understanding* information relevant to the condition and the recommended treatment, *reasoning* about potential risks and benefits of the choices, *appreciating* the nature of the situation and the consequences of choices, and *expressing a choice*. The advantages of using a systematic approach such as the MacCAT-T, particularly in high-risk or difficult situations, are that it ensures evaluation of a full range of capacities, provides documentation, and helps structure clinical conclusions.

Numerous other instruments have been developed to assess decisional abilities (Carney et al., 2001; Dymek et al., 2001; Janofsky et al., 1992; Kim et al., 2002). The Hopkins Competency Assessment Test (HCAT) consists of a brief essay about durable power of attorney (DPA) and a questionnaire to determine patients' understanding of the essay (Janofsky et al., 1992). The Capacity to Consent to Treatment Instrument (CCTI) (Dymek et al., 2001) tests competency performance and assigns outcomes (capable, marginally capable, incapable) according to 4 different legal standards. Instruments should be considered as aids in capacity evaluations, complementing rather than substituting for the full clinical examination. The further development and refinement of instruments for decisional ability is an area of intensive research.

Improving Capacity. It is the obligation of the clinician to maximize patients' abilities to participate in the informed consent process and to prevent older persons from being inappropriately judged as incapacitated. Decisional incapacity may be transient and reversible, fluctuating with the course of illness, with the setting and manner in which information is disclosed, and with transient stress reactions that can occur when the person is overwhelmed. Among the wide array of interventions found to significantly improve decisional abilities are improving the disclosure process by using smaller items of disclosure information or written memory aids, recognizing and remediating sensory impairments, including trusted others in the process, involving translators, addressing emotional issues, and evaluating decisional capacity over time (Grisso, 1998; Roberts & Roberts, 1999; Sugarman et al., 1998).

Identification of the specific neuropsychological processes involved in decisional incapacity may prove useful in enhancing capacity by providing specific remediation to that impairment or utilizing remaining strengths to bypass the impairment (Carpenter et al., 2000; Dunn & Jeste, 2001; Taub & Sturr, 1990). For example, a patient with short-term memory impairments can be helped by written memory aids; the patient's choices will still be honored as long as the patient consistently makes the same choice when presented with the same options and information (Stanley et al., 1984). Recent studies showed significant improvements in comprehension with repetition of consent information (Palmer et al., 2002), and Dunn and colleagues (2001, 2002) showed that an enhanced consent procedure (consisting of computerized slide show bullet points and key information) improved the comprehension of consent for older patients with psychosis. Ongoing research will further develop capacity improvement techniques and determine the scope and limits of their effectiveness.

Depression and Decisional Capacity. Geropsychiatrists confront difficult ethical problems when a depressed patient refuses life-sustaining treatment. A judgment must be made as to whether such refusal represents a long-standing autonomous desire or whether it derives from hopelessness, worthlessness, apathy, anger, or the death wish of depression. Much of the attention in capacity assessments has focused on cognitive capacities, but the meaning and weight that a patient gives to risks and benefits is influenced and possibly distorted by affective states (Blank et al., 2001; Bursztajn et al., 1991).

Seriously depressed patients, particularly if they are hopeless, overestimate the risks and underestimate the benefits of treatment (Ganzini et al., 1994) and may refuse treatment as an occult suicidal act. Less is known about the impact of mild-to-moderate depression on life-sustaining treatment decisions, although it appears to be more limited (Ganzini et al., 1994; Lee & Ganzini, 1992, 1994).

When the outcomes of decisions involve substantial risk, careful, systematic assessment of capacity should focus on the emotional components as well as the traditional cognitive components. The consequence of erroneously presuming depression as the cause of incapacity is that patients may be exposed to weeks of unwanted life-sustaining treatment while waiting for an antidepressant response. It is important for psychiatrists to keep in mind that, in the context of intractable suffering, hopelessness and helplessness may not be pathological in origin; some patients refuse treatment out of a sense that their quality of life is intolerable (Sullivan & Youngner, 1994). Further empirical work on the effects of depression on decisional capacity in a range of clinical situations is needed to inform clinical practice.

Consent for Electroconvulsive Therapy. Prejudices against electroconvulsive therapy (ECT) have resulted in the majority of states implementing additional regulations for ECT. Questions have been particularly focused on the adequacy of procedural safeguards for patients with compromised consent capacity (Levine et al., 1991). Formal regulations in some locations limit the conditions under which ECT can be provided and may require involvement of the court in treatment decisions. The clinician must be knowledgeable about any state and local laws regarding informed consent for ECT and the procedures required if the patient is involuntarily hospitalized or lacks capacity to give informed consent (American Psychiatric Association, 1990).

Informed Consent, Truth Telling, and Alzheimer's Disease. Until recently, AD was the prototype of a terminal, degenerative, and untreatable disorder. Some had argued that, without beneficial treatment to offer, informed consent was not relevant, and that there were psychological interests in withholding such information. The availability of effective medications has dramatically increased the importance of early diagnosis and truth telling for patients and their families (Kapp, 2002; Post & Whitehouse, 1998). Early diagnosis enables the patient to (1) plan to optimize experiences and relationships while relatively intact; (2) prepare advance directives, including durable power of attorney; (3) consider possible participation in AD research; (4) participate in AD support groups; (5) make an informed decision about antidementia agents; and (6) attend to estate and will issues (Post, 2001).

Informed consent is critical when considering the prescription of anti-dementia medications and genetic testing. While antidementia agents often provide benefit, for moderately demented individuals who have already adjusted to cognitive loss, the introduction of donepezil may result in temporary partial "awakenings" that force the patient and caregiver to cope with the crises of decline a second time (Post & Whitehouse, 1998).

In addition, if agents such as vitamin E and selegiline extend life, questions are raised as to whether this is a moral or reasonable outcome. Genetic testing in Alzheimer's disease is another area that requires careful informed consent. Clinical and research use of apolipoprotein E genotyping raises concerns about privacy, discrimination in access to insurance (particularly long-term care), employment, social stigma, and impact on family dynamics (National Institute on Aging/Alzheimer's Association Working Group, 1996; Post et al., 1997).

Cultural/Ethnic Considerations and Informed Consent. The informed consent doctrine, with its central principle of autonomy, reflects the rugged individualism inherent in traditional American culture and character. A growing body of national and cross-national literature suggests that autonomy should be balanced against culturally relevant moral concepts (Blackhall et al., 1995; Carrese & Rhodes, 1995; Gostin, 1995). The concept of respect for an individual's autonomy, codified by the informed consent doctrine, can be at odds with cultures that define persons by their relations to others and emphasize the embeddedness of the individual within society (Gostin, 1995).

Similarly, some cultures have ways of considering health and illness that are divergent from Western bioethics. Disclosure of "negative" information, such as discussing the risks of death or encouraging end-of-life care planning, may be regarded as harmful in cultures that believe that speaking of negative outcomes can shape reality (Carrese & Rhodes, 1995).

Geropsychiatrists work in an increasingly culturally pluralistic society and are likely to evaluate older persons of varied backgrounds. Genuine respect requires weighing other values along with autonomy, obtaining consent in ways that are comprehensible and consistent with the person's language and culture, and encouraging family and community participation in decision making when indicated.

Exceptions to Informed Consent. While courts hold that informed consent is central to the doctor-patient relationship, there is some flexibility in its application in certain circumstances. Among the recognized exceptions to informed consent are emergency situations (for which immediate medical treatment is required to preserve life or to prevent serious health impairments), waiver, and therapeutic privilege. In a true medical emergency, treatment may be initiated without informed consent, but only if there is no serious indication that the treatment would be refused were the patient able to make personal wishes known (Kapp, 1999).

In a waiver, a patient may surrender the right to make the decision and delegate responsibility to another person, including the physician. Current cohorts of elderly persons are less familiar with having an active role in medical decision making and, when stressed, are perhaps more prone to use this option, although generally it should be discouraged. The patient who waives the right to be informed essentially gives the physician permission to act paternalistically. Ideally, this waiver should be expressed (and carefully documented) rather than implied and should be accepted only after the physician has made clear that there exist risks and alternatives to the intervention and that the doctor is available to discuss them (Kapp, 1999).

The exception known as therapeutic privilege is the most controversial exception to informed consent. It allows some therapeutic discretion in the degree or manner of disclosure when the physician can document that the person is severely emotionally unstable or imminently imperiled, and that disclosure would likely "complicate or hinder necessary treatment" and "cause severe psychological harm" (Kapp, 1999, p. 35). Patients with dementia, for example, may respond to an overwhelming cognitive task with a catastrophic reaction of agitation and helpless panic. In this circumstance, temporary withholding of potentially harmful information is permissible, but disclosure should follow at a time when it is safer to do so. The use of therapeutic privilege has been construed very narrowly by the courts and, generally, should be avoided. If utilized, it is recommended that the clinician first seeks independent consultation, carefully document the rationale, and when possible, give full disclosure to next of kin (Kapp, 1999).

Surrogate Decision Making

The two broad types of formal surrogate decision-making arrangements are those that are established by the person before becoming incapacitated and those established by someone else for the already-incapacitated person.

BEFORE INCAPACITY Advance directives executed by the still-competent person are of two types: instructional directives, such as living wills and "do not" orders (do not resuscitate, do not intubate, etc.), and proxy directives, which include health care agents and durable power of attorney for health care (Grossberg, 1998).

Instructional directives express a competent person's desires and provide instructions that can be used in the event the person becomes incapacitated and cannot form or convey personal wishes. According to the provisions of the Patient Self-Determination Act (PSDA) of 1991, all persons entering a health care facility must be asked if they have an advance directive, and the directive (or documentation that none exists) must be entered into the record. The facility is also responsible for informing the person about its policy concerning which directives it will and will not honor. A shortcoming of the PSDA is that it does not apply to outpatient settings, which would be more suitable for discussion and encouragement of advance directives (Grossberg, 1998). Ideally, a health care directive will combine the person's "values history," goals, and "treatment specific directives" (Emanuel, 1991; Emanuel & Emanuel, 1989). Because even the most well thought out written directive cannot anticipate all possible circumstances, the advance directive should also designate a proxy decision maker.

Proxy directives are the various forms of power of attorney (POA) and must be prepared while the person is competent. General POA takes effect when the person (the principal or maker) is competent, but ceases if incompetency occurs. In a durable power of attorney (DPA), the principal delegates decision-making authority to a person of his or her choice (the agent or attorney-in-fact) with the transfer of decision making to be effective either immediately (immediate DPA) or on some specified occurrence (springing PDA), such as a physician's determination of the principal's incapacity (Kapp, 1999).

Joint ownership and trusts are often instituted by a competent person and the person's family and enable two or more people to co-own any investment that has a title. Each person has full control and rights of ownership, and thus this arrangement can be subject to abuse. Competent elderly persons can arrange for assets to be transferred legally to a trustee according to terms set forth in a trust document. Trusts continue to function after the person becomes incompetent.

Wills are the best-known advance directive and are discussed below with other specific competencies.

AFTER INCAPACITY   When incapacity is present, it is the responsibility of the clinician to seek valid proxy consent. State laws and regulations delineate who can make decisions for incapacitated persons. Informal arrangements involving the families and close friends are the most common means of providing surrogate decision making for incapacitated persons (Grossberg, 1996). When no decision maker is available or the incapacitated person objects to family involvement or is at risk because of the surrogate's incapacity or possible maltreatment, formal surrogate arrangements such as court-appointed guardianship should be considered.

Guardianship involves the judicial appointment of a guardian empowered to make personal or financial decisions for an incompetent individual (referred to as the ward). The judge determines that a person is fully or partially incompetent, with limited forms of guardianship taking over only the compromised areas of decision making. An example is the appointment of a conservator, whose control is usually limited to the ward's estate (Kapp, 1999).

General guardianship, also called a committee of the person or plenary guardian (depending on the jurisdiction), involves complete control over the ward. Appointment of a general guardian requires that the court be provided clear and convincing evidence of a substantial incapacity to manage one's affairs or to provide for oneself due to a specific disability (Ciccone, 1994). The ward loses most legal and civil rights and is reduced to the legal status of a child. The guardian makes decisions about medical treatment, living arrangements, finances, and contracts. The guardianship process can have far-reaching practical and emotional consequences for the patient and family (Gutheil & Appelbaum, 2000). In addition, it is often expensive and time consuming, usually requiring an attorney, court time, and monitoring.

Thorough capacity evaluations should include a comprehensive medical history; review of medical records and medications; physical, neurological, and psychiatric examinations, including formal mental status testing; and relevant laboratory tests (Grossberg, 1998). Functional abilities should be evaluated in the context of the demands on the patient in the patient's environment, that is, with attention to that person's responsibilities and supports. Individualized functional evaluation might focus on abilities for activities of daily living (ADLs), including household ADLs (meal preparation and kitchen safety, shopping, housework) and more advanced ADLs, including financial capacities. There is a surprising paucity of research to inform decisions regarding financial capacities, and instruments specific to financial capacities are in the development stage (Marson et al., 2000). Evaluations should include the ability to handle money, conduct cash transactions, use checks, pay bills, and manage finances with reasonable judgment so that self-interest is protected (Marson et al., 2000). Psychiatrists are well advised to check with objective corroborating sources when conducting such evaluations and to consider the extent of demands on the patient.

The steps in the guardianship process vary from state to state, but generally involve a petition filed with the court, a physician's deposition, service of notice to the respondent and interested parties, a court hearing, adjudication and appointment of a guardian, and in most states, monitoring.

Termination of guardianship can occur when the ward requests a hearing and convinces the court that personal competence is restored. Some jurisdictions require periodic reviews of incompetence, and others have automatic restoration of competence unless the guardian petitions for reappointment (Ciccone, 1994).

A representative payee is established to receive and manage, on the behalf of an incapacitated beneficiary, regular benefit payments from government institutions, such as pension and disability checks from the Veterans Administration or Social Security checks.

COMPLEXITIES OF MAKING DECISIONS FOR INCAPACITATED PERSONS When a surrogate makes a decision on behalf of an incapacitated person, two models guide the process: the substituted judgment model and the best interest model. Substituted judgment is the recognized legal and ethical model of surrogate decision making for incompetent patients (American Academy of Neurology Ethics and Humanities Subcommittee, 1996). Substituted judgment is an attempt to reproduce the decisions the patient would have chosen if competent. This model of decision making is geared toward preserving the right of self-determination, including the right to refuse treatment, for incompetent patients. While substituted judgment is the recognized legal/ethical standard for practice, its supremacy has been debated (Dresser, 1995; Fellows, 1998). Implementation may be complex even in the presence of written evidence of the patient's prior expressed wishes in the form of an advance directive. Enacting advance directives often requires degrees of extrapolation or brings ethical principles, particularly beneficence and respect for autonomy, into conflict.

Some ethicists argue that strict adherence to advance directives values the patient's past expressed views more than the experience the patient currently faces (Dresser, 1995; Emanuel, 1996; Fellows, 1998). The formulation of the advance directive may have been based on insufficient information and mistaken assumptions about hypothetical future situations. The sentiment made concrete by the advance directive, "I wouldn't want to live like that," does not allow for a change in perspective or the possibility that experiencing the disability may turn out to be more positive than the person had predicted. As Fellows (1998) wrote: "The advance directive standard ends as a riddle: the competent patient can decide but can't know the circumstances of the decision; the incompetent patient experiences these circumstances intimately but can no longer decide" (p. 925).

Best interest determinations may be necessary to prevent suffering, but can be highly subjective and value laden. When the best interest standard is used, the surrogate gives added weight to the cognitively impaired person's subjective experience and quality of life (Fellows, 1998). The many difficulties inherent in making judgments based on best interest may cast doubts on the legitimacy of this approach (Dresser & Whitehouse, 1994; Fellows, 1998; Sullivan, 2002). There is the danger that the surrogate's conclusions will reflect more about personal biases than the patient's interests. Evidence exists that physicians underestimate their older patients' quality-of-life ratings compared to the patients' views (Uhlmann & Pearlman, 1991).

Caution should be exercised in situations for which the outcome of a best interest judgment invalidates previously stated patient preferences. Although these situations often involve caring and protective wishes, there is the risk of reverting to paternalism, obviating the original purpose of the advance directive. While many patients may feel comfortable with their proxies having discretion to override their advance directives, for others this possibility could seriously undermine the trust they need to have in their system of care and

leave them fearful that their integrity will not be honored. The surrogate decision maker and clinician should seek balance, guided by the advance directive
and the principle of substituted judgment as much as possible but considering
the patient's best interests as necessary. Post's (1995) concept of stewardship
makes the previously capable "then" self one of the stewards, along with concerned friends and thoughtful caregivers, of the incapacitated "now" self.
Respecting prior competent wishes through advance directives should never
result in families and health care professionals standing by while the incompetent person suffers harm (Post, 1995; Sullivan, 2002).

It is especially difficult for proxies when decisions for the patient are in
conflict with the proxies' personal interests (Gutheil & Appelbaum 1983). Caring for a patient with dementia often becomes the center of the caregiver's
existence, so vastly altering their quality of life that it becomes difficult to separate the interests of each. Medical decisions often have dramatic impact on
both the patient and the caregiver. Obviously, families are more than surrogate
decision makers; for example, they are also crucial persons in relationship to
the patient with dementia (Holstein, 1998; Post, 1998). However, in situations
when the physician becomes concerned about the caregiver's motives, consultation should be sought with social workers, ethics committees, adult protective
services, or other appropriate professionals.

RESEARCH PARTICIPATION

Research participation involves many ethical principles, including justice (allowing older people to receive their fair share of potential benefits of clinical
research), nonmaleficence (causing no harm), respect (protecting autonomy),
and fidelity (privacy and confidentiality). Most older potential research subjects do not substantially differ from those who are younger and require no
additional protections. But two special populations deserve attention, those
with decisional incapacity from neuropsychiatric impairments and those residing in long-term care settings.

While many persons with neuropsychiatric illnesses retain capacity to consent to research or can make competent decisions with educational interventions (Carpenter et al., 2000), neuropsychiatric illnesses increase the likelihood
of decisional incapacity. Federal regulations allow consent to research by the
participant or by the "legally authorized representative" and defer to states on
the issue of who is a legally authorized representative for surrogate consent for
treatment and various activities. State laws, however, generally do not address
the question of when one can enroll another person in research (Appelbaum,
2002).

Geriatric psychiatry researchers have commonly approached persons
closely affiliated with the subject, usually a family member, for research consent, a practice sanctioned by the American Geriatrics Society Ethics Committee (AGS Ethics Committee, 1998). In the case of subjects with dementia,

family consent is often in conjunction with the subjects' assent. Appelbaum (2002) points out, however, that a legal gray zone currently exists because of lack of explicit definition of what constitutes a legally authorized representative for surrogate consent in the research context.

In addition, many questions exist regarding the extent and limits of the authority of surrogate decision makers in permitting research. In the treatment realm, there are clearly limits to what families can authorize; they are expected to make treatment choices that are consistent with the patient's interests and cannot authorize treatments that are of no benefit. The closer research resembles ordinary treatment, the more justification exists for allowing surrogate consent. But research often diverges from ordinary clinical treatment in important ways; there are often no direct benefits, discomforts or risks may be introduced, placebos may be utilized, and the personal care associated with clinical care can be sacrificed. Disagreement exists regarding whether it is ethically justifiable to include decisionally impaired subjects in research that offers no direct medical benefit or has greater than minimal risk.

It has been suggested that advance directives offer potential for research participation, as is the practice at the National Institutes of Health's Clinical Center (NIH, 1987), but research advance directives are a very partial solution at best (Appelbaum, 2002). The number of persons who would actually formulate them is expected to be very low, and they would have to be formulated before decisional capacity is lost. Much needed attention, including legislative change, is being drawn to creating solutions and safeguards to permit the enrollment of decisionally impaired subjects in appropriate research (Appelbaum, 2002; Oldham et al., 1999)

Nursing home residents considered for research participation are particularly vulnerable to exploitation. In addition to the concerns about decisional capacity, valid informed consent is jeopardized by encroachments on autonomy inherent in the institutional setting (Hayley et al., 1996; Roberts, 2002). Life within a "total institution" challenges the ability of even the cognitively intact persons to make free, voluntary decisions (Roberts, 2002). Can residents easily refuse to participate in a research project when they are profoundly dependent on staff? This is also problematic if the nursing home staff or doctors conduct the research and recruit the subjects. Clear safeguards need to be in place both to facilitate nursing home residents' participation in appropriate research and to protect them. Finally, regardless of setting, the objections of the decisionally incapacitated patient to participation should always be honored (at a minimum, the participation must be halted while the patient's objections are assessed), even over the consent of a surrogate.

NURSING HOME PLACEMENT

Most people hope not to become nursing home residents when they grow old. Geropsychiatrists are obliged to be patient advocates in the process of nursing home placement decisions. Becoming a nursing home resident can radically change a person's self-definition, may result in iatrogenic morbidity and mortality, and often deleteriously affects others' perceptions of the person. Fear of nursing home placement can precipitate depression, desperation, and suicide (Loebel et al., 1991). The increased dependency and diminished efficacy that results from institutionalization can markedly compromise the resident's capacity to function as an autonomous adult (Hayley et al., 1996; Kapp, 1998). Such erosions of status should be carefully weighed against whatever benefits to physical care derive from placement. Placements must be based on actual demonstrated, rather than predicted, failures to manage at home.

In theory, the process of nursing home admission is clearly defined and requires either the present decisional capacity of the resident or explicit, documented legal authority on the part of the surrogate. In reality, however, individuals sometimes have been "voluntarily" admitted even though they apparently lacked decisional capacity to participate fully in the decision, had not been formally found incompetent, and had no formally authorized surrogate decision maker (Kapp, 1998).

Typically, nursing home admission decisions occur in times of tremendous emotional and intellectual turmoil, acute illness, spousal death, or unraveling of support networks. Before the placement of an unwilling, incapacitated person, proper legal authority and protections must be in place. Involvement of the local long-term care ombudsman may be beneficial in ensuring that less restrictive alternatives have not been overlooked or discarded prematurely, and that the potential resident's interests are respected as much as possible. Ultimately, however, despite respect for personal autonomy, painful choices may be unavoidable, and the support of survival and physical functioning may come at the cost of greatly compromising the patient's enjoyment of life.

Physicians who provide care for nursing home residents are regularly challenged by numerous ethical and legal issues and regulatory requirements. Issues frequently encountered in this area include advance directives, capacity, life-sustaining treatment decisions, resident abuse, chemical and physical restraints, risk management, and participation in research. There are many excellent references that discuss the unique presentations of legal and ethical issues in long-term care (American Academy of Neurology Ethics and Humanities Subcommittee, 1996; Dawkins, 1998; Dodds, 1996; Goodwin et al., 1995; Hayley et al., 1996; Iwasiw et al., 1996; Kapp, 1998; Tinetti et al., 1991).

OTHER SPECIFIC CAPACITIES

Testamentary Capacity

Testamentary capacity refers to an individual's capacity to make or alter a will. To have testamentary capacity, persons must know and understand that they are making a will, the extent of their bounty, and the natural objects of their bounty (Ciccone, 1994). Because questions of testamentary capacity are more often raised with elderly than with younger persons, the testator or attorney should consider having a psychiatric evaluation or videotape made at the time of the will's preparation or signing (Grossberg, 1996).

When wills are contested, the geropsychiatrist may be requested to perform the difficult task of a posthumous assessment of the assumed competency of the testator. The usual questions here involve whether there is evidence of significant incapacity, and whether there is evidence that the testator was the subject of undue influence by others. Undue influence is frequently the basis on which wills are contested and is defined as "manipulation or deception in engaging the affections of the testator, significantly impairing the ability of the testator to freely decide on the distribution of his property" (Ciccone, 1994, p. 254).

Contractual Capacity

The law presumes competence of any adult who enters into a contract, but proof of decisional incapacity can void a transaction. To be found lacking contractual capacity, evidence must be presented to the court that the mental disability prevented the individual from understanding the nature of the transaction and acting in a reasonable manner (Ciccone, 1994). As with testamentary capacity, contractual capacity provides a mechanism for the protection of incapacitated individuals.

The Capacity to Work

Psychiatrists are sometimes involved in determining the "competency" of elderly persons to work productively or safely in a particular job. Boards of medicine, for instance, may refer elderly doctors for mandatory psychiatric evaluation when their continued skill or capacity is brought into doubt (Sprehe, 1994). These evaluations almost always require information from collateral sources about actual job performance.

Driving "Capacity"

Driving is a complex task that makes demands on attention, visual processing, judgment, memory, sequencing, and motor processing. Many age-related and illness factors contribute to decrements in the ability to operate a vehicle safely (Hunt et al., 1997; Marottoli et al., 1998). Although the majority of older persons have good driving records, the number of crashes, severity of injuries, and fatalities increase significantly after age 65 years (Ball & Owsley, 2000).

Current evidence demonstrates that car crashes of cognitively impaired older drivers often occur because of failure to notice other drivers at intersections or failure to yield (Rizzo et al., 2001). Drivers with Alzheimer's disease at a severity of Clinical Dementia Rating (CDR) 1 were found to pose a significant traffic safety problem both from crashes and from driving performance measurements. (Carr, 1997; Carr et al., 2000; Dubinsky et al., 2000; Hunt et al., 1993). Studies of the risk of accidents among drivers with early Alzheimer's disease CDR 0.5 (possible AD, slight forgetfulness, and slight impairment of activities) have yielded highly variable results. Some studies conclude that these individuals pose a danger and should be advised not to drive (Bonn, 2000), but other studies show mild impairments that are not measurably greater than those tolerated in other segments of the driving population (e.g., drivers aged 16 to 21 years and those driving under the influence of alcohol at a blood alcohol concentration less than 0.08%) (Dubinsky et al., 2000). More research is needed to determine methods to identify subsets of people with mild AD who can drive safely with certain restrictions.

It is essential that some reliable means be developed to identify those at high risk of motor vehicle accidents. Several medical conditions (history of stroke, transient ischemic attack, arthritis, falls), medications, and everyday functioning characteristics have been found to be correlated with driving risk (McGwin et al., 2000; Owsley et al., 1999; Sims et al. 2000). Efforts are being made to design neuropsychological batteries that test functions relevant to driving (Carr et al., 1998; Johansson et al., 1996; Lundberg et al., 1998; Marottoli et al., 1998). Objective tests need further development to capture and identify more reliably those who are at risk (Ball & Owsley, 2000; Lundqvist, 2001).

Revoking an elderly person's driving privileges is difficult, often drastically damaging the person's self-esteem, limiting daily functioning, and disadvantaging the ability to perform self-maintenance tasks, such as shopping and going to doctor appointments. Most states do not have systematic procedures to evaluate and prevent "unsafe" elderly drivers from driving (Hunt et al., 1997). The responsibility of geropsychiatrists with regard to compromised drivers is imprecisely delineated. Physicians should be alert to the possibility of impaired driving skills, identify and address reversible causes of impairment (including psychotropic medications), recommend driving evaluation when available, and inform and advise patients and families when there is a safety concern.

States vary tremendously in the criteria and required degree of detail for reporting motorists to the Department of Motor Vehicles. Some state statutes involve mandatory physician reporting of unsafe drivers, others require more frequent testing of older drivers, and still others require older drivers to provide medical documentation of their fitness to drive. The continuing development of driver competency assessment techniques and refinements of reporting requirements are needed to provide clinicians with guidelines that address public safety needs while attending to confidentiality concerns.

CONFIDENTIALITY

As a general ethical principle and legal rule, physicians have the duty to hold confidential all personal patient information. Older patients, who came of age prior to computers and mass communication, may assign an even higher value to privacy than do younger generations (Kapp, 1999). Unfortunately, elderly persons are particularly vulnerable to violations of confidentiality. This happens more often when they are dependent on others and when they receive care from health care teams or in congregate settings. But loss of mental capacity or physical independence should not include loss of privacy and respect.

As a general rule, physicians should be careful to ask elderly persons for permission to discuss their condition with family members. Some older persons may oppose disclosure of information about cognitive decline to family members, perhaps fearing that others will use it to undermine their self-determination. Also, it is optimal if physicians explain to patients that the team approach involves an expansion of the circle of confidentiality. In privileged communication, the privilege belongs to the patient, not to the therapist, and prohibits the therapist from disclosing information in court without the patient's permission or a court order.

SUMMARY

The care of older patients is intimately interwoven with legal and ethical challenges. Geropsychiatrists need to work knowledgeably with relevant legal and ethical issues that they encounter in clinical practice. In difficult situations, consultation should be sought from an attorney, ombudsman, or hospital ethics committee. When professionals skillfully and responsibly address the legal and ethical dimensions, the care of older persons is optimized and more humane.

REFERENCES

AGS Ethics Committee. Informed consent for research on human subjects with dementia. *J Am Geriatr Soc.* 1998;46:1308–1310.

American Academy of Neurology Ethics and Humanities Subcommittee. Ethical issues in the management of the demented patient. *Neurology.* 1996;46:1180–1183.

American Psychiatric Association. *The Practice of Electroconvulsive Therapy: Recommendations for Treatment, Training and Privileging. A Task Force Report.* Washington, DC: American Psychiatric Association; 1990.

Appelbaum PS. Involving decisionally impaired subjects in research: the need for legislation. *Am J Geriatr Psychiatry.* 2002;10:120–124.

Appelbaum PS, Grisso T. The MacArthur treatment competence study. I: Mental illness and competence to consent to treatment. *Law Hum Behav.* 1995;19:105–126.

Ball K, Owsley C. Increasing mobility and reducing accidents of older drivers. In: Shaie KW, Pietrucha M, eds. *Mobility and Transportation in the Elderly.* New York, NY: Springer; 2000:213–250.

Bassett SS. Attention: neuropsychological predictor of competency in Alzheimer's disease. *J Geriatr Psychiatry Neurol.* 1999;12:200–205.

Blackhall LJ, Murphy ST, Frank G, et al. Ethnicity and attitudes toward patient autonomy. *JAMA.* 1995;274:820–825.

Blank K, Robison J, Doherty E, et al. Life-sustaining treatment and assisted death choices in depressed older patients. *J Am Geriatr Soc.* 2001;49:153–161.

Bonn D. Patients with mild Alzheimer's disease should not drive. *Lancet.* 2000;356:49.

Buchanan AE, Brock DW. *Deciding for Others. The Ethics of Surrogate Decision Making.* Cambridge, UK: Cambridge University Press; 1989.

Bursztajn HJ, Harding HP Jr, Gutheil TG, et al. Beyond cognition: the role of disordered affective states in impairing competence to consent to treatment. *Bull Am Acad Psychiatry Law.* 1991;19:383–388.

Carney MT, Neugroschl J, Morrison RS, et al. The development and piloting of a capacity assessment tool. *J Clin Ethics.* 2001;12:17–23.

Carpenter WT, Gold JM, Lahti AC, et al. Decisional capacity for informed consent in schizophrenia research. *Arch Gen Psychiatry.* 2000;57:533–538.

Carr DB. Motor vehicle crashes and drivers with DAT. *Alzheimer Dis Assoc Disord.* 1997;11(suppl 1):38–41.

Carr DB, Duchek J, Morris JC. Characteristics of motor vehicle crashes of drivers with dementia of the Alzheimer type. *J Am Geriatr Soc.* 2000;48:18–22.

Carr DB, LaBarge E, Dunnigan K, et al. Differentiating drivers with dementia of the Alzheimer type from healthy older persons with a Traffic Sign Naming test. *J Gerontol A Biol Sci Med Sci.* 1998;53:M135–M139.

Carrese JA, Rhodes LA. Western bioethics on the Navajo reservation. Benefit or harm? *JAMA.* 1995;274:826–829.

Ciccone RJ. Testamentary capacity and guardianship. In: Rosner R, ed. *Principles and Practice of Forensic Psychiatry.* New York, NY: Chapman and Hall; 1994:252–257.

Dawkins VH. Restraints and the elderly with mental illness: ethical issues and moral reasoning. *J Psychosoc Nurs Ment Health Serv.* 1998;36:22–27.

Dodds S. Exercising restraint: autonomy, welfare and elderly patients. *J Med Ethics.* 1996;22:160–163.

Drane JF. The many faces of competency. *Hastings Cent Rep.* 1985;15:17–21.

Dresser R. Dworkin on dementia. Elegant theory, questionable policy. *Hastings Cent Rep.* 1995;25:32–38.

Dresser R, Whitehouse PJ. The incompetent patient on the slippery slope. *Hastings Cent Rep.* 1994;24:6–12.

Dubinsky RM, Stein AC, Lyons K. Practice parameter: risk of driving and Alzheimer's disease (an evidence-based review): report of the quality standards subcommittee of the American Academy of Neurology. *Neurology.* 2000;54:2205–2211.

Dukoff R, Sunderland T. Durable power of attorney and informed consent with Alzheimer's disease patients: a clinical study. *Am J Psychiatry.* 1997;154:1070–1075.

Dunn LB, Jeste DV. Enhancing informed consent for research and treatment. *Neuropsychopharmacology.* 2001;24:595–607.

Dunn LB, Lindamer LA, Palmer BW, et al. Enhancing comprehension of consent for research in older patients with psychosis: a randomized study of a novel consent procedure. *Am J Psychiatry.* 2001;158:1911–1913.

Dunn LB, Lindamer LA, Palmer BW, et al. Improving understanding of research consent in middle-aged and elderly patients with psychotic disorders. *Am J Geriatr Psychiatry.* 2002;10:142–150.

Dymek MP, Atchison P, Harrell L, et al. Competency to consent to medical treatment in cognitively impaired patients with Parkinson's disease. *Neurology.* 2001;56:17–24.

Emanuel L. The health care directive: learning how to draft advance care documents. *J Am Geriatr Soc.* 1991;39:1221–1228.

Emanuel L. Patients' advance directives for health care in case of incapacity. In: Cassel CK, Cohen HJ, Larson EB, eds. *Geriatric Medicine.* 3rd ed. New York, NY: Springer; 1996:993–1023.

Emanuel LL, Emanuel EJ. The medical directive. A new comprehensive advance care document. *JAMA.* 1989;261:3288–3293.

Fellows LK. Competency and consent in dementia. *J Am Geriatr Soc.* 1998;46:922–926.

Ganzini L, Lee MA, Heintz RT, et al. The effect of depression treatment on elderly patients' preferences for life-sustaining medical therapy. *Am J Psychiatry.* 1994; 151:1631–1636.

Goodwin PE, Smyer MA, Lair TI. Decision-making incapacity among nursing home residents: results from the 1987 NMES survey. National Medical Expenditure Survey. *Behav Sci Law.* 1995;13:405–414.

Gostin LO. Informed consent, cultural sensitivity, and respect for persons. *JAMA.* 1995; 274:844–845.

Grisso T, Appelbaum, PS. *Assessing Competence to Consent to Treatment: A Guide for Physicians and Other Health Professionals.* New York, NY: Oxford University Press; 1998a.

Grisso T, Appelbaum PS, eds. *MacArthur Competence Assessment Tool for Treatment (MacCAT-T).* Sarasota, FL: Professional Resource Press; 1998b.

Grisso T, Appelbaum PS. The MacArthur treatment competence study. III: Abilities of patients to consent to psychiatric and medical treatments. *Law Hum Behav.* 1995; 19:149–174.

Grisso T, Appelbaum PS, Hill-Fotouhi C. The MacCAT-T: a clinical tool to assess patients' capacities to make treatment decisions. *Psychiatr Serv.* 1997;48:1415–1419.

Grisso T, Appelbaum PS, Mulvey EP, et al. The MacArthur treatment competence study. II: Measures of abilities related to competence to consent to treatment. *Law Hum Behav.* 1995;19:127–148.

Grossberg GT. Advance directives, competency evaluation, and surrogate management in elderly patients. *Am J Geriatr Psychiatry.* 1998;6:S79–S84.

Grossberg GT. Medical-legal issues. In: Sadavoy J, Lazarus LW, Jarvik LF, et al., eds. *Comprehensive Review of Geriatriac Psychiatry.* 2nd ed. Washington, DC: American Psychiatric Press; 1996:1037–1049.

Gutheil TG, Appelbaum PS. *Clinical Handbook of Psychiatry and the Law.* Philadelphia, PA: Lippincott Williams & Wilkins; 2000.

Gutheil TG, Appelbaum PS. Substituted judgment: best interests in disguise. *Hastings Cent Rep.* 1983;13:8–11.

Gutheil TG, Bursztajn H. Clinicians' guidelines for assessing and presenting subtle forms of patient incompetence in legal settings. *Am J Psychiatry.* 1986;143:1020–1023.

Gutheil TG, Duckworth K. The psychiatrist as informed consent technician: a problem for the professions. *Bull Menninger Clin.* 1992;56:87–94.

Hayley DC, Cassel CK, Snyder L, et al. Ethical and legal issues in nursing home care. *Arch Intern Med.* 1996;156:249–256.

Holstein MB. Ethics and Alzheimer's disease: widening the lens. *J Clin Ethics.* 1998;9: 13–22.

Hunt L, Morris JC, Edwards D, et al. Driving performance in persons with mild senile dementia of the Alzheimer type. *J Am Geriatr Soc.* 1993;41:747–752.

Hunt LA, Murphy CF, Carr D, et al. Reliability of the Washington University Road Test. A performance-based assessment for drivers with dementia of the Alzheimer type. *Arch Neurol.* 1997;54:707–712.

Iwasiw C, Goldenberg D, MacMaster E, et al. Residents' perspectives of their first 2 weeks in a long-term care facility. *J Clin Nurs.* 1996;5:381–388.

Janofsky JS, McCarthy RJ, Folstein MF. The Hopkins Competency Assessment Test: a brief method for evaluating patients' capacity to give informed consent. *Hosp Community Psychiatry.* 1992;43:132–136.

Johansson K, Bronge L, Lundberg C, et al. Can a physician recognize an older driver with increased crash risk potential? *J Am Geriatr Soc.* 1996;44:1198–1204.

Kapp M. *Geriatrics and the Law.* 3rd ed. New York, NY: Springer; 1999.

Kapp M. "A place like that," advance directives and nursing home admissions. *Psychology Public Policy Law.* 1998;4:805–828.

Kapp MB. Legal standards for the medical diagnosis and treatment of dementia. *J Legal Med.* 2002;23:359–402.

Kapp MB. Medical treatment and the physician's legal duties. In: Cassel CK, Cohen HJ, Larson EB, eds. *Geriatric Medicine.* 3rd ed. New York, NY: Springer; 1996: 979–991.

Kapp MB. Proxy decision making in Alzheimer disease research: durable powers of attorney, guardianship, and other alternatives. *Alzheimer Dis Assoc Disord.* 1994; 8(suppl 4):28–37.

Kim SY, Caine ED, Currier GW, et al. Assessing the competence of persons with Alzheimer's disease in providing informed consent for participation in research. *Am J Psychiatry.* 2001;158:712–717.

Kim SYH, Karlawish JHT, Caine ED. Current state of research on decision-making competence of cognitively impaired elderly persons. *Am J Geriatr Psychiatry.* 2002;10: 151–165.

Lee M, Ganzini L. The effect of recovery from depression on preferences for life-sustaining therapy in older patients. *J Gerontol.* 1994;49:M15–M21.

Lee MA, Ganzini L. Depression in the elderly: effect on patient attitudes toward life-sustaining therapy. *J Am Geriatr Soc.* 1992;40:983–988.

Levine SB, Blank K, Schwartz HI, et al. Informed consent in the electroconvulsive treatment of geriatric patients. *Bull Am Acad Psychiatry Law.* 1991;19:395–403.

Lidz CW, Appelbaum PS, Meisel A. Two models of implementing informed consent. *Arch Intern Med.* 1988;148:1385–1389.

Loebel JP, Loebel JS, Dager SR, et al. Anticipation of nursing home placement may be a precipitant of suicide among the elderly. *J Am Geriatr Soc.* 1991;39:407–408.

Lundberg C, Hakamies-Blomqvist L, Almkvist O, et al. Impairments of some cognitive functions are common in crash-involved older drivers. *Accid Anal Prev.* 1998;30: 371–377.

Lundqvist A. Neuropsychological aspects of driving characteristics. *Brain Inj.* 2001;15: 981–994.

Marottoli RA, Richardson ED, Stowe MH, et al. Development of a test battery to identify older drivers at risk for self-reported adverse driving events. *J Am Geriatr Soc.* 1998;46:562–568.

Marson DC, Chatterjee A, Ingram KK, et al. Toward a neurologic model of competency: cognitive predictors of capacity to consent in Alzheimer's disease using three different legal standards. *Neurology.* 1996;46:666–672.

Marson DC, Cody HA, Ingram KK, et al. Neuropsychologic predictors of competency in Alzheimer's disease using a rational reasons legal standard. *Arch Neurol.* 1995; 52:955–959.

Marson DC, Hawkins L, McInturff B, et al. Cognitive models that predict physician judgments of capacity to consent in mild Alzheimer's disease. *J Am Geriatr Soc.* 1997;45:458–464.

Marson DC, Ingram KK, Cody HA, et al. Assessing the competency of patients with Alzheimer's disease under different legal standards. A prototype instrument. *Arch Neurol.* 1995;52:949–954.

Marson DC, Sawrie SM, Snyder S, et al. Assessing financial capacity in patients with Alzheimer disease: a conceptual model and prototype instrument. *Arch Neurol.* 2000;57:877–884.

McGwin G Jr, Sims R, Pulley L, et al. Relations among chronic medical conditions, medications, and automobile crashes in the elderly: a population-based case-control study. *Am J Epidemiol.* 2000;152:424–431.

National Institute on Aging/Alzheimer's Association Working Group. Apolipoprotein E genotyping in Alzheimer's disease. *Lancet.* 1996;347:1091–1095.

National Institutes of Health (NIH). *Report and Recommendations: Research Involving Those Institutionalized as Mentally Infirm.* 1987 National Commission for the Protection of Human Subjects of Biomedical and Behavioral Research. Washington, DC: Author; 1987.

Oldham JM, Haimowitz S, Delano SJ. Protection of persons with mental disorders from research risk: a response to the report of the National Bioethics Advisory Commission. *Arch Gen Psychiatry.* 1999;56:688–693.

Owsley C, Stalvey B, Wells J, et al. Older drivers and cataract: driving habits and crash risk. *J Gerontol A Biol Sci Med Sci.* 1999;54A:M203–M211.

Palmer BW, Nayak GV, Dunn LB, et al. Treatment-related decision-making capacity in middle-aged and older patients with psychosis: a preliminary study using the Mac-CAT-T and HCAT. *Am J Geriatr Psychiatry.* 2002;10:207–211.

Post SG. Alzheimer disease and the "then" self. *Kennedy Inst Ethics J.* 1995;5:307–321.

Post SG. Dementia care ethics. In: Weisstub DN, Thomasma DC, Gauthier S, et al., eds. *Caring for Our Elders.* Dordrecht, Netherlands: Kluwer Academic; 2001:177–190.

Post SG. The fear of forgetfulness: a grassroots approach to an ethics of Alzheimer's disease. *J Clin Ethics.* 1998;9:71–80.

Post SG, Whitehouse PJ. Emerging antidementia drugs: a preliminary ethical view. *J Am Geriatr Soc.* 1998;46:784–787.

Post SG, Whitehouse PJ, Binstock RH, et al. The clinical introduction of genetic testing for Alzheimer disease. An ethical perspective. *JAMA.* 1997;277:832–836.

Rizzo M, McGehee DV, Dawson JD, et al. Simulated car crashes at intersections in drivers with Alzheimer disease. *Alzheimer Dis Assoc Disord.* 2001;15:10–20.

Roberts LW. Informed consent and the capacity for voluntarism. *Am J Psychiatry.* 2002; 159:705–712.

Roberts LW, Roberts B. Psychiatric research ethics: an overview of evolving guidelines and current ethical dilemmas in the study of mental illness. *Biol Psychiatry.* 1999; 46:1025–1038.

Royall DR, Mahurin RK, Gray KF. Bedside assessment of executive cognitive impairment: the executive interview. *J Am Geriatr Soc.* 1992;40:1221–1226.

Saks ER, Dunn LB, Marshall BJ, et al. The California Scale of Appreciation: a new instrument to measure the appreciation component of capacity to consent to research. *Am J Geriatr Psychiatry.* 2002;10:166–174.

Schwartz HI, Roth LH. Informed consent and competency in psychiatric practice. In: Tasman A, Hales E, Frances A, eds. *American Psychiatric Press Review of Psychiatry.* Washington, DC: American Psychiatric Press; 1989:409–431.

Sims RV, McGwim G Jr, Allman RM, et al. Exploratory study of incident vehicle crashes among older drivers. *J Gerontol A Biol Sci Med Sci.* 2000;55A:M22–M27.

Sprehe DJ. Geriatric psychiatry and the law. In: Rosner R, ed. *Principles and Practice of Forensic Psychiatry.* New York, NY: Chapman and Hall; 1994:501–507.

Stanley B, Guido J, Stanley M, et al. The elderly patient and informed consent. Empirical findings. *JAMA.* 1984;252:1302–1306.

Stanley B, Stanley M, Guido J, et al. The functional competency of elderly at risk. *Gerontologist.* 1988;28:53–58.

Sugarman J, McCrory DC, Hubal RC. Getting meaningful informed consent from older adults: a structured literature review of empirical research. *J Am Geriatr Soc.* 1998; 46:517–524.

Sullivan MD. The illusion of patient choice in end-of-life decisions. *Am J Geriatr Psychiatry.* 2002;10:365–372.

Sullivan MD, Youngner SJ. Depression, competence, and the right to refuse lifesaving medical treatment. *Am J Psychiatry.* 1994;151:971–978.

Taub HA, Sturr JF. Evaluating informed consent for research: a methodological study with older adults. *Educ Gerontol.* 1990;16:273–281.

Tinetti ME, Liu WL, Marottoli RA, et al. Mechanical restraint use among residents of skilled nursing facilities. Prevalence, patterns, and predictors. *JAMA.* 1991;265: 468–471.

Uhlmann RF, Pearlman RA. Perceived quality of life and preferences for life-sustaining treatment in older adults. *Arch Intern Med.* 1991;151:495–497.

39

Financial Issues

Helen H. Kyomen, MD, MS
Gary L. Gottlieb, MD, MBA

INTRODUCTION

In this chapter, we examine key financial issues that affect the psychiatric care of older adults. Essential details specific to reimbursement of geropsychiatric services are provided, and relatively recent changes in third-party payment mechanisms are described. An understanding of the terminology and subtleties of these financing mechanisms should help providers cope with some of the systematic barriers to the care of this exceptionally needy population.

Financing strategies have closely shaped the development of psychiatric services for older adults (Goldman et al., 1987; Goldman & Frank, 1990). Mental health benefit structure, payment mechanisms, and associated policy have influenced patient and provider incentives, which have had an impact on the identification of patient populations, the organization of services, the sites of service delivery, the mix and behavior patterns of providers, and the process of evaluation and treatment. Therefore, it is reasonable to infer that outcomes of geropsychiatric care depend on reimbursement for service delivery. Beginning in 1965, with the implementation of Medicare and Medicaid, a substantial proportion of the financial responsibility for the psychiatric care of elderly persons in the United States shifted to the federal government (Medicare) or to shared responsibility between the states (Medicaid) and the federal government.

In 1965, before the initiation of Medicare, only about half the population aged 65 years or older in the United States had health insurance. Today, 96%

of the elderly are enrolled in the Medicare program (Moon, 2001). Most acute psychiatric inpatient services provided to elderly patients, together with limited outpatient geropsychiatric specialty services, are paid for via the Medicare system and its various supplemental coverages, including Medicaid. In 2000, health care spending by federal, state, and local governments rose to $587 billion, or 45% of the nation's total health care expenses, an increase from 40% in 1990 (Levit et al., 2002).

The substantial growth in recent years in psychiatric services in private and general hospital settings was stimulated by the fee-for-service framework of these programs and changes in private indemnity insurance coverage. The massive state hospital deinstitutionalization movement of the 1950s and 1960s, combined with the availability of shared federal-state financing via the Medicare and Medicaid programs, resulted in a shift of the primary venue for chronic geropsychiatric care from state hospitals to privately owned and managed, largely Medicaid-financed, nursing homes. Limitations in Medicare reimbursement, changes in the nursing home industry, and insurance reforms continue to affect the process and content of psychiatric care for elderly patients.

A working knowledge of the organization of the geriatric mental health delivery system and the mechanisms for payment for health and mental health services for elderly individuals in the United States is fundamental for optimizing geropsychiatric service delivery. Both individual practitioners and organized care systems providing psychiatric services to elderly persons must understand the financing system and how to use it effectively if they wish to provide geropsychiatric services of the highest quality achievable within the prevailing structure.

DEMOGRAPHIC TRENDS AND THE ECONOMICS OF AGING

The elderly are a fast-growing population for whom financial access may pose a significant barrier to mental health care. Financial barriers may impose a particular burden for some groups, such as women and ethnic minorities, due to lower incomes and, in some instances, greater need.

The size, diversity, and need of the aging population shape the economic environment of geriatric mental health care. In the mid-1950s, only 1 of every 11 Americans was older than 65 years. By the end of the 1980s, about 1 in 8 Americans was older than 65 years. In 2003, about 1 in 7 Americans was 65 years or older. The American elderly population grew by 23% to nearly 31 million during the 1980s. As a result of relatively small Depression era birth rates, the older population grew more slowly in the 1990s; still, there were over 35 million people older than 65 years living in the United States in 2000 (US Bureau of the Census, 2000). Projected expansion rates suggest that there will be about 39 million older Americans by 2010. Shortly thereafter, the aging of the post–World War II baby boom cohort will cause dramatic growth in the population segment older than 65 years. By the year 2030, about one fourth of the population (approximately 66 million people) will be in this age group.

Gender differences in life expectancy and the distribution of minorities among the elderly have important economic consequences. There are approximately 1.5 women for every man older than 65; this trend continues for those older than 85 years (US Bureau of the Census, 2000). Surviving women are adversely affected by lower educational levels, traditional work roles, and diminished Social Security and pension provisions compared to men (Pamuk et al., 1998; Vartanian & McNamara, 2002). In general, continued earning potential from work throughout the life span and from fixed sources of income in late life are less for women than for men. Generally, older women have more limited financial resources than older men. Inasmuch as they usually live longer than their spouses, women are more likely than men to become dependent on adult children and on government-related resources to meet social and medical needs (Soldo et al., 1997).

Ethnic minorities make up a growing segment of the older population. In 1990, about 11% of persons older than 65 years were nonwhite. By the year 2025, about 25% of elderly individuals are expected to be from minority groups (US Bureau of the Census, 2000). Life expectancy at birth for whites exceeds that for African Americans by about 8%, and at 65–74 years of age, mortality rates for African Americans are higher than those for whites (Minino & Smith, 2001). Elderly African Americans have considerably higher rates of poverty and illness than whites in the same age group (Hobbs, 2001). Economic and social discrimination and the underprivileged standing associated with minority status in the United States are exacerbated by the socioeconomic realities of older age: Accrued social and financial resources are limited, barriers to preventive and acute health care are more substantial, and access to non–health care governmental services, including housing, transportation, meals, and income maintenance, is compromised. Cultural differences may also affect the expression of illness and the ways in which American health care, designed for a predominantly white population, is accessed by non-white Americans (Crose & Minear, 1998; Minear & Crose, 1996).

The distribution of wealth and income among older adults is highly variable. Examined cross-sectionally, postretirement incomes in 1998 in households with the head of household aged 65 years or older averaged only 48% of preretirement incomes in households with the head of household aged 47 to 64 years (Wolff, 2002). Most older adults derive postretirement income from a combination of Social Security benefits, public or private pensions, and income from savings or investments (Soldo & Agree, 1988; Wolff, 2002). The magnitude of these earnings depends almost entirely on preretirement income. After age 70, only about 10% of men and 4% of women are in the labor force (Wolff, 2002). In addition to these financial consequences of retirement, leaving the workforce may affect health insurance premium costs, the types of insurance available, and the possibility of participating in some health delivery systems (e.g., some health maintenance organizations [HMOs] and other managed-care systems).

For many, reduction of income associated with retirement may affect the standard of living adversely. Older adults may suffer the consequences of poverty for the first time in their lives (Furino & Fogel, 1990; Wolff, 2002). In 2000, 3.4 million elderly (10.2%) in the United States had incomes below the poverty level. Another 2.2 million, or 6.7% of the elderly, were "near poor" (with incomes between the poverty level and 125% of this level). These rates are even more dramatic for women and for minorities. Older women had a higher poverty rate (12.2%) than older men (7.5%) in 2000. One of 12 (8.9%) elderly whites were poor in 2000, compared to 22.3% of elderly African Americans and 18.8% of elderly Hispanics. Above-average poverty rates for elderly were found for those who lived in central cities (12.4%), in rural areas (13.2%), and in the South (12.7%) (Dalaker, 2001). Poverty and aging are not synonymous, however. Indeed, almost 13% of households headed by individuals older than 65 years have net assets in the top 5% of American families.

This disparity in distribution of wealth has an important effect on health and welfare policy. Lawmakers frequently do not recognize the socioeconomic heterogeneity of the older population. As a consequence, social welfare programs such as Social Security and Medicare do not address completely the financial and health care needs of all older adults. Resulting gaps are filled unevenly by programs for indigent individuals. These inequities are particularly important in mental health and long-term care, for which out-of-pocket payments make up a substantial component of costs to consumers (Letsch, 1993).

Since 1970, the older population has grown twice as rapidly as the rest of the population. Because many of the programs that benefit older adults depend on contributions from the younger population, the growing ratio of older Americans to younger persons may affect society's ability to supply the goods, services, and payments necessary to meet this expanding demand. There are currently about 19 Americans older than 65 years per 100 people aged 18 to 64 years. This so-called dependency ratio is expected to double by 2050 (Hollmann et al., 2000). Emerging policy is likely to require the older generation to support a larger share of its own needs. Elimination of mandatory retirement age policies and the shift of the American economy from heavy industry to less physically demanding service and technology production may extend the working longevity of the population.

Medicare, the predominant payor for medical and psychiatric services for the elderly, has been based on a shared financial risk policy throughout its history. Medicare beneficiaries pay a substantial share of the cost of their health care services out of pocket. These circumstances have substantial relevance to the provision of psychiatric services to elderly Medicare beneficiaries.

THE MEDICARE SYSTEM

Enacted in 1965 and initiated on July 1, 1966, under Title XVIII of the Social Security Act, Medicare is a social insurance program first designed to provide medical care benefits for Americans older than 65 years (Cutler & Fine, 1985; Iglehart, 1992; US Senate Committee on Finance, 1978). The program was developed in response to years of debate regarding national health insurance policy, supported with data derived from a comprehensive evaluation of the needs of elderly individuals provided by the Senate Select Committee on Aging. In 1972, the program was expanded to include younger disabled individuals and older individuals not eligible for social security, but willing to pay a monthly premium for coverage. In 1973, Medicare coverage was extended to provide medical coverage for individuals experiencing end-stage renal disease. Of Americans aged 65 years or older, 96% are currently enrolled in the Medicare program (Moon, 2001).

The Medicare program consists of two principal components, Parts A and B. Eligible Medicare beneficiaries are entitled to Medicare Part A (hospital insurance) at no premium cost and are able to supplement it with Medicare Part B (supplementary insurance) and private "Medigap" insurance.

Medicare benefits are designed to cover acute care services primarily. Long-term care and outpatient prescription medications are among the excluded benefits. Some services, including outpatient mental health care, are subject to limitations in coverage and substantial copayments.

Medicare and Medicare-Supplemental Financing Mechanisms

MEDICARE PART A   By virtue of participation in the Social Security system, most Americans older than 65 years are entitled to Medicare Part A coverage, which was originally funded by a 0.7% payroll tax, shared equally by employers and employees. The maximum taxable amount of annual earnings in 1966 was $6,600. Today, the Medicare payroll tax is 2.9%, and all earnings, with no earnings cap, are taxable (Centers for Medicare and Medicaid Services, 2003).

Part A covers inpatient hospital services, skilled nursing facility (SNF) benefits following a hospital visit of at least 3 days, home health visits following a hospital or SNF stay, hospice care, and blood provided in the hospital (after the member has paid for the first three pints).

Hospital-Based Coverage for General Medical Services.   Part A hospital coverage is intentionally limited to coverage of relatively brief inpatient stays, presumably for stabilization of acute conditions. Regulations provide coverage for spells of illness. A *spell* is defined as an inpatient episode that begins with inpatient admission and ends with the close of the first period of 60 consecutive days after discharge. It is possible for a patient to be discharged and readmitted on several occasions during a given episode of illness and still be considered to be in the same spell as long as 60 days have not elapsed between discharge and admission. For admission to general hospitals, there is no limit on the number of spells or "total lifetime" days covered. However, the maximum number of covered days during a single spell is 150.

There are different levels of coverage for various lengths of hospitalization. These are delineated in Table 39-1.

Skilled Nursing Facility–Based Coverage.   Part A also provides limited coverage for care in SNFs. Services provided by domiciliary, personal care, and intermediate care facilities are not reimbursable by Medicare. To obtain SNF benefits, an individual must have been hospitalized for at least 3 consecutive days, and admission must occur within 30 days of hospital discharge. Hospital Insurance covers up to 100 days of SNF care. SNF care costs the beneficiary nothing during the first 20 days, after which a copay of $105 (in 2003) per day is required until SNF day 100, after which the beneficiary pays all costs (Centers for Medicare and Medicaid Services, 2003). For beneficiaries receiving SNF care, the need for continued skilled care must be reassessed and documented regularly. Similarly, home health care services are limited and must be related to acute and remediable conditions (Centers for Medicare and Medicaid Services, 2003).

Development of the Prospective Payment System and Diagnosis Related Groups.   There are two main mechanisms for reimbursing hospital-based care

TABLE 39-1.   Medicare coverage by length of hospitalization

Days of hospitalization	Medicare coverage/patient costs
Days 1–60	Medicare pays in full after a deductible equal to the average cost of 1 day of hospitalization ($840 in 2003) has been paid by patient
Days 61–90	Patient covers 25% per hospital day copayment
Days 91–150 (lifetime reserve days)*	Patient covers 50% per hospital day copayment
Days beyond 150	Patient covers all costs†

*Coverage for these days may be used electively during any episode, but can be used only once during a patient's lifetime. For example, if a patient requires three hospitalizations totaling 110 days with no period of discharge as long as 60 days, the patient would have 40 reserve days of remaining coverage in his or her lifetime for subsequent spells lasting longer than 90 days. Patients may elect to save these days for future prolonged hospitalizations and use other financial resources for payment of any part of the costs of days 91–150.

†With the exception of a brief period during 1989–1990, at which time the Catastrophic Coverage Act of 1988 was in effect, there has been no annual limitation on the out-of-pocket liability of Medicare recipients (Centers for Medicare and Medicaid Services, 2003).

that have an impact on psychiatric treatment: (1) a prospective payment system (PPS) based on diagnosis related groups (DRGs), which largely applies to psychiatric treatment for patients in beds scattered throughout general hospitals; and (2) a retrospective payment system with Tax Equity and Fiscal Responsibility Act (TEFRA) capitation rates that are based on payment patterns derived from the first fiscal year after 1982, which mainly applies to freestanding psychiatric hospitals and general hospital psychiatric units.

From 1966 to late 1983, Medicare Part A paid for all inpatient care through a retrospective, cost-based reimbursement system. To prevent depletion of the Hospital Insurance trust fund, Congress and the Reagan administration enacted TEFRA in 1982. TEFRA emphasized cost containment, providing for limits on all inpatient operating costs and establishing target rates for cost increases. Incentives were developed to provide reduced hospital reimbursement if cost limitation targets were not met and extra payments if limits were not exceeded. Reimbursement limits were adjusted to reflect patient mix, geographic location, and training costs. TEFRA mandated replacement of the system of cost-based reimbursement with a PPS (English et al., 1986; Frazier et al., 1986; Scherl et al., 1988; Wells et al., 1993).

Public Law 98-21 of the Social Security Amendments of 1983 (Public Law 98-21, 1983) established a PPS for Medicare payments for inpatient services. The PPS is based on a patient-discharge classification system using DRGs to cluster patients who presumably require similar care. The DRG system categorizes patients into 23 general major diagnostic categories and then assigns each discharge to one of 468 DRGs derived from principal and secondary diagnoses, procedures rendered, and to a lesser degree, age, sex, comorbidity, complications, and discharge status. Hospitals are paid a predetermined amount for each case according to the DRG assigned. This sum essentially is independent of actual costs incurred. Therefore, the payment system is considered to provide incentives for efficient utilization of resources. If patients consume extraordinary resources or require prolonged inpatient care, they are classified as *outliers*, and Medicare provides additional payments to the hospital, but at rates considerably less than actual cost.

Of the DRGs, 14 apply to discharges related to treatment of psychiatric disorders. Concerns regarding the ability of DRGs to accurately predict resource consumption for psychiatric disorders led to exemptions from this payment method for freestanding psychiatric hospitals and for distinct psychiatric units in general hospitals. However, treatment of primary psychiatric patients in "scatter" beds on general medical and surgical units is reimbursed through the DRG system.

Research on the Application of Diagnosis Related Groups to Psychiatric Treatments. Research regarding the application of DRGs to treatment of patients with principal psychiatric diagnoses has substantiated their inaccuracy in prediction of resource consumption. DRGs have been shown to account for only a limited proportion (16%–40%) of the variation in individual length of stay for all diagnoses. Moreover, they are considerably less accurate in predicting psychiatric utilization, generally accounting for less than 8% of the variance (English et al., 1986; Frank & Lave, 1985; Goldman, 1988).

A comprehensive assessment by the American Psychiatric Association of DRG data (English et al., 1986) suggested that similarities among patients within a given psychiatric DRG are extremely limited. Patients who require very brief psychiatric hospitalizations are frequently clustered by the DRG system with individuals in need of much longer hospital stays. Analysis of study data indicated that DRGs favor less severely ill patients and settings that provide short-term evaluation and limited treatment (English et al., 1986).

Medicare Reimbursement for Treatment in Freestanding Psychiatric Hospitals and General Hospital Psychiatric Units. Although there is no limit on the total number of hospitalizations or inpatient days covered for medical or surgical diagnoses or for psychiatric care in general hospitals, coverage for inpatient psychiatric care in facilities recognized by the Centers for Medicare and Medicaid Services (until 2001 known as the Health Care Financing Administration [HCFA]) as freestanding psychiatric hospitals is limited to a total of 190 days during an individual's lifetime. In addition, if an individual becomes eligible for Medicare during the course of a first episode of psychiatric hospitalization, Medicare's local intermediary may elect to cover less than the full 150 benefit days of that spell of illness. This provision is designed to restrict Part A psychiatric benefits to the active component of treatment and to avoid full reimbursement for a person who may have been institutionalized for long periods of time.

Freestanding psychiatric hospitals and exempted psychiatric units in general hospitals continue to be paid retrospectively by Medicare, subject to caps established under TEFRA that were originally based on payment patterns derived from the first full fiscal year after 1982. The Balanced Budget Act of 1997 (BBA 1997) modified and substantially limited these reimbursements. Under TEFRA, Medicare reimbursement for treatment at these sites was capped at a target rate established for each facility based on resource utilization during a "base" year (the first full fiscal year of operation after October 1, 1983). If the actual cost per case exceeds the target rate, the hospital must absorb this loss. Until 1998, if the cost was less than the TEFRA capped rate, the hospital could retain 50% of the difference up to 5% of the target rate. Based on a series of adjustments specified in the BBA 1997, differential caps, with or without wage adjustment, were established based on different percentiles of the national median of the target amount for hospitals in the same class for cost-reporting periods ending during fiscal year 1996. The BBA also put into place less-generous bonus and relief payments for PPS-exempt facilities.

The Balanced Budget Refinement Act of 1999 (BBRA 1999) addressed some of the flawed policy and excessive payment reductions resulting from BBA 1997. The BBRA 1999 provided for wage adjustments, amounting to payments at the 75th percentile limit established by the BBA 1997 for PPS-exempt facilities that received their first Medicare payment before October 1, 1997. In addition, BBRA 1999 provided increased bonus payments for psychiatric hospitals, from 1.0% to 1.5% for cost-reporting periods beginning on or after October 1, 2000, and before September 30, 2001, and 2.0% for cost-reporting periods beginning on or after October 1, 2001, and before September 30, 2002.

Implications of Medicare Payments Under Prospective Diagnosis Related Groups and Retrospective Tax Equity and Fiscal Responsibility Act Caps for Geriatric Psychiatry. For hospitals that care for a substantial number of geriatric patients with complex problems, the payment scheme is even more arbitrary than DRGs. As geriatric psychiatry expands as a field, recognition and aggressive treatment of acute mental disorders in Medicare recipients are more widespread. This likely will translate into greater resource consumption in acute care settings. Therefore, the employment of relatively old utilization experience (i.e., 1984 or 1985 for established institutions) to set payment limits for geriatric psychiatry may result in de facto per-case reimbursement at rates that have little correspondence with patient needs or diagnoses.

The nature of psychiatric disorders in elderly individuals makes these incentives worrisome. Incomplete evaluation of complicated patients in settings that are discouraged from employing expensive, but often necessary, diagnostic technologies may result in preventable disability and ultimately generate substantially greater costs (Fogel et al., 1990). In addition, the high prevalence of medical disorders among older adults with psychiatric diagnoses makes both DRGs and TEFRA caps even less appropriate. The presence of active medical diagnoses among patients treated by psychiatric personnel in scatter beds or in exempt units has not been examined in research assessing the validity of these payment mechanisms.

Wells and coworkers (1993) evaluated the effects of the PPS on various aspects of quality of care and other outcomes for older adult patients with depression who required hospitalization. They compared data for patients who were hospitalized for depression in acute care general medical hospitals just prior to TEFRA (1981–1982) with those collected shortly after its full implementation (1985–1986). This analysis determined that the quality of "psychological" components of care improved after implementation of the PPS. However, even in light of the improvements noted, the authors determined that the overall quality of care received by geriatric patients with depression was in the low-to-moderate range. The authors recognized that some of the improvement noted could have been attributable to the development of geriatric psychiatry as a field and to various significant improvements in treatment technology. These authors found no improvement in the quality of nonpsychological medical care provided. Additional research is needed, and new data that assess the effectiveness of care and focus on long-term functional and psychiatric outcomes are necessary.

A number of alternative mechanisms have been proposed to allow implementation of an effective PPS for inpatient psychiatry. Although several analytic methods that substantially improve predictability of length of stay and other measures of resource consumption are now available, no system has yet been tested with adequately large data sets in a way that reflects the extremely differentiated nature of the mental health care delivery system (Bartels, 2002; Goldman, 1988). Research in this area remains active, and potential improvements in policy in the near future are possible. Final rules regarding implementation of a PPS for inpatient psychiatry are pending.

MEDICARE PART B   Medicare Part B covers doctors' services, outpatient care, diagnostic tests, ambulatory services, durable medical equipment, outpatient and occupational therapy, clinical laboratory services, limited home health care, outpatient hospital services, blood provided on an outpatient basis, and of primary interest here, specialty mental health services. Medicare Part B also covers a number of preventive services, such as screenings for breast, cervical, vaginal, colorectal, and prostate cancer; testing for loss of bone mass; diabetes monitoring and self-management; and influenza, pneumonia, and hepatitis B vaccinations.

Coverage for Psychiatric Services Provided by Physicians.   Medicare Part B is partially financed by beneficiary premiums that originally covered 50% of the program's costs. General tax revenues finance the balance of Part B. Persons choosing Part B services in 2003 pay a premium of $58.70 per month (Centers for Medicare and Medicaid Services, 2003) or approximately one quarter of the actual cost of the coverage. In addition, most of Medicare Part B services, including psychiatric services, are subject to an annual deductible of $100 (Centers for Medicare and Medicaid Services, 2003) and a variably determined copayment. For nonpsychiatric physician services and psychiatric inpatient services, a 20% copayment is required. For outpatient initial psychiatric evaluation and for outpatient management of psychotropic drugs, the copayment rate is 20%; a 50% copayment is required for other outpatient psychiatric services. This provision is prejudicial for psychiatry in comparison with other services. Coverage of medical and surgical visits has never been limited by number of visits or costs of resources consumed. However, when Part B psychiatric benefits were designed, mental illness was depicted as "lacking precise diagnostics and established treatment protocols expected to lead to specified outcomes within a defined period of time" (Cutler & Fine, 1985, p. 20). Therefore, coverage for outpatient psychiatric treatment was limited severely. From the initiation of Medicare in 1966 through early 1988, total annual reasonable charges for mental health services were set at $500 per beneficiary, and the law required that the maximum annual Medicare reimbursement for outpatient psychiatric services was $312.50 per person or 62.5% of reasonable charges, whichever was lower. The 80% federal share, which was the maximum amount paid by Medicare to the psychiatrist, was only $250 per beneficiary per year.

The Omnibus Budget Reconciliation Act of 1987 (OBRA 87; Pub L No. 100-203) recognized, in part, the discrimination against services for mental disorders inherent in the Supplemental Medical Insurance benefit. Coverage for outpatient psychiatric services was increased to $2,200 annually in 1989. However, the 50% copayment for these outpatient services remained. In addition, services for the medical management of psychiatric disorders were exempted from the $2,200 limit and made subject to the same 20% copayment required for nonpsychiatric outpatient services. The Omnibus Budget Reconciliation Act of 1989 (OBRA 89; Pub L No. 101-239) provided further improvement of the psychiatric benefit. Effective July 1, 1990, the annual dollar limit for outpatient mental health services was eliminated by OBRA 89. However, the discriminatory 50% copayment and 190-day lifetime psychiatric hospital utilization limit were unaffected by the new law.

Coverage for Nonphysician Mental Health Services Under Medicare. OBRA 89 was also revolutionary in its expansion of coverage provided by nonphysician providers. Until the enactment of this legislation, necessary mental health services delivered by psychologists, social workers, therapists, nurses, and aides were reimbursable only if performed under the "direct supervision" of a physician. Direct supervision had been defined as immediate availability to provide assistance at the time of service. Exceptions to this rule included psychological testing and services provided by psychologists in some community mental health settings.

The new OBRA legislation provided for direct reimbursement of psychologists in all settings. Also mandated was direct reimbursement of clinical social worker services at a rate of 80% of the actual charge or 75% of the amount paid to a psychologist, whichever was less, except for services provided to an inpatient of a hospital or SNF as required for the facility's participation in Medicare. OBRA 89 specified criteria regarding consultation with a physician for these nonphysician providers. These criteria were vague and somewhat superficial: The provider must document that the patient has been informed of the desirability of consultation with the patient's primary care physician to consider potential medical conditions that may contribute to the patient's condition. In addition, the provider must document written or verbal communication with the primary physician regarding the patient's treatment unless the patient specifically refuses such contact. The law made no provision for assessment or consultation with a psychiatrist. Under OBRA 89, reimbursement for services provided by psychiatric nurses and other therapists continued to require direct physician supervision. However, under BBA 1997, physician assistants and nurse practitioners were allowed to bill Medicare Part B directly, as authorized under state licensure laws, with reimbursement set at 85% of the Physician Fee Schedule effective January 1, 1998 (BBA 1997).

Under OBRA 89, for payment for direct patient treatment or evaluation, it is required that Medicare be billed. Services rendered by telephone and patient contacts that do not involve evaluation of patient status (e.g., renewing a prescription) are not reimbursable. However, charges for obtaining treatment information from relatives or close associates of a patient who is unreliable or uncommunicative are allowable. Family counseling services are covered only when the purpose of counseling is to facilitate treatment of the identified patient.

Provider Options Under Medicare. There are currently two procedures available for Medicare beneficiaries to receive benefits for provider services under Part B:

1. A provider may agree to accept assignment from Supplemental Medical Insurance and thereby accept the Medicare-approved fee as payment in full. The fiscal intermediary (FI) pays the approved amount, less copayment and deductible, to the provider directly. The copayment and deductible must be collected from the patient. Physicians who are Medicare participants are required to accept the Medicare-approved level of assigned payment. Physicians who are not Medicare participants may elect to accept assignment on a claim-to-claim basis.

2. A Medicare nonparticipating provider may elect not to accept assignment. Nonparticipating providers may charge up to 115% of the Medicare-approved fee for the procedures they perform. However, Medicare pays unassigned claims at a rate that is 95% of the Medicare-approved fee, less copayments and deductibles. Providers must bill patients directly for the entire service charge as Medicare makes unassigned claim payments to the patient. In addition, since April 1, 1990, all providers are required to accept assignment from Medicare beneficiaries who are also recipients of Medicaid and from all Medicare recipients who are at or below the federal poverty level (OBRA 89).

Medicare offers several incentives for physicians to participate, including a 5% higher payment rate than for nonparticipating physicians and provision of directories of participating physicians to senior citizen groups and the public. However, payment reductions (5.4% in 2002) may cause more physicians to deselect Medicare participation and refuse assignment due to the overall decreases in Medicare reimbursement relative to cost. The recent declines in Medicare reimbursement have been associated with a multiplier system, linked to the gross national product (GNP), that has been used to implement rate changes. The effects of this multiplier system were ameliorated, to some extent, by corrections to this reimbursement formula that were proposed and passed in Omnibus Appropriations bill House Joint Resolution 2 (H.J. Res. 2) in February 2003. As a result, an increase of approximately 1.6% in physician fees for the remainder of 2003 was estimated.

Medicare Methodology for Establishing Procedure Codes: The Resource-Based Relative Value Scale System. Since Medicare implementation of the PPS for hospital services, the annual growth rate for costs of physicians' services has been more than twice the rate of growth for inpatient hospital services. Part B expenditures currently account for about one third of Medicare expenditures (Letsch, 1993).

OBRA 89 provided for the development of expenditure targets, or volume performance standards, to control growth in physician services. The volume performance standards are based on fee increases, growth in the size of the Medicare population, changes in service volume and intensity, and a volume performance factor.

In addition, OBRA 89 provided for the development of a uniform Medicare fee schedule to replace Medicare's traditional method of payment based on determination of customary, prevailing, and reasonable charges ascertained for individual physicians. The OBRA 89 fee schedule is based on a resource-based relative value scale (RBRVS), developed after extensive research led by Hsiao and colleagues (1988, 1992) and substantial input from the Physician Payment Review Commission (1989) and professional groups nationally. The RBRVS system was used to determine the relative values of about 7,000 physician services, based on three measurable components: the work required to perform the procedure, associated practice and malpractice insurance expenses, and the amortized value of the opportunity costs for training in a specialty. (This last component is not included in fee determination.) Fee schedule amounts are based on a weighted average of specialty-specific practice expense and malpractice insurance premium cost data, with approximately 60% of each fee adjusted for geographic variations in cost (Hsiao et al., 1992). The product of each relative value and a monetary conversion factor determines the fee for each service.

The transition to the new fee schedule began in 1990 with reductions in payments for "overvalued procedures." Existing fee schedules for anesthesia and radiology were adjusted to conform to the RBRVS fee schedule. For most other specialties, the RBRVS fee schedule was implemented in 1992, with a gradual phase-in of adjustments occurring until 1996.

In an effort to correct for perceived overvaluation of noncognitive procedures, the RBRVS placed strong emphasis on cognitive assessment, patient management, and caring activities performed by providers (Hsiao et al., 1988, 1992). Procedure codes from the Current Procedural Terminology (CPT) (American Medical Association, 1990) were then employed to describe the procedure performed.

Unfortunately, efforts to apply the RBRVS system to psychiatry were seriously flawed. The case vignettes employed to assess time and intensity of required services were simplistic and unrepresentative of psychiatric practice. Measurements of clinical work performed and of practice costs were inconsistent, and efforts to develop work scenarios comparable to those encountered in other specialties considered the circumstances of psychiatric care unrealistically. In addition, the CPT codes for psychiatry were extremely broad and therefore difficult to map onto the activities associated with specific vignettes (Fogel et al., 1990; Sharfstein, 1990). Despite several technical surveys, the

Medicare fee schedule for psychiatric services did not result in improved valuations for these predominantly cognitive services. Notably, just prior to the implementation of RBRVs, a modification in the fee schedule resulted in increased payment for psychotherapy codes, although without adjustment in other psychiatric codes that reflect similar work.

A summary of the mental health services covered under Medicare Part A and Part B is provided in Table 39-2.

HEALTH MAINTENANCE ORGANIZATION AND MEDICARE + CHOICE (MEDICARE PART C) OPTIONS
Since the mid-1980s, Medicare beneficiaries have been able to enroll in private HMOs as an alternative to remaining in the traditional Medicare fee-for-service program. The percentage of individuals in managed Medicare plans increased into the mid-1990s, but has been declining since then due to departure of numerous health plans from the Medicare managed-care market because of declining reimbursement rates. As of July 1, 2000, there were 6.3 million Medicare HMO enrollees, down 2.8% from 6.4 million enrollees on July 1, 1999 (InterStudy Publications, 2001). On average, the service costs have been higher for Medicare HMO enrollees than they would have been if the same enrollees had remained in the traditional fee-for-service program (General Accounting Office, 2002). Managed Medicare accounts for a relatively small proportion of overall Medicare expenditures, particularly within mental health managed care.

As part of the 1997 Balanced Budget Act, Congress created Medicare + Choice (so-called Part C) to increase beneficiary choice of health plan and to attempt to control rising spending for Medicare benefits (Balanced Budget Act of 1997). Medicare Part C built on the Medicare HMO program by expanding the type of plans beneficiaries could choose; it also reformed the payment system affecting some of these plans. The Part C plans generally allow members to visit only health care providers agreeing to treat members of the plan and often require members to obtain a referral to see specialists. Medicare makes a set payment every month to the care plan private insurer or HMO that the Medicare beneficiary chooses. Some plans offered by private insurers and HMOs provide benefits that are not covered by traditional Medicare, such as outpatient prescription drugs, and these plans are allowed to charge additional monthly premiums for these added benefits. Medicare + Choice provides extensive benefit options for Medicare beneficiaries, including the following:

Private fee-for-service (private FFS) plans

Medical savings account (MSA) plans

Preferred provider organizations (PPOs)

HMOs

Provider-sponsored organizations (PSOs)

For eligible persons who make application, Medicare/Medicaid dual coverage (DUAL coverage)

TABLE 39-2. Beneficiary payments for psychiatric services in the traditional Medicare fee-for-service system

Service	2003 Payment by Patient
Part A	
Psychiatric inpatient	
Deductible for each illness episode	$840
Copayment, days 61–90	$210/day
Copayments for lifetime reserve days 91–150	$420/day
Lifetime limit	190 days
Skilled nursing facility	
Days 21–100	$105.00/day
Beyond 100 days	All costs
Home health care	
Durable medical equipment	20% of approved amount
Blood, after first 3 pints	All costs
Part B	
Medical expenses	$100 annual deductible
Outpatient mental health services*	50% of approved charges*
Outpatient substance abuse services	50% of approved charges†
Physician (non–mental health) services	20% of approved charges
Physician not accepting assignment	100% allowable excess charges
Monthly premium	$58.70/month
Other costs not covered by Medicare	
Routine medical examinations	All costs
Outpatient prescription drugs‡	All costs‡
Long-term care	All costs
Care outside the United States	All costs
Services not medically necessary	All costs
Dental, hearing, and vision care	All costs

Source: http://www.medicare.gov/Coverage.

*Medicare covers outpatient mental health services provided by a physician, psychologist, clinical social worker, clinical nurse specialist, or physician's assistant.

†Covered when provided at a Medicare-certified treatment center.

‡Medicare covers a limited number of drugs and antigens that cannot be self-administered. These are erythropoietin, pneumococcal vaccine and flu shots, immunosuppressive drugs connected with covered organ transplants, and oral anticancer drugs if they are of the same chemical entity as similar drugs that are administered intravenously.

Medicare basically pays all of the Medicare + Choice plans the same amount per beneficiary. Each plan must provide at least the same level of benefit as the original Medicare program. The benefits available under any of these options do not replace the original program, but instead provide for additions that supplement basic Medicare.

The private FFS plans are regular indemnity insurance plans with their own fee schedules, which may be higher or lower than Medicare's schedule. These plans typically have higher payment schedules than basic Medicare so that enrollees will have access to physicians and facilities that otherwise would not accept current Medicare fee schedules. It was expected that this arrangement would broaden access to physicians and other providers for Medicare beneficiaries.

The MSA program is a 4-year pilot program that combines a savings account and a catastrophic medical plan option. The difference between the catastrophic plan premium and the Medicare health plan payment goes into a savings account that the retiree can subsequently use to pay for any expenses related to health care. If all of the funds are not used in a given year, the following year's deposit is added to the balance. The MSA plan operates very much like the popular flexible health care spending accounts to which many workers have access during their years of employment. The catastrophic plan component is similar to the private fee-for-service plan, with the exception that there is a high deductible for catastrophic coverage.

The PPO option is similar in concept to what many pre-retirees currently have as a health benefit through their employment. The beneficiary electing PPO coverage has access to a PPO network of providers and is charged according to PPO-negotiated discounted rates. Retirees also have the option to go outside the PPO network of providers to obtain treatment, but then the beneficiary payments (coinsurance and deductibles) are typically higher than if network providers were used.

The HMO option is a continuation of the pre–Balanced Budget Act 1997 Medicare HMO option that attracted many Medicare beneficiaries, especially in the 5-year period prior to enactment of the 1997 law. Generally, under these HMO plans, Medicare beneficiaries must use the HMO's network of providers to receive a benefit, although exceptions are made in emergency circumstances.

The PSOs, a newly available option under BBA 1997, may be the fastest-growing Medicare option in certain locations. Hospital and physician groups sponsor these plans. They are expected to be especially popular in rural areas, particularly in communities in which only a single hospital/physician group is available.

With DUAL coverage, the Medicare/Medicaid beneficiary participates in a structured plan very similar in its organization and operation to the PPO/HMO/PSO plans, with the main difference that both basic and supplemental coverage are paid with public funds.

For elderly persons in managed-care plans, an additional mechanism intended to control health care expenditures is the mental health "carve out" (Frank et al., 1996). This mechanism provides for a separate preapproval and service limitation system, administered by a third-party contractor, for treatment of psychiatric conditions. These carve-out contractors are most commonly large, for-profit companies or group practices specializing in managed mental health care. Psychiatric carve outs may focus on utilization control, without prioritizing patient care and outcomes, and this may have a disproportionate impact on certain covered subgroups that are primarily elderly (Kihlstrom, 1998).

To our knowledge, no data quantifying whether these carve-out programs significantly affect the quality of care provided to Medicare/Medicaid beneficiaries with psychiatric conditions are yet available. However, these programs have been put into operation to attempt to control putative overutilization, so it seems likely that their net effect will be to reduce the volume of services provided to elders with problems with psychiatric illness. A review of carve-out programs available to Medicare beneficiaries demonstrates a consistent lack of required training in the care of the elderly, lack of specific protocols for older adult care, and a paucity of special services for institutionalized older persons. In addition, the disconnection of psychiatric and medical care in this population is potentially perilous (Gottlieb, 1998).

The Medicare + Choice program essentially has created a whole new level of government-sponsored health care. In many regions, Medicare beneficiaries have several options that were not previously available. The Balanced Budget Act of 1997 also established a new method of determining Medicare reimbursements to health plans that, in most areas, has resulted in lower increases in aggregate cost from year to year. Indeed, in many areas, increases in Medicare payment to health plans are limited to 2% per year. However, this can result in larger increases in beneficiary payments. Table 39-3, which uses example data for 1999 and 2000, illustrates how this "leveraging" effect works.

Prior to the initiation of Medicare + Choice, the federal government's strategy for managing growing Medicare costs had been to encourage Medicare beneficiaries to enroll in HMO senior plans. As recently as 1998, senior plan HMO enrollment was growing at a rate of about 80,000 new members per

TABLE 39-3. The leveraging effect of Medicare

	1999	2000	Change, %
Total cost of care	$500	$520	4
Payment by Medicare	$460	$469	2
Beneficiary's Medicare + Choice premium rate	$40	$51	27.5

month nationally. Changes in Medicare's formula for paying HMO senior plans, brought about by the Balanced Budget Act of 1997, resulted in substantial cutbacks in Medicare payments to HMOs, and numerous HMOs across the nation closed their senior plans during 1998 and 1999. This forced hundreds of thousands of Medicare beneficiaries who had elected HMO senior plans to select a non-HMO Medicare option.

Summary of Medicare-Covered Mental Health Services

Specialty mental health services for older adults account for only a relatively small fraction of Medicare expenditures. In 1997, outlays for treatment of psychiatric and substance abuse disorders were about 4.7% of total Medicare spending, excluding dementia care (Coffey et al., 2000). The relative underutilization of specialty mental health services by older Medicare beneficiaries results from the reinforcement of longstanding provider- and patient-induced barriers to care by economic disincentives and systematic stigmatization.

Currently, Medicare mental health benefits include the following (US Department of Health and Human Services, 1999a):

- Inpatient psychiatric care if in a general hospital or psychiatric unit of a general hospital (few limits). In a freestanding psychiatric hospital, coverage is for 190 days (lifetime).
- Outpatient psychotherapy that requires a 50% copayment, while a 20% copayment is required for medical management, diagnostic services, and professional services for evaluation.
- Partial hospitalization in a structured program of intensive services for those in acute psychiatric distress who would be hospitalized without these services. Certification by a physician is required. This benefit is unlimited. A 20% copayment is required. Services can be provided by approved community-based mental health centers, hospital-based programs, or freestanding partial hospital programs. There are about 1,150 Medicare-certified community mental health centers and about 1,000 hospital outpatient departments that provide these services (HCFA, 1998; National Alliance for the Mentally Ill [NAMI], 2000).
- Previously, based on a systematic identification of this diagnosis, Medicare routinely rejected charges for psychiatric services for patients with Alzheimer's disease. These actions were rooted in the incorrect belief that an individual with Alzheimer's disease could not benefit from various interventions. In September 2001, the Centers for Medicare and Medicaid Services issued a memorandum with instructions directing Medicare contractors not to install system edits that would automatically deny claims for reimbursement for Medicare-covered services based solely on a diagnosis of dementia. Instead, Medicare carriers were advised to judge, on a case-by-case evaluation of the patient's needs and

capabilities, the appropriateness of billings for services provided to patients with Alzheimer's disease.

The most important gaps in Medicare's mental health benefits include the following (NAMI, 2000):

- Lack of prescription drug coverage. The new generations of psychotropic medications (e.g., atypical antipsychotic and selective serotonin reuptake inhibitor medications) represent major advances in treatment technology for the mental health field. Some Medicare managed-care and Medigap plans cover prescription drugs, but many beneficiaries have no prescription drug coverage. Congress is debating various proposals that would add a prescription drug benefit to Medicare, and legislation, if it develops from this debate, would address this issue.
- Differences in copayments. A 50% copayment is required for beneficiaries who use outpatient psychotherapy services, while the required copayment is only 20% for most other outpatient health services. HCFA estimates that about 33% of Medicare beneficiaries have secondary coverage for this additional coinsurance from Medigap or Medicaid plans.
- Limited coverage of community-based services. Community care programs such as crisis intervention teams, assertive community treatment teams, psychosocial rehabilitation, wraparound services, or intensive case management for persons with severe mental illnesses are not covered under Medicare. These kinds of care coordination approaches have been successful in helping older adults remain in their homes and preventing or delaying their admission to costly acute care or extended care institutions.

In addition, there is significant variation in local intermediary interpretation of Medicare policy, resulting in dramatically different levels of reimbursement or types of covered services regionally.

INSURANCE COVERAGE SUPPLEMENTING MEDICARE

Medicare provides broad coverage of basic health care services, including mental health services, but it does not cover outpatient prescription drugs, has relatively high deductibles, and has no cap on out-of-pocket spending. To help with Medicare's cost-sharing requirements and fill gaps in the benefit package, most beneficiaries have supplemental insurance (Figure 39-1). In 1999, of all Medicare beneficiaries, 9% had basic Medicare coverage only. More than 90% had supplemental Medicare coverage, including 36% with employer-sponsored retiree health benefits, 27% with Medigap policies, 17% with Medicare + Choice coverage (including Medicare HMO enrollment), and 11% with dual Medicaid-Medicare coverage (Rice & Bernstein, 1999).

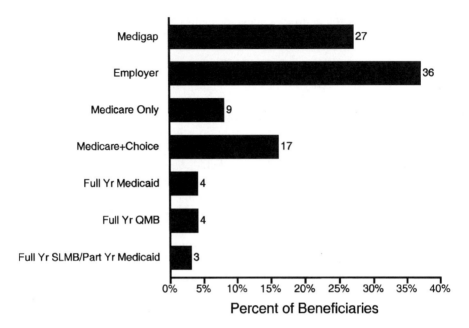

FIGURE 39-1. Supplemental coverage of Medicare beneficiaries, 1999. (QMB, qualified Medicare beneficiary; SLMB, specified low-income Medicare beneficiary.)

Supplemental coverage varies substantially by income level. About half of poor beneficiaries (49%) have Medicaid assistance; in addition, about 12% of the near poor have Medicaid. There are 1 in 6 (16%) Medicare beneficiaries with incomes below twice the poverty level who have no supplemental coverage, compared with 7% of higher income beneficiaries. Over half (52%) of the group with incomes over 200% of the poverty level have retiree health benefits, twice the rate in the near-poor subgroup.

Medigap Insurance

Medicare beneficiaries can purchase Medigap policies to cover some or all of the deductibles and copayments associated with receipt of Part A or B Medicare services, as well as some additional services. Federal legislation, known as the Baucus amendment, enacted in the Omnibus Reconciliation Act of 1980 (OBRA 80) established criteria for a voluntary certification program that most states implemented. Under the Baucus amendment, Medigap plans were to provide minimum benefits and meet minimum loss ratios, as well as provide information to prospective purchasers and prohibit abusive marketing practices of agents and their companies.

Congress later enacted the Omnibus Budget Reconciliation Act of 1990 (OBRA 90), which replaced voluntary state certification with national requirements that all Medigap policies sold after July 1992 conform to 1 of 10 standardized sets of benefits that the National Association of Insurance Commissioners developed as "model" policies. These policies encompass various combinations of benefits, including (1) core benefits that include coverage of all Medicare Part A coinsurance for stays longer than 60 days, the 20% Medicare Part B coinsurance, and the Parts A and B blood deductible; (2) SNF coinsurance; (3) Medicare Part A deductible; (4) Medicare Part B deductible; (5) Medicare Part B excessive charges; (6) foreign travel; (7) at-home recovery; (8) prescription drugs; and (9) preventive medical care (Rice et al., 1997).

Medigap premium costs vary widely by market location and underwriting category. Underwriting categories include such factors as sex, age, and past health status. The average premium for these Medigap policies increased significantly in the 1990s. From 1994 through 1998, the average price of one of the most commonly purchased Medigap policies rose an estimated 41% (Lieberman, 1998). For a large proportion of retired couples, buying Medigap policies may add up to 10% of the total household income (Rice & Bernstein, 1999). Medigap plans offering prescription drug coverage commonly are extremely expensive due to adverse selection.

Mental Health Parity Within Supplemental Insurance Coverage

Until the enactment of the Mental Health Parity Act (MHPA) of 1996 through the Health Insurance and Portability and Accountability Act of 1996 (HIPAA), psychiatric and other mental health services were consistently reimbursed at lower rates than most other medical or surgical benefits. The MHPA is a federal law that prohibits group health plans sponsored by companies with more than 50 employees from placing annual or lifetime dollar limits on mental health benefits that are lower or less favorable than annual or lifetime financial limits for medical and surgical benefits offered under the benefits packages. Although the law requires "parity," or equivalence, with regard to dollar limits, there are significant limitations to the MHPA.

For example, the MHPA does not require group health plans and their health insurance issuers to include mental health coverage in their benefits package. If the group health plan has separate dollar limits for mental health benefits, the dollar amounts that the plan has for treatment of substance abuse or chemical dependency (both of which can affect mental health adversely) are not included when totaling the limits for mental health benefits and medical and surgical benefits to determine if there is parity. Coverage under MHPA does not apply to group health plans sponsored by employers with fewer than 51 workers or to individual health insurance coverage.

Group health plans may impose some restrictions on mental health benefits and still comply with the law. For example, MHPA does not prohibit group health plans from increasing copayments or limiting the number of covered visits for mental health benefits, even if the plan does not impose similar visit limits for medical and surgical benefits; MHPA does not prohibit different cost-sharing arrangements, such as higher coinsurance payments, for mental health benefits compared to medical and surgical benefits. These and other specifications greatly hinder the effectiveness of MHPA in achieving true parity of mental health benefits for patients. Medicare regulations implementing the MHPA were effective at the beginning of 1998.

BENEFICIARY OUT-OF-POCKET
PAYMENTS UNDER MEDICARE

Eligible Medicare beneficiaries are entitled to Medicare Part A (hospital insurance) at no premium cost and are able to supplement it with Medicare Part B and private supplementary insurance. Persons choosing Part B services in 2003 paid a premium of $58.70 per month or approximately one quarter of the actual cost of the coverage. In 1965, elderly persons spent, on average, about 19% of their income on health care. That share fell to about 11% in 1968; in 2001, it was estimated to be more than 20% (Maxwell et al., 2001). The most vulnerable beneficiaries spend an even higher percentage; those with incomes below poverty spend over a third of their income on health services; those in fair/poor health spend over a quarter of household income on health services (Maxwell et al., 2001).

In the 1990s, Medicare out-of-pocket charges to beneficiaries (including the Medicare Part B premium) rose about 9% per year, on average, a much faster rate of growth than that of income among beneficiaries (US Department of Health and Human Services, 1999b). In 1999, estimated aggregate out-of-pocket expenditures for health services for noninstitutionalized Medicare beneficiaries over 65 years old totaled an average of $2,430 per person, approximately 19% of the income for the average beneficiary (Gross & Brangan, 1999).

Lack of prescription drug coverage contributes substantially to high out-of-pocket spending. Over a third of all beneficiaries have no supplemental coverage to help pay for medications. In 1997, beneficiaries who used prescription drugs spent an average of $440 out of pocket for their medications, with 10% of beneficiaries spending over $1,200 out of pocket annually for drugs (Maxwell et al., 2001).

Expenditures for long-term care services for older adults represent a large share of total health care spending in the United States. This is an area of major concern for state policymakers. Nursing home and home health care accounted for almost 12% of personal health expenditures in 1995 and approximately 14% of all state and local health care spending in that year. Importantly, neither private insurance nor Medicare cover long-term care to any significant extent, and few older adults have private long-term care insurance. The disabled elderly must rely on their own resources or, when these are depleted, turn to Medicaid or state-funded programs to pay for their long-term care. Because of the high cost of long-term care, Medicaid coverage for these services provides a safety net for the middle class as well as the poor. Medicaid long-term care expenditures for the elderly are projected to more than double in inflation-adjusted dollars between 1993 and 2018 due to the aging of the population and to price increases in excess of general inflation (Weiner et al., 1998).

THE MEDICAID PROGRAM

Medicaid is a joint federal and state program that covers medical costs for some people with low incomes and limited resources. It is the principal source of funding for long-term care for the elderly and those of all ages with disabilities, covering 77.7% of nursing home long-term care services (HCFA, 2000a). In 1998, Medicaid served 3.9 million elderly beneficiaries (HCFA, 2000b).

Within broad federal guidelines, each state determines the amount and duration of services offered under its Medicaid program. While Medicaid is more likely than Medicare to provide reimbursement for community care services, there is considerable flexibility at the state level as to whether, and at what rate, such services will be reimbursed (Cohen et al., 2000). Medicare beneficiaries who have low incomes and limited resources or who meet other eligibility criteria may receive help paying for their out-of-pocket expenses for health services through the Medicaid program in their state.

In addition, there are various benefits available to *dual eligibles*, those qualified to receive both Medicare and Medicaid. Services covered by both programs are paid first by Medicare, with the balance paid by Medicaid up to the state's payment limits as specified in the state's Medicaid program. Medicaid also covers additional services, including nursing facility care beyond the 100-day Medicare limit, prescription drugs, eyeglasses, and hearing aids (HCFA, 1999b).

States have the option of providing Medicaid coverage for certain other categorically needy groups who meet eligibility criteria more liberally defined than for the mandatory coverage categories. These groups include certain aged, blind, or disabled adults, institutionalized individuals, and persons who would be eligible if institutionalized, but are receiving care under home- and community-based services waivers. In addition, a state may choose to include the medically needy population or those whose income is too high for them to qualify under the mandatory or optional categorically needy groups. These persons, who may be aged, blind, or disabled, may "spend down" to Medicaid eligibility by incurring medical expenses so that their income is below the maximum allowed by the state (HCFA, 1999b).

A number of basic Medicaid services are mandatory and must be offered to the categorically needy, who include persons receiving federally assisted income maintenance payments such as Supplemental Security Income (SSI) available to the aged, blind, and disabled; low-income families with children; and certain other Medicare beneficiaries. Mandatory health care services include inpatient hospital services, outpatient hospital services, physician services, nursing facility services for those older than 21 years, and home health care for persons eligible for nursing facility services (HCFA, 1999b).

The mandatory Medicaid services most relevant to the mental health of older persons are described below (HCFA, 2000a).

- Nursing facility services, including skilled nursing care, rehabilitation services, and health-related services. The facility must maintain an ongoing treatment program directed by a qualified professional designed to meet the physical, mental, and psychosocial well-being of each resident, as well as treatment required by mentally ill and mentally retarded residents not otherwise provided for by the state (HCFA, 1999c).
- Home health services for individuals entitled to nursing facility services. Services must be provided at a recipient's place of residence and must be ordered by a physician and reviewed every 60 days. These services include nursing and home health aide services provided by a home health agency and medical supplies or equipment suitable for use in the home (HCFA, 1999a).

Medicaid optional services most relevant to mental health include rehabilitation services, which may be provided in any setting and generally include mental health services such as individual and group therapies; psychosocial services; and physical, occupational, and speech therapies. These benefits, which must be recommended by a physician (HCFA, 1999d), target case management services to assist an individual to gain access to needed medical, social, educational, and other services, including, for example, housing or legal services. The state Medicaid programs must submit a separate plan amendment for each target group.

Medicaid is a major resource for providing indigent elderly or disabled persons with access to mental health services in both the private and public sectors. Factors that restrict Medicaid coverage of community treatment models include (Taube et al., 1990)

- Uneven optional benefits. States have the option of offering minimal or no optional mental health benefits. Thus, Medicaid beneficiaries who need certain services may not have access to them if their state does not cover these services.
- Reimbursement policies. The Medicaid program, in general, sets rates lower than those paid by commercial and other third-party insurers. Medicaid payments may not reflect the cost of caring for the behavioral and mental health problems that occur in nursing homes and other settings. Furthermore, states determine the payment rates for providers. If these reimbursements are low, psychiatrists and other highly

trained mental health professionals may be reluctant to serve Medicaid beneficiaries.

Medicaid is 50% funded through state sources. Many states are struggling to finance their Medicaid programs because of declining state revenue sources. As well, Medicaid-funded long-term care and pharmaceutical costs have been escalating. Several states have been attempting to contain pharmacy costs through pharmacy benefit management (PBM) mechanisms and other prior authorization approaches. There also has been a substantial increase in managed Medicaid programs across the United States as states struggle to contain Medicaid costs.

Medicare-Medicaid Dual Coverage

Since the early years of the Medicare program, certain low-income beneficiaries have been eligible for both Medicare and Medicaid. They account for a disproportionately large amount of the overall costs. These persons (dual eligibles) are jointly Medicare/Medicaid eligible either because they qualify for SSI (the case assistance program for aged, blind, or disabled people with low incomes) or because they otherwise are considered medically needy. The medically needy group comprises the aged and disabled, many of whom are in nursing homes, who are ineligible for SSI, but whose health bills are so high that their net incomes put them near or below the poverty level ($8,860 for a single person in 2002 in the 48 contiguous states) (Department of Health and Human Services, 2002a). Although some low-income elderly receive assistance from Medicaid, numerous poor and near-poor Medicare beneficiaries do not qualify for these assistance programs. Brief descriptions of these dual coverage programs follow.

THE QUALIFIED MEDICARE BENEFICIARY AND SPECIFIED LOW-INCOME MEDICARE BENEFICIARY PROGRAMS The Qualified Medicare Beneficiary (QMB) program was set up under the Medicare Catastrophic Coverage Act of 1988 (this law was largely repealed in 1989, but the QMB program was retained). Under QMB, state Medicaid programs are required to pay Medicare's Part B premium and cost sharing for Medicare beneficiaries with incomes below the poverty level and assets not exceeding twice the limits set for SSI. Federal matching funds are provided for QMBs.

Since 1995, the states have also been required under the Specified Low-Income Medicare Beneficiary (SLMB) program to pay the Part B premium for Medicare beneficiaries with incomes from 100% to 120% of poverty levels and assets not exceeding twice the SSI limits. As in the QMB program, SLMB benefits are treated as part of Medicaid and are partially supported with federal matching funds.

The 1997 Balanced Budget Act introduced further provisions for low-income Medicare beneficiaries, specifically those with incomes between 120%

and 175% of poverty levels, to help shield them from short-term increases in Medicare's Part B premium. Under the Balanced Budget Act of 1997, $1.5 billion was made available to states to cover these premium costs from 1998 to 2002. After 2002, absent an extension of this provision of the law, this coverage is scheduled to be discontinued.

Many nominally eligible Medicare beneficiaries do not participate in the QMB/SLMB programs. Of some 5.7 million people who were potentially eligible for the QMB program in early 1998, only about 4.5 million (79%) were participating (Moon et al., 1998). For the SLMB program in that year, only about 270,000 of 1.6 million eligibles (17%) were participating in it (Moon et al., 1998). The reasons for the low rates of QMB and SLMB participation are not fully known, but it is believed that many Medicare beneficiaries are either unaware of the programs or unwilling to participate in them. This may be due to the complexity of the enrollment process, the requirement to apply at a welfare office, and the long lag time before QMB eligibility is activated.

THE QUALIFYING INDIVIDUALS PROGRAMS   The Balanced Budget Act of 1997 created two new groups of Medicare beneficiaries who will receive aid: Qualifying Individuals-1 (QI-1s), who have incomes from 120% to 135% of poverty levels; and Qualifying Individuals-2 (QI-2s), who have incomes from 135% to 175% of poverty. Medicaid will pay the full Medicare premium for QI-1s. For QI-2s, the Medicaid subsidy will be limited to that portion of the Part B premium increase directly attributable to the transfer of payment responsibility for home health visits to the Part B program (a provision of the Balanced Budget Act of 1997).

Both QI-1s and QI-2s will receive assistance only as long as funds are available through the program's federal block grant.

Table 39-4 summarizes estimated costs of Medicaid supplement programs for 2002. The large difference in QMB/SLMB/QI participation levels between

TABLE 39-4.   Estimated costs of existing QMB/SLMB/QI programs, 1998

	Participants (millions)	Federal costs (billion $)	Total costs (billion $)
Program			
Part B	4.5	1.4	2.4
Part A	0.3	4.4	7.7
Cost sharing			
Total QMB	4.5	4.4	7.7
SLMB	0.3	0.1	0.1
QIs	N/A	0.3	0.3
Total	4.8	4.8	8.2

Source: Moon et al. (1998).
QMB, qualified Medicare beneficiary; SLMB, specified low-income Medicare beneficiary; QI, qualified individuals, 1 and 2; N/A, not applicable.

Part A (.3 million) and Part B (4.5 million) indicated in Table 39-4 is due to the circumstance that only a small fraction of patients to whom Medicare coverage was extended through the QMB/SLMB/QI programs received Medicare Part A services, while a much larger fraction received Medicare Part B services, in 1998.

CONCLUSION

The economic and health care needs of older adults are extensive and diverse. Health and mental health policy for elderly individuals has been a patchwork that has left extraordinary gaps despite massive and growing expenditures. For nearly 30 years, Medicare policy has been the most important force in the organization and delivery of geriatric psychiatric services. Stigmatization and discrimination, reflected in exceptionally poor reimbursement of mental health services and perverse incentives to employ expensive inpatient services, have reinforced existing barriers to care for this important and needy population.

Numerous areas of health care policy with respect to mental health care reimbursement and financing pose controversial challenges for future mental health policy changes for older Americans. Until recently, mental health services for Alzheimer's disease and other dementias were not compensated by Medicare because of the mistaken belief that patients with these conditions could not be helped due to the progressive, chronic, and incurable nature of Alzheimer's disease.

Also, the debate over parity for mental health care continues, and it is not clear whether achieving this will increase health care costs or potentially save money through cost offsets. It may be that a legitimate cost offset would result from effective mental health service leading to decreased utilization of medical care services. However, available data are insufficient for documentation. The dispute over Medicare prescription drug coverage, with concerns over escalating costs and advocacy for differing methods of cost containment, persists.

There is debate over how to protect the integrity of Medicare and prevent the Medicare fund from becoming depleted, especially as managed-care programs have been found unable to contain costs and ensure quality health care consistently. Indeed, many individual and managed-care program providers currently are fleeing the Medicare market due to reimbursement reductions. A current important policy issue is how to retain incentives so that these providers will remain Medicare providers.

There is also controversy over the extent to which Medicare should be supplementing or offsetting the costs of training within America's teaching hospitals. Changes in Medicare policy in this area may have made such training more difficult and less desirable to prospective geriatric psychiatrists.

Recent legislation has provided somewhat improved access to mental health services for older adults. Innovative cost containment methods may supply incentives that result in greater continuity of mental health care services. However, limited scrutiny by policymakers of the quality of managed mental health care may put some of the improvements in psychiatric care created by the growth of the field of geriatric psychiatry at substantial risk. The greatest challenges in this dynamic environment lie ahead. It is hoped that proactive policy development and improved financing arrangements will facilitate the delivery of higher quality mental health services to this population as it grows rapidly in the next several years.

REFERENCES

American Medical Association. *Current Procedural Terminology*. 4th ed. Chicago, IL: American Medical Association; 1990.

Balanced Budget Act of 1997, Pub L No. 105-33 110 Stat. 2023 (1997), 43 USC.

Balanced Budget Refinement Act of 1999, Pub L No. 106-113 (1999).

Bartels SJ. Quality, costs, and effectiveness of services for older adults with mental disorders: a selective overview of recent advances in geriatric mental health services research. *Curr Opin Psychiatry*. 2002;15:411–416.

Centers for Medicare and Medicaid Services. 2003. Available at: http://cms.hhs.gov/.

Coffey RM, Mark T, King E, et al. *National Estimates of Expenditures for Mental Health and Substance Abuse Treatment, 1997*. Rockville, MD: Center for Substance Abuse Treatment and Center for Mental Health Services, Substance Abuse and Mental Health Services Administration; July 2000. SAMHSA Publication SMA-00–3499.

Cohen CI, Cohen GD, Blank K, et al. Schizophrenia and older adults. *Am J Geriatr Psychiatry*. 2000;8:19–28.

Crose R, Minear M. Project CARE: a model for establishing neighborhood centers to increase access to services by low-income, minority elders. *J Gerontol Soc Work*. 1998;30:73–82.

Cutler J, Fine T. Federal health care financing of mental illness: a failure of public policy. In: Sharfstein SS, Beigel A, eds. *The New Economics of Psychiatric Care*. Washington, DC: American Psychiatric Press; 1985:17–37.

Dalaker J. *Poverty in the United States: 2000*. Washington, DC: US Government Printing Office; 2001. US Census Bureau, Current Population Reports, Series P60-214.

English JT, Sharfstein SS, Scherl DJ, Astrachan B, Muszynski IL. Diagnosis-related groups and general hospital psychiatry: the APA study. *Am J Psychiatry*. 1986;143: 131–139.

Fogel BS, Gottlieb GL, Furino A. Present and future solutions. In: Fogel BS, Furino A, Gottlieb GL, eds. *Mental Health Policy for Older Americans: Protecting Minds at Risk*. Washington, DC: American Psychiatric Press; 1990:257–277.

Frank RG, Huskamp HA, McGuire TG, Newhouse JP. Some economics of mental health "carve-outs." *Arch Gen Psychiatry*. 1996;53:933–937.

Frank RG, Lave JL. The psychiatric DRGs: are they different? *Med Care*. 1985;23: 1148–1155.

Frazier SH, Goldman H, Taube CA. Psychiatry, Medicare, and prospective payment [editorial]. *Am J Psychiatry*. 1986;143:198–200.

Furino AF, Fogel BS. The economic perspective. In: Fogel BS, Furino A, Gottlieb GL, eds. *Mental Health Policy for Older Americans: Protecting Minds at Risk*. Washington, DC: American Psychiatric Press; 1990:23–36.

General Accounting Office. *Budget Issues: Budgetary Implications of Selected GAO*

Work for Fiscal Year 2001. Washington, DC: US Government Printing Office; 2002.

Goldman HH. Overview of studies on psychiatric hospital care under a prospective payment system. In: Scherl DJ, English JT, Sharfstein SS, eds. *Prospective Payment in Psychiatric Care.* Washington, DC: American Psychiatric Association; 1988:81–89.

Goldman HH, Frank RG. Division of responsibility among payors. In: Fogel BS, Furino A, Gottlieb GL, eds. *Mental Health Policy for Older Americans: Protecting Minds at Risk.* Washington, DC: American Psychiatric Press; 1990:85–95.

Goldman HH, Taube CA, Jencks SJ. The organization of the psychiatric inpatient services system. *Med Care.* 1987;25(9 suppl):S6–S21.

Gottlieb GL. *Managed Behavioral Healthcare Standards, Guidelines, and Competencies for Older Adults with Mental Illness.* Rockville, MD: Center for Mental Health Services, Substance Abuse and Mental Health Services Administration; 1998.

Gross DJ, Brangan N. *Out-of-Pocket Spending on Health Care by Medicare Beneficiaries Age 65 and Older: 1999 Projections.* Washington, DC: AARP Public Policy Institute; December 1999.

Health Care Financing Administration. Protecting Medicare's partial hospitalization benefit in community mental health centers. 1998. Available at: http://www.hcfa.gov/facts/f092998.htm. Accessed February 2002.

Health Care Financing Administration. Home health services. 1999a. Available at: http://www.hcfa.gov/medicaid/ltc9.htm. Accessed February 2002.

Health Care Financing Administration. Medicaid eligibility. 1999b. Available at: http://www.hcfa.gov/medicaid/meligib.htm. Accessed February 2002.

Health Care Financing Administration. Nursing facility services for individuals age 21 and older. 1999c. Available at: http://www.hcfa.gov/medicaid/ltc1.htm. Accessed February 2002.

Health Care Financing Administration. Rehabilitation services. 1999d. Available at: http://www.hcfa.gov/medicaid/ltc3.htm. Accessed February 2002.

Health Care Financing Administration. Medicaid long term care services. 2000a. Available at: http://www.hcfa.gov/medicaid/ltchomep.htm. Accessed February 2002.

Health Care Financing Administration. *A Profile of Medicaid: Chartbook 2000.* Washington, DC: US Dept of Health and Human Services; 2000b.

Health Insurance Portability and Accountability Act of 1996, Pub L No. 104-191, 110 Stat. 2023 (1996), 42 USC.

Hobbs FB. *The Elderly Population.* Washington, DC: US Bureau of the Census, Population Division and Housing and Household Economic Statistics Division, US Government Printing Office; 2001.

Hollmann FW, Mulder TJ, Kallan JE. *Methodology and Assumptions for the Population Projections of the United States: 1999 to 2100.* Washington, DC: US Census Bureau Population Projections Branch, Population Division, Department of Commerce, US Government Printing Office; 2000. Population Division Working Paper 38.

Hsiao WC, Braun P, Dunn D, Becker ER. Resource-based relative values: an overview. *JAMA.* 1988;260:2347–2353.

Hsiao WC, Braun P, Dunn DL, et al. An overview of the development and refinement of the resource-based relative value scale: the foundation for reform of US physician payment. *Med Care.* 1992;30(11 suppl):NS1–NS12.

Iglehart JK. Health policy report: the American health care system. *N Engl J Med.* 1992; 327:1467–1472.

InterStudy Publications. HMO enrollment continues to decrease. May 7, 2001. Available at: http://www.interstudypublications.com.

Kihlstrom LC. Managed care and medication compliance: implications for chronic depression. *J Behav Health Serv Res.* 1998;25:367–376.

Letsch SW. National health care spending in 1991. *Health Aff.* 1993;12:94–110.

Levit K, Smith C, Cowan C, Lazenby H, Martin A. Inflation spurs health spending in 2000. *Health Aff.* 2002;21:172–181.

Lieberman T. Medicare: new choices, new worries. *Consumer Reports.* 1998;63:27.

Maxwell S, Moon M, Segal M. *Growth in Medicare and Out-of-Pocket Spending: Impact on Vulnerable Beneficiaries.* New York, NY: Commonwealth Fund; 2001.

Minear M, Crose R. Identifying barriers to services for low-income frail elders. *J Gerontol Soc Work.* 1996;26:57–64.

Minino AM, Smith BL. Deaths: preliminary data for 2000. *Natl Vital Stat Rep.* 2001; 49(12):7–13.

Moon M. Medicare: health policy 2001. *N Engl J Med.* 2001;344:928–931.

Moon M, Brennan N, Segal M. *Improving Coverage for Low-Income Medicare Beneficiaries, Policy Brief.* New York, NY: Commonwealth Fund; 1998.

National Alliance for the Mentally Ill. The Medicare partial hospitalization benefit. 2000. Available at: http://www.nami.org/updte/unitedpartial.html.

Omnibus Reconciliation Act of 1980, HR 7765, Pub L No. 96-499.

Omnibus Budget Reconciliation Act of 1987, HR 3545, Pub L No. 100-203.

Omnibus Budget Reconciliation Act of 1989, HR 3299, Pub L No. 101-239.

Omnibus Budget Reconciliation Act of 1990, HR 5835, Pub L No. 101-508.

Pacala JT, Boult C, Hepburn KW, et al. Case management of older adults in health maintenance organizations. *J Am Geriatr Soc.* 1995;43:538–542.

Pamuk E, Makuc D, Heck K, Reuben C, Lochner K. *Socioeconomic Status and Health Chartbook. Health, United States, 1998.* Hyattsville, MD: National Center for Health Statistics; 1998.

Physician Payment Review Commission. *Annual Report to Congress.* Washington, DC: US Government Printing Office; 1989:7–28.

Rice T, Bernstein J. *Supplemental Health Insurance for Medicare Beneficiaries.* Washington, DC: National Academy of Social Insurance; November 1999. Medicare Brief 6.

Rice T, Graham ML, Fox PD. The impact of policy standardization on the Medigap market. *Inquiry.* 1997;34:106–116.

Scherl DJ, English JT, Sharfstein SS, eds. Preface. In: Scherl DJ, English JT, Sharfstein SS, eds. *Prospective Payment and Psychiatric Care.* Washington, DC: American Psychiatric Association; 1988:xv–xxii.

Sharfstein SS. Payment for services: a provider's perspective. In: Fogel BS, Furino A, Gottlieb GL, eds. *Mental Health Policy for Older Americans: Protecting Minds at Risk.* Washington, DC: American Psychiatric Press; 1990:97–107.

Social Security Amendments of 1983, Pub L No. 98-21 (1983).

Soldo BJ, Agree EM. America's elderly population. *Popul Bull.* 1988;43(3):1–53.

Soldo BJ, Hurd MD, Rodgers WL, Wallace RB. Asset and health dynamics among the oldest old: an overview of the AHEAD study. *J Gerontol B Psychol Sci Soc Sci.* 1997;52(special issue SI):1–20.

Taube CA, Goldman HH, Salkever D. Medicaid coverage for mental illness: balancing access and costs. *Health Aff.* 1990;9:5–18.

US Bureau of the Census. *Projections of the Resident Population by Age, Sex, Race, and Hispanic Origin: 1999–2100.* Washington, DC: US Government Printing Office; 2000. Series NP-D1-A.

US Department of Health and Human Services. *Health Care Financing Review Medicare and Medicaid Statistical Supplement, 1999.* Baltimore, MD: US Dept of Health and Human Services; 1999b.

US Department of Health and Human Services. *Mental Health: A Report of the Surgeon General.* Rockville, MD: US Dept of Health and Human Services, Substance Abuse and Mental Health Services Administration, Center for Mental Health Services, National Institutes of Health, National Institute of Mental Health; 1999a.

US Department of Health and Human Services. Annual update of the HHS poverty guidelines. 67 *Federal Register* 6931–6933 (2002a).

US Department of Health and Human Services. Medicare program; revisions to payment policies under the physician fee schedule for calendar year 2003 and inclusion of registered nurses in the personnel provision of the critical access hospital emergency services requirement for frontier areas and remote locations; final rule. 67 *Federal Register* 79966–80184 (2002b).

US Senate Committee on Finance. *Background Material on Health Insurance.* Washington, DC: US Government Printing Office; 1978.

Vartanian TP, McNamara JM. Older women in poverty: the impact of midlife factors. *J Marriage Family.* 2002;64:532–548.

Weiner JM, Stevenson DC. *Long-Term Care for the Elderly: Profiles of the 13. Assessing the New Federalism States.* Washington, DC: Urban Institute; August 1998.

Wells KB, Rogers WH, Davis LM, et al. Quality of care for hospitalized, depressed elderly patients before and after implementation of the Medicare prospective payment system. *Am J Psychiatry.* 1993;150:1799–1805.

Wolff EN. *Retirement Insecurity: The Income Shortfalls Awaiting the Soon-to-Retire.* Washington, DC: Economic Policy Institute; 2002.

40

Private Practice Issues

Elliot Martin Stein, MD

Provision of psychiatric services to the elderly does not happen in a vacuum. This chapter explores aspects of the support structure and environment that allow those clinical services to be provided in a private practice. Many of the rules, regulations, laws, and policies governing these areas are in frequent flux and are affected by multiple regional and state variations in the legal regulations and financial reimbursements. Although only a limited number of references in this area focus on private practice in geriatric psychiatry (Crossett, 1995; Greene et al., 2000; Siegal et al., 1997; Stein, 1983a, 1983b; Stein & Moak, 2002), additional sources are available that provide general psychiatric resources (American Psychiatric Association [APA] Web site for early career psychiatrists, www.psych.org/ecp/index.html; Klein et al., 1984; Logsdon, 1985) and medical practice information (American Medical Association [AMA] Web site Young Physician's Section, www.ama-assn.org/ama/pub/category/16.html), as well as many general business resources. Readers contemplating setting up a private practice should consider consulting with a variety of advisors, including an attorney, an accountant, a banker, and a business planner.

More than 80% of psychiatric income derives from direct patient care (Zarin et al., 1998). Fee for service is the primary payment mechanism for these patient care services, accounting for more than 50% of this income (Zarin et al., 1998). Even for those psychiatrists who are receiving salaries, reimbursements for their services by third-party payers are becoming increasingly important as supplements to their salaries. It is therefore vital to understand that a private practice is a business, a business created and maintained for the purpose of providing services (in this case, psychogeriatric services) and in turn generating income for the provider. Consequently, this chapter focuses on the following points:

- The current nature and demographics of the geriatric psychiatric business in the United States
- The creation of this type of business
- The provision of service and generating income
- Maintaining the business

Although these areas are discussed separately, obviously there is synergy and overlap among them.

NATURE AND DEMOGRAPHICS OF THE GERIATRIC PSYCHIATRIC BUSINESS IN THE UNITED STATES

The demographics of elderly individuals and the projected pattern of aging in the future are well described elsewhere in this text (see Chapter 6).

Current Number and Income of Psychiatrists Providing Services

Although most American psychiatrists see few or no geriatric patients, this trend is changing. During their 1997–1998 Professional Activities (Biographical) Survey, the APA found that over 5,400 of more than 36,000 members expressed an interest in geriatrics (APA, unpublished data, 2000). Membership in the American Association for Geriatric Psychiatry (AAGP) has grown to over 1,800 (AAGP, unpublished data, 2003), and interest in geriatric psychiatry among general psychiatrists is increasing. In 1991, the American Board of Psychiatry and Neurology (ABPN) first administered a board certifying subspecialty examination (at first called "added qualifications") in geriatric psychiatry. As of February 2003, 2,595 individuals had passed this examination (ABPN, unpublished data, 2003).

Only limited data are available on income and workload for geriatric psychiatrists as a group (Colenda et al., 1999; Dorwart et al., 1992; Olfson & Goldman, 1992; Pincus et al., 1999; Stein & Moak, 2002; Zarin et al., 1998). For psychiatrists in general, 1999 median annual gross income was $167,090 (a 2.6% decrease from 1998), but annual net income was $125,790, a 6.0% increase from 1998 (Goldberg, 1999). Nonetheless, this was, once again, the second lowest income of the 17 largest office-based specialties surveyed by the journal *Medical Economics* that year.

Medicare has historically been perceived by psychiatrists as paying poorly for treatment. The advent and growth of managed care has imposed restrictions on both service provision and reimbursements for psychiatric treatment. Making Medicare coverage attractive to providers is an essential factor for encouraging more psychiatrists to furnish treatment to the elderly.

Demographics of Provision of Services

In 1996, 18% of American psychiatrists had geriatric caseloads exceeding 20% of their practices (Colenda et al., 1999). Overall, in this 1996 survey, of the 970 responders, an average of 14.0% to 17.7% of their psychiatric patients were older than 65 years of age (Colenda et al., 1999), compared to 8.4% found in a 1987 study (Loran et al., 1987). Psychiatrists who provide a higher proportion of geriatric services (greater than 20% of their caseload) have been found to spend proportionately less time in office-based practices and more time in hospitals and nursing homes than those who see lower proportions of geriatric patients (Colenda et al., 1999). In 1997, a further patient survey of 531 psychiatrist members of the APA who spent at least 15 hours per week in direct face-to-face patient care found 14.8% of patients older than 65 years (Colenda et al., 2002). For these patients, Medicare was the principal payor for 69.6%, private/commercial insurance paid for 10.5%, Medicaid paid for 1.1%, self-pay or no charge was used by 0.9%, and 12.5% used other sources of payment.

CREATION OF A GERIATRIC PSYCHIATRIC BUSINESS

Types of Practice

Several important philosophical and practical parameters help structure the creation of a psychiatric business. Private practice can be based in an office or in other locations, can be full time or part time, can be solo or shared with others, and can focus primarily on geriatric patients or on a heterogeneous mixed-aged population.

FULL-TIME VERSUS PART-TIME   Many psychiatrists work at more than one setting. A private practice may often be started while working part time in an employed position (such as for a private or public sector agency). This can help provide a steady income while building a practice. Also, an employed position can provide professional interactions and stimulation, which an independent practice may not. It may also serve as a source of referrals to the private practice.

SOLO PRACTICE VERSUS SHARED PRACTICE   Individual practice is the traditional model for psychiatric and other mental health private practitioners. A shared practice can consist of two or more independent practitioners who share office space and overhead, or it can be a partnership or incorporated practice with shared caseloads, finances, and medical-legal responsibility. Even independent solo practitioners can benefit from creating formal or informal relationships with other private practitioners for purposes such as mutual support, consultation, and cross coverage (evenings, weekends, vacations, etc.). A shared practice may be in the form of a psychiatric group, a multidisciplinary mental health group, or a multispecialty medical group (Zarin et al., 1998). Psychiatrists may hire or establish relationships with other medical or nonmedical clinical staff. The creation of a partnership or a corporate relationship with other health care providers requires agreement on multiple issues, including generating and dividing income, division of labor, coverage, policies for bringing in future new partners, and procedures for eventually ending the partnership or buying out a partner.

INCORPORATION PLUSES AND MINUSES   Accountants and attorneys can provide full information about the pros and cons of incorporation and partnerships. Incorporation may have tax-related, retirement planning, or other advantages for either solo or group practices. Although in most states the corporate structure will not protect against individual malpractice liability judgments, it may protect against other legal risks. There are different types of partnerships and corporations. Incorporation and some forms of partnership require additional legal and accounting expenses.

PATIENT POPULATIONS AND SERVICES   Although it is entirely possible to have a practice solely devoted to treating the elderly, many practitioners see a mixed-age patient population. There are differing characteristics in the practitioners and practices of those who see larger numbers of older patients compared to those who see fewer (Colenda et al., 1999, 2002; Olfson et al., 1999). There may be varying points of view on the advantages and disadvantages of seeing a geriatric versus mixed-age patient population, but it can be difficult keeping up with developments, journals, conferences, and treatment needs for a wide range of patients. Younger patients are also more likely to be insured with a managed-care organization (MCO). In view of relatively low numbers of psychiatrists with a specific interest in treating the elderly, when the medical and general communities know that a particular psychiatrist is a geriatric specialist, there is usually no shortage of patients needing these services.

In addition to direct clinical services to patients, other sources of income may include consultation to programs and facilities, administrative services (e.g., to an inpatient unit, partial hospital program [PHP], nursing home [NH]), and forensic work. Contracts with managed-care organizations, although possible, typically only form a small proportion of the patient care provided by a geriatric psychiatrist (Colenda et al., 1999).

OFFICE-BASED VERSUS OTHER LOCATIONS   Although an office is the most common venue for the provision of geriatric psychiatric services, many private practitioners may also spend some or all of their time in inpatient or outpatient hospital locations, nursing homes, adult living facilities, or even making home visits (Colenda et al., 1999). In the 1997 survey of APA members (Colenda et al., 2002), 49.36% of patients older than 65 years were seen in an outpatient setting, 31.96% as inpatients, and 15.95% in nursing homes.

In selecting a location for a geriatric psychiatric practice, assess the demographics of the local elderly population, both at present and projected future trends. Also, consider the locations of other physicians and hospitals providing services to these elders. Also, review the locations of other elderly-related services, such as senior centers, social security offices, nursing homes, adult living facilities, retirement communities, and the PHPs that serve older populations. Before deciding where to establish a practice, also assess the number of other geriatric psychiatrists who currently practice in that location and whether there is room for another.

Establishment of an Office

Office space availability and costs are major considerations. Office space is often the second most costly element of overhead after salaries. Options may include buying versus renting and the costs of renovation under each option. When starting out in a new private practice, it may be cost-effective to share or sublet space in the office of another health care provider. Some assisted-living facilities, senior centers, hospitals, medical clinics, or NHs may have space available to rent, which can also help ensure ready access to and for patients in a familiar environment.

TRANSPORTATION   The choice of location requires consideration of the availability of transportation, convenient parking, and proximity to major roadways and to public transportation (Stein, 1983a, 1983b; Stein & Moak, 2002). Selection of an office location in a rural community or in an area with poor public transportation can prevent patients from attending appointments. Some communities, hospitals, senior centers, adult living facilities, or senior retirement communities have senior transportation services that will take people with limited mobility and handicapping conditions to physicians' offices.

OFFICE DESIGN   For patient areas, a geriatric-friendly office includes considerations of access such as the availability of ramps, elevators rather than stairs, a short distance from parking or bus stops, the length of the corridors that must be traversed, and doorways wide enough for wheelchairs. The office must have enough room for patients and the people who accompany them, including multiple family members, nurses, aides, or guardians. If patients are seen for shorter visits, such as medication management or brief psychotherapy visits, there should be sufficient waiting room space for the current patient and the next two or three scheduled patients (and the respective accompanying persons). The seating should be appropriate for the elderly, including sturdy, stain-proof chairs with arms to assist in sitting or standing and firm seats at an appropriate height (not low, "comfortable" chairs that an older person will have difficulty getting in and out of). There should be a conveniently located, handicapped accessible lavatory for patients.

In the patient areas, the lighting should be bright enough to allow people with poor vision to see adequately. Flooring should have a nonskid surface. Area rugs, low tables, spring-loaded doors, and other potential obstacles can be hazardous. Adequate sources of diversion in the waiting room such as music, a television, or reading material (including large-print material) should be available for waiting patients and their accompanying people.

In addition to the standard equipment required in the business areas of the office, optional equipment could include a wheelchair, scale, stethoscope, thermometer, sphygmomanometer, and psychological/neuropsychological testing equipment.

LICENSES, REGISTRATIONS, FEES, AND MEMBERSHIPS All appropriate licenses and payment of fees are required in setting up an office. These include city and county occupational licenses, fire department office occupancy certificates, property insurance, office liability (slip-and-fall) insurance, and malpractice insurance. Business names that are other than the physician's own (e.g., Geriatric Psychiatry Clinic of Centerville) may have to be registered with the county or state, including the requirement of a public notice in a local newspaper or registration as a trademark with the state. If forming a partnership or incorporating, appropriate documents will have to be filed with the state and Internal Revenue Service; additional licenses, insurance policies, and the like in the name of the business may be required.

A separate Medicare number is required for each office address where services are provided. Generally, separate numbers for services provided in locations where the psychiatrist does not have an office, such as in the hospital, nursing home, or assisted-living facility, are not needed unless this is the primary location of the business. Similarly, registration is required with the state Medicaid carrier and each of the other insurance carriers with whom the doctor will be doing business. MCOs require application to their provider panels. These may be "full" and may not always accept new providers, but sometimes a "closed" panel will accept someone who can demonstrate expertise in geriatric psychiatry. Every hospital and various nursing homes require an application for privileges.

MALPRACTICE INSURANCE Malpractice insurance is typically available in two forms: *occurrence policies* provide coverage for any incident that occurs while the policy is in force; *claims-made insurance* covers any liability claim made against the physician while the policy is in force. If a claims-made policy is purchased, there will be a need later to purchase a "tail" insurance policy that protects from future liability when the doctor stops purchasing the claims-made insurance. This may occur at retirement, when leaving practice, or when changing insurance companies. If practicing in a potentially litigious community or if there are other concerns about medical liability, it would probably be wise to purchase a policy with high limits.

OFFICE REFERENCES The needed resource material includes clinically oriented references, business-oriented references, and community resources (see also Chapter 37).

Clinically Oriented References. It is useful to have both the bound copy and the CD-ROM version of the annually updated *Physicians Desk Reference* (*PDR*; 2003) or other similar pharmacological reference texts (Fuller, 1999) and similar references for a personal digital assistant (PDA), as well as a reasonable selection of professional journals. Compilations of useful forms are available. These include sample patient registration forms, HIPAA forms, psychiatric evaluations, medication monitoring sheets, and standardized cognitive assessment and symptom rating forms. Additional forms include patient information sheets, informed consent to take medication, and medication information sheets (Goldberg, 2000; Greene et al., 2000; Siegal et al., 1997; Wyatt, 1998; Zuckerman, 1992), which may be modified or customized. Having a selection of such organized, structured forms can improve comprehensiveness and efficiency while instilling confidence in patients.

Business-Oriented References. All Medicare intermediaries and most other insurers utilize the coding terminology in the *Current Procedural Terminology* (*CPT*) and *International Classification of Diseases, Ninth Revision* (*ICD-9*) books exclusively for reimbursement for services. The American Medical Association's *CPT* books (AMA, 2003) are updated, and should be purchased, annually. The *ICD-9-CM* (*International Classification of Diseases, Ninth Revision, Clinical Modification*; World Health Organization, 2002) is the standard coding nomenclature for diseases (*ICD-10* is in preparation and will supplant *ICD-9*).

After registration with Medicare, the local Medicare carrier sends (usually in December) an annual update of reimbursement rates for the forthcoming year for all Medicare-eligible services. A carrier Medicare bulletin (Medicare B, 2000), which includes updates of Medicare policies, procedures, and announcements, is sent monthly or bimonthly and should be reviewed regularly. The local Medicare carrier can provide copies of their policies manual for psychiatric services (Health Care Financing Administration [HCFA], 1999). Policy manuals are also available for other areas, such as guidelines for coverage of nurse practitioners and other nonphysician practitioners. Note that these policy manuals will be different for each Medicare carrier. Although all Medicare carriers fall under the authority of the Centers for Medicare and Medicaid Services (CMS), the carriers have flexibility in their interpretation of Medicare policy and regulations.

Community and Other Resources. The consultation room should have ready access to telephone directories; directories of local hospitals or medical and psychiatric society physician membership directories, including the AAGP directory; and the directory of the local Alzheimer's Association, home health agencies, visiting nurse associations, senior transportation services, nurses aide employment agencies, as well as addresses and phone numbers of the local Social Security office, senior centers, adult and elderly protective services, the local guardianship programs, the local community mental health center, and crisis intervention centers. These and similar resource materials are invaluable to psychiatrist and patient alike.

Often, some of the most important therapeutic interventions a psychiatrist can make will be to give information on available resources to patients, to their families, to caregivers, or to referring sources. Families will ask for advice on placement in an adult living facility or nursing home. Recommendations may include that the patient obtain a hearing aid or attend classes at the local Lighthouse for the Blind, purchase a 7-day pillbox, or investigate which pharmacies in the community tend to be less expensive. The geriatric psychiatrist is often afforded the role of the patients' overall case manager, as well as focusing on their mental health care.

Many pharmaceutical companies have programs to provide free or low-cost medications to people in need who cannot afford them and who are not covered by medication plans. Similarly, some third-party payers (such as state Medicaid programs) may provide medications, but have limitations on the number or amount of medications they will typically provide. Provision of other types of health information, such as patient information brochures published by AAGP, the APA, governmental agencies, and others (AAGP, no date; APA, no date; Florida Highway Patrol, no date; Department of Health and Human Services, 1993; Jefferson, 1996) is a valuable service for patients (and can be valuable marketing tools for the physician's business). They tell the patient and family that the psychiatrist is concerned about them in a "take home" format (a business card can be stapled to the back of the brochure). The patient or family can be directed to online resources for health information or to the psychiatrist's own Web site.

OFFICE STAFF   Guidebooks are available and can be important references on creating a business and running an office, including information on employer-employee relationships (Greenspan, 1996; Weidner et al., 1993). In considering the hiring of staff, it should be remembered that an appropriate infrastructure will be cost-efficient. Each individual has specific roles to play, which will allow the physician, the member of the office team whose work generates the operating revenue, to focus on patient care activities.

Staff Functions   Although the beginning private practitioner many start out answering his or her own calls and making appointments, the tasks required to run the office can quickly grow beyond the time availability of the clinician. Some of the functions of an office staff can be outsourced, such as by the use of an answering service, a billing service, or transcription service.

Basic staff functions include answering and responding to telephone calls and front desk/reception area functions such as greeting patients, filling out basic forms, photocopying insurance cards, making and changing appointments, handling correspondence, receiving and sending mail, and handling such routine patient-oriented tasks as calling for a taxi, making an appointment with another physician, or sending for medical records. Other tasks can include dictation, transcription, billing and bookkeeping, filing, and office maintenance chores such as purchasing, payroll, banking, ordering supplies, and so on.

Hiring office staff necessitates basic decisions regarding duties, workdays, work hours, and frequency of salary payments. In determining an appropriate salary and benefits, it may be helpful to consult with colleagues or their office managers. In addition to direct costs of salaries, payment of local, state, and federal taxes is required. Accountants or legal advisors can provide information about these responsibilities.

Benefits offered to employees can include such things as parking, vacation time, sick leave, paid holidays, educational opportunities, and the like. Other possible benefits, depending on community standards and employment market, include health insurance or disability or life insurance. Some of these benefits can be phased in after a trial period or after the first anniversary date. Worker's compensation insurance and/or unemployment insurance are typically required by the state.

It is common when hiring employees that they be given an initial temporary probationary period of 1 to 3 months before they are considered regular employee. Depending on state regulations, employees can be fired during this period of time "at will" (without specific cause) and without adverse consequence to the employer. People fired after they are established, full-time employees may be eligible, depending on the location, to collect unemployment compensation from the state (which is then reflected in the unemployment compensation taxes for which the employer may be liable in the future).

Employee Relations. Employee training should be offered, particularly in areas that help improve the functioning of an office. This training can include classes in various computer programs, Medicare guidelines, Medicare compliance issues, Health Insurance and Portability and Accountability Act of 1996 (HIPAA) regulations, emergency resuscitation, or basic medical procedures, such as how to assess blood pressure and pulse. The psychiatrist should delineate the issues of particular importance for which he or she wishes to be consulted, and staff should be encouraged to request guidance and instruction.

In addition to ongoing employee feedback throughout the year, employee evaluations should be regularly scheduled, typically at the end of the initial trial period and on each annual anniversary date of employment. Performance reviews should provide the employee with formal comments assessing their functioning, productivity, initiative, and achievement. Salary increases or other additional compensation can be awarded during this time. Often a postdiscussion written evaluation is signed by employer and employee.

It may be helpful to have an employee handbook to serve as formal notification of the rules, policies, and procedures of the office, including confidentiality, duties, expectations, and so on. However, before creating a handbook, the psychiatrist should review available models and consult business and legal advisors. Statements in an employee handbook may be construed as formal contractual language between employer and employee and as such may contain pitfalls or problems for the employer.

Employee Positions. Good interpersonal skills of a front desk receptionist will help create a positive image of the psychiatrist and the office and a favorable experience for patients and families. The receptionist often functions as "gatekeeper," responding to questions and engaging in some triage activities. Responsibilities include making appointments, inquiring as to the reasons for the request to be seen, the age of the prospective patient, the referring source, and the status of insurance coverage, including clarifying whether the physician participates in the patient's managed-care plan.

BILLING AND BOOKKEEPING Bookkeeping and billing are complex tasks that require attention to detail and consistent follow-up. It is critically important that the physician be directly involved in overseeing billing. Staff involved in billing must learn about Medicare policies and procedures, *CPT* and *ICD-9-CM* codes and help ensure compliance with appropriate documentation of services to be billed (Gardiner, 2000; Grant, 2002; HCFA, 1999; *Medicare B*, 2000). Hiring a medical billing company can be an efficient option. However, it is essential that the billing company be psychiatrically oriented and thoroughly understand Medicare psychiatric billing issues and procedures. The psychiatrist must be fully cognizant of personal responsibility for the accuracy of all billing and claims data. It is the physician, and not the staff, who is legally accountable.

GENERATING INCOME

Medicare

HISTORY The history of Medicare and its legislative history are summarized in Chapter 39 (also see Grant, 2002). This chapter focuses on the impact of Medicare regulations on psychiatrist billing. Medicare was created in 1965 by Congress as an amendment to the Social Security Act, adding Title 18: Health Insurance for the Aged and Disabled. Initially designed as a hospital benefit for the elderly (Medicare Part A), a physician's benefit (Medicare Part B) was "added on" (Ball, 1996). Part B contained restrictions, including a 50% co-payment requirement and a $250 annual Medicare expenditure limit for psychiatric treatment services, except for those provided to hospital inpatients. Although the annual limit was gradually increased and then eliminated in 1990 as part of the Omnibus Budget Reconciliation Act of 1989 Reform (OBRA 89), the 50% copayment requirement for many psychiatric services remains.

As of mid-2003, as has been tried on multiple occasions over the past several years, legislation has been introduced in Congress to eliminate this 50% psychiatric reduction and establish payment parity with other medical treatments. The fate of this legislation is unresolved at this writing.

Supplemental Medigap insurance policies and private Medigap policies were developed to provide coverage for copayments and were standardized as of July 30, 1992 (Grimaldi, 1992). Among the requirements for the core benefits package was the mandate for payment for the full 50% copayment requirement for outpatient psychiatric services. However, some insurance intermediaries have not fully implemented this provision, declaring that elderly individuals who initially purchased their coinsurance policies prior to that date are not covered by these provisions. In December 2002, CMS again clarified that a Medigap issuer is generally responsible for payment of 50% of the Medicare "allowed" amount for psychiatric treatment services (CMS, 2002). Additional coverage restrictions apply to patients covered by Medicaid (see below).

Some supplemental insurance policies are not considered "true Medigap policies" (e.g., some plans provided by former employers, labor unions, or pension plans). These might have different psychiatric coverage rules and may pay only 12.5% of the Medicare allowed amount (see below). Similarly, managed care organization secondary policies may have various payment restrictions.

MEDICARE COVERAGE AND LIMITATIONS Medicare will make payments to providers who have signed contracts to abide by Medicare rules. On signing the contract, the provider receives a Medicare number, which allows for reimbursement by local companies that are designated as the carriers of the federal insurance. Signing a Medicare contract allows providers and their patients to utilize Medicare benefits, but requires that the provider adhere to the contract for all Medicare patients treated. Individualized "private" arrangements are not allowed.

Medicare pays for four kinds of physicians' services: diagnosis, therapy, surgery, and consultations/concurrent care. In performing a covered Medicare service, a health care provider must either (1) examine a patient in person or (2) evaluate the patient's condition using technology alone (for example, examine and interpret an x-ray). Medicare pays only for services that are considered "medically necessary" and only for "covered" services. Determinations of medical necessity are based on federal guidelines, but are subject to the interpretation of local insurance carriers. Chart documentation is integral to demonstrating medical necessity, but may be insufficient if a local carrier deems a particular service as given more frequently than is needed or for diagnoses that are not considered appropriate.

MEDICARE PARTICIPATION Physicians are given the option annually to become Medicare participating providers. Agreement to participate in Medicare involves signing a contract agreeing that the doctor will always accept assignment for the amount Medicare sets as the payment for the Medicare covered services provided to Medicare recipients during the coming year. This means that Medicare pays the provider 80% (or 50%, depending on the service and place of service) of this Medicare allowable. The patient can be billed no more than the remaining 20% (or 50%) copayment, no matter what the physician's usual fee schedule is.

There are several advantages to participating in Medicare. These include higher fee schedule payments than nonparticipating providers receive; many of the claims will be automatically sent to the patient's Medigap insurer (crossover), which diminishes paperwork; and publication of the doctor's name in a Medicare participating physician/supplier directory. Participating providers receive basic payments for services rendered from Medicare, but can and are expected to bill patients for copayments that are not covered by coinsurance.

A nonparticipating provider is allowed to accept assignment on a case-by-case basis. However, when assignment is accepted by a nonparticipating provider, it is paid at 5% less than the Medicare allowed amount paid to participators. The advantage is that a nonparticipating provider is not required to accept assignment. This means that the patient can be billed more than the Medicare allowable amount (up to a limiting charge or *balance billing limit*) when the provider chooses to do so. This limiting charge is capped at 115% of the nonparticipating fee schedule payment (which is 95% of the participating allowable amount); this equals 109.25% of the Medicare allowed amount.

Billing the patient for more than the limiting charge is considered a breach of the basic Medicare contract that all providers who bill under Medicare have signed. Billing beyond the allowable limiting charge can trigger a warning or investigation and result in punitive fines. Some state laws further restrict balance billing of Medicare patients below the federally mandated limiting charges. (These states include Connecticut, Massachusetts, New York, Pennsylvania, Rhode Island, and Vermont; Grant, 2002.) Both participating and nonparticipating providers must accept assignment from Medicare beneficiaries who are also Medicaid recipients or who are at or below the federal poverty level (OBRA 89).

CLAIMS FILING   Whether or not they elect to become a participating provider, for all Medicare claims, assigned or unassigned, the physician and not the patient is required to fill out the Medicare claim form and submit it for payment. Payment for assigned claims is sent by the Medicare carrier to the physician. Payment for unassigned claims is sent to the patient. The patient may not be charged by the physician for the service of filling out and submitting the claim. Although claims may be sent to the Medicare carrier on paper (the HCFA 1500 form) or electronically, Medicare is encouraging electronic submission and may charge a fee for the submission of paper claims.

FEE SCHEDULE   Each year, Medicare publishes a fee schedule for all Medicare covered services in the forthcoming year. It is distributed to all registered providers in December. Listed in numerical order by *CPT* code numbers, these are the allowable fees for each of these services. There is some regional variation based on geographic and other factors.

Psychiatric Coverage Limitations. Medicare sets a fee schedule for all psychiatric services (the 908xx series of *CPT* codes), just as it does for all other medical services. However, as noted, there is a limitation of payment by Medicare for all therapeutic services for treatment performed outside an acute care inpatient setting for all "mental and emotional disorders."

The original Medicare legislation limited payment for these therapeutic services to 50% of the allowable amount. Because the structure of the Medicare payment system also dictates a payment of 80% of an allowed amount, Medicare calculated that the legislated 50% must be equal to 80% of something and created the 62.5% psychiatric payment limitation (80% × 62.5% = 50%). Note that the limitation applies to treatment services provided when the diagnosis is for mental or emotional disorders. Therefore, the limitation applies even when the service is an evaluation and management (E&M) therapeutic service. This 62.5% psychiatric limitation does not apply when therapeutic services are provided in an inpatient hospital, inpatient psychiatric facility, or comprehensive inpatient rehabilitation facility. It also does not apply in a hospital emergency room when the 99xxx procedure codes are used (Grant, 2002).

There is no such payment limitation for diagnostic, consultative, and testing services. This applies whether the diagnostic services are from the E&M series (new patient, hospital admission, consultations, confirmatory consultation), for a psychiatric diagnostic service (90801), or for psychological testing or neuropsychological testing.

Brief psychiatric office visits for the sole purpose of monitoring or changing prescriptions (coded M0064) are not subject to the 62.5% payment limitation (Grant, 2002). Many Medicare carriers consider the psychiatric medication management code (90862) as a service that is subject to the 50% limitation, but some do not. Also, local carriers may differ in the frequency with which they deem that medication management is medically necessary in a particular setting or for a particular diagnosis. This level of local variability requires psychiatrists to be informed of the guidelines used by their local Medicare carriers despite the fact that this information may be difficult to obtain.

Medicare reduces the amount paid for services (with the same procedure code) performed in certain facilities to compensate for "lower practice expenses" physicians have when providing services in the facilities. For example, treatment provided at an outpatient hospital is reimbursed at a lower rate than the same service rendered at the psychiatrist's office.

Psychotherapy. There are 24 codes to describe psychotherapy services (codes 90804–90829). These are divided by duration of time: briefer (20–30 minutes), longer (45–50 minutes), and extended (75–80 minutes). They are also divided by place of service: inpatient (which in this case is considered to include general hospital, psychiatric hospital, inpatient rehabilitation facilities, and nursing home locations) and outpatient (all other locations). They are divided into those services that include or do not include E&M services and into those that use or do not use interactive techniques. Interactive techniques involve the use of physical aids and nonverbal communication to overcome barriers to therapeutic interaction in patients who have lost or not yet developed either the expressive or receptive language communication skills required to explain symptoms and response to treatment. Interactive codes are commonly used to describe play therapy with children, but could also be used to describe work with a patient suffering from aphasia or deafness.

Some patients receive psychotherapeutic services alone, and some receive psychotherapy with medical E&M services. Although E&M codes are most commonly used by medical practitioners to describe the assessment and management of their patients, these codes may be used appropriately by psychiatrists to describe their clinical work (see the next section on evaluation and management). Each of the psychotherapy codes has an assigned allowed fee. A slightly higher fee is paid for the psychotherapy services provided with the E&M code format, but documentation of the assessment and intervention procedures is required.

E&M services can include ongoing medical diagnostic evaluation; interim history taking; medication management; physician's orders; interpretation of laboratory or other medical diagnostic studies; counseling or coordination of care with nursing or other service providers or with facilities, caregivers, or family; or examination of the patient (including any elements of a physical examination or a single-system examination, including a mental status examination). Provision and documentation of any of these additional services can be sufficient to warrant billing for the higher fee service than is provided by the conventional psychotherapy codes.

Evaluation and Management: The E&M Codes. The Centers for Medicare and Medicaid Services (CMS, formerly HCFA), in conjunction with the AMA, has created documentation guidelines for E&M services. These were originally described in 1995 and revised in 1997. Either documentation scheme can be utilized by a provider. The *CPT* codes for these services are in the 99xxx series. Each includes three "key" components (history, examination, and medical decision making) and four subsidiary components (counseling, coordination of care, nature of presenting problem, and time). Various combinations of these factors establish the *level* of the service for billing purposes. Time is only considered in establishing a level of care provided during an E&M service when more than 50% of the service involves counseling or coordination of care.

E&M codes can be used for initial visits with a patient or follow-up visits for ongoing evaluation and management. They can be used for patients of the doctor's own or patients of another physician who are seen in consultation. Many of the service codes are place specific, and there are subseries of E&M codes for the office, hospital, nursing home, domiciliary services, and emergency room.

Although psychiatrists may use E&M service codes, they must be aware of documentation requirements. To be reimbursable at a specific E&M level, the service must be medically necessary for the identified problem. For example, the use of a complex E&M code may be considered unnecessary for the ongoing management of a minor problem. Also, components of the service must be appropriately documented. Psychiatrists can provide services up to the highest level (comprehensive) if they perform a complete single-system (e.g., psychiatric) examination or a complete multisystem examination together with a comprehensive history, including a review of systems and a complete past (medical and surgical, personal and family, and social) history obtained at that visit. In the case of a previously established patient, it is acceptable for the physician to refer to an existing record reflecting the changes in the patient's medical, family, and social history from the last encounter. The definitions of what constitutes a brief, extended, or comprehensive history or examination and the other aspects of the E&M coding system are included in the information about the documentation guidelines for evaluation and management services in the *CPT* codebook and at the Web site for the Centers for Medicare and Medicaid Services (cms.hhs.gov/medlearn/emdoc.asp; AMA, 2002).

When a psychiatrist sees a new patient, the service might be billed as an initial psychiatric visit (90801), as an initial E&M visit by a new patient in the office, as an admission to the hospital, as an office consultation, or as an inpatient consultation. The differences among these are in the nature of the questions asked, the examination done, the place of service, whether another physician requested the consultation, and in the manner of documentation. Consultations also require that correspondence or other (preferably written) communication be sent to the requesting physician to assist in their treatment of the patient. Medicare payment for evaluation and diagnosis is paid at 80% of the Medicare allowed amount regardless of which of these services is performed.

Reimbursement for medication management of psychiatric disorders, especially of dementias, was to be exempted from the 50% copayment requirement (OBRA 87). Nevertheless, many Medicare intermediaries have not implemented this change and continue to reimburse at the 50% copayment for all psychiatric service codes (908xx series), including the 90862 code for psychiatric medication management of a mental disorder *CPT* code (290–319). However, services provided using E&M codes (99xxx series), which do not use mental disorder series *CPT* codes, may be reimbursable at 80% by some Medicare carriers. These nonmental disorder series *CPT* codes, which a psychiatrist, like any other physician, may use, include the diseases of the nervous system and sense organs (including "hereditary and degenerative diseases of the central nervous system 330–337," such as 331.0 for Alzheimer's disease or 331.1 for Pick's disease) or diseases of the circulatory system (which includes 438.0, late effects of cerebrovascular disease, cognitive deficits) (*ICD-9-CM*).

Medicare Copayment. Regarding the Medicare copayment requirement to bill the patient for the 50% copayment balance or the 37.5% residual balance, some Medigap or supplemental insurance policies pay the full amount of the 50% copayment. All Medigap policies, except for those issued prior to the implementation of OBRA 90 in July 1991, must cover mental health services. Such policies must pay the entire beneficiary share, generally 50% of the total Medicare allowed amount for outpatient services (CMS, 2002). Other patients have policies, such as secondary insurance issued by employers, that pay only 12.5% (the equivalent of the 20% these policies pay for all Medicare copayments), for a total received of 62.5%.

Some patients have no secondary coverage. Where the patient does not have a secondary insurance policy that pays the full balance of the 50% copayment, the psychiatrist is required by Medicare to bill the patient for the remaining amount (although not required to collect it). The physician is allowed to waive the collection of the copayment in selected cases if discussion with the patient determines that paying the copayment would be a financial hardship. Documentation of the discussion and rationale for waiving the copayment is recommended, and forgiving the copayment must be justified by particular circumstances. Waiving copayments for groups of patients is forbidden. However, doctors are not allowed to bill copayment balances to Medicare beneficiaries who are also Medicaid recipients or who are at or below the federal poverty level.

Patients may be surprised when billed for copayment of psychiatric services. It is, therefore, recommended that the psychiatrist explain this fact to patients at the beginning of treatment, including the fact that Medicare will only pay for 50% of the allowable fee for treating emotional disorders outside the hospital setting.

Deductibles. Medicare has an annual deductible of $100 per beneficiary that the patient is expected to pay. This is generally charged against (deducted from the payment made to) the provider of services that year whose claims are received first by the Medicare carrier regardless of whether that provider was the first physician who saw the patient that year. To avoid having too many deductibles subtracted from her or his fees, doctors may delay billing some Medicare claims in the beginning of the year, especially for those patients from whom it may be difficult to collect the deductible. Some of the Medicare legislative proposals considered by Congress in 2003 include provisions to increase the amount of the annual deductible.

Noncovered Services. Medicare only covers those services considered "reasonable and necessary for the diagnosis and treatment of illness or injury" or "to improve the functioning of a malformed body member" (Grant, 2002, p. 12303). Medicare has developed rules to protect patients from liability when a claim is denied as not medically necessary. These rules, which apply to assigned claims, are called *waiver of liability* provisions. The patient is only liable if the patient signed a statement (called an Advance Beneficiary Notice) agreeing to pay for a service that the physician informed him or her would be denied by Medicare as a noncovered service. The statements to the patient must be specific and individualized so that the patient has a clear idea of why the doctor is predicting that Medicare will not pay. This should be put in writing as part of the statement the patient signs (Grant, 2002). This applies to services that Medicare might pay for at times, but that might not be paid on this occasion (e.g., a psychotherapy session when there is no diagnosed mental disorder). It does not apply to services that are never covered by Medicare and for which, therefore, the physician may charge a fee directly to the patient (e.g., psychiatric legal or forensic services).

TOOLS AND RESOURCES

Software. Billing and bookkeeping software can enhance efficiency. When evaluating the purchase of such software, there must be consideration of its ease of use, its comprehensiveness, and its cost. Such software should be able to electronically transmit bills directly to the Medicare carrier. It may also be possible to electronically transmit directly to the Medicaid carrier. CMS and the Medicare intermediaries have instituted a nationally standardized protocol for electronic transmission of all claims.

The software should also have the ability to print out standard insurance forms, especially the HCFA 1500, which is the form Medicare uses. In addition, it should be able to print out one or more styles of patient billing letters, including form letters that the psychiatrist designs. Alternatively, providers may pay a fee to have a billing service submit their Medicare and secondary insurance bills electronically. Providers remain responsible for the accuracy of claims that are submitted.

The software should provide reports on the status of billings, receipts, outstanding balances, unpaid claims, and the like as well as daily, weekly, monthly, and yearly reports of various kinds. It should include features to prevent the entry of incorrect data and to prevent the failure to enter necessary data. Often, the software will include electronic entry of payments from the Medicare carrier. The vendor of the software should include training, support, and upgrades (although there may be extra charges for these).

Other Resources. Other necessary resource materials (as mentioned above) include the annually updated *CPT* codebook, the annually updated Medicare carrier fee schedule, the current year's version of the *ICD-9-CM* codebook, the Medicare carrier policies and procedures manuals (which include descriptions of the covered codes and their documentation requirements), and the monthly Medicare update bulletin. It would also be helpful for the doctor or the office staff to attend some of the Medicare carrier's periodic classes and seminars.

Each Medicare carrier is required by CMS to have a carrier advisory committee (CAC) consisting of representatives of providers, including one representative for each specialty and for most subspecialties. Although there are psychiatric representatives appointed to most CACs, representation by psychiatric subspecialties, such as by a geriatric psychiatrist, is highly unusual. These provider representatives are generally appointed by the state specialty societies. Knowing the psychiatric representative to the CAC, volunteering to serve as a representative or alternate, and helping the CAC respond to specific questions can increase sensitivity to issues pertaining to geriatric psychiatry.

DOCUMENTATION   It is vitally important to correctly and appropriately document the provision of services in a manner that accurately describes what was done and that meets coding documentation guidelines for this service (cms.hhs.gov/medlearn/emdoc.asp; AMA, 2002; Gardiner, 2000; Grant, 2002; HCFA, 1999). Services must be documented prior to billing for those services. Documentation must be legible. The documentation must follow appropriate medical procedure, the Medicare carrier's policies/procedures manual, *and* (where appropriate) the CMS E&M coding guidelines. The coding of services must be consistent with the documentation, and the reimbursement is contingent on the coding. In the absence of a note, it is assumed the service did not occur.

The psychiatrist might find it helpful to create templates for initial evaluations, progress notes, medication tracking log, and other useful records. This may be especially helpful if providing any E&M services that require specific types and styles of documentation. These forms could include some checklists or blank areas (if either of these is done, additional blank spaces are needed for other information). Software can be purchased that provides standard templates for entering Medicare notes. The primary advantages of creating or using electronic forms is to assist in documentation, including ensuring that collection and recording of important data are not forgotten and helping reduce writing time.

COMPLIANCE PLANS   There is a continuing and growing emphasis from CMS and the local Medicare intermediaries and carriers to reduce fraud and abuse by providers. Their efforts to do this include instituting prepayment reviews, postpayment reviews, overt and undercover investigations by the Office of the Investigator General (OIG), the "correct coding initiative," and the creation of "compliance plans." The guidelines for compliance plans for small physicians' practices are considered voluntary, but physicians are strongly urged to have a compliance plan in place. Having a Medicare compliance plan provides documentation of the physician's earnestness in helping avoid fraud and abuse. This can be of assistance in defending a physician in an OIG or carrier investigation (OIG, 2000; Tengesdal, 2000). As part of this, the physician must educate staff members in practice ethics and the importance of the relationship between service documentation and correct billing.

OPTING OUT OF THE MEDICARE SYSTEM   Under the Balanced Budget Act of 1997 (BBA 97), a physician can drop out of Medicare. The physician must file an affidavit with Medicare to this effect. This allows the physician to enter into private contracts with patients for payment for the physician's services. However, by doing so the physician is prohibited from billing Medicare for any services (except emergency treatment) provided to any patient for a period of 2 years. No services provided by that physician to any patient are reimbursable by Medicare. A written agreement between the physician and each patient, signed by each, ensures that patients cannot claim subsequently that they expected the services to be covered by Medicare and to be subject to its fee limitations. The agreement should state clearly that the beneficiary gives up all Medicare coverage for the services provided and agrees not to bill Medicare or their Medigap insurer for these services. This agreement does not limit the right of the patient to have Medicare coverage for services from other providers. Physicians who opt out of the Medicare system are allowed to create a fee-for-service relationship with patients unrestricted by the Medicare fee schedule (Grant, 2002). Renewing the agreement every 2 years ensures that the contract remains valid.

Other Insurance Carriers

COINSURANCE AND MEDIGAP POLICIES Medigap insurance policies are sold by private insurers to Medicare beneficiaries. These pay for Medicare coinsurance and, in some cases, deductible charges. As an incentive for doctors to become participating providers in Medicare, carriers automatically send a patient's claim to the Medigap insurer when assignment is accepted. The Medigap insurers automatically pay claims directly to participating physicians under the following circumstances: (1) the plan is a true Medigap plan as defined by the Social Security Act and not a supplemental insurance plan provided by an employer, pension plan, or labor union; and (2) the claim is on behalf of a participating provider. A Medigap carrier may send payment to the patient (even when assignment is accepted) when the physician is a nonparticipating provider (Grant, 2002).

MEDICAID

Medicaid as a Secondary Payer. When Medicaid is the secondary insurer (after Medicare), they may not pay the usual Medicare copayment. Many states have declared that, when the dollar payment by Medicare for a service exceeds the amount that Medicaid allows for that service, payment will be restricted to the Medicare allowable amount. If the Medicare dollar payment is less than the allowed Medicaid payment, payment is equal to the difference between the Medicare payment and the Medicaid allowable. In some (but not all) states, Medicaid will pay the annual Medicare deductible, but may pay it at the Medicaid fee schedule (BBA 97).

Medicaid as a Primary Payer. Some seniors only have Medicaid and not

Medicare Parts A or B. For these individuals, services will be paid according the Medicaid fee schedule. Providers must register with Medicaid to receive Medicaid payments and must accept the Medicaid fee schedule as payment for the services. The Medicaid fee schedule varies from state to state. Providers are forbidden from billing patients who have Medicaid for any services, even an unpaid balance of copayment or for coinsurance in the case of a patient with Medicare who has Medicaid as a secondary payer.

MANAGED-CARE ORGANIZATIONS   Many Medicare MCOs and health maintenance organizations (HMOs) "carve out" psychiatric and other mental health services. The limitations inherent in this may prevent many geriatric psychiatrists from working for those provider panels (Stein & Moak, 2002). It is necessary for a psychiatrist to apply for admission to a provider panel and to sign a contract with the MCO. MCOs may also have other barriers to provision of services, such as requiring preauthorization or repeated authorization for ongoing treatment and by strictly limiting the availability of inpatient or partial hospitalization services.

These obstacles may explain the dearth of psychiatrists available to care for elderly persons in health maintenance organizations. Among those psychiatrists who have more than 20% of their caseload devoted to treating the elderly, a mean of only 1% (with a standard deviation of 7.9%) of their caseload is devoted to treating elderly HMO patients (Colenda et al., 1999). Mental health carve-outs create disincentives for psychiatric services, such as limiting the number of providers or locations where care is available (Bartels & Colenda, 1998).

There is now a reported tendency to carve in (reintegrate) psychiatric services into the general medical milieu of managed-care plans. Mental health services under managed-care organizations may be reimbursed through contracts with the providers for negotiated fees for services (for example, a fee schedule) or by capitated arrangements. It may be possible to negotiate a contracted fee for providing services (for example, to all of the HMOs elderly patients in a facility such a nursing home) (Jackson, 1997; Weidner, 1996).

Insurance Payment Errors

Insurance carriers may make errors in reimbursement policy and in reimbursing for services. Carriers may not explain why the errors are made. The doctor's office should monitor the receipt of payments and resubmit if bills have been lost or never paid. This follow-up should not be delayed as many insurers have requirements regarding timeliness of claims submissions. Claims denied or "down-coded" in error can be appealed successfully, providing that the service is medically necessary and that a note documents the level of service.

Medicare has instituted a series of prepayment, postpayment, and random reviews of services. Medicare will ask for copies of medical records for those services. If documentation of the need and the service provided is considered unjustified, the service may be down-coded and paid at a lower rate or denied entirely. If payment has already been made, the carrier may ask that payment be returned. Such determinations can be appealed. A consistent pattern of over-billing for services that are not adequately documented may lead to additional reviews and, in more extreme cases, to penalties.

A common cause of billing error and nonpayment for services can occur when a patient changes insurance (e.g., Medigap, HMO, etc.). Patients should be asked regularly whether their insurance has changed, and a copy of their new insurance card (including the back of the card, which includes the phone number of the insurance company) should be obtained. Also, the insurance company should be contacted (starting at the beginning of treatment) to verify the patient's eligibility, the correctness of the insurance number and the extent of coverage, whether there is any deductible or other limitation, whether payment will be made to the doctor or to the patient, the correct billing address, and any necessary authorization for treatment. It is becoming increasingly common for Medicare secondary payors to behave like primary managed-care companies in requiring authorization, justification, and information about treatment, even when Medicare has paid its portion of the claim.

MAINTAINING THE BUSINESS

Building and maintaining a geriatric psychiatry business includes the areas of customer relations, development of relationships with referring sources, and marketing and public relations (Bernstein & Freiermuth, 1992; Sachs, 1991).

Physicians are accustomed to thinking of the patient as the customer of medical services. However, in the business context, the definition requires expansion. In some cases, customers may be the patient's family insofar as they may be the ones encouraging and supporting the receipt of services by the identified patient. Other potential customers include those who refer patients: physicians and other medical providers; other mental health clinicians; facilities (nursing homes, assisted living facilities, senior centers, hospitals, partial hospital programs, etc.); attorneys or accountants who provide services to the elderly; judges; or governmental or quasi-governmental programs (e.g., a guardianship program).

In each case, it is important for the geriatric psychiatrist to satisfy these customers by addressing the needs and causes for the referral. To do so, it is important to clarify the reasons the referral was made. These may be simple or complex, and in some cases, there may be multiple reasons. For example, the family may bring a senior who is depressed and yet is reluctant to seek treatment, or they may have just become aware of a cognitive disturbance. On the other hand, there may be an underlying family conflict between elderly spouses or between parent and child or between children. If those issues are not addressed, they may interfere with the patient's ability to obtain treatment. Physicians may refer a patient for a number of reasons, including the patient's medical complexity, failure of the patient to respond to conventional treatment, or an inordinate proportion of time spent on management of the patient. A facility or program may refer a patient because the patient is disruptive within the program setting. The psychiatrist may see the problem as manageable, but the referring program may insist on or expect hospitalization to reduce inconvenience to the facility. If the program's concerns are not addressed, the treatment may fail, and future referrals may be unlikely. Attorneys or accountants may request an assessment for competence to sign documents or engage in business or respond to concerns about protecting an individual's assets.

Referring Sources

A related topic is the creation and development of relationships with referring sources. In addition to those mentioned, sources of referral can include clergy, the Alzheimer's Association, community hotlines, social service agencies, medical and professional society offices, hospital or nursing home social workers, hospital and nursing home nursing staff, and psychologists working in the hospital or community. Relationships can be developed through shared working experiences, such as care of patients. In addition, interacting in the setting of charitable or committee work (for example, serving on the medical advisory board for the local Alzheimer's Association chapter), in professional organizations, or in community or religious organization activities can all contribute to business marketing.

Marketing and Public Relations

Public relations activities, which can be crucial to developing a private practice, are generally directed at the groups of people noted in the section on referring sources and at others who may be sources of referral, particularly satisfied patients and their families (Bernstein & Freiermuth, 1992; Sachs, 1991).

The opportunities for this type of public relations include optimizing the design of business cards and stationary. The font on business cards should be large enough for seniors with impaired vision to read clearly. Develop a personal practice brochure or information sheet that is given to patients or is available in the waiting room. The brochure should describe the physician's background, credentials, achievements and honors, special interests, and treatments offered in clear and readily understandable language (for example, "Specializing in the care of older individuals who are suffering from problems with depression and anxiety, forgetfulness, or the stresses that naturally occur after losses, retirement, or illness"). It should also clearly indicate whether Medicare assignment is accepted and include address office hours, phone number, fax number, and the address of the doctor's Web site if there is one. Other opportunities for practice-enhancing public relations include writing articles for local or regional newspapers or appearing on local radio and television shows. Participation in the geriatric section of the district branch of the American Psychiatric Association or of the local or state medical society will inform colleagues of the geriatric psychiatrist's special expertise.

Yellow page listings and advertisements can be expensive and may not be cost-effective. Consider listings under "Physicians—Psychiatry" and possibly under such areas as the general physician listings and under "Physicians—Geriatrics" (if such exists in the local yellow pages).

In many cases, other medical and mental health providers will be the most frequent referrers of new patients. Therefore, advertising/public relations directed toward them will probably have the greatest yield. Every consultation report sent to a referring physician should be an opportunity to enhance the potential for future referrals. For example, consider using such phrases as "thank you for your continuing confidence in me" or "as always, I very much appreciated the opportunity to see Mrs. Jones in consultation." Timeliness in responding to physician requests for consultations or appointments and in providing feedback or ongoing information and advice are also inherently good customer relations, as well as good patient care.

Additional public relations devices include sending holiday cards to physicians and other referring sources or mailing or displaying copies of articles that the psychiatrist has written, of articles written about the psychiatrist, or of notices of awards won or honors achieved. Articles that cover the overlap between geriatric psychiatry and other areas of medicine can be sent to colleagues (with a personalized cover letter or handwritten note such as, "Dear Dr. Jones, I ran across this article and thought you might find it interesting").

Marketing and public relations, whether overt or in more subtle forms as noted, are ongoing. There may be many people who would refer patients, but they may not think of it at the time the opportunity (and the patient) presents itself. Optimally, they would be repeatedly, but not intrusively, reminded of the geriatric psychiatrist's existence, expertise, and services so that when the prospective patient is with them, the information will come to mind.

Beginning, managing, and maintaining a successful private practice is a complex task. However, it also can be a gratifying and rewarding experience.

REFERENCES

American Association for Geriatric Psychiatry. *Depression in Late Life, Not a Natural Part of Aging.* Bethesda, MD: American Association for Geriatric Psychiatry; no date.

American Medical Association. *CPT-2003, Current Procedural Terminology, 2003.* Chicago, IL: American Medical Association; 2002.

American Psychiatric Association. *Let's Talk Facts About . . .* Pamphlet series, various titles. Washington, DC: American Psychiatric Association; no date.

Ball RM. Medicare's roots, what Medicare's architects had in mind. *Generations.* 1996; 20(2):13–18.

Bartels SJ, Colenda CC. Mental health services for Alzheimer's disease: current trends in reimbursement and public policy, and the future under managed care. *Am J Geriatr Psychiatry*. 1998;6:S85–S100.

BBA 97. *Balanced Budget Act of 1997*. Washington, DC: US Government Printing Office; 1997.

Bernstein A, Freiermuth D. *The Practice Builder, Complete Marketing Library of $1,000,000 Strategies*. Englewood Cliffs, NJ: Prentice Hall; 1992.

Center for Medicare and Medicaid Services. *Program Memorandum: Medigap Coverage of Outpatient Mental Health Services That Are Subject to the Mental Health Payment Reduction*. Baltimore, MD: CMS; December 2002. Transmittal No. 02–02.

Colenda CC, Mickus MA, Marcus SC, et al. Comparison of adult and geriatric psychiatric practice patterns; findings for the American Psychiatric Association's Practice Research Network. *Am J Geriatr Psychiatry*. 2002;10:609–617.

Colenda CC, Pincus H, Tanielian TL, et al. Update of geriatric psychiatry practices among American psychiatrists; analysis of the 1996 National Survey of Psychiatric Practice. *Am J Geriatr Psychiatry*. 1999;7:279–288.

Crossett JHW. Practice of geriatric psychiatry. In: Silberman EK, ed. *Successful Psychiatric Practice, Current Dilemmas, Choices and Solutions*. Washington, DC: American Psychiatric Press; 1995:175–186.

Department of Health and Human Services. *Depression Is a Treatable Illness, a Patient's Guide*. Rockville, MD: Dept. of Health and Human Services, Public Health Service, Agency for Health Care Policy and Research; 1993. Publication AHCPR 93–0553.

Dorwart RA, Chartock LR, Dial T, et al. A national study of psychiatrists? Professional activities. *Am J Psychiatry*. 1992;149:1499–1505.

Florida Highway Patrol. *Driving Safely for Aging Floridians*. Tallahassee, FL: Florida Highway Patrol; no date.

Fuller MA. *Drug Information Handbook for Psychiatry, 1999–2000, American Pharmaceutical Association*. Hudson, OH: Lex-Comp; 1999.

Gardiner J. *Physician Practice Coder* [monthly newsletter]. Rockville, MD: Part B News Group; 2000.

Goldberg J. Doctor's earnings: you call this progress? *Med Econ*. 1999;18:172.

Goldberg RJ. *The Brown University Geriatric Psychopharmacology Update* [monthly newsletter]. Providence, RI: Manisses Communications Group; 2000.

Grant DW. *Part B Answer Book*. Rockville, MD: Part B News Group; 2002.

Greene J, Loebel P, Banazak D, et al. *Manual of Nursing Home Practice for Psychiatrists*. Washington, DC: American Psychiatric Press; 2000.

Greenspan AL. *Medical Employers Guide: A Handbook of Employment Laws and Regulations*. 3rd ed. Forth Worth, TX: Summers Press; 1996.

Grimaldi P. Medigap insurance policies standardized. *Nurs Manag*. 1992;23:20–24.

Health Care Financing Administration. *Medicare Guidelines for Mental Health Services*. Jacksonville, FL: First Coast Service Options; 1999.

Jackson JN. Managed Medicare. In: Siegal A, Jackson J, Moak G, eds. *Geriatric Psychiatry Practice Management Handbook*. Bethesda, MD: American Association for Geriatric Psychiatry; 1997:5-1–5-80.

Jefferson JW. *Lithium and Manic Depression: A Guide*. Middletown, WI: Lithium Information Center, Dean Foundation for Health, Research and Education; 1996.

Klein JI, MacBeth JE, Onek JN. *Legal Issues in the Private Practice of Psychiatry*. Washington, DC: American Psychiatric Press; 1984.

Logsdon L. *Establishing a Psychiatric Private Practice*. Washington, DC: American Psychiatric Press; 1985.

Loran LM, Taintor Z, Mairza M. Patient characteristics and treatment modalities. In: Loran LM, ed. *The Nation's Psychiatrists*. Washington, DC: American Psychiatric Association; 1987:97–112.

Medicare B Update [monthly newsletter of the Florida Medicare carrier]. Jacksonville, FL: First Coast Service Options; 2000.

Office of the Inspector General. Department of Health and Human Services, Office of the Inspector General Web site. Available at: http://oig.hhs.gov/authorities/docs/physician.pdf; 2000.

Olfson M, Goldman HH. Psychiatric outpatient practice: patterns and policies. *Am J Psychiatry*. 1992;149:1492–1498.

Olfson M, Marcus SC, Pincus HA. Trends in office based psychiatric practice. *Am J Psychiatry*. 1999;156:451–457.

Physicians' Desk Reference. 57th ed. Montvale, NJ: Medical Economics; 2003.

Pincus HA, Zarin DA, Tanielian TL, et al. Psychiatric patients and treatments in 1997: findings from the American Psychiatric Practice Research Network. *Arch Gen Psychiatry*. 1999;56:441–449.

Sachs L. *The Professional Practice Problem Solver—Do It Yourself Strategies That Really Work*. Englewood Cliffs, NJ: Prentice Hall; 1991.

Siegal A, Jackson J, Moak G, eds. *Geriatric Psychiatry Practice Management Handbook*. Bethesda, MD: American Association for Geriatric Psychiatry; 1997.

Seigler EL, Messett E. Nurse practitioner and physician assistants in the health care system. *Ann Long-Term Care*. 2000;8:56–57.

Stein EM. Geriatric psychiatry in office and clinic. *J Appl Gerontol.*; 1983a;2:102–111.

Stein EM. Some practical considerations in the private practice of psycho-geriatrics. *Clin Gerontol*. 1983b;2:56–58.

Stein EM, Moak GS. Community-based psychiatric ambulatory care: the private practice model. In: Copeland J, Abou-Saleh M, Blazer D, eds. *The Principles and Practice of Geriatric Psychiatry*. 2nd ed. Sussex, UK: John Wiley and Sons; 2002:697–703.

Tengesdal S. *Physician Compliance Alert* [monthly newsletter]. Rockville, MD: Part B News Group; 2000.

Weidner DW. *Physician's Desk Guide to Managed Care and Contracting*. Jacksonville, FL: Florida Physician's Association; 1996.

Weidner DW, Bobo T, Spicer, et al. *Florida Physician's Desk Guide to Law and Medicine*. Jacksonville, FL: Florida Physicians Association; 1993.

World Health Organization. *International Classification of Diseases, Ninth Revision—Clinical Modification, 2003 edition*. Dover, DE: American Medical Association; 2002.

Wyatt RJ. *Practical Psychiatric Practice, Forms and Protocols for Clinical Use*. 2nd ed. Washington, DC: American Psychiatric Press; 1998.

Zarin DA, Pincus HA, Peterson BD, et al. Characterizing psychiatry with findings from the 1996 National Survey of Psychiatric Practice. *Am J Psychiatry*. 1998;155:397–404.

Zuckerman EL. *The Paper Office 1, Forms, Guidelines and Resources*. Pittsburgh, PA: Clinician's Toolbox; 1992.

41

Psychiatry at the End of Life

Linda Ganzini, MD, MPH
Harvey Max Chochinov, MD, PhD, FRCP (C)

In 1998, 75% of all deaths in the United States occurred in persons older than 65 years (Martin et al., 1999). Many deaths in old age are foreseeable, occurring in the context of chronic progressive or terminal illness. Geriatric psychiatrists, who experience the death of many of their patients, have much to offer in assisting these patients and their families in the final months of life. Significant themes in the psychiatric care of elderly dying patients include the importance of differentiating normative from pathological changes, respect for patients' and families' values in the dying process, careful definition of realistic and appropriate goals of care, keen awareness of diminished life expectancy in setting those goals, focus on treatment of symptoms more than diseases, high priority on comfort as a short-term objective, and assiduous avoidance of interventions that may worsen suffering. This chapter reviews the important principles of palliative care in psychiatry as applied to the elderly.

Palliative care is the active total care of patients whose diseases are not responsive to curative treatments. Palliative care addresses physical, psychological, social, and spiritual domains with the goal of improvement in quality of life for patients and for their families (World Health Organization, 1990). A major goal of palliative care is *a good death*. The Institute of Medicine defines a good death as one that is free of avoidable distress and suffering for patients, families, and caregivers; in general accord with patients' and families' wishes; and reasonably consistent with clinical, cultural, and ethical standards (Field & Cassel, 1997).

Studies have highlighted that many deaths in the United States do not meet this definition. For example, the Study to Understand Prognoses and Preferences for Outcomes and Risks of Treatment (SUPPORT) investigated outcomes across five US academic medical centers for over 4,000 seriously ill, hospitalized patients who died. Notably, 38% of these patients spent 10 days or more in an intensive care unit, and 46% of do-not-resuscitate orders were written within 2 days of death (SUPPORT Principal Investigators, 1995). Aggressive care was received by 1 in 10 patients even when, according to the family, comfort care was preferred. Further, 40% had moderate to extreme pain, and over half had dyspnea at least half of the time in the last 3 days of life. Psychiatric symptoms were also common: In the last 3 days of life, dysphoria, anxiety, and confusion were experienced at least half of the time by 25% of the study participants who died (Lynn et al., 1997).

In 2002, half of deaths in the United States occurred in hospitals, 25% in nursing homes, and 25% in residences (National Hospice and Palliative Care Organization, 2003). The most common causes of death in persons older than 65 years were heart disease, cancer, stroke, and chronic obstructive pulmonary disease (Martin et al., 1999). High-quality care for the dying is delivered through community hospice organizations for patients living at home, in residential treatment facilities, or skilled nursing facilities. Hospice care is practically defined by the Medicare hospice benefit, which pays for physician services, in-home nursing services, home health aide services, and medications for patients who have less than 6 months to live and are not receiving life-sustaining medical treatments. This benefit also pays for respite care and bereavement counseling for patients' families (Medicare Rights Center, 1998). In 2002, 25% (an estimated 600,000) of people who died in the United States received hospice services, although there are wide geographic variations (National Hospice and Palliative Care Organization, 2003); 60% were age 75 or older. Increasingly, health care systems have palliative care consultation teams (Bascom, 1997; Weissman & Griffie, 1994).

Prognostication has assumed increasing importance both for helping determine the focus of care and more practically because hospice requires certification that patients have a 6-month life expectancy. Obtaining prognostic information is a high priority for many patients; giving prognostic information is very uncomfortable for physicians (Christakis & Lamont, 2000). The median stay in hospice is 3 weeks (National Hospice and Palliative Care Organization, 2003), yet experts believe patients and families maximally benefit from hospice stays longer than 3 months. Late referrals from physicians deny both patients and families many of the benefits of hospice.

Christakis and Lamont (2000) asked 343 physicians to predict survival of 468 terminally ill patients at the time of hospice referral. Median survival was 24 days, and only 20% of predictions of survival were accurate. Overall, physicians overestimated survival by a factor of 5.3. Prognostic accuracy decreased as the duration of the doctor-patient relationship increased and time since last contact decreased.

Singer and coworkers (1999) found that the most important concerns of ill and dying patients are to receive adequate pain and symptom management, avoid inappropriate prolongation of dying, achieve a sense of control, relieve their loved ones' burden, and strengthen relationships with loved ones. Steinhauser and colleagues (2000) used focus group discussions with patients, families, and providers to explore components of a good death. Participants identified pain and symptom management, clear decision making, preparation for death, completion, contributing to others, and affirmation of the whole person. Physicians' definition of a good death differed from that of other providers and family members, offering a more biomedical perspective. Geriatric psychiatrists' appreciation of the biopsychosocial model, human development and the life cycle, the power of reminiscence and review, and integration of the family makes them potent allies in assisting dying patients to reach their goals.

DELIRIUM

Delirium is marked by disturbances of consciousness, primarily reduced ability to attend and concentrate, as well as other cognitive and perceptual disturbances (American Psychiatric Association, 1994). The disorder often develops over a short period of time, fluctuates during the course of the day, and is usually secondary to a general medical condition. Delirium is comprehensively reviewed in Chapter 18; we restrict this discussion to aspects of delirium in dying persons that differ from usual geropsychiatric care.

There are few studies of the epidemiology of delirium in dying patients; these comprised few subjects and were biased toward hospitalized patients as opposed to patients dying in homes or nursing facilities. Despite these limitations, delirium appears to be the most common mental disorder in the dying, with a point prevalence of 20% to 61% in hospitalized cancer patients or hospice inpatients, and an incidence of 33% to 85% in terminal care (Bruera, Miller, et al., 1992; Gagnon et al., 2000; Massie et al., 1983; Minagawa et al., 1996; Pereira et al., 1997). Within palliative care, health care providers frequently do not recognize delirium unless they systematically examine for it. Bruera, Miller, and coworkers (1992) reported that, among cancer patients in an inpatient hospice who had acute cognitive failure (as defined by a Mini-Mental State Examination [MMSE] score of less than 24 or decline of 30% or more on the MMSE), physicians did not detect mental status changes on daily rounds in 23% of patients.

We are not aware of any studies that have examined for qualitative differences in clinical manifestations of delirium between patients who do and do not die. As in all delirious patients, mild delirium may be misdiagnosed as depression, anxiety, or another psychological problem, leading to inappropriate and ineffective psychopharmacological or psychotherapeutic interventions (Farrell & Ganzini, 1995).

Delirium has been subtyped into hyperactive, hypoactive, and mixed states. Hyperactive or agitated delirium is characterized by increased psychomotor activity, restlessness, and excitability (Lipowski, 1990). Although studies have not clearly validated these subtypes, agitated delirium, which in palliative care is termed *terminal restlessness* or *terminal agitation*, has received special attention and is often a hallmark of a "bad death" (Breibart et al., 1998). The agitated, restless, and wandering patient can be a danger to himself or herself, increase family members' emotional distress and exhaustion, and impede the family members' preparation for death (Fainsinger et al., 1993).

Pain and symptom control are much more difficult in delirious patients (Fainsinger et al., 1993; Gagnon et al., 2000). In inpatient palliative care settings, before death about 10% to 26% of patients experience agitated delirium that requires sedation (Fainsinger et al., 1991, 1998).

In contrast, the patient with hypoactive delirium is quiet, lethargic, and listless. Within palliative care, quiet delirium is expected, considered part of the dying process, and often consistent with a peaceful, unanxious death. Treatment of hypoactive delirium is controversial. Particularly, visual hallucinations of a spiritual nature in the final days of life are considered normative by some and consistent with *decathexis*, or the letting go of life (Farber et al., 2000). More research is needed to determine how often such experiences occur outside the context of delirium and if patients and families would be more comfortable with active treatment of these symptoms. As underscored by Breitbart and Strout (2000), hallucinations that are pleasant at one point may become menacing.

As in usual geriatric care, the most effective approach to delirium is to find and treat the underlying cause and support the patient as necessary until the delirium is resolved. The most common causes of delirium in terminally ill may not differ from those in other delirious patients: infections, drugs, metabolic disturbances, dehydration, end-organ failure, and central nervous system disease (Breitbart et al., 1998). There may be a higher prevalence of delirium for which no etiology is found.

Bruera, Miller, and colleagues (1992) completed a workup of delirious hospice inpatients with cancer; the workup included a complete medical examination, laboratory evaluation, review of medications, and neuroimaging. Among patients who developed delirium a mean of 16 days before death, no cause of the delirium was found in 56% of cases.

Drugs used for symptom management in dying patients, including opiates, anticholinergic medications, and steroids, are commonly implicated as causes of delirium. The frequency of some causes can be inferred by effective interventions. Bruera, Franco, and coworkers (1995) found that hydration by hypodermoclysis and *opioid rotation* (changing to a different opioid) reduced the incidence of agitated delirium from 26% to 10% in an inpatient hospice.

Delirium is often not reversible in the final few days of life if related to organ failure or primary central nervous system disease or when decreased medications result in unacceptable resurgence of symptoms. On the other hand, between one third and one half of patients in palliative care settings who develop delirium will improve significantly before death, many without intervention (Bruera, Miller, et al., 1992; Gagnon et al., 2000). Diagnostic evaluations are often limited in home hospice, and treatments that are painful and require hospitalization are not consistent with a focus on patient comfort, especially in moribund patients for whom there is little realistic hope of altering their course.

Psychopharmacological interventions are indicated in patients who are agitated, psychotic, or appear distressed. Breitbart and coworkers (1998) recommended high-potency neuroleptics to treat agitation and psychosis and to improve cognition. Haloperidol delivered orally or subcutaneously is an option in home care. Haloperidol, an antipsychotic with little anticholinergic potency, and chlorpromazine, an antipsychotic with high anticholinergic potency, were reported to be equally effective in delirious hospitalized patients with acquired immunodeficiency syndrome (AIDS). Although anticholinergic medications may worsen delirium, patients receiving chlorpromazine had improved cognition (Breitbart, Marotta, et al., 1996).

Concern about long-term consequences of neuroleptics, such as tardive dyskinesia, is unwarranted in patients with only a few weeks to live. The incidence of akathisia and drug-induced parkinsonism is low (Breitbart, Marotta, et al., 1996). There is increasing clinical experience with risperidone and olanzapine for patients for whom extrapyramidal syndromes are a concern, but no systematic studies have been performed (Breitbart et al., 1998; Breitbart & Strout, 2000).

At times, for agitated patients in the final hours to days of life, the focus of treatment is appropriately "quiet sedation." Quiet sedation is considered for patients when more conservative interventions have not been effective, and patient comfort is given a higher priority than patient awareness or clear cognition.

In rare cases, constant infusions of midazolam, a short-acting benzodiazepine, or propofol, a general anesthetic, are administrated to induce light anesthesia (Krakauer et al., 2000). Family members should be involved in determining whether quiet sedation should be a goal of care and reassured that there is no intent to hasten death (Breitbart & Strout, 2000; Krakauer et al., 2000).

DEPRESSION

Reports of the prevalence of depressive syndromes in terminally ill patients vary widely, ranging from 23% to 58% (Chochinov, 2000), depending on the characteristics of the populations, method of diagnosis, inclusion versus exclusion of neurovegetative signs such as fatigue and weight loss, and severity threshold for psychological criteria. For decades, controversy has surrounded the diagnosis of depression in patients with severe medical illness (Lynch, 1995). Among the terminally ill, diagnosis is made more difficult by the presence of normal anticipatory grief and sadness (Lander et al., 2000). As in geriatric patients in general, emphasis on depressed mood, loss of interest or pleasure in activities disproportional to functional impairment, inappropriate hopelessness, and sense of worthlessness or guilt is more likely to result in an accurate diagnosis.

Chochinov and colleagues (1997) reported that a single item that asked, "Are you depressed?" was more effective than the Beck Depression Inventory or a visual analogue scale in screening for depression in cancer patients receiving palliative care. Bukberg and colleagues (1984) found that excluding fatigue and weight loss from diagnostic criteria halved the point prevalence of depression in cancer patients from 42% to 24%.

Chochinov and associates (1994) demonstrated that, when using high-severity thresholds for psychological criteria (that is, only counting the mood symptoms toward the diagnosis if they are at least moderately severe), classification of somatic signs and symptoms ceased to influence the diagnosis. They reported that, when using these thresholds, the prevalence of major depressive disorders in hospice inpatients was 9%. On the other hand, application of high symptom severity thresholds may result in failure to identify and treat many suffering patients.

Advanced disease, pain, poor social support, and functional disability are important risk factors for depression in terminally ill patients (Chochinov, 2000; Lynch, 1995), but type of disease, gender, and age are less influential. The relationship between depression and socioeconomic factors and marital status, which are risk factors for depression in general geriatric populations, is less clear in terminally ill groups. Cancer chemotherapeutic agents, narcotic analgesics, H_2 blockers, corticosteroids, and sedatives have been implicated as causes of depression in both ill and general populations (Lynch, 1995). There are no longitudinal studies clarifying the course of depression and the outcomes in treated and undertreated groups of palliative care patients.

Several studies have confirmed that, although primary care physicians' assessment of depression is often accurate, there is substantial underdiagnosis of treatable depressive syndromes. Passik and colleagues (1998) reported that oncologists underestimated the level of depression in the most severely depressed cancer patients, missing about half of all depressive cases, even when the oncologists were aware that the concordance between their diagnosis and research diagnosis was under examination. These oncologists were most influenced by symptoms such as depressed mood and crying episodes, but failed to probe for anhedonia, guilt, and hopelessness. Reasons for failure to diagnose depression in primary and subspecialist care may include that patients are reluctant to discuss symptoms or have so many physical concerns that depression is simply a lower priority; health care providers are reluctant to ask about symptoms for fear of upsetting the patient; and beliefs that depression associated with terminal illness is normal or untreatable (Passik et al., 1998).

Psychotherapeutic interventions must be tailored to the patient's energy level, cognitive abilities, and life expectancy. Active coping strategies should be encouraged; these focus on maintaining level of function and mastery and working through feelings related to the disease. Reassurance of nonabandonment is crucial. Psychodynamic approaches that focus on developmental issues and psychological understanding are often less practical in dying patients (Chochinov, 2000).

Most terminally ill patients with a major depressive disorder should be started on an antidepressant medication. Shortened life expectancy often precludes a plan that proposes a trial of psychotherapy before medication and may deprive a patient of the chance to have the depression remit before death. The choice of antidepressant is also influenced by life expectancy. For patients with an expected life of longer than 2 months, selective serotonin reuptake inhibitors (SSRIs) are recommended because their side-effect profile makes them more tolerable than tricyclic antidepressants. Because of its long half-life, fluoxetine is not recommended; if adverse effects develop, they may persist, and metabolites with a long half-life may preclude other medication treatments (Breitbart et al., 1998). A study of mirtazepine for pain in cancer patients found the medication well tolerated with minimal analgesia, but substantial improvement in depressive symptoms, sleep, and appetite (Steve Passik, PhD, unpublished data, 2002).

Patients with a life expectancy of less than 2 months may not have an opportunity to respond to an SSRI if intolerance occurs or response takes several weeks. The importance of considering life expectancy was demonstrated in a study by Lloyd-Williams and coworkers (1999) of over 1,000 patients admitted to a palliative care team. Physicians prescribed antidepressants for 10%, but 76% of these patients received antidepressants in the final 2 weeks of life; 96% were prescribed either a tricyclic antidepressant or an SSRI. There are several advantages to psychostimulants, such as amphetamine, methylphenidate, or pemoline. Response can be seen within 2 days, and side effects resulting in discontinuation are uncommon (10%) (Olin & Masand, 1996). Pemoline can be chewed, an advantage in patients with dysphagia (Breitbart & Strout, 2000). Psychostimulants both augment opioid analgesia and diminish opioid sedation (Breitbart & Strout, 2000). Concerns about abuse or dependence are, for the most part, irrelevant. Noncontrolled studies in cancer patients demonstrated response rates of 73% (Olin & Masand, 1996). Macleod (1998), in a retrospective study of 26 hospice inpatients with advanced malignancy, reported a 46% response rate to methylphenidate (mean 18 mg day). However, only 7% of patients within 6 weeks of death improved. Prospective randomized trials of psychostimulants are needed to verify their effectiveness in this population.

SUICIDE AND DESIRE FOR HASTENED DEATH

Cancer is a risk factor for suicide, especially when the disease is advanced and the prognosis is poor (Goldblatt, 2000). Depression, anxiety disorders, and alcohol abuse are the most common psychiatric disorders in cancer patients who complete suicide (Henrikkson et al., 1995). Efforts to understand dying patient attitudes toward assisted suicide and hastened death have been spurred in North America by increased publicity of persons who request and receive physician aid in dying and legalization, in 1994, of physician-assisted suicide in Oregon. Many (although not all) studies of patients with cancer, AIDS, and amyotrophic lateral sclerosis showed a relationship between desire for hastened death or interest in assisted suicide and depression, hopelessness, poor social support, male gender, and low religiousness. These studies less consistently showed a relationship between pain and interest in assisted suicide (Breitbart, Rosenfeld, et al., 1996; Chochinov et al., 1995; Emanuel et al., 1996; Ganzini et al., 1998; Wilson et al., 2000). In Oregon, physicians reported that patients who request assisted suicide place a high value on independence and desire for control. Palliative interventions, especially hospice referral, resulted in a substantial number of patients withdrawing their request for assisted suicide (Ganzini et al., 2000). However, among those who died by legalized assisted suicide in Oregon, three quarters were in hospice for a median of 7 weeks before death (Sullivan et al., 2000).

SUBSTANCE ABUSE

The presence of alcohol abuse has been identified in some studies as a prognostic factor for poor pain control and poor patient and family coping (Bruera, Moyano, et al., 1995). Alcohol abuse is diagnosed in 13% of cancer patients who complete suicide (Henriksson et al., 1995). Some studies reported overall prevalence of substance abuse in cancer patients of 3% to 5%, lower than the general population (Passik et al., 2002). Bruera, Moyano, and coworkers (1995) reported that the prevalence of past or current alcohol dependence was 28% on an inpatient palliative care unit.

Opioid abuse and addiction are rare in patients dying of cancer, although dependence is common, and many patients will require very high dosages of morphine or an equivalent medication. Fears of addiction by ill patients and their physicians remain an unfortunate barrier to good pain control in dying patients (Passik et al., 2002).

DEMENTIA

Many dementias are progressive and untreatable, and eventually patients succumb to the complications of their disease. Studies have challenged the benefit of life-prolonging therapies in patients terminally ill with dementia and called attention to the underuse of palliative approaches.

An estimated 1.8 million people in the United States are in the final stages of a dementing illness such as Alzheimer's disease, with their course marked by inexorable loss of independence in dressing, bathing, communication, and ambulation (Morrison & Sui, 2000). Medical complications become more frequent, including malnutrition, dysphagia, aspiration pneumonia, urinary tract infections, decubitus ulcers, and septicemia. In the final stage of the illness, patients are mute, dependent in all activities of daily living, and unable to have relationships with other people.

Luchins and associates (1997) demonstrated that, among patients who lost function in an ordinal progression on the Functional Assessment Staging Scale (FAST), the median life expectancy was 3 months at the point the patients were mute and dependent in all activities, including ambulation (FAST level 7C). Morrison and Sui (2000) reported that the 6-month mortality for patients with end-stage dementia and pneumonia was 53%, and it was 55% for patients with end-stage dementia and hip fracture. Cohen-Mansfield and colleagues (1999) found that, among nursing home residents with cognitive impairments, older age, impaired activities of daily living, and screaming behavior at a high frequency were predictive of mortality.

The medical benefit of aggressive life-sustaining treatment for end-stage dementia patients has been challenged. Fabiszewski and coworkers (1990) demonstrated that patients with Alzheimer's disease who received antibiotics for fevers had no survival advantage over those treated with palliative measures. Treatment of fevers was associated with transfer to the hospital, sputum inductions, mechanical restraints, and in 20% of patients, repeated painful intramuscular injections. Hanrahan and associates (1999) reported that the use of antibiotics did not change survival in end-stage dementia, and Foley catheters were associated with decreased survival.

Tube feeding of severely cognitively impaired nursing home residents does not appear to improve nutrition enough to prevent either decubitus ulcers or aspiration and its complications, or to prolong survival (Gillick, 2000; Mitchell et al., 1997; Peck et al., 1990). Tube feeding, including permanent gastrostomy, puts the patient at serious risk of need for mechanical restraints to prevent the patient from pulling the tube out and chemical restraints to treat the agitation that results from mechanical restraints (Gillick, 2000). As a consequence, tube feeding of patients with advanced dementia may significantly worsen quality of life and increase suffering for unclear medical benefit. Studies suggested greater medical benefit in persons who have gastrostomy following a stroke, but even in these patients, over 50% died within 6 months (Huang & Ahronheim, 2000). Although aspiration and choking are common and patient appetite is frequently diminished, the literature indicates that, with systematic evaluation of feeding difficulties and efforts to overcome them, comfort feeding can continue in many cases (Frissoni et al., 1998).

Decisions about palliative care are complicated in demented patients because, unlike other terminal illnesses in which the patient retains decision-making capacity, patients may have lost decision-making capacity for many years and may not have clarified their wishes or completed an advance directive before the onset of dementia. Unlike other terminal illnesses, changes are so gradual and insidious that it is often not clear when the patient became "terminal." The health care team, providers, and family may need assistance in stepping back and reevaluating the goals of care. In most states, families can decide to pursue a palliative approach even if the patient did not execute an advance directive. The bioethical literature supports, and the US Supreme Court has confirmed, that even artificial food and hydration constitute medical treatment that can be forgone (see Chapter 38). However, some states, such as Missouri and New York, require a higher standard of proof regarding the patient's wishes before allowing the surrogate to withhold or withdraw artificial hydration or nutrition from a patient who lacks decision-making capacity.

Despite arguments for lack of medical benefit and, in some cases, worse quality of life resulting from these treatments, not instituting them can be perceived by both families and professional caregivers as a limitation of care. Decisions about tube feeding can be especially difficult. The family and staff may worry that, in not offering a feeding tube, they are failing to offer care or even starving the patient. There may be a perception of legal, institutional, and ethical barriers to not offering food and hydration in this manner. A consensus-based approach to palliative care in demented patients has been recommended that includes a dialogue with the family about the patient's disease state, the expected course of disease, an exploration of the patients' and families' values and perceptions, explanations of the role of palliative care, advocacy for improving quality of life and dignity, and professional guidance based on clinical data and expertise. Appeals to withholding of treatment because of poor quality of life or futility should be avoided; this message may inadvertently convey that "nothing more can be done" or that the demented patient's "life has no value" (Karlawish et al., 1999).

Among severely demented patients, aggressiveness, resistance to care, and disruptive vocalizations are the most problematic behavioral difficulties. Obvious psychosis, paranoia, and wandering diminish as language and ambulation dysfunction increase (Burns et al., 1990; Jeste et al., 1992). Although antipsychotics have been somewhat effective for psychotic features in dementia and aggressiveness, their role in palliative care is less clear. Even mild drug-induced parkinsonism at this stage of the illness may worsen remaining feeding and ambulation. As at any stage of the illness, antipsychotic-induced akathisia may worsen agitation.

Clinicians should consider underlying pain syndromes in severely demented patients with behavioral disorders. Pain assessment can be difficult in patients with severe language impairments and inability to report symptoms. Ferrell and colleagues (1995) reported that, among nursing home residents with a mean MMSE of 12, 83% were able to complete at least one of five pain intensity rating scales, and 62% had pain complaints. Scales have been developed for nonverbal patients with dementia (Feldt et al., 1998). Demented patients are less likely than nondemented patients to receive pain medications after hip fractures. Feldt and coworkers (1998) reported that, although pain intensity measurement did not differ between cognitively impaired and cognitively intact patients after hip fracture repair, cognitively impaired subjects received significantly less opioid analgesics than cognitively intact subjects. Clinicians caring for demented patients in long-term care settings increasingly advocate for liberal use of analgesics, but there are no published empirical trials of pain control for disruptive behaviors.

For the terminally ill demented patient, emphasis should be placed on comfort. Any interventions, even routine care, must be balanced by the fact that the patient cannot understand the benefit and may respond with agitation. Although hospice care may seem fitting for the patient with end-stage dementia, only 1% to 2% of all hospice patients have dementia listed as the terminal illness (Christakis & Escarce, 1996). Surveys of geriatric health providers and families suggest strong support for hospice care. Difficulties in predicting survival, however, have constituted a major impediment to enrollment (Luchins & Hanrahan, 1993). Some hospices have developed prehospice programs that provide limited service to these patients (Volicer, 1997). The National Hospice Organization has issued guidelines on criteria for enrollment of patients with end-stage dementia in hospice (Stuart et al., 1995).

CONCLUSION

Geriatric psychiatrists have much to offer in understanding the complex emotional experiences of dying elderly patients, facilitating the patient's and the family's transition, and ensuring quality of care. Further research is needed on the best treatments for the most common psychiatric disorders in the dying and amelioration of emotional and existential suffering.

REFERENCES

American Psychiatric Association. *Diagnostic and Statistical Manual of Mental Disorders*. 4th ed. Washington, DC: American Psychiatric Press; 1994.

Bascom PB. A hospital-based comfort care team: consultation for seriously ill and dying patients. *Am J Hosp Palliat Care*. 1997;14:57–60.

Breitbart W, Chochinov HM, Passik S. Psychiatric aspects of palliative care. In: Doyle D, Hanks GWC, MacDonald N, eds. *Oxford Textbook of Palliative Medicine*. 2nd ed. Oxford, UK: Oxford University Press; 1998:933–956.

Breitbart W, Marotta R, Platt MM, et al. A double-blind trial of haloperidol, chlorpromazine, and lorazepam in the treatment of delirium in hospitalized AIDS patients. *Am J Psychiatry.* 1996;153:231–237.

Breitbart W, Rosenfeld BD, Passik SD. Interest in physician-assisted suicide among ambulatory HIV infected patients. *Am J Psychiatry.* 1996;153:238–242.

Breitbart W, Strout D. Delirium in the terminally ill. *Clin Geriatr Med.* 2000;16:357–372.

Bruera E, Fainsinger RL, Miller MJ, Kuehn N. The assessment of pain intensity in patients with cognitive failure: a preliminary report. *J Pain Symptom Manage.* 1992; 7:267–270.

Bruera E, Franco JJ, Maltoni M, Watanabe S, Suarez-Almazor M. Changing pattern of agitated impaired mental status in patients with advanced cancer: association with cognitive monitoring, hydration, and opioid rotation. *J Pain Symptom Manage.* 1995;10:287–291.

Bruera E, Miller L, McCallion J, Macmillan K, Krefting L, Hanson J. Cognitive failure in patients with terminal cancer: a prospective study. *J Pain Symptom Manage.* 1992;7:192–195.

Bruera E, Moyano J, Seifert L, Fainsinger RL, Hanson J, Suarez-Almazor M. The frequency of alcoholism among patients with pain due to terminal cancer. *J Pain Symptom Manage.* 1995;10:599–603.

Bukberg J, Penman D, Holland JC. Depression in hospitalized cancer patients. *Psychosom Med.* 1984;46:199–212.

Burns A, Jacoby R, Levy R. Psychiatric phenomena in Alzheimer's disease. I. Disorders of thought content. *Br J Psychiatry.* 1990;157:72–76.

Chochinov HM. Psychiatry and terminal illness. *Can J Psychiatry.* 2000;45:143–150.

Chochinov HM, Wilson K, Enns M, et al. Correlates of desire for death among the terminally ill. *Am J Psychiatry.* 1995;152:1185–1191.

Chochinov HM, Wilson KG, Enns M, Lander S. Prevalence of depression in the terminally ill: effects of diagnostic criteria and symptom threshold judgments. *Am J Psychiatry.* 1994;151:537–540.

Chochinov HM, Wilson KG, Enns M, Lander S. "Are you depressed?" Screening for depression in the terminally ill. *Am J Psychiatry.* 1997;154:674–676.

Christakis NA, Escarce JJ. Survival of Medicare patients after enrollment in hospice programs. *N Engl J Med.* 1996;335:172–178.

Christakis NA, Lamont EB. Extent and determinants of error in doctors' prognoses in terminally ill patients: prospective cohort study. *Br Med J.* 2000;320:469–473.

Cohen-Mansfield J, Marx MS, Lipson S, Werner P. Predictors of mortality in nursing home residents. *J Clin Epidemiol.* 1999;52:273–280.

Emanuel EJ, Fairclough DL, Daniels ER, Clarridge BR. Euthanasia and physician-assisted suicide: attitudes and experiences of oncology patients, oncologists, and the public. *Lancet.* 1996;347:1805–1810.

Fabiszewski KJ, Volicer B, Volicer L. Effect of antibiotic treatment on outcome of fevers in institutionalized Alzheimer patients. *JAMA.* 1990;263:3168–3172.

Fainsinger R, Miller MJ, Bruera E, et al. Symptom control during the last week of life on a palliative care unit. *J Palliat Care.* 1991;7:5–11.

Fainsinger RL, Landman W, Hoskings M, Bruera E. Sedation for uncontrolled symptoms in a South African hospice. *J Pain Symptom Manage.* 1998;16:145–152.

Fainsinger RL, Tapper M, Bruera E. A perspective on the management of delirium in terminally ill patients on a palliative care unit. *J Palliat Care*. 1993;9:4–8.

Farber S, Egnew TR, Stempel J, Vleck J. *End-of-Life Care: AAFP Home Study Self-Assessment*. American Academy of Family Physicians; 2000. Monograph 250/251.

Farrell K, Ganzini L. Misdiagnosing delirium as depression in medically ill elderly patients. *Arch Intern Med*. 1995;155:2459–2464.

Feldt KS, Warne MA, Ryden MB. Examining pain in aggressive cognitively impaired older adults. *J Gerontol Nurs*. 1998;24:14–22.

Ferrell BA, Ferrell BR, Rivera L. Pain in cognitively impaired nursing home patients. *J Pain Symptom Manage*. 1995;10:591–598.

Field MJ, Cassel CK. *Approaching Death: Improving Care at the End of Life*. Washington, DC: National Academy Press; 1997:24.

Frissoni GB, Franzoni S, Bellelli G, Morris J, Warden V. Overcoming eating difficulties in the severely demented. In: Volicer L, Hurley A, eds. *Hospice Care for Patients With Advanced Progressive Dementia*. New York, NY: Springer; 1998:48–67.

Gagnon P, Allard P, Masse B, DeSerres M. Delirium in terminal cancer: a prospective study using daily screening, early diagnosis and continuous monitoring. *J Pain Symptom Manage*. 2000;19:412–426.

Ganzini L, Johnston WS, McFarland BH, Tolle SW, Lee MA. Attitudes of patients with amyotrophic lateral sclerosis and their care givers toward assisted suicide. *N Engl J Med*. 1998;339:967–973.

Ganzini L, Nelson HD, Schmidt TA, Kraemer DF, Delorit MA, Lee MA. Physicians' experiences with the Oregon Death with Dignity Act. *N Engl J Med*. 2000;342:557–563.

Gillick MR. Rethinking the role of tube feeding in patients with advanced dementia. *N Engl J Med*. 2000;342:206–210.

Goldblatt MJ. Physical illness and suicide. In: Maris RW, Berman AL, Silverman MM, eds. *Comprehensive Textbook of Suicidology*. New York, NY: Guilford Press; 2000:342–356.

Hanrahan P, Raymond M, McGowan E, Luchins DJ. Criteria for enrolling dementia patients in hospice: a replication. *Am J Hospice Palliat Care*. 1999;16:395–400.

Henriksson MM, Isometsa ET, Hietanen PS, Aro HM, Lonnqvist JK. Mental disorders in cancer suicides. *J Affect Disord*. 1995;36:11–20.

Huang Z, Ahronheim JC. Nutrition and hydration in terminally ill patients: an update. *Clin Geriatr Med*. 2000;16:313–325.

Jeste DV, Wragg RE, Salmon DP, et al. Cognitive deficits of patients with Alzheimer's disease with and without delusions. *Am J Psychiatry*. 1992;149:184–189.

Karlawish JHT, Quill T, Meier DE. A consensus-based approach to providing palliative care to patients who lack decision-making capacity. *Ann Intern Med*. 1999;130:835–840.

Krakauer EL, Penson RT, Truog RD, King LA, Chabner BA, Lynch TJ. Sedation for intractable distress of a dying patient: acute palliative care and the principle of double effect. *Oncologist*. 2000;5:53–62.

Lander M, Wilson K, Chochinov HM. Depression and the dying older patient. *Clin Geriatr Med*. 2000;16:335–356.

Lipowski ZJ. *Delirium: Acute Confusional States*. New York, NY: Oxford University Press; 1990:175–188.

Lloyd-Williams M, Friedman T, Rudd N. A survey of antidepressant prescribing in the terminally ill. *Palliat Med.* 1999;13:243–248.

Luchins DJ, Hanrahan P. What is the appropriate level of health care for end-stage dementia patients? *J Am Geriatr Soc.* 1993;41:25–30.

Luchins DJ, Hanrahan P, Murphy K. Criteria for enrolling dementia patients in hospice. *J Am Geriatr Soc.* 1997;45:1054–1059.

Lynch ME. The assessment and prevalence of affective disorders in advanced cancer. *J Palliat Care.* 1995;11:10–18.

Lynn J, Teno JM, Phillips RS, et al. Perceptions by family members of the dying experience of older and seriously ill patients: SUPPORT investigators. Study to understand prognoses and preferences for outcomes and risks of treatments. *Ann Intern Med.* 1997;126:97–106.

Macleod AD. Methylphenidate in terminal depression. *J Pain Symptom Manage.* 1998; 16:193–198.

Martin JA, Smith BL, Mathews TJ, Ventura SJ. Births and deaths: preliminary data for 1998. *Natl Vital Stat Rep.* 1999;47:1–45.

Massie MJ, Holland J, Glass E. Delirium in terminally ill cancer patients. *Am J Psychiatry.* 1983;140:1048–1050.

Medicare Rights Center. *A Technical Guide to the Medicare Home Health Benefits: Care for People With Advanced Illnesses.* New York, NY: Medicare Rights Center; 1998.

Minagawa H, Uchitomi Y, Yamawaki S, Ishitani K. Psychiatric morbidity in terminally ill cancer patients: a prospective study. *Cancer.* 1996;78:1131–1137.

Mitchell SL, Kiely DK, Lipsitz LA. The risk factors and impact on survival of feeding tube placement in nursing home residents with severe cognitive impairment. *Arch Intern Med.* 1997;157:327–332.

Morrison RS, Siu AL. Survival in end-stage dementia following acute illness. *JAMA.* 2000;284:47–52.

National Hospice and Palliative Care Organization. *Facts and Figures on Hospice Care in America.* Alexandria, VA: National Hospice and Palliative Care Organization; September 2003.

Olin J, Masand P. Psychostimulants for depression in hospitalized cancer patients. *Psychosomatics.* 1996;37:57–62.

Passik SD, Dugan W, McDonald MV, Rosenfeld B, Theobald DE, Edgerton S. Oncologists' recognition of depression in their patients with cancer. *J Clin Oncol.* 1998; 16:1594–1600.

Passik SD, Kirsch KL, Portenoy RK. Substance abuse issues in palliative care. In: Berger A, Portenoy RK, Weissman DE, eds. *Principles and Practice of Palliative Care and Supportive Oncology.* 2nd ed. Philadelphia, PA: Williams and Wilkins; 2002:593–606.

Peck A, Cohen CE, Mulvihill MN. Long-term enteral feeding of aged demented nursing home patients. *J Am Geriatr Soc.* 1990;38:1195–1198.

Pereira J, Hanson J, Bruera E. The frequency and clinical course of cognitive impairment in patients with terminal cancer. *Cancer.* 1997;79:835–842.

Singer PA, Martin DK, Kelner M. Quality end-of-life care: patients' perspectives. *JAMA.* 1999;281:163–168.

Steinhauser KE, Clipp EC, McNeilly M, Christakis NA, McIntyre LM, Tulsky JA. In search of a good death: observations of patients, families, and providers. *Ann Intern Med.* 2000;132:825–832.

Stuart B, Herbst L, Kinbrunner B, et al. *Medical Guidelines for Determining Prognosis in Selected Non-Cancer Diseases.* Arlington, VA: National Hospice Organization; 1995.

Sullivan AD, Hedberg K, Fleming DW. Legalized physician-assisted suicide in Oregon—the second year. *N Engl J Med.* 2000;342:598–604.

SUPPORT Principal Investigators. A controlled trial to improve care for seriously ill hospitalized patients: study to understand prognoses and preferences for outcomes and risks of treatments. *JAMA.* 1995;274:1591–1598.

Volicer L. Hospice care for dementia patients. *J Am Geriatr Soc.* 1997;45:1147–1149.

Weissman DE, Griffie J. The Palliative Care Consultation Service of the Medical College of Wisconsin. *J Pain Symptom Manage.* 1994;9:474–479.

Wilson KG, Scott JF, Graham ID, et al. Attitudes of terminally ill patients toward euthanasia and physician-assisted suicide. *Arch Intern Med.* 2000;160:2454–2460.

World Health Organization. *Cancer Pain Relief and Palliative Care.* Geneva, Switzerland: World Health Organization; 1990. Technical Report Series 804.

Index

change, assessment instruments for documenting, 272
chloral hydrate, 779–780, 782t
choice(s)
appreciating one's situation and consequences of, 1189
expressing a, 1189
see also autonomy; decision making
cholinesterase inhibitors, 488–489, 540, 661, 958–959
for dementias, 959, 960t, 961–962
efficacy, 959, 960t, 961–962
for neuropsychiatric disturbances associated with dementia, 962–963
pharmacokinetics, dosing, and drug-drug interactions, 963–964
pretreatment assessment and clinical monitoring, 963
properties, 959, 960t
tolerability, 959, 960t, 961
see also anticholinergic side effects
chorea, 68
chore services, 1155
chromosome 17, 60–61
chromosome 1 gene. *see presenilin 2*
chromosome 14 gene. *see presenilin 1*
circadian rhythms, 106, 769; *see also* diurnal rhythm disturbance
clearance (pharmacokinetics), 905t, 908–909
clergy, recognizing the role of, 219–220
Clinical Dementia Rating (CDR), 1200
clozapine, 660; *see also* antipsychotic drugs
coagulopathy, 513t
Cochrane Collaboration, 831
cognitive abulia, 467t
cognitive assessment, 115, 116f, 377, 385t
format, 267t
principles, 266–271
purpose, 265–266
screening tests, 273–274
cognitive-behavioral, social skills training (CBSST), 670–671
cognitive-behavioral group therapy, 1031–1033, 1047
cognitive-behavioral therapy (CBT), 634, 635, 670, 693, 825, 1010–1012, 1031
cognitive change
aging and, 131–141, 320
neurological disorders and, 343
cognitive impairment, 13, 16
alcohol abuse and, 734–735
personality disorders and, 711, 715
vascular, 483
see also dementia(s); intellectual abilities; mild cognitive impairment
cognitively impaired individuals
psychotherapy with, 1007–1009
verbal-centered groups for, 1036–1037

cognitive processing measures across lifespan, 115, 116f
Cognitive subscale of Alzheimer's Disease Assessment Scale (ADAS-Cog), 959
collaboration and coordination of treatment, 716, 829, 1124–1125; *see also* consultation
collaborative care model (CCM), 1127
coma
hyperglycemic hyperosmolar nonketotic, 290
myxedema, 297
community care, 1153
community housing, 1174–1175
long-term care facilities, 1167 (*see also* hospice; nursing homes)
planned housing, 1167–1174
community mental health center (CMHC), 1113
community mental health services, 1157–1159
community outreach, 1158–1159
community resources, 1245–1246
community services, 1143–1144, 1174–1175
assistance and protection, 1145, 1150–1153
case or care management, 1151–1152
how to access, 1145, 1150–1151
principal governmental programs relevant to, 1144–1145, 1148–1149t
types of, 1144, 1146–1147t; *see also specific services*
competency, 264–265, 1186
assessment of, 1129–1130
standards of, 1186–1187
depression and decisional capacity, 1190
global vs. specific incapacities, 1188
improving capacity, 1189–1190
structured instruments and decision-making abilities, 1188–1189
see also informed consent
complicated grief reaction. *see* traumatic grief
compulsions, 690; *see also* obsessive-compulsive disorder
concentration, 267–268
concrete thinking, 271
confidentiality, 1200–1201
confrontation naming, 268
confusional states, 17
Confusion Assessment Method (CAM), 534
congregate housing, 1171
constipation, 290–292
causes, 291t
constructional ability, 269–270